Essentials of Nursing: Care of Adults and Children

Barbara K. Timby, RN, BC, BSN, MA

Nursing Professor, Medical Surgical Nursing
Glen Oaks Community College
Centreville, Michigan

Nancy E. Smith, MS, RN

Professor and Chair, Department of Nursing
Southern Maine Community College
South Portland, Maine

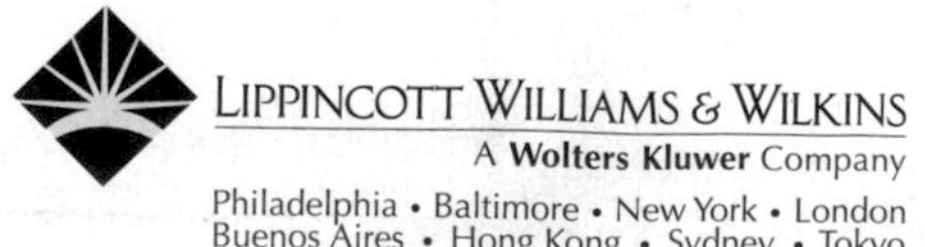

Acquisitions Editor: Elizabeth Nieginski
Developmental Editor: Renee Gagliardi
Editorial Assistant: Josh Levandoski
Senior Production Editor: Debra Schiff
Director of Nursing Production: Helen Ewan
Managing Editor/Production: Erika Kors
Art Director: Brett MacNaughton
Interior Designer: Melissa Olson
Cover Designer: Melissa Walter
Senior Manufacturing Manager: William Alberti
Indexer: Angie Wiley
Compositor: Circle Graphics
Printer: Quebecor

9 8 7 6 5 4 3 2 1

Library of Congress Cataloging-in-Publication Data

Timby, Barbara Kuhn.
Essentials of nursing : care of adults and children / Barbara K. Timby, Nancy E. Smith.
p. ; cm.
Includes bibliographical references and index.
ISBN 0-7817-5098-9
1. Nursing. 2. Pediatric nursing. I. Smith, Nancy E. (Nancy Ellen), 1949- II. Title.
[DNLM: 1. Nursing Care—methods—Adult. 2. Nursing Care—methods—Child. 3. Nursing Care—methods—Infant. WY 100 T583e 2005]
RT41.T537 2005
610.73—dc22
2004001663

LWW.com

Dedication

We dedicate this textbook to the nurses of the armed forces who care for men and women all over the world and represent what is best in the nursing profession. Where there is a soldier, there is a nurse ready to care for the casualties of war and peace. We salute you.

Contributors

Therese M. Bower, EdD, RN, MSN, CNS
Nursing Instructor
Firelands Regional Medical Center
School of Nursing
Sandusky, Ohio

Ann Carmack, RN, BSN
Former Director of Educational Services
Assessment Technologies
Overland Park, Kansas

Myrth C. Condon, RNCS, MSN, FNP
Family Nurse Practitioner
Battle Creek Family Center
Battle Creek, Michigan

Nancy T. Hatfield, MA, BSN, RN
Director/Department Chairperson
Practical Nursing/Health Occupations
Albuquerque Public Schools
Career Enrichment Center
Albuquerque, New Mexico

Diana Rupert, RNC, MSN
Nursing Instructor
Conemaugh School of Nursing
Johnstown, Pennsylvania

Reviewers

LeVon Barrett, RN, BSN
Instructor of Vocational Nursing
Division of Nursing
Amarillo College
Amarillo, Texas

Mary Ann Cosgarea, RN, BSN, BA
Coordinator
W. Howard Nicol School of Practical Nursing
Portage Lakes Career Center
Green, Ohio

Karen D. Danielson, RN, MSN
Associate Professor
Practical Nursing
North Central State College
Mansfield, Ohio

Janet Grace, RN
Director, Practical Nursing Program
Southern Arkansas University Tech
Camden, Arkansas

Pamela Gwin, RNC
Director, Vocational Nursing Program
Brazosport College
Lake Jackson, Texas

Rebecca A. Kelly, MSN, RN, CS
Coordinator, PN Program
Greater Altoona Career and Technology Center
Altoona, Pennsylvania

Debra A. Menshouse, RN, BSN
Nursing Faculty
Ashland Technical College
Ashland, Kentucky

Sally Powers, MS, RN
Associate Professor of Nursing
Department of Nursing
Southern Maine Community College
South Portland, Maine

Pamela Rutar, RN, Cm, BSN, MSN
Instructor
Firelands Regional Medical Center School of Nursing
Sandusky, Ohio

Judy Stauder, MSN, RN
Coordinator
Practical Nurse Program of Canton City Schools
Canton, Ohio

Deborah Theysohn, RN, BSN, MS
Licensed Practical Nursing Coordinator/Instructor
Sullivan County Board of Cooperative Educational Services
Liberty, New York

Roselena Thorpe, PhD, RN
Department Chairperson and Professor of Nursing
Community College of Allegheny County
Allegheny Campus
Pittsburgh, Pennsylvania

Kynthia Williams, RN, BSN
Instructor
Practical Nursing Program
Southwest Georgia Technical College–Grady County
Cairo, Georgia

Linda S. Wood, RN, MSN
Director of Practical Nursing
Massanutten Technical Center
Harrisonburg, Virginia

Regina Wrenn, PNEP
Department Head
Kaynor RVTS
Waterbury, Connecticut

Preface

In today's changing health care environment, nurses face many challenges and opportunities. *Essentials of Nursing: Care of Adults and Children* was written to help nurses meet these challenges and take advantage of continually growing and expanding opportunities.

STRUCTURE AND PHILOSOPHY OF THE TEXT

This book is designed to address the needs of various client populations across the health care continuum in succinct but comprehensive and adequately detailed chapters. The content is organized to teach nurses the appropriate care of clients across the life span, using the following format:

- Unit 1, *Maternity Nursing,* starts where life begins! It covers appropriate care of the maternity client, newborn, and family throughout pregnancy, labor, delivery, and the postpartum period. The four chapters in this unit explore such care under normal and high-risk circumstances.
- Unit 2, *Pediatric Nursing,* progresses to care of children and adolescents. It begins with Chapter 5, *Introduction to Pediatric Nursing,* which focuses on aspects of care that differ specifically and significantly for the pediatric population. Chapter 6, *Biopsychosocial Aspects of Caring for Children and Adolescents,* explores growth and development from infancy through the teen years. Chapter 7, *Caring for the Child or Adolescent With a Psychobiologic Disorder,* describes common pediatric problems in the realm of mental health. Chapters 8 and 9 focus on common pediatric medical–surgical conditions. The presentation of content in these chapters is similar to the order and structure of chapters found in Units 6 to 17, which focus on adult medical–surgical conditions.
- Unit 3, *Adult Growth and Development,* considers the stages of growth and development and common problems confronted by young, middle, and older adults.
- Unit 4, *Caring for Adults With Psychobiologic Disorders,* explores issues pertinent to adult psychiatric–mental health nursing care. Chapter 12, *Interaction of Body and Mind,* explores the nature of stress and the growing field of complementary and alternative medicine. Chapters 13 to 18 explore major categories of psychiatric disorders and appropriate nursing care for clients and families encountering these problems.
- Unit 5, *Caring for Adults With Common Medical–Surgical Problems,* addresses the critical issues of cancer and shock and their appropriate medical, surgical, and nursing management.
- Units 6 through 17 present information on adult medical–surgical disorders according to body systems. Each unit begins with an introductory chapter for that body system that reviews anatomy and physiology, discusses pertinent assessments, and highlights common diagnostic and laboratory tests. The remaining chapters in the unit focus on a disorder or disorder group within that body system, exploring pathophysiology and etiology, assessment findings, medical and surgical management, and nursing management.
- Unit 18, *Moving Forward as a Nurse,* teaches students about roles beyond those of the basic licensed practical/vocational nurse (LPN/LVN). By exploring issues related to leadership, management, and career preparation and transitions, readers will be better prepared to meet the challenges of the rapidly evolving health care industry as well as to consider their own futures.

Several philosophical concepts are the basis for this text:

- The human experience is a composite of physiologic, emotional, social, and spiritual aspects that affect health and healing.
- Caring is the essence of nursing and is extended to every client.
- Each client is unique, and nurses must adapt their care to meet the individual needs of every person without compromising safety or achievement of desired outcomes.
- A supportive network of health care providers, family, and friends promotes health restoration and

health promotion. Therefore, including a client's significant others in teaching, formal discussions, and provision of services is essential.
- Licensed and student nurses are accountable for their actions and clinical decisions; consequently, each must be aware of legislation as it affects nursing practice.

BOOK HIGHLIGHTS

- **Full, four-color art program.** This book contains a brilliant design with illustrations and photographs **in full color** to assist visual learners to understand important concepts.
- **Words to Know.** These words are listed at the beginning of each chapter and set in bold type within the text where they appear with or near their definitions. Additional technical terms are italicized throughout the text.
- **Learning Objectives.** These student-oriented objectives appear at the beginning of each chapter to serve as guidelines for acquiring specific information.
- **Stop, Think, and Respond boxes.** Found in all chapters, these boxes ask students to consider scenarios related to pertinent topics and to respond quickly based on their understanding. They are numbered for quick reference, with answers provided on the back-of-book CD-ROM so students can check their learning.
- **Client and Family Teaching boxes.** These specially numbered boxes highlight essential education points for nurses to communicate to clients and their families.
- **Nursing Guidelines.** These boxed displays present essential nursing information related to caring for a client with a specific disorder or requiring a special treatment, skill, or measure.
- **Nursing Care Plans.** Numerous Care Plans address the care of clients with such diverse issues and problems as rape, Alzheimer's disease, cancer, myocardial infarction, cerebrovascular accident, diabetes mellitus, modified radical mastectomy, and chronic renal failure.
- **Drug Therapy Tables.** These clearly labeled and numbered medication charts address the major categories of medications prescribed to treat common disorders discussed. They include categories of drugs, an example of generic and trade names, their mechanism of action, common side effects, and nursing considerations. This feature reinforces and coordinates pharmacology information in an easy-to-understand and consistent style.
- **Nursing Process.** These sections are found throughout the text. Within each, the steps are separated visibly, with diagnoses and expected outcomes clearly related to interventions and rationales. The text has incorporated diagnoses from the most recently approved NANDA list, a copy of which is found in the back end page of the text.
- **General Gerontologic Considerations.** The older adult population comprises the fastest-growing age group in the United States and is most representative of the clients for whom nursing students care. This section found at the end of most chapters addresses unique characteristics and problems of aging adults as they pertain to the chapter content.
- **Critical Thinking Exercises.** These questions aim to facilitate application of the material contained within the chapter, using clinical situations or rhetorical questions.
- **NCLEX-Style Review Questions.** Found at the end of each chapter, these questions are written in accordance with NCLEX standards and will help students master chapter content as well as prepare for tests and examinations. Correct answers with full rationales appear on the back-of-book CD-ROM so students can check their work.
- **References and Selected Readings.** These are intended to provide a guide to current literature that has been cited within chapters or to encourage further independent learning.

USE WITH *FUNDAMENTAL NURSING SKILLS AND CONCEPTS*, EIGHTH EDITION

Essentials of Nursing may be adopted as a single text for students in a nursing program. Additionally, the text may be adopted in conjunction with the eighth edition of *Fundamental Nursing Skills and Concepts. Essentials of Nursing* builds on the foundational concepts and skills discussed in the companion text, showing students how to apply those principles and techniques in the fields of maternity, pediatric, psychiatric, and adult health nursing. The design, style, and features of both texts have been coordinated closely for a consistent and familiar presentation that enhances student understanding. Additionally, the following icon highlights key content areas in this book discussed from a different perspective in *Fundamental Nursing Skills and Concepts,* for students who want to find more information: 📖. Together, these excellent texts and their accompanying ancillary materials provide a foundation of learning that spans the entire LPN/LVN curriculum!

BACK-OF-BOOK CD-ROM

The student back-of-book CD-ROM contains Review Questions, the Glossary, General Nutritional and Pharmacological Considerations, Clinical Simulations, A mations, Printable Drug Tables and Client and Family Teaching Boxes, and Math Review and English as a Second Language (ESL) material. It also contains the answers to the Stop, Think, and Respond boxes and NCLEX-Style Review questions found throughout the text. In the text itself, the following icon alerts and reminds students that related valuable material is found on the accompanying CD-ROM: .

ANCILLARY PACKAGE

The ancillary package includes the *Instructor's Resource CD-ROM to Accompany Essentials of Nursing.* The Instructor's Manual portion contains Chapter Overviews, Lesson Plans, Words to Know, Teaching/Learning Activities, and Case Study exercises. The CD-ROM also provides multiple-choice test-bank questions, a PowerPoint Presentation, and English as a Second Language (ESL) Common Words, Phrases, and Resources for Spanish-speaking students.

The *Study Guide to Accompany Essentials of Nursing* designed for use with this text includes practice exercises of all question types and an answer key. All questions in the study guide are based on information in the textbook.

Acknowledgments

When writing and preparing a textbook, so many people are involved that acknowledging them all is difficult. In fact, we have not met most of them! Nevertheless, we are most thankful that they are skilled and knowledgeable in their craft and are true professionals. They certainly help to keep us on track.

Many at Lippincott Williams & Wilkins we can name and thank personally. The first are Acquisition Editors Lisa Stead, who developed the initial ideas for this textbook, and Elizabeth Nieginski, who provided leadership for the process and oversaw a remarkable team. In particular, Renee A. Gagliardi, Senior Development Editor, has been such an important asset to this work that words are inadequate. Thank you is a mere acknowledgment for the time, dedication, and support that Renee provided, and we are especially grateful that she could be part of this project. And we also thank Debra Schiff, Senior Production Editor, for her insight and perseverance in the final editing. It was a pleasure to work with her again.

We express our gratitude to the contributors who supplied new content under tight deadlines and met high standards of consistency, quality, and accuracy. Thanks to Therese M. Bower, EdD, RN, MSN, CNS; Ann Carmack, RN, BSN; Myrth C. Condon, RNCS, MSN, FNP; Nancy T. Hatfield, MA, BSN, RN; and Diana Rupert, RNC, MSN. We also thank the many text reviewers who supplied useful insights during the planning phase of this text and offered valuable suggestions for refinement throughout.

We are excited about this new book. We hope that *Essentials of Nursing: Care of Adults and Children* provides readers with the necessary skills and knowledge to care for clients of all ages in today's health care environment.

May your nursing journey be one of great rewards and opportunities!

Barbara K. Timby, RN, BC, BSN, MA
Nancy E. Smith, MS, RN

Contents

chapter 1

Caring for Clients During Normal Pregnancy, Labor, and Delivery

Words to Know

abortion
amenorrhea
amniotic fluid
antepartal
bloody show
Braxton Hicks contractions
certified nurse midwife
Chadwick's sign
chorion
chorionic villi
colostrum
conception
crowning
deceleration
dilate
ductus arteriosus
ductus venosus
efface
embryo
engagement
epidural
episiotomy
fertilization
fetal attitude
fetus
fontanelles
foramen ovale
gestation
gravida
labor
lie
lightening
molding
natural childbirth
obstetrician
obstetrics
oxytocic
para
perinatal
position
postpartal
preconceptual care
presentation
quickening
station
surfactant
sutures
tocodynamometer
trimester
viability
zygote

Learning Objectives

On completion of this chapter, the reader will:

- Identify the presumptive, probable, and positive signs of pregnancy.
- Define key terms related to pregnancy, gestation, labor, and delivery.
- Describe the processes of fertilization, implantation, and placental development.
- Describe maternal physical changes during each trimester of pregnancy.
- Identify at least four concepts related to prenatal care important for client teaching.
- Identify recommended nutritional guidelines during pregnancy.
- Explore anticipatory guidance and ways to support the growing family.
- Identify at least three differences between true labor and false labor.
- Discuss potential variations in lie, presentation, station, and position.
- Identify three nursing considerations for the latent, active, and transitional phases of labor.
- Explain the significance of involution and three related nursing considerations.

Few experiences in life are as exciting, highly anticipated, and challenging as childbearing. The woman's body is designed to conceive and bear children. A complex system of hormonal and physical changes enables her to release an egg and support a pregnancy. When pregnancy does not occur, the woman has a regular menstrual period. Pregnancy is a normal physiologic process, not a disease.

This chapter describes the overall process of a normal healthy pregnancy and associated maternal physiological changes. It explores the process of human fetal development and the stages of labor that result in the birth of a healthy infant. It also provides information about how nurses can help their clients experience a healthy preg- nancy and provide vital instruction about accompan[illegible] changes for the evolving family.

PREGNANCY

Signs of Pregnan[illegible]

Different sign[illegible] ...s of certainty can help confir[illegible] ...ptive signs indicate pregnancy but may also signify disease. They include the following:

- **Amenorrhea** (absence of menstruation)
- Nausea and vomiting
- Frequent urination
- Swelling, tingling, or tenderness of the breasts
- Changes in abdominal shape
- **Quickening** (sensation of fetal movement)
- Skin changes
- **Chadwick's sign** (a violet or purplish discoloration in the vagina, cervix, and vulva)

Probable signs indicate a high likelihood that a woman is pregnant but are not 100% reliable. They include:

- Enlargement of the uterus
- Positive pregnancy tests (using urine or blood to measure the level of human-chorionic gonadotropin [HCG])

Positive signs of pregnancy occur only with pregnancy. They include:

- Visualization of the fetal skeleton on x-ray or ultrasound
- Fetal movement felt by an examiner
- Auscultation of fetal heartbeat via Doppler at 10 to 12 weeks or fetoscope after 18 weeks

Stop, Think, and Respond ● BOX 1-1

A client comes to the clinic stating that her menstrual period is more than 2 weeks late. What questions would the nurse ask to gather further information?

Terminology of Pregnancy

Gestation is the time from when sperm fertilizes an egg until a baby is born. The uniting of sperm and egg is called **fertilization** (also called **conception**) and usually occurs 2 weeks after a women's last normal menstrual period (LMP or LNMP). Specific cells (ova or eggs in females and sperm in males) carry genetic messages to offspring. A woman's ovum and a man's sperm combine esult in a new individual or **zygote** with a unique makeup.

9 c peri al length of a full-term gestation is 40 weeks or mate nths. Gestation is divided into three 3-month tal (be rimesters. Pregnancy, also termed the labor), p divided into three periods: antepar- placenta), ption and ends with the onset of 6 weeks late ning of labor to delivery of the to prepregna (delivery of the placenta to tive organs have returned

Throughout her pregnancy, a woman is referred to as a **gravida** (pregnant woman). Latin numerical prefixes indicate the number of pregnancies, such as *nulligravida* (none), *primigravida* (one), and *multigravida* (multiple). The term **para** refers to mother and baby and is used to denote the number of actual births. Examples include *nullipara* (none), *primipara* (one), and *multipara* (multiple). A woman who has given birth five times or more is called a *grand multipara.* A shorthand method of keeping track of a client's obstetric history is to record the gravida/para (Box 1-1).

Abortion is the term used to indicate loss of the fetus before the age of **viability** (capability of living), whether spontaneous or induced.

Obstetrics is the branch of medicine concerned with reproductive health, pregnancy, and birth. An **obstetrician** is a physician who practices obstetrics. A registered nurse with specialized training in the management of labor and birth who works with healthy women during pregnancy is called a **certified nurse midwife (CNM)**. These nurses provide assessment and detailed instruction on maintaining wellness and attend at vaginal births. They refer women with health risks before or during pregnancy to obstetricians (see Chap. 2).

Preconceptual care means care of the woman before she is pregnant. Components include balanced nutrition, vitamins (especially folic acid), and adequate rest. Such measures make pregnancy safer for the woman and fetus. Preconceptual care should begin early, because the first trimester is the most critical time in human development. Many couples also elect genetic counseling to reduce the

BOX 1-1 ● Classifying Pregnancy History

Nurses use a set of numbers and letters to classify a woman's pregnancy history.

G–Gravida: the total number of pregnancies a woman has had, including the current pregnancy, regardless of the outcome (e.g., term birth, miscarriage, abortion)

P–Para: the total number of babies born after 20 weeks' gestation (including multiples)

For example, a pregnant woman has had two babies before, one at 39 weeks and the other at 32 weeks. The nurse would write G3 P2.

Para can be broken down further, using the acronym FPAL.

F–Full term: the total number of babies born at 37 weeks' gestation or more

P–Preterm: the total number of babies born between 20 and 37 weeks' gestation

A–Abortions: the total number of abortions (spontaneous and elective) before 20 weeks' gestation

L–Living: the total number of children currently alive

For example, a woman is not pregnant but has been pregnant three times before. One baby was born at term, twins were born preterm, and one pregnancy ended in miscarriage at 14 weeks. G = 3, F = 1, P = 2, A = 1, L = 3. Thus, the nurse would write G3 P1213.

Adapted from Rosdahl, C. B., & Kowalski, M. T. (2003). *Textbook of basic nursing* (8th ed.). Philadelphia: Lippincott Williams & Wilkins.

risk of genetic disorders or to estimate the risk of having a child with a genetic defect.

Pregnancy Physiology

Fertilization and Implantation

Fertilization occurs in the outer third of the fallopian tube. The resulting zygote carries 46 chromosomes (44 autosomes and 2 sex chromosomes). Sperm determines the sex, because ova have two X sex chromosomes, whereas sperm may carry an X or Y sex chromosome. If the sperm carrying a Y chromosome fertilizes an ovum, a boy (XY) will result; if the sperm carries an X chromosome, a girl will result (XX).

Ciliary and peristaltic activity 7 to 9 days after fertilization moves the zygote through the fallopian tubes to arrive in the uterus. The uterine lining, or endometrium, has become rich in nutrients in preparation for pregnancy. The zygote continues its rapid phase of cell division and burrows or implants into the endometrium. At this time, some women experience implantation bleeding, which is bloody discharge. It rarely is more than slight spotting, but it does cause some women to think they have had a short and light menstrual cycle when they are actually pregnant. When implantation is successful, the developing organism now is called an **embryo.**

The outermost cell layer surrounding the embryo and fluid cavity is called the **chorion.** Some of the outer cells send out projections (**chorionic villi**), which are the roots through which the embryo receives oxygen and nourishment from the mother. Chorionic villi also secrete human HCG, which is tested for in serum pregnancy tests. See Figure 1.1.

Embryonic and Fetal Development

The period of the embryo lasts until the 8th week after conception. This embryonic phase is critical, because all major body systems develop during this time, as does the placenta. The embryo is especially vulnerable to substances the mother consumes. A simple heart begins beating, and the embryo acquires a human appearance by the end of 8 weeks. **Amniotic fluid** surrounds the embryo, cushioning against injury, regulating fetal temperature, and allowing room for growth. The amount of fluid changes from 30 mL (1 oz) to as much as 1 L at delivery. In late pregnancy, amniotic fluid is primarily fetal urine and lung fluid.

From the beginning of the 9th week until birth, the embryo is called a **fetus.** Fetal development is a period of increasing growth, differentiation, and functional tissue development. Normal fetal growth and development follows a definite and predictable head-to-toe pattern (Fig. 1.2). Viability is estimated to begin at approximately the 20th week of gestation.

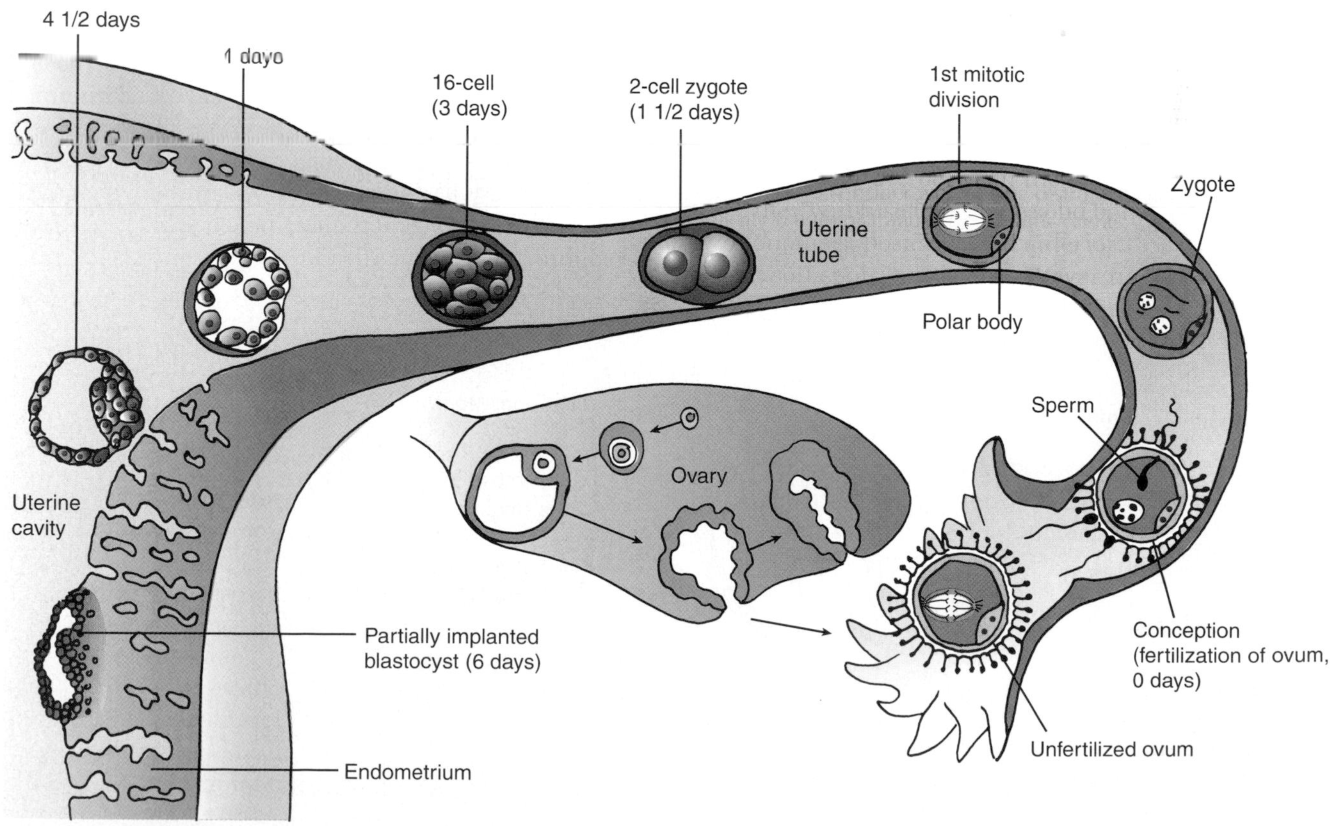

FIGURE 1.1 Fertilization and implantation.

Fetal Development

1st Lunar Month

The fetus is 0.75 cm to 1 cm in length.
Trophoblasts embed in decidua.
Chorionic villi form.
Foundations for nervous system, genitourinary system, skin, bones, and lungs are formed.
Buds of arms and legs begin to form.
Rudiments of eyes, ears, and nose appear.

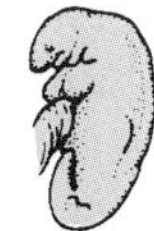
4 weeks

2nd Lunar Month

The fetus is 2.5 cm in length and weighs 4 g.
Fetus is markedly bent.
Head is disproportionately large, owing to brain development.
Sex differentiation begins.
Centers of bone begin to ossify.
Heart pulsates.

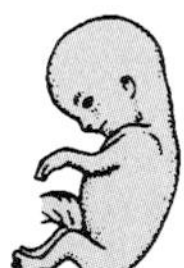
8 weeks

3rd Lunar Month

The fetus is 7 cm to 9 cm in length and weighs 28 g.
Fingers and toes are distinct.
Placenta is complete.
Fetal circulation is complete.
Organ systems are complete.

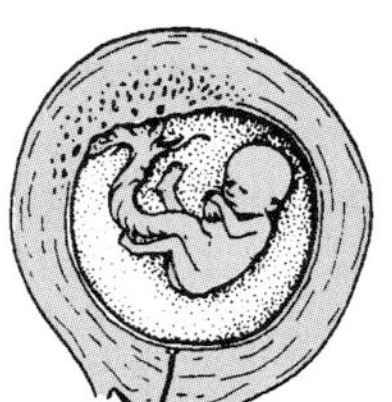
12 weeks

4th Lunar Month

The fetus is 10 cm to 17 cm in length and weighs 55 g to 120 g.
Sex is differentiated.
Rudimentary kidneys secrete urine.
Heartbeat is present.
Nasal septum and palate close.

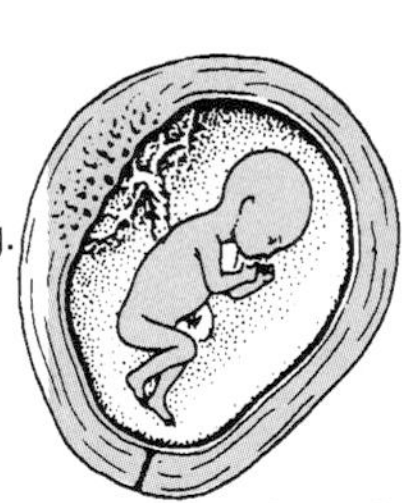
16 weeks

5th Lunar Month

The fetus is 25 cm in length and weighs 223 g.
Lanugo covers entire body.
Fetal movements are felt by mother.
Heart sounds are perceptible by auscultation.

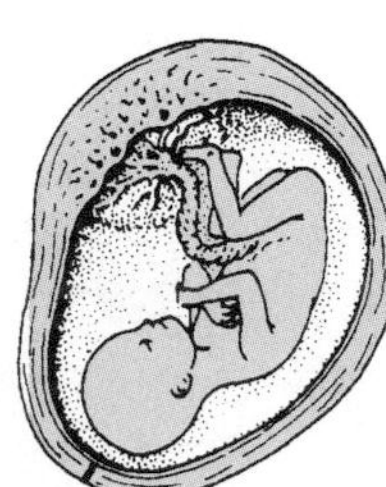
20 weeks

6th Lunar Month

The fetus is 28 cm to 36 cm in length and weighs 680 g.
Skin appears wrinkled.
Vernix caseosa appears.
Eyebrows and fingernails develop.

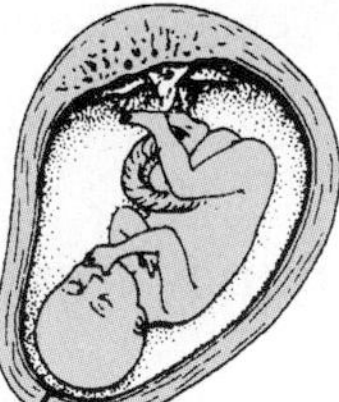
24 weeks

7th Lunar Month

The fetus is 35 cm to 38 cm in length and weighs to 1200 g.
Skin is red.
Pupillary membrane disappears from eyes.
The fetus has an excellent chance of survival.
Eyes open and close.

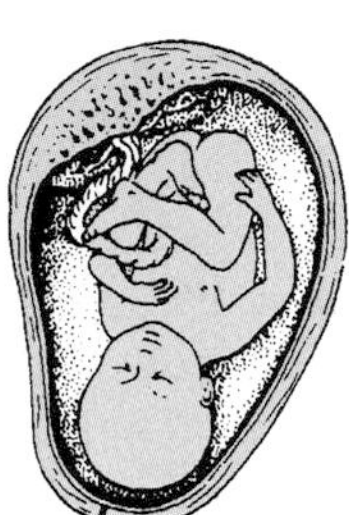
28 weeks

8th Lunar Month

The fetus is 38 cm to 43 cm in length and weighs 1500-2500 g.
Fetus is viable.
Eyelids open.
Fingerprints are set.
Vigorous fetal movement occurs.

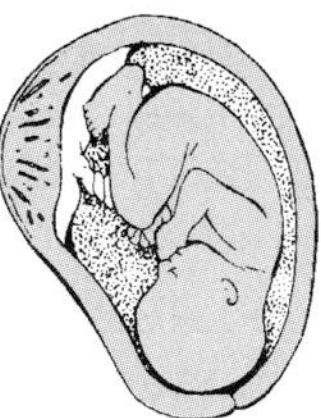
32 weeks

9th Lunar Month

The fetus is 42 cm to 49 cm in length and weighs 1900 g to 2700 g.
Face and body have a loose wrinkled appearance because of subcutaneous fat deposit.
Lanugo disappears.
Amniotic fluid decreases.

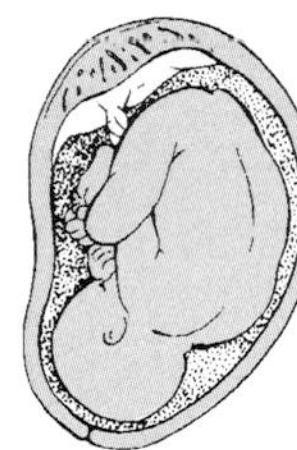
36 weeks

10th Lunar Month

The fetus is 48 cm to 52 cm in length and weighs 3000 g.
Skin is smooth.
Eyes are uniformly slate colored.
Bones of skull are ossified and nearly together at sutures.

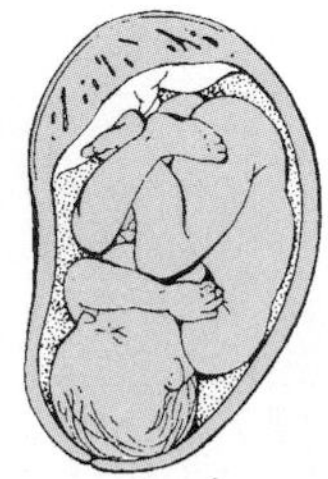
40 weeks

FIGURE 1.2 Monthly diagram of fetal development.

Placenta and Umbilical Cord

A properly functioning placenta and umbilical cord are essential to fetal growth and development. The placenta:

- Functions as an endocrine gland, secreting HCG, estrogen, and progesterone, which maintain the pregnancy
- Supplies food and oxygen to the developing fetus
- Carries wastes away for excretion by the mother
- Slows maternal immune response so that her body does not reject fetal tissue

The placenta normally weighs 400 to 600 g. After delivery, it is of no further use and is expelled. The side attached to the uterine wall is dark red with a rough surface and is documented as the "Dirty Duncan." The side against the fetus is smooth and shiny and called the "Shiny Schultze."

The umbilical cord joins the embryo/fetus to the placenta. It normally is 20 to 22 inches long and attaches to the center of the placenta. Most of the cord is a pale, white gelatinous-mucoid substance called *Wharton's jelly,* which prevents compression of the blood vessels. Normally, two arteries and one vein give the cord a rope-like appearance. The vein carries oxygenated blood to the fetus, while the arteries return deoxygenated blood to the placenta. The blood vessels are inspected after delivery of the placenta and umbilical cord. The cord has no pain receptors, so cutting it after delivery causes no discomfort. Frequently, the woman's partner in the delivery room is offered the experience of "cutting the cord."

Fetal Circulation

As early as the 3rd week of gestation, fetal blood has started to exchange nutrients with maternal circulation across the chorionic villi (Fig. 1.3). Fetal circulation differs from newborn and adult circulation in several ways. The fetus derives oxygen and excretes carbon dioxide via the placenta. Blood is shunted away from the fetal lungs to supply the most important organs: brain, liver, heart, and kidneys.

Fetal circulation is complex. A system of arteries, veins, and accessory structures exchanges oxygen and nutrients; this system closes after birth. Blood arriving to the fetus from the placenta is highly oxygenated. It enters the

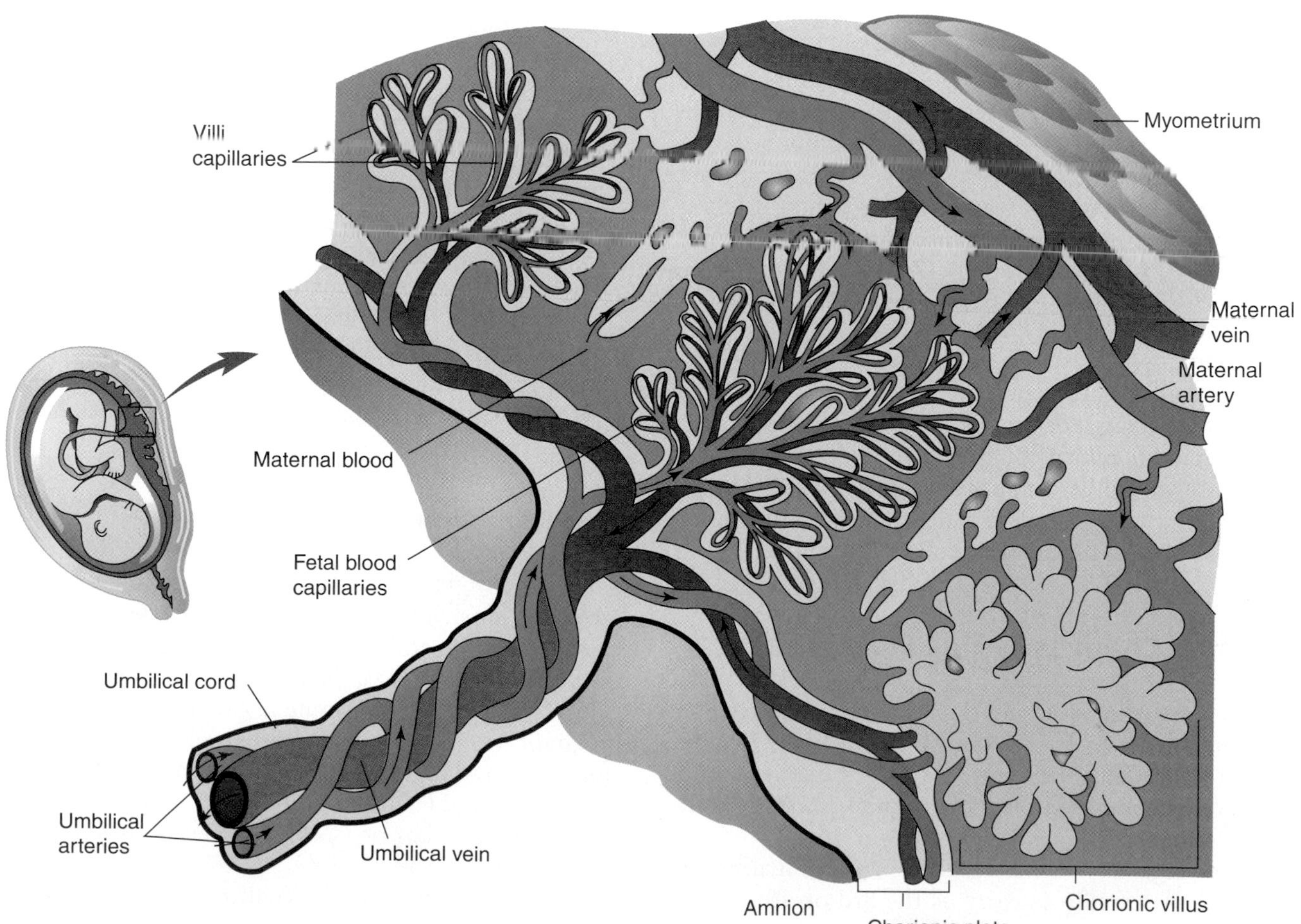

FIGURE 1.3 Fetal circulation.

fetus through the umbilical vein (called a vein even though it carries oxygenated blood), which carries blood to the inferior vena cava through an accessory structure called the **ductus venosus.** This short duct is found only in the fetus. It supplies the fetal liver with blood and atrophies after birth. From the inferior vena cava, a septum between the atria called the **foramen ovale** carries blood to the right atrium and shunts it through to the left atrium. The foramen ovale allows most blood to bypass the right ventricle. From the left atrium, blood follows the course of normal circulation into the left ventricle and then through the aorta. A small amount passes from the right atrium to the right ventricle and makes its way to the pulmonary artery. Thus, a small amount of blood services lung tissue but is not for oxygen exchange. The blood is then shunted through the **ductus arteriosus,** a connection between the pulmonary artery and aorta that allows blood to shunt around the fetal lungs.

Normally, the lungs expand with the newborn's first few respirations as soon as pressure within the chest alters. The foramen ovale closes, and the ductus arteriosus and ductus venosus become fibrous ligaments. Failure to resolve the fetal circulation results in congenital heart defects (see Chaps. 4 and 8).

Fetal Respiratory System

Development of the respiratory system is an important consideration in assessing fetal viability. Initially, the respiratory and digestive tracts are a single tube. By the end of the fourth week of gestation, a septum begins to divide the esophagus from the trachea. At the same time, lung buds appear on the trachea. Respiratory developmental milestones include the following:

- Development of the alveoli and capillaries enables gas exchange.
- Spontaneous respiratory movements begin as early as 3 months of pregnancy.
- Low surface tension and viscosity of respiratory fluid aid in expansion of alveoli after birth.
- At 24 weeks' gestation, **surfactant** excreted by the alveolar cells decreases surface tension on expiration, preventing alveolar collapse.

Maternal Changes During Pregnancy

Diagnosis of pregnancy marks a major life milestone. If pregnancy was planned, the woman is likely to experience feelings of fulfillment and achievement. An unplanned or undesired pregnancy may cause extreme stress.

Many pregnancy-related changes in the woman's body are visible externally as early as the 3rd or 4th month, depending on body type. The abdomen becomes more round and contoured as the fetus grows. The woman must pay more attention to balance, because her center of gravity shifts forward and an inward curvature of the lower back called *lordosis* develops. During late pregnancy, the rib cage flares outward, making more room for the growing fetus.

Breast changes are gradual and often subtle. They result from estrogen and progesterone and may begin to be noticeable at approximately 6 weeks' gestation. The woman may note breast fullness, tenderness, and tingling as a result of increased estrogen levels. The areolae and nipples darken and increase. As breast vascularity increases, blue veins are visible over the surface. By 16 weeks, the nipples may expel **colostrum,** a thin, watery, high-protein fluid that is the precursor to human milk.

Many changes also are taking place internally from a unique hormonal environment. Levels of estrogen and progesterone rise steadily from early pregnancy until near term when they begin to decline slowly. Other hormones such as human placental lactogen (HPL) and HCG drop during the second trimester. These reproductive hormones and other normal body hormones create an environment that supports the pregnancy throughout the 40 weeks. Some of the most important hormonal effects include the following:

- Developing the endometrium so that the embryo can implant
- Creating changes in maternal metabolism so that nutrients are available for mother and fetus
- Increasing maternal blood volume and red blood cell mass to provide extra oxygen needed for the fetus and increased maternal demands
- Increasing blood supply to the gastrointestinal tract while slowing peristaltic waves, which increase absorption of nutrients
- Relaxing the ligaments that connect the pelvic bones to allow passage of the baby during labor
- Preparing the breasts for lactation

Cultural Beliefs

Noting the woman's ethnic, cultural, and religious background is important to anticipate client-specific nursing interventions to add to or to eliminate from the plan of care. Mattson (2000) explains that many cultures consider it unacceptable for a male caregiver to examine a pregnant woman; some cultures believe that an episiotomy allows the woman's spirit to leave her body. Cultural beliefs and values can influence a woman's reliance on her obstetrician or CNM and decisions she makes about receiving care.

When assessing a woman's cultural and religious preferences regarding care, Callister (1995) suggests that nurses ask questions about:

- Value and meaning the client places on the birth experience
- View of childbirth experience
- Practices regarding diet, medications, activity, and emotional and physical support
- Appropriate maternal and paternal behaviors
- Birth companions (who are they and what should they do)
- Views regarding the newborn and his or her care immediately after birth

Antepartal Care

Antepartal care is essential for the overall health of woman and fetus. Unfortunately, many people do not receive regular, routine healthcare. Promoting antepartal healthcare has been a national initiative through radio and television advertisements, hospital brochures, outreach community education, and emphasis from healthcare and insurance industries.

Choosing a healthcare provider is an important step in planning for care throughout pregnancy. Above all else, the provider should be someone who genuinely listens to the woman and her concerns.

The initial antepartal health visit is the time to establish baseline data and perform a risk assessment. The goal of risk assessment is to identify women and fetuses at risk for complications during pregnancy, labor, birth, or the neonatal period (directly after birth). Findings may indicate a need for genetic testing. The initial visit includes a health history, complete physical examination (including a pelvic examination to estimate pelvic size), and laboratory tests for Rh factor and blood type, complete blood count (CBC), syphilis, antibody screen, and rubella titer. Some practitioners also include an HIV test. An indirect Coombs test is completed and generally repeated at 28 weeks to determine if Rh antibodies are present, indicating Rh incompatibility. In addition, a pregnancy test is completed to confirm pregnancy. The practitioner will establish an estimated date of delivery (EDD) (Box 1-2).

Pregnant women usually return to their practitioners for monthly visits until the last trimester. These visits include checks of weight; blood pressure; urine dipstick for protein, glucose, and sometimes nitrites and leukocytes; measurement of the uterus (Fig 1.4); fetal heart tones; edema in the face, hands, legs, and feet; and continuing risk assessments.

Between 15 and 19 weeks, a blood test called the maternal serum-alpha fetoprotein (MS-AFP) is done to screen for fetal neural tube defects. Many women undergo an ultrasound between 16 and 20 weeks to establish gestational age and to examine the fetus for normal development. Between 24 and 28 weeks, women usually are screened for gestational diabetes with a 1-hour random glucose tolerance test (see Chap. 52).

BOX 1-2 ● Estimating the Date of Delivery

Healthcare practitioners commonly use Nagele's rule to determine an estimated date of delivery (EDD) for pregnant women. The steps involved are as follows:

- Determine the first day of the woman's last normal menstrual period (LNMP). The LNMP should have arrived on schedule and been of normal duration and flow.
- Add 7 days.
- Subtract 3 months.
- Add 1 year.

The outcome is the EDD.

For example, a pregnant woman's LNMP began on May 5, 2003. Adding 7 days is May 12, 2003. Subtracting 3 months is February 12, 2003. Adding 1 year is February 12, 2004, which is her EDD.

After the 8th month, the schedule of visits changes from monthly to every 2 weeks for that month. In the 9th month, the schedule changes to weekly visits until birth.

Stop, Think, and Respond ● BOX 1-2

You are assigned to follow a primigravida through her pregnancy. She is currently at 12 weeks' gestation. What anticipatory guidance would be most appropriate as she enters the second trimester?

Health Promotion

Most pregnant women want to learn more about pregnancy, childbirth, motherhood, and associated changes. Pregnancy is one time when most women, physicians, and insurance providers recognize and value the importance of regular medical supervision and preventive and diagnostic measures. Most pregnant women think of

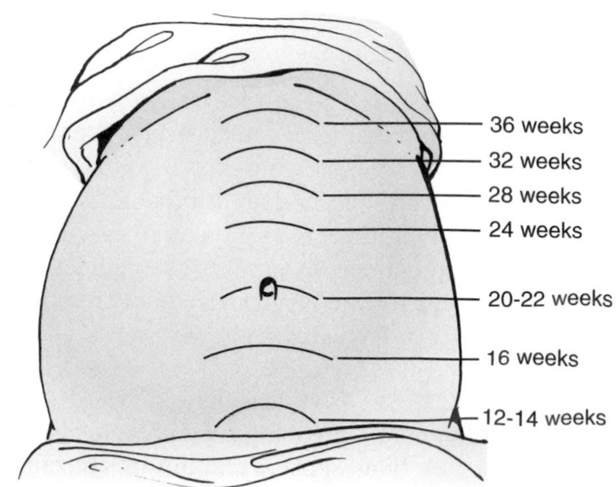

FIGURE 1.4 Fundal height.

their baby first and do everything advised to ensure the child's health. The following discussions focus on common health promotion measures for healthcare professionals to communicate to pregnant women and their families.

NUTRITION. One of the earliest and most important considerations of antepartal care is adequate nutrition to support the woman and growing fetus. Nutritional requirements for pregnant women differ from those for nonpregnant women. Caloric needs increase during pregnancy; however, quality, not quantity, of food should be the focus. Women should select foods from all food groups to obtain the necessary distribution of nutrients. In addition to the requirements of the basic food guide pyramid, pregnant women should follow these suggestions:

- Increase daily caloric intake by approximately 300 calories.
- Increase calcium intake (3 to 4 cups daily) before the last half of pregnancy to ensure proper development of fetal bones and teeth and for blood clotting.
- Maintain intake of iron and folic acid as well as most vitamins. Prenatal vitamins are regularly prescribed during pregnancy.
- Increase protein intake to build and repair body tissues and to aid in milk production for the nursing mother.
- Avoid empty calories such as alcohol, sugared soda drinks, sweets, and salty foods.
- Limit use of salt.
- Increase fluid intake to 10 glasses daily to assist in kidney and bowel function.
- Avoid laxatives and enemas. Use fiber in the diet or a stool softener, if needed.
- Avoid *pica,* the craving and eating of substances not normally considered edible (e.g., clay, dirt, cornstarch).

All pregnant women should gain weight during pregnancy. Recommended weight gain is based on height and pre-pregnancy weight. A general rule is a total weight gain of 25 to 35 pounds in the average-sized woman.

- By the 20th week of gestation, weight gain is generally 10 pounds for the average-sized woman.
- Any woman who loses more than 8 pounds during the first trimester (as a result of pregnancy-related nausea and vomiting) is at increased risk. Weight loss during pregnancy is never recommended.
- Although weight gain is normal, equally important is the quality of food leading to weight gain.

ACTIVITY AND EXERCISE. Women should continue normal activities throughout an uncomplicated pregnancy. Routine fitness programs and sports generally are considered safe; however, women should discuss their exercise routines with healthcare personnel. Discourage high-risk activities or those requiring balance and coordination. Consultation with the provider and use of common sense are the best steps. See Client and Family Teaching 1-1.

REST AND SLEEP. Women will note few changes in maternal sleep patterns in the first trimester. They may feel more tired than usual and need rest periods or naps during the day with the feet elevated. Placing pillows under the abdomen and legs will promote proper body alignment and rest.

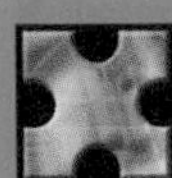

1-1 *Client and Family Teaching*
Exercise in Pregnancy

The nurse advises the pregnant woman as follows:

- Work with your provider to determine a routine appropriate for your endurance.
  - Sedentary women should begin exercise very gradually.
  - Women with uncomplicated pregnancies who regularly engage in moderate exercise can continue their routines, provided that they reduce exercise intensity by approximately 25% and limit strenuous exercise to 15 to 20 minutes.
  - Women used to extreme activity should reduce their usual levels of exertion.
- Decrease the intensity of weight-bearing exercise. Safe forms of exercise with solid overall benefits to health include walking and swimming.
- Avoid dangerous or potentially risky forms of exercise. Examples include contact sports such as football, sports that could result in damage to joints and ligaments (e.g., gymnastics, volleyball), mountain climbing, sky diving, surfing, and horseback riding.
- Continue relaxation, stretching, and yoga exercises.
- Light weight lifting is safe to continue, but avoid heavy resistance on machines and use of heavy free weights.
- Do not exercise or play sports in conditions of extreme heat or cold, high humidity, air pollution or high altitudes.
- Ensure proper hydration by drinking plenty of water before, during, and after exercise.
- Be sure to properly warm up before and cool down after exercise.
- Wear a supportive bra and comfortable, supportive sports shoes.
- Stop exercise immediately if numbness, dizziness, abdominal pain, vaginal bleeding, or shortness of breath develop. Immediately contact your healthcare provider.

As abdominal size increases, women may find it increasingly difficult to rest in a comfortable position, particularly those who prefer to sleep prone. The supine position is not recommended as the woman approaches her due date, because it may cause excessive pressure on the aorta and vena cava. A side-lying position is recommended.

COMMON DISCOMFORTS. Even in normal pregnancy, women commonly experience unusual, and sometimes uncomfortable, events and sensations. Most are minor and do not threaten the fetus or mother. Distinguishing between a truly common discomfort and a warning sign of a more serious problem may be difficult. Table 1.1 provides a list of common discomforts of pregnancy with relief measures.

MEDICATION USE IN PREGNANCY. A standard guide is that pregnant woman should **not** take any medications, herbs, or nutritional supplements unless absolutely necessary and ordered by her healthcare provider. The safety of any drug during pregnancy is unpredictable. The U.S. Food and Drug Administration (FDA) has established five categories of drugs based on their potential teratogenic effects in humans (Box 1-3). When providers prescribe a medication for a pregnant woman, they carefully assess the medication and maintain the smallest effective dose.

Preparation for Childbirth

As the final trimester approaches, the woman focuses more on labor and birth and arrangements for the baby following arrival. Safety for herself and the fetus is an overriding concern. Planning for the birth may include choosing a site for delivery, an attendant, and a plan for analgesia and positioning. Frequently, the woman and her partner have attended childbirth classes in preparation.

Only the woman herself can decide what alternatives she wants to explore to meet her needs during labor and delivery. Many of these alternatives focus on the woman's values, beliefs, and goals. The nurse's task is to support the woman's choices.

Natural childbirth consists of progressive relaxation and abdominal breathing techniques taught to the expec-

TABLE 1.1 COMMON DISCOMFORTS OF PREGNANCY AND ASSOCIATED RELIEF MEASURES

DISCOMFORT	RELIEF MEASURES
Back pain	Wear shoes with a slight heel that provide good support. Change position frequently. Limit time spent on feet.
Breast tenderness	Wear a bra with good support. Ensure good posture.
Constipation	Increase fluids, fiber intake, and activity.
Heartburn	Eat small, frequent meals. Avoid caffeine intake. Do not lie down after meals.
Insomnia	Place a pillow under the abdomen, between the legs, or both to help improve body positioning during sleep. Do not eat heavy meals before bedtime. Eliminate caffeine intake. Take a warm bath or shower before retiring.
Itching	Bathe with baking soda, cornstarch, or colloidal oatmeal. Do not use soap on affected areas. Use moisturizer.
Mood swings	Engage in relaxation exercises (e.g., meditate, listen to soothing music). Ask friends and family for support, understanding, and help.
Nausea and vomiting	Avoid heavy and fatty meals. Drink peppermint or ginger tea.
Skin pigment changes	Minimize sun exposure. Use sunblock.
Stretch marks	Apply coconut, olive, or vitamin E oil to affected areas.
Swollen feet and legs	Elevate legs when sitting. Ensure adequate calcium and potassium intake.
Urinary frequency	Void whenever needed. Decrease fluid intake before bedtime.
Vaginal discharge	Do not use soap on vulva.

BOX 1-3 ● Categories of Drug Safety in Pregnancy

The FDA has rated drugs according to their relative safety during pregnancy as follows:

Category A: Controlled studies in women do not demonstrate a risk; possibility of fetal harm appears remote.

Category B: Animal studies fail to demonstrate fetal risks, and there are no controlled studies in women; *or* animal studies show an adverse effect, but the same effect was not confirmed in studies in women.

Category C: Animal studies have demonstrated fetal risks, but no controlled human studies are available; *or* studies in women and animals are not available. Drugs in this category should be given only if the potential benefit to the mother outweighs the possible risk to the fetus.

Category D: Human fetal risks exist, but the benefits of use in pregnant women may be acceptable despite the risk—such as when a life-threatening situation exists, or for a serious disease for which safer drugs cannot be used or are not effective.

Category X: Proven fetal risks exist; drug is contraindicated in women who are or may become pregnant.

tant mother and a birth attendant. Relaxing, focusing, and working through contractions as labor progresses are common. The *Lamaze method* is the best-known model of childbirth preparation and includes education and training. Expectant women learn toning and relaxation exercises and breathing techniques, which change for the different stages of labor. A birth attendant or "coach" provides support and encourages the woman throughout labor and delivery. Several other options for coping with the stress and pain of childbirth include massage therapy, water therapy, relaxing music and lighting, and aromatherapy.

Medications to ease the pain of labor include IV and epidural medications. Medications and techniques have been successful at providing more comfort while allowing the woman to work with the contractions, continuing the labor process.

NORMAL LABOR AND DELIVERY

As stated at the beginning of the chapter, the woman's body is designed for conceiving, carrying, and bearing children. Even though this process is normal, most women experience it only a few times in their lives. In most pregnancies, the fetus reaches maturity and the uterus begins the process of labor at exactly the right time. Although the process has been repeated throughout history, researchers are still trying to discover the exact cause for the onset of labor. This section focuses on promotion of normal labor progression through the postpartum period.

Signs of Impending Labor

Labor is a series of events during which the woman's uterus contracts and expels the fetus. Although the cause of labor remains unknown, certain signs indicate its imminent onset. **Lightening** is when the fetus seems to settle into the pelvis and usually means labor will begin in approximately 2 weeks. After lightening, the woman usually notices urinary frequency and some relief from dyspnea as the fetus is no longer directly under her rib cage.

The **bloody show** typically consists of blood-tinged vaginal mucus and indicates that the cervix has begun to change in consistency. The cervix begins to soften, become thin (**efface**), and open (**dilate**).

Backache and **Braxton Hicks contractions** (irregular tightening of the pregnant uterus that begins in the first trimester and increases in frequency, duration, and intensity as pregnancy progresses) are common as pregnancy reaches term. Braxton Hicks contractions remain irregular and do not dilate the cervix.

Onset of Labor

Labor progresses through four stages in which the uterus:

- Undergoes rhythmic contractions (labor contractions) that open the cervical os and move the fetus downward into the birth canal
- Continues contracting until the baby is delivered through the vaginal opening
- Expels the placenta
- Contracts again to prevent any excessive blood loss

Table 1.2 compares the signs of true labor and false labor.

TABLE 1.2 TRUE VERSUS FALSE LABOR

TRUE LABOR CONTRACTIONS	FALSE LABOR CONTRACTIONS
Become regular with progression of labor	Remain irregular and short
Strengthen over time and with walking	Do not strengthen or change with walking
Do not disappear with rest	May be relieved with rest
Start in the back and radiate to the front	Usually occur in the front
Are accompanied by dilation and effacement of the cervix	Are not accompanied by significant cervical changes
Become longer and more frequent with labor (every 20 to 30 minutes or more)	Do not lengthen, become more frequent, or happen close together

chapter 1

Caring for Clients During Normal Pregnancy, Labor, and Delivery

Words to Know 

abortion
amenorrhea
amniotic fluid
antepartal
bloody show
Braxton Hicks contractions
certified nurse midwife
Chadwick's sign
chorion
chorionic villi
colostrum
conception
crowning
deceleration
dilate
ductus arteriosus
ductus venosus
efface
embryo
engagement
epidural
episiotomy
fertilization
fetal attitude
fetus
fontanelles
foramen ovale
gestation
gravida
labor
lie
lightening
molding
natural childbirth
obstetrician
obstetrics
oxytocic
para
perinatal
position
postpartal
preconceptual care
presentation
quickening
station
surfactant
sutures
tocodynamometer
trimester
viability
zygote

Learning Objectives

On completion of this chapter, the reader will:

- Identify the presumptive, probable, and positive signs of pregnancy.
- Define key terms related to pregnancy, gestation, labor, and delivery.
- Describe the processes of fertilization, implantation, and placental development.
- Describe maternal physical changes during each trimester of pregnancy.
- Identify at least four concepts related to prenatal care important for client teaching.
- Identify recommended nutritional guidelines during pregnancy.
- Explore anticipatory guidance and ways to support the growing family.
- Identify at least three differences between true labor and false labor.
- Discuss potential variations in lie, presentation, station, and position.
- Identify three nursing considerations for the latent, active, and transitional phases of labor.
- Explain the significance of involution and three related nursing considerations.

Few experiences in life are as exciting, highly anticipated, and challenging as childbearing. The woman's body is designed to conceive and bear children. A complex system of hormonal and physical changes enables her to release an egg and support a pregnancy. When pregnancy does not occur, the woman has a regular menstrual period. Pregnancy is a normal physiologic process, not a disease.

This chapter describes the overall process of a normal healthy pregnancy and associated maternal physiological changes. It explores the process of human fetal development and the stages of labor that result in the birth of a healthy infant. It also provides information about how nurses can help their clients experience a healthy pregnancy and provide vital instruction about accompanying changes for the evolving family.

PREGNANCY

Signs of Pregnancy

Different signs with varying degrees of certainty can help confirm pregnancy. *Presumptive signs* indicate pregnancy but may also signify disease. They include the following:

- **Amenorrhea** (absence of menstruation)
- Nausea and vomiting
- Frequent urination
- Swelling, tingling, or tenderness of the breasts
- Changes in abdominal shape
- **Quickening** (sensation of fetal movement)
- Skin changes
- **Chadwick's sign** (a violet or purplish discoloration in the vagina, cervix, and vulva)

Probable signs indicate a high likelihood that a woman is pregnant but are not 100% reliable. They include:

- Enlargement of the uterus
- Positive pregnancy tests (using urine or blood to measure the level of human-chorionic gonadotropin [HCG])

Positive signs of pregnancy occur only with pregnancy. They include:

- Visualization of the fetal skeleton on x-ray or ultrasound
- Fetal movement felt by an examiner
- Auscultation of fetal heartbeat via Doppler at 10 to 12 weeks or fetoscope after 18 weeks

Stop, Think, and Respond ● BOX 1-1

A client comes to the clinic stating that her menstrual period is more than 2 weeks late. What questions would the nurse ask to gather further information?

Terminology of Pregnancy

Gestation is the time from when sperm fertilizes an egg until a baby is born. The uniting of sperm and egg is called **fertilization** (also called **conception**) and usually occurs 2 weeks after a women's last normal menstrual period (LMP or LNMP). Specific cells (ova or eggs in females and sperm in males) carry genetic messages to offspring. A woman's ovum and a man's sperm combine to result in a new individual or **zygote** with a unique genetic makeup.

The total length of a full-term gestation is 40 weeks or 9 calendar months. Gestation is divided into three 3-month periods called **trimesters.** Pregnancy, also termed the maternity cycle, is divided into three periods: **antepartal** (begins with conception and ends with the onset of labor), **perinatal** (beginning of labor to delivery of the placenta), and **postpartal** (delivery of the placenta to 6 weeks later or when reproductive organs have returned to prepregnancy state).

Throughout her pregnancy, a woman is referred to as a **gravida** (pregnant woman). Latin numerical prefixes indicate the number of pregnancies, such as *nulligravida* (none), *primigravida* (one), and *multigravida* (multiple). The term **para** refers to mother and baby and is used to denote the number of actual births. Examples include *nullipara* (none), *primipara* (one), and *multipara* (multiple). A woman who has given birth five times or more is called a *grand multipara.* A shorthand method of keeping track of a client's obstetric history is to record the gravida/para (Box 1-1).

Abortion is the term used to indicate loss of the fetus before the age of **viability** (capability of living), whether spontaneous or induced.

Obstetrics is the branch of medicine concerned with reproductive health, pregnancy, and birth. An **obstetrician** is a physician who practices obstetrics. A registered nurse with specialized training in the management of labor and birth who works with healthy women during pregnancy is called a **certified nurse midwife (CNM).** These nurses provide assessment and detailed instruction on maintaining wellness and attend at vaginal births. They refer women with health risks before or during pregnancy to obstetricians (see Chap. 2).

Preconceptual care means care of the woman before she is pregnant. Components include balanced nutrition, vitamins (especially folic acid), and adequate rest. Such measures make pregnancy safer for the woman and fetus. Preconceptual care should begin early, because the first trimester is the most critical time in human development. Many couples also elect genetic counseling to reduce the

BOX 1-1 ● Classifying Pregnancy History

Nurses use a set of numbers and letters to classify a woman's pregnancy history.

G–Gravida: the total number of pregnancies a woman has had, including the current pregnancy, regardless of the outcome (e.g., term birth, miscarriage, abortion)

P–Para: the total number of babies born after 20 weeks' gestation (including multiples)

For example, a pregnant woman has had two babies before, one at 39 weeks and the other at 32 weeks. The nurse would write G3 P2.

Para can be broken down further, using the acronym FPAL.

F–Full term: the total number of babies born at 37 weeks' gestation or more

P–Preterm: the total number of babies born between 20 and 37 weeks' gestation

A–Abortions: the total number of abortions (spontaneous and elective) before 20 weeks' gestation

L–Living: the total number of children currently alive

For example, a woman is not pregnant but has been pregnant three times before. One baby was born at term, twins were born preterm, and one pregnancy ended in miscarriage at 14 weeks. G = 3, F = 1, P = 2, A = 1, L = 3. Thus, the nurse would write G3 P1213.

Adapted from Rosdahl, C. B., & Kowalski, M. T. (2003). *Textbook of basic nursing* (8th ed.). Philadelphia: Lippincott Williams & Wilkins.

their baby first and do everything advised to ensure the child's health. The following discussions focus on common health promotion measures for healthcare professionals to communicate to pregnant women and their families.

NUTRITION. One of the earliest and most important considerations of antepartal care is adequate nutrition to support the woman and growing fetus. Nutritional requirements for pregnant women differ from those for nonpregnant women. Caloric needs increase during pregnancy; however, quality, not quantity, of food should be the focus. Women should select foods from all food groups to obtain the necessary distribution of nutrients. In addition to the requirements of the basic food guide pyramid, pregnant women should follow these suggestions:

- Increase daily caloric intake by approximately 300 calories.
- Increase calcium intake (3 to 4 cups daily) before the last half of pregnancy to ensure proper development of fetal bones and teeth and for blood clotting.
- Maintain intake of iron and folic acid as well as most vitamins. Prenatal vitamins are regularly prescribed during pregnancy.
- Increase protein intake to build and repair body tissues and to aid in milk production for the nursing mother.
- Avoid empty calories such as alcohol, sugared soda drinks, sweets, and salty foods.
- Limit use of salt.
- Increase fluid intake to 10 glasses daily to assist in kidney and bowel function.
- Avoid laxatives and enemas. Use fiber in the diet or a stool softener, if needed.
- Avoid *pica,* the craving and eating of substances not normally considered edible (e.g., clay, dirt, cornstarch).

All pregnant women should gain weight during pregnancy. Recommended weight gain is based on height and pre-pregnancy weight. A general rule is a total weight gain of 25 to 35 pounds in the average-sized woman.

- By the 20th week of gestation, weight gain is generally 10 pounds for the average-sized woman.
- Any woman who loses more than 8 pounds during the first trimester (as a result of pregnancy-related nausea and vomiting) is at increased risk. Weight loss during pregnancy is never recommended.

[illegible]lthough weight gain is normal, equally important [illegible]e quality of food leading to weight gain.

AC[illegible] EXERCISE. Women should continue normal acti[illegible] [illegible]hout an uncomplicated pregnancy. Routine [illegible]s and sports generally are considered safe; h[illegible]n should discuss their exercise routines [illegible] personnel. Discourage high-risk activities or those requiring balance and coordination. Consultation with the provider and use of common sense are the best steps. See Client and Family Teaching 1-1.

REST AND SLEEP. Women will note few changes in maternal sleep patterns in the first trimester. They may feel more tired than usual and need rest periods or naps during the day with the feet elevated. Placing pillows under the abdomen and legs will promote proper body alignment and rest.

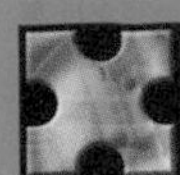

1-1 *Client and Family Teaching* Exercise in Pregnancy

The nurse advises the pregnant woman as follows:

- Work with your provider to determine a routine appropriate for your endurance.
  - Sedentary women should begin exercise very gradually.
  - Women with uncomplicated pregnancies who regularly engage in moderate exercise can continue their routines, provided that they reduce exercise intensity by approximately 25% and limit strenuous exercise to 15 to 20 minutes.
  - Women used to extreme activity should reduce their usual levels of exertion.
- Decrease the intensity of weight-bearing exercise. Safe forms of exercise with solid overall benefits to health include walking and swimming.
- Avoid dangerous or potentially risky forms of exercise. Examples include contact sports such as football, sports that could result in damage to joints and ligaments (e.g., gymnastics, volleyball), mountain climbing, sky diving, surfing, and horseback riding.
- Continue relaxation, stretching, and yoga exercises.
- Light weight lifting is safe to continue, but avoid heavy resistance on machines and use of heavy free weights.
- Do not exercise or play sports in conditions of extreme heat or cold, high humidity, air pollution or high altitudes.
- Ensure proper hydration by drinking plenty of water before, during, and after exercise.
- Be sure to properly warm up before and cool down after exercise.
- Wear a supportive bra and comfortable, supportive sports shoes.
- Stop exercise immediately if numbness, dizziness, abdominal pain, vaginal bleeding, or shortness of breath develop. Immediately contact your healthcare provider.

BOX 1-3 ● Categories of Drug Safety in Pregnancy

The FDA has rated drugs according to their relative safety during pregnancy as follows:

Category A: Controlled studies in women do not demonstrate a risk; possibility of fetal harm appears remote.

Category B: Animal studies fail to demonstrate fetal risks, and there are no controlled studies in women; *or* animal studies show an adverse effect, but the same effect was not confirmed in studies in women.

Category C: Animal studies have demonstrated fetal risks, but no controlled human studies are available; *or* studies in women and animals are not available. Drugs in this category should be given only if the potential benefit to the mother outweighs the possible risk to the fetus.

Category D: Human fetal risks exist, but the benefits of use in pregnant women may be acceptable despite the risk—such as when a life-threatening situation exists, or for a serious disease for which safer drugs cannot be used or are not effective.

Category X: Proven fetal risks exist; drug is contraindicated in women who are or may become pregnant.

tant mother and a birth attendant. Relaxing, focusing, and working through contractions as labor progresses are common. The *Lamaze method* is the best-known model of childbirth preparation and includes education and training. Expectant women learn toning and relaxation exercises and breathing techniques, which change for the different stages of labor. A birth attendant or "coach" provides support and encourages the woman throughout labor and delivery. Several other options for coping with the stress and pain of childbirth include massage therapy, water therapy, relaxing music and lighting, and aromatherapy.

Medications to ease the pain of labor include IV and epidural medications. Medications and techniques have been successful at providing more comfort while allowing the woman to work with the contractions, continuing the labor process.

NORMAL LABOR AND DELIVERY

As stated at the beginning of the chapter, the woman's body is designed for conceiving, carrying, and bearing children. Even though this process is normal, most women experience it only a few times in their lives. In most pregnancies, the fetus reaches maturity and the uterus begins the process of labor at exactly the right time. Although the process has been repeated throughout history, researchers are still trying to discover the exact cause for the onset of labor. This section focuses on promotion of normal labor progression through the postpartum period.

Signs of Impending Labor

Labor is a series of events during which the woman's uterus contracts and expels the fetus. Although the cause of labor remains unknown, certain signs indicate its imminent onset. **Lightening** is when the fetus seems to settle into the pelvis and usually means labor will begin in approximately 2 weeks. After lightening, the woman usually notices urinary frequency and some relief from dyspnea as the fetus is no longer directly under her rib cage.

The **bloody show** typically consists of blood-tinged vaginal mucus and indicates that the cervix has begun to change in consistency. The cervix begins to soften, become thin (**efface**), and open (**dilate**).

Backache and **Braxton Hicks contractions** (irregular tightening of the pregnant uterus that begins in the first trimester and increases in frequency, duration, and intensity as pregnancy progresses) are common as pregnancy reaches term. Braxton Hicks contractions remain irregular and do not dilate the cervix.

Onset of Labor

Labor progresses through four stages in which the uterus:

- Undergoes rhythmic contractions (labor contractions) that open the cervical os and move the fetus downward into the birth canal
- Continues contracting until the baby is delivered through the vaginal opening
- Expels the placenta
- Contracts again to prevent any excessive blood loss

Table 1.2 compares the signs of true labor and false labor.

[illegible]ABLE 1.2 TRUE VERSUS FALSE LABOR

[illegible]OR CONTRACTIONS	FALSE LABOR CONTRACTIONS
Str[illegible] Do [illegible]lar with progression of labor	Remain irregular and short
Start [illegible] time and with walking	Do not strengthen or change with walking
Are acc[illegible] with rest	May be relieved with rest
Become [illegible] radiate to the front	Usually occur in the front
30 minu[illegible]ilation and effacement of the cervix	Are not accompanied by significant cervical changes
[illegible] frequent with labor (every 20 to	Do not lengthen, become more frequent, or happen close together

Sites for Labor and Delivery

Just as women choose their birth attendants from husbands, boyfriends, mothers, sisters, and friends, so they have various options for birth setting. Most women choose to deliver in hospitals because that is where most practitioners practice. Some hospitals assign women to one room where they labor and then another room for the delivery. Other hospitals admit women directly to a birthing room, in which both labor and delivery take place.

An alternative to a hospital is a freestanding birthing center. This structured establishment promotes the concept of safe and cost-effective childbirth. The National Association of Childbirth Centers uses standards and criteria for care and safety at childbirth centers. Women can arrange for home births, commonly with the assistance of a CNM. Only women in good health with uncomplicated pregnancies are candidates for birth outside hospitals.

Maternal Considerations

Pelvis

A woman's pelvic size is important for the ability of the fetus to pass through the birth canal. The superior portion of the pelvis (iliac segment of the innominate bones) supports the uterus and fetus during late pregnancy. These bones help direct the fetus into the lower portion of the pelvis called the *true pelvis.* The fetus must be able to pass through the true pelvis during birth. The true pelvis is divided into three segments: cavity, midpelvis, and outlet. The pelvis may be evaluated by *palpation* (determining the distance between the ischial tuberosities by palpating the bony prominences), *pelvimetry* (using x-rays from different views to determine pelvic size), and *ultrasonography* (sound waves used to estimate pelvic size). The adequacy of the pelvis needs to be determined before labor.

Soft Tissues

During labor, the uterus, cervix, vagina, and perineal muscles change in consistency and shape to allow passage of the fetus. The upper uterus has a thickened musculature that provides the force for contractions. The muscle walls of the lower segment thin and act as a band of tissue. As contractions of the upper muscular segment apply downward pressure, the uterine contents press, causing effacement and dilation of the cervix. In response to hormonal changes during pregnancy, increased blood supply and loosening of the connective tissue with enlargement of the smooth muscle cells make the vagina capable of stretching (dilating) to allow passage of the fetus. Pressure of the presenting fetal part stretches and thins the muscles of the pelvic floor (perineum). The anus may appear dilated and bulging.

Fetal Considerations

Another important consideration during labor is the relationship of the fetal body to the maternal body. Several terms are used to describe fetal positioning within the mother.

Fetal Lie, Attitude, and Presentation

Lie is the term used to compare the position of the fetal and maternal spinal cords. Normal fetal lie is longitudinal (up and down), placing the spine parallel to the mother's. In transverse lie, the fetus lies crosswise in the uterus and cannot be vaginally delivered without alteration. A cesarean birth may be required.

Fetal attitude is the relationship of the fetal body parts to one another. The fetus assumes a characteristic posture (attitude) within the uterus partly because of how he or she conforms to the shape of the uterine cavity.

Fetal **presentation** (part of the fetus that first enters the pelvis and lies over the inlet) determines the fetal body part that will be in contact with the cervix. The presenting part can be the head or face, breech, or shoulders. See Figure 1.5. In most vaginal deliveries, the presenting part is the head (*cephalic presentation*). The four types of cephalic presentations are vertex (region between the fontanelles), brow, face, and mentum (chin). When the presenting part is the face, the presentation is noted as *vertex presentation.*

In the *breech presentation,* either the buttocks or legs are in contact with the cervix. The four types of breech presentations are:

- Complete—the buttocks present and the thighs are flexed on the abdomen.
- Frank—the buttocks present and the thighs extend across the abdomen and chest.
- Footling—either one or both legs are extended both at the hip and the knee.
- Kneeling—the legs extend at the hip but are flexed at the knee.

In the *shoulder presentation,* the fetus is on a transverse lie. The shoulder, arm, backside, or abdomen may be the presenting part.

Fetal Skull

Because the fetal skull is usually the largest part of the body, delivery of the head poses the greatest concern. **Crowning** occurs when the fetal head presents at the vulva. The bones of the skull have not joined (fused), allowing the bony plates to overlap during progression through the maternal pelvis. The reshaping of the skull bones in response to pressure against the maternal pelvis during birth is called **molding.**

The major bones of the fetal skull are the two frontal bones, two parietal bones, two temporal bones, and occiput. These are joined by membranous spaces called

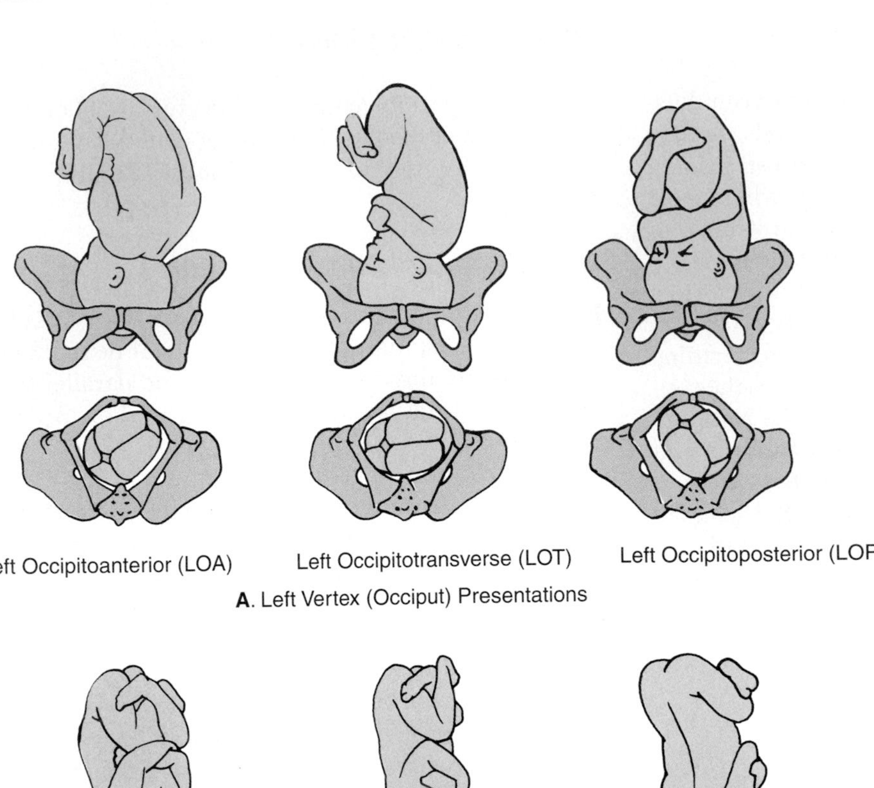

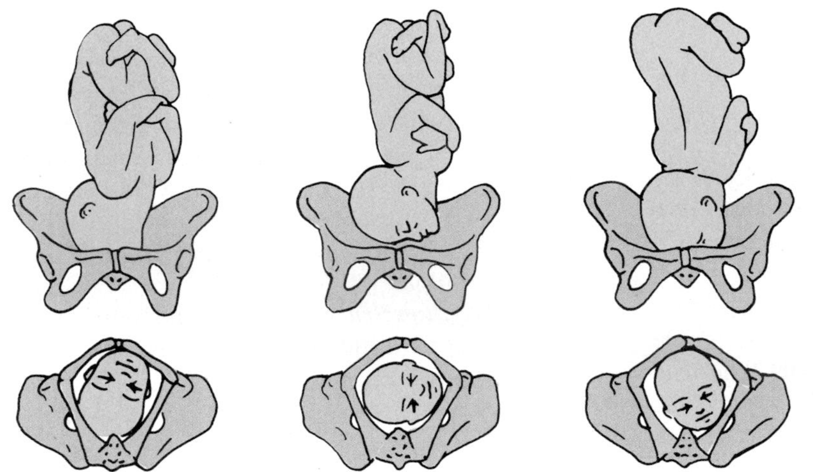

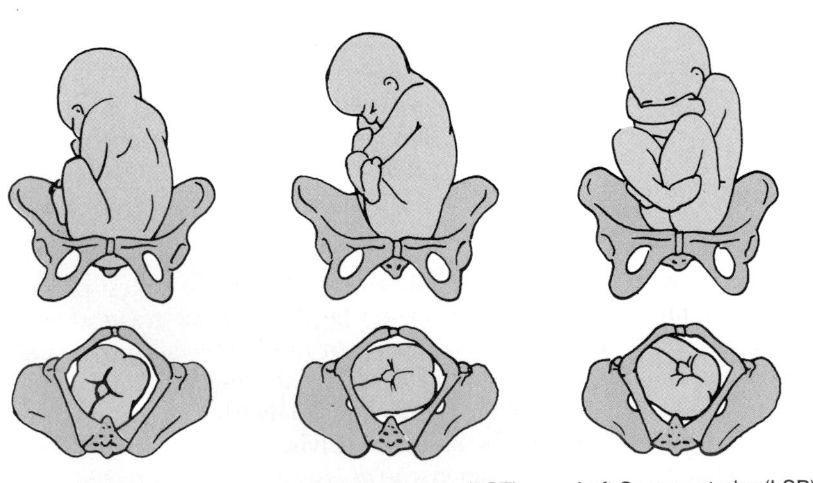

FIGURE 1.5 Presentation positions.

sutures. The sutures meet at large membranous areas called **fontanelles.** The two fontanelles (anterior and posterior) can allow the healthcare provider to determine fetal presentation during labor. The largest transverse diameter of the skull can be biparietally measured to ensure that the fetal head can pass through the maternal pelvis. The shoulders and pelvis may be turned and rotated and do not often cause a problem during birth.

Fetal Positions

Position is the relationship of the presenting part to the four quadrants of the mother's pelvis. Position is denoted by a three-letter abbreviation:

- The first letter denotes the location of the presenting part in the right (R) or left (L) side of the mother's pelvis.
- The middle letter denotes the specific presenting part of the fetus (O for occiput, S for sacrum, M for mentum, and Sc for scapula).
- The third letter denotes the location of the presenting part in relation to the anterior (A), posterior (P), or transverse (T) portion of the maternal pelvis.

Station is the relationship of the presenting part to an imaginary line drawn between the maternal ischial spines. It is a measure of the degree of descent of the presenting part through the birth canal. Placement of the presenting part is measured in centimeters above and below the ischial spines. Station should be determined when labor begins so that the rate of descent of the fetus during labor can be accurately determined (Fig 1.6).

Engagement is the term used to indicate that the largest transverse diameter of the presenting part (usually the biparietal diameter) has passed through the maternal pelvic brim or inlet into the true pelvis and corresponds with station 0. Engagement often occurs in the weeks before labor in primigravidas; it may occur before or during labor in multigravidas. Engagement can be determined by abdominal or vaginal examination.

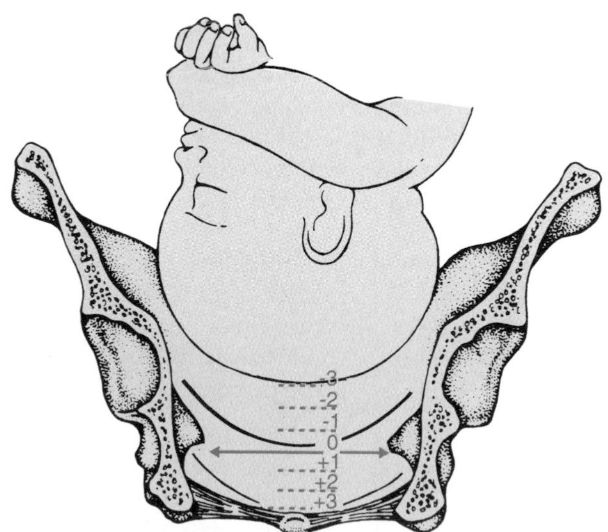

FIGURE 1.6 Stations of the presenting part.

Monitoring

The fetus is monitored continuously during labor. Fetal heart rate (FHR) is a good indicator of fetal condition and normally ranges between 120 to 160 beats per minute (bpm). An increase or decrease of 30 bpm may indicate fetal distress and should be reported immediately (Gabbe, Niebyl, & Simpson, 2002).

Nurses use fetoscopes, Dopplers, or continuous internal or external heart monitors to monitor FHR. Monitor the heart rate every 15 to 30 minutes during the first stage of labor and every 5 minutes during the second stage. Assess FHR immediately after rupture of the membranes, particularly if the head is not engaged.

Frequently in the hospital and birthing center settings, personnel apply continuous electronic monitors, either internal or external. They are more accurate in detecting subtle changes in condition. External monitors are also useful in monitoring the frequency and duration of contractions by use of a **tocodynamometer.** When a tocodynamometer is placed directly over a woman's uterus, the device transfers an electrical impulse to the monitor, creating a readout. A strip chart prints out both FHR (upper part of the strip) and uterine activity (lower part of the strip). If an external monitor reports a potential fetal or maternal problem, an internal or direct monitor is used because it is more accurate. An internal monitor places an electrode on the fetal presenting part. It can provide precise information, including a fetal electrocardiogram.

Fetal heart monitoring is assessed in relation to contractions during labor. A decrease in FHR in response to a contraction is called a **deceleration** and can indicate fetal distress. Decelerations can be early, late, or variable in relation to the contractions.

Nurses are responsible for interpreting fetal monitoring information. Some terms used to assess monitor strips include:

- *Accelerations:* Accelerations are brief increases in FHR of 15 bpm or more. They are healthy if they occur after stimulation or with movement. Any acceleration over 60 bpm is considered a complication.
- *Decelerations:* Decelerations of FHR are linked to the timing of a contraction. An early deceleration begins early in the contraction and returns to baseline by the end of the contraction, mirroring the contraction pattern. Early decelerations are attributed to vagal nerve stimulation, resulting from pressure on the fetal head, and are considered norm[al] during labor. Variable decelerations can occu[r]

time and can indicate umbilical cord compression. The FHR should not fall below 100 bpm.

- *Decreased variability:* Little or no fluctuation is a dangerous sign and may indicate an abnormality of the fetal nervous system. It also may indicate that the mother has been given a central nervous system depressant that has crossed to the fetus.

Stop, Think, and Respond ● BOX 1-3

Identify procedures that evaluate the location and status of the fetus.

Powers of Delivery

Involuntary and voluntary powers combine to expel the fetus and placenta from the uterus. Involuntary uterine contractions, termed the *primary powers,* signal the beginning of labor. Once the cervix is dilated, voluntary "bearing down" efforts by the mother, termed the *secondary powers,* augment the force of involuntary contractions.

Primary Powers

Involuntary contractions originate in the thickened muscle layers of the upper uterine segment. Contractions move downward in waves over the uterus and are separated by short rest periods. Contractions may be 15 to 30 minutes apart during early labor to as frequent as every 2 to 3 minutes in active labor. The frequency (time from the beginning of one contraction to the beginning of the next), duration (length of the contraction), and intensity (strength of the contraction) are noted.

The primary powers are responsible for cervical effacement and dilation. Only a thin edge of the cervix is palpable when effacement is complete. Dilation is complete when the diameter of the cervix increases from less than 1 cm to full dilation at approximately 10 cm.

Secondary Powers

As soon as the presenting part reaches the pelvic floor, contractions change in character and become expulsive. The laboring woman experiences an involuntary urge to push. By using the secondary powers (bearing-down efforts) as the uterus contracts, intraabdominal pressure compresses the uterus from all sides and aids the expulsive forces.

The secondary powers have no effect on cervical dilation. Studies have shown that pushing during the second stage of labor is more effective because the woman is less tired than when she begins to push only after she has progressed to the period of having the urge to push (Roberts & Woolley, 1996).

Stages of Labor

Labor is considered "normal" when the mother is at or near term, with no pregnancy complications; there is a single fetus with a vertex presentation; and the labor is completed within 24 hours. The labor process is to have regular uterine contractions, effacement, and progressive dilation of the cervix and progress of the descending part.

First Stage of Labor

The first stage of labor is from the onset of the first regular contractions to full dilation of the cervix. This stage is generally the longest and difficult to estimate. The woman may be admitted to the labor unit just before birth, or the timing of regular contractions may be difficult to estimate. In primiparas, this stage averages 10 to 12 hours; in multiparas, it averages 6 to 8 hours. The first stage is divided into three phases:

- Early latent phase. The cervix is 0 to 3 cm dilated; contractions are 5 to 8 minutes apart, lasting 20 to 35 seconds each. The woman is generally alert and talkative and tends to be receptive to coaching on breathing techniques. Pain is mild and controlled. Backache is the most common complaint. Many women prefer to be at home during this phase. Frequent position changes enhance the progress of labor.
- Mid/active phase. The cervix is 4 to 7 cm dilated; contractions are 3 to 5 minutes apart, lasting 40 to 60 seconds each. The woman is more focused and less talkative. Pain intensity increases but still may be manageable without medication.
- Transitional phase. The cervix is 7 to 10 cm dilated; contractions are 2 to 3 minutes apart, lasting up to 80 seconds. This is a time of deep focus in which the woman may not wish to communicate with the birth attendant or nurse. She may experience nausea and request pain medication.

Alleviation of pain is important. Women may choose to deal with childbirth pain through nonpharmacologic methods or a combination of nonpharmacologic and pharmacologic methods. Nonpharmacologic methods frequently are taught at childbirth classes and include such strategies as conscious relaxation, music, massage, breathing techniques, diversional activities, water therapy, and aromatherapy.

Pharmacologic management includes sedatives, analgesia (alleviation of the sensation of pain), and anesthesia (abolishes the pain perception). Opioid (narcotic) agonist administration is most commonly administered intravenously. Nerve blocks or spinal and **epidural** blocks are also an option.

Second Stage of Labor

DELIVERY OF INFANT. This stage begins with complete dilation and ends with birth of the baby. It lasts an average of

20 minutes for a multipara and 50 minutes for a primipara. Contractions continue to last 80 to 90 seconds, but they may be slightly less frequent. Generally, the woman experiences the urge to push and is anxious to do so. The woman needs support, for pushing is hard work. Resting between contractions helps conserve energy. She should be discouraged from using the Valsalva maneuver (holding her breath and tightening the abdominal muscles) for pushing. This activity increases intrathoracic pressure, reduces venous return, and increases venous pressure. During the Valsalva maneuver, fetal hypoxia may occur.

The primary care provider may provide anesthesia and perform an **episiotomy** (surgical incision of the perineum to facilitate delivery and to avoid a laceration of the perineum). The most common type of episiotomy is midline in which the tissues of the perineum are separated at an anatomic junction. If the perineum is too small, a mediolateral incision that cuts the muscle is performed. This is generally more uncomfortable and has a longer recovery period, so it is performed only when necessary. The rate of performing episiotomies, in general, in the United States has declined over the past 20 years (Cleary-Goldman, 2003). Research has noted less infection with perineal tearing than episiotomies.

Immediately after delivery of the newborn, the airway is established and maintained and the umbilical cord is clamped with two clamps and then severed between them. If everything is normal, the baby is shown to the parents and generally placed on the mother's chest.

NURSING MANAGEMENT. Assess vital signs every 15 to 30 minutes. Assess every contraction, and look for vaginal show every 15 minutes. Monitor FHR every 15 minutes. Check for signs of fetal descent (i.e., urge to bear down and push, perineal bulging, and crowning) every 10 to 15 minutes.

Change perineal pads hourly as needed. Encourage the birth attendant to support the woman, and facilitate breathing and relaxation techniques. Begin room preparation for the baby by having a warming isolette available, as well as supplies and equipment for delivery and neonatal resuscitation equipment.

Assist the woman to an effective position, which may be lying, sitting, side lying, or squatting. Coach her in effective pushing and breathing techniques. She should bear down and take panting breaths to ensure proper rate of delivery.

Third Stage of Labor

DELIVERY OF THE PLACENTA. The third stage begins with delivery of the infant and ends with delivery of the placenta. The average time to deliver the placenta is 5 to 20 minutes. Risk of hemorrhage increases with the duration of this stage. The mother is more focused on the newborn than the placenta. Many women do not wish to see the placenta.

When the placenta detaches from the uterine wall, a sudden outpouring of blood appears from the vagina. The cord protruding from the vagina lengthens, and the uterine shape becomes more round and firm. The woman may again experience more contractions. Usually the placenta is delivered with one or two contractions. At this time, the episiotomy is repaired, if needed.

Total blood loss is normally between 200 to 300 mL. Excessive blood loss is more than 500 mL. An **oxytocic** (hormone produced by the pituitary gland) may be administered to stimulate uterine contractions, thus accelerating childbirth and preventing postdelivery hemorrhage. This medication causes the uterus to contract firmly, compressing the blood vessels inside and minimizing blood loss.

NURSING MANAGEMENT. Assess vital signs every 15 minutes. Look for placental separation. Assess bleeding until the woman has expelled the placenta.

Change perineal pads as needed. Notify the obstetrician or midwife of labor progression. Gather supplies and equipment needed for delivery of the placenta.

Assist the woman to an effective position. Usually she is in the lithotomy position following childbirth. Instruct on contractions for placental delivery.

The Fourth Stage of Labor: Postpartum

The fourth stage of labor arbitrarily lasts approximately 2 to 4 hours after delivery of the placenta. The mother is monitored closely following the birth process. During this period of immediate recovery, homeostasis is reestablished. Some women are exhausted and wish only to rest. Others appear euphoric and wish to talk about their experience or spend time with the baby and loved ones.

It is important to monitor vital signs, signs of abnormal bleeding, and the perineal tissue. During the first hour, document assessments every 15 minutes, then every 30 minutes for the next hour. If all findings are within normal limits, assessments decrease in frequency.

Critical Thinking Exercises

1. *Develop a teaching plan for a 37-week primigravida who is anxious about labor and delivery. What decisions can she make before labor?*
2. *You are an on-call nursing consultant for an obstetric practice. A woman phones stating she is unsure if she is in labor. What questions would you ask? How would you advise her?*

• NCLEX-STYLE REVIEW QUESTIONS 

1. A woman of normal weight for her height and age comes to the clinic for an initial prenatal visit. The nurse informs the client that the recommended amount of weight gain during pregnancy is:
   1. 10 to 15 pounds
   2. 15 to 20 pounds

3. 25 to 35 pounds
4. 40 to 50 pounds

2. The nurse notes that a fetus is having decelerations during contractions. The fetal heart rate is 90 beats/min. What is the nurse's most appropriate action?
1. Phone the physician.
2. Check for effacement and dilation.
3. Assist the client to a sitting position.
4. Assess the client's need for pain medication.

3. During the immediate postpartum period, which of the following nursing interventions is most important?
1. Assess for hemorrhage.
2. Provide the client with food and water.
3. Observe the intravenous site for infiltration.
4. Provide hygiene needs for the client.

connection

Visit the Connection site at **http://connection.lww.com/go/timbyEssentials** for links to chapter-related resources on the Internet.

References and Suggested Readings

Callister, L. (1995). Cultural meanings of childbirth. *Journal of Obstetric, Gynecological, and Neonatal Nursing, 24*(4), 327–331.

Cleary-Goldman, J. (2003). The role of episiotomy in current obstetric practice. *Perinatology, 2*(1), 3–7.

Cunningham, F., et al. (2001). *Williams obstetrics* (21st ed.). New York: McGraw-Hill.

Gabbe, S., Niebyl, J., & Simpson, J. (Eds.) (2002). *Obstetrics: Normal and problem pregnancies* (4th ed.). New York: Churchill Livingstone.

Hilton, J. (2002). Folic acid intake of young woman. *Journal of Obstetric, Gynecological, and Neonatal Nursing, 31*(2), 172–177.

Hunter, L. (2002). Being with woman: A guiding concept for the care of laboring women. *Journal of Obstetric, Gynecological, and Neonatal Nursing, 31*(6), 650–657.

Mattson, S. (2000). Working toward cultural competence: Making first steps through cultural assessment. *AWHONN Lifelines, 4*(4), 41–43.

Miltner, R. (2002). More than support: Nursing interventions provided to women in labor. *Journal of Obstetric, Gynecological, and Neonatal Nursing, 31*(6), 753–761.

Minato, J. (2000). Is it time to push? Examining rest in the second stage of labor. *Lifelines, 4*(6), 20–23.

Ramer, L., & Frank, B. (2001). *Pregnancy: Psychosocial perspectives* (3rd ed.). White Plains, NY: March of Dimes.

Roberts, J., & Woolley, D. (1996). A second look at the second stage of labor. *Journal of Obstetric, Gynecological, and Neonatal Nursing, 25*(5), 415–423.

Walker, L., & Grobe, S. (1999). The construct of thriving in pregnancy and postpartum. *Nursing Science Quarterly, 12*(2), 151–157.

chapter 2

Caring for Clients During High-Risk Pregnancy, Labor, and Delivery

Words to Know

abruptio placenta
amniocentesis
biophysical profile
cervical incompetence
diabetes mellitus
ectopic pregnancy
fetal dystocia
HELLP syndrome
hematoma
hyperemesis gravidarum
maternal dystocia
molar pregnancy
multiple pregnancies
nonstress test
nuchal cord
oxytocin challenge test
placenta accreta
placenta previa
polyhydramnios
preeclampsia
pregnancy-induced hypertension
premature (preterm) labor
premature rupture of membranes
prolapsed cord
spontaneous abortion
thrombophlebitis
uterine rupture

Learning Objectives

On completion of this chapter, the reader will:

- Describe the tests used to assess fetal well-being.
- Explain ectopic and molar pregnancies, spontaneous abortion, and incompetent cervix.
- Discuss maternal pre-existing medical conditions and their effects on pregnancy.
- Explain placental and amniotic complications and their effects on the fetus.
- Explain the increased risks of pregnancy for adolescents and women older than 40 years.
- Discuss nursing interventions and responsibilities related to emergency delivery.
- Define the nursing responsibilities when labor is induced.
- Discuss operative obstetrics.
- Describe physiologic and psychological conditions that cause postpartum problems.
- Identify complications during labor and delivery and their effects on mother and fetus.

The processes of gestation and birth are normal. Nevertheless, many complications can occur during pregnancy, labor, and delivery that place the health of the mother, fetus, or both at risk. Before a woman even discovers she is pregnant, she may be at risk for complications.

Advances in technology have improved the ability to assess a fetus for complications and to provide treatments to improve chances for the best outcome. Early diagnosis and frequent monitoring also have improved the odds for a healthy mother and baby.

A pregnancy diagnosed as high risk may be the result of maternal or fetal conditions. Maternal factors are those associated with labor and delivery, placenta, psychological disorders, and pre-existing or newly acquired medical conditions. Fetal factors include those of a genetic or environmental nature. The goal of antepartal care is to ensure the best possible environment for the fetus to develop with the least risk to the mother as her body adapts to pregnancy.

FETAL TESTING

Maternal, fetal, or psychological factors are used to determine a high-risk pregnancy. Several diagnostic tools are available to identify pregnancy risks based on fetal factors. The easiest test is simply having the woman count the number of fetal movements in 1 hour. If fetal movements are less than three, decreased, or absent over 1 hour, additional testing is warranted. Ultrasound is a noninvasive test that presents an image of the fetus through the use of sound waves. Another diagnostic tool is the **nonstress test,** which requires the mother to identify when she feels fetal movements while being monitored with an external fetal monitor. When the fetus moves and fetal heart rate (FHR) changes in response to maternal activity or with Braxton Hicks contractions, test results are determined to be positive. If there is little activity or change in FHR, further testing of fetal well-being is done. A well-oxygenated fetus maintains a normal FHR without significant alterations following a contraction. A hypoxic fetus will respond with late u-shaped heart rate decelerations between contractions (see Chap. 1).

A **biophysical profile** is the combination of four to six of the following diagnostic tests: ultrasound, FHR, fetal breathing movements, gross body movement, fetal tone, FHR variability, and amniotic fluid volume. Results are given a score similar to the APGAR system (see Chap. 3). The biophysical profile has been found to yield more accurate results than any single test.

Amniocentesis is an invasive procedure using sonography to guide placement of a needle into the uterus to obtain amniotic fluid for laboratory testing. This procedure carries a risk of complications, of which the nurse or physician must inform the client. Such complications include contractions, labor, and hemorrhage if the placenta was nicked. A mixture of maternal and fetal blood with an Rh^- mother and an Rh^+ baby could increase risks to the pregnancy. Invasion of the sterile uterine environment by introducing instrumentation during the procedure could cause infection and potentially lethal complications.

Another diagnostic test of fetal well-being is the **oxytocin challenge test** (also called a *contraction stress test*). It uses the hormone oxytocin to induce uterine contractions. Having the client roll her nipples, which stimulates release of oxytocin, also can induce uterine contractions. The FHR is monitored for decelerations during the contraction. This test carries the risk of being unable to stop the contractions. The client will need to remain in the healthcare facility for at least 30 minutes after completing the test to ensure that contractions have stopped.

Stop, Think, and Respond ● BOX 2-1

What tests would you expect the physician to order for a 41-year-old woman who wants to know if her fetus has any abnormalities?

COMPLICATIONS OF PREGNANCY

● ECTOPIC PREGNANCY

As discussed in Chapter 1, after egg and sperm unite, the newly formed zygote divides and makes its way into the uterus for implantation into the uterine wall. The placenta forms to provide nutrition and elimination of waste necessary for the fetus to survive.

A zygote that implants outside the uterus is known as an **ectopic pregnancy.** The fallopian tube is the major site of extrauterine zygote implantation (Fig. 2.1). The client with an ectopic pregnancy may report amenorrhea or abnormal menses, pain, and some bleeding. With rupture of the fallopian tube, the client may complain of sharp lower abdominal pain radiating to the shoulders. In this case, immediate surgical removal of the tube is necessary to prevent hemorrhage. Nursing responsibilities include a detailed history of the client's symptoms, including monitoring of vital signs and strict measurement of output to determine fluid loss.

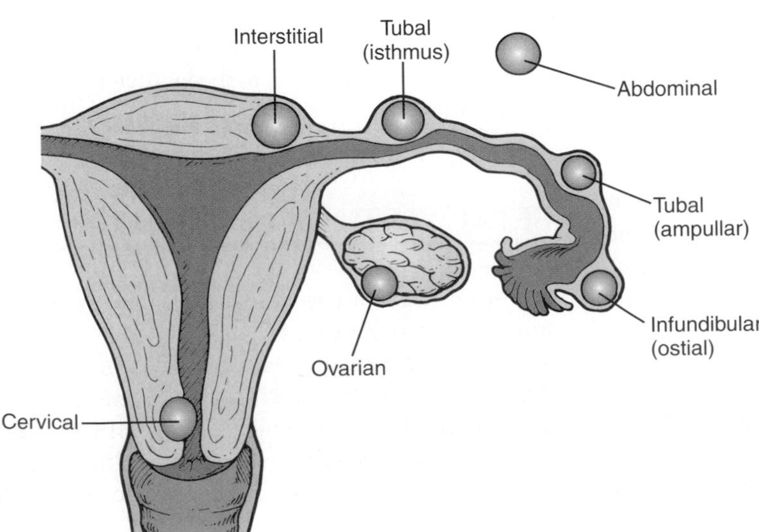

FIGURE 2.1 Sites of ectopic pregnancy.

• MOLAR PREGNANCY

Pathophysiology and Etiology

Molar pregnancy is also called gestational trophoblastic tumor or hydatidiform mole. The cause is related to abnormal chromosomes, folic acid deficiency, or hormonal imbalance.

Assessment Findings

Early symptoms are often similar to pregnancy and include a high human chorionic gonadotropin (HCG) level. The client presents with bleeding, hyperemesis, no fetal heart tones, palpable ovaries, and abdominal pain. Ultrasound reveals hyperplasia of trophoblast cells connected by fibrous strands, which may (incomplete mole) or may not (complete mole) contain a fetus. The type of mole determines diagnosis and risk of choriocarcinoma or trophoblastic tumor.

Medical Management

Treatment includes dilation and curettage (D and C) to remove diseased products and involved tissue. Frequent monitoring of the client's HCG levels for 1 year following molar pregnancy is necessary; a chest x-ray is obtained to rule out lung metastasis. Birth control to prevent possible pregnancy during follow-up care is strongly suggested.

• SPONTANEOUS ABORTION

Pathophysiology and Etiology

Spontaneous abortion is the expulsion of the uterine products of conception before the age of fetal viability. Several different types of spontaneous abortion are classified by probable cause (fetal, placental, or maternal) and fetal age. Abortion resulting from fetal flaws occurs during 6 to 10 weeks' gestation and usually is related to improper implantation of the fetal sac to the uterine wall, leading to an inability of the fetus to grow and survive. Spontaneous abortion at approximately 14 weeks is thought to be associated with defective implantation of the placenta into the uterine wall, separation of the placenta from the uterine wall, or an error of hormone production by the placenta. Maternal factors are thought to be the cause between weeks 11 and 19 and are associated with abnormal endocrine functions, infectious processes, maternal malnutrition, incompetent cervix, or abdominal trauma. See Box 2-1.

BOX 2-1 ● Classifying Spontaneous Abortions

Spontaneous abortions are further defined by the level of expulsion of the fetus:

- A *complete abortion* is when the fetus is expelled completely; no products of conception remain in the uterus.
- An *incomplete abortion* is the partial expulsion of the uterine contents.
- A *missed abortion* is when fetal products remain in the uterus and are not expelled.
- The term *threatened abortion* is used when any bloody discharge occurs during the pregnancy, because the fetus may or may not be expelled.
- An *inevitable abortion* is when amniotic membranes rupture and cervical dilation begins.
- A *septic abortion* is associated with an infectious process resulting from a break in the sterile environment during a procedure.

Cervical incompetence, a possible cause of spontaneous abortion, is when the cervix prematurely dilates, with rupture of the membranes and premature loss of the products of conception. Questioning the client about her gynecological history, including cervical problems, surgery, and any previous history of spontaneous abortion, is appropriate (see Chap. 53).

Assessment Findings

Symptoms include painless contractions, bleeding, cervical dilation, and rupture of the membranes prior to expulsion of the fetus. If a diagnosis of cervical incompetence is made during ultrasound or vaginal examination before rupture of the membranes, the physician performs a cerclage procedure (cervical closure with a suture). The suture is removed prior to delivery, usually at approximately 37 to 38 weeks' gestation, when the fetus has reached maturity.

Nursing Management

Nursing responsibilities for a client who has experienced a spontaneous abortion include monitoring of vital signs and detailed documentation of the amount and color of bleeding. Provide comfort and emotional support to client and family during this time. Offer them the names and numbers of support or grief groups to help them cope with the loss.

• HYPEREMESIS GRAVIDARUM

Many women experience nausea and vomiting in the first trimester of pregnancy. Provided that these women are not losing significant amounts of weight and are receiving adequate nutrition and prenatal vitamins, such nausea and vomiting usually is not problematic. **Hyperemesis gravidarum** is severe vomiting causing altered nutritional status, dehydration, electrolyte imbalance, weight loss, ketoacidosis, and acetonuria.

Pathophysiology and Etiology

Hyperemesis gravidarum is more prevalent in Caucasians than in African Americans. Women with hyperemesis gravidarum frequently require hospitalization for treatment. The cause is unknown but linked to altered thyroid hormones, vitamin deficiency, pancreatitis, biliary tract disease, decreased hydrochloric acid secretions, decreased gastrointestinal tract motility, and psychological factors.

Assessment Findings

Symptoms are severe nausea and vomiting extending beyond the common "morning sickness" of the first trimester. Evaluation and laboratory findings support the severely compromised status and increased nutritional needs of the woman and fetus. If the condition is unresolved, vomiting of undigested food and mucus can progress to a coffee-ground emesis. A positive hemoccult test for suspected gastrointestinal bleeding requires further action.

Medical and Nursing Management

Treatment depends on identification of an underlying cause, severity of the disease, and physical condition of the woman. It may include prescribed antiemetic therapy, strict monitoring of intake and output, and restoration of fluid and electrolyte balance. Tube feedings may be initiated to supply nutrition to the mother and fetus, with hospitalization or home healthcare.

• PREGNANCY-INDUCED HYPERTENSION

Pregnancy-induced hypertension (PIH) is elevation in maternal blood pressure after the 20th week of gestation, presenting risks to both mother and fetus. It is the leading cause of maternal death; if left untreated, PIH can progress to strokes, cardiac decompensation, renal failure, and possibly maternal death.

Pathophysiology and Etiology

Incidence of PIH is increased with adolescent pregnancy, pregnancy after age 35 years, nulliparity, multiple gestation, history of vascular disease, low socioeconomic status, increased body mass index, abnormal placenta, and molar gestation. It can result in premature labor necessitating premature delivery, because delivery is the only successful cure. Complications cause the fetus to suffer intrauterine growth retardation and intrauterine death from chronic hypoxia.

Preeclampsia

Preeclampsia is PIH with proteinuria, characterized by a sudden increase in blood pressure. It can progress to eclampsia, a condition that involves seizures of the central nervous system. Potential complications of both are abnormal liver enzymes, thrombocytopenia, HELLP (*h*emolysis, *e*levated *l*iver function, *l*ow *p*latelets) syndrome, and fetal and maternal death.

HELLP Syndrome

HELLP syndrome is a severe condition of hepatic disorders. It leads to hemolysis, elevated liver enzymes, decreased platelet count, decreased perfusion to all organs (including uteroplacental perfusion), ischemia, and altered maternal vascular endothelium.

Assessment Findings

Diagnosis of gestational PIH is based on elevation in blood pressure only, without any other signs or symptoms. PIH is categorized as mild if blood pressure is 140/90 mm Hg. It is classified as severe above 160/110 mm Hg. Although symptoms are not necessary for diagnosis, clients with PIH may experience headaches, oliguria, blurred vision (indicating possibly increased intracranial pressure), heartburn (which may mean pancreatic edema and impending convulsion), increased irritability, and emotional tension. They may show signs of edema of the face and hands, pitting edema of the legs and feet, and hyperreflexia of the deep tendons.

Medical and Nursing Management

Frequent monitoring of the client with PIH is essential for the best possible outcome for mother and fetus. Treatment may include bed rest, antihypertensive medication, and hospitalization for IV magnesium sulfate to gain control of the blood pressure. If PIH is not controlled, it can lead to multiorgan system failure and convulsions, so seizure precautions are initiated. A toxemia tray will need to be in the room with preparations for a cesarean section and emergency resuscitation in place.

PRE-EXISTING MATERNAL COMPLICATIONS •

Pre-existing medical conditions can contribute to a diagnosis of high-risk pregnancy. Examples include diabetes, cardiac disease, and substance abuse.

DIABETES MELLITUS

Diabetes mellitus, a metabolic disorder of the pancreas, affects carbohydrate, fat, and protein metabolism (see Chap. 52). It can lead to complications during pregnancy. When poorly controlled, diabetes can lead to infertility and polycystic ovarian syndrome. Pregnant women suffering from type 1 diabetes are especially at increased risk during pregnancy because of the lack of endogenous insulin production. Poor control of maternal circulating blood glucose directly affects the fetus. The fetus is dependent on glucose, amino acids, and lipids for energy, protein synthesis, and new tissue production. The fetal endocrine system removes glucose from the maternal circulation, leading to hyperinsulinemia.

Gestational diabetes, or diabetes occurring in a woman for the first time during pregnancy, usually develops during the second trimester as a result of metabolic changes associated with the growing fetus and placental production of hormones, which increase insulin resistance. Gestational diabetes increases the risk of the mother developing complications such as PIH and infections.

The oral glucose tolerance test (OGTT) is one diagnostic test used to identify gestational diabetes in any woman older than 25 years between 24 and 28 weeks' gestation. The test is repeated later if the client is older or obese. If the level is 126 mg/dL or higher after the first hour, the woman is considered to have diabetes and an HbA_{1C} is done.

Gestational diabetes usually is controlled with blood glucose monitoring, diet, and exercise. Insulin may be added later during the pregnancy when the demands on the body decrease insulin sensitivity. The higher the HbA_{1C} level, the higher the risk for maternal and fetal complications.

Educational needs for a woman with diabetes include understanding signs and symptoms of hyperglycemia and hypoglycemia, demonstration of blood glucose monitoring, and testing of the urine for ketones to avoid reactions that may harm the fetus (see Chap. 52). Assessing fetal movement daily, ultrasound, nonstress test, and contraction stress testing often are done to determine fetal well-being.

CARDIAC DISEASE

Pregnancy in women with pre-existing cardiac disease is increasing as technology advances allow more women with cardiac problems a chance to conceive and sustain a pregnancy. Women who have previously not shown signs of cardiac disease may suddenly develop cardiac problems and symptoms because of the additional stress pregnancy places on the heart. The type and the severity of the condition affect the level of risk.

There are four degrees of cardiac disease severity, based on the heart's ability to perfuse and supply the vital organs and placenta with enough oxygen and nutrients to sustain maternal and fetal needs (Table 2.1). Signs and symptoms depend on the area of the heart defect. Some medications used to control heart disease have teratogenic effects, so counseling and education prior to conception help identify potential problems and options for a couple.

Frequent monitoring of the pregnant client's cardiac status is essential for maternal and fetal well-being. Adjusting medication, monitoring weight gain, and pacing activity will help conserve energy and decrease cardiac workload to increase the heart's ability to handle the stress of the pregnancy. Labor is another concern because it places great stress on the heart; epidurals are recommended for clients with cardiac conditions to conserve energy and decrease the workload on the heart. A congenital heart defect in the mother increases the possibility of a similar defect in the fetus.

TABLE 2.1 CLASSIFICATIONS OF CARDIAC DISEASE SEVERITY

CLASS	NEW YORK HEART ASSOCIATION FUNCTIONAL CLASSIFICATION
I	Patients have cardiac disease but *without* the resulting *limitations* of physical activity. Ordinary physical activity does not cause undue fatigue, palpitation, dyspnea, or anginal pain.
II	Patients have cardiac disease resulting in *slight limitation* of physical activity. They are comfortable at rest. Ordinary physical activity results in fatigue, palpitation, dyspnea, or anginal pain.
III	Patients have cardiac disease resulting in *marked limitation* of physical activity. They are comfortable at rest. Less than ordinary physical activity causes fatigue, palpitation, dyspnea, or anginal pain.
IV	Patients have cardiac disease resulting in *inability* to carry on any physical activity without discomfort. Symptoms of cardiac insufficiency or of the anginal syndrome may be present even at rest. If any physical activity is undertaken, discomfort is increased.

From http://www.cochranfoundation.com/docs/nyha-class.htm.

● SUBSTANCE ABUSE

Substance abuse during pregnancy has the potential of greatly affecting the fetus. Drugs, alcohol, and tobacco are known toxins to the fetus and can lead to low birth weight, growth and mental retardation, or malformations. The infant of a woman with substance abuse may experience symptoms of withdrawal. Illicit drug use and risky lifestyles increase the neonate's risk of sexually transmitted infections (STIs; see Chap. 56), Hepatitis B, and HIV. Effects of various commonly abused substances in infants are discussed in more detail in Chapters 4 and 9.

Signs of substance abuse in a pregnant woman may include fatigue, erratic appetite, missed appointments or starting prenatal care late in pregnancy, a history of frequent miscarriages or stillbirths, previous abruptio placenta, and signs and symptoms of intoxication (see Chap. 17). Maternal complications include anemia, hypertension, premature rupture of membranes, placental problems, hemorrhage, STIs, nutritional deficits, and low self-esteem. Substance abuse may lead to increased difficulty in maternal-newborn bonding.

PLACENTAL AND AMNIOTIC COMPLICATIONS

Abnormalities of the placenta are classified and defined according to the portion of cervix involved and effect on the fetus. Causes of abnormal placenta formation include trophoblastic and vascular endometrial disorders.

● PLACENTA PREVIA

Placenta previa is a potentially life-threatening condition occurring the third trimester. In placenta previa the placenta is implanted and covers the cervix totally, partially, or marginally (Fig 2.2).

Pathophysiology and Etiology

Risk factors include a previous history, uterine scars or anomalies, short time intervals between pregnancies, cigarette smoking, and multiple gestations. Symptoms include painless vaginal bleeding at least once during the pregnancy, with the amount of bleeding determining severity. Severe cases can lead to shock, coagulopathy, and uterine rupture, with the FHR responding to the degree of hypoxia.

The diagnosis is usually made during the second or, more commonly, the third trimester. Ultrasound can be used to identify the position of the placenta; a placenta found low in the uterus presents symptoms similar to placenta accreta.

Medical and Nursing Management

Once diagnosed, the client may be instructed to refrain from intercourse and limit activity. Cesarean section usually is performed as soon as the fetus is considered mature (approximately the 37th week of gestation). Prepare for an emergency cesarean delivery. A type and crossmatch for blood should be done. Vaginal examinations are contraindicated because of the risk of hemorrhage.

● PLACENTA ACCRETA

Placenta accreta is the term used when decidual formation (lining of the uterus during pregnancy) is defective, with the placenta attached firmly to the wall over a uterine scar or the lower segment. Often placenta accreta is associated with placenta previa. An inability to control bleeding increases the risk of hemorrhage, perforation of the uterus, infection, and hysterectomy. Treatment measures involve maintenance of maternal blood volume and provision of oxygen to the fetus until an emergency cesarean delivery can be performed. Inform the client and family of possible outcomes, including fetal death.

● ABRUPTIO PLACENTA

Pathophysiology and Etiology

Abruptio placenta is premature separation of the placenta (prior to delivery), causing hemorrhage into the deciduas basalis (the part of the decidua that helps to form the placenta) and forming a hematoma. Risk factors include PIH, cigarette smoking, multigravida, illicit drug use, chronic renal disease, and abdominal trauma.

Assessment Findings

The client experiences blood loss, an enlarging uterus, and a firm, painful abdomen with or without contractions. Fetal heart tones mirror the amount of hypoxia.

The size of the placental area involved in the separation determines the diagnosis. Separation is defined in degrees:

- Marginal means a slow gradual bleed.
- Moderate means approximately 50% separated.
- Severe is 70% separation or more, which causes severe pain and rapid progression to maternal shock and fetal death.

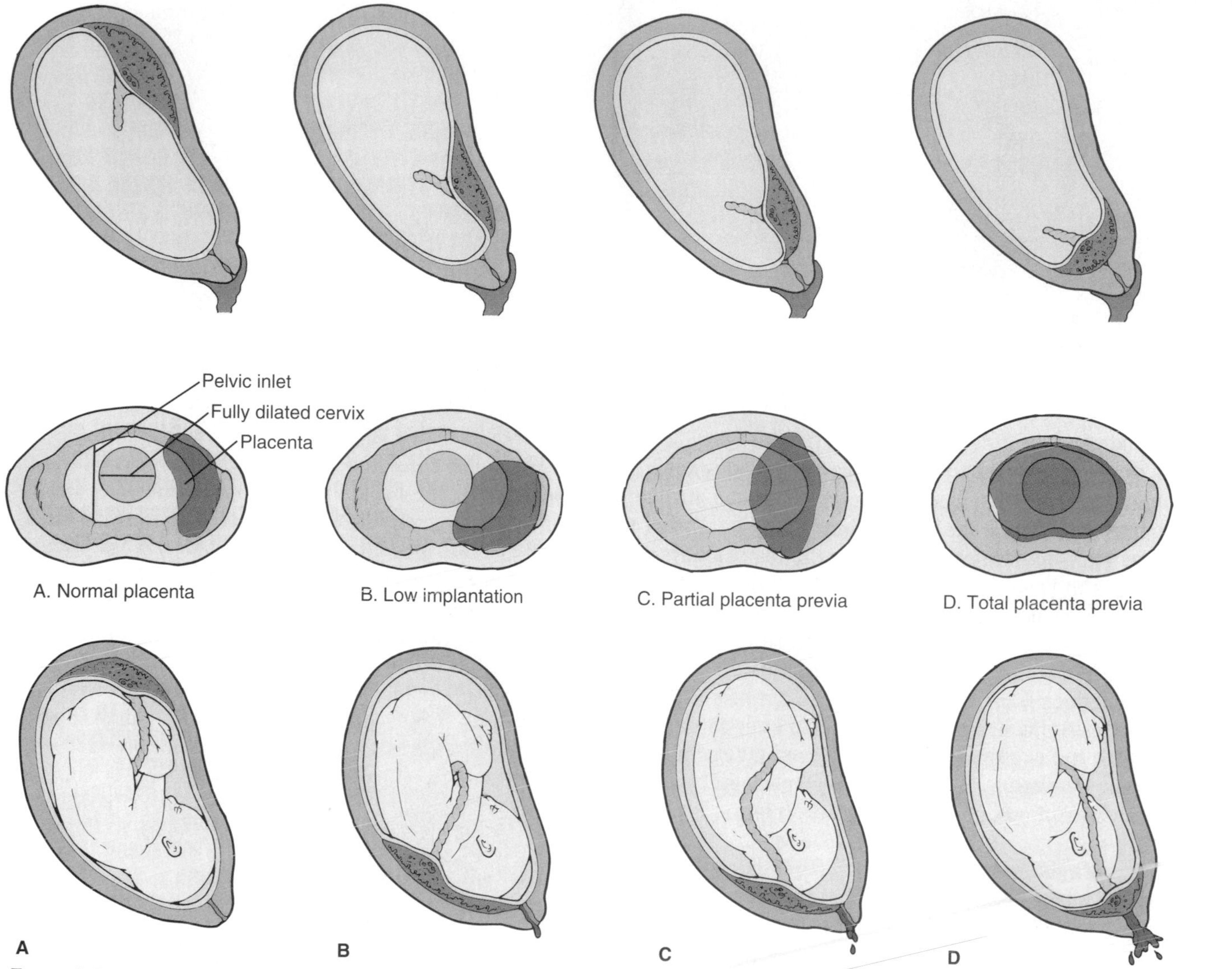

FIGURE 2.2 Variations of placenta previa. (**A**) Normal placenta. (**B**) Low implantation. (**C**) Partial placenta previa. (**D**) Total placenta previa.

As the placenta separates and the area of separation increases, bleeding, pain, and the likelihood of mortality also increase (Fig. 2.3).

Medical and Nursing Management

Monitoring of the client and fetus is essential. Fluids and oxygen are administered. Preparations are made for cesarean delivery. Vaginal examinations must be avoided. Comfort and support to the client are crucial.

• POLYHYDRAMNIOS

Polyhydramnios is abnormal amniotic fluid (2 L between 32 and 36 weeks' gestation). Risk of preterm delivery and prolapsed cord is increased. The cause is unknown, but polyhydramnios is more common with Rh-sensitized pregnancies, insulin-dependent diabetes mellitus, defective fluid transfer mechanism, and fetal gastrointestinal obstructions.

Stop, Think, and Respond ● BOX 2-2

What action would you take if a pregnant woman has bright red vaginal drainage? 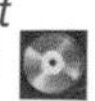

OTHER COMPLICATIONS

• INFECTIONS

No significant increases in infection have been found during pregnancy, but susceptibility to certain infections, especially viruses, may be increased. Urinary tract infections are more common because of pregnancy-rela

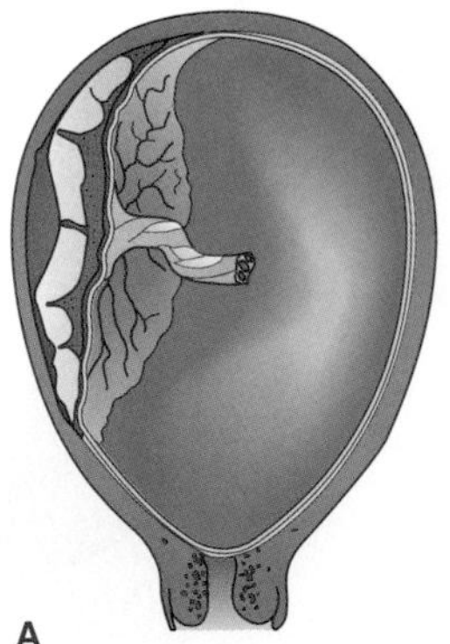

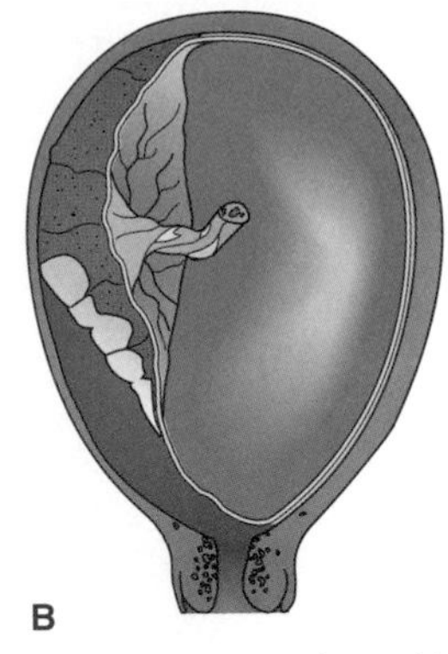

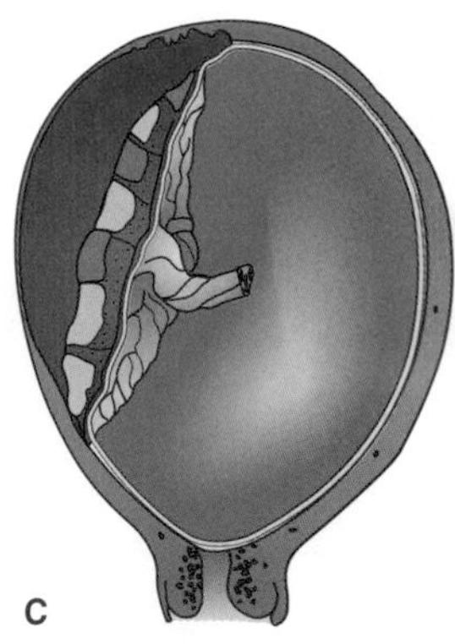

FIGURE 2.3 Abruptio placentae. (**A**) Low and incomplete separation, with vaginal hemorrhage. (**B**) High separation, with no external hemorrhage but internal bleeding. Fetus is in grave danger. (**C**) Complete abruption, posing grave danger to fetus.

anatomical changes in the urinary tract, leading to urinary stasis. Fungal infections such as candidiasis are more prevalent as hormone production increases during the third trimester. Viral infections during pregnancy are more severe and have a longer recuperation time. Acute infection with high fever leads to the release of catecholamine and corticotropin hormones. Both can result in an irritable uterus, causing contractions to begin.

Infections during pregnancy may be a cause of preterm labor. Assessment and identification of infection is important for high-risk clients so that treatment begins early. Immunizations with active viruses or bacteria are dangerous as the potential for fetal malformation is unclear. Only when the mother or fetus is exposed to a preventable disease is the immunization recommended, because the disease may cause more harm than the immunization.

• MULTIPLE PREGNANCIES

Advances in technology and fertility medications have helped contribute to a growing number of **multiple pregnancies** (pregnancies with two or more fetuses) in recent years. Twin pregnancies are most common. Monozygotic twins result when one egg is fertilized by one sperm and the initial cells divide into two separate beings. Dizygotic twins result when two separate ova are fertilized by two separate sperm (Fig. 2.4). Other types of multiple pregnancies are triplets, quadruplets, and quintuplets.

The first indication of a multiple pregnancy may be when assessment reveals a uterus that is larger than expected for gestational age. When gestation dates and uterine measurement are inconsistent with norms, an ultrasound is used to determine the possibility of multiple pregnancy. If not found early, the woman carrying two or more fetuses may report increased activity compared to gestational date or activity felt simultaneously in different abdominal areas.

Confirmation of multiple pregnancy means an increased risk to the mother and fetuses. Risk factors include increased uterine size and the mother's health status and physical ability to handle the added workload of multiple pregnancies. Multiple pregnancies increase the risk of PIH, abruptio placentae, preterm labor, hydramnios, anemia, and intrauterine growth retardation (IUGR) during pregnancy, with increased risk of postpartum bleeding because the uterus is stretched much more than is common during a single delivery. The woman with multiple pregnancies needs frequent assessments of fetal growth. Fetal risks occur when one twin is larger than the other, or with twin-to-twin transfusion syndrome, in which one twin grows larger while the other is lacking in size. If a single amnion is present, risk is increased for the umbilical cords to twist or knot, leading to fetal distress or birthing complications.

• AGE-RELATED CONCERNS

Many factors influence a woman's acceptance of her pregnancy. An important influence for both the woman and her family and friends is her age. In many cases, a woman and those close to her may react negatively if they believe the woman is too young or old to have a child.

Pregnancy during adolescence can be very stressful. It interferes with the teen's potential to graduate from high school. The adolescent may face numerous challenges trying to support herself and the child. Family members may respond poorly if they fear they will become caregivers of the child. Religious beliefs may influence the family's acceptance or rejection of the pregnancy and their decision as to whether to provide support for mother and child. Risks to the adolescent include unfinished maternal bone growth, because pregnancy-related hormones can lead to growth cessation. Delivery by cesarean section may then be required as a result of cephalopelvic disproportion (CPD). Other risks to the pregnant teen include PIH, nutritional deficiencies, immature uterine vascular development, low birth weight infants, IUGR, and increased uterine infection.

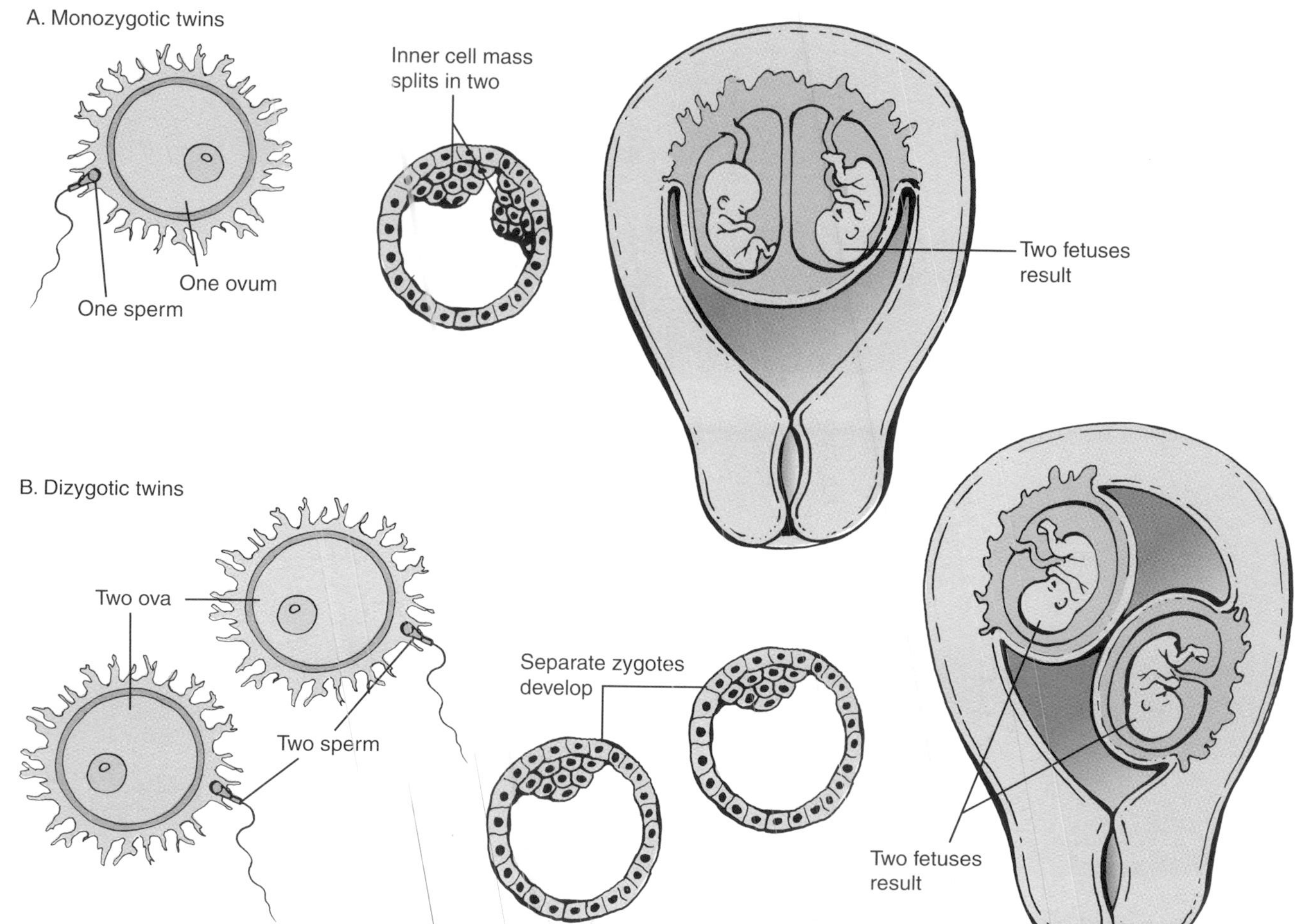

FIGURE 2.4 Monozygotic and dizygotic twins. (**A**) In monozygotic twins, one ovum and one sperm split to develop into two babies. (**B**) In dizygotic twins, two sperm fertilize two eggs, both of which develop into two babies.

At the other end of the spectrum, many women choose to pursue education, travel, and careers for many years before beginning a family. This can increase the responsibilities and stress placed on them during and after pregnancy. Chronic diseases increase with age; conditions such as diabetes, arthritis, and hypertension add additional challenges toward a healthy pregnancy and birth. The incidence of genetic and chromosomal disorders increases in women who are pregnant after 35 years of age.

When working with teenage or older pregnant clients, tailor care to promote the best possible outcomes. Teach principles of solid nutrition and appropriate stress management and rest. Discuss with clients the importance of diagnostic testing, such as chorionic villi sampling and amniocentesis, for detecting fetal abnormalities. Offer support and encourage parenting classes and resources to help women of all ages to develop strategies to cope with the increased energy needed to care for a newborn.

COMPLICATIONS OF LABOR AND DELIVERY

• HEMORRHAGE

Hemorrhage may occur early in labor or during delivery as the fetus passes through the birth canal, resulting in tears in the cervix, vagina, or perineum. Risk of hemorrhage increases when the uterus is overstretched as with multiple pregnancies, polyhydramnios, dystocia, previous history of hemorrhage, infection, injury from trauma during birth, use of drugs or anesthesia prior to or during delivery, and retention of placental fragments. Disseminated intravascular coagulation (DIC) should be considered when all other causes have been ruled out. DIC is diagnosed by prolonged clotting times and a decrease in fibrinogen and platelet levels.

Assessment for hemorrhage includes the duration, amount, and color of the blood. Hemorrhage during labor or delivery requires continuous monitoring of vital signs for signs of shock. Provide support and comfort measures. Be sure to evaluate intake and output carefully and replace fluid volume.

• PREMATURE RUPTURE OF MEMBRANES

Pathophysiology and Etiology

Premature rupture of membranes (PROM) is spontaneous rupture of the membranes before labor begins in pregnancies over 20 weeks' gestation. PROM places the fetus younger than 37 weeks at risk, because labor usually begins within 24 hours of rupture. Increased risk of PROM is associated with maternal infectious processes. While the exact cause of PROM is unknown, it is thought to be associated with a malpresentation. PROM has a greater risk of prolapsed cord involved if the fetus is in a nonvertex position.

Medical Management

In the absence of signs of infection (e.g., elevated temperature or white blood cell [WBC] count, change in amniotic color or odor) and contractions, the woman usually will be hospitalized if the fetus is younger than 34 weeks. The fetus will then be allowed to mature in utero as long as no signs or symptoms of maternal infection appear and the FHR shows no signs of distress during monitoring.

Nursing Management

Monitor signs and symptoms of infection at least every 4 hours. Provide support and education on signs and symptoms of infection and possible outcomes if the fetus is younger than 34 weeks.

• PREMATURE LABOR

Pathophysiology and Etiology

With or without rupture of the membranes, contractions and labor could begin prematurely. **Premature (preterm) labor** is rhythmic uterine contractions causing cervical changes and dilation after the 20th but before the 37th week of gestation. Risk of fetal death in cases of preterm labor is high. Thus, educating the client about risk factors associated with premature labor is essential in making an early diagnosis so prompt treatment can begin.

Causes of preterm labor include PROM, uterine anomalies, PIH, multiple gestation, polyhydramnios, maternal age younger than 16 years or older than 40 years, cigarette smoking, substance abuse, trauma, previous history, low socioeconomic status, placenta abruptio and previa, incompetent cervix, abdominal surgery, infectious processes, and fetal death. Conceptual models have been developed proposing preterm delivery pathways. A group of maternal and fetal factors is responsible for preterm labor including stress, inflammation, decidual hemorrhage, and pathologic uterine distention.

Assessment Findings

Diagnostic studies may reveal an elevated WBC count and urinary tract infection. Ultrasound examination may be performed to monitor risk for preterm labor.

Medical Management

Treatment focuses on stopping contractions in a fetus with fetal lung immaturity and a cervical dilation less than 4 cm unless otherwise contraindicated. Regular prenatal care, adequate diet and rest, and fetal monitoring are the best preventions for preterm labor. Once preterm labor begins, administration of tocolytic or beta-adrenergic drugs to stop uterine contractions are given when necessary. Tocolytic drugs are effective in stopping labor for 48 to 72 hours, allowing delivery of glucocorticoids in an effort to enhance fetal lung maturity.

Nursing Management

Listen carefully and be alert when the client complains of low back pain, flank pain, urgency, gastrointestinal complaints, dysuria, elevation in temperature, confusion, stress, and fear associated with loss of the fetus. Monitor the client so that prompt treatment can achieve the best outcome possible.

• RUPTURED UTERUS

Ruptured uterus is a rare but devastating event that often results in fetal death. **Uterine rupture** occurs when a scar in the uterus from trauma (D and C or instrumented abortion) or an incision from a previous cesarean section is under enough strain to cause a rupture. If untreated, the uterine rupture leads to massive maternal hemorrhage and possible fetal death. Classification is based on the extent of the rupture:

- Complete is a laceration directly into the peritoneal cavity.
- Incomplete is a laceration separated by the visceral peritoneum.
- Uterine scar dehiscence is when a previous scar begins to separate.

Uterine rupture is rare with normal spontaneous contractions, but prolonged labor, multiple gestation, malpresentation, oxytocin induction, obstruction, previous cesarean section, uterine anomalies, or traumatic use of forceps or traction could cause a rupture.

Be alert for signs and symptoms of rupture and the presence of retraction rings. Bandl's ring is a visible line between the upper and lower uterine segments. When a vaginal birth after cesarean is attempted, and when oxytocin is necessary to induce contractions, the result can be prolonged contractions that place added strain on the uterus, increasing the chance for rupture.

If rupture occurs, monitor vital signs and observe for signs of maternal shock and fetal distress. Prepare for an emergency cesarean section as soon as uterine rupture is suspected. Administer fluids to replace circulating blood volume. Provide support related to the fear and anxiety that accompany the threat to maternal and fetal life.

• DYSTOCIA

Dystocia means dysfunctional (long, difficult, and abnormal) labor resulting from maternal or fetal factors. **Maternal dystocia** results from ineffective uterine contractions, alterations in the pelvic structure or maternal position during labor, or psychologic responses during labor based on past experiences, culture, preparation, or support person. **Fetal dystocia** is based on abnormal presentation or position, multiple fetuses, or fetus size. Other causes include a small maternal pelvis, fatigue, dehydration, fear of a long labor, too early or too much analgesic administration, and uterine anomalies.

Provide education and information on the risk and complications. Perform assessments at least every 30 minutes. Monitor intake and output. Offer support to the client to help decrease feelings of stress.

• PROLAPSED CORD

When the fetal head is not engaged prior to rupture of the membranes or at the beginning of labor, incidence of **prolapsed cord** is increased. This condition is more common with a premature fetus, hydramnios, multiple gestation, placenta previa, malpresentation, PROM, and conditions that prevent the fetal head from engaging into the pelvis. It usually is suspected when the FHR decelerates because cord compression causes hypoxia. The cord may be visible or found on examination.

A cesarean section is the preferred method of delivery. Releasing pressure on the cord until a cesarean is performed is essential.

Position the client in the knee–chest or Trendelenburg position, and administer oxygen. Maintain continuous fetal monitoring until the cesarean section is performed.

• NUCHAL CORD

An umbilical cord found to be looped around the newborn's neck is known as a **nuchal cord.** If looped loosely, the cord is removed to decrease traction during delivery of the shoulders or body. A single loop is usually not a problem. If there is more than one loop or the loop is too tight and cannot be removed easily, the cord must be clamped and cut before the delivery of the shoulders to ensure adequate oxygen supply to the fetus.

Stop, Think, and Respond ● BOX 2-3

Discuss complications that may occur with active labor.

EMERGENCY DELIVERY

In the event of conditions that cause complications and compromise the fetus or mother, it is sometimes necessary to induce or artificially begin labor to correct the problem. As discussed earlier, PIH and diabetes lead to additional complications if the pregnancy continues. Post-term pregnancies (beyond 42 weeks' gestation) are induced because normal mechanisms are not initiating labor. Nurses monitor maternal and fetal heart rates frequently during induction of labor and check for any complications (e.g., hypertension, cardiovascular difficulties, diabetes) that might cause further complications. See Nursing Guidelines 2-1.

If a vaginal delivery is prolonged and threatens the health, safety, or life of the infant or mother, an emergency cesarean section is performed. The classical vertical incision is used because it can be performed quickly. Healing and recuperation are the same as for any other cesarean but decrease the chance for a vaginal birth with subsequent pregnancies.

NURSING GUIDELINES 2-1

Assisting With an Emergency Delivery

- Stay calm and provide support for the woman. *A calm presence can reassure the mother.*
- Perform handwashing and don sterile gloves, if available. *These measures reduce transfer of microorganisms.*
- Try to find a large, flat surface (e.g., table, bed) covered with a clean sheet or towels to use for birthing. Help to provide good lighting and warmth. *A suitable environment provides comfort to the client and facilitates ease of delivery.*
- Do not attempt to delay or prevent delivery. *Measures to stop delivery can seriously injure the baby.*
- Remove uncomfortable clothing from the woman. Provide pillows. *This helps show concern for the client's comfort.*
- Have the mother take deep, slow breaths, particularly during contractions. *Breathing helps ease the pain of contractions.*
- At the time of delivery, assist the woman to lie on her back with her knees bent and spread apart. If possible, place a folded towel or blanket under the mother's right hip. *Proper positioning will ease the birth process.*
- Help provide comfort and support during the delivery—hold the woman's hand, encourage her to breathe, apply a cool towel to her head. *The client will appreciate the nurse's concern.*
- Once the newborn has arrived, keep the baby warm and ensure that he or she is breathing. *Thermoregulation and respiration require major transitions from newborns and need careful assessment and, sometimes, assistance by nurses.*
- Tie off the umbilical cord in two places and have the woman hold the baby to her breast.
- Get medical assistance immediately. *Proper care ensures the health and well-being of mother and child.*
- Write down the time of birth and of delivery of the placenta, along with the name and address of the woman.

POSTPARTAL COMPLICATIONS

● HEMATOMA

A **hematoma** results from trauma during labor or delivery. Blood becomes trapped between the tissue and skin; it may be drained or allowed to absorb. A hematoma is evident in the perineal area with inspection, and the client complaints of pain and pressure unrelieved by routine medication.

Treatment is ice for the first 24 hours followed by warm, moist heat. Depending on the amount of extravasated blood, the client may have limited activity.

● HEMORRHAGE

During the birth process, normal blood loss may be as much as 500 mL for a vaginal birth and 1200 mL for a cesarean birth. Anything more is considered hemorrhage with increased risk of maternal death. The greatest period of hemorrhage is within the first hour after birth. Postpartal assessments of the client's vital signs and amount of vaginal or operative drainage at least every 15 minutes are essential to detect hemorrhage at the earliest stage possible. Early postpartum hemorrhage occurs within the first 24 hours; late postpartum hemorrhage is beyond the first 24 hours but within 6 weeks of delivery. The cause of early postpartum hemorrhage is uterine atony making the uterus unable to contract, which inhibits loss from the vascular area where the placenta was attached to the uterine wall. Any complication of birth (abruptio placentae, placenta accreta or previa, missed abortion, fetal death, inverted uterus, or preeclampsia) can lead to increased risk for postpartal hemorrhage.

• INFECTION

Postpartum or puerperal infection occurs immediately after birth and is a frequent cause of newborn death. The best treatment is prevention, so standard precautions and sterile and aseptic techniques are essential components of care.

Pathophysiology and Etiology

Rupture of membranes past 24 hours, prolonged and difficult labor, or any break in the skin could allow organisms to enter the body, as could any condition that weakens the body's natural defense mechanisms. *Anaerobic streptococci, Clostridia, beta-hemolytic streptococcus, Escherichia coli,* and *Klebsiella* are the most common causes of infections.

Assessment Findings

The most common sites of puerperal infection are the reproductive system, urinary tract, and breasts. The first sign is increased temperature within 10 days of delivery, lasting 24 hours, with chills and headache. Other signs and symptoms depend on the site and whether the infection is localized or systemic. Diagnostic tests include culture and sensitivity of lochia (see Chap. 3), cesarean incision, and vaginal tissue; WBC count; and sedimentation rate.

Medical and Surgical Management

Treatment is initiated with a broad-spectrum IV antibiotic until cultures isolate the causative organism. Isolation is necessary if the infection is contagious; otherwise, standard precautions are sufficient. Hygiene and handwashing must be reinforced with the client.

• THROMBOPHLEBITIS

Thrombophlebitis is an infection in a vessel lining with a clot attached (see Chap 25). The most common site is the veins in the legs or pelvis, usually between 10 and 20 days postpartum. Clients with thrombophlebitis are at risk for pulmonary embolism, which could result in death.

Thrombophlebitis may be superficial, involving the venous system only. Superficial thrombophlebitis is thought to result from the lithotomy position used during labor. Deep vein thrombophlebitis has an increased risk of embolism from pressure on the veins during delivery.

Prevention is the best course of management, with early and frequent ambulation after delivery. Should thrombophlebitis develop, treatment is strict bed rest, anticoagulant therapy, and antibiotics if ordered.

Monitor for edema of the leg or groin, stiffness, chills, and pain (a positive Homans' sign; see Chap. 27). Educate the client on bleeding precautions. Monitor vital signs at least every 4 hours. Check coagulation studies and measurements of the leg. Assess the lungs and mental status and provide emotional support.

• PSYCHOLOGICAL PROBLEMS

The incidence of psychological disorders increases during and after pregnancy related to increased hormone production. Throughout pregnancy and during the postpartum period, the client requires assessment for signs or verbalization of increased stress, difficulty coping, or depression.

The postpartum period is a time of transition and adjustment to the new family member. The woman experiences three distinct phases during this period: taking in, taking hold, and letting go. Feelings of dependency immediately after birth change as the mother takes her child home and can care for herself and her infant and adapt to motherhood. She begins to recognize the infant as a separate being. If the woman feels overwhelmed, and is crying, complaining of headache, insomnia, fatigue, depression, and anger, she may be experiencing *postpartum blues* or *postpartum depression.* In postpartum blues, such symptoms begin immediately after birth and disappear within a few days. In postpartum depression, women experience these feelings as more severe and they last beyond a few weeks, impairing activities of daily living. Treatment is essential and consists of observing the client for signs and symptoms of depression, providing support to the woman and her family, and administering prescribed medications.

Stop, Think, and Respond ● BOX 2-4

What would you say to a woman who presents with signs and symptoms of postpartum depression?

Critical Thinking Exercises

1. *How would you respond to a 41-year-old pregnant woman who asks for your opinion about whether she should have an amniocentesis?*
2. *Discuss the risks for a pregnant teenager diagnosed with PIH and her fetus.*

• NCLEX-STYLE REVIEW QUESTIONS

1. A client with uncontrolled pregnancy-induced hypertension is hospitalized. To ensure the client's safety, the nurse should:
    1. Maintain the client's NPO status.
    2. Implement seizure precautions.

3. Perform daily neurological checks.
4. Assist the client to walk to the bathroom as needed.

2. A woman in her 26th week of pregnancy is diagnosed with gestational diabetes. The nurse discusses ways to control the condition. Which instruction is most appropriate?
1. "You need to monitor your blood glucose level frequently."
2. "You need to include more carbohydrates in your diet."
3. "You should maintain your current weight for the rest of the pregnancy."
4. "You must remember to exercise at least twice every week."

3. A pregnant client is diagnosed with severe abruptio placenta. Which nursing intervention is most important initially?
1. Prepare for a cesarean section.
2. Monitor the fetal heart rate.
3. Perform a sterile vaginal examination.
4. Administer pain medication.

connection

Visit the Connection site at **http://connection.lww.com/go/timbyEssentials** for links to chapter-related resources on the Internet.

References and Suggested Readings

Beck, C. (2002). Theoretical perspectives of postpartum depression and their treatment implications. *Maternal Child Nursing, 23,* 282–287.

Blackburn, S. (2003). *Maternal fetal, & neonatal physiology* (2nd ed.). Philadelphia: W. B. Saunders.

Burrow, G., & Duffy, T. (1999). Medical complications during pregnancy (5th ed.). Philadelphia: W. B. Saunders.

Deacon, J., & O'Neill, P. (Eds.) (1999). *Core curriculum for neonatal intensive care nursing* (2nd ed.). Philadelphia: W. B. Saunders.

Evans, A., & Niswander, K. (2000). *Manual of obstetrics* (6th ed.). Philadelphia: Lippincott Williams & Wilkins.

Gupton, A., Heaman, M., & Cheung, L. (2001). Complicated and uncomplicated pregnancies: Women's perception of risk. *Journal of Obstetric, Gynecological, and Neonatal Nursing, 30,* 192–201.

Hayes, B., Kaiser, K., McMahon, C., & Kaup, K. (2000). Building the knowledge base for high-risk prenatal clients. *Maternal Child Nursing, 25,* 151–163.

Maloni, J., Brezinski-Tomasi, J., & Johnson, L. (2001). Antepartum bed rest: Effect upon the family. *Journal of Obstetric, Gynecological, and Neonatal Nursing, 30,* 165–173.

Mattson, S., & Smith, J. (eds.) (2000). *A WHONN core curriculum for maternal-newborn nursing* (2nd ed.). Philadelphia: W. B. Saunders.

Patrick, T. (1999). Current concepts in preeclampsia. *Maternal Child Nursing, 24,* 193–200.

Pillitteri, A. (2003). *Maternal & child health nursing* (4th ed.). Philadelphia: Lippincott Williams & Wilkins.

Poole, J., & Thorsen, M. (1999). Acute renal failure in pregnancy. *American Journal of Maternal/Child Nursing, 24*(2), 66–72.

Steele, N., French, J., Gatherer-Boyles, J., Newman, S., & Leclaire, S. (2001). Effect of acupressure by Sea-Bands on nausea and vomiting of pregnancy. *Journal of Obstetric, Gynecological, and Neonatal Nursing,* 30, 61–68.

Weitz, B. (2001). Premature rupture of the fetal membranes. *Maternal Child Nursing, 26,* 86–92.

chapter 3

Caring for the Normal Newborn and Family

Words to Know

acrocyanosis
Apgar score
autolysis
brown fat
caput succedaneum
cephalhematoma
colostrum
ductus arteriosus
en face
engorgement
epispadias
Epstein's pearls
erythema toxicum neonatorum
foramen ovale
foremilk
frenulum
harlequin sign
hindmilk
hypospadias
involution
lanugo
lochia alba
lochia rubra
lochia serosa
meconium
milia
mongolian spot
mottling
ophthalmia neonatorum
petechiae
phimosis
polydactyly
port-wine stain
stork bite
strawberry hemangioma
subconjunctival hematoma
vernix

Learning Objectives

On completion of this chapter, the reader will:

- Explain changes in body systems that occur in newborns as they adapt to extrauterine life.
- Understand how to assign an Apgar score to a newborn.
- Explain how nurses measure and weigh newborns.
- Explain the importance of giving erythromycin and vitamin K to newborns.
- Discuss the concept of bonding.
- Describe the gestational age assessment process.
- Name unique physical assessment findings in newborns related to the delivery process.
- Identify the newborn reflexes.
- Discuss normal ranges for newborn vital signs.
- Describe the process for bathing a newborn.
- Describe the nurse's role in circumcision and related care.
- Describe normal formula-feeding.
- Explain how nurses can promote and assist mothers with breastfeeding.
- Describe nursing management for engorgement, nipple soreness, and mastitis.
- Explain physical changes in the postpartum woman.
- Identify key areas of assessment in postpartum women.
- Discuss pain management strategies for new mothers.
- Name important client teaching topics for new parents.

This chapter focuses on care of the normal newborn at delivery and for the first 24 to 48 hours of life as well as postpartum care of the new mother. It also covers client teaching for mothers regarding newborn and self-care, with special attention to bonding and parenting skills.

DELIVERY PREPARATION

When planning for delivery, nurses must ensure that all needed equipment is available and working properly. A warmer is important; its head often is in a slight Trendelenburg position to help facilitate drainage of airway secretions. Also needed are pre-warmed blankets, cord clamp, wall suction with a mucous trap, bulb syringe, timer with alarms at 1 and 5 minutes, infant stethoscope, measuring tape, scale, erythromycin eye ointment, vitamin K, and identification bands. Other emergency resuscitation equipment should be available, including oxygen mask and tubing; Ambu bag and mask; laryngoscope with both 0 and 1 blades; endotracheal tubes sizes 2.5, 3.0, 3.5, and 4.0; and resuscitation drugs including Narcan. Narcan is used in newborns to reverse respiratory suppression resulting from maternal pain medication. It has a very short half-life, and infants receiving it require close monitoring. Narcan can wear off before the respiratory suppressive effects of maternal pain medication subside. Occasionally, nurses may need to administer Narcan a second time.

Before a delivery, review information about the mother's prenatal history and labor to assess for potential risks during delivery. This information include length of rupture of membranes, any meconium staining to the amniotic fluid, any signs of maternal infections prenatally or during labor, fetal heart monitoring such as decelerations, estimated gestational age, single or multiple gestation, and any maternal pain medications and when they were last dosed.

Most healthcare facilities provide scrubs for all obstetric personnel to wear and usually have scrubbing procedures to follow. Nurses always adhere to standard precautions by wearing gloves and possibly face masks with eye shields depending on policy and personal preference.

TRANSITION OF THE NEWBORN

For the first 28 days of life, the baby is considered a *newborn* or *neonate.* At delivery, newborns face the challenge of adapting to extrauterine life. As a result, various body systems must undergo major changes. First are changes in the respiratory and circulatory systems. The gastrointestinal system begins working to take in nutrition and get rid of waste. The renal system also adapts. Finally, neonates must maintain their own thermoregulation. Because of all these changes, newborns require close monitoring for the first several days of life.

Respiratory Changes

After delivery, newborns can no longer rely on the placenta for oxygen and nutrients. They also cannot rid themselves of carbon dioxide and waste products via transplacental exchange. They must breathe on their own. Several factors stimulate the first inspiration:

- Change in pressure
- Decreased blood levels of oxygen and pH
- Increased level of carbon dioxide
- Sensory changes in response to bright lights, noises, and a cooler temperature

With the first inspiration, the diaphragm contracts and causes negative intrathoracic pressure. This in turn leads to expansion of the alveoli. Surfactant, a substance made in the lungs, contributes to breathing by decreasing surface tension. If surface tension of the alveoli decreases, then they can remain open during expiration. Thus, the second inspiration needs much less effort that the first. As respirations continue, each becomes easier.

The lungs develop with fluid in them; however, it is not amniotic fluid but fluid that the lungs make. Delivery compresses the chest cavity, which eliminates approximately one third of the total fluid volume. The rest is removed through reabsorption by the lymph and circulatory systems, by the neonate through swallowing, or through drainage or suctioning.

Circulatory Changes

Fetal circulation depends on patency of the **foramen ovale** (an opening between the right and left atria) and **ductus arteriosus** (an opening that allows blood to flow from the pulmonary artery into the aorta). These two openings allow most blood volume to bypass the dormant lungs and instead to move through the fetal side of the placenta, providing oxygen and eliminating carbon dioxide and wastes. At birth, once the cord is clamped, these two communicating openings must close for proper circulation.

Newborn color at birth is typically pale or even cyanotic. As newborns begin breathing and circulation changes, oxygen-rich blood reaches the extremities, causing overall body color to become pinker. Even so, it is still common for neonates to have acrocyanosis or mottling. With **acrocyanosis,** the trunk remains pink, but the extremities appear cyanotic (Fig. 3.1). Acrocyanosis usually resolves after the first 24 hours. **Mottling** is a marbled appearance to the skin that often occurs when neonates are chilled slightly, such as when being undressed. Mottling also is related to circulatory lability and dissipates over time.

Thermoregulation

Babies are born with a substance in the upper back called **brown fat,** which is a stored energy that they can use to generate heat. Term infants have more brown fat than preterm babies (see Chap. 4). All babies have a finite amount, however, and once they use it, they produce no more. Therefore, keeping newborns warm and avoiding cold stressing them are essential.

The four types of heat loss in newborns are evaporative, conductive, radiant, and convective. Evaporation occurs immediately as the neonate's wet body makes contact with air temperature. Therefore, drying newborns immediately after birth is critical. Conduction occurs

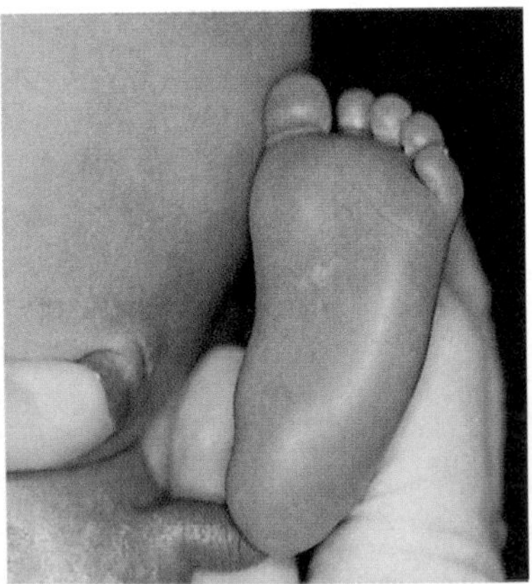

FIGURE 3.1 Acrocyanosis in a newborn.

when heat from a warm object transfers to a cooler object through direct contact. An example is placement of an infant into a cold crib. To prevent this, healthcare agencies use pre-warmed blankets and equipment. Radiation occurs when heat is lost from a warm object to a cooler one not in contact with each other. An example is the use of radiant warmers, which lose heat to help warm cool neonates. Finally, convection occurs when neonates lose heat to cooler air. It is important to keep infants away from currents such as air conditioners and fans.

The surface area of the newborn's head is very large compared to the surface area of the body. Placing a hat on the head can reduce heat loss. For the first few days of life, keeping the hands and feet warm with booties and mittens may be necessary until circulation is stable.

POSTPARTUM CARE OF THE NEWBORN

For several years, the healthcare industry has worked to make delivery a more family-oriented experience. Consequently, many facilities have changed their approach to care. Gone are labor and delivery units and separate postpartum floors. In many facilities, new mothers labor, deliver, recover, and spend their entire postpartum time in one room. Also, many babies room in with their mothers; as a result, traditional newborn nurseries have decreased. Nurses are now prepared to take care of both mothers and infants in new birthing centers. Delivery may take place in a traditional delivery room or in a labor, delivery, recovery, and postpartum (LDRP) room.

Immediate Nursing Care

Drying and Suctioning

Following delivery, the obstetrician or certified nurse midwife either may place the newborn directly on the mother's abdomen or clamp and cut the cord right away to place the baby on the warmer. Briefly dry the baby and take off the wet blanket. Then position the infant's head in the sniffing position and suction the airway. Next, assess respiratory effort and provide stimulation if necessary. The exception is if there is meconium-stained fluid. **Meconium** is the first stool that the neonate passes; it is very thick and sticky. Usually, infants pass meconium after delivery, but a stressed fetus may do so earlier. Newborns can aspirate meconium, so if it is present, suction before stimulating the baby to breathe by wiping. Also, if meconium is present, someone trained to view the infant's cords and suction meconium from them should be at the delivery.

Always suction the mouth first and the nose second. The rationale is that suctioning the nose first may stimulate respirations and the infant can aspirate secretions still in the mouth. If the neonate is starting to respire independently, ascertain the heart rate by auscultating the heart or holding the clamped cord to palpate the pulse. Count this rate for 6 seconds and multiply by 10 to equal the beats per minute (bpm) rate. Target heart rate is greater than 100 bpm (or more than a count of 10 beats for 6 seconds).

If the infant is breathing well and the heart rate is above 100 bpm, then direct attention at continuing to dry the child. Rapidly remove wet blankets and replace them with warm dry ones. The drying process stimulates respirations or crying.

Apgar Scoring

Dr. Virginia Apgar devised a quick method of assessment to use on neonates after delivery to evaluate their status and need for resuscitation. The **Apgar score** consists of five different items: appearance (color), pulse (heart rate), grimace (irritability to suctioning), activity (muscle tone), and respiration (breathing efforts). Each of these five items is scored as 0, 1, or 2 for a maximum total of 10. Apgar scores are given 1 and 5 minutes after birth. Although this quick assessment can aid in determining the need for resuscitation, never wait until 1 minute to decide if a neonate needs resuscitation (Fig. 3.2).

After determining a 1-minute Apgar score, continue drying, suctioning, and stimulating the infant as needed. At 5 minutes, ascertain the second Apgar score. This second score typically is higher, indicating improved respiration and circulation. After these 5 minutes, if the neonate is stable, continue with delivery room care.

Measurements and Weight

Obtaining an accurate length of the baby in both inches and centimeters is important. Measure length from the top of the head to the bottom of the foot with the child's leg extended fully (Fig. 3.3). Average length of full-term neonates ranges from 18 to 22 inches (46 to 56 cm). Measure head circumference around the forehead to the posterior part of the occiput. Normal range for term neonates is 13 to 14.5 inches (33 to 37 cm). Weigh the baby in both pounds and grams. Because they must be naked during weighing, take care not to chill newborns. Normal term range for weight is 5 pounds, 8 ounces to 9 pounds, 8 ounces (2500 to 4250 g). Over the first several days of life, neonates usually lose weight. A loss of up to 10% of body weight is considered normal. They usually regain this weight within the first 8 to 12 days.

Eye Prophylaxis

Ophthalmia neonatorum is an eye infection in newborns resulting from exposure to chlamydia or gonorrhea in the mother. Both chlamydia and gonorrhea can be covert maternal genital tract infections. Therefore, all

	0	1	2
Appearance (color)	Blue, pale	Body pink, extremities blue	Completely pink
Pulse (heart rate)	Absent	Less than 100 bpm	More than 100 bpm
Grimace (reflex irritability)	No response	Weak cry, grimace	Vigorous cry
Activity (muscle tone)	Flaccid	Some flexion of extremities	Active motion
Respiratory effort (crying)	Absent	Slow, irregular	Good, crying

FIGURE 3.2 Apgar scoring system.

infants receive eye prophylaxis with erythromycin ophthalmic ointment, whether delivery is vaginal or cesarean.

Before instillation of the ointment, wipe any remaining blood or body fluids from the baby's eyelids. Gently open the eyelids and instill a ribbon of ointment 0.5 to 1 cm long. After a few minutes, wipe excess ointment from the lids or surrounding skin to prevent possible irritation.

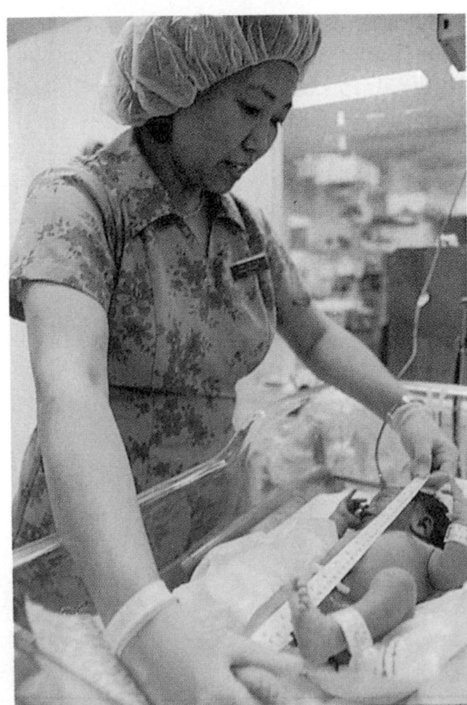

FIGURE 3.3 The nurse measures the length of a newborn.

Vitamin K Administration

Vitamin K, a fat-soluble vitamin made by the colon, is an important component in blood clotting. Neonates are born with a sterile gut. After some time, normal flora will colonize the colon, and neonates will begin to produce vitamin K. Before then, however, they are at risk for bleeding problems. Newborns therefore require an intramuscular injection of 0.5 to 1.0 mL of vitamin K (aqua Mephyton). This injection usually is given into one of the anterolateral thighs.

Identification and Safety

Soon after delivery, the neonate needs to be identified with the mother. Hospitals use identification bracelets with corresponding numbers. These bracelets usually come in sets of three or four. One is put on the mother's wrist. The other two are put on the neonate. If a fourth band is used, it may be put on the father or another person the mother chooses. Many hospitals take footprints of the newborn and a thumbprint of the mother for identification purposes. To decrease the chances of baby abduction, some facilities place an electronic bracelet device on the infant. If the infant is taken beyond a certain designated point, an alarm sounds to alert staff.

Personnel identification badges are another safety item used in units. Nurses working in OB units must properly identify themselves to parents. They must teach mothers to ask to see the identification badge of anyone who comes to take the baby away for any reason.

Suctioning of Stomach Contents

One other common procedure in most institutions is suctioning the stomach contents. In this procedure, nurses pass a suction catheter down the newborn's throat into the stomach and suction the gastric contents into a mucous trap. Removal of gastric contents helps prevent potential aspiration and can aid in feedings.

When doing this procedure, observe the contents and note the volume. Passing a catheter into the stomach can cause vagal nerve stimulation, which in turn can decrease heart rate. Therefore, assess the heart rate after the procedure and do not do this procedure before giving the 5-minute Apgar score.

Documentation

After completing delivery room care, assess the neonate's condition one more time. Auscultate heart rate for up to 1 full minute and lung sounds. Assess respiratory effort, color, and muscle tone. If all is well, bundle up the child and give him or her to the mother for some quality bonding time (discussed next).

The delivery room record often has an area for both maternal and infant information. Infant information includes time of delivery, presentation part (e.g., cephalic, breech), if a cord was around the neck, and, if so, how many times it was wrapped. It also should include the presence of any meconium-stained fluid, 1- and 5-minute Apgar scores, and if the baby required oxygen or other resuscitative efforts. Document administration of erythromycin eye ointment and vitamin K as well as length, head circumference, weight, identification band numbers, and sex.

Newborn Assessment

Gestational Age

Newborns require thorough assessment shortly after birth, including gestational age. Before birth, practitioners based the due date on the mother's last menstrual period or according to measurements of fetal parts by ultrasound. These methods, however, are estimates. After birth, a gestational age assessment can determine how many weeks the infant was in gestation.

An infant considered "term" is born between 38 to 41 gestational weeks. A preterm infant is born at 37 weeks or less. A postterm infant is born at 42 weeks or more. Potential complications are related to both preterm and postterm gestations (see Chap. 4).

Different assessment forms have been designed to determine gestational age. They consider different areas, consisting of movements and muscle tone, reflexes, and neurobehavior. The Dubowitz assessment is one example; the Ballard is another. A third example, the Maturational Assessment of Gestational Age (New Ballard Score), considers neuromuscular and physical maturity (Fig. 3.4). This form can be used to evaluate gestational age for all infants, even very premature babies.

Most hospitals specify the form they want staff members to use when assessing gestational age. To learn how to perform accurate gestational age assessments, it is advisable to observe a skilled nurse do several for many infants of differing gestational ages.

Head-to-Toe Physical Assessment

The full head-to-toe physical assessment usually occurs within the first 1 to 2 hours of life. It may be done before or after bathing the infant. If the parents are present, this can be a good opportunity to teach them about the newborn. It is best to do this examination with the infant on a radiant warmer to protect against chilling while affording the best possible view.

HEAD. The neonate's head consists of the two halves of the frontal bone, the occipital bone, and two parietal and two temporal bones. At birth, these six bones have not yet fused together, allowing for their mobility when the head passes through the maternal pelvis during delivery. If the active pushing stage of labor took some time, molding of the infant's head can be significant, leading to a very cone-shaped appearance. Reassure parents that this cone shape will disappear in a few days without any intervention.

Suture lines are between the six bones. As the baby ages, they will fuse to become solid bone. Of note are the two fontanels, posterior and anterior. No bone exists in these "soft spots" in the head. Over time, bone material will grow and fill these two areas. The posterior fontanel is located along the posterior upper edge of the two parietal bones and the superior edge of the occipital bone. It is triangle shaped. The anterior fontanel is larger and diamond shaped. It is located between the posterior corners of the frontal bones and the anterior corners of the parietal bones. The posterior fontanel closes usually by 12 months, and the anterior fontanel closes by 18 months. Normally, they feel soft and fairly flat to the touch.

With the intense pressure of the head traversing the pelvis at delivery, two forms of head trauma are possible. **Caput succedaneum** is a collection of blood or serum above the periosteum that can cross suture lines. Its appearance resembles a skullcap across the back of the infant's head. **Cephalhematoma,** a rarer type of trauma, is a collection of blood between the bone and periosteum that cannot cross suture lines. Cephalhematoma appears as a swollen area on one side of the head in the posterior

MATURATIONAL ASSESSMENT OF GESTATIONAL AGE (New Ballard Score)

NAME ____________ SEX ____________

HOSPITAL NO. ____________ BIRTH WEIGHT ____________

RACE ____________ LENGTH ____________

DATE/TIME OF BIRTH ____________ HEAD CIRC. ____________

DATE/TIME OF EXAM ____________ EXAMINER ____________

AGE WHEN EXAMINED ____________

APGAR SCORE: 1 MINUTE ________ 5 MINUTES ________ 10 MINUTES ________

NEUROMUSCULAR MATURITY

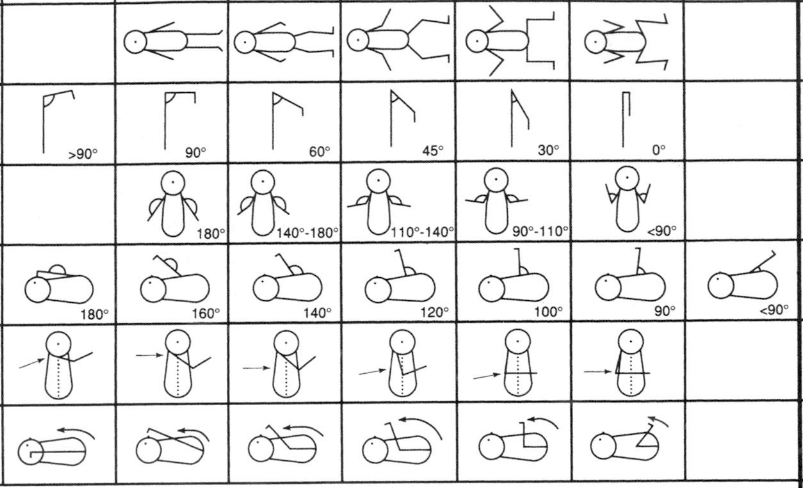

NEUROMUSCULAR MATURITY SIGN	SCORE -1	0	1	2	3	4	5	RECORD SCORE HERE
POSTURE								
SQUARE WINDOW (Wrist)	>90°	90°	60°	45°	30°	0°		
ARM RECOIL		180°	140°-180°	110°-140°	90°-110°	<90°		
POPLITEAL ANGLE	180°	160°	140°	120°	100°	90°	<90°	
SCARF SIGN								
HEEL TO EAR								

TOTAL NEUROMUSCULAR MATURITY SCORE ____

PHYSICAL MATURITY

PHYSICAL MATURITY SIGN	SCORE -1	0	1	2	3	4	5	RECORD SCORE HERE
SKIN	sticky friable transparent	gelatinous red translucent	smooth pink visible veins	superficial peeling &/or rash, few veins	cracking pale areas rare veins	parchment deep cracking no vessels	leathery cracked wrinkled	
LANUGO	none	sparse	abundant	thinning	bald areas	mostly bald		
PLANTAR SURFACE	heel-toe 40-50 mm:-1 <40 mm:-2	>50 mm no crease	faint red marks	anterior transverse crease only	creases ant. 2/3	creases over entire sole		
BREAST	imperceptible	barely perceptible	flat areola no bud	stippled areola 1-2 mm bud	raised areola 3-4 mm bud	full areola 5-10 mm bud		
EYE/EAR	lids fused loosely: -1 tightly: -2	lids open pinna flat stays folded	sl. curved pinna; soft; slow recoil	well-curved pinna; soft but ready recoil	formed & firm instant recoil	thick cartilage ear stiff		
GENITALS (Male)	scrotum flat, smooth	scrotum empty faint rugae	testes in upper canal rare rugae	testes descending few rugae	testes down good rugae	testes pendulous deep rugae		
GENITALS (Female)	clitoris prominent & labia flat	prominent clitoris & small labia minora	prominent clitoris & enlarging minora	majora & minora equally prominent	majora large minora small	majora cover clitoris & minora		

TOTAL PHYSICAL MATURITY SCORE ____

SCORE

Neuromuscular ________

Physical ________

Total ________

MATURITY RATING

score	weeks
-10	20
-5	22
0	24
5	26
10	28
15	30
20	32
25	34
30	36
35	38
40	40
45	42
50	44

GESTATIONAL AGE (weeks)

By dates ________

By ultrasound ________

By exam ________

FIGURE 3.4 The Maturational Assessment of Gestational Age (New Ballard Score).

region. As with molding, both conditions are self-resolving. Be sure to tell parents this also.

EYES. Eye examination includes assessment of the pupils, which should be round and equal in size and reactive to constriction by light. Use of an ophthalmoscope to view the retina should reveal a red reflex. The iris of Caucasian infants is blue or grey; over time the color may change. The iris of African American, Hispanic, and Asian infants is brown. Corneas should be clear; sclera should be white. As a result of pressure on the head during delivery, however, blood vessels in the sclera can break, giving the sclera a red color. This condition is referred to as a **subconjunctival hematoma.** This bruise of the eye retains a red color because of oxygen in the air that penetrates through the thin layers of cells in the eye. This red color usually is curved as the iris is, and it is near but never crosses the iris.

Newborns have relatively weak eye muscles, and the eyes do not always move together. Thus, some babies look cross-eyed. The eye muscles strengthen over time.

EARS. Positioning of the ears should be viewed in relation to the head. If an imaginary line were drawn from the outer corner of the eye posteriorly, the top of the ear should touch this line. An ear that does not touch this line is said to be "low set" and may indicate that the child has certain syndromes. Check the ears for patency and view the tympanic membrane with an otoscope.

NOSE. The nose should be midline with both nares patent. When the infant is at rest, the nares should not flare out with normal respirations. Nasal flaring at rest is a sign of respiratory distress. The tight squeeze through the pelvis during birth may push the nose to one side of the face or bruise it. This should be self-correcting over time.

MOUTH. The tongue should be midline. The **frenulum** is a thin membrane that attaches vertically from the bottom of the tongue to the base of the inner lower jaw. If the frenulum is too short, the infant is said to be "tongue-tied." In some cases, this interferes with the infant's ability to breastfeed.

Normally, no teeth are present. Any teeth that appear are removed to prevent potential aspiration. Small, white, pearl-like bumps called **Epstein's pearls** may be on the palate; these are of no concern. The lips sometimes have a white, thick, blister-like appearance, referred to as a "sucking blister." These are not true blisters and should cause no alarm.

THORAX. The throat should be midline. Palpate the clavicles to assess for fracture. Infants large for gestational age sometimes fracture their clavicles during birth. The chest should rise and fall equally with respiration. At rest, the ribs should show no signs of retraction. Grunting is defined as a grunt sound made with every expiration. Report grunting, retractions, and nasal flaring immediately, as they are all signs of respiratory distress. Auscultate the lung sounds.

Auscultate the heart with an infant stethoscope. Normal heart rate is usually 100 to 160 bpm; it increases with activity and decreases with sleep. Note S1 and S2 sounds as well as any murmurs. Sometimes the ductus arteriosus remains open after birth for a short time, making a murmur audible. Monitor this finding, noting the disappearance or persistence of the murmur. As infants can cry loudly, checking both apical rate and lung sounds before disturbing them is advisable.

Enlargement of breast tissue can occur in both male and female infants in response to maternal hormones. They also may have some nipple discharge. Reassure parents that such findings will resolve within a few weeks.

ABDOMEN. The abdomen should be rounded and soft. Auscultate bowel sounds before palpating the abdomen. The cord normally contains three vessels. Note if there are only two vessels; this finding is associated with internal anomalies. Firmly attach the cord clamp.

GENITALIA. Genitalia in term newborn girls can be slightly pink and swollen for a few days. The labia majora should cover the labia minora. Sometimes the vagina has a whitish or blood-tinged discharge, which results from maternal hormones and will disappear over several days.

The male infant's scrotum is slightly darker in color. Palpate the testicles bilaterally. Male infants can be born with one or both testicles undescended (see Chap. 9). Sometimes they can be palpated in the inguinal canal and brought down into the scrotum. The foreskin of the penis tends to be quite tight and small. **Phimosis** is a condition in which the foreskin cannot be retracted to expose the glans penis. Note the location of the urethral meatus, normally at the tip of the penis. A meatus located on the upper outer side is called **epispadias.** A meatus located on the underside is called **hypospadias.**

Check the anus for patency. Some institutions assess patency by taking a rectal temperature routinely on every newborn. Other hospitals use documentation of passage of stool as demonstration of patency. If performing a rectal temperature, gently insert the tip of the thermometer probe no more than one half inch. Hold the probe with one hand while holding the legs of the infant with the other hand.

EXTREMITIES. Term infants should have good flexed muscle tone and full range of motion in all extremities. Capillary refill should be immediate. Palpate peripheral pulses at the brachial arteries and at the groin. Examine all fingers and toes. Note any extra digits or skin tags on hands and feet, referred to as **polydactyly.**

SKIN. Newborn skin is usually soft and smooth with little or no peeling. Postterm infants tend to have more cracking and peeling. **Vernix,** a white cheese-like substance, protects the fetal skin from the amniotic fluid. At approximately 36 weeks' gestation, vernix starts to decrease. By term, newborns usually have only small amounts of vernix on the body, mainly in the axilla and groin.

Lanugo is fine downy hair on the body of the fetus. It begins to disappear at 28 weeks' gestation from the face first, then from the anterior trunk, and finally from the back and rest of the body. A term infant may have some lanugo across the upper back.

Skin color in Caucasian infants is quite pink. African American infants have a light gray or brown complexion, which darkens over time. Some infants are very ruddy because of their high red blood cell concentration. They need close monitoring for jaundice, a yellowish color of the skin (see Chap. 4). Assess for jaundice by pressing a finger over the sternum or nose to blanch the skin and lifting the finger quickly to see if the blanched skin is yellow. If an infant is jaundiced, check bilirubin levels and the records for any possible ABO or Rh incompatibilities. Jaundice also may be seen in the sclera.

A transient and benign variation in normal coloration is a **harlequin sign.** This occurs when half of the infant is quite pink while the other half is pale (as if a line were drawn down the body bisecting it from head to toe). This sign often lasts only a few minutes but is quite interesting to view.

Small, white, raised areas on the face approximately 1 mm in diameter are called **milia** and are self-resolving. **Petechiae,** small, flat, red or purple dots anywhere on the body, are tiny pinpoint bruises caused by pressure during labor. They will fade over several days. A **mongolian spot** looks like a large bruised area over the buttocks and coccyx. It is in no way related to Down syndrome. It is totally benign and nontender and may fade as the child grows. All these findings are common among non-Caucasian infants.

A **stork bite** (telangiectatic nevus) is a flat red mark usually on the face or neck. Stork bites are benign and fade over the first 1 to 2 years of life. A **strawberry hemangioma** is a raised cherry red area caused by capillaries being close to the skin surface. It can enlarge, but over time usually shrinks and disappears. A **port-wine stain** is a flat reddish-purple skin patch, usually on the face. It does not disappear and may need medical attention. A red raised rash with vesicles over the entire body is called **erythema toxicum neonatorum.** This is benign and will resolve with no treatment.

Assessment of Reflexes

Certain reflexes in term infants indicate normal neurologic functioning. Their nervous system, however, remains immature. Neurologic development continues until approximately 2 years of age, when myelination is complete. Some reflexes persist throughout life: sneezing, coughing, and blinking. The following reflexes present at birth disappear over time:

- *Rooting reflex:* The infant turns the head toward the stimulus when the mouth is stroked.
- *Palmar grasp:* The infant automatically grasps an object placed into the hand (Fig. 3.5A).
- *Moro reflex:* The infant flails out the arms and then pulls them back when startled (Fig. 3.5B).
- *Tonic neck reflex:* The infant responds to turning of the head to one side by extending the leg and arm on the same side and flexing the opposite arm and leg (Fig. 3.5C).
- *Babinski reflex:* The infant splays out the toes in response to the foot being scraped from heel to toe on the sole. An adult responds to this same stimulus by flexing toes inward (Fig. 3.5D).
- *Stepping reflex:* The infant steps with alternating feet when held in a standing position with the feet touching a surface (Fig. 3.5E).
- *Sucking reflex:* The infant automatically sucks when a nipple is placed at the lips.

Ongoing Nursing Care

The following section discusses newborn care during the remainder of the hospital stay. This care, which nurses usually document on a daily flow sheet, includes assessment and monitoring, bathing, cord care, assistance with elimination, screening tests, circumcision care, and assistance with feeding.

Assessment and Monitoring

Periodic assessments of the infant's condition include evaluation of vital signs. Normal pulse rate ranges from 110 to 160 bpm, depending on activity. Measure by auscultating an apical pulse for 1 minute. Normal respiratory rate ranges from 30 to 60 breaths per minute. Take respiratory rate by counting how often the chest rises and falls in 1 minute. Note whether the infant was at rest or active or crying during evaluation of pulse and respiratory rates.

Normal temperature ranges from 97.6° to 98.6°F (36.6° to 37.0°C). Take axillary temperature by placing the tip of the thermometer probe firmly in the axilla and holding it there for 3 minutes. A digital thermometer may take less time. Facilities commonly use tympanic temperature probes, which have a probe that is inserted into the ear canal pointing toward the tympanic membrane. Hold the infant's head still while performing a tympanic temperature. Monitor the infant's thermoregulation throughout the hospital stay and strive to prevent cold stress.

Blood pressure is normally low. Systolic readings can range from 50 to 80 mm Hg; diastolic readings can range

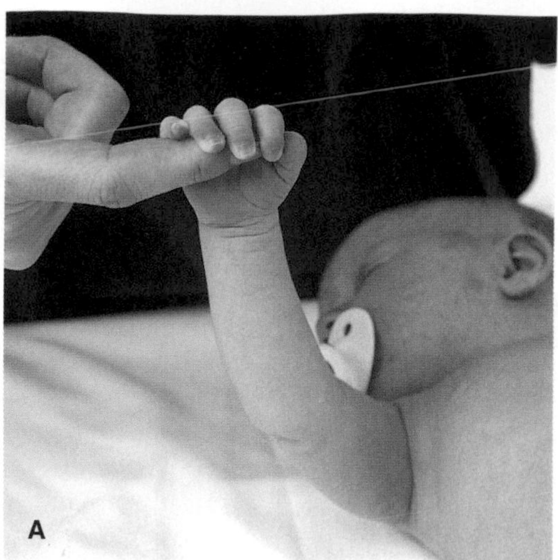

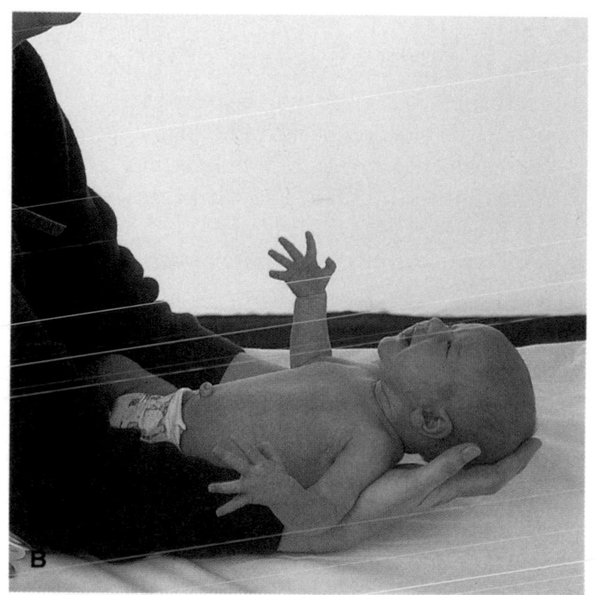

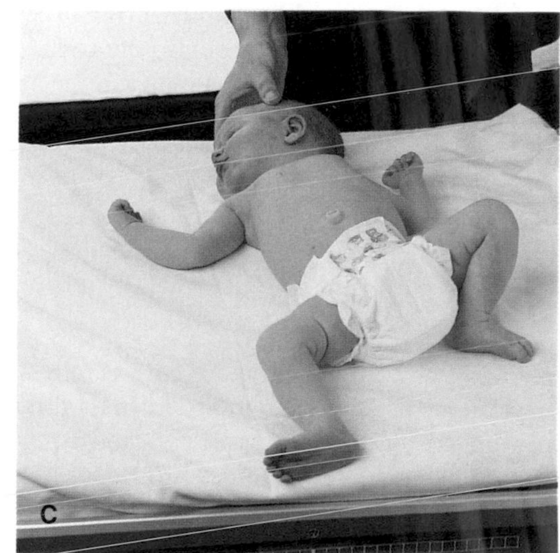

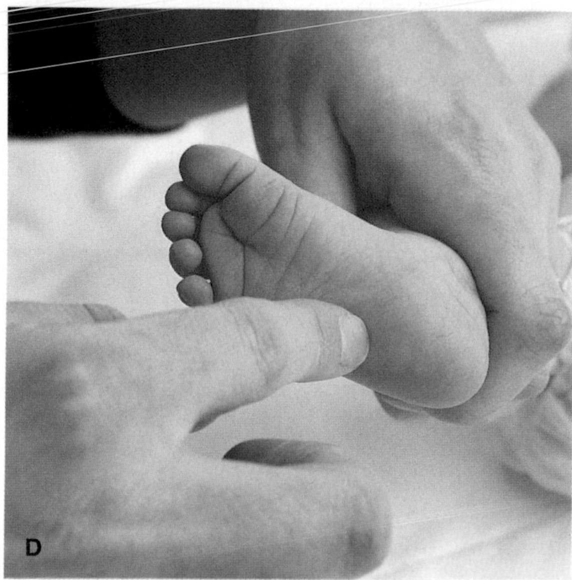

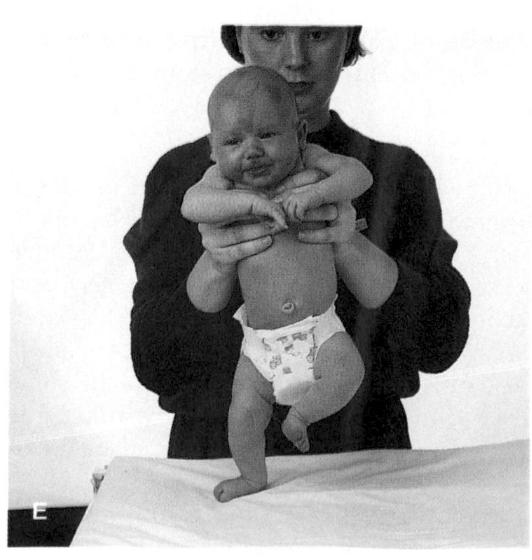

FIGURE 3.5 Newborn reflexes: (**A**) Palmar grasp. (**B**) Moro. (**C**) Tonic neck. (**D**) Babinski. (**E**) Stepping.

from 30 to 50 mm Hg. Measure blood pressure using an appropriately sized cuff and machine. The usual site used is the leg.

Agencies may have certain protocols regarding when to measure and how often to check blood glucose level. Nurses may perform a heel stick or toe prick to obtain a small drop of blood. A heel stick is done by using a lancet to stick either the lateral or medial solar surface of the heel. A standard glucose monitor may be used. Hypoglycemia occurs if the reading is less than 40 mg/dL. Usual treatment for hypoglycemia is an immediate feeding, followed by re-evaluation for persistence of the condition.

Bathing

The infant needs bathing to remove blood and body fluids. Bathe the infant on a radiant warmer to prevent heat loss. Use warm water in a basin. Wipe the eyes clean first using warm water. Then wash the face. Use an infant body wash soap on the rest of the body. When washing the head, using a soft scrub brush to remove blood and debris can be helpful. Washing proceeds down the body to the neck, chest, abdomen, back, arms, and legs. Finally, wash the bottom area—first the genitals and then the anus. After washing each area, dry it to prevent heat loss before progressing to the next body part.

After the initial bath, give the infant sponge baths until the cord has fallen off. Then, tub baths are appropriate.

Cord Care

After 24 to 48 hours, removal of the cord clamp is safe. Cord care consists of putting rubbing alcohol on the cord with every diaper change. Take care to fold the front of the diaper down to leave the cord outside the diaper. A cord tucked into the diaper can remain moist. The cord will dry and usually fall off in 10 to 14 days. Once it falls off, yellowish or greenish drainage may appear from the umbilicus. To help dry this drainage, continue to apply alcohol. Some facilities use triple dye on the cord to facilitate drying and prevent infection. This purple dye requires careful application, because it also can stain the skin purple.

Elimination

Infants normally have 6 to 10 wet diapers per day. Document the time and number of wet diapers every day on the flow sheet. Usually the diaper is wet at every feeding time. The first stool is meconium (discussed earlier). A transitional stool follows, which is greenish to yellow and often seedy. Within a few days, the stool changes to mushy yellow or golden. The stool of a breastfed infant is somewhat less offensive in odor than that of a formula-fed infant. Also document the time, type of stool, and amount on the daily flow sheet.

Teach parents that they must change diapers fairly frequently to limit skin exposure to urine and stool to help prevent diaper rashes. Cleanse the infant's bottom with moist wipes from anterior to posterior. Discourage use of powder, which can pose an aspiration risk, trap moisture, and promote rashes.

Screening Tests

Individual states determine which blood tests will be done for all infants to screen for diseases. Most states require testing for phenylketonuria (PKU), galactosemia, maple syrup urine disease, hypothyroidism, glucose-6-phosphate dehydrogenase deficiency, biotinidase deficiency, hemoglobinopathy, and congenital adrenal hyperplasia. Some check for sickle cell trait. Test for sickle cell trait should not be done before 24 hours of life, and results are more accurate after 48 to 72 hours of life. If the screen is drawn before 24 hours, a redraw may be necessary by 2 weeks of age. This may become an issue with early discharge.

The nurse is the usual person to draw the newborn screen. In some hospitals, laboratory phlebotomists draw the screen. A heel stick with a special testing card is used to obtain the blood. If performing such a screen, be sure to place the blood on the card in the specified areas and allow it to soak into the card. Pre-warm the heel to increase blood flow to the area. One method of pre-warming is to wrap a warm compress (a diaper with warm water in it) around the foot. Once warmed, clean the heel with alcohol and allow it to dry. Then stick the lateral outer edge with a lancet. Most infants' heels need to be squeezed a bit to encourage blood flow. Take care not to bruise the foot. Use standard precautions during the procedure.

Most institutions give the first hepatitis B vaccination before discharge. This intramuscular injection is given similarly as the vitamin K injection. Commonly used brands are Engerix-B and Recombivax HB. If the infant's mother was found to be positive for hepatitis B, then the infant also receives an injection of hepatitis B immune globulin (HBIG). Document these injections in the infant's chart. Also, document the hepatitis B immunization on an immunization record card and give it to the mother.

Circumcision

Circumcision is surgical removal of the foreskin of the penis. It is done for various reasons, including beliefs about cleanliness and religious reasons. Staff members should not make any judgment regarding the parents' decision to circumcise or not. Those who want their sons to be circumcised must complete a consent form before surgery. Nurses must be well versed in the procedure to be able to discuss it with parents and answer their questions.

Anesthesia may be used, usually in the form of a penile nerve block with lidocaine. Do not feed the infant right before the procedure, because feeding can lead to possible regurgitation and potential aspiration. Assist the physician or midwife who performs the circumcision; monitor the infant's status during the procedure. The physician or midwife may use a Gomco or Mogen circumcision or the newer disposable Plastibell circumcision. If he or she uses a Gomco or Mogen, then he or she will wrap sterile petroleum gauze around the end of the penis. This gauze remains in place for 24 hours. If using a Plastibell, a plastic bell remains of the end of the penis. Both the Plastibell and the petroleum gauze help protect the skin from sticking to the diaper. A dried yellow exudate will form over the first 24 hours after the procedure. This is part of the normal healing process and should not be removed. It may persist for up to 2 to 3 days.

Inspect the site for bleeding often for the first few hours. If bleeding is persistent, apply pressure and notify the physician or midwife. Provide comfort measures for the infant after the procedure. Also assess for voiding. Do not lay the infant on his abdomen for several hours after the procedure.

At every diaper change, examine the circumcision for bleeding. Gently clean the penis to remove urine or stool. Apply a new dose of petroleum jelly liberally to the site to help prevent sticking to the diaper. Total healing takes approximately 1 week. Circumcisions often are performed right before discharge, so parents need to be comfortable with postprocedure care.

Stop, Think, and Respond ● BOX 3-1

A client asks you if she should have her newborn son circumcised. How would you respond?

Feeding

Feedings often are initiated shortly after birth as part of the bonding process, especially if the infant is breastfed. Certain anomalies could cause aspiration. Therefore, some hospitals have protocols stating that the first thing an infant can receive is sterile water. Other hospitals allow breastfeeding but state that if an infant is to be bottle-fed, he or she is to receive sterile water before formula.

Newborns are fed "on demand." That means when they are hungry, feed them. Usually, most newborns awaken every 2 to 4 hours to eat. If the newborn is rooming in with the mother, she may readily feed the baby. If the newborn is in a nursery, staff needs to monitor the infant's activity and get him or her ready to visit the mother for feedings if she so desires, or the nurse may feed the infant.

FORMULA-FEEDING. Many good formulas are available today. Different kinds include cow's milk, soy, lactose-free, and special formulas to treat certain digestive disorders such as maple syrup urine disease. Formulas made for premature infants have more calories per ounce to meet their higher caloric requirements. Several different companies make formulas, which provide competition that helps keep consumer costs low. Some formulas are in a ready-to-feed state; others are available in powder or concentrated liquid forms. Both powder and concentrate forms need mixing with water before they are ready to feed. All formulas usually are fed at room temperature or warmed slightly.

Different types of nipples and bottles are available. Some nipples are shaped to imitate the breast. Some bottles and nipples are designed to decrease the air that the infant swallows. Certain infants do better with specific types of nipples or bottles. Make parents aware of this so that they can try different variations if infants have problems with feedings.

Most newborns eat 1 to 3 ounces per feeding, often every 3 hours. Over a few weeks, the amount per feeding increases; the infant may drop a nighttime feeding.

When feeding an infant, first wash your hands. Feedings are a clean, not sterile, procedure. Begin with the properly prepared formula. Cradle the infant in one arm with the baby's head slightly elevated. Hold the bottle with your other hand, making sure the nipple is down so that formula is in the neck of the bottle. This prevents the baby from swallowing excess air. The infant must coordinate sucking, swallowing, and breathing. The infant takes several sucks and swallows then may pause to breathe. Infants are obligate nose breathers, meaning they must breathe from the nose. Therefore, any nasal congestion can cause feeding problems.

Burp the infant after he or she has taken approximately 0.5 to 1 ounce of formula. Continue this burping pattern throughout the feeding. Burp by placing the infant upright against your shoulder and chest and gently patting or rubbing the baby's back, or sit the infant upright on your lap. Support the infant's head by holding onto his or her jaw and use your other hand to gently pat or rub the back. Some infants burp very easily, while others do not.

Hiccoughs are frequent in newborns. The phrenic nerve, which affects the diaphragm, lies in close approximation to the esophagus. The act of swallowing or burping can disturb the phrenic nerve and cause hiccoughs. Conversely, if an infant has hiccoughs, an additional swallow or burp can make them stop. As the infant grows, hiccoughs are much less frequent.

Feeding time is much more than just when infants get their nutrition. It is a time of socialization for babies. During feeding, they can interact with parents and others. They receive both visual and auditory stimulation. People usually talk to infants during feeding. Rocking provides vestibular stimulation. Babies gain a sense of security being bundled and held. Those feeding babies always should hold infants—they should NEVER prop bottles.

Parents may choose formula feeding for various reasons. Medical reasons include a premature infant or an infant with physical anomalies that interfere with breastfeeding. Mothers may need to take certain medications not recommended with breastfeeding. Parents may simply want the father or others to be able to feed the infant.

Whatever the reason, nurses should support the parent's decision. In their enthusiasm to promote breastfeeding, nurses should never make mothers feel guilty for choosing to bottle-feed, nor should they ever goad women into breastfeeding.

BREASTFEEDING. "Breast is best" is the current catch phrase. Promotion of breastfeeding in the United States has been extensive over the past few decades. Many hospitals have changed their policies to encourage early breastfeeding and to increase contact between infant and mother. Facilities have changed the physical space and layout of labor, delivery, and postpartum units to promote breastfeeding.

Breastfeeding has several advantages. First, it costs much less than buying formula and bottles. Breast milk is always available at the right temperature and needs no mixing. It protects the infant's immune system through transfer of maternal antibodies. It may reduce the chances of the infant developing allergies later in life. Studies have shown that breastfeeding can reduce ear infections in infants. It can enhance infant–maternal bonding and help the uterus return to its normal size and shape. It also can delay ovulation.

Breast milk is the perfect nutrition for a newborn. **Colostrum,** the first breast milk the woman produces after delivery, is thick and yellowish. It contains many vitamins, minerals, protein, and fats and is high in antibodies.

Infants should breastfeed frequently, often every 2 hours. Frequent feedings help stimulate milk production. The more the demand is, the more the supply increases. Women also can increase rest and both fluid and protein intake to increase breast milk supply.

Engorgement. Within 2 to 4 days, true breast milk replaces colostrum. True milk is thinner and light colored, often bluish white. When true milk "comes in," its volume tends to be greater than that with colostrum. At this point, mothers may find that their breasts become larger, more firm, and tender. This is referred to as **engorgement** and typically lasts 24 to 48 hours. The best treatment for engorgement is to prevent it as much as possible through frequent and regular breastfeeding. If mothers experience engorgement, the goal is to remove milk and relieve the discomfort. Massaging the breasts before feeding helps increase circulation and softens the breast, which makes it easier for the infant to latch onto the nipple. Applying heat to the breast is another method to increase milk flow. Women can use a warm compress or a warm shower before breastfeeding. Finally, expressing some milk can give relief. The woman can manually express milk or use a manual or electric breast pump. It is important that nursing mothers wear a good supportive bra at all times. If she experiences much pain, the woman can apply ice packs between feedings. A physician or midwife may order pain medications such as acetaminophen or even codeine in severe cases.

Beginning Breastfeeding. Nurses should be available to help mothers initiate breastfeeding. Starting when the infant is alert and hungry is best. Teach the mother how to hold the infant to support the baby while maintaining personal comfort. The woman can use pillows and blankets for positioning. The cradle and football holds are the most common positions for breastfeeding.

For the cradle hold, place the infant into the woman's arm with the baby's head in the bend of the mother's elbow. The woman's forearm should support the baby's back; her hand should support the child's bottom or thigh. The infant's body should face the mother's body. The woman can then use her other hand to support her breast. If the woman is holding the infant in her left arm, then she can use her right hand to hold her breast. She may form a "C" by placing her right thumb on top of her breast with her fingers extended around the underside of the breast. Alternatively, she may place her right hand on the end of the breast with the nipple and areola between her index and middle fingers (Fig 3.6A).

The football hold places the infant's head in the mother's hand while the baby's body and feet extend posteriorly behind the mother (Fig 3.6B). The woman holds the baby with the body facing hers. Positioning this way allows the infant to grasp the nipple and areola in a different position. Using different positions may help avoid nipple soreness for the mother.

Stroking the infant's mouth will induce the rooting reflex. When the infant's mouth is open wide, the woman should place the nipple and areola far into the mouth past the baby's jaws. The infant usually then begins to suck and swallow. The infant uses the jaws to compress and empty the sinuses. He or she uses the tongue to pull the nipple to the back of the palate and suck milk from the nipple. The milk stimulates the infant's swallow reflex. Observe the infant's lower jaw moving up and down with effective sucking and hear audible swallowing sounds. If sucking and swallowing seem ineffective, reposition the infant. To break the infant's suction, simply place a finger into the side of the infant's mouth and move the breast from it. Never just pull an infant off the breast, because doing so will cause nipple soreness. Help the woman reposition the infant and facilitate latching on. A large or engorged breast can block the infant's nose, so the woman should continue to support her breast while the infant is feeding to prevent this.

As with bottle-feeding, the infant will take several sucks and swallows and then pause to breathe. Allow the infant to feed for at least 5 to 7 minutes. After this time, burp the infant. After burping, reposition the infant at the other breast. As the stomach gets larger, infants may feed for up to 10 minutes per side. When they first eat,

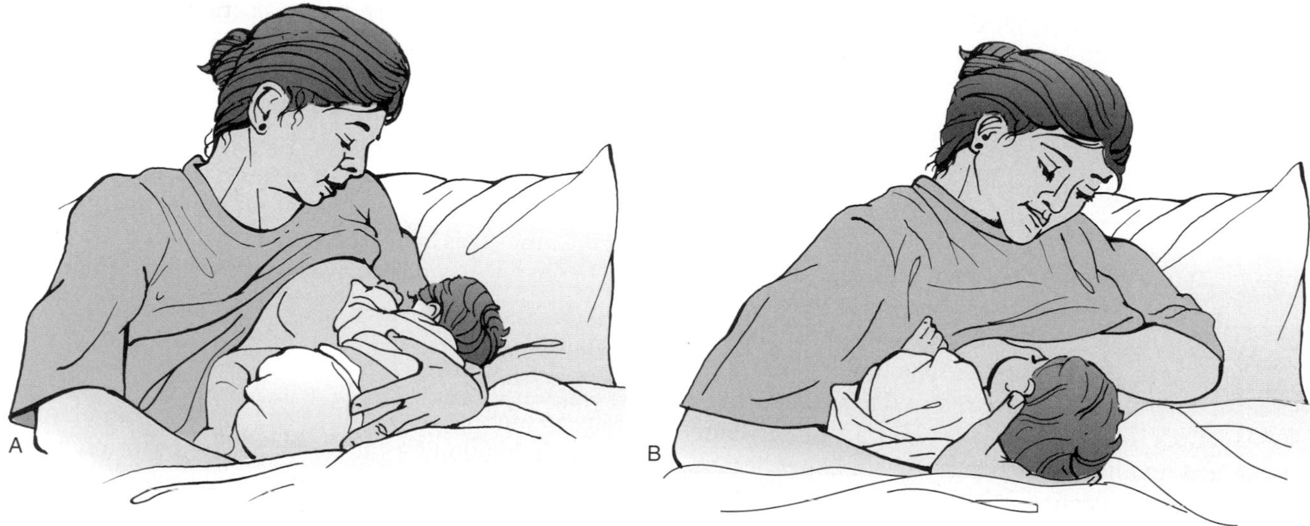

FIGURE 3.6 Two holds for breastfeeding. (**A**) Cradle hold. (**B**) Football hold.

they are hungriest and may suck more eagerly on the first side. After repositioning to the second side, they may suck less intensely and for a shorter period. At the beginning of the feeding, the infant receives **foremilk,** which is relatively low in fat. At the end of the feeding, the infant receives **hindmilk,** which is higher in both fat and calories. For these reasons, it is important to alternate breasts and to offer the opposite breast first at the next feeding. Sometimes women place a safety pin or ribbon on their bra straps to remind them which breast to offer at the next feeding.

Let-Down Reflex. The let-down reflex is a tingling sensation that the woman feels in both breasts when the infant sucks at one breast. With the let-down reflex, milk flows much more freely. The woman may notice milk dripping from her opposite nipple. The infant's suck and swallow pattern may change, because the baby may not have to suck as hard. When a breastfeeding pattern is established, the woman may not need nipple stimulation and may notice the let-down reflex when a normal feeding time approaches or when she hears her infant cry.

Sore Nipples. Nipples can become sore and cracked. The most common cause is improper positioning of the infant that leads the woman to place only the nipple in the child's mouth. This compresses the nipple against the jaws, causing pain. It is important to get much of the areola into the infant's mouth so that the nipple is well beyond the jaws. Treatment of sore nipples includes proper positioning, using different positions, limiting time of feeding on the sore side, and offering the side that is not sore first, when the infant has the most vigorous suck. The woman may rub some breast milk on the nipples after breastfeeding and allow it to air-dry. She also always should let her nipples air-dry after feedings before closing the flap on the nursing bra. Women should wear cotton bras. They may use breast pads but must change these frequently to prevent constant moisture against the skin. Women should not use soap on the nipple because it is drying. They can rub vitamin E oil on the nipples sparingly; however, they need to wash it off before the infant feeds. Tannic acid is thought to help skin heal, so women may place a cooled used tea bag on the sore nipples after feedings.

Mastitis. Mastitis is a bacterial infection of the breast. Symptoms include redness, swelling, tenderness, feeling warm to the touch, and fever. The typical cause is bacteria from the infant's mouth entering the breast through a crack on the nipple. Treatment is with antibiotics; the infant can continue to breastfeed.

Supplemental Feedings. Occasions may arise when breastfeeding is impossible and an infant must receive formula or a supplemental feeding. In such cases, concern on the part of the mother, nurse, or physician often exists about nipple confusion. Breastfeeding and bottle-feeding use different sucking techniques; however, infants are capable of learning both. Breastfeeding is harder for an infant and takes more energy. If offered both bottle-feeding and breastfeeding, the infant may form a preference for one over the other. If there is great concern that bottle-feeding can undermine breastfeeding efforts, then caregivers can provide supplemental feedings using a cup, spoon, or dropper.

NON-NUTRITIVE SUCKING. Infants need to suck as a mechanism for self-calming. With non-nutritive sucking, an infant sucks but does not swallow. Infants will suck their own fingers or fists. Some parents prefer them to suck a pacifier.

POSTPARTUM CARE OF THE WOMAN

The postpartum period is the time following delivery of the placenta until the woman's body and reproductive organs return to her normal pre-pregnant state. That period usually takes up to 6 weeks. The first 6 hours of the postpartum period usually are referred to as the recovery stage or fourth stage of labor (see Chap. 1). Closely monitor the new mother during these first 6 hours because many changes are occurring in her body.

Physical Changes

Uterus

The uterus undergoes extraordinary changes during the postpartum period. Immediately after delivery of the placenta, the uterus flattens out through muscle fiber contraction, which occurs as a response to oxytocin. The muscle contraction helps compress blood vessels and stops bleeding from the uterine wall at the site where the placenta once was. Failure of the muscles to contract can cause excessive bleeding (see Chap. 2).

The uterus decreases dramatically over the first few postpartum weeks. This reduction is part of the normal process called **involution.** Another process called autolysis promotes involution. **Autolysis** is self-digestion or self-destruction of cells and develops from the sudden drop in estrogen and progesterone levels. Autolysis assists the downward growth of the endometrium. The net effect is that the 2-pound (1000-g) uterus at delivery decreases to approximately 1 pound (500 g) at the end of the first postpartum week. At the end of the second week, the uterus weighs approximately 12 ounces (350 g). By the end of the postpartum period, the uterus weighs approximately 1½ to 2 ounces (45–60 g).

Involution can be observed by palpating the height of the uterine fundus. Right after delivery of the placenta, the top of the fundus is palpable halfway between the umbilicus and symphysis pubis. After approximately 12 hours, the top of the fundus can be felt at the level of the umbilicus. It then slowly falls. By 1 week postpartum, it is barely palpable at the level of the symphysis pubis.

The size of the area where the placenta had been attached to the uterus is approximately 3 to 4 inches (8–10 cm) in diameter. A tissue layer remains attached here from the placenta. This tissue layer will be sloughed off along with some mucus and blood. This sloughing, or exfoliation, will leave a healthy layer of endometrial tissue, which is important for subsequent pregnancies. The sloughed material and blood is called **lochia rubra,** as it consists mainly of blood. It usually lasts approximately 3 days. As the uterine wall heals, the bleeding diminishes. The character of the discharge becomes more watery and lightens to pink. This discharge is referred to as **lochia serosa** and may last from 3 to 10 days postpartum. Finally, the discharge becomes thinner and clear and is called **lochia alba.** This final discharge can persist up to 3 weeks. Lochia has a very distinctive scent and should normally never be foul smelling.

Cervix and Vagina

Delivery often causes swelling and small lacerations of the cervix. Involution for the cervix makes it shorter, firmer, and thicker. After delivery the vagina is smooth and swollen and has poor tone and lubrication. By 4 weeks, vaginal rugae return and lubrication increases with the estrogen level.

Perineum

The perineum also may have suffered damage such as swelling, bruising, and lacerations. Lacerations can be classified as first-, second-, third-, or fourth-degree tears. A first-degree tear is the mildest; a fourth-degree tear is the worst and extends into the rectum. An episiotomy may have been made to avoid lacerations. Both an episiotomy and a laceration are sutured and will heal during the early postpartum period.

Menstruation and Ovulation

Breastfeeding affects the return of ovulation and menstrual cycles. The return of normal menstrual cycles happens faster for nonlactating women, usually at approximately 10 weeks postpartum. Any cycles before 6 weeks are typically anovulatory. For lactating women, ovulation may be delayed for 3 to 6 months, depending upon the length of lactation.

Breasts

Changes in the breasts occur throughout pregnancy. Many hormones play a role, but prolactin, released by the anterior pituitary gland, is very important. Prolactin causes breast size to increase by increasing the amount and complexity of the ducts and alveoli. Estrogen and progesterone also stimulate duct size and alveolar growth but to a lesser degree. Both estrogen and progesterone also inhibit secretion of milk. After delivery of the placenta, estrogen and progesterone levels drop dramatically, but prolactin level continues to remain high. Prolactin seems most important to initiate lactation. Continued prolactin is not as important to sustain lactation.

For women who choose not to breastfeed, lactation needs to be suppressed. The easiest way to do so is to avoid stimulation of the breasts. Many women can suppress lactation by wearing a tight bra and not manipulating their nipples or breasts. Bromocriptine (Parlodel), an ergotamine derivative, is a drug that used to be given to all nonlactating women to suppress milk production. Rare cases of seizures were associated with this medication, however, so its use was discontinued.

Cardiovascular System

Bradycardia is common for the first 24 to 48 hours after delivery. Normally, blood pressure remains unchanged. The increased blood volume experienced with pregnancy decreases over the first 1 to 2 weeks postpartum. With the immediate loss of the placenta, however, the blood that would have circulated there normally now rejoins the woman's regular circulation. This along with increased venous return causes a transitory increase in circulating blood volume in the first 48 to 72 hours after delivery. Thus, the hematocrit level can fall, leading to profound diuresis. This increases cardiac output by approximately 35%. With all these changes, the woman is at risk in the early postpartum period for heart failure and thrombus formation and requires close monitoring.

The total pregnant blood volume is 5 to 6 L. A normal vaginal delivery usually has a net loss of 400 mL of blood; 600 to 800 mL can be lost in a cesarean section. Other volume loss is in the form of diuresis and diaphoresis.

Bladder

After delivery the bladder mucosa is swollen and has diminished tone. Bladder distention and urinary retention are common. If the woman empties her bladder regularly, normal bladder tone will return within 1 week.

Gastrointestinal System

Pregnancy slows gastrointestinal motility, which returns to normal within 2 weeks of delivery. Appetite is typically good following delivery. Women are also often thirsty for 2 to 3 days, probably as a result of the intense diuresis and diaphoresis and the effects of fluid restrictions during labor, if there were any. Many women are constipated for the first few days after delivery. Common causes include fluid restrictions, pain, and pain medication, such as codeine. Pain from lacerations or an episiotomy or hemorrhoids may deter the desire to defecate. The use of stool softeners and laxatives are common in the early postpartum period.

Neuromuscular System

Many women find that certain discomforts they experienced during pregnancy leave during the postpartum period. Nerve compression of the arms and legs from edema or fluid retention and pressure of the enlarged uterus usually are relieved early in the postpartum period. The hormone effects of relaxed cartilage, tendons, and other connective tissue are reversed. Over 6 to 8 weeks the pelvis regains its normal stability. With the loss of the large uterus and the weight of the fetus and amniotic fluid, the body's normal center of gravity returns and decreases the strain on the lower back. Women may still complain of back pain, however, because of the new strain of toting an infant, car seat, and diaper bag.

Integumentary System

The darker pigmented areas of the body associated with pregnancy tend to fade over time but usually do not disappear completely. These areas are the hyperpigmented areolas and nipples, linea nigra (the dark line from umbilicus to symphysis pubis), and chloasma (the dark "mask" of pregnancy). Abdominal striae, or stretch marks, tend to fade but usually do not leave completely. Many pregnant women develop varicose veins and small spider veins in the legs. These usually do not disappear; if bothersome, they may require further treatment.

Nursing Care

Nursing care for new mothers aims at monitoring the body for potential problems, such as infection, hemorrhage, or cardiovascular problems. Providing information about physical changes is another important nursing function. Pain management and comfort measures are very important, as is attention to the woman's personal hygiene. Another essential nursing task is teaching the woman to care for her new infant and herself and getting them ready for discharge.

Vital Signs

Vital signs frequently require monitoring for the first few hours after delivery. Hospitals usually have certain protocols. The pulse rate may be normally low for the first week (60 bpm or less). Blood pressure should remain normal. New mothers may experience orthostatic hypotension, which is when the blood pressure drops suddenly in response to a change in positioning (usually from lying or sitting to standing). This may make the woman feel suddenly faint. Respiratory rate should be within the normal range. Temperature may be elevated for the first 24 hours after delivery. It may reach 100.4°F (38°C). If the elevated temperature lasts for more than 24 hours, check the woman for sources of infection. Dehydration also can play a role in elevated temperature. Report abnormalities in the vital signs, which should be stable within 2 hours of delivery. If not, continue to monitor them and notify the physician or midwife as necessary.

Fundus and Lochia Checks

During the first 2 hours after delivery, assessment of uterine tone and bleeding amount is very important. These usually are checked every 15 minutes along with vital signs. Palpate the woman's abdomen to assess the location and tone of the uterine fundus. The uterus should feel firm. If the uterus is not firm, too much bleeding will occur. If the nurse palpates the fundus and it feels spongy or boggy, she needs to massage it until it feels firm again. To massage the fundus, place one hand above the symphysis pubis and the other hand on the lower abdomen. Use the second hand to rub gently in a circular motion around the lower abdomen over the fundus. Take care not to overmassage the uterus, because this can cause complications. This process is usually uncomfortable for the woman and causes cramping. Explain the importance of this massage to the woman. There are also usually a lot of blood clots expelled after massaging the fundus. If the fundus does not contract with massaging, notify the physician or midwife. Sometimes oxytocin (Pitocin) or methylergonovine (Methergine) is given. These are oxytocics and cause contraction of the uterine muscle. These medications also can cause bradycardia, increased blood pressure, nausea, headache, and dizziness. Monitor the woman for these side effects. A full or distended bladder can interfere with uterine tone and promote bleeding. Assess for bladder distention and help the woman empty her bladder frequently as needed.

Check the amount of lochia frequently over the first few hours after delivery. Look at the peri pads and assess the character and amount of lochia present (Fig. 3.7). Heavy bleeding is considered as completely soaking a peri pad within 1 hour. Moderate bleeding is a bloodstain of 6 inches or less on a pad. Light bleeding is an area of 4 inches or less. Scant bleeding is an area of 1 inch or less. Occasionally, blood can trickle from the vagina and pool under the woman's bottom, missing the peri pad altogether. Be aware of and check for this potential. Estimate the amount of blood loss. If excessive, report this finding to the physician or midwife.

Certain factors can put a woman at risk for postpartum bleeding. Women who are multiparous with multiple deliveries are at increased risk for bleeding. A woman who has had much uterine distention from a very large infant, multiple pregnancy, or hydramnios is at increased risk. It has been observed that red-haired women tend to bleed more easily.

Toileting

After considering the woman's status, determine when she is ready to get up to ambulate. This first trip is usually short, such as to the bathroom and back. The woman should sit at the edge of the bed a moment and rise slowly to help prevent orthostatic hypotension. Have an ammonia ampule handy as well as a wheelchair, in case the woman feels faint while in the bathroom. Assist the mother to the bathroom and get her situated. Leave the bathroom to provide some privacy, but remain outside the door and verbally check on the woman every few minutes. If the woman had either an episiotomy or lacerations, she needs to use a spray bottle to rinse her bottom after voiding. Help with this rinsing and changing her peri pads if needed. If a woman cannot void in the bathroom or use a bedpan, she may require straight catheterization to empty the bladder. This is done the same way as for any other type of client, but take care not to contaminate the urinary meatus with lochia after cleaning it.

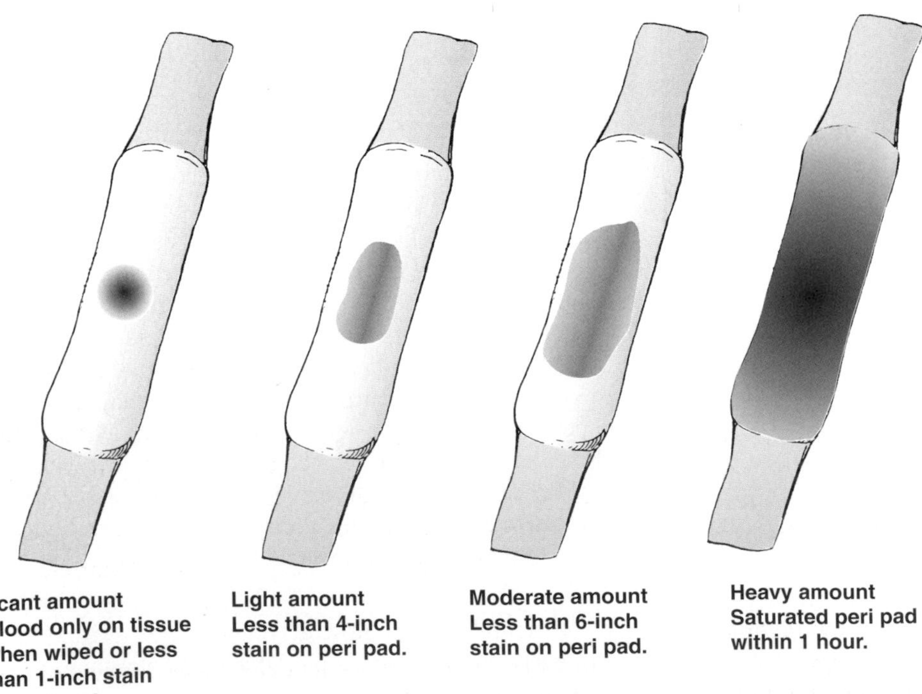

FIGURE 3.7 Variations in lochia.

After the first few hours postpartum, if the mother is stable, the frequency of taking vital signs and fundus and lochia checks can decrease to every few hours, depending upon hospital policy. Any woman who delivered by cesarean section also should be considered a surgical client. Agencies will employ typical postoperative nursing care as well as postpartum care for this woman. Such postoperative care includes deep breathing and early ambulation.

Ambulation

Early ambulation is important for the postpartum woman for the same reasons as it is for all clients after surgery. Ambulation helps decrease the chances of developing thrombophlebitis. It promotes gastric motility, increases circulation, and enhances respirations to help diminish chances of developing pneumonia.

The type of pain medication or anesthesia used during delivery can greatly affect a woman's capability for early ambulation. Epidural blocks commonly are used for both vaginal and cesarean deliveries. Assess the woman for the return of feeling in her feet and legs before she gets up to ambulate. Other oral pain medications can make the woman very drowsy and unsteady on her feet.

Physical Assessment

Nurses should perform a head-to-toe physical assessment every shift. The following need assessment: vital signs, heart and lung sounds, breasts, fundus and lochia, episiotomy or laceration repairs, abdominal incision if a cesarean section was done, bladder and bowel function, and circulation including a check for thrombus formation in the calves by checking for Homans' sign (see Chap. 27). Also assess the new mother's emotional status. A simple pneumonic can help nurses remember the important parts of the postpartum assessment: BUBBLE-HE. It stands for **b**reast, **u**terus, **b**ladder, **b**owel, **l**ochia, **e**pisiotomy, **H**omans' sign, and **e**motional status. Most hospitals have charting forms available for documenting normal findings. Abnormal findings are usually noted in a longer narrative note. If any abnormal findings are identified, notify the physician or midwife.

Pain Management

Include assessment of pain level during the physical examination. Many oral or injectable medications are available for mothers to manage pain. Discuss their use with the mother. Topical ointments or Tucks pads can help decrease perineal pain. Stool softeners and laxatives can make bowel movements easier if there are hemorrhoids, lacerations, or episiotomies.

Nonpharmacologic methods for pain management can be offered. Heat may help engorged breasts. For a nonlactating woman, ice may help the pain from engorgement. An ice pack may ease perineal pain. A sitz bath may help hemorrhoidal or perineal pain. A sitz bath is a special tub designed to allow the woman to sit in warm water and soak her bottom without getting the rest of her body wet. The average sitz bath lasts 20 minutes. Place a nurse call light within the woman's reach while she has a sitz bath. Ambulation can help ease abdominal gas pains. A warm shower can provide some overall relaxation, as can a back rub.

After delivery the uterus continues to contract as part of involution. These contractions cause pain similar to menstrual cramps and are referred to as afterpains. These are more prevalent in women who have had many deliveries or who had great uterine distention. Breastfeeding women also experience afterpains. Infant sucking stimulates release of oxytocin, which causes uterine contractions.

Personal Hygiene

Assist the new mother with her personal hygiene until she can do it for herself. After delivery the mom should receive a sponge bath. This will help remove the sweat from labor and any blood and body fluids that may have gotten on her skin during delivery. By the next day, if she is up and steady on her feet, she may shower on her own. If not, help her with a bed bath. If the woman is not breastfeeding, she may wash her breasts with mild soap and water. If breastfeeding, then she can cleanse the breasts with clear water only. She may need assistance in changing her peri pads for 1 or 2 days. Changes should be fairly frequent to keep the perineum clean. Rinse her buttocks with the squirt bottle after every void to help prevent infection.

Activity

Normally the new mother is allowed to get up as often as she wants as long as she is stable and the nurse has observed her several times. While it is important for the woman to ambulate, it is also important for her to rest. Many new mothers are very excited and try to do too much after delivery. While in the hospital, a woman can and should take advantage of having reliable help to watch her infant while she sleeps. Once she is home she may have a whole family demanding her attention and energy. Facilitate rest by making the room quiet and comfortable. Limit the number of visitors. Minimize causes of stress or worry. Offer to watch and feed the infant for the mother to allow her several hours of uninterrupted sleep.

Proper nutrition is important for recovering moms. If breastfeeding, the woman needs adequate calories, vitamins, and liquids. She should continue to consume about the same caloric amount as when she was pregnant. Women often will continue taking prenatal vitamins into the postpartum period.

Emotional Status

By giving birth, the new mother has just experienced a major life event filled with joy, excitement, anxiety, fear, and fatigue. She also is enduring dramatic changes in hormone levels. As a result, many women experience postpartum blues or postpartum depression. Both of these conditions can begin 2 to 7 days after delivery.

Talk with the new mother and monitor her for depression. One sign may include a lack of interest in anything related to the newborn. The woman may react negatively to the newborn, spouse, or other visitors. She may have problems with her body image. She may cry often. Also, she may have no or few social support systems. If depression is suspected, notify the physician or midwife for appropriate intervention.

Stop, Think, and Respond ● BOX 3-2

A woman has given birth a few hours ago and is resting quietly in her room. She looks slightly sad and worried. You ask her if anything is wrong. She sighs and says she just wonders if her body will ever return to normal. What information can you give the client?

EDUCATING PARENTS

Parenting is a learned behavior, not instinctive. New mothers and fathers are influenced by how they were raised and parented when they were children. They watch friends or relatives and learn vicariously how to parent. Nurses also can influence new parents. They must role model appropriate care and provide instruction about infant behavior.

Nurses can provide parent education in different ways. They may give written materials to parents to read and take home. Many educational videos are available for parents to view; when used, nurses should talk with parents after viewing to answer any questions. Nurses often demonstrate procedures for the mother or father. Another method is to have the parent return demonstrate the same procedure to ensure that he or she can perform it.

Be sure to document any parent education that occurs. This documentation may be as simple as a checklist, or it may involve narrative long notes in the chart. See Client and Family Teaching 3-1.

Promoting Bonding

Bonding refers to the initial attachment process between newborn and parents. It should begin soon after delivery. Current trends are to promote early and extended bonding time.

Be attentive to the environment to allow for quiet and privacy. Assess both the mother's and baby's physical needs; provide any needed care for both. Point out all the right body parts (ten toes, ten fingers). Have the mother hold the infant in the **en face** position (the baby is in the mother's arms, and baby and mother look at each other face-to-face). The distance from the mother's face to the infant is also the distance that a newborn can best focus. Note that when first placed in the eyes, erythromycin eye ointment can interfere with the infant's focusing ability. For this reason, some facilities delay instillation until after the infant and mother have had time to focus on each other. Nurses also may choose to place the infant's naked body against the mother's naked chest for skin-to-skin contact. This provides warmth for the infant and a sense of attachment between mother and child.

Be alert to cues parents give about their needs at this point. For example, a couple experiencing the birth of their first child may need more support and information than a couple with several children. Either way, provide information about the infant when they are ready for it. Give accurate details about the infant's behavior, physical care, and social needs. Parents most often are concerned that everything is "OK" with the baby. Reassure them verbally and explain procedures to them before or as they occur.

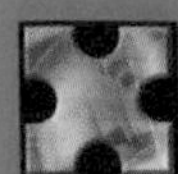

3-1 *Client and Family Teaching* Postpartum Care

The nurse reviews the following topics with the family as follows:

INFANT CARE	
Use of bulb syringe	Bathing
Cord care	Diapering
Circumcision care	Temperature taking
Infant positioning (back to sleep)	Bottle-feeding and formula prep
Infant comfort measures	Breastfeeding
Hepatitis B immunization	Using breast pump
Newborn screen	Home safety measures
Car seat	Appropriate dressing
Infant behavior	Recognize signs of illness

MOTHER'S SELF CARE	
Showering or bathing	Perineal care
Breast support	Sitz baths
Cracked nipples	Medication use
Signs of mastitis	Rest and exercise
Nutrition	Follow-up visit with provider
Recognize signs of illness	

Observe infant–parent interactions and assess for positive attachment. Positive parental signs include cuddling the infant, gently touching and stroking the baby, and softly talking (often in a singsong high-pitched voice). Lack of such signs may indicate a need for intervention.

Instructing in Physical Care

Teach parents how to physically care for the infant. Basics include feeding the infant (bottle, breast, or both), caring for the cord, changing diapers, giving care after circumcision (if applicable), bathing, and appropriately clothing and wrapping the infant for warmth. See earlier discussions of these topics for more information.

Providing Safety

Parent also must learn how to provide a safe environment for their child. Teach parents never to place the infant on the abdomen to sleep at night. They must place the baby on the back to prevent sudden infant death syndrome (SIDS) (see Chap. 8). There are times that infants can be placed on the abdomen, such as when they are continuously monitored by adults. Being on the abdomen is actually good for motor development and should be encouraged, but it needs to be done safely. Other factors include making the crib safe by avoiding lots of stuffed toys and pillows and loose-fitting mattresses to reduce the risk of suffocation. Teach parents not to place a crib by windows with blinds or curtain cords that could cause strangulation. Parents need to avoid toys with small pieces or loose parts that babies could place in the mouth, leading to choking.

As the infant's ability for self-locomotion increases, focus needs to include other areas of the home. Parents should cover electrical outlets and place childproof latches on cupboards. They must store harmful cleaning solutions or chemicals in out-of-reach areas. They need to pick up and put away small items. Placement of the infant also becomes an issue. When infants learn to roll over, parents must be very careful not to place them in an area from which they could roll and hurt themselves.

All infants must have an approved car seat that parents know how to use properly. Many hospitals have policies related to car seat use at discharge. Hospital staff may accompany parents and infant to the car to ensure proper securing of the infant into the car seat. This is then documented in the record.

Explaining Infant Behavior

Over the past 40 years, many studies of newborns have been done. One important finding is that newborns prefer to look at their mothers' faces over those of strangers. When the mother and a stranger each speak into one of the newborn's ears, the newborn will turn the head toward the mother's voice. Newborns prefer to look at moving objects versus still objects. They prefer to gaze upon faces instead of shapes. They see high contrasting colors such as white, black, and red better than soft pastel colors. Human infants are totally dependent on others. They cry to communicate their needs, which include hunger, a wet diaper, pain or discomfort, or boredom. Parents must learn to respond to infant cry patterns.

Newborns spend most of a 24-hour day sleeping; however, they go through different states of arousal. They can progress from deep to light sleep to drowsiness to a quiet alert state. They then may go from an active alert state to a hyperalert state to a crying state. Alert states are quite short in comparison to sleep states. As infants age, alert states lengthen. Holding newborns upright tends to result in a longer period of alertness. Parents should try to interact with newborns in the quiet and active alert states.

Once a newborn is in the hyperalert state, parents should tone down the interaction to avoid overstimulation, the end result of which is crying. Newborns will give early cues of being overstimulated before crying. Teach parents to watch for these cues and respond accordingly. They include averting the gaze, extending the arm and placing the hand between self and the stimulus, turning the head away from the stimulus, or shutting the eyes. Identify these for parents and show them how to decrease the stimulus to allow the infant to regroup and again be in the quiet or active alert state and be ready for stimulation.

Assisting With Emotional Adjustments

Mothers typically go through three phases after delivery. The first phase, "taking in," occurs immediately after delivery. The woman may be very passive and dependent on others for care; she may sleep a lot. She also usually recounts the labor and delivery events to others over and over. She tends to focus on her own needs during this time. The second phase is "taking hold." During this phase, she is very interested in learning everything there is to know about her infant's care. She is also very concerned about her own health and the status of her infant's health. The third phase is "letting go." This phase occurs a little later in the postpartum period. In this phase, she will reestablish relationships with family and friends.

The woman now has a new role to add to her list of mother and primary caregiver to a new baby. Before delivery, she may have worked a full-time job outside the house. With the new role comes many stresses and worries. There may be financial stress related to being away from work and the addition of another person to the family who requires clothes, diapers, and formula. The woman may plan to return to work, but this adds the stress of finding adequate day care, which also costs money. She may experience guilt feelings for not being with her newborn. Other women may choose to stay home, but then there may be only one source of income.

Men also get a new role as dad. Obviously, men do not have the physical contact that women do with the fetus during pregnancy. So for men, the first contact is the initial time that they hold the newborn. At this point, many fathers realize their new role. They may share the same stress and worries that women have related to finances and time away from the infant.

Involve fathers in the care of the infant. Newborns may intimidate some men, who fear that they will hurt the infant. Teach how to properly handle the newborn. Show fathers how to change the diaper and bottle-feed the infant, if bottle-feeding is the method of choice. Learning these skills will aid in infant–father bonding.

Having a baby is a life-altering event. The parents will no longer have the freedoms that they once had. Their lives will become more structured and routine. As a result, couples often put their own intimacy on hold. Women may have no desire for sexual relations for a various reasons from pain and lack of healing time to body image issues to concerns about the baby. Men may be concerned about not hurting their partners; at other times, they may feel resentment or jealousy because the baby is getting all of the woman's attention. It is important for couples to communicate with each other about their feelings and needs during this time.

DISCHARGE PLANNING

In the current climate of shortened hospital stays, discharge planning starts with admission to the hospital. Hospitals usually follow clinical pathways or some other plan of care or protocol to ensure delivery of proper care at the appropriate time during the hospital stay, so that mother and infant are ready for discharge. Following these clinical pathways also ensures that the woman receives all necessary teaching about self and infant care. Before mother and baby leave the hospital, a postdischarge follow-up office appointment is often scheduled for the infant to see the provider within a few days. The mother usually sees her physician or midwife 6 weeks after delivery. If delivery was by cesarean section, an earlier visit is scheduled to remove abdominal staples or sutures and to evaluate her condition. The woman is given a list of instructions of what to look for if something goes wrong with her or the infant. She should receive the name and number of whom to call if she needs help or has questions.

Critical Thinking Exercise

1. *Identify how nurses can help prevent heat loss for newborns in the delivery room, while conducting the physical assessment, and when providing care during the infant's hospital stay.*

● NCLEX-STYLE REVIEW QUESTIONS 

1. A nurse is preparing to administer an aqua Mephyton injection to a newborn. The baby's parents refuse to allow the nurse to "put that shot in his leg." Which explanation for giving the injection is most appropriate?
   1. "This shot causes bacteria to grow in the bowel, which helps digestion."
   2. "Your pediatrician ordered this, and every baby must have a shot."
   3. "The shot doesn't hurt much, and the baby won't remember it."
   4. "The shot helps blood clotting until the baby makes his own vitamin K."
2. Prior to discharge, the nurse instructs a new mother about cord care. Which statement made by the mother indicates a need for further instruction?
   1. "I will apply alcohol to the cord whenever I change her diaper."
   2. "I should tuck the cord inside the diaper when I change her."
   3. "I expect the cord to fall off in about 10 days."
   4. "I'll give my baby a tub bath after the cord falls off."
3. The nurse is providing instructions regarding circumcision care to the mother of a newborn. Which information given by the nurse to the mother is most accurate?
   1. "Lay the infant on his abdomen after the circumcision."
   2. "Closely count wet diapers for the first 2 days after circumcision."
   3. "Clean off the yellow drainage when giving your baby his tub bath."
   4. "Call the pediatrician if the Plastibell falls off in 7 to 10 days."

connection

Visit the Connection site at **http://connection.lww.com/go/timbyEssentials** for links to chapter-related resources on the Internet.

References and Suggested Readings

Deacon, J., & O'Neill, P. (Eds.) (1999). *Core curriculum for neonatal intensive care nursing* (2nd ed.). Philadelphia: W. B. Saunders Company.

Gunn, V., & Nechyba, C. (2002). *The Harriet Lane handbook* (16th ed.). St. Louis: Mosby.

chapter 4

Caring for the High-Risk Newborn and Family

Words to Know

ambiguous genitalia
anencephaly
apnea
average for gestational age
Bell's palsy
choanal atresia
congenital dislocated hip
diaphragmatic hernia
duodenal atresia
encephalocele
Erb's palsy
erythroblastosis fetalis
esophageal atresia
exstrophy of the bladder
galactosemia
gastroschisis
Hirschsprung's disease
hydrocephaly
imperforate anus
kernicterous
Klinefelter's syndrome
large for gestational age
low birth weight
L/S ratio
macrosomic
meconium aspiration syndrome
meconium ileus
meningocele
microcephaly
myelomeningocele
necrotizing enterocolitis
opisthotonic posturing
phenylketonuria
phototherapy
physiologic jaundice
postterm
preterm
respiratory distress syndrome
retinopathy of prematurity
RhoGAM
small for gestational age
syndactyly
term
TORCH screen
toxoplasmosis
tracheoesophageal fistula
trisomy 13
trisomy 18
Turner's syndrome
very low birth weight

Learning Objectives

On completion of this chapter, the reader will:

- Identify maternal factors that place infants at risk.
- Explain differences in small for gestational age, large for gestational age, preterm, and postterm infants.
- Identify nursing care for premature infants.
- Explain the difference between physiologic and pathologic jaundice.
- Describe at least 10 different congenital anomalies and their treatments.
- Identify chromosomal anomalies and the typical outcome of each.
- Identify the different infectious diseases tested with the TORCH screen.
- Explain how group B beta streptococci are involved in neonatal sepsis.
- Explain typical behaviors for infants exposed to heroin and cocaine during pregnancy.
- Identify how nurses can help parents of infants with congenital anomalies.

Newborns can be at risk for problems with various causes. Risks can be related to maternal factors. A woman who smokes, drinks alcohol, or uses illegal drugs during pregnancy places her fetus at risk for physical anomalies, low birth weight, premature delivery, asphyxia, and even death. If a woman contracts infections during pregnancy, the fetus or newborn also can contract them and be at risk for associated problems. Nonmaternal factors also can pose problems. A woman can have a perfectly normal pregnancy, and yet the infant can be at risk related to size, gestational age, or congenital anomalies.

This chapter examines infant risk and subsequent potential problems. It discusses some nursing care that infants with problems require. The infant's condition and need for special care will affect the mother and other family members. Thus, this chapter also explores the family unit and discusses how nurses can help families cope with such problems.

NEWBORN CLASSIFICATIONS

At birth infants are classified by size as **small for gestational age** (SGA), **average for gestational age** (AGA), or **large for gestational age** (LGA). The birth weight of an SGA infant is below the 10th percentile for gestational age. The birth weight of an AGA infant is in the 11th to 90th percentile. The birth weight of an LGA infant is greater than the 90th percentile. The infant's size is determined after assessment of gestational age using a Dubowitz or Ballard form (see Chap. 3). The healthcare provider uses a graph to plot the infant's size according to length, head circumference, and weight (Fig. 4.1). Two other classifications related to size are **low birth weight** (LBW), defined as birth weight less than 5½ pounds (2500 g), and **very low birth weight** (VLBW), defined as birth weight between 1 to 3½ pounds (500–1499 g).

Infants also can be classified according to gestational age. **Term** infants are born between 38 to 41 weeks. **Preterm** is the classification used for infants born at less than 37 weeks' gestation. **Postterm** is the classification for infants born after 41 weeks.

Infants may have risks related to size, age, or both. Most LBW infants also are preterm. An SGA infant, however, may be postterm. An LGA infant may be term. Both types of infants may have unique risks and problems.

The following section discusses some risk factors for SGA, LGA, postterm, and preterm infants. It examines problems that are fairly common for each group. Some problems are common for several of these groups of infants. For example, hypothermia is common in SGA, preterm, and postterm babies. Many problems discussed for preterm infants apply to the other groups as well and require similar care.

Small-for-Gestational-Age Infants

Factors that contribute to decreased oxygen supply to the placenta or impaired nutrition can result in an SGA infant. Examples include maternal smoking, poor nutrition, alcohol use, illegal drug use, pregnancy-induced hypertension (PIH), maternal infection, multiple gestation (such as twins), congenital anomalies, and placental abnormalities (see Chap. 2).

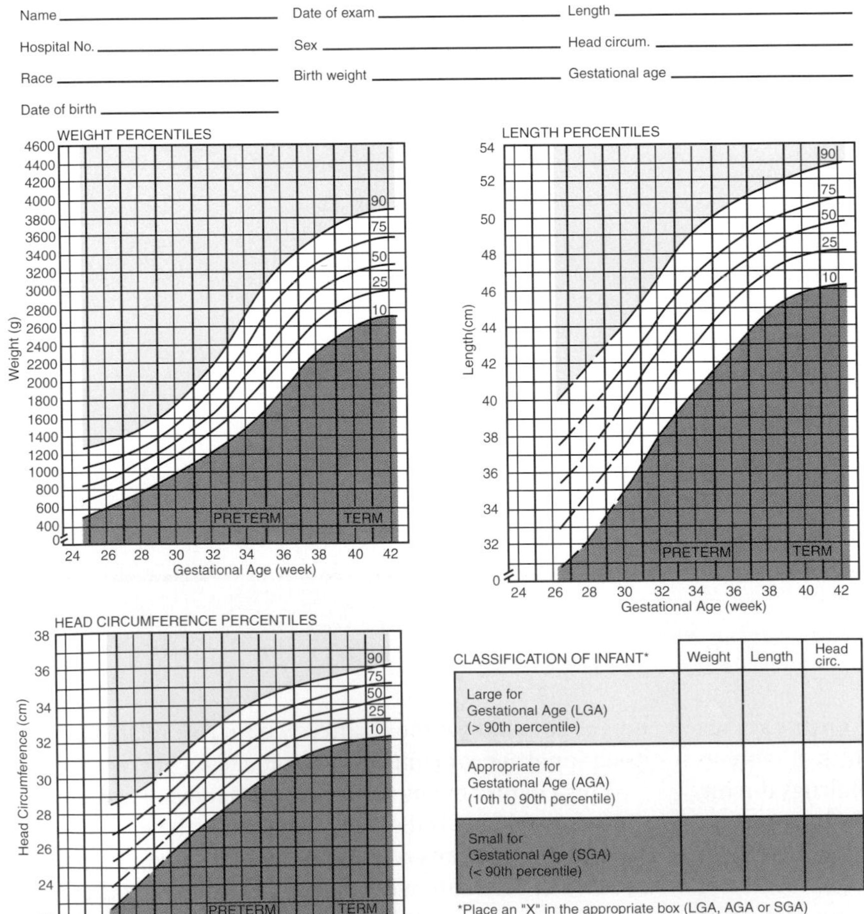

FIGURE 4.1 Chart for classification of newborns by intrauterine growth and gestational age.

Because of their small size and few reserves, SGA infants are at risk for hypothermia, hypoglycemia, and respiratory problems such as apnea, respiratory distress, and sudden infant death syndrome (SIDS). Monitor them closely for any signs of these problems; take corrective measures quickly. A postterm infant may be SGA. If the placenta is breaking down because of advanced fetal age, he or she may not be getting enough nutrients and oxygen and can actually start to lose weight. This infant is at risk for meconium aspiration (see Chap. 3).

Large-for-Gestational-Age Infants

Infants who are LGA also are called **macrosomic.** They commonly are born to women with diabetes. The woman with diabetes transfers her blood glucose level to the fetus via the placenta, causing the infant to grow quite large. In response, the infant increases insulin production to maintain a normal blood glucose level. At birth, this high source of glucose is cut off, but excessive insulin remains in the baby. As a result, the infant's blood glucose level can drop too low, causing hypoglycemia. Careful monitoring and prompt treatment are necessary to prevent further complications.

Because of their size in relation to the normal birthing process, LGA infants are at risk for physical trauma. The baby's size may contribute to dystocia (difficult labor) (see Chap. 2). Skull fractures and related brain injuries are possible. Fractured clavicles are fairly common because these infants simply are too large to be delivered normally. When the infant's head has been delivered and the shoulder is stuck, it is referred to as *shoulder dystocia.* The obstetrician or midwife sometimes deliberately breaks the clavicle to deliver the infant.

Brachial nerve palsy can result from irritation or damage to the brachial plexus during the birthing process. The most common palsy is **Erb's palsy,** which affects the C-5 through C-7 nerve roots, causing problems with the shoulder, upper arm, and biceps reflex. The infant does not move the upper arm; however, palmar grasp is normal. Treatment for Erb's palsy includes immobilization for the first 7 to 10 days, followed by passive range-of-motion exercises. Most cases of Erb's palsy recover fully by 1 year. **Bell's palsy** affects cranial nerve VII (the facial nerve), leading to paralysis on one side of the face. One corner of the mouth does not move with crying, and the eye of the same side does not blink. Bell's palsy can result from forceps delivery. In most cases, the palsy is temporary and resolves spontaneously. Nursing care may include instilling saline eye drops into the affected eye to provide lubrication. Also, be aware of potential feeding problems with a weak suck resulting from the mouth paralysis.

The LGA infant is at risk for respiratory problems. If the labor was long and delivery difficult, the infant may have endured some hypoxia. In such a case, the rectal sphincter relaxes and meconium can pass. The infant can then aspirate meconium while in utero or during delivery. If meconium is found in the amniotic fluid at or before delivery, someone skilled at viewing the vocal cords and suctioning them must attend the delivery. This condition is called **meconium aspiration syndrome** (MAS) and is best treated by prevention. Infants with MAS usually receive care in a special nursery or neonatal intensive care unit (NICU). They often need oxygen and sometimes mechanical ventilation.

Postterm Infants

Postterm infants are at risk for respiratory problems. As gestation progresses, the placenta ages, breaks down, and fails to provide sufficient oxygen and nutrients to the infant. Thus, the postterm infant can be SGA and have respiratory distress at birth. He or she also is at risk for MAS. Postterm infants tend to have wrinkled, cracked, or peeling skin and can have an "old person" appearance. Usually, the skin has little to no vernix or lanugo.

Stop, Think, and Respond ● BOX 4-1

A client is at 43 weeks' gestation and preparations are being made to induce labor. She does not understand why it is important to deliver the fetus, stating "Isn't it better for my child to be born when ready? Maybe he needs a little extra time!" What information would you give this client to help her understand the risks that postterm infants can face?

Preterm Infants

Preterm infants are at risk for many problems, depending on how many weeks premature they are. Prematurity can result from several maternal factors: poor nutrition, smoking, illegal drug use, alcohol use, infections, trauma, uterine anomalies, incompetent cervix, poor maternal health, age younger than 19 years or older than 35 years, lack of prenatal care, and poor socioeconomic status.

Medical and nursing care of premature infants has greatly improved over the last 2 decades. With the development of new medications, infants can survive at much younger ages. Many providers now consider the age of fetal viability to be 23 to 25 weeks' gestation. Nevertheless, many premature infants who survive have long-term health problems as a result of their immaturity and size. The following section discusses these problems and some medical treatments and nursing care required for them.

Hypothermia

Premature infants have very few glucose reserves, little subcutaneous fat, and a large surface area to body weight ratio. As a result, they are at increased risk for hypothermia. They also have very little brown fat available, which helps older newborns create body heat (see Chap. 3). A cold-stressed infant can become hypoglycemic, lose weight, and develop respiratory distress. Thus, these newborns need much assistance to preserve body heat. They must be warmly bundled in many layers of blankets. They must wear hats (Fig. 4.2). If these measures are not enough to help maintain normal body temperature, then infants usually are placed in an isolette (incubator). This plexiglas-enclosed bed is heated to maintain a neutral environment. It contains portholes so nurses can reach in to provide care. It also has a door that can be opened to gain access to the infant.

Hypoglycemia

Premature infants are at risk for low blood glucose level related to a lack of reserves. Their digestive tract is immature and may not be able to absorb nutrients. Some premature infants have immature nervous systems, causing their suck and swallow coordination to remain undeveloped. Premature infants can experience respiratory distress, with a respiratory rate greater than 60 breaths per minute. Infants with respiratory distress should not attempt bottle-feeding because of the potential for aspiration. Many premature infants can neither bottle-feed nor breastfeed and are instead given gavage feedings or tube feedings. If an infant is having trouble regulating blood glucose level with feedings, an intravenous line may be started to provide a stable intake of glucose. Monitor the infant closely and check the blood glucose level every few hours. Many hospitals have a flow chart or an algorithm that delineates which interventions are appropriate for the different blood glucose readings.

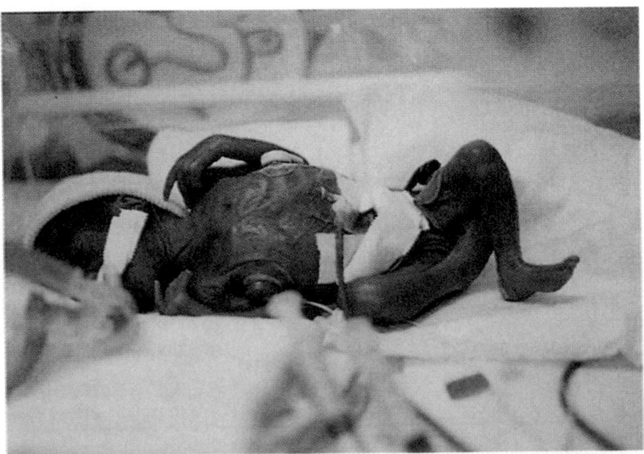

FIGURE 4.2 A hat is placed on the preterm newborn's head to help the baby conserve heat.

Problems With Intake and Output

Most premature infants require close monitoring of their fluid intake and output. Intake can consist of oral or gavage feedings and IV fluids. Output consists of urine and stool. Usually nurses remove diapers and weigh them on a scale. Subtract the weight of the diaper from the total weight. Of the weight left, 1 g in weight is equal to approximately 1 mL of output. Occasionally, nurses also monitor the amount of blood removed from various blood draws, as this figure contributes to output and can cause hemoglobin to fall. Insensible water loss occurs, especially if the infant has any respiratory distress and the respiratory rate is increased.

Electrolyte balance is very important and must be monitored and corrected with the use of IV fluids. Nurses usually are responsible for starting, maintaining, and monitoring IV lines.

Respiratory Distress

Premature infants can be born with very immature lungs and often develop **respiratory distress syndrome** (RDS). Prenatally, one of the best indicators of fetal lung maturation is the ratio of lecithin to sphingomyelin, also called the **L/S ratio.** The fluid made in the lungs contains lecithin, which can be first detected at 22 weeks' gestation. This fluid passes from the mouth into the amniotic fluid. The greater the amount of lecithin in the amniotic fluid, the more mature the lungs are. The L/S ratio should be 2:1 or greater to demonstrate maturity. Some factors that affect this ratio and hasten fetal lung maturation are premature or prolonged rupture of membranes (more that 48 hours), fetal hypoxia from placental insufficiency or an abruptio placentae, maternal toxemia, maternal heroin use, and prenatal administration of glucocorticoids (betamethasone). From 24 to 40 weeks' gestation, the lungs continue to develop with new alveoli and alveolar ducts. At 34 to 36 weeks' gestation, surfactant dramatically increases. Remember from Chapter 3 that surfactant decreases the amount of pressure the alveoli need to stay open for breathing. Most infants born before 34 weeks have some form of RDS. Some need support for breathing with an oxygen hood; others need mechanical ventilation.

OXYGEN USE. Infants who require oxygen, whether delivered by hood or ventilator, need close monitoring. A chest x-ray usually is done shortly after delivery to assess lung status. A pulse oximeter is a noninvasive monitoring device that uses a light passing through the skin on a finger or toe to read the oxygen saturation in the blood. Arterial or venous blood gasses also are used frequently to monitor treatment and to make changes. If blood gasses need to be checked frequently, an arterial line usually is placed. Good sites for newborns are the umbilical vein and artery. A physician or neonatal nurse practitioner (NNP) places these central lines. Monitor the lines for patency and give IV fluids. Nurses usually are responsible for blood draws from the lines. A radial artery line also can be used, usually if the umbilical venous catheter (UVC) or umbilical arterial catheter (UAC) site is not available. Other monitoring includes taking hourly vital signs consisting of heart rate, respiratory rate, temperature, and oxygen saturation (usually read off the monitor); checking glucose levels every few hours; measuring intake and output; checking daily weights; and looking for signs of respiratory distress such as grunting, nasal flaring, retractions, and cyanosis.

Oxygen delivered by hood needs to be warmed and humidified. Monitor the infant's temperature and check for condensation inside the hood (Fig. 4.3). A wet or damp infant can be cold stressed. Oxygen warmed too much through humidification can cause the infant to become overheated. Elevate the head of the infant's bed. If there was any aspiration of fluid in the lungs, the infant may require chest percussion every few hours.

Room air is 21% oxygen. Some infants who require help with breathing can maintain normal oxygen saturation (95%–100%) with oxygen delivered into a hood at 30% to 40%. If the oxygen requirements increase above 40% to 50%, the infant usually is intubated and put on a ventilator. The ventilator "breathes" for the infant and provides oxygen at levels greater than room air. It also provides positive airway pressure to help keep the alveoli open between breaths (see Chap. 23).

As discussed earlier, surfactant is the substance in the lungs that helps keep the alveoli open. With surfactant, the infant needs less air pressure to keep the alveoli open and breathing is easier. Without surfactant, the infant needs a much higher air pressure to keep the alveoli open; this higher pressure increases the risk of pneumothorax. With preterm infants, surfactant often is not yet present or is not enough to be effective. Newer medications called Exosurf and Survanta serve as artificial surfactants. These are given to infants through an endotracheal tube. Since the advent of these medications, the typical duration of mechanical ventilation is much shorter and the amount of pressure required to keep the airway open has decreased greatly. In addition, infants can survive at much younger gestational ages.

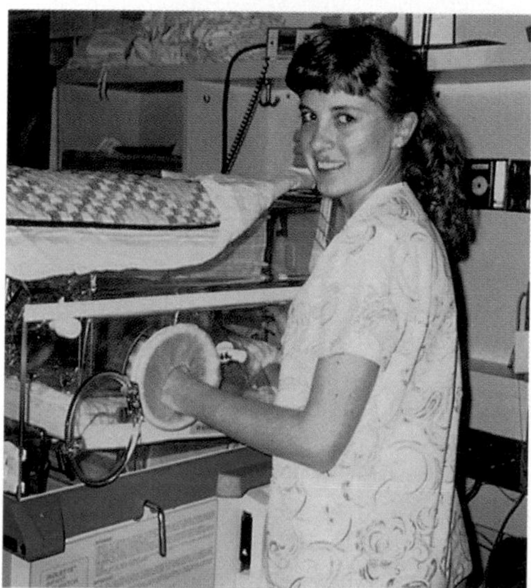

FIGURE 4.3 The nurse checks for condensation inside the oxygen hood for a newborn.

An infant who is intubated and on mechanical ventilation will need the same monitoring and care mentioned for an infant receiving hood oxygen. Endotracheal tube patency is of utmost importance. Thus, monitoring for tube patency and suctioning the endotracheal tube are very important nursing responsibilities.

APNEA. **Apnea** is defined as an absence of breathing for at least 20 seconds. It is common in preterm infants. It is not clear why, but the cause is thought to be related to an immature nervous system. Apnea is most frequent when the infant is sleeping, especially in the REM cycle. Premature infants are monitored for heart and respiratory rates. Usually when the respirations stop, the heart rate falls. The monitors are set to alarm to alert about this problem. Stimulate the infant—usually all he or she will need are a few pats on the bottom. If apnea is frequent, the physician may order a stimulant medication such as theophylline or caffeine. Monitor blood levels of these medications periodically. Infants receiving these medications can get very irritable. Decrease environmental stimulation by minimizing noise and dimming the lights in the nursery.

NECROTIZING ENTEROCOLITIS. Any infant who endures hypoxia can suffer intestinal damage. If hypoxia occurs, blood-carrying oxygen is shunted away from the gastrointestinal tract to the more important organs of the heart, brain, and lungs. This lack of intestinal oxygen can result in **necrotizing enterocolitis** (NEC). NEC develops when part of the bowel necroses or dies, which happens more commonly in preterm infants. Nurses must monitor vigilantly for any signs of NEC, including abdominal distention with or without bowel loops visible under the skin, irritability, temperature instability, jaundice, increased gastric residuals noted with gavage tube feedings, vomiting, and blood in the stools. Care of NEC includes NPO status with nutrients given through IV fluids or total parenteral nutrition (TPN). Often a nasogastric or orogastric tube is placed to decompress the bowel with intermittent suction. The gut is then allowed to rest. Sometimes surgery is required to remove the dead part of the gut. Ostomy care is required until a resection can be done. Infection can play a role in NEC; antibiotics are an important part of treatment.

Retinopathy of Prematurity

High concentrations of oxygen can lead to **retinopathy of prematurity** (ROP) in which retinal blood flow is hampered, resulting in damage to the retina. The ability to monitor how much oxygen an infant is receiving with the use of the pulse oximeter has greatly reduced incidence of ROP. In the past there was no treatment for ROP. Currently, use of cryotherapy to correct the damage of ROP has been successful.

Parental Involvement

Having a premature infant can be very frightening for parents. These babies are most often cared for in NICUs, with many monitors, wires, IV lines, tubes, and all their accompanying noises. The sights and sounds of the NICU can be very intimidating and overwhelming. It is important that nurses take time to talk with and prepare parents before they enter the NICU. Most NICUs have scrubbing and gowning policies. Show the parents how to do this properly. Once the parents are in the nursery, show them their infant. Explain the purpose of all tubes and monitors being used. Give information about the infant's condition and answer questions. Most parents do not remember much of what is said in this first visit, so expect to repeat information during subsequent visits.

Parents with premature infants incur many stressors. Physical separation and being unable to hold or console the infant can be very difficult. Mothers going home empty-handed after their postpartum stay may feel sad, cheated, angry, and worried. Other stressors can include labor and delivery issues, concerns about the infant's health, the NICU environment, communications with doctors and nurses, and job and home issues. Be aware of such issues and consider them when working with parents. Be supportive of parental needs.

Premature infants are often in the NICU for a long time. NICU nurses usually have a good opportunity to bond with parents and become trusted educators and mentors to them in the care of their infant. Encourage parents to visit often and to call for progress reports if they cannot. As the infant becomes more stable, encourage the parents to participate in care as much as possible. Gentle human touch of the infant can be a positive stimulus. Teach parents how to gently touch their infant to assist the bonding process. "Kangaroo care" involves a parent holding the infant with skin-to-skin contact. The parent usually holds the naked infant against his or her naked chest and covers the baby with blankets. Kangaroo care aids in the bonding process for both parent and infant. Kangaroo care is appropriate if the infant is stable. Over time, teach parents how to help with gavage and bottle-feedings. Encourage mothers to pump and store breast milk if they are able and so desire. Parents can change diapers. When the infant is stable, they can bring clothing from home and dress their infant. They can bring appropriate toys. Musical toys provide auditory stimulation; other toys can provide visual stimulation. Parents can bring books to read to their infant while holding and rocking him or her.

HYPERBILIRUBINEMIA

Hyperbilirubinemia can affect any infant, whether he or she is preterm, term, or postterm. Jaundice is the yellowing of the skin observed when an infant has an elevated bilirubin level.

Causes

Physiologic Jaundice

The infant's body breaks down red blood cells into a by-product called *bilirubin.* Bilirubin is in the blood and flows into the liver to be conjugated. Liver function can be immature, causing bilirubin to accumulate. **Physiologic jaundice** is defined as a rise in the unconjugated or indirect bilirubin level during the first week of life. Bilirubin level tends to peak at 6 to 8 mg/dL by the third or fourth day of life for term infants. In preterm infants, liver function is more immature and bilirubin level can peak at 10 to 12 mg/dL, usually by the fifth day of life. Jaundice can be more pronounced in premature infants. Approximately 40% to 60% of term infants develop jaundice; this percentage is even higher in preterm infants, because of their more immature liver function. If jaundice occurs in the first 24 hours of life, the conjugated or direct bilirubin level is greater than 1.5 to 2 mg/dL, or if jaundice persists for more than 1 week for a term infant (or more than 2 weeks for a preterm infant), then it is no longer considered normal physiologic jaundice.

Pathologic Jaundice

Nonphysiologic jaundice can result from several different causes. If ecchymosis is excessive from delivery or a cephalhematoma, then there are more red blood cells for the infant to break down, causing jaundice. A deficiency in an enzyme called glucose-6-phosphate dehydrogenase (G6PD) causes hemolytic anemia, which involves red blood cell breakdown and jaundice. Two other causes of jaundice are an Rh or an ABO incompatibility.

Rh INCOMPATIBILITY. Rh is an inherited trait, with Rh positive being dominant over Rh negative. An Rh incompatibility occurs when the biological mother is Rh negative, or lacks antigens, and the biological father is Rh positive and has antigens. During this couple's first pregnancy, assuming the fetus is Rh positive, the woman is sensitized or exposed to the antigens through the placenta, where some fetal cells can enter her circulation and some maternal cells can enter the fetal circulation. The woman's body recognizes the antigens as foreign and thus begins to make antibodies. This process takes time, and usually no harm is done to this first fetus. The problem may occur with the next pregnancy. Again assuming that the fetus is Rh positive during the second pregnancy, the mother receives some fetal cells and some of her cells enter the fetus. Her cells now contain antibodies and these antibodies immediately start to attack and destroy the fetal red blood cells. This destruction results in a fetal anemia that can kill the fetus. This is referred to as **erythroblastosis fetalis** (formerly, hydrops fetalis). It is possible for erythroblastosis fetalis to happen with the first fetus if the woman was sensitized earlier (e.g., a prior miscarriage or abortion).

Erythroblastosis fetalis is quite rare since the use of anti-D gamma globulin (**RhoGAM**), which is given to all Rh-negative women at 28 weeks' gestation or after any invasive procedures that could cause mixing of maternal and fetal blood (e.g., amniocentesis, abortion). RhoGAM clears fetal cells and also may depress the woman's immune system. Rh incompatibility can still be seen with women who do not receive prenatal care.

ABO INCOMPATIBILITY. ABO incompatibility can occur when the mother is blood type O and the infant is A, B, or AB; or if the mother is A and the infant is B or AB; or if the mother is B and the infant is A or AB. This incompatibility acts similarly to that of Rh. The A and B antibodies that the mother's body makes are large and do not readily cross the placental barrier. An ABO incompatibility is always milder, usually causing jaundice and an enlarged spleen. ABO incompatibilities cannot be prevented.

Treatment

Treatment for an infant with jaundice and hyperbilirubinemia includes the use of **phototherapy,** or light therapy. Phototherapy was discovered after researchers observed that infants exposed to sunlight when their cribs were positioned by windows were less jaundiced than those who were not. Phototherapy has been used widely since the late 1950s. It consists of a bank of four to eight cool white or special blue fluorescent lights or a single quartz halogen lamp. The lights shine through the top of an isolette onto the skin of a naked infant. Through the use of the lights, bilirubin is made more water soluble and can be excreted in bile and urine. The infant usually wears a diaper, or if the diaper covers a significant area of skin, the diaper may be laid out flat and the infant lies atop. The infant's eyes need to be covered to prevent any possible damage from the light. Bili masks are available that use Velcro sticky patches applied to the infant's temples. The outer Velcro side of the patches holds the mask that is shaped to cover the infant's eyes without obstructing the nares. The infant remains under the light as much as possible. At feeding times, the light is turned off and the mask can be removed. This is a good time for bonding with parents and for infant en face interaction. A newer form of phototherapy uses a photoblanket wrapped around the infant. This allows for the light therapy to continue during feedings or holding.

After initiating phototherapy, monitor blood levels of bilirubin frequently, every 4 to 12 hours. The degree of jaundice decreases when the phototherapy is started, so the degree of jaundice is no longer a valid indicator. During phototherapy, the infant's insensible water loss increases, as does the water content of the stool, so fluid balance becomes important. Monitor intake and output, and check the specific gravity of the urine frequently. Carefully monitor the infant's temperature, because the phototherapy light can artificially heat the isolette or interfere with heat sensors. Infants with a high bilirubin level are often fussy and hard to console. This may be because of not feeling well, not being bundled or cuddled, not having unobstructed vision, and a lack of parental contact. Try to address these needs for the infant as best as possible. Musical toys may calm these infants. Rolling up a blanket and wrapping it around the outer side of the infant can provide boundaries and reassurance to help calm him or her. Offer a pacifier. The reassuring touch of a hand on the infant's back or bottom can help. Encourage the parents to come for feeding times as much as possible.

Untreated hyperbilirubinemia can lead to **kernicterus,** a toxic high level of bilirubin that accumulates in the central nervous system. Kernicterus can cause nerve damage, brain damage, and even death. Signs are a poor Moro reflex, poor suck and feeding ability, vomiting, a high-pitched cry, hypotonia, and **opisthotonic posturing.** Opisthotonic posturing is when the infant lies with the back arched so that the head points back to the toes. There is no specific bilirubin level at which kernicterus occurs. Most providers agree that if the bilirubin level is kept below 20 mg/dL, kernicterus is unlikely. Many providers initiate phototherapy when the bilirubin level reaches 10 to 15 mg/dL.

Use of phototherapy has greatly decreased the incidence of kernicterus. Before phototherapy was widely used, bilirubin levels increased dramatically and the treatment was an *exchange transfusion,* which involved repeatedly removing small amounts of the infant's blood and infusing new antibody-free blood. Exchange transfusions are rare but still used if the bilirubin level becomes quite high.

CONGENITAL ANOMALIES

Congenital anomalies are abnormalities present at birth. A possible cause is a *teratogen,* which is any substance that causes birth defects. Examples of teratogens include certain medications, alcohol, smoking, and illegal drug use. Congenital anomalies may have no apparent cause.

The next section identifies several congenital anomalies affecting many different body systems.

Neural Tube Defects and Anomalies of the Head

Before the 26th day of fetal development, failure of the neural tube to close properly results in an opening on the posterior side of the tube. Common neural tube defects are anencephaly, encephalocele, and myelomeningocele:

- **Anencephaly** is a lack of normal brain tissue above the brain stem. It can result in fetal demise or death of the infant shortly after birth.
- **Encephalocele** occurs when the neural tube does not close at the head end. Part of the meninges or brain tissue is visible outside the skull.
- **Myelomeningocele,** also known as *spina bifida,* is caused by the neural tube failing to close at the tail end (Fig. 4.4). The infant is born with an opening at the lower lumbar region. A sac comprised of the meninges is filled with cerebrospinal fluid, and part of the spinal cord can protrude (see Chap. 8). If only the sac filled with cerebrospinal fluid and none of the spinal cord is present, then it is called **meningocele.** Alternatively, it can be an occult case. In an occult case, a small dimple with an open sinus track is noted. Often a small tuft of hair is present on the skin overlying the dimple in the lumbar area. If the defect is small, surgical repair can be done. However, many infants have complications and death is possible. In the case of an infant with a membrane-enclosed sac, positioning is very important so as not to damage any contents within. Keep a moist covering over the sac to prevent it from drying out.

Hydrocephaly is a head abnormality that results from an overaccumulation of fluid in the ventricles of the brain. This extra fluid causes the skull bones to separate and the head to enlarge abnormally. Cesarean delivery of infants with hydrocephaly is common. On physical examination, along with enlarged head circumference, they have eyes set low in the sockets, referred to as "sunset" eyes. They often have a high-pitched cry. Take care to position these infants to avoid trauma to the head and neck and to ensure a patent airway. Treatment involves surgically placing shunts to drain fluid from the head into the abdominal cavity. Infants may have other anomalies and can have mental retardation.

Microcephaly is an abnormally small head. This often results from maternal viral infections, exposure to x-rays, or chromosomal anomalies. Brain matter is decreased, and mental retardation is common. There is no treatment.

Respiratory Anomalies

In **choanal atresia,** the posterior nasal passages are blocked. The blockage can consist of soft tissue or bone and can be unilateral or bilateral. Infants are obligate nose breathers, so infants with choanal atresia display respiratory distress at rest or with feedings. Infants breathe through their mouths when crying; thus, stimulating an infant with choanal atresia to cry can be very helpful. Insertion of an oral airway can maintain respirations until the atresia can be corrected. Diagnosis can be made by failure to pass a catheter through the nares to the pharynx. Treatment involves surgical repair.

Diaphragmatic hernia is another respiratory problem more common on the left side. During fetal development, the gut can pass through the diaphragm into the chest cavity, which subsequently interferes with lung development on the affected side. Depending on the degree of intestinal involvement, little lung tissue may be available at birth. After birth the infant usually has respiratory distress within the first few hours. On assessment, breath sounds on the affected side are diminished or nonexistent. Bowel sounds can be auscultated over the chest on the

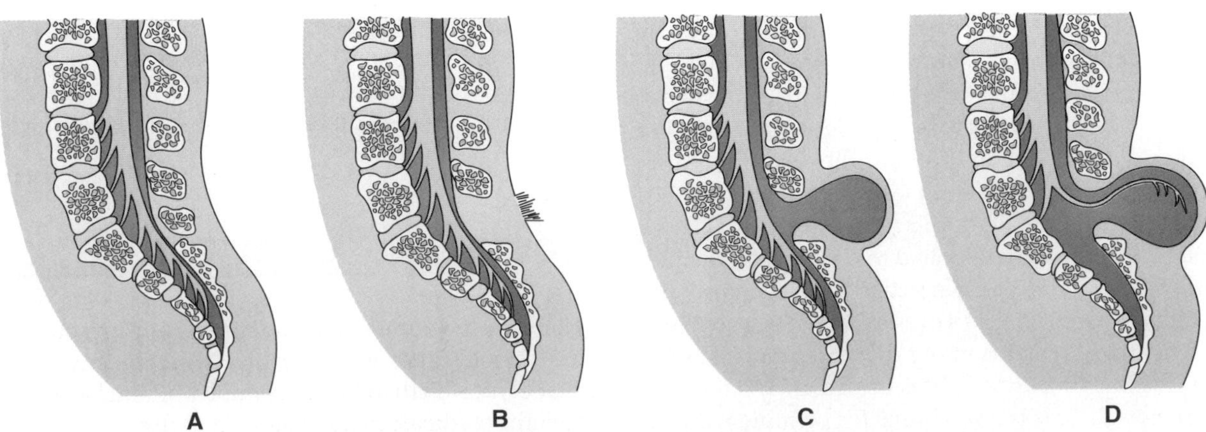

FIGURE 4.4 Variations in spinal cord anomalies. (**A**) Normal. (**B**) Spina bifida occulta. (**C**) Meningocele. (**D**) Myelomeningocele.

affected side, and there is usually a scaphoid abdomen. Diagnosis is made by x-ray. Gas and bowel patterns are seen in the chest cavity. The infant is usually intubated, placed on mechanical ventilation, and left NPO. Surgical treatment is required, but the infant may still not survive if little lung tissue is left. Infants with diaphragmatic hernia also tend to have persistent fetal circulation with the cardiac anomalies of a patent foramen ovale and ductus arteriosus.

Gastrointestinal Anomalies

Cleft lip and cleft palate are fairly common anomalies in which a split occurs in the lip or palate tissue. This condition is discussed in detail in Chapter 9.

Various anomalies affect the esophagus and trachea. **Esophageal atresia,** the most common, occurs when the esophagus simply ends in a blind pouch. The anomaly usually is located closely below the separation of the trachea and esophagus. When the infant is fed, formula/breast milk quickly fills the pouch and spills into the trachea, causing aspiration. The infant can have trouble with his or her own secretions and saliva. There tends to be much drooling, coughing, gagging, and respiratory distress during feedings. Esophageal atresia requires surgical correction.

Esophageal atresia has three other variations. In the first, the esophagus has an upper blind pouch; a distal piece of the esophagus comes up from the stomach and ends in another blind pouch. The second variation consists of one continuous esophagus that is extremely narrow in the middle. In the last variation, referred to as **tracheoesophageal fistula,** a communicating piece connects the esophagus and trachea, making the two tubes looks like an "H." All these problems require surgical correction (Fig. 4.5).

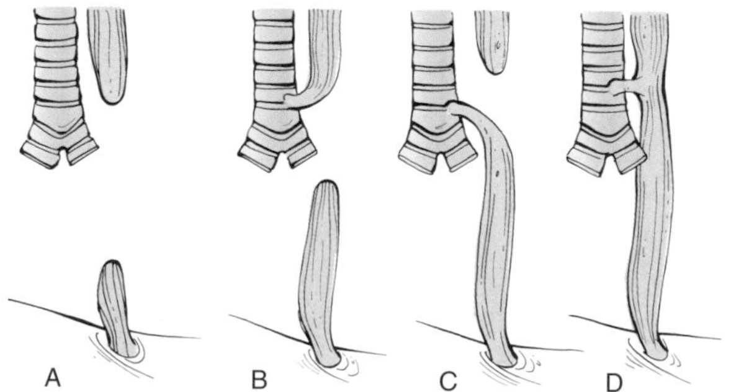

FIGURE 4.5 Esophageal atresia and tracheoesophageal fistula. (**A**) The upper and lower segments are blind and do not connect to the air passages. (**B**) The upper segment opens into the trachea, while the other remains a blind pouch. (**C**) In this most common variation, the upper segment of the esophagus ends in a blind pouch near the level of the bifurcation of the trachea. A short fistulous tract connects the lower segment from the stomach to the trachea. (**D**) The esophagus and trachea share a common fistulous tract in the "H" type.

Gastroschisis and omphalocele are anomalies affecting the abdominal wall. With **gastroschisis,** an opening in the abdomen usually 2 to 4 cm in diameter, causes the intestines to extrude. The intestines never have any membrane or covering tissue; the liver, spleen, and other organs remain internal. The lesion is located to the side of the umbilical cord. An *omphalocele* develops between 8 to 10 weeks' gestation; in this condition, the intestines extrude. See Chapter 9 for more discussion.

An **imperforate anus** results in the rectum ending in a blind pouch with no external anal opening. This can be seen on physical examination. Female infants also can have a fistula, with stool passing from the rectum into the vagina or bladder. Male infants can have a fistula connecting to the bladder. Surgical intervention is necessary.

Meconium ileus involves a very sticky meconium plug of the ileum. It is most often seen in infants with cystic fibrosis, a disease in which intestinal enzymes needed to break down proteins from the amniotic fluid swallowed in utero are missing. As a result, the meconium forms a very sticky plug. Meconium ileus can be seen on x-ray as a "soap bubble" pattern in the right lower quadrant. Treatment consists of enemas. See Chapter 8 for more discussion.

Hirschsprung's disease, caused by a lack of ganglia in the bowel wall, starts at the anus and extends proximally. Without ganglia, the bowel remains in a constantly contracted state, creating a functional bowel obstruction. Infants with Hirschsprung's disease usually have no stool within the first 48 hours of life. They may have abdominal distention and begin to vomit. Usually a digital rectal examination will produce stool and the infant may be discharged home without a diagnosis. Over time the infant will have poor weight gain, abdominal distention, and difficulty passing stool. X-rays and barium enemas are used in diagnosis. Treatment involves surgery to remove the aganglionic colon and an ostomy. Hirschsprung's disease is usually genetic and sometimes occurs in conjunction with Down syndrome.

Duodenal atresia or stenosis involves narrowing or total closure of the duodenal intestine. Infants develop feeding problems and abdominal distention within the first 1 to 2 days of life. On x-ray the classic "double bubble" (an air or fluid pattern in the stomach and duodenum) is seen. Treatment is surgical repair.

The final two gastrointestinal problems are genetic. The first is **phenylketonuria** (PKU), which results from an inability to metabolize certain amino acids. It has no cure, and treatment consists of a special diet. All infants are tested for PKU before discharge from the healthcare facility. If treatment with diet is not used, the infant will develop mental and behavioral problems. The second problem is **galactosemia.** Infants with galactosemia lack an enzyme needed to metabolize galactose. They experience weight loss, vomiting, and diarrhea. Treatment is eliminating lactose and galactose from the diet.

Cardiac Anomalies

Six main cardiac problems can occur in newborns. Chapter 9 presents more detailed discussion of these congenital heart defects; to summarize:

- With *atrial septal defect* (ASD), an opening remains between the right and left atria, causing left to right shunting of blood.
- In *ventricular septal defect* (VSD), a hole remains between the right and left ventricles, also usually with left to right shunting of blood. If pulmonary pressure is increased, however, blood can flow from right to left.
- The third cardiac anomaly is *patent ductus arteriosus* (PDA). The ductus, a connection between the aorta and pulmonary artery, is important in fetal circulation to bypass the pulmonary circuit. After delivery it soon closes. On occasion the ductus can remain patent and allow for shunting of blood from the aorta into the pulmonary artery.
- The fourth cardiac anomaly is *transposition of the great arteries.* The aorta exits the right ventricle and the pulmonary artery exits the left ventricle. This creates two independent circulatory systems. Treatment involves surgery, but before that can happen, it is vital to keep the PDA and any ASDs or VSDs open.
- In *coarctation of the aorta,* the aorta has a narrowed area that increases left ventricular pressure. The coarctated area can occur proximal or distal to a PDA.
- With *tetralogy of Fallot,* four different defects occur: VSD, hypertrophy of the right ventricle, an overriding aorta, and pulmonary stenosis.

Infants with cardiac anomalies usually have cyanosis and murmurs upon chest auscultation and some form of respiratory distress. Treatment consists of respiratory support and usually surgery to correct the anomalies.

Urogenital Anomalies

Exstrophy of the bladder occurs when the bladder is exposed on the outside of the body. Surgery is usually done within the first 2 to 3 days of life while the sacroiliac joints are very pliable. *Epispadias* describes the urethral meatus being located on the upper side of the penis. *Hypospadias* is when the meatus is located on the underside of the penis. It can occur in female infants with the meatus opening onto the perineum. If epispadias occurs in a female infant, there is also usually exstrophy of the bladder. In male infants, a *hydrocele* occurs when an opening in the peritoneal cavity allows peritoneal fluid to enter the scrotum. Inguinal hernias are common with hydroceles. Hydroceles and inguinal hernias are surgically repaired. In male infants, the testicles can be undescended at birth. This condition often resolves within the first few months after birth. If by 18 to 24 months they have not descended, then surgery is done. All these conditions are discussed in detail in Chapter 9.

A condition known as **ambiguous genitalia** can occur in newborns. In this instance, genitalia look abnormal, causing an inability to determine if the infant is truly male or female. Cases need further evaluation by chromosomal studies, hormonal tests, or both. It is very important not to label the infant as a "he" or "she" prematurely until the gender can be determined definitively. This can be very distressing to parents; provide the family with needed support.

Orthopedic Anomalies

Infants can be born with certain malformations of the joints and extremities. A **congenital dislocated hip** can involve one or both hips. If unilateral, the left hip is affected more commonly. Degrees of dislocation vary. Treatment aims at keeping the hips abducted by triple diapering or use of a splint or brace. The problem usually resolves in 3 to 4 months. On physical examination the infant may have an audible or palpable click heard or felt when the hip is abducted and adducted. The length of the infant's thighs may be visibly different. More fat rolls or skin folds may be seen in one thigh than the other.

Infants can be born with extra fingers and toes or webbed fingers and toes. *Polydactyly* refers to extra fingers or toes (see Chap. 3). These extra digits often contain no bone material and usually are treated by using suturing thread to tie them off at the base. They dry up and fall off within a few days. X-rays can be done to check for bone material. If bone material exists, surgery is required. **Syndactyly** occurs when the toes or fingers are joined with a webbed appearance. Surgery may be done to correct syndactyly.

CHROMOSOMAL ANOMALIES

Several chromosomal syndromes have multiple congenital anomalies. The first is *Down syndrome,* also called trisomy 21, and discussed in detail in Chapter 7. Typical physical features observed in infants with Down syndrome include a small head, a flattened appearance to the posterior side of the head, eyes set close together, low-set ears, flattened nose, large tongue that protrudes from the mouth, short wide neck, short hands, simian creases in the palms, and mental deficiency. Other anomalies common in infants with Down syndrome include heart defects, duodenal atresia, esophageal atresia, imperforate anus, poor muscle development, and loose joints. These infants are at increased risk for infection. Survival rates are high, assuming surgical correction of any heart defects or other anomalies.

Edwards' syndrome, also called **trisomy 18,** is another chromosomal syndrome. Infants born with this syndrome tend to have micrognathia (small lower jaw), corneal opacities, ptosis, overlapping digits, rocker-bottom feet, increased muscle tone, and heart defects. They rarely live beyond 3 months.

Patau's syndrome is also called **trisomy 13.** Physical features common with this syndrome include cleft lip and palate, microthalmia, polydactyly, and congenital heart defects. Like with trisomy 18, infants born with trisomy 13 rarely survive beyond 3 months.

Another chromosomal syndrome is **Turner's syndrome** (45, X) in female infants. Girls born with Turner's syndrome lack an X chromosome. At birth physical features include webbing of the neck and edema of the feet and neck. If the fetus reaches term gestation, then the infant usually has a very good survival rate. With maturation, the female child has an ovarian failure so normal sexual maturation does not occur.

Finally, **Klinefelter's syndrome** is seen in males who have an extra X chromosome (47, XXY). They are born with male genitalia. Often Klinefelter's syndrome is undiagnosed until puberty. With this syndrome testicular failure results in small and firm testicles, gynecomastia, abnormally long legs, and lowered intelligence.

INFECTIONS

Maternal infections during pregnancy can have devastating effects on the fetus. Prenatally, mothers are screened for different infections. One screen, called a **TORCH screen,** checks for the following infections: *t*oxoplasmosis, *o*ther (syphilis, hepatitis B, and varicella zoster), *r*ubella, *c*ytomegalovirus, and *h*erpes simplex virus. Sexually transmitted infections (STIs) in the mother can have long-term sequela in the fetus (see Chap. 56). Prenatally, women are screened for STIs and treated as necessary. Other infections that can affect newborns are group B streptococci, sepsis, and *Candida albicans.* Women who receive little or no prenatal care miss these screenings and any needed treatment, so risk for their infants is increased at delivery.

TORCH Infections

Toxoplasma gondii is a protozoon found in many birds and mammals, especially cats. Pregnant women should not change cat litter because of the potential presence of *T. gondii* in cat feces. *T. gondii* also may be found in raw meats and eggs. *T. gondii* causes **toxoplasmosis,** which mothers can transmit transplacentally to the fetus. Infants with toxoplasmosis can be born with microcephaly or hydrocephaly, cerebrospinal fluid abnormalities, seizures, intracranial calcifications, anemia and other bleeding problems, hyperbilirubinemia, chorioretinitis, cataracts, glaucoma, hepatosplenomegaly, vomiting, diarrhea, hypothermia, fever, rash, and pneumonia. The infant may have many of these symptoms or a subclinical infection. If a woman tests positive for infection with *T. gondii,* medical treatment is available. Prevention remains the best treatment.

The organism *Treponema pallidum* causes syphilis, an STI (see Chap. 56). If a mother has syphilis prenatally and is not treated, there is a 50% chance that the infant will be stillborn or premature and die in the immediate neonatal period. The other 50% of infants who do not die will develop congenital syphilis. Symptoms of congenital syphilis are snuffles, serosanguinous rhinitis, fissures of the lips, skin rash, hepatosplenomegaly, lymphadenopathy, anemia, bone abnormalities seen on x-ray, and other central nervous system signs. For positive infants, treatment is penicillin and strict isolation.

Hepatitis B, a viral infection, can be transmitted to the fetus in utero, but it is more commonly transmitted during birth with exposure to contaminated maternal blood. Hepatitis B can be transmitted to infants postpartally through infected saliva, serum, breast milk, urine, or feces. Infants born to mothers with a positive hepatitis screen should receive hepatitis B immune globulin (HBIG) soon after delivery and the hepatitis B immunization injection (see Chap. 3). Nurses must follow strict standard precautions when caring for these infants.

Varicella zoster is the virus that causes chickenpox. Transmission of varicella zoster to the fetus can cause various defects of the eye, skin lesions, defects of the limbs including missing digits, muscle atrophy and paralysis, and central nervous system problems such as seizures, encephalitis, and mental retardation. Varicella zoster can infect the mother at the end of the gestational period and the infant can develop congenital varicella zoster. In this case, if the woman is infected within 5 days of delivery, the infant has a 30% chance of death. If the woman is infected more that 5 days before delivery, then the infant usually has a less severe infection.

Rubella is another viral infection. With widespread use of vaccines, rubella infections are relatively rare in the United States. Pregnant women have a titer tested prenatally to see if they are immune to rubella. A woman who is not immune needs to be careful to avoid contact with any person with rubella; after delivery she needs to receive a booster immunization. The earlier in the prenatal period that the mother is infected with rubella, the worse the fetal outcome. Fetal death is common. Newborns who survive commonly have cardiac defects, cataracts, and deafness. Other problems include growth retardation, glaucoma, hepatic problems, meningitis, bone lesions, and pneumonia. Rubella has no specific treatment; care is supportive.

Cytomegalovirus (CMV) infections are quite common and occur in 6 to 34 of 1000 live births. Infants can be infected with CMV postnatally. Postnatal rates of transmission are 20 in 1000 live births. Infants can be asymptomatic at birth. CMV causes many problems for the infant. At birth, jaundice and hepatosplenomegaly are the most common. Other problems include low birth weight, heart problems, pneumonia, anemia, petechiae, cataracts, chorioretinitis, microcephaly or hydrocephaly, intracranial calcifications, encephalitis, and bone lesions. Treatment is supportive.

The last TORCH infection is herpes simplex virus (HSV), another STI. HSV type 1 usually affects the lip and nasal area, and HSV type 2 affects the genitalia. HSV type 1 has been cultured from lesions on the genitalia and vice versa. The most common mode of transmission is that the infant comes into contact with HSV during a vaginal delivery. Delivery by cesarean section can decrease the chance of contact with HSV. Transmission can occur if membranes are ruptured for more than 6 hours and the virus ascends upward to the fetus. If a woman has an outbreak with visible lesions or if the membranes have been ruptured for less than 4 to 6 hours, a cesarean section usually is performed to help prevent transmission of HSV.

Other Sexually Transmitted Infections

Neisseria gonorrhoeae and *Chlamydia trachomatis* are two sexually transmitted organisms that can be transmitted during vaginal delivery. Gonorrhea commonly causes conjunctivitis, which leads to swelling and redness of the eyelids and purulent discharge. Gonorrhea can cause damage to the corneas; if left untreated, blindness may ensue (ophthalmia neonatorum). Treatment consists of parenteral penicillin, irrigation of the eyes, and antibiotic eye ointment.

Chlamydia also can infect the eye. Symptoms are the same as seen with a gonorrheal infection; however, the corneas usually are spared. Treatment is with the drug of choice, erythromycin. Silver nitrate is not effective with chlamydia. Infants who get conjunctivitis caused by chlamydia also may develop pneumonia. An infant with pneumonia needs antibiotic therapy and respiratory support.

HIV can be transmitted to the fetus transplacentally or during delivery. Almost all infants born to HIV-positive mothers also test positive. Some of these infants also test positive for the HIV antigen. These infants who are antigen positive are thought to develop AIDS later. Positive infants also may be started on antiviral treatments.

Other Infections

Thrush is an infection of the oral cavity caused by *Candida albicans,* a yeast or fungus that can reside on the skin. The baby can acquire the infection from the mother during birth or postnatally by a lack of asepsis during feedings or from the woman's nipples during breastfeeding. The infant's immune system is often not sufficient to fight this organism, and the infant will develop a thick white exudate on the tongue and mucous membranes of the mouth. Treatment consists of nystatin applied topically many times per day or Diflucan suspension given orally once per day. Infants with thrush can be irritable and feed poorly because of oral discomfort.

Newborn infants can develop sepsis; group B streptococci is the most common cause. Incidence of sepsis is 1 to 3 in 1000 live births. Group B streptococci commonly can be cultured from the genital tract, stools, and throat. Transmission usually is through the birth canal, especially with prolonged rupture of membranes and premature labor and delivery. Most infants are colonized at delivery, but actual infection rates are relatively low comparatively. Infants born with infection tend to develop respiratory distress, fever, glucose instability, feeding intolerance, and lethargy. The infant is screened for infection with a complete blood count and differential, a C-reactive protein test, blood cultures, and urine cultures. Treatment includes antibiotic therapy, respiratory support, and other care as required.

MATERNAL SUBSTANCE USE

Maternal substance use during pregnancy can have devastating effects on an infant. Outcomes depend on the types of substances used, how much, and at what part of the gestational period. Women who abuse substances often use multiple drugs, alcohol, and tobacco products. Knowing what substances an infant was exposed to during pregnancy can facilitate appropriate postpartum care. See Chapter 17 for more information on substance abuse and treatment.

The woman can be tested with a urine drug screen to identify what is in her system at the time the screen is done. This test is of limited help, however, because many illegal substances are present in the urine only for a few days and the drug screen then cannot detect what substances she used earlier in the pregnancy (Table 4.1). Newborns can have a urine drug screen as well, but this will show what the infant was exposed to only within the last few days to few weeks. Drug testing can be done on meconium to identify drug exposure much longer into the gestational period and can give a broader picture of exposure.

Women who abuse substances need special care. Usually a multidisciplinary team approach is helpful. A mother may need to be admitted to an inpatient program for substance abuse. A social worker can help find child care for the infant. The family will need follow-up counselors after discharge from the inpatient program. Home health nurses

SUBSTANCE	METABOLITES STILL PRESENT AFTER LAST USE FOR...
Cocaine	3 days after use (up to 2 weeks in habitual user)
Opiates	
Heroin	up to 2 days
Methadone	up to 3 days
Marijuana	up to 2 weeks
Methamphetamine	up to 2 days

TABLE 4.1 URINE DRUG SCREEN

can teach the woman how to interact with and appropriately care for the infant. The infant also needs follow-up care to evaluate normal development, identify problems, and be placed into early intervention programs.

Stop, Think, and Respond ● BOX 4-2

A woman who has recently given birth comes to the healthcare facility for follow-up care for her infant. She admitted to using drugs "once or twice" during her pregnancy; fortunately, her baby seems to be doing well. The woman is contemplating trying for another child "soon." What teaching and information can you provide to help deter the woman from substance abuse during a subsequent pregnancy?

Cocaine

Cocaine inhibits nerve conduction and prevents uptake of norepinephrine. The result is excessive norepinephrine, leading to vasoconstriction, tachycardia, and increased blood pressure. Consequences include heart dysrhythmias, seizures, strokes, respiratory and cardiac arrest, and sudden death. When a pregnant woman uses cocaine, all the above can happen; most importantly, there is vasoconstriction of placental blood flow. Maternal cocaine use causes increased rates of spontaneous abortions, placental abruptions, and stillbirths. It also may lead to premature labor and delivery, growth retardation, low birth weight, microcephaly, fetal hypertension, and strokes.

A baby born to a woman who used cocaine during pregnancy can be at risk for problems long after gestation and delivery. Infants exposed to cocaine tend to have tremors, increased muscle tone, tachycardia, tachypnea, abnormal sleep respiratory pattern with apnea and periodic breathing, poor feeding patterns, and increased risk of SIDS. They tend to be very irritable with an increased startle response to stimuli. Upon awakening from a deep sleep state, they may immediately be in an active crying state. Because of this abnormal state regulation, they tend to not be able to handle normal stimulation. This severely interferes with normal parent–infant bonding. This lack of bonding and other long-term problems put these infants at risk for developmental delays and abuse. Postdischarge home follow-up is a must.

When working with these infants, diminish environmental stimuli. Bundle the infant to promote muscle flexion, which can help decrease potential contractures from muscle hypertonicity. Looking at the nurse's face can be too much stimulation for the infant. To decrease stimulation during feedings, hold the infant facing a blank wall for the baby to focus on while eating. These infants often have poor suck and swallow coordination. Monitor feeding ability closely. They do not tolerate normal rocking and actually tolerate vertical rocking better. Teach the infant's mother about behaviors in her child that differ from those of babies who were not exposed to cocaine. The mother must learn how to care for the infant appropriately to help promote mother–infant bonding.

Opioids

Opioids include heroin and methadone. Infants can become opioid dependent during gestation. Such infants have a set of commonly observed symptoms called the *neonatal abstinence syndrome.* These symptoms include tremors and jitteriness, hyperactive reflexes, increased muscle tone, sweating, fever, mottling, decreased sleep, irritability, high-pitched and excessive crying, frantic nonproductive sucking and rooting behavior, poor feeding, vomiting, diarrhea, tachypnea, sneezing, nasal stuffiness, abrupt state changes, and gaze aversion. Symptoms range in severity among infants and usually begin within the first 24 to 72 hours of life. Onset can be a bit later for methadone (as much as 96 hours). Duration of symptoms is approximately 8 weeks; however, irritability can continue for 3 to 4 months. Neonatal abstinence syndrome interferes with normal parent–infant bonding. Educate the mother on how to interact with her infant. It important for these infants to receive follow-up home evaluation and care.

Marijuana

In pregnant women, use of marijuana can cause tachycardia, hypertension, altered placental perfusion, increased appetite, dry mouth, and altered mind functioning. It may lead to fetal death, premature labor and delivery, and low birth weight. Infants exposed to marijuana in utero often display nervous system abnormalities.

Alcohol

Women who use alcohol during pregnancy put their fetus at great risk for problems. Some infants exposed to alcohol have few to no noticeable problems, while others have a host of problems such as fetal alcohol syndrome (FAS), which is discussed in detail in Chapter 7. The level of drinking that causes FAS is unknown, so pregnant women are strongly encouraged to consume no alcohol whatsoever during their pregnancies.

Smoking

It has been well documented that maternal smoking contributes to LBW. It also can cause premature labor and delivery, placental abruption and previa, and fetal deaths. Encourage pregnant women who smoke to quit.

FAMILY TEACHING FOR FAMILIES WITH INFANTS WHO HAVE COMPLICATIONS

Infants born with congenital and chromosomal anomalies often spend time in special care nurseries or NICUs. If they require surgeries over time, they can be admitted to various pediatric units. Parents of these infants have many of the same concerns and anxieties as parents with premature infants. They go through a grieving process with the loss of their "perfect child." Just like with grieving the loss of a loved one, they experience stages of grief: shock, denial, anger, and acceptance. They go through phases of ups and downs. Some conditions deteriorate quickly; whereas other conditions improve over time. Roller-coaster patterns may continue for weeks and months. Finally, parents prepare for discharge. This final phase can be full of stressors. Help teach parents to care for their infants and to meet any special needs that their babies have. Try to instill confidence that parents are indeed capable of independently caring for their infant.

Stop, Think, and Respond ● BOX 4-3

How would you provide support and comfort to a family who has given birth to a child with a disorder in which the child will live but will face ongoing developmental and physical challenges?

PERINATAL LOSS

Despite many advances in technology and medical treatments, infants still die. Perinatal loss can be devastating for families. It may be in the form of miscarriage, stillbirth, or death of a preterm or term infant. Parents of children born with potentially fatal problems may go through two grieving processes: once for the loss of the "perfect child" and another with the actual physical loss of the infant.

Mothers and fathers may grieve differently. Mothers may have a greater bond established with the infant because they had more physical contact with the fetus during gestation. They may have a harder time dealing with grief. The couple may develop communication problems, which can lead to other difficulties in their relationship. Rather than providing support and nurturing, the relationship can become full of animosity. Support from family and friends may be less readily available for parents with a perinatal loss as compared to loss of an older child. One contributing factor may be that family members and friends had no bonding with the infant.

Many healthcare agencies have perinatal loss programs that provide parents with support. Clergy members can visit the parents and perform baptism if the parents so desire it. Some parents send their infant's body to a funeral home. In the case of a miscarriage or stillbirth, the healthcare agency may cremate the products of conception or body. In this case, the facility may have a special burial spot or memorial garden for placing the remains or setting a marker. Often, agencies provide special boxes for parents to place mementos, such as a lock of the infant's hair, foot and hand prints, plaster castings of the foot or hand, photos of the infant, crib or isolette name tags, identification bracelets, hat, booties, and receiving blanket. Of course, parents should take home any personal belongings.

If the infant was in the NICU for some time, many nurses and doctors become attached to the infant and parents. These people often can provide comfort to the parents. Nurses can offer a listening ear and encourage parents to still call the NICU to talk if they want. If appropriate, nurses who felt close to the parents can attend any funeral or memorial services for the baby.

Critical Thinking Exercise

1. *Verbally explain to a nursing classmate the differences between physiologic and pathologic jaundice. Develop a nursing plan of care for an infant with hyperbilirubinemia who is going to be placed under phototherapy, acting irritable, and having feeding problems demonstrated by a poor suck and vomiting.*

● NCLEX-STYLE REVIEW QUESTIONS 

1. The nurse is assessing an SGA newborn in the hospital nursery. As the nurse provides care, which action is the highest priority?
    1. Check the infant's temperature every 2 hours.
    2. Auscultate the infant's bowel sounds every day.
    3. Listen for heart murmurs every shift.
    4. Assess for jaundice with every diaper change.

2. A 3-day-old newborn is diagnosed with hyperbilirubinemia. The nurse explains to the mother that the infant will need phototherapy. Which statement by the mother indicates a need for further instruction?
   1. "I need to cover my baby's eyes while the lights are on."
   2. "I need to cover my baby with a blanket while in the isolette."
   3. "I need to leave off the diaper when I put my baby under the lights."
   4. "I need to save any wet diapers when I change my baby."

3. A newborn whose mother has admitted to cocaine use throughout pregnancy is irritable and cannot be consoled. In addition to decreasing the infant's stimulation, which of the following nursing interventions should be the priority?
   1. Document the infant's weight daily.
   2. Document the infant's sleep and wake cycles.
   3. Document the infant's behavior during rocking.
   4. Document the infant's blood glucose levels.

connection

Visit the Connection site at **http://connection.lww.com/go/timbyEssentials** for links to chapter-related resources on the Internet.

References and Suggested Readings

Deacon, J., & O'Neill, P. (Eds.) (1999). *Core curriculum for neonatal intensive care nursing* (2nd ed.). Philadelphia: W. B. Saunders Company.

Gunn, V., & Nechyba, C. (2002). *The Harriet Lane handbook* (16th ed.). St. Louis: Mosby.

Merenstein, G., & Gardner, S. (2002). *Handbook of neonatal intensive care* (5th ed.). St. Louis: Mosby.

chapter 5

Introduction to Pediatric Nursing

Words to Know 

family caregivers
malocclusion
orthodontia
point of maximum impulse
scoliosis
symmetry
therapeutic play

Learning Objectives

On completion of this chapter, the reader will:

- Discuss the role of the nurse in communicating with the child and family caregivers.
- Explain the importance of routine physical and dental examinations.
- List 12 communicable diseases against which children are commonly immunized.
- Describe the process for collecting subjective data from children and adolescents and their caregivers.
- Discuss the role of the nurse in assisting with the physical examination.
- Explain the role of family caregivers when a child is hospitalized.
- Describe how health professionals can assist with the adjustment of a child scheduled for surgery.
- Discuss the purpose of a hospital play program.
- Explain the reason for monitoring accurate intake and output when caring for children.
- Describe the use of gavage or gastrostomy feedings in children.
- Discuss preventive measures for each of the leading causes of accidents in children.
- Identify behavioral characteristics that may indicate an infant or a young child has pain.
- List the methods used to administer oxygen to children.
- Describe four methods of collecting a urine specimen in children.
- List safety measures to consider when using restraints or holding a child.
- Discuss medication administration for pediatric clients.

Communication is an important role of the nurse working with children and families. Often the nurse explains, teaches, and clarifies information for the child and family. Whether the setting is outpatient, community or hospital, nurses must understand how to adapt nursing care and interventions to pediatric clients.

COMMUNICATION

An important role for pediatric nurses in all settings is communicating with both children and their family caregivers. Developing good communication skills enables nurses to provide better care to children and their families.

Communicating With Children

Infants and Young Children

Communicating with infants and children can be challenging. Infants respond to sounds and actions, so they must be handled and spoken to in a quiet, secure manner. The child who is old enough to distinguish between people (generally after 6 months of age) tends to be frightened of strangers. Sudden, abrupt, or noisy approaches may upset them. They need time to evaluate the situation while still secure in a caregiver's familiar arms. Do not rush the situation but allow time for the child to initiate the relationship. Often, a nurse may start the conversation with the child's doll or stuffed animal. Distrust of strangers may last through the first 3 or 4 years of life. A casual approach with reluctant children is usually most effective. Children who are anxious or hostile are often putting up a defense against their own fears and feelings. This behavior can be ignored unless it threatens the child's or someone else's well-being.

When speaking with small or young children, get down on their eye level. Speak in a slow, clear, positive voice, using simple words and short sentences. Choices should be simple and offered only if they actually exist. Listen to the child's fears and worries and be honest in your answers. The perceptions of young children are literal. Be careful to use positive explanations in familiar and nonthreatening terms.

School-Age Children

School-age children are interested in knowing what and why. Simple explanations that help them understand how equipment works are important. These children will ask more questions if their curiosity is not satisfied.

Adolescents

Communicating with adolescents may be challenging. Young teenagers frequently waver between thinking like children and like adults. Sometimes adolescents do not want to reveal much if a parent is present. Teens may need to relate information that they do not wish others to know, and a discussion about confidentiality may set their concerns at ease. They need to know that the nurse will listen attentively in an open-minded, nonjudgmental way. The adolescent and the family may not view a problem in the same way, and the nurse may need to define the problem more clearly to facilitate an agreement, if possible.

Communicating With Family Caregivers

The people who care for the child in the home setting are known as **family caregivers.** These people are usually the child's parents or other family members. It is important for the nurse to identify who the child's family caregivers are so they can participate in providing information relevant to the child's care and help with planning for the child's healthcare needs. Conferring with family caregivers and other members of the healthcare team helps form a clearer picture of the child, promotes better understanding of his or her behavior, and presents an opportunity to consider differing types of treatment and relationships. It is most important to keep family caregivers well informed about what is happening and being planned for their child. When a procedure is planned, tell caregivers what will happen and invite them to help, if practical. No caregiver who is reluctant to help with or observe a procedure, however, should be urged to stay or made to feel that involvement is a duty.

Some caregivers are so anxious and apprehensive that they communicate their concerns and negative reactions to the child rather than provide support. Listening and communication skills are extremely important when working with caregivers. Giving them time to discuss anxieties and concerns, exploring such problems, and demonstrating genuine caring help ease these feelings.

An older child may feel self-sufficient and may view the family caregiver's presence as being treated "like a baby." It is normal to regress during illness, however, and most children of any age appreciate the presence of a reassuring, self-controlled person during trying, uncomfortable times.

HEALTH MAINTENANCE

Routine physical and dental checkups and examinations are important aspects of health maintenance in infants and children. In addition, keeping a child's immunizations current offers the best possible protection against preventable diseases.

Routine Checkups

Routine well-baby or well-child visits are recommended throughout childhood (Agency for Health Care Policy and Research, 2003). During these visits, nurses collect data about the child's growth and development, nutrition, hygiene, and sleep; the caregiver–child relationship; and any potential problems. They document the child's growth information and give immunizations. Routine checkups offer an opportunity for family teaching, which is an integral part of health promotion and maintenance. Screening procedures include urinalysis, hematocrit, lead level, tuberculin skin testing, and Denver Developmental Screening Test.

During the first year of life, usually six well-baby visits are recommended (Agency for Health Care Policy and Research, 2003). The child is seen at 15 months for immunization boosters and at least annually thereafter. Preschoolers seen for routine checkups will need immunization boosters, which are required for entrance into kindergarten. Family caregivers should tell preschoolers and older children in advance about upcoming examinations to provide them with an opportunity to ask questions and voice anxieties. Several books available through public libraries are excellent for teaching children about visits to the pediatrician. Vision and hearing should be checked during a preschool well-child check and periodically (annually or biannually) thereafter so that any problems can be treated before the child enters school at 5 or 6 years.

Elementary school children generally are healthy with only minor illnesses, so the yearly routine check may be the only time they visit a practitioner. School, family, or behavioral problems are discussed at these visits. During a physical examination at approximately 10 to 11 years, the child is examined initially for signs of **scoliosis** (lateral curvature of the spine). The child is monitored on an ongoing basis and re-examined during adolescence. The school nurse often conducts these examinations.

A routine annual physical examination is encouraged during adolescence. Nurses must recognize and acknowledge that adolescents may feel uncomfortable and out of place in a pediatrician's waiting room. Adolescents must be given privacy, individualized attention, confidentiality, and the right to participate in decisions about their healthcare. Tuberculin testing is included. Thyroid enlargement should be checked through 14 years of age. A routine physical is an excellent time to counsel teens about sexual activity and sexually transmitted infections (STIs), including human immunodeficiency virus (HIV). Sexually active girls must have a pelvic examination, screening for STIs, and a Pap smear. Urinalysis is performed on all female adolescents, and a urine culture is performed if the girl has any symptoms of a urinary tract infection.

Body piercing and tattoos are becoming more common in adolescents. See Chap. 10 for more discussion of nursing interventions for clients with these.

Dental Care/Checkups

Dental caries (cavities) are a major health problem in children and adolescents. Development of dental caries is linked to the effect of diet on the oral environment. Bacteria can combine with sugar and form a film, or dental plaque, on the teeth, resulting in tooth decay. Children who eat sweet foods frequently accumulate plaque easily and are prone to dental caries; therefore, dental checkups and examinations are important during childhood. To help prevent tooth decay, encourage children to eat healthy snacks such as fruits, raw vegetables, and natural cheeses rather than candy, cakes, or sugar-filled gum.

Children of low-income families often have poor dental hygiene and care, both because of the costs involved and parental lack of knowledge about proper care and nutrition. Some caregivers may believe it is unnecessary to take proper care of baby teeth because "they fall out anyway." Nevertheless, the care and condition of the baby teeth affect the normal growth of permanent teeth, which form in the jaw under the baby teeth. Teach caregivers the importance of proper care of the child's baby teeth (see Chap. 6).

When the child is approximately 2 years of age, he or she should learn to brush the teeth or at least to rinse the mouth after each meal or snack. Toddlers like to imitate others, so they learn best by example. Plain water should be used for brushing until the child has learned how to spit out toothpaste. An adult also should brush the child's teeth until the child becomes experienced; even then, the adult should check the cleanliness of the teeth. The caregiver should be responsible for flossing the child's teeth until the child has attained the necessary motor skills.

Fluoride toothpaste strengthens tooth enamel and helps prevent tooth decay, particularly in communities with unfluoridated water. An adult should supervise the use of fluoride toothpaste; the child should use only a pea-sized amount. The provider may recommend supplemental fluoride, but families on limited incomes may find this difficult to afford. A fluoride supplement is a medication and should be treated and stored as such. Fluoride also can be applied during regular visits to the dentist, but the greatest benefit to the tooth enamel occurs before teeth erupt.

The first visit to the dentist should occur at approximately 2 years of age to give the child a chance to get acquainted with the dentist, staff, and office. A second visit might be a good time for a preliminary examination, with subsequent visits twice a year for checkups, cleaning, and fluoride application. During visits, allowing a younger child to watch an older sibling can help the younger child overcome the fear of a strange setting.

Adolescents need continued regular dental checkups every 6 months. Dental **malocclusion** (improper alignment of the teeth) is a common condition that affects the way the teeth and jaws function. **Orthodontia,** or correction of the malocclusion with dental braces, improves chewing ability and appearance. Such treatment usually begins in late school age or early adolescence.

Tongue piercing among adolescents has increased. For teens with such piercing, dental checkups are a good opportunity to discuss concerns of possible infections and tooth damage.

Immunizations

Every child is entitled to the best possible protection against disease. Protection in the form of immunizations is available against several serious or disabling diseases such as diphtheria, tetanus, pertussis, hepatitis A and B, polio, measles, mumps, German measles (rubella), varicella (chickenpox), *Haemophilus influenzae* meningitis, and pneumococcal disease.

The Academy of Pediatrics and the Centers for Disease Control and Prevention (CDC) have recommended a schedule of immunizations for healthy children living in normal conditions (Figure 5.1). Additional recommendations are made for children who live in certain regions and areas or who have certain risk factors. Immunizations should be given within the prescribed timetable unless the child's physical condition makes doing so impossible. An immunization need not be postponed if the child has a cold but should be postponed if the child has an acute febrile condition or a condition causing immunosuppression or if he or she is receiving corticosteroids, radiation, or antimetabolites. A urine pregnancy screening is advisable before administration of the rubella vaccine to a girl of childbearing age because such administration during pregnancy can cause serious risks to the developing fetus.

Side effects vary with the type of immunization. The most common side effect is a fever within the first 24 to 48 hours and possibly a local reaction at the injection site. These reactions are treated symptomatically with acetaminophen for the fever and warm compresses to the injection site.

Many children do not get their initial immunizations in infancy and may not get them until they reach school age, when most states require immunizations for school entrance. Healthcare personnel should make every effort to encourage parents to have their children immunized in infancy to avoid the danger of possible epidemic outbreaks. Answer any questions the caregiver may have about immunizations. Remember, however, that the caregiver has a right to refuse immunizations if he or she has been fully informed about them and any possible reactions. Maintain a nonjudgmental viewpoint throughout the discussion.

Stop, Think, and Respond ● BOX 5-1

What diseases should the child be immunized against before he or she starts school?

PEDIATRIC ASSESSMENT

Gathering information about the child's history and current status is important. Subjective and objective data collection is continuous throughout a child's care, but most data are collected during the interview and the physical examination.

Collecting Subjective Data

Information spoken by the child or family is called *subjective data.* Interviewing the family caregiver and child allows the nurse to collect information to help develop an appropriate plan of care. The interview process is goal-directed.

Conducting the Client and Family Interview

Nurses collect most subjective data during the interview with the family caregiver and child. The interview helps establish a relationship between the nurse and the child and family. Listening and using appropriate communication techniques help promote a good interview. Past experiences with healthcare may influence the interview. The younger child may sit on the caregiver's lap, or the nurse may offer age-appropriate toys and activities to occupy the child. The family caregiver provides most of the information needed in caring for the child, especially the infant or toddler. It is helpful to observe the reactions of the child and caregiver as they interact.

It is important for nurses to include preschoolers and older children in the interview by using age-appropriate questions during discussion. Using a doll or familiar stuffed animal can help involve them.

Adolescents can provide information about themselves; interviewing them in private often encourages them to share information that they might not contribute in front of their caregivers. This is especially true when asking sensitive questions such as information regarding drug use or sexual practices.

Obtaining a Client History

In any healthcare setting, gathering information about the child's current condition as well as past medical history is essential. Collect and record identifying information including the child's name, address, and phone number as well as information regarding the caregiver. This information is part of the legal record and requires confidential treatment. A questionnaire often is used to gather information such as the child's nickname, feeding habits, food likes and dislikes, allergies, sleeping schedule, and toilet-training status. Any special words the child uses or understands to indicate needs or desires, such as words used for urinating and bowel movements, are helpful.

The reason for the child's visit to the healthcare setting is called the chief complaint. To best care for the child, it is important to get the most complete explanation of what brought the child to the healthcare setting.

Elicit information about the current situation, including the child's symptoms; when they began; how long they have been present; their description, intensity, and frequency; and treatments to this time.

Obtaining a past health history for the child includes information about the pregnancy and delivery as well as common childhood, serious, or chronic illnesses; immunizations and health maintenance; feeding and nutrition; as well as hospitalizations and injuries.

The caregiver usually can provide information regarding family health history. Use this information to do preventative teaching with the child and family.

Ask the caregiver or child questions about each body system. Using a head-to-toe approach, gather information

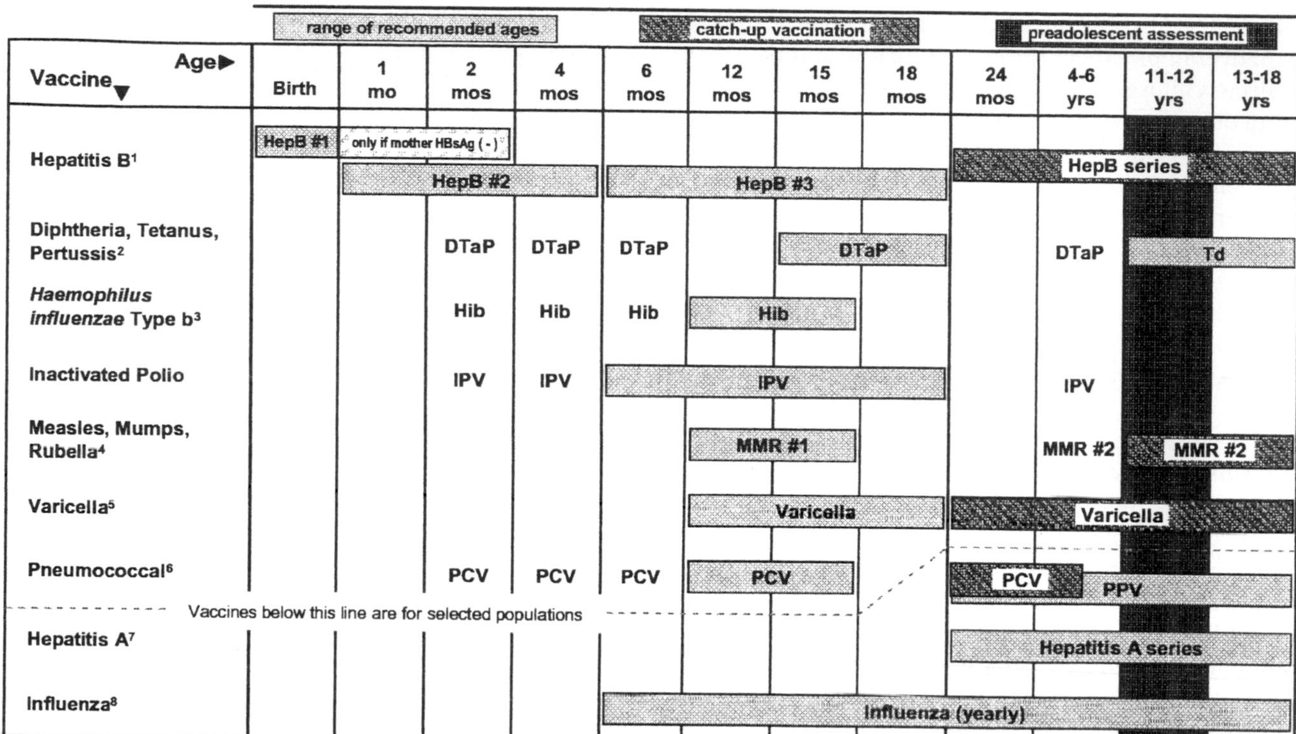

This schedule indicates the recommended ages for routine administration of currently licensed childhood vaccines, as of December 1, 2002, for children through age 18 years. Any dose not given at the recommended age should be given at any subsequent visit when indicated and feasible. ▒ Indicates age groups that warrant special effort to administer those vaccines not previously given. Additional vaccines may be licensed and recommended during the year. Licensed combination vaccines may be used whenever any components of the combination are indicated and the vaccine's other components are not contraindicated. Providers should consult the manufacturers' package inserts for detailed recommendations.

1. Hepatitis B vaccine (HepB). All infants should receive the first dose of hepatitis B vaccine soon after birth and before hospital discharge; the first dose may also be given by age 2 months if the infant's mother is HBsAg-negative. Only monovalent HepB can be used for the birth dose. Monovalent or combination vaccine containing HepB may be used to complete the series. Four doses of vaccine may be administered when a birth dose is given. The second dose should be given at least 4 weeks after the first dose, except for combination vaccines which cannot be administered before age 6 weeks. The third dose should be given at least 16 weeks after the first dose and at least 8 weeks after the second dose. The last dose in the vaccination series (third or fourth dose) should not be administered before age 6 months.

Infants born to HBsAg-positive mothers should receive HepB and 0.5 mL Hepatitis B Immune Globulin (HBIG) within 12 hours of birth at separate sites. The second dose is recommended at age 1-2 months. The last dose in the vaccination series should not be administered before age 6 months. These infants should be tested for HBsAg and anti-HBs at 9-15 months of age.

Infants born to mothers whose HBsAg status is unknown should receive the first dose of the HepB series within 12 hours of birth. Maternal blood should be drawn as soon as possible to determine the mother's HBsAg status; if the HBsAg test is positive, the infant should receive HBIG as soon as possible (no later than age 1 week). The second dose is recommended at age 1-2 months. The last dose in the vaccination series should not be administered before age 6 months.

2. Diphtheria and tetanus toxoids and acellular pertussis vaccine (DTaP). The fourth dose of DTaP may be administered as early as age 12 months, provided 6 months have elapsed since the third dose and the child is unlikely to return at age 15-18 months. **Tetanus and diphtheria toxoids (Td)** is recommended at age 11-12 years if at least 5 years have elapsed since the last dose of tetanus and diphtheria toxoid-containing vaccine. Subsequent routine Td boosters are recommended every 10 years.

3. *Haemophilus influenzae* type b (Hib) conjugate vaccine. Three Hib conjugate vaccines are licensed for infant use. If PRP-OMP (PedvaxHIB® or ComVax® [Merck]) is administered at ages 2 and 4 months, a dose at age 6 months is not required. DTaP/Hib combination products should not be used for primary immunization in infants at ages 2, 4 or 6 months, but can be used as boosters following any Hib vaccine.

4. Measles, mumps, and rubella vaccine (MMR). The second dose of MMR is recommended routinely at age 4-6 years but may be administered during any visit, provided at least 4 weeks have elapsed since the first dose and that both doses are administered beginning at or after age 12 months. Those who have not previously received the second dose should complete the schedule by the 11-12 year old visit.

5. Varicella vaccine. Varicella vaccine is recommended at any visit at or after age 12 months for susceptible children, i.e. those who lack a reliable history of chickenpox. Susceptible persons aged ≥13 years should receive two doses, given at least 4 weeks apart.

6. Pneumococcal vaccine. The heptavalent **pneumococcal conjugate vaccine (PCV)** is recommended for all children age 2-23 months. It is also recommended for certain children age 24-59 months. **Pneumococcal polysaccharide vaccine (PPV)** is recommended in addition to PCV for certain high-risk groups. See *MMWR* 2000;49(RR-9);1-38.

7. Hepatitis A vaccine. Hepatitis A vaccine is recommended for children and adolescents in selected states and regions, and for certain high-risk groups; consult your local public health authority. Children and adolescents in these states, regions, and high risk groups who have not been immunized against hepatitis A can begin the hepatitis A vaccination series during any visit. The two doses in the series should be administered at least 6 months apart. See *MMWR* 1999;48(RR-12);1-37.

8. Influenza vaccine. Influenza vaccine is recommended annually for children age ≥6 months with certain risk factors (including but not limited to asthma, cardiac disease, sickle cell disease, HIV, diabetes, and household members of persons in groups at high risk; see *MMWR* 2002;51(RR-3);1-31), and can be administered to all others wishing to obtain immunity. In addition, healthy children age 6-23 months are encouraged to receive influenza vaccine if feasible because children in this age group are at substantially increased risk for influenza-related hospitalizations. Children aged ≤12 years should receive vaccine in a dosage appropriate for their age (0.25 mL if age 6-35 months or 0.5 mL if aged ≥3 years). Children aged ≤8 years who are receiving influenza vaccine for the first time should receive two doses separated by at least 4 weeks.

For additional information about vaccines, including precautions and contraindications for immunization and vaccine shortages, please visit the National Immunization Program Website at www.cdc.gov/nip or call the National Immunization Information Hotline at 800-232-2522 (English) or 800-232-0233 (Spanish).

Approved by the Advisory Committee on Immunization Practices (www.cdc.gov/nip/acip), the American Academy of Pediatrics (www.aap.org), and the American Academy of Family Physicians (www.aafp.org).

FIGURE 5.1 Recommended childhood and adolescent immunization schedule—United States, 2003.

that helps to focus the physical examination as well as to get an overall picture of the child's current status.

Discuss allergic reactions to any foods, medications, or any other known allergens to prevent the child from receiving any problematic medications or substances. Record medications the child is taking or has taken. In the adolescent, ask questions to assess the use of tobacco, alcohol, and illegal drugs. Other important areas are school and social history as well as personal and nutritional issues.

Collecting Objective Data

The collection of objective data includes the nurse doing a baseline measurement of the child's height, weight, temperature, pulse, respiration, and blood pressure. Data also are collected by examination of the body systems. Often the examination of a child is not done in a head-to-toe manner as in adults but rather in an order that considers the child's age and developmental needs. Aspects of the examination that might be more traumatic or uncomfortable for the child, such as examining the nose or mouth, are saved for last. The procedure of the physical examination may be familiar from previous healthcare visits. If comfortable with helping, the caregiver may be involved with the data collection. For example, he or she might help take a young child's temperature and obtain a urine specimen. Arrangements should be made so that the caregiver also may be present, if possible, for tests or examinations that need to be performed. Included in this initial examination is an inspection of the child's body. All observations are recorded. Carefully document any finding that is not within normal limits and describe in detail any unusual findings.

Nurses conduct or assist with a complete physical examination with special attention to any symptoms that the caregiver has identified. Their primary role in the complete assessment may be to support the child. All the information gathered is used to plan the child's care.

General Status

Use knowledge of normal growth and development to note if the child appears to fit the characteristics of the stated age. Interactions the child has with caregivers and siblings provide information about these relationships. Note the child's overall general appearance, facial expressions, speech, and behavior.

OBSERVING GENERAL APPEARANCE. Observing physical appearance and condition can give clues to the child's overall health. The infant or child's face and body should be symmetrical (i.e., well-balanced). Observe for nutritional status, hygiene, mental alertness, and body posture and movements. Examine the skin for color, lesions, bruises, scars, and birthmarks. Also observe hair texture, thickness, and distribution.

NOTING PSYCHOLOGICAL STATUS AND BEHAVIOR. Carefully observing the child's behavior and recording those observations provide vital clues to a child's condition. Observation of behavior should include factors that influenced the behavior and how often the child repeats it. Note physical behavior as well as emotional and intellectual responses; also consider the child's age and developmental level, the abnormal environment of the healthcare facility, and if the child has been hospitalized previously or otherwise separated from family caregivers. It is important to note if the behavior is consistent or unpredictable and any apparent reasons for changes.

Measuring Height and Weight

The child's height and weight are helpful indicators of growth and development. Measure and record height and weight each time the child has a routine physical examination as well as at other healthcare visits. Chart these measurements and compare them with norms for the child's age. Plotting the child's growth on a growth chart gives a good indication of the child's health status. This process gives a picture of how the child is progressing and often indicates wellness. Although the charts are indicators, the size of other family members, the child's illnesses, general nutritional status, and developmental milestones also must be considered. In a hospital setting, weigh the infant or child at the same time each day on the same scales while wearing the same amount of clothing. Weigh the infant while he or she is nude, lying on an infant scale; when the infant is big enough to sit, the nurse can weigh the child while sitting. Keep a hand within 1 inch of the child at all times to protect against injury. To measure the height of a child who cannot stand alone steadily (usually younger than 2 years), place the child flat, with the knees held flat, on an examining table. Determine height by straightening the infant's body and measuring from the top of the head to the bottom of the foot. Sometimes, nurses make marks on the paper table covering and then measure between the marks. Weigh a child who can stand alone steadily on a platform-type scale and measure for height at the same time.

Measuring Head Circumference

The head circumference is measured routinely in children up to 2 or 3 years or in any child with a neurologic concern. Place a paper or plastic tape measure around the largest part of the head just above the eyebrows and around the most prominent part of the back of the head. Record this measurement and plot it on a growth chart.

Vital Signs

Vital signs, including temperature, pulse, respirations, and blood pressure, are taken at each visit and compared to the normal values for children of the same age as well as to that child's previous recordings. In a hospital setting, monitor closely and record the vital signs; report any changes. Keeping in mind the child's developmental needs will increase the nurse's ability to take accurate vital sign measurements. It usually will be less traumatic for the infant if the nurse counts the respirations before the child is disturbed, then takes the pulse and the temperature.

TEMPERATURE. The policy of the healthcare setting commonly sets the method of measuring a child's temperature. The temperature can be measured by oral, rectal, axillary, or tympanic method. A normal oral temperature range is 97.6°F to 99.3°F (36.4°C to 37.4°C). A rectal temperature is usually 0.5° to 1.0° higher than the oral measurement. An axillary temperature usually measures 0.5° to 1.0° lower than the oral measurement. The temperature measurement taken by the tympanic method is in the same range as the oral method. Report any deviation from the normal range of temperature. It is important to record the method of temperature measurement as well as the measured temperature. In pediatrics, oral temperatures usually are taken only on conscious and cooperative children older than 4 to 6 years. Place the oral thermometer in the side of the child's mouth. Leave no child unattended while taking any temperature.

Many healthcare settings now use tympanic thermometers to measure temperature. The tympanic thermometer records the temperature rapidly (registering in about 2 seconds), is noninvasive, and causes little disturbance to the child.

Rectal temperatures are measured in infants and children younger than 4 to 6 years. They are not desirable in newborns because of the danger of irritation to the rectal mucosa. When taking a rectal temperature, lubricate the end of the thermometer with a water-soluble lubricant.

Axillary temperatures are taken on newborns and on infants and children with diarrhea or when a rectal temperature is contraindicated. Check to ensure that there is skin-to-skin contact with no clothing in the way. Leave the thermometer in place for 10 minutes or until the electronic thermometer signals.

PULSE. Counting an apical rate is the preferred method to determine the pulse in an infant or young child. Try to accomplish this while the child is quiet. The apical pulse should be counted before the child is disturbed for other procedures. A child can be held on the caregiver's lap for security for the full minute that the pulse is counted. A radial pulse may be taken on an older child. Pulse rates vary with age (Table 5.1).

RESPIRATIONS. Respirations of an infant or young child also must be counted during a quiet time. Observe the child while he or she is lying or sitting quietly. Infants are abdominal breathers; therefore, observe the movement of the infant's abdomen to count respirations. Observe the older child's chest much as you would an adult's. The infant's respirations must be counted for a full minute because of normal irregularity. The chest of the infant or young child must be observed for retractions that indicate respiratory distress. Retractions are noted as substernal (below the sternum), subcostal (below the ribs), intercostal (between the ribs), suprasternal (above the sternum), or supraclavicular (above the clavicle) (Fig. 5.2).

TABLE 5.1 NORMAL PULSE RANGES IN CHILDREN

AGE	NORMAL RANGE	AVERAGE
0 to 24 hours	70 to 170 bpm	120 bpm
1 to 7 days	100 to 180 bpm	140 bpm
1 month	110 to 188 bpm	160 bpm
2 months to 1 year	80 to 180 bpm	120 to 130 bpm
2 years	80 to 140 bpm	110 bpm
4 years	80 to 120 bpm	100 bpm
6 years	70 to 115 bpm	100 bpm
10 years	70 to 110 bpm	90 bpm
12 to 14 years	60 to 110 bpm	85 to 90 bpm
15 to 18 years	50 to 95 bpm	70 to 75 bpm

bpm = beats per minute.

BLOOD PRESSURE. For children 3 years and older, blood pressure monitoring is part of routine and ongoing data collection. Children of any age should have a baseline blood pressure taken. It is important to offer the child an

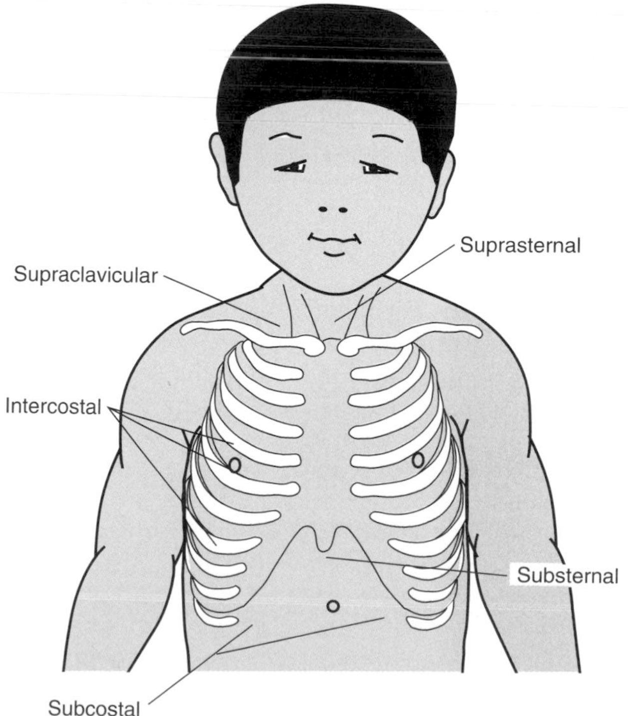

FIGURE 5.2 Sites of respiratory retraction.

explanation of the procedure in understandable terms. Referring to the blood pressure cuff as "giving your arm a hug" will help in the explanation. First taking a blood pressure on a stuffed animal or doll will further show the child the procedure is not one to fear. Obtaining a blood pressure measurement in an infant or small child is difficult, but equipment of the proper size helps ease the problem. The cuff should be wide enough to cover about two thirds of the upper arm and long enough to encircle the upper arm without overlapping. The Doppler method is used with increasing frequency to monitor pediatric blood pressure, but the cuff still must be the correct size. Blood pressures also can be taken using the child's thigh, calf, or ankle.

Conducting a Physical Examination

Data are also collected by examining the child's body systems. Nurses provide or assist the healthcare provider with the physical examination.

HEAD AND NECK. Observe the head's general shape and movement. **Symmetry** or a balance should be noted in the features of the face and in the head. Observe the child's ability to control the head and the range of motion. To see full range of motion, ask the older child to move the head in all directions. In the infant, gently move the head to observe for any stiffness in the neck. Feel the skull to determine if the fontanels are open or closed and to check for any swelling or depression.

Eyes. Observe the eyes for symmetry and location in relationship to the nose. Note any redness, evidence of rubbing, or drainage. Ask the older child to follow a light to observe his or her ability to focus. An infant also will follow a light with his or her eyes. Observe pupils for equality, roundness, and reaction to light. Neurologic considerations are discussed later in this chapter. Routine vision screening is done in school settings. Screening helps identify vision concerns in children; with early detection, appropriate visual aids can be provided.

Ears. Note the alignment of the ears by drawing an imaginary line from the outside corner of the eye to the prominent part of the child's skull; the top of the ear, known as the *pinna,* should cross this line. Ears that are set low often indicate mental retardation. Note the child's ability to hear during normal conversation. A child who speaks loudly, responds inappropriately, or does not speak clearly may have hearing difficulties that should be explored. Note any drainage or swelling.

Nose, Mouth, and Throat. The nose is in the middle of the face. If an imaginary line were drawn down the middle, both sides of the nose should be symmetrical. Flaring of the nostrils might indicate respiratory distress and should be reported immediately. Observe for swelling, drainage, or bleeding. To observe the mouth and throat, have the older child hold the mouth wide open and move the tongue from side to side. With the infant or toddler, use a tongue blade to see the mouth and throat. Gently place the tongue blade on the side of the tongue to hold it down. Observe the mucous membranes for color, moisture, and any patchy areas that might indicate infection. Observe the number and condition of the child's teeth. The lips should be moist and pink. Note any difficulty in swallowing.

CHEST AND LUNGS. Chest measurements are done on infants and children to determine normal growth rate. Take the measurement at the nipple level with a tape measure. Observe the chest for size, shape, movement of the chest with breathing, and any retractions (see respirations in this chapter). In the older school-age child or adolescent, note evidence of breast development. Evaluate respiratory rate, rhythm, and depth. Report any noisy or grunting respirations. Using a stethoscope, listen to breath sounds in each lobe of the lung, anterior and posterior, while the child inhales and exhales. Describe, document, and report absent or diminished breath sounds as well as unusual sounds such as crackling or wheezing. If the child is coughing or bringing up sputum, record its frequency, color, and consistency.

HEART. In some infants and children, a visible pulsation in the chest indicates the heartbeat. This point is called the **point of maximum impulse** (PMI) and is where the heartbeat can be heard the best with a stethoscope. Listen for the rhythm of the heart sounds and count the rate for 1 full minute. Abnormal or unusual heart sounds or irregular rhythms might indicate the child has a heart murmur, heart condition, or other abnormality that should be reported. The heart is responsible for circulating blood to the body. To determine the heart function's effectiveness, assess the pulses in various parts of the body (see Ch. 24).

ABDOMEN. The abdomen may protrude slightly in infants and small children. To describe the abdomen, divide the area into four sections and label them with the terms left upper quadrant (LUQ), left lower quadrant (LLQ), right upper quadrant (RUQ), and right lower quadrant (RLQ). Using a stethoscope, listen for bowel sounds or evidence of peristalsis in each section and record what you hear. Observe the umbilicus for cleanliness and any abnormalities. Infants and young children sometimes have protrusions in the umbilicus or inguinal canal called hernias. Report a tense or firm abdomen or unusual tenderness.

GENITALIA AND RECTUM. When inspecting the genitalia and rectum, it is important to respect the child's privacy and consider the child's age and stage of growth and development. Keeping the child covered as much as possible is important. While wearing gloves, inspect the genitalia and rectum. Observe the area for any sores or lesions, swelling, or discharge. In male children, the testes descend at varying times during childhood; if the testes are not palpable, report this information. Be aware that *unusual findings,* such as bruises in soft tissue or with a clear outline of an object, or unexplained injuries might indicate child abuse and require further investigation (see Chap. 7).

BACK AND EXTREMITIES. Observe the back for symmetry and curvature of the spine. In infants the spine is rounded and flexible. As the child grows and develops motor skills, the spine further develops. Screening is done in school-age children to detect abnormal curvatures such as scoliosis. Note gait and posture when the child enters or is walking in the room. The extremities should be warm, have good color, and be symmetrical. By observing the child's movements during the examination, note range of motion, movement of the joints, and muscle strength. In infants, examine the hips and report any dislocation or asymmetry of gluteal skin folds. These could indicate a congenital hip dislocation.

NEUROLOGIC. Assessing neurologic status of the infant and child is the most complex aspect of the physical examination. All the body systems function in relationship to the nervous system. Practitioners in the healthcare setting assess the neurologic status of the child by doing a complete neurological examination, which includes detailed examination of the reflex responses as well as the functioning of each of the cranial nerves. Nurses often are responsible for using neurologic assessment tools to monitor a child's neurologic status following the initial neurologic examination. They use a neurologic assessment tool such as the Glasgow Coma Scale for this (see Chap. 38). Use of a standard scale permits the comparison of results from one time to another and from one examiner to another.

HOSPITALIZED CHILD

Caring for the hospitalized child requires an understanding of many different aspects of the pediatric unit. Additional considerations include infection control, caregiver participation, the child undergoing surgery, and the need for play and activities on the unit. Children often are cared for in the home, but in some cases may be hospitalized for serious illness, surgery, or treatment that cannot be done in the home setting.

Pediatric Unit

An effort by pediatric units and hospitals to create friendly, warm surroundings for children has produced many attractive pediatric settings. Walls and curtains are colorful; furniture is attractive, appropriate in size, and designed with safety in mind. Staff members on the pediatric unit often wear colorful uniforms and encourage children to wear their own clothing or colorful printed pajamas.

Treatments are performed in a treatment room, not in the child's room, to promote the concept that the child's bed is a "safe" place. A playroom or play area is a vital part of all pediatric units and should be a place safe from all procedures. Some hospitals provide a person trained in therapeutic play to coordinate and direct the play activities.

Most pediatric settings provide rooming-in facilities (where the caregiver can stay in the room with the child) and encourage parents or family caregivers to visit as frequently as possible. This helps minimize the separation anxiety of the young child in particular. Caregivers are involved in much of the young child's care to provide comfort and reassurance. As much as possible, the same nurse cares for the child, thus giving him or her the opportunity to establish a trusting relationship with the child.

Planning meals that include the child's favorite foods, within the limitations of any special dietary restrictions, may perk up a poor appetite. When space permits, several children may eat together at a small table. Younger children can be seated in high chairs or other suitable seats and should be supervised by an adult. Meals should be served out of bed, if possible, and in a pleasant atmosphere.

Infection Control

Infection control is important in the pediatric setting, as it is in any healthcare setting. The ill child may be especially vulnerable to pathogenic (disease-carrying) microorganisms and contagious diseases. 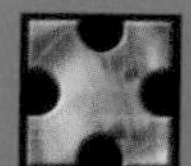 Precautions must be taken to prevent the spread of microorganisms and to protect children, families, and personnel (Client and Family Teaching 5-1).

5-1 *Client and Family Teaching*
Preventing Infections

The nurse teaches the client and family as follows:

- Cover your mouth when coughing or sneezing.
- Throw away tissues used for nose blowing.
- Wipe carefully after bowel movements (girls wipe front to back).
- Wash hands after going to bathroom or blowing your nose.
- Wash hands before eating.
- Do not share food that you've partly eaten.
- If food or an eating utensil falls on the floor, wash it right away.
- Do not drink from another person's cup.
- Do not share a toothbrush with someone else.

Standard precautions are geared toward reducing the risk of transmission of microorganisms. Transmission-based precautions pertain to clients documented or suspected to have highly transmissible or other pathogens that require additional precautions. Handwashing is the cornerstone of all infection control. Wash your hands between seeing each client, even when wearing gloves for a procedure. Gowns and masks often are used to decrease the spread of infection, and caregivers may need to have precaution measures reviewed including handwashing, gowning, and masking as necessary. Gloves prevent the child from experiencing skin-to-skin contact; explain at the child's level of understanding why gloves are necessary.

The child who is segregated by transmission-based precautions is subject to social isolation and may have feelings of loneliness and depression. Work to try to reduce these feelings by spending extra time in the room when performing treatments and procedures. Encourage family caregivers to spend time with the child, as well as encouraging communication with friends and siblings.

Stop, Think, and Respond ● BOX 5-2

What are some characteristics of pediatric units that make them appealing and comfortable for children?

Caregiver Participation

Research has shown that separating young children from their family caregivers, especially during times of stress, may have damaging effects. Because young children have no concept of time, separation is especially difficult for them. Three characteristic stages of response to separation have been identified: protest, despair, and denial. During *protest,* the first stage, the young child cries, often refuses to be comforted by others, and seeks the primary caregiver at every sight and sound. When the caregiver does not appear, the child enters the second stage—*despair*—and becomes apathetic and listless. Healthcare personnel often interpret this as a sign that the child is accepting the situation, but this is not the case; the child has given up. In the third stage—*denial*—the child begins taking interest in the surroundings and appears to accept the situation. The damage is revealed, however, when the caregivers do visit: the child often turns away from them, showing distrust and rejection. It may take a long time before the child accepts them again, and even then remnants of the damage linger. The child may always have a memory of being abandoned at the hospital. Regardless of how mistaken they may be, childhood impressions have a deep effect.

Encouraging the caregiver to participate and to stay with the child helps remove the young hospitalized child's hurt and depression. Although separation from primary caregivers is thought to cause the greatest upset in children younger than 5 years, children of all ages feel more secure as a result of the caregiver's attention and involvement. The caregiver may participate in many aspects of care and treatments. Special chairs or beds in the child's room add to the caregiver's comfort. The caregiver's basic role is to provide security and stability for the child, and nursing staff should be careful to avoid creating a situation in which they appear to expect primary caregivers to perform as healthcare technicians. It is important to encourage caregivers to take a break, leave for a meal, or occasionally go home, if possible, for a shower and rest. When the caregiver leaves, the child needs a familiar frame of reference to understand when something is going to happen. For example, the parent or caregiver may say, "I will be back when your lunch comes" or "I will be back when the cartoons come on TV." Explaining that it is time for "Mommy and Daddy to go to work" might help an unhappy child realize that the parent or caregiver is not leaving because of any negative behavior of the child's. Many pediatric units also have recognized the importance of allowing siblings to visit the ill child. This policy benefits both the ill child and the sibling.

Child Undergoing Surgery

Surgery may be frightening to children because they may not understand why it is necessary and how it will help them. If properly prepared, older children and adolescents are capable of understanding the need for surgery and what it will accomplish. Outpatient surgery facilities are used for minor procedures and permit clients to return home the day of the operation, which helps reduce the separation of parents and children, one of the most stressful factors in surgery for children.

Preoperative care and teaching are important. With young children, direct explanations to family caregivers help to relieve their anxiety and to prepare them to participate in the child's care after surgery. Preparation varies according to the type of surgery planned and may include client teaching, skin preparation, preparation of the gastrointestinal system, and preoperative medication. The health professionals involved in the child's care must determine how much the child and family knows and is capable of learning, help correct any misunderstandings, explain the preparation for surgery and what the surgery will "fix," and how the child will feel after surgery. This preparation may be done prior to admission and must be based on the child's age, developmental level, previous experiences, and caregiver support. Explanations should be clear and honest and expressed in terms the child and the family caregivers can understand.

Therapeutic play, discussed later in this chapter, is useful in preparing the child for surgery. Using drawings to identify the area of the body to be operated on helps the child have a better understanding of what will happen.

Children need to be prepared for standard preoperative tests and procedures. Explain the reason for withholding food and fluids before surgery so children do not feel they are being neglected or punished when others receive meal trays.

Children sometimes interpret surgery as punishment. Reassure them that they did not cause the condition. Children also fear mutilation or death and must be able to explore those feelings. It is important to emphasize that the child will not feel anything during surgery because of the special sleep that anesthesia causes. Describing the postanesthesia care unit (PACU or wake-up room) and any tubes, bandages, or appliances that will be in place after surgery lets the child know what to expect.

Role playing, adjusted to the child's age and understanding, is helpful. This approach may include a trip on a stretcher and pretending to go to surgery.

The older child or adolescent may have a greater interest in the surgery itself, what is wrong and why, how the repair is done, and the expected postoperative results. Models or drawings of a child's internal organs or individual organs, such as a heart, are useful for demonstration.

A child needs to understand that several people will be involved in preoperative, surgical, and postoperative care; if possible, these staff members should visit the child preoperatively. Explaining what the people will be wearing (caps, masks, and gloves) and what equipment will be used (including bright lights) helps make the operating room experience less frightening. A preoperative tour of the ICU or PACU is also helpful.

Children should be prepared for postoperative pain. They need to know when they may expect to be allowed to have fluids and food after surgery. Children should be taught to practice coughing and deep-breathing exercises. Using games that encourage blowing makes this exercise fun. Teaching children to splint the operative site with a pillow helps reassure them that the sutures will not break and allow the wound to open.

Tell children where their family will be during and after surgery, and make every effort to minimize separation. Encourage family caregivers to be present when the child leaves for the operating room.

A cleansing enema the night before surgery may be ordered. An enema is an intrusive procedure and must be explained to the child before it is given. If old enough, the child should understand the reason for the enema.

Children usually receive nothing by mouth (NPO) 4 to 12 hours before surgery to decrease the chances of vomiting and aspiration, particularly during general anesthesia. Explain to the child that food and drink are being withheld to prevent an upset stomach. The NPO period varies according to the child's age. Infants become dehydrated more rapidly than older children and thus require a shorter NPO period before surgery. Intravenous (IV) fluids usually are started when the child is NPO. Loose teeth are a potential hazard; count and record them according to hospital policy.

Preoperative medications may be given in two stages: a sedative, administered about 1.5 to 2 hours before surgery, and an analgesic–atropine mixture administered immediately before the client leaves for the operating room. When the sedative has been given, dim the lights and minimize noise to help the child relax and rest. Family caregivers and the child should be aware that atropine could cause a blotchy rash and a flushed face.

Family caregivers sometimes can accompany the child to the operating room and wait until the child is anesthetized.

During the immediate postoperative period, the child is cared for in the PACU or the surgical ICU. When the child returns to his or her room, nursing care focuses on careful observation for any signs or symptoms of complications. Monitor and record vital signs. Note and observe dressings, IV apparatus and sites, urinary catheters, and any other appliances. Also monitor intake and output closely. The first voiding is important in the child postoperatively to monitor for urinary retention. Note, record, and report the voiding. Notify the provider if anuria (absence of urine) persists longer than 6 hours.

Postoperative orders may provide for ice chips or clear liquids to prevent dehydration; administer them with a spoon or in a small medicine cup.

As with all procedures, explain to the child what will be done and why before beginning the dressing change. Some dressing changes are painful; if so, tell the child that it will hurt and praise him or her for behavior that shows courage and cooperation.

Postoperative teaching is as important as preoperative teaching. Repeat some explanations and instructions given earlier during postoperative care because the child's earlier anxiety may have prevented thorough understanding. Now that tubes, restraints, and dressings are part of the child's reality, they need discussion again: why they are important and how they affect the child's activities.

Family caregivers want to know how they can help care for the child and what limitations are placed on the child's activity. If caregivers know what to expect and how to aid in their child's recovery, they will be cooperative during the postoperative period.

As the child recuperates, encourage caregivers and child to share their feelings about the surgery, any changes in body image, and their expectations for recovery and rehabilitation.

When the sutures are removed, reassure the child that the opening has healed and the child's insides will not "fall out," which is a common fear.

Before the child is discharged from the hospital, teaching focuses on home care, use of any special equipment or appliances, medications, diet, restrictions on activities, and therapeutic exercise. Caregivers should demonstrate the procedures or repeat information so the nurse can determine if learning has occurred.

Play

Play is the business of children and a principal way in which they learn, grow, develop, and act out feelings and problems. Playing is a normal activity; when it is a part of hospital care, the child will be more comfortable and secure. In the hospital playroom, children may express their feelings through play without the fear of being scolded. Children, however, must not be allowed to harm themselves or others.

An organized and well-planned play area is considerably important to the overall care of the hospitalized child. It should provide a variety of play materials suitable for the ages and needs of all children. If possible, adolescents should have a separate recreation room or area. Although a well-equipped playroom is of major importance in any pediatric department, some children cannot be brought to the playroom. In these situations, nurses must be creative in providing play opportunities for children and bring materials to their rooms. Children in isolation may be given play material, providing infection control precautions are strictly followed.

Nurses must understand the difference between play therapy and therapeutic play. *Play therapy* is a technique of psychoanalysis used to uncover a disturbed child's underlying thoughts, feelings, and motivations to help understand them better. The therapist might have the child act out experiences using dolls as the participants in the experience. **Therapeutic play** is a play technique that may be used to help the child have a better understanding of what will be happening to them in a specific situation. For instance, the child who will be having an IV started before surgery might be given the materials and encouraged to "start" an IV on a stuffed animal or doll. By observing the child, the nurse can often note concerns, fears and anxieties the child might express.

Nurses choose play material with safety in mind; there should be no sharp edges and no small parts that can be swallowed or aspirated. They inspect toys and equipment regularly for broken parts or sharp edges. Constant supervision of children while they are playing is necessary for safety.

One important playroom function is that it gives the child opportunities to dramatize hospital experiences. One section of the playroom containing hospital equipment, miniature or real, gives the child an opportunity to act out feelings about the hospital environment and treatments. Stethoscopes, simulated thermometers, stretchers, wheelchairs, examining tables, instruments, bandages, and other medical and hospital equipment are useful for this purpose.

Dolls or puppets can be dressed to represent the people with whom the child comes in contact, including nurses and hospital staff. Hospital scrub suits, scrub caps, isolation-type gowns, masks, or other types of uniforms may be provided for children to use in acting out their hospital experiences. These simulated hospitals also serve an educational purpose: they may help a child who is to have surgery, tests, or special treatments to understand the procedures and why they are done. Books and other materials allow the child to be creative as well as entertained. Sometimes only a little imagination is needed to initiate an interesting playtime.

ASSISTING WITH BASIC NEEDS

Nutrition

Measuring intake and assisting with specialized feeding methods (including gavage and gastrostomy feedings) are important roles of the pediatric nurse. The nutritional needs of and variations in each age and stage of growth and development are discussed in Chapter 6.

Intake Measurement

Accurately measuring and recording intake and output are especially important in working with ill or hospitalized children. In many settings, nurses record these measurements as often as every hour and keep a running total to closely monitor the child. They measure and record oral fluids, feeding tube intake, IV fluids, and foods that become liquid at room temperature.

Gavage Feeding

Sometimes infants or children who have had surgery or have a chronic or serious condition cannot take adequate food and fluid by mouth and must receive nourishment by gavage feeding. Gavage feedings provide nourishment directly through a tube passed into the stomach. This procedure is particularly appropriate for infants. A feeding syringe is inserted into the tube, and the feeding, which has been warmed to room temperature, is allowed to flow by gravity. The entire feeding takes 15 to 20 minutes, after which the infant must be burped and positioned on the right side for at least 1 hour to prevent regurgitation and aspiration. Following the feeding, if the tube will be left in position for further use, it should be secured to the infant's nose using adhesive tape. The correct position of the tube must be verified before each feeding.

Gastrostomy Feeding

Children who must receive tube feedings over a long period may have a gastrostomy tube surgically inserted through the abdominal wall into the stomach. It also is used in children who have obstructions or surgical repairs in the mouth, pharynx, esophagus, or cardiac sphincter of the stomach or who are respirator-dependent. The child may need to be restrained to prevent pulling on the tube, which may cause leakage of caustic gastric juices. When regular oral feedings are resumed, the tube is surgically removed, and the opening usually closes spontaneously.

For long-term gastrostomy feedings, a gastrostomy button may be inserted. Some advantages of buttons are that they are more desirable cosmetically, are simple to care for, and cause less skin irritation.

Safety

Accidents involving motor vehicles, aspiration, suffocation, ingestion of toxic substances, drowning, and burns are the most common causes of death in children. Discussing safety issues and providing information for caregivers are important. Older children in the family should learn to be watchful for possible dangers to infants, and caregivers must be alert to potential dangers that siblings may introduce, such as unsafe toys, rough play, or jealous harmful behavior. A child's curiosity often exceeds his or her judgment. All children should know their full name, home address and telephone number, and caregivers' names. Children should learn the appropriate way to call for emergency help. A pediatric nurse can include safety and accident prevention teaching in any discussion with children and family caregivers. See Client and Family Teaching 5-2.

Pain Management

Pain is a concern for all clients. Infants and young children cannot adequately express themselves and need help to tell where or how great pain is. Longstanding beliefs that children do not have the same amount of pain that adults have, and that they tolerate pain better than adults have contributed to undermedicating infants and children in pain. Research has shown that infants and children do experience pain (Gallo, 2003).

Be alert to indications of pain, especially in young clients. Careful assessment is necessary—for example, noting changes in behavior such as rigidity, thrashing, facial expressions, loud crying or screaming, flexion of knees (indicating abdominal pain), restlessness, and irritability. Physiologic changes, such as increased pulse rate and blood pressure, sweating palms, dilated pupils, flushed or moist skin, and loss of appetite, also may indicate pain. Some children may try to hide pain because they fear an injection or are afraid that admitting to pain will increase the time they have to stay in the hospital.

Various tools have been devised to help children express the amount of pain they feel and allow nurses to measure the effectiveness of pain management efforts. These tools include the numeric scale, the FACES pain rating scale, and the color scale. The numeric scale is used primarily with children 7 years of age and older. The FACES scale is used for those 3 years of age and older. To use the color scale, the young child is given crayons ranging from yellow to red or black. Yellow represents no pain, and the darkest color (or red) represents the most pain. The child selects the color that represents the amount of pain felt.

Pain medication may be administered orally, intramuscularly, or by IV routes, including patient-controlled analgesia (PCA), a programmed IV infusion of narcotic analgesia that the child may control within set limits. Patient-controlled analgesia may be used for children 7 years of age or older who have no cognitive impairment and undergo a careful evaluation. Intramuscular injections are avoided if possible, since injections can be traumatic and painful for the child. Monitor the child's vital signs and document level of consciousness frequently following the standards of the facility when administering pain medications.

Nurses should use comfort measures along with the administration of analgesics. Encouraging the child to become involved in activities that may provide distraction is important. Such activities must be appropriate for the child's age, level of development, and interests. No child should be allowed to suffer pain unnecessarily. Appropriate nonpharmacologic comfort measures may include position changes, massage, distraction, play, soothing touch, talk, coddling, and affection.

Oxygenation

Oxygen is administered to treat symptoms of respiratory distress or when the oxygen saturation level in the blood is below normal. Depending on the child's age and oxygen needs, many different methods are used for delivery. The infant often receives oxygen while in an isolette or incubator. Infants as well as older children might have oxygen administered by nasal cannula or prongs, mask, or via an oxygen hood (Table 5.2). Oxygen tents also may be used to deliver oxygen. An advantage of using an oxygen tent for the toddler and school-age child is that no device has to be put over the child's nose or face. The oxygen concentration is more difficult to maintain in the tent because it is opened many times throughout the day. The tent is frightening to children, so they must be reassured frequently. Whatever equipment is used to administer oxygen, explain the procedure and equipment to the child and caregiver. Letting the child hold and feel the equipment and flow of oxygen through the device helps decrease the child's fear and anxiety about the procedure. The device warms and humidifies oxygen to prevent the recipient's nasal passages from becoming dry. Closely monitor children receiving oxygen therapy; when

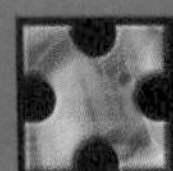

5-2 *Client and Family Teaching* Accident Prevention

The nurse teaches the client and family as follows:

Motor Vehicle Accidents

- Place infant in an approved car carrier when in the car.
- Start the car only when children and passengers are securely in the car seat or seat belt.
- Never permit a child to stand in a car that is in motion.
- Obey traffic signals and safe pedestrian practices; stop at a curb, look both ways for traffic, cross at corners or crosswalks, escort child across street.
- Teach children to never play behind a car or truck or run into the street after a ball.
- Teach children never to walk between parked cars to cross.
- Be alert for children running into the street when driving in a residential area.
- When riding a bicycle, wear a helmet, use hand signals, ride with traffic, not against it, and ride as far to the right as possible.
- Stop at all stop signs and red lights.
- Don't ride when it's dark, and if riding at dusk, dawn, or in the evening, wear reflective material on clothing or bike and use lights on the bike.
- Wear a helmet and elbow and knee pads when skating or riding a skateboard or scooter.

Aspiration/Suffocation

- Crib and playpen bars should be spaced less than $2\frac{1}{2}$ inches apart.
- Choose toys carefully; watch for loose or sharp parts and avoid small buttons or parts that can come off.
- Check toys for toxic material.
- Close safety pins and keep out of infant's reach.
- Keep plastic bags out of child's reach.

Poisoning

- Move all toxic substances (cleaning fluids, detergents, insecticides) out of reach and keep them locked up.
- Remove any houseplants that may be poisonous.
- Protect infant from inhaling lead paint dust (from remodeling) or chewing on surfaces painted with lead paint.
- Place medicines in locked cupboards; don't rely on a high shelf being out of a child's reach; remind family and friends to do the same.
- Take only medicine that your caregiver gives you.
- Keep medicines in their original containers in a locked cupboard; never refer to medicines as candy.
- Discard unused medicines by a method that eliminates any possibility of access by children, other persons, or animals (e.g., flush them down the toilet).
- Replace safety caps properly, but do not depend on them to be childproof, children can sometimes open them more easily than adults can.
- Keep a bottle of syrup of ipecac in a locked cupboard to induce vomiting if recommended by the poison control center.
- Keep the telephone number of the nearest poison control center posted near the telephone.
- Keep a chart with emergency treatment for poisoning in a handy permanent spot.
- Never put kerosene or other household fluids in soda bottles or other drink containers.

Drowning

- Never leave infant alone in the bath or in the bathroom.
- Teach children not to run near a swimming pool.
- Teach children to swim.
- Always swim with someone else, only let children swim with an adult.
- Always know the water depth.
- Don't dive headfirst.
- Use a life jacket when boating.

Burns

- Turn household hot water to a safe temperature—120°F (48.8°C).
- Supervise small children at all times in the bathtub.
- Teach children to never play with matches or lighters.
- Place matches in metal containers and lighters out of reach of children.
- Teach children to stay away from fires.
- Cover electrical wall outlets with safety caps.
- Keep electrical cords out of sight; don't let electrical cords dangle over a counter or table; repair frayed cords.
- Turn handles of pans on the stove toward the back of the stove; place pans on back burners out of the child's reach.
- Place cups of hot liquid out of reach; do not use overhanging tablecloths that children can pull.
- Use caution when serving foods heated in the microwave; they can be hotter than is apparent.

TABLE 5.2 METHODS OF OXYGEN ADMINISTRATION

METHOD	AGE OR REASON TO USE	NURSING CONCERNS WHEN USING
Isolette/Incubator	Newborn or infant	
Nasal prongs/cannula	Many sizes available Nasal prongs fit into child's nose Toddlers may pull out of nose, other method better	Not humidified; causes dryness Keep nasal prongs clean and clear of secretions Monitor nostrils for irritation
Mask	Various sizes available Covers mouth and nose, not eyes Humidified; decreases dryness	Not used in comatose children
Hood	Fits over head and neck of child Clear so child can be seen	May be frightening for child
Oxygen tent/croupette	Equipment does not come in contact with face Allows for movement inside tent	Difficult to see child in tent Difficult for child to see out Child feels isolated Change clothing and linen often Keep side rails up
Tracheostomy	Used in emergencies or when long-term oxygen is needed	Must be kept clean with airway patent Suction when needed

oxygen is to be discontinued, it is done gradually. Exposure to high concentrations of oxygen can be dangerous to small infants and children with other respiratory diseases. Many times children are cared for in a home setting while on oxygen. Teach the family caregiver regarding oxygen administration, equipment, and safety measures (Client and Family Teaching 5-3).

Elimination

Output Measurement

Accurately measuring and recording intake and output are especially important in working with the ill or hospitalized child. In many settings nurses record these measurements as often as every hour and keep a running total to closely monitor the child.

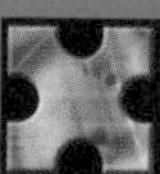

5-3 *Client and Family Teaching* Oxygen Safety

The nurse teaches the client and family as follows:

- Keep equipment clean; dirty equipment can be a source of bacteria.
- Use signs noting that oxygen is in use.
- Give good mouth care; use swabs and mouthwash.
- Offer fluids frequently.
- Keep nose clean.
- Don't use electric or battery-powered toys.
- Don't allow smoking, matches, or lighters nearby.
- Don't keep flammable solutions in room.
- Don't use wool or synthetic blankets.

Measure urine, vomitus, diarrhea, gastric suctioning, and any other liquid drainage, all of which are considered output. Describe and record the color and characteristics of the output.

To measure the output of an infant wearing a diaper, weigh the wet diaper and subtract the weight of the dry diaper before recording the amount. To monitor the intake and output, collect and measure all urine whether voided into a diaper, urinal, bedpan, or toilet collection device.

Specimen Collection

Urine is collected for various reasons; nurses can use several methods to obtain specimens. They can place cotton balls in the diaper of an infant; they can collect and use the urine squeezed from the cotton ball for many urine tests. Because toddlers and young children cannot usually void on command, offer them fluids 15 to 20 minutes before the urine specimen is needed. When requesting a specimen, use the word the child knows to identify urination, such as "pee-pee" or "potty," so the child will understand. Offering privacy to the older child and adolescent is important when obtaining a urine specimen. In preparation for collecting a urine specimen, position the infant or child so that the genitalia are exposed and the area can be cleansed.

To collect a urine specimen from infants and toddlers who are not potty trained, nurses use a pediatric urine collection bag (Fig. 5.3). The device is a small, plastic bag with a self-adhesive material to apply it to the child's skin. For the collection bag to stay in place, the skin must be clean, dry, and free of lotions, oils, and powder. Remove the paper backing from the urine collection container and apply the adhesive surface over the penis in the male and the vulva in the female. Replace the child's diaper. Remove the collection device as soon as the child voids.

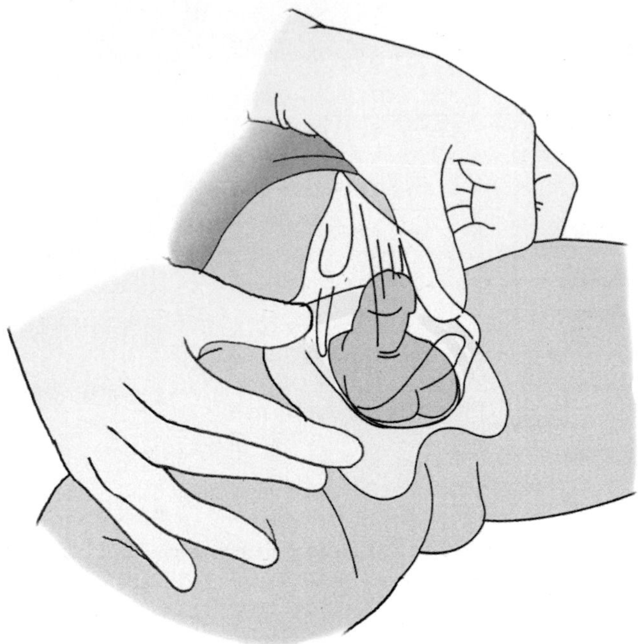

Figure 5.3 The skin must be clean and dry in order for the urine collection bag to adhere to the child's skin.

If a urine specimen is needed for a culture, the older child may be able to cooperate in the collection of a midstream specimen. Instruct the child as to the procedure and clean the genital area. The child urinates a small amount, stops the flow, and then continues to void into a specimen container.

Occasionally children must be catheterized to obtain a specimen, particularly if a sterile specimen is required. If the catheter is needed only to get a specimen, often a small sterile feeding tube is used.

Positioning

Safety is the nurse's most important responsibility when performing procedures related to positioning such as using restraints, transporting, holding, or positioning children for sleep.

Restraints

Restraints often are needed to protect a child from injury during a procedure or an examination or to ensure the infant's or child's safety and comfort. Restraints should never be used as a form of punishment. Nurses must follow the procedure for the healthcare setting when using restraints. Many settings require a written order and have a set procedure of releasing the restraint at least every 2 hours and documenting this. When possible, restraining by hand is the best method. Mechanical restraints must be used to secure a child during IV infusions, to protect a surgical site from injury such as cleft lip and cleft palate, or when restraint by hand is impractical.

Various types of restraints may be used (Fig. 5.4). Whatever the type of restraint, however, caution is essential. Close and conscientious observation is a necessary part of nursing care. Also be alert to family concerns when the child is in restraints. Explanations about the need for restraints will help the family understand and be cooperative. The caregiver may wish to restrain the child physically to prevent use of restraints, and this action is often possible.

MUMMY RESTRAINTS AND PAPOOSE BOARDS. Mummy restraints are used for an infant or small child during a procedure. This device is a snug wrap that is effective when performing procedures that involve only the head or neck. Papoose boards are used with toddlers or preschoolers.

CLOVE HITCH RESTRAINTS. These are used to secure an arm or leg, most often when a child is receiving an IV infusion. They are made of soft cloth formed in a figure eight. Padding under the restraint is desirable if the child puts any pull on it. Check and loosen the site at least every 2 hours. Commercial restraints also are available for this purpose. This restraint should be secured to the lower part of the crib or bed, not to the side rail, to avoid possibly causing injury when the side rail is raised or lowered.

ELBOW RESTRAINTS. Elbow restraints often are made of muslin in two layers. Pockets wide enough to hold tongue depressors are placed vertically in the width of the fabric. The top flap folds over to close the pockets. The restraint is wrapped around the child's arm and tied securely to prevent the child from bending the elbow. Care must be taken that the elbow restraints fit the child properly. They should not be too high under the axillae. They may be pinned to the child's shirt to keep them from slipping. Commercially made elbow restraints also may be used.

JACKET RESTRAINTS. Jacket restraints are used to secure the child from climbing out of bed or a chair or to keep the child in a horizontal position. The restraint must be the correct size for the child. Check the child in a jacket restraint frequently to prevent him or her from slipping and choking on the neck of the jacket. Ties must be secure to the bed frame, not the sides, so that the jacket is not pulled when the sides are moved up and down.

Transporting

When moving infants and small children in a healthcare setting, the safety of the child is the biggest concern. It is best to carry the infant or place him or her in a crib or bassinet. Often, pediatric settings use wagons to transport children; the wagon ride is functional as well as enjoyable for the child. The toddler may be transported in a crib with high siderails or a high-topped crib. Strollers or wheelchairs are used when the child can sit. Older children are

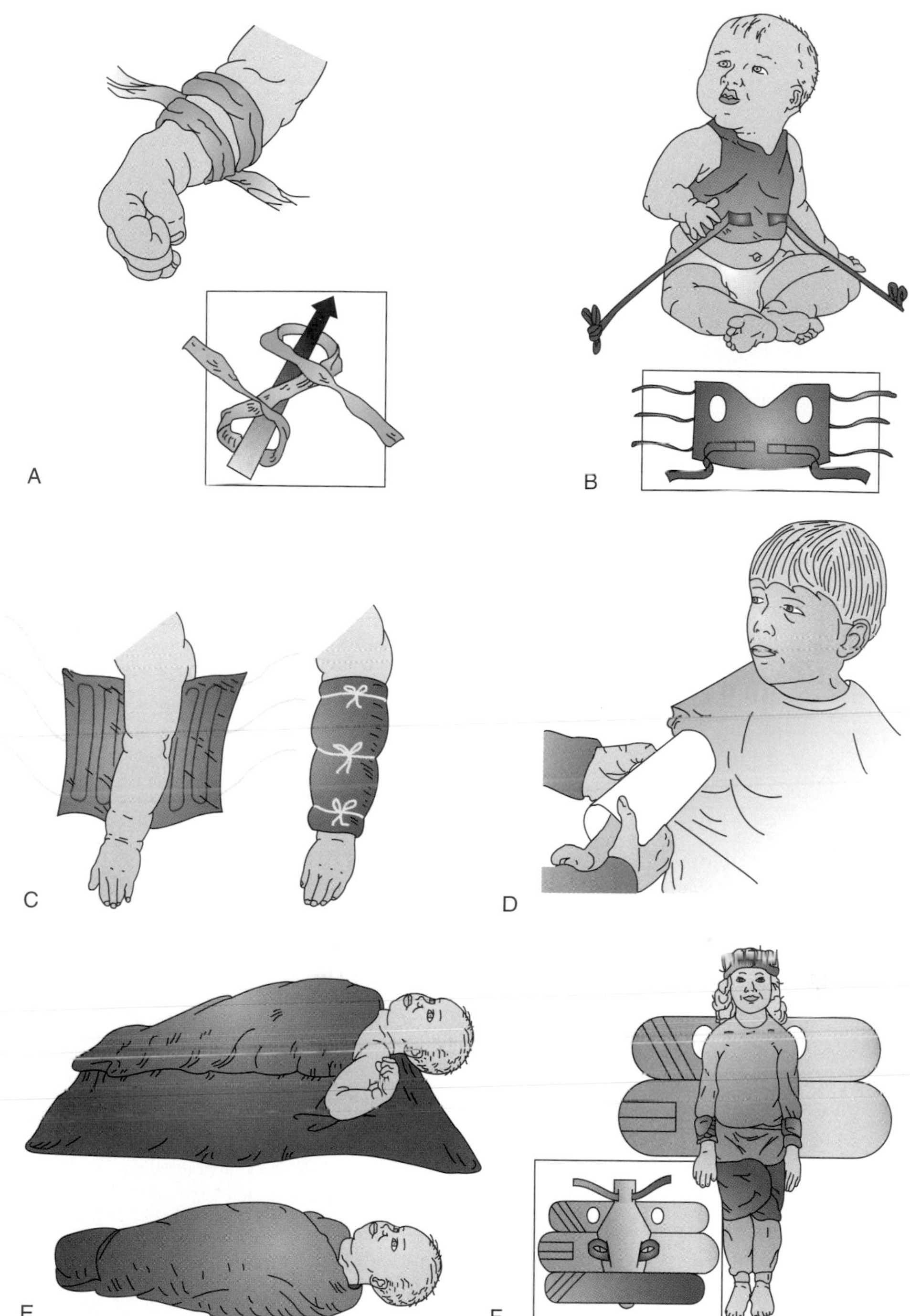

FIGURE 5.4 (**A**) Clove hitch restraint. (**B**) Jacket restraint. (**C**) Elbow restraint. (**D**) Commercial elbow restraint. (**E**) Mummy restraint. (**F**) Papoose board.

placed on stretchers or may be moved in their beds. Seat belts or safety straps should be used when the child is being transported using a wagon, stroller, wheelchair or stretcher. Often a hospitalized child who is in traction, which cannot be removed, can go to the playroom or other areas in the hospital in this manner.

Holding

When holding a child, it is most important to be sure the child is safe and feels secure. The three most common methods of holding are the horizontal position, upright position, and football hold (Fig. 5.5). When holding an infant, always support the head and back. During and after feedings, nurses sometimes hold the infant to be burped in a sitting position on the lap. The infant should lean forward against the nurse's hand while the nurse's thumb and finger support the infant's head. This leaves the other hand free to gently pat the infant's back.

Sleeping

Infants should be positioned on their backs or supported on their sides for sleeping. The nurse working with family

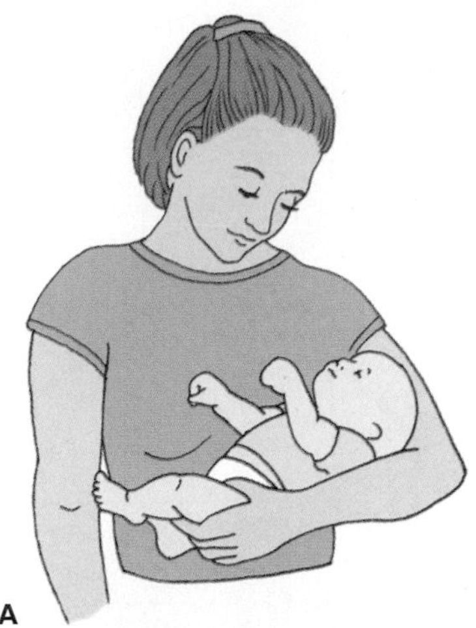

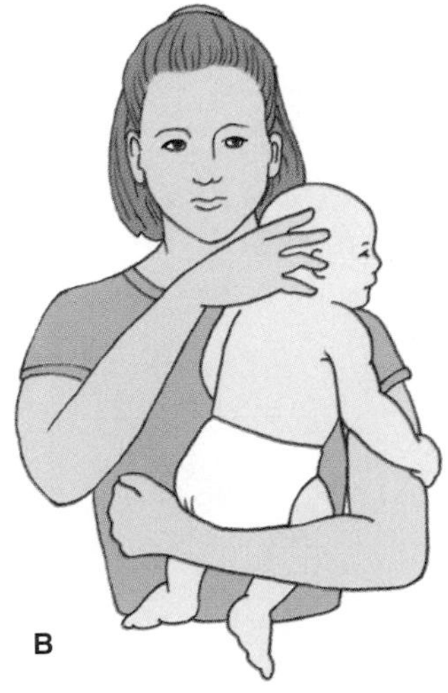

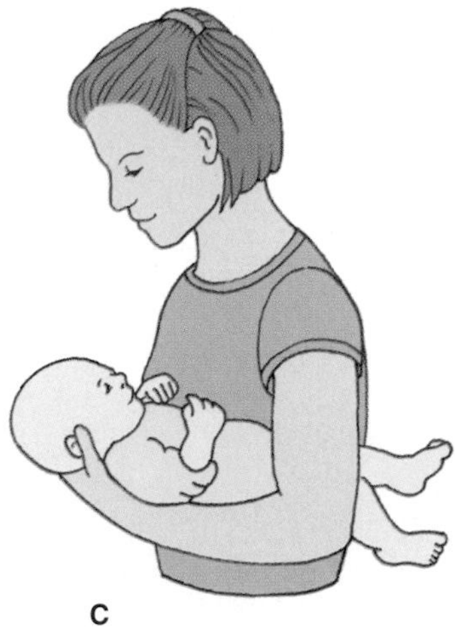

FIGURE 5.5 Positions to hold an infant or child: (**A**) horizontal position, (**B**) upright position, (**C**) football hold.

caregivers teaches and reinforces this information. These positions seem to have decreased the incidence of crib death or SIDS in infants (Carroll & Loughlin, 1999).

MEDICATION ADMINISTRATION

Administering medications is one of the most important pediatric nursing responsibilities, calling for accuracy, precision, and considerable psychological skill. Accurate administration of medications to children is especially critical because of the variable responses to drugs that children have as a result of immature body systems. Understand the factors that influence or alter how the child absorbs, metabolizes, and excretes the medication, and any allergies that the child has. It is also important to teach the client and family caregivers about the effects and possible side effects of medications.

Rules to guide the nurse in administering medications are presented in Box 5-1. Evaluate each child from a developmental point of view to administer medications successfully. Always calculate the drug dosage to ensure administration of the correct dosage.

Oral medications may be given to infants through a nipple, with a medicine dropper, or with an oral syringe. When using a syringe, place it on the side of the tongue and slowly drip it into the mouth. Chewable tablets work well for preschoolers. Medications should not be given in food because if the child does not consume the entire amount of food, the dosage of medication will not be accurate. In addition, if given with food, the child may eventually associate the bad taste of the medication with food and may refuse to eat that food. If the child objects to the taste of the medication, mix in a small amount of corn syrup to disguise the taste.

Critical Thinking Exercises

1. *During a routine checkup for an adolescent, what assessments are necessary? What is the best approach when dealing with adolescents?*
2. *Why might restraints be used when caring for children? What are some important factors to be aware of when using restraints?*

● NCLEX-STYLE REVIEW QUESTIONS 

1. The nurse is assessing temperature, pulse, and respirations of a hospitalized 2-year-old client. Which set of

BOX 5-1 ● Rules of Medication Administration in Children

- Never give a child a choice of whether or not to receive medicine. The medication is ordered and is necessary for recovery; therefore, there is no choice to be made.
- Do give choices that allow the child some control over the situation such as the kind of juice or the number of bandages.
- Never lie. Do not tell a child that an injection will not hurt.
- Keep explanations simple and brief. Use words that the child will understand.
- Assure the child that it is all right to be afraid and that it is okay to cry.
- Do not talk in front of the child as though he or she were not there. Include the child in the conversation when talking to family caregivers.
- Be positive in approaching the child. Be firm and assertive when explaining to the child what will happen.
- Keep the time between explanation and execution to a minimum. The younger the child, the shorter the time should be.
- Preparations such as setting up an injection, solutions, or instrument trays should be done out of the child's sight.
- Obtain cooperation from family caregivers. They may be able to calm a frightened child, persuade the child to take the medication, and achieve cooperation for care.

findings is considered within normal limits for a child of this age?
1. 98.1°F, 136 beats/min, 44 breaths/min
2. 96.8°F, 84 beats/min, 32 breaths/min
3. 99°F, 110 beats/min, 28 breaths/min
4. 99.4°F, 124 beats/min, 60 breaths/min

2. The nurse is doing a physical examination of a quiet and content 6-month-old. Which of the following does the nurse perform first?
1. Palpation of the abdomen and kidneys
2. Examination of the ears and throat
3. Inspection of the genitals and legs
4. Auscultation of the heart and lungs

3. Which method of oral medication administration is most appropriate for infants?
1. Using a nipple or medicine dropper
2. Using chewable, flavored tablets
3. Placing medication in a bottle of juice
4. Dissolving medication in pudding

connection—

Visit the Connection site at **http://connection.lww.com/go/timbyEssentials** for links to chapter-related resources on the Internet.

References and Suggested Readings

Agency for Healthcare Policy and Research. (2003). *Child health guide: Put prevention into practice. Consumer information.* Rockville, MD: Author. [On-line.] Available: http://www.ahrq.gov/ppip/ppchild.htm.

Barone, M. A., & Rowe, P. C. (1999). Pediatric procedures. In *Oski's pediatrics: Principles and practice* (3rd ed). Philadelphia: Lippincott Williams & Wilkins.

Carroll, J. L., & Loughlin, G. M. (1999). Sudden infant death syndrome. In *Oski's pediatrics: Principles and practice* (3rd ed). Philadelphia: Lippincott Williams & Wilkins.

Gallo, A. M. (2003). The fifth vital sign: Implementation of the Neonatal Infant Pain Scale. *Journal of Obstetrics, Gynecologic and Neonatal Nursing, 32*(2), 199–206.

Kristensson-Hallstrom, I. (2001). Parental participation in pediatric surgical care. *AORN Journal, 73*(3).

Mera, K. E., & Hackley, B. (2003). Childhood vaccines: How safe are they? *American Journal of Nursing, 103*(2), 79.

O'Connor-Von, S. (2001). Preparing children for surgery–an integrative research review. *AORN Journal, 73*(3).

Pasero, C. (2002). Assessment in infants and young children: Premature infant pain profile. *American Journal of Nursing, 102*(9), 105.

Pillitteri, A. (2002). *Maternal and child health nursing* (4th ed.). Philadelphia: Lippincott Williams & Wilkins.

Salantera, L. S. (2000). Nursing students' knowledge of and views about children in pain. *Nurse Education Today, 20*(7), 539–547.

Wong, D. L., Perry, S., & Hockenberry, M. (2002). *Maternal child nursing care* (2nd ed.). St. Louis: Mosby.

VanHulle, V. C. (2001). Nurses' analgesic practices with hospitalized children. *Journal of Child and Family Nursing, 4*(2), 79.

chapter 6

Biopsychosocial Aspects of Caring for Children and Adolescents

Words to Know 

associative play
autonomous
bottle mouth caries
classification
conservation
cooperative play
dawdling
decentration
deciduous teeth
deliriants
development
developmental tasks
discipline
doubt
dramatic play
epiphyses
extrusion (protrusion) reflex
growth
heterosexual
hierarchical arrangement
homosexual
identity
industry
inferiority
inhalants
magical thinking
menarche
mistrust
negativism
nocturnal emission
nursing bottle caries
parallel play
pedodontists
punishment
reversibility
ritualism
role confusion
shame
temper tantrums
trust

Learning Objectives

On completion of this chapter, the reader will:

- State the major developmental task of the infant, toddler, preschooler, school-age child, and adolescent according to Erikson.
- Describe skeletal growth rate and physical characteristics observed in the child from infancy through adolescence.
- Describe the social characteristics observed in the child from infancy through adolescence.
- Discuss the pattern of eruption of teeth in the child and adolescent.
- Discuss nutritional needs, patterns, and concerns of children from infancy through adolescence.
- State the physiologic development required for bowel and bladder control and the typical age when this development occurs.
- Discuss the progression of language development in children.
- Discuss the role of magical thinking, imagination, and play in the development of children.
- Discuss topics (including health, sex, and substance abuse) that nurses should include in the education of family caregivers and children of all ages.
- Discuss factors that may affect the child's experience of hospitalization at each age and related nursing implications.

Growth and development refer to the total growth of the child from birth toward maturity. **Growth** is the physical increase in the body's size and appearance caused by increasing numbers of new cells. **Development** is the progressive change in the child's maturation. How a helpless infant grows and develops into a fully functioning independent adult has fascinated scientists for years. Erik Erikson formulated a series of eight **developmental tasks** or crises. The first five pertain to children and youth; the other three pertain to adulthood and are discussed in Chapters 10 and 11. In each task, the person must master the central problem before moving to the next one. Each task holds positive and negative counterparts.

INFANT: 28 DAYS TO 1 YEAR

Infants who have lived through the first month of life have a busy year ahead. During this year, they grow and develop skills more rapidly than they ever will again. Table 6.1 summarizes the accepted norms in physical, psychosocial, motor, language, and cognitive growth and development in the first year of life.

Developmental Stage and Task: Trust Versus Mistrust

Infants have no way to control the world other than crying for help and hoping for rescue. During the first year, they learn whether the world can be trusted to give love and concern or only frustration, fear, and despair. Infants who are fed on demand learn to **trust** that others will answer their cries communicating their needs. Babies fed according to the nurse or caregiver's schedule do not understand the importance of routine. They learn only that these cries may go unanswered, and thus learn to **mistrust** the world.

Physical Characteristics

Although such factors as genetic background, environment, health, gender, and race influence growth in the first year of life, healthy infants progress in a predictable pattern.

Head and Chest Measurement

At birth, head circumference averages approximately 13.75 inches (35 cm) and is usually slightly larger than the chest circumference. The chest measures approximately the same as the abdomen at birth. By 1 year of age, the head circumference has grown to approximately 18 inches (47 cm). The chest also grows rapidly, catching up to the head circumference at approximately 5 to 7 months. From then on, the chest can be expected to exceed the head in circumference.

The posterior fontanelle usually closes by 2 to 3 months. The anterior fontanelle may increase slightly in size during the first few months of life. After 6 months it begins to decrease, closing between 12 and 18 months. The sutures between the cranial bones do not ossify until later childhood.

Skeletal Growth and Maturation

During fetal life, the skeletal system is completely formed in cartilage by the end of 3 months' gestation. Bone ossification and growth occur during the remainder of fetal life and throughout childhood. The pattern of maturation is so regular that radiologic examination can determine the "bone age." When the bone age matches the child's chronological age, the skeletal structure is maturing at a normal rate.

Eruption of Deciduous Teeth

Calcification of the **deciduous** (primary) **teeth** starts early in fetal life. Shortly before birth, calcification begins in the permanent teeth, which first erupt in later childhood. The first deciduous teeth, usually the lower central incisors, usually erupt between 6 and 8 months. Babies differ in the timing of tooth eruption; some families show a tendency toward very early or very late eruption without other signs of early or late development. Some infants may become restless or fussy from swollen, inflamed gums during teething, but teething is a normal developmental process and does not cause high fever or upper respiratory conditions.

Nutritional deficiency or prolonged illness in infancy may interfere with calcification of both deciduous and permanent teeth. The role of fluoride in strengthening calcification has been well documented. Fluoride should be administered to infants and children in areas where the fluoride content of drinking water is inadequate or absent (Kula & Wright, 1999).

Cardiovascular System

In the first year of life, the circulatory system undergoes several changes. After birth, when oxygen is supplied through the respiratory system as opposed to being supplied via the placenta during fetal life, hemoglobin decreases in volume, and red blood cells gradually decrease until 3 months. Thereafter, the hemoglobin level gradually increases until reaching adult levels. Average blood pressure during the first year is 85/60 mm Hg, with expected variations. Also during the first year, the average apical rate ranges from 70 (asleep) to 150 (awake) beats per minute and as high as 180 beats per minute while the infant is crying.

Body Temperature and Respiratory Rate

Body temperature follows the average normal range after the initial adjustment to postnatal living. Respirations average 30 breaths per minute with a wide range (20 to 50 breaths per minute) according to the infant's activity.

Neuromuscular Development

As infants grow, nerve cells mature and fine muscles begin to coordinate in an orderly pattern of development. Average rates of growth and development are useful for purposes of comparison. A small time lag may be insignificant in the overall neuromuscular development of the infant, but a large time lag may require greater stimulation from the environment or a watchful attitude to discover how overall development is proceeding.

Social Characteristics

Infants begin to develop a sense of trust when fed on demand. Nevertheless, they eventually learn that not every need is met immediately. Gradually, they understand that the environment responds to desires expressed

TABLE 6.1 GROWTH AND DEVELOPMENT: THE INFANT

AGE	PHYSICAL	PSYCHOSOCIAL	FINE MOTOR	GROSS MOTOR	LANGUAGE	COGNITION
Birth–4 weeks	Weight gain of 5–7 oz (150–270 g) per wk Height gain of 1″ per month first 6 months Head circumference increase ½″ per month Moro, Babinski, rooting, and tonic neck reflexes present	Some smiling Begins Erikson's stage of "trust vs. mistrust"	Grasp reflex very strong Hands flexed	Catches and holds objects in sight that cross visual field Can turn head from side to side when lying in a prone position When prone, body in a flexed position When prone, moves extremities in a crawling fashion	Cries when upset Makes enjoyment sounds during mealtimes	At 1 month, sucking activity associated with pleasurable sensations
6 weeks	Tears appear	Smiling in response to familiar stimuli	Hands open Less flexion noted	Tries to raise shoulders and arms when stimulated Holds head up when prone Less flexion of entire body when prone	Cooing predominant Smiles to familiar voices Babbling	**Primary Circular Reactions** Begins to repeat actions
10–12 weeks	Posterior fontanelle closes	Aware of new environment Less crying Smiles at significant others	No longer has grasp reflex Pulls on clothes, blanket, but does not reach for them	No longer has Moro reflex Symmetric body positioning Pumps arms, shoulders, and head from prone position	Makes noises when spoken to	Beginning of coordinated responses to different kinds of stimuli
16 weeks	Moro, rooting, and tonic neck reflexes disappear; drooling begins	Responds to stimulus Sees bottle, squeals, laughs Aware of new environment and shows interest	Grasps objects with two hands Grasps objects in crib voluntarily and brings them to mouth Eye–hand coordination beginning	Plays with hands Brings objects to mouth Balances head and body for short periods in sitting position	Laughs aloud Sounds "n," "k," "g," and "b"	Likes social situations Defiant, bored if unattended

20 weeks	May show signs of teething	Smiles at self in mirror Cries when limits are set or when objects are taken away	Holds one object while looking for another one Grasps objects wanted	Able to sit up Can roll over Can bear weight on legs when held in a standing position Able to control head movements	Cooing noises Squeals with delight	Visually looks for an object that has fallen
24 weeks	Birth weight doubles; weight gain slows to 3–5 oz (90–150 g) per wk Height slows to ½″ per month Teething begins with lower central incisors	Likes to be picked up Knows family from strangers Plays "Peek-a-Boo" Knows likes and dislikes Fear of strangers	Holds a bottle fairly well Tries to retrieve a dropped article	Tonic neck reflex disappears Sits alone in high chair, back erect Rolls over and back to abdomen	Makes sounds "guh," "bah" Sounds "p," "m," "b," and "t" are pronounced Bubbling sounds	**Secondary Circular Reactions** Repeats actions that affect an object Beginning of object permanence
28 weeks	Lower lateral incisors are followed in the next month by upper central incisors	Imitates simple acts Responds to "no" Shows preferences and dislikes for food	Holds cup Transfers objects from one hand to the other	Reaches without visual guidance Can lift head up when in a supine position	Babbling decreases Duplicates "ma-ma" and "pa-pa" sounds	
32 weeks	Teething continues	Dislikes diaper and clothing change Afraid of strangers Fear of separating from mother	Adjusts body position to be able to reach for an object May stand up while holding on	Crawls around Pulls toy toward self	Combines syllables but has trouble attributing meaning to them	
40 weeks–1 year	Birth weight triples; has six teeth; Babinski reflex disappears Anterior fontanelle closes between now and 18 months	Does things to attract attention Tries to follow when being read to Imitates parents Looks for objects not in sight	Holds tools with one hand and works on it with another Puts toy in box after demonstration Starts blocks Holds crayon to scribble on paper	Stands alone; begins to walk alone Can change self from prone to sitting to standing position	Words emerge Says "da-da" and "ma-ma" with meaning	Coordination of secondary schemes; masters barrier to reach goal, symbolic meanings

through their own efforts and signals and become aware that the environment is separate from self.

Caregivers who expect too much too soon are not encouraging optimal development. Rather than teaching the rules of life before infants have learned to trust the environment, the caregivers actually teach that nothing is gained by activity and that the world does not respond to needs. Conversely, caregivers who rush to anticipate every need give infants no opportunity to test the environment and to discover that through personal actions, they may manipulate the environment. Client and Family Teaching 6-1 suggests healthy childrearing patterns during infancy.

Infant development depends on a mutual relationship between infant and environment, in which family caregivers play the most important role. Infants soon connect the smiling face looking down with the pleasure of being picked up, fed, or bathed. In only a few weeks, they learn that one particular person is the main source of comfort and pleasure. Infants cannot apply abstract reasoning but understand only through the five senses. As they mature enough to recognize the mother or primary caregiver, infants become fearful when this person disappears. To them, out of sight means out of existence, and infants cannot tolerate this. For infants, self-assurance is necessary to confirm that objects and people do not cease to exist when out of sight. This is a learning experience on which the infant's entire attitude toward life depends. The ancient game of "peek-a-boo" is a universal example of this learning technique. It is also one of the joys of infancy as babies affirm their ability to control the disappearance and reappearance of self. In the same manner, it confirms the existence of others even when temporarily out of sight.

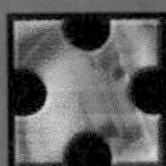

6-1 *Client and Family Teaching* Infants From Birth to 1 Year

The nurse teaches the client and family as follows:

- *First 6 weeks:* Frequent holding of infant gives infant feeling of being loved and cared for. Rocking and soothing baby are important.
- *6 weeks to 3½ months:* Respond to cries; provide visual stimulation with toys, pictures, mobiles, and auditory stimulation by talking and singing to baby.
- *3½ to 5 months:* Play regularly with baby; give child variety of things to look at; offer a variety of items to touch—soft, fuzzy, smooth, and rough—to provide tactile stimulation, move baby around home to provide additional stimulation; begin placing infant on floor to provide freedom of movement.
- *5 to 8 months:* Continue to give infant feeling of being loved and cared for by holding, cuddling, and responding to needs; talk to infant; put infant on floor more often to roll and move about; fear of strangers is common at this age.
- *8 to 12 months:* Accident-proof the house; give the infant maximum access to living area: supply infant with toys; stay close by to support infant in difficult situations; continue to talk to infant to provide language stimulation. The baby at this age loves surprise toys like jack-in-the-box and separation games like "peek-a-boo"; loves putting-in and taking-out activities.

Nursing Implications

Nurses working with infants and family caregivers must recognize the importance of good nutrition and meeting nutritional needs. Often they must do teaching regarding breast or bottle-feeding, the addition of solid foods, and the process of weaning. When infants enter a healthcare setting or are hospitalized, they need much of their energies to cope with the illness. It is important to work with infants and families to promote normal growth and development.

Nutrition

Rapid growth in infancy creates a need for more nutrients than at any other time of life. The Academy of Pediatrics Committee on Nutrition (2003) has endorsed breastfeeding as the best method of feeding infants. Either breast milk or commercial infant formulas supply most of the infant's requirements for the first 4 to 6 months. Nutrients that may need to be supplemented are vitamins C and D, iron, and fluoride. Fluoride is needed in small amounts for strengthening tooth calcification and preventing tooth decay. Vitamin preparations combined with fluoride are available.

ADDITION OF SOLID FOODS. At about 4 to 6 months, iron supply becomes low, and infants need supplements of iron-rich foods. They know only one way to take food: namely, to thrust the tongue forward as if to suck. This is called the **extrusion (protrusion) reflex** and has the effect of pushing solid food from the mouth. The process of transferring food from the front of the mouth to the throat for swallowing is a complicated skill that must be learned. A small spoon fits the infant's mouth better than a large one and makes it easier to put food further back on the tongue. Babies soon learn to manipulate the tongue and come to enjoy this way of eating. To avoid the danger of aspiration, caregivers must quiet an upset or crying baby before proceeding with feeding. They should start foods in small amounts (1 or 2 tsp daily), and foods should be smooth, thin, lukewarm, and bland. Offering one new food at a time is best. This method helps determine which food is responsible if the baby has a reaction to a new food. When teeth start erupting, infants appreciate a piece of zwieback or hard toast to practice chewing.

After a few teeth have erupted, caregivers can substitute chopped foods for pureed foods. They gradually replace breast milk or formula with whole milk as infants learn to drink from a cup.

PREPARATION OF FOODS. Pureed baby foods, chopped junior foods, and prepared milk formulas are available, but many families cannot afford them. Advise caregivers to read food labels carefully to avoid foods with undesirable additives, especially sugar and salt. Baby foods can be prepared at home from fresh foods, not canned, to avoid commercial additives. Preparation and storage of baby food at home require careful sanitary practices. Equipment used to prepare an infant's food must be cleaned carefully with hot, soapy water and rinsed thoroughly. Most infants do not like strongly flavored or bitter foods.

SELF-FEEDING. At approximately 7 or 8 months, babies may grab the spoon from the caregiver, examine it, and mouth it. They also stick fingers in the food to feel the texture and to bring it to the mouth for tasting. This is an essential, although messy, part of the learning experience. The next task is to try self-feeding. Babies may find that getting a spoon right side up into the mouth is complex, so they favor fingers over the spoon. Eventually, they succeed in getting some food from spoon to mouth at least part of the time.

WEANING. Caregiver must attempt weaning, either from breast or bottle, gradually without fuss or strain. The abrupt removal of a main source of satisfaction—sucking—before the baby has conquered basic mistrust of the environment may prove detrimental to normal development. At 5 or 6 months, infants who have watched others drink from a cup usually are ready to try a sip when it is offered. Infants who take food from a dish and milk from a cup during the day may still be reluctant to give up a bedtime bottle. A child never should take a bottle of formula, milk, or juice to bed. **Pedodontists** (dentists who specialize in the care and treatment of children's teeth) discourage bedtime bottles because the sugar from formula or sweetened juice coats the infant's teeth for long periods and causes erosion of the enamel on the deciduous teeth, resulting in a condition known as **"bottle mouth"** or **"nursing bottle" caries.** If the caregiver does give a bedtime bottle, only water should be given. It is important to teach that in addition to tooth damage, liquids can pool in the mouth and flow into the eustachian tube, causing otitis media (ear infection) if the infant falls asleep with the bottle.

Stop, Think, and Respond ● BOX 6-1

What is the reason it is suggested that bedtime bottles be discouraged? If a bottle is given at bedtime, what fluids are acceptable for the child to drink?

Infant in the Healthcare Facility

Hospitalization hampers the infant's normal pattern of living. Long-term hospitalization may present serious problems, even with the best of care. If the hospital atmosphere is emotionally unresponsive, infants may fail to respond to treatment. Touching, rocking, and cuddling are essential elements of nursing care. The small infant matures largely as a result of physical development. If hindered from reaching out and responding to the environment, infants become apathetic and cease to learn. This situation is particularly apparent when restraints are necessary to keep children from undoing surgical procedures or dressings or to prevent injury. Children in restraints need extra love and attention and the use of every possible method to provide comfort (see Chap. 5). Spending time with them, playing music in the room, or encouraging someone to stay with them might help to make infants more comfortable.

TODDLER: 1 TO 3 YEARS

Soon after a child's first birthday, important and sometimes dramatic changes occur. Physical growth slows considerably; mobility and communication skills improve rapidly; and a determined, often stubborn little person begins to create a new set of challenges for caregivers. During this transition, children learn many new physical and social skills. Significant landmarks in the toddler's growth and development are summarized in Table 6.2.

Developmental Stage and Task: Autonomy Versus Shame and Doubt

Even the smallest child wants to feel in control and needs to learn to perform tasks independently, or as an **autonomous** person. The task may take a long time or make a mess, but toddlers gain reassurance and self-respect from self-feeding, crawling, or walking alone. Toddlers exploring the environment begin to explore and learn about their bodies, too. If caregivers shame children for behavior or natural curiosity, toddlers may develop and sustain a belief or sense of **doubt** or **shame** and think that somehow they are dirty, nasty, and bad.

Physical Characteristics

Toddlerhood is a time of slowed growth and rapid development. Each year toddlers gain 5 to 10 pounds (2.26 to 4.53 kg) and approximately 3 inches (7.62 cm). Continued eruption of teeth, particularly the molars, helps toddlers learn to chew food. They learn to stand alone and to walk between 1 and 2 years. During this time, most

TABLE 6.2 GROWTH AND DEVELOPMENT: THE TODDLER

AGE (MONTHS)	PERSONAL–SOCIAL	FINE MOTOR	GROSS MOTOR	LANGUAGE	COGNITION
12–15	Begins Erikson's stage of "autonomy versus shame and doubt" Seeks novel ways to pursue new experiences Imitations of people are more advanced	Builds with blocks; finger paints Able to reach out with hands and bring food to mouth Holds a spoon Drinks from a cup	Movements become more voluntary Postural control improves; able to stand and may take few independent steps	First words are not generally classified as true language. They are generally associated with the concrete and are usually activity-oriented.	Begins to accommodate to the environment, and the adaptive process evolves
18	Extremely curious Becomes a communicative social being Parallel play Fleeting contacts with other children "Make-believe" play begins	Better control of spoon; good control when drinking from cup	Walks alone; gait may still be a bit unsteady Begins to walk sideways and backward	Begins to use language in a symbolic form to represent images or ideas that reflect the thinking process Uses some meaningful words such as "hi," "bye-bye," and "all gone" Comprehension is significantly greater	Demonstrates foresight and can discover solutions to problems without excessive trial-and-error procedures Can imitate without the presence of a model (deferred limitation)
24	Language facilitates autonomy Sense of power from saying "no" and "mine" Increased independence from mother	Turns page of a book Places objects in holes or slots Turns pages of a book singly Adept at building a tower of six or seven cubes When drawing, attempts to enclose a space	Runs well with little falling Throws and kicks a ball Walks up and down stairs one step at a time	Begins to use words to explain past events or to discuss objects not observably present Rapidly expands vocabulary to about 300 words; uses plurals	Enters preconceptual phase of cognitive development State of continuous investigations Primary focus is egocentric
36	Basic concepts of sexuality are established Separates from mother more easily Attends to toilet needs	Copies a circle and a straight line Grasps spoon between thumb and index finger Holds cup by handle	Balances on one foot; jumps in place; pedals tricycles	Quest for information furthered by questions like "why," "when," "where," and "how" Has acquired the language that will be used in the course of simple conversation during adult years	Preconceptual phase continues; can think of only one idea at a time; cannot think of all parts in terms of the whole

children say their first words and continue to improve and refine their language skills. By the end of this period, toddlers may have learned partial or total toilet training. To be able to cooperate in toilet training, the child's rectal and urethral sphincter muscles must have developed to the stage when the child can control them. An understanding by the child of holding urine and stool until they are in the appropriate place is also necessary. The child must be able to postpone the urge to defecate until reaching the toilet or potty and must be able to signal the need before the event. This level of maturation seldom takes place before the age of 18 to 24 months. See Client and Family Teaching 6-2.

The rate of development varies with each child, depending on individual personality and opportunities available to test, explore, and learn.

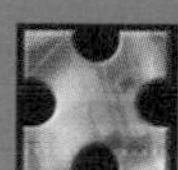

6-2 *Client and Family Teaching* Toilet Training

The nurse teaches the family as follows:

- Use a potty chair in which a child can comfortably sit with the feet on the floor. Most small children are afraid of a flush toilet.
- Leave the child on the potty chair for only a short time. Be readily available but do not hover anxiously over the child. If urination or defecation occurs, approval is in order; if not, no comment is necessary.
- During the beginning stages of training, the child is likely to have an accident soon after leaving the potty. This is not willful defiance and need not be mentioned.
- Empty the potty unobtrusively after the child has resumed playing. The child has cooperated and produced the desired result. If caregivers immediately throw away the potty contents, the child may be confused and not so eager to please the next time.
- The ability to feel shame and self-doubt appears at this age. Therefore, do not tease the child about reluctance or inability to conform. This teasing can shake the child's confidence and cause feelings of doubt in self-worth.
- Do not expect perfection, even after the child has achieved control. Lapses are inevitable, perhaps because the child is completely absorbed in play or has a temporary episode of loose stools. Occasionally a child feels aggression, frustration, or anger and may use this method to "get even." As long as lapses are occasional, caregivers should ignore them. If frequent and persistent, however, the cause should be sought.

Social Characteristics

Toddlers develop a growing awareness of self as a being, separate from other people or objects. Children tend to test personal independence to the limit. This age has been called an age of **negativism.** The toddler's response to nearly everything is a firm "no," but this is more an assertion of individuality than an intention to disobey.

Ritualism, dawdling, and temper tantrums also characterize this stage. **Ritualism,** employed by young children to help develop security, involves following routines that make rituals of even simple tasks. **Dawdling,** wasting or whiling away time, serves much the same purpose. Young children must decide between following the wishes and routines of the caregiver and asserting independence by following personal desires. If the task to be done is important, caregivers should help children to follow along the way they should go; otherwise, caregivers usually can ignore dawdling. **Temper tantrums** are behaviors that spring from the many frustrations that are natural results of a child's urge to be independent. Even the best of caregivers may lose patience and show a temporary lack of understanding. Children react with enthusiastic rebellion. Reasoning, scolding, or punishing during a tantrum is useless. A trusted person who remains calm and patient needs to be nearby until the child gains self-control. After the tantrum is over, diverting attention with a toy or some other distraction helps the child relax. Head-banging and breath-holding can accompany these tantrums. Head-banging can cause injury, so the caregiver needs to provide protection. Breath holding can be frightening to the caregiver, but the child will shortly lose consciousness and begin breathing.

Toys and Play

Play moves from the solitary play of the infant to **parallel play,** in which toddlers play alongside, but not with, other children. Much of the playtime is filled with imitation of the people children see as role models: adults around them, siblings, and other children. Toys that involve the toddler's new gross motor skills, such as push–pull toys, rocking horses, large blocks, and balls, are popular. Toddlers develop fine motor skills by use of thick crayons, finger paints, wooden puzzles with large pieces, toys that fit pieces into shaped holes, and cloth books. They enjoy talking on a play telephone and like pots, pans, and toys that help them imitate the adults in their environment. Children cannot share toys until the later stage of toddlerhood. Adults should not make an issue of sharing at this early stage.

Guidance and Discipline

To **discipline** means to train or instruct to produce a particular behavior pattern, especially moral or mental improvement and self-control. **Punishment** means penalizing someone for wrongdoing. Although all small children need discipline, they need punishment much less frequently. Toddlers learn self-control gradually. Two year olds begin to show some signs of accepting responsibility for their own actions, but they lack inner controls because of their egocentricity. They still want the forbidden thing but may repeat, "no, no, no" while reaching for a desired treasure, recognizing that the act is not approved. Even at this age, children want and need limits. When no limits are set, they develop a feeling of insecurity and fear. Consistency and timing are important in the approach that caregivers use when disciplining children. This period can be challenging to adults. Toddlers need to learn that the adults are in control and will help children gain self-control while learning to be independent. A useful method for a child who is not cooperating or is out of control is to send the child to a "time out" chair, where the child can be alone but observed without other distractions. Parents should praise children for good behavior and, when possible, ignore negative behavior. "Extinction" is another discipline technique effective with this age group. If a child has certain undesirable behaviors that occur frequently, parents ignore the behavior as long as it is not harmful to the child or others. When the child responds acceptably in a situation in which the undesirable behavior was the usual response, caregivers should be sure to compliment the child. Spanking or other physical punishment usually does not work well, because the child merely learns that hitting or other physical violence is acceptable.

Sharing With a Sibling

The first child in a family has the caregivers' undivided attention until a new baby arrives, often when the first child is a toddler. Toddlers can feel the mother's abdomen and understand that this is where the new baby lives; this alone does not adequately prepare them for the baby's arrival. This real baby represents a rival for the mother's affection. Toddlers frequently regress to more infantile behavior when a new baby appears. Toilet training may regress, with toddlers having episodes of soiling and wetting. Moving the older child to a larger bed some time before the new baby appears helps the toddler take pride in being "grown up" now.

Many books are available to help prepare young children for the birth of a sibling. Displaced toddlers almost certainly will feel some jealousy, but helping to care for the baby, according to the child's ability, contributes to a feeling of continuing importance and self-worth. Parents should not shame toddlers for reverting to babyish behavior. Positive time and attention from the mother and other family members help toddlers feel special.

Nursing Implications

Toddlers present many challenges for family caregivers as well as nurses working with the family. Eating problems and nutritional needs are important nursing considerations. When toddlers enter a healthcare setting, it is necessary for the healthcare provider to be aware of growth and development concerns.

Nutrition

Eating problems commonly appear between 1 and 3 years. These problems occur for several reasons:

- Growth rate has slowed; therefore, toddlers may want and need less food than before. Family caregivers need to know that this is normal.
- A strong drive for independence and autonomy compels an assertion of will for the child to prove his or her individuality both to self and others.
- Appetite varies according to the kind of foods offered. "Food jags," the desire for only one kind of food for awhile, are common.

To minimize these eating problems, parents should plan meals with an understanding of the toddler's developing feeding skills. At 15 months, toddlers can sit through meals, prefer finger feeding, and want to self-feed. By 18 months, appetite decreases, control of the spoon improves, and children hold cups with both hands. At 24 months, toddlers have clearly defined likes, dislikes, and food jags. By 30 months, some toddlers hold the spoon and cup in an adult manner.

The Toddler in the Healthcare Facility

The developmental stage of the toddler intensifies the anxiety of hospitalization. Toddlers fear strangers and show anxiety when separated from family. Unfamiliar people and surroundings make their reaction to hospitalization understandable. As part of the child's admission procedure, nurses use a social assessment that covers eating habits and food preferences, toileting habits and terms used for toileting, family members, pets, favorite toys, sleeping or napping patterns, and other significant information to help the staff plan appropriate care. Separation anxiety is high during toddlerhood, and encouraging family members to stay with children is helpful.

If assigned to a toddler, maintain as much as possible the toddler's pattern and schedule. Recognize that the toddler may use a favorite blanket or stuffed animal to provide self-comfort.

Toddlers just learning to use the toilet, self-feed, and be disciplined present a unique challenge. Toddlers learning sphincter control are still dependent on familiar surroundings and the family caregiver's support. For this reason, some pediatric personnel automatically put toddlers back in diapers when they are admitted. This practice should be discouraged and the child should be given a chance to maintain control. Potty chairs can be provided for the child when appropriate. The nursing staff must know the method and times of accomplishing toilet training used at home and must try to comply with them as closely as possible in the hospital.

A toddler's eating habits may loom large in the nurse's mind as a potential problem. In the hospital or clinic as at home, food can assume an importance out of proportion to its value and create unnecessary problems. Some helpful hints to minimize potential problems are as follows:

- View mealtime as a social event; allow others to eat with the child.
- Encourage self-feeding; offer finger foods.
- Do not push the child to eat; serve small portions
- Offer familiar foods, served warm or cool, *not* hot or cold.
- Provide fluids in small, but frequent amounts.

Safety promotion for toddlers may be challenging. Curious toddlers need to be watched with extra care but should not be unnecessarily prohibited from exploring and moving about freely.

PRESCHOOL CHILD: 3 TO 6 YEARS

Preschoolers are fascinating individuals. As their social circles enlarge, preschoolers' language, play patterns, and appearance change markedly. Their curiosity about the world around them grows, as does their ability to explore that world in greater detail. Important milestones for growth and development of the preschool child are summarized in Table 6.3.

Developmental Stage and Task: Initiative Versus Guilt

The developmental task of the preschool age is initiative versus guilt. Preschoolers often try to find ways to do things to help, but they may feel guilty if scolded when they fail because of inexperience or lack of skill.

During this period, children engage in active, assertive play. Steadily improving physical coordination and expanding social skills encourage "showing off" to gain adult attention and, they hope, approval. Preschoolers, still self-centered, play alone, although in the company of other children; interaction comes later. These children want to know what the rules are and enjoy "being good" and the adult approval that action gains. During this time, children develop a conscience and accept punishment for doing wrong because it relieves feelings of guilt. Children in this phase of development generally do not have a concept of time. These children need a familiar frame of reference to understand when something is going to happen. For example, the parent or caregiver may say, "I will be back when your lunch comes" or "I will be back when the cartoons come on TV."

Physical Characteristics

The preschool period is one of slow physical growth, but changes in dentition and visual development are significant during this time.

Growth Rate

Preschoolers gain approximately 3 to 5 pounds each year (1.4 to 2.3 kg) and grow about 2.5 inches (6.3 cm). Because the increase in height is proportionately greater than the increase in weight, 5-year-olds appear much thinner and less babyish than 3-year-olds. Boys tend to be leaner than girls are during this time. Gross and fine motor skills continue to develop rapidly. By 5 years, children generally can throw and catch a ball well, climb effectively, and ride a bicycle.

Dentition

The deciduous teeth have completely emerged by the beginning of the preschool period. Toward the end of the preschool stage, permanent teeth begin to replace these teeth. The age at which a child loses the deciduous teeth varies, but the central incisors are usually the first to go, just as they were the first to erupt in infancy.

Visual Development

Visual development is still immature at 3 years. Eye–hand coordination is good, but judgment of distances generally is faulty, leading to many bumps and falls. During the preschool years, vision should be checked to screen for *amblyopia* or reduced vision. Usually by 6 years, children have achieved 20/20 vision, but mature depth perception may not occur in some children until 8 to 10 years.

Skeletal Growth

Between the third and sixth birthdays, the greatest amount of skeletal growth occurs in the feet and legs. This contributes to the change from the wide-gaited, pot-bellied look of the toddler into the slim, taller figure of the 6-year-old. In addition, the carpals and tarsals mature in the hands and feet, which contribute to better hand and foot control.

TABLE 6.3 GROWTH AND DEVELOPMENT: THE PRESCHOOLER

AGE (YEAR)	PERSONAL–SOCIAL	FINE MOTOR	GROSS MOTOR	LANGUAGE	COGNITION
3	Begins Erikson's stage of "initiative vs. guilt." Conscience develops. Shy with strangers and inept with peers. Sufficiently independent to be interested in group experiences with age mates (e.g., nursery school)	Able to button clothes Copies O and + Uses pencils, crayons, paints Shows preference for right or left hand	Tends to watch motor activities before attempting them Can jump several feet Uses hands in broad movements Rides tricycle Negotiates stairs well	Vocabulary up to 1000 words Articulates vowels accurately Talks a lot Sings and recites Asks many questions	Continues in preoperational state (2–7 years) characterized by: 1. *Centration,* or the inability to attend to more than one aspect of a situation 2. *Egocentricity,* or the inability to consider the perception of others 3. The static and irreversible quality of thought that makes the child unable to perceive the processes of change
4	Boisterous and inflammatory Aggressive physically and verbally but developing behaviors to become socially acceptable Becomes socially acceptable Accepts punishment for wrongdoing because it relieves guilt	Can use scissors; copies a square Adds three parts to stick figures	Has some hesitation but tends to try feats beyond ability Greater powers of balance and accuracy Hops on one foot; can control movements of hands	Vocabulary of about 1500 words Constant questions Sentences of four or five words Uses profanity Reports fantasies as truth	Reality and fantasy are not always clear to the preschooler. Believes that words make things real—"magical thinking"
5	Initiates contacts with strangers and relates interesting little tales Interested in telling and comparing stories about self Peer relations are important ("best friends" abound) Responds to social values by assuming sex roles with rigidity	Ties shoelaces Copies a diamond and a triangle Prints a few letters or numbers May print first name Cuts food	Will not attempt feats beyond ability Throws and catches ball well Jumps rope Walks backward with heel to toe Skips and hops Adept on bicycle and climbing equipment	Vocabulary of 3000 words Speech is intelligible Asks meanings of words Enjoys telling stories	Thinks feelings and thoughts can happen Intrusions into the body cause fear and anxiety (fear of mutilation and castration)

Social Characteristics

Between 3 and 5 years, language development is generally rapid. Children develop a vivid imagination and imitate the adults around them. Preschoolers enjoy playing and spending time with others the same age. They learn about the body and become aware of their sexuality.

Language Development

Most 3-year-olds can construct simple sentences, but their speech has many hesitations and repetitions as they search for the right word or try to make the right sound. Stuttering can develop during this period but usually disappears within 3 to 6 months. By the end of the fifth year, preschoolers use long, rather complex sentences; their vocabulary will have increased by more than 1500 words since 2 years. Preschoolers' use of language changes during this period. Three-year-olds love to talk and often talk to themselves or to their toys or pets without any apparent purpose. By 4 years, children use words to transmit information other than their own needs and feelings. Four- and 5-year-olds delight in using "naughty" words or swearing.

Hearing impairment or another physical problem, lack of stimulation, overprotection, or lack of parental interest or rejection by parents may cause delays or other difficulties in language development. Children develop good language skills as they engage regularly in conversation with caregivers and others. Reading and talking with children about pictures in storybooks can enhance language development. Family and cultural patterns may influence language development (e.g., children from bilingual families try to learn the rules of both languages).

Development of Imagination

Preschoolers have learned to think about something without actually seeing it—to visualize or imagine. This normal development, sometimes called **magical thinking,** makes it difficult for them to separate fantasy from reality. Preschoolers believe that words or thoughts can make things real, and this belief can have either positive or negative results. For example, in a moment of anger, a child may wish that a parent or a sibling would die; if that person later is hurt, the child feels responsible and suffers guilt. The child needs reassurance that this is not so. During this stage, children often have imaginary playmates that are very real to them. The imaginary friend often has the characteristics that the child might wish for. Sometimes children blame the imaginary friend for breaking a toy or engaging in another act that they do not want to take responsibility for. Caregivers need assurance that this behavior is normal. The preschooler's active imagination often leads to a fear of the dark or nightmares; consequently, problems with sleep are common. It is important to acknowledge the child's fears. Providing a small night light and reassurance helps to decrease these fears.

Sexual Development

Preschool children become acutely aware of their sexuality including sexual roles and organs. They generally develop a strong emotional attachment to the parent of the opposite sex. Children's curiosity about their own genitalia and those of peers and adults may make parents uncomfortable and evoke responses that indicate to children that sex is dirty and something to be ashamed and guilty about. Many families find dealing with young children's questions and actions difficult. Nurses can help caregivers understand that sexual curiosity is a normal, natural part of total curiosity about oneself and the surrounding world. In addition to responsible teaching of sexual information, caregivers also should teach children about "good touch" and "bad touch." Children need to understand that no one should touch their bodies in a way that is unpleasant.

Exploration of the genitalia is normal for preschoolers. It is one way they learn to perceive the body as a possible source of pleasure and is the beginning of the acceptance of sex as natural and pleasurable. Reassure caregivers that this behavior is not uncommon, and that a calm, matter-of-fact response to children found masturbating is the most effective approach.

Social Development

Preschoolers are outgoing, imaginative, social beings. They play vigorously and, in the process, learn about the world in which they live. As they gain control over their environment, preschoolers try to manipulate it, and this may lead to conflict with caregivers. Generally, however, preschoolers are delightful to watch as they go about the business of growing and learning.

PLAY. Play activities are one way that children learn. By 3 years, children begin imitative play, pretending to be mommy, daddy, a policeman, an astronaut, or some well-known person or television character. Listening to a preschooler scold a doll or stuffed animal lets the adults hear how they sound to the child. **Dramatic play** allows a child to act out troubling situations and to control the solution to the problem. Drawing is another form of play; as fine motor skills improve, children's drawings become much more complex and controlled. The pictures can reveal insight about the child's self-concept and perception of the environment. Preschoolers may engage in **cooperative play,** in which children play in an organized group with one another, as in team sports. **Associative play** occurs when children play together and are engaged in a similar activity but without organization, rules, or a leader, and each child does what she or he wishes. In parallel play, children play alongside each other but independently. Although common among toddlers, parallel play exists in all age groups—for example, in a scout troop where each member works on an individual project or craft. Children need all types of play to aid in their total development.

> **Stop, Think, and Respond ● BOX 6-2**
>
> *What types of play are seen in children? How does play affect the child?*

AGGRESSION. Temper tantrums are an early form of aggression. Preschoolers with newly developed language skills use words aggressively in name-calling and threats. Four-year-olds use physical aggression as well; they push, hit, and kick in an effort to manipulate the environment. The task of family caregivers during these years is to help children understand that the anger and frustration that result in aggressive behavior are normal but need to be handled differently because aggressive behavior is not socially acceptable.

DISCIPLINE. Family caregivers need to remember that preschoolers want to be good and follow instructions, and they feel bad when they do not, even if they are not physically punished. Discipline during this time should strive to teach a sense of responsibility and inner control. All caregivers must understand and agree to the limits and discipline measures for the child. Taking away a privilege from a child who has misbehaved until he or she can demonstrate that behavior has improved is effective.

NURSERY SCHOOL OR DAY CARE EXPERIENCE. Group experiences with peers and adults outside the immediate family are important to a child's development. The transition to new experiences, people, and surroundings can be threatening to some preschoolers. If preschoolers spend time in nursery school or other day care programs, the family should understand that this probably means that children will demand more of their attention during the hours when they are together.

Nursing Implications

Preschoolers watch and copy older children as well as adults. The examples that family caregivers as well as the nurse illustrate to preschoolers are important. When preschoolers enter the healthcare facility, it is important for nurses to support them and recognize their normal growth and development needs.

Nutrition

The preschool period is not a time of rapid growth, so children do not need large quantities of food. Protein needs continue to remain high to provide for muscle growth. Appetite is erratic. Portions are smaller than adult-sized portions, so children may need frequent, small meals with nutritious snacks in between. Preschoolers need guidance in choosing foods and are strongly influenced by the example of family members and peers. Families should never use food as a reward or bribe. Preschoolers have definite food preferences; they may accept new foods, but families should introduce them one at a time to avoid overwhelming children. Preschoolers show growing independence and skill in eating. They try to mimic adult behavior; 4-year-olds are more skilled with the use of utensils, and 5-year-olds often can cut their own food and practice table manners. Rituals may become important to mealtime happiness.

The Preschooler in the Healthcare Facility

Preschoolers may view hospitalization as an exciting new adventure or as a frightening, dangerous experience depending on preparation by caregivers and health professionals. Play is an effective way to let children act out their anxieties and to learn what to expect from the hospital situation. Preschoolers are frightened about intrusive procedures. Children are less anxious about procedures if they are explained in appropriate words. Encouraging children to handle equipment beforehand and perhaps "use" it on a doll or another toy lessens anxiety. Hospitalized preschoolers may revert to bedwetting but should not be scolded for it, and the family should be assured that this is normal. If a child is afraid of the dark, a night-light can be provided. Hospital routines should follow home routines as closely as possible, and children should be allowed to participate in care. If the child is ambulatory and not on infection-control precautions, the playroom can offer diversionary activities. If not, play materials can be provided for use in bed.

SCHOOL-AGE CHILD: 6 TO 10 YEARS

The first day of school marks a major milestone in a child's development, opening a new world of learning and growth. Most children reach school age with the necessary skills, abilities, and independence to function successfully in this new environment. Growth and development of the school-age child is summarized in Table 6.4.

Developmental Stage and Task: Industry Versus Inferiority

Children begin to seek achievement in this phase. They learn to interact with others and sometimes to compete with them. They like activities they can follow through

TABLE 6.4 GROWTH AND DEVELOPMENT: THE SCHOOL-AGE CHILD

AGE (YEAR)	PHYSICAL	MOTOR	SOCIAL	LANGUAGE	PERCEPTUAL	COGNITIVE
6	Average height 45 inches (116 cm) Average weight 46 lb (21 kg) Loses first tooth (upper incisors) Six-year molars erupt Food "jags" Appetite increased	Ties shoes Can use scissors Runs, jumps, climbs, skips Can ride bicycle Can't sit for long periods Cuts, pastes, prints, draws with some detail	Increased need to socialize with same sex Egocentric—believes everyone thinks as they do Still in pre-operational stage until age 7	Uses every form of sentence structure Vocabulary of 2,500 words Sentence length about 5 words	Knows right from left May reverse letters Can discriminate vertical, horizontal, and oblique Perceives pictures in parts or whole but not both	Recognizes simple words Conservation of number Defines objects by use Can group according to an attribute to form subclasses
7	Weight is seven times birth weight Gains 4.4–6.6 lb/yr (2–3 kg) Grows 2–2.5 inches/yr (5–6 cm)	More cautious Swims Printing smaller than 6-year-old's Activity level lower than 6-year-old's	More cooperative Same-sex play group and friends Less egocentric	Can name day, month, season Produces all language sounds	b, p, d, q confusion resolved Can copy a diamond	Begins to use simple logic Can group in ascending order Grasps basic idea of addition and subtraction Conservation of substance Can tell time
8	Average height 49.5 inches (127 cm) Average weight 55 lb (25 kg)	Movements more graceful Writes in cursive Can throw and hit a baseball Has symmetric balance and can hop	Adheres to simple rules Hero worship begins Same-sex peer group	Gives precise definitions Articulation near adult level	Can catch a ball Visual acuity 20/20 Perceives pictures in parts and whole	Increasing memory span Interest in causal relation Conservation of length
9–10	Average height 51.5–53.5 inches (132–137 cm) Average weight 59.5–77 lb (27–35 kg)	Good coordination Can achieve the strength and speed needed for most sports	Enjoys team competition Moves from group to best friend Hero worship intensifies	Can use language to convey thoughts and look at other's point of view	Eye–hand coordination almost perfect	Classifies objects Understands explanations Conservation of area and weight Describes characteristics of objects Can group in descending order

to completion and tangible results, thus developing the sense of **industry.** If standards are so high that children feel there is no chance of winning, or if they receive criticism, not praise, they develop feelings of **inferiority.** It is important to emphasize that everyone is a unique person and deserves to be appreciated for his or her own special qualities.

Physical Characteristics

Physical development includes changes in weight and height. Skeletal growth is evident in the changing appearance of school-age children. During this time they have changes in dentition, and permanent teeth begin to erupt.

Skeletal Growth

Between 6 and 10 years, growth is slow and steady. Average annual weight gain is approximately 5 to 6 pounds (2 to 3 kg). By 7 years, children weigh approximately seven times as much as at birth. Annual height increase is about 2.5 inches (6 cm). This period ends in the preadolescent growth spurt in girls at approximately 10 years and in boys at approximately 12 years. A protruding abdomen and lordosis ("swayback") characterize the 6-year-old's silhouette. By the time a child reaches 10 years, the spine is straighter, the abdomen flatter, and the body generally more slender and long-legged. Bone growth occurs mostly in the long bones and is gradual during the school years. Bone replaces cartilage at the **epiphyses** (growth centers at the end of long bones and at the wrists). Skeletal maturation is more rapid in girls than in boys.

Dentition

At approximately 6 years, children start to lose the deciduous ("baby") teeth, usually beginning with the lower incisors. At about the same time, the first permanent teeth, the 6-year molars, appear directly behind the deciduous molars. These 6-year molars are important; they help to shape the jaw and affect the alignment of the permanent teeth. If these molars are allowed to decay so severely that they must be removed, children will have dental problems later.

Social Characteristics

A sense of duty and accomplishment occupies the years from 6 to 12. Children apply the energies earlier put into play toward accomplishing tasks and often spend numerous sessions on one project. With these attempts come the refinement of motor, cognitive, and social skills and the development of a positive sense of self. Some school-age children, however, are not ready for this stage because of environmental deprivation, a dysfunctional family, insecure attachment to parents, immaturity, or other reasons. Entering school at a disadvantage, these children may not be ready to be productive. Excessive or unrealistic goals set by a teacher or caregiver who is insensitive to a child's needs will defeat such a child and possibly lead to the child's feeling of inferiority rather than self-confidence. When environmental support is adequate, school-age children develop coping mechanisms, a sense of right and wrong, feelings of self-esteem, and an ability to care for themselves.

During the school-age years, cognitive skills develop; at approximately 7 years, children enter the concrete operational stage identified by Piaget (Berger, 2001). The skills of **conservation** (the ability to recognize that a change in shape does not necessarily mean a change in amount or mass) are significant. This begins with the conservation of numbers, when the child understands that the number of cookies does not change even though they may be rearranged, along with the conservation of mass, when the child can see that an amount of cookie dough is the same whether in ball form or flattened for baking. This is followed by conservation of weight, in which the child recognizes that a pound is a pound regardless of whether plastic or bricks are weighed. Conservation of volume (for instance, a half-cup of water is the same amount regardless of the shape of the container) does not come until late in the concrete operational stage at approximately 11 or 12 years.

Each child is a product of personal heredity, environment, cognitive ability, and physical health. All children need love and acceptance, with understanding, support, and concern when they make a mistake. Children thrive on praise and recognition and will work to earn them (Client and Family Teaching 6-3).

Children From 6 to 7 Years

Children 6 to 7 years old are still characterized by magical thinking—believing in the tooth fairy, Santa Claus, the Easter bunny, and others. Keen imaginations contribute to fears, especially at night. Trouble distinguishing fantasy from reality can contribute to lying to escape punishment or to boost self-confidence.

Children who have attended a day care center, preschool, kindergarten, or Head Start program usually make the transition into first grade with excitement and little anxiety. Those without that experience may find it helpful to visit the school to experience separation from home and caregivers and to try getting along with other children on a trial basis. Most 6-year-olds can sit still for short periods and understand about taking turns.

Group activities are important to most 6-year-olds, even if the group is only a few children. They delight in learning and show an interest in every experience. Judgment about acceptable and unacceptable behavior is not well developed and possibly results in name-calling and the use of vulgar words.

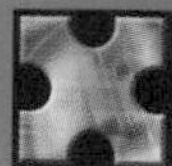

6-3 *Client and Family Teaching* Guiding Your School-Age Child

The nurse teaches the client and family as follows:

- Give your child consistent love, attention, and respect. Try to see the situation through your child's eyes. Do your best to avoid a hostile or angry reaction toward your child.
- Know where your child is at all times and who his or her friends are. Never leave your child home alone.
- Encourage your child to become involved in school and community activities. Become involved with your child's activities whenever possible. Encourage fair play and good sportsmanship.
- Show your children good examples by your behavior toward others.
- Never hit your children. Physical punishment shows them that it is all right to hit others and that they can solve problems in that way.
- Use positive nonphysical methods of discipline such as
  - "Time out"—1 minute per year of age is an appropriate amount of time.
  - Grounding"—don't permit them to play with friends or take part in a special activity.
  - Take away a special privilege.
- Set these limits for brief periods only. Be consistent. Make a reasonable rule, let your child know the rule, and then stick with it. You can involve your children in helping to set rules.
- Find the "positives" and praise the child for those behaviors.
- Let the child know what you expect of him or her. Children who have responsibilities (age-appropriate) learn self-discipline and self-control.
- When you have a problem with your child, try to sit down and solve it together. Help him or her figure out ways to solve problems nonviolently.

Between 6 and 8 years, children begin to enjoy participating in real-life activities such as helping with gardening, housework, and other chores. They love making things such as drawings, paintings, and craft projects.

Children From 7 to 10 Years

Between the seventh and eighth birthdays, children begin to shake off their acceptance of parental standards as the ultimate authority and become more impressed by the behavior of their peers. Interest in group play increases, and acceptance by the group or gang is important. These groups quickly become all-boy or all-girl groups and are often project-oriented, such as scout troops. Private clubs with homemade clubhouses, secret codes, and languages are popular. Individual friendships also are formed, and "best friends" are intensely loyal, if only for short periods. Table games, arts and crafts requiring skill and dexterity, computer games, and school science projects and fairs are popular. This period includes the beginning of many neighborhood team sports including Little League, softball, football, and soccer. Both boys and girls are actively involved in many of these sports.

Even though parents are no longer considered the ultimate authority, their standards have become part of the child's personality and conscience. Although children may cheat, lie, or steal occasionally, they suffer considerable guilt if they have learned that these behaviors are unacceptable.

Important changes occur in thinking processes at approximately 7 years, when there is movement from preoperational, egocentric thinking to concrete, operational, decentered thought. For the first time, children can see the world from someone else's point of view. **Decentration** means being able to see several aspects of a problem at the same time and to understand the relation of various parts to the whole situation. Cause-and-effect relations become clear; consequently, magical thinking begins to disappear. During the seventh or eighth year, understanding of the conservation of continuous quantity increases. Understanding conservation depends on **reversibility,** the ability to think in either direction. Seven-year-olds can add and subtract, count forward and backward, and see how it is possible to put something back the way it was. A 7- or 8-year-old can understand that illness is probably only temporary, whereas a 6-year-old may think it is permanent.

Another important change in thinking during this period is **classification,** the ability to group objects into a **hierarchical arrangement** (grouping by some common system). Children in this age group love to collect sports cards, insects, rocks, stamps, coins, or anything else that strikes their fancy. These collections may be only a short-term interest, but some can develop into lifetime hobbies.

Nursing Implications

School-age children have developed many skills as well as the increased ability to learn. In many settings, nurses have opportunities to teach information concerning good nutrition, the human body, health, sex, and substance abuse education.

Nutrition

As coordination improves, children become increasingly active and require more food to supply necessary energy. Increased appetite and a tendency to go on food "jags" are typical of 6-year-olds. Allowing them to express food dislikes and permitting refusal of disliked food items are usually the best ways to handle this phase.

Children learn by example and they will accept more readily the importance of manners, calm voices, appropriate table conversation, and courtesy if they see others carry them out consistently at home. Caregivers never should use mealtimes for nagging, finding fault, correcting manners, or discussing a poor report card. They should teach hygiene in a cheerful but firm manner, even if children must leave the table more than once to wash their hands adequately. Most children prefer simple, plain foods. Forcing children to eat is not helpful and can have harmful effects. Caregivers must carefully supervise children's snacking habits to be sure that snacks are nutritious and not too frequent. They should encourage children to eat a good breakfast to provide the energy and nutrients needed to perform well in school.

Obesity can be a concern during this age. A genetic tendency, environmental factors, and a sedentary lifestyle may contribute. Other children, especially in the later elementary grades, can be unkind to overweight children. Overweight children often are miserable. Encouraging physical activity and limiting dietary fat intake will help control weight. Health teaching at school reinforces the importance of a proper diet.

Stop, Think, and Respond ● BOX 6-3

What factors contribute to childhood obesity? What can help the school-age child with weight control?

Health Education

Health teaching in the home and at school is essential. Caregivers have a responsibility to teach children about basic hygiene, sexual functioning, substance abuse, and accident prevention. Schools must include these topics in the curriculum, because many families are not informed enough to cover them adequately. Some schools offer health classes taught by a health educator at each grade level. Other schools integrate health and sex education into the curriculum, with different classroom teachers covering these topics. Nurses should become active in their community to ensure that these kinds of programs are available to children.

SEX EDUCATION. Children learn about femininity and masculinity starting at birth. Behaviors, attitudes, and actions of the men and women in the child's life, especially their actions toward the child and each other, form impressions that last a lifetime. The proper time and place for formal sex education have been very controversial. Part of the problem seems to be that many people automatically think that sex education means adult sexuality and reproduction. Sex education, however, includes helping children develop positive attitudes toward their own bodies, their own sex, and their own sexual role to achieve optimum satisfaction in being a boy or a girl.

Some schools limit sex education to one class, usually in the fifth grade, in which children see films about menstruation and their developing bodies. Often these topics are taught in separate classes for boys and girls. Some health educators strongly recommend starting sex education in kindergarten and developing topics gradually over the successive grades.

Learning about reproduction of plants and animals, about birth and nurturing in other animals, and about the roles of the male and the female in family units can lead to the natural introduction of human reproduction, male and female roles, families, and nurturing. If all children grew up in secure, loving, ideal families, much of this could be learned at home. Many children do not have this type of home, however, so they need healthy, positive information to help them develop healthy attitudes about their own sexuality. Books or pamphlets are available for various age groups that caregivers or nurses can use to provide children with information. Feelings of self-worth woven into these lessons help children feel good about themselves and who they are.

At a young age, children are exposed to sexually provocative information through the media. Children who do not get accurate information at home or at school will learn what they want to know from their peers; this information often is inaccurate, which makes sex education even more urgent. In addition, the U.S. Centers for Disease Control currently recommends that elementary school children learn about AIDS and how it is spread. Many school districts are working hard to integrate this information into the health curriculum at all grade levels in a sensitive, age-appropriate manner.

SUBSTANCE ABUSE. In addition to nutrition, health practices, safety, and sex education, school-age children also need substance abuse education. Programs that teach children to "just say no" are one way that children can learn that they are in control of the choices they make regarding substance abuse. Teaching children the unhealthy aspects of tobacco and alcohol use and drug abuse should start in elementary school as a good foundation for more advanced information in adolescence.

Children may experiment with **inhalants** (substances whose volatile vapors can be abused) because they are readily available and may seem no more threatening than an innocent prank. Inhalants classified as **deliriants** are commonly found in the home and include model glue, rubber cement, paint, and hair spray. The fumes are mind-altering when inhaled. Overdose can cause loss of consciousness and possible death. Children who experiment with inhalants may proceed to abuse other drugs in an attempt to get similar effects. Addiction occurs in younger children more rapidly than in adults.

Family caregivers must work to develop a strong, loving relationship with the children in the family. They must teach family values and the difference between right and wrong, set and enforce rules for acceptable behavior, teach facts about drugs and alcohol, and actively listen to the children in the family. An excellent reference for family caregivers is *The Parents Guide to Drug Prevention: Growing Up Drug Free,* which is published by the United States Department of Education and can be ordered free by calling the Department of Education's toll-free number, (800) 624-0100, or via the Internet at *http://www.ed.gov/offices/OESE/SDFS.*

The School-age Child in the Healthcare Facility

Increased understanding of their bodies, continuing curiosity about how things work, and the development of concrete thinking all contribute to helping school-age children understand and accept a healthcare experience more easily than younger children can. They can communicate better with healthcare providers, understand cause and effect, and tolerate longer separations from their family.

Nurses who care for school-age children should understand that concepts about birth, death, the body, health, and illness change between 6 and 10 years. Explain all procedures to children and their families; showing the equipment and materials to be used (or pictures of them) and outlining realistic expectations of procedures and treatments are helpful. Answer children's questions including those about pain truthfully. Children of this age have anxieties about looking different from other children. An opportunity to verbalize these anxieties will help them cope. School-age children need privacy more than younger children do and this should be respected.

Family caregivers may feel guilty about the child's need for hospitalization and, as a result, may overindulge the child. The child may regress in response to this, but this regression should not be encouraged. Sometimes the family needs as much reassurance as the child does. Discipline and rules have a place on a pediatric unit. Inform families and children about the rules as part of the admission routine. Opportunities for interaction with peers, learning situations, and doing crafts and projects can help make the child's experience more tolerable.

PREADOLESCENT: 10 TO 12 YEARS

During the period between 10 and 12 years, the rate of growth varies greatly in boys and girls. This variability in growth and maturation can be a concern to children who develop rapidly or to those who develop more slowly than peers. Children at these ages do not want to be different from their friends. The developmental characteristics of preadolescents overlap with those of early adolescence; nevertheless, unique characteristics set this stage apart (Table 6.5).

Physical Characteristics

Preadolescence begins in females between ages of 9 and 11 years and is marked by a growth spurt that lasts for about 18 months. Girls grow about 3 inches each year until **menarche** (the beginning of menstruation), after which growth slows considerably. Early in adolescence, girls begin to develop a figure, the pelvis broadens, and axillary and pubic hair begins to appear along with many changes in hormone levels. The variation between girls is great and often is a cause for much concern by the "early bloomer" or the "late bloomer." Physical changes often embarrass young girls who begin to develop physically as early as 9 years. In girls, the onset of menarche marks the end of the preadolescent period.

Boys enter preadolescence a little later, usually between 11 and 13 years, and grow generally at a slower, steadier rate than do girls. During this time, the scrotum and testes begin to enlarge, the skin of the scrotum begins to change in coloring and texture, and sparse hair begins to show at the base of the penis. Boys who start their growth spurt later often are concerned about being shorter than their peers. In boys, the appearance of **nocturnal emissions** ("wet dreams") is often used as the indication that the preadolescent period has ended.

Preparation for Adolescence

Preadolescents need information about their changing bodies and feelings. Sex education includes information about the hormonal changes that are or will be occurring. Girls need information that will help them handle their early menstrual periods; irregular periods, which may occur for the first year or so; as well as questions about protection during the menstrual period and the advisability of using sanitary pads or tampons. They need to be allowed to express their anxieties and concerns.

Boys also need information about their bodies. Erections and nocturnal emissions are topics they need to discuss, as well as the development of other male secondary sex characteristics. Both boys and girls need information about changes in the opposite sex, including discussions that address their questions. This kind of information helps them increase their understanding of human sexuality.

Preadolescence is appropriate for discussions that will help the young teen resist pressures to become sexually active too early. Perhaps the most important aspect of discussions about sexuality is to give honest, straightforward answers in an atmosphere of caring concern.

TABLE 6.5 GROWTH AND DEVELOPMENT: THE PREADOLESCENT

PHYSICAL	MOTOR	PERSONAL–SOCIAL	LANGUAGE	PERCEPTUAL	COGNITIVE
Average height $56\frac{3}{4}$ inches–59 inches (144–150 cm) Average weight 77–88 lb (35–40 kg) Pubescence may begin Girls may surpass boys in height Remaining permanent teeth erupt	Refines gross and fine motor skills May have difficulty with some fine motor coordination due to growth of large muscles before that of small muscle growth; hands and feet are first structures to increase in size; thus, actions may appear uncoordinated during early preadolescence Can do crafts Uses tools increasingly well	Attends school primarily for peer association Peer relationships of greatest importance Intolerant of violation of group norms Can follow rules of group and adapt to another point of view Can use stored knowledge to make independent judgments	Fluent in spoken language Vocabulary 50,000 words for reading; oral vocabulary of 7200 words Uses slang words and terms, vulgarities, jeers, jokes, and sayings	Can catch or intercept ball thrown from a distance Possible growth spurts may cause myopia	Begins abstract thinking Conservation of volume Understands relation among time, speed, and distance Ability to sympathize, love, and reason are all evolving Right and wrong become logically clear

ADOLESCENT: 12 TO 18 YEARS

The adolescent is maturing physically and emotionally, growing from childhood toward adulthood, and seeking to understand what it means to be grown up.

Developmental Stage and Task: Ego Identity Versus Role Confusion

Adolescents confront marked physical and emotional changes and the knowledge that soon they will be responsible for their own lives. They develop a sense of being independent people with unique ideals and goals. During this period, teens are engaged in a struggle to master the developmental tasks that lead to successful completion of this stage and the development of their own personal **identity.** If parents, caregivers, and other adults refuse to grant that independence, adolescents may break rules just to prove that they can. Stress, anxiety, and mood swings are typical of this phase and add to the feelings of **role confusion.**

Physical Characteristics

Rapid growth occurs during adolescence. Girls begin growing during the preadolescent period and achieve 98% of their adult height by 16 years. Boys start growing at approximately 13 years and may continue to grow until 20 years. The skeletal system's rapid growth, which outpaces muscular system growth, causes the long and lanky appearance of many teens and contributes to the clumsiness often seen during this age. Bone growth is completed during adolescence, and a person's height will remain basically the same throughout adult life even though weight can fluctuate greatly.

At 13 to 15 years, the menstrual cycle becomes ovulatory and pregnancy is possible. The girl's breasts take on an adult appearance by 16 years, and pubic hair is curly and abundant.

By 16 years in boys, the penis, testes, and scrotum are adult in size and shape, and mature spermatozoa are produced. Male pubic hair also is adult in appearance and amount. After 13 years, muscle strength and coordination develop rapidly. The larynx and vocal cords enlarge, and the voice deepens. The "change of voice" makes the teenage male's voice vary unexpectedly, which occasionally causes embarrassment for him.

Social Characteristics

Adolescence is a time of transition and the development of a sense of moral judgment and a system of values and beliefs. The foundation provided by family, religious groups, school, and community experiences is still a strong influence, but the peer group exerts tremendous power. Trends and fads among adolescents dictate clothing choices, hairstyles, music, and other recreational choices. Peer pressure to experiment with potentially dangerous practices such as drugs, alcohol, and reckless driving also can be strong; adolescents may need careful guidance and understanding support to help resist this peer influence.

Personality Development

Adolescents confront a greater variety of choices than ever before. Sex role stereotypes have been shattered in most careers and professions. Transportation has made greater geographic mobility possible, so adolescents may go to school in a foreign country, attend college thousands of miles from home, and begin a career in an even more remote location. Making decisions and choices is never simple. Adolescents often are preoccupied with their own concerns and may seek intimate relationships usually with members of the opposite sex. Most intimate relationships during adolescence are **heterosexual,** or between members of the opposite sex. Sometimes, however, young people form intimate attachments with members of the same sex, or **homosexual** relationships. Because our culture is predominately heterosexual and is still struggling with trying to understand homosexual relationships, these relationships can cause great anxiety for family caregivers and children.

Body Image

Body image is closely related to self-esteem. Seeing one's body as attractive and functional contributes to a positive sense of self-esteem. During adolescence, the desire not to be different can extend to feelings about one's body and can cause adolescents to feel that their bodies are inadequate even though they are actually healthy and attractive. Adolescents, particularly males, who feel that they are underdeveloped, suffer great anxiety. Girls in this age group often feel that they are too fat and try strange, nutritionally unsound diets to reduce their weight. They may develop a condition called anorexia nervosa (see Chap. 16).

Nursing Implications

Nurses working with adolescents must recognize the increased caloric needs of teens as well as their sometimes erratic eating habits. Give adolescents adequate and complete information regarding their own personal health. Often nurses are called on to teach as well as to support adolescents. Recognizing their growth and development needs and allowing them to participate in their own healthcare is essential.

Nutrition

Nutritional requirements greatly increase during periods of rapid growth in adolescence. Adolescent boys need more calories than do girls throughout the growth period. Appetites increase, and most teens eat frequently. Nutritional needs are related to growth, physical activities, and sexual maturity rather than age. Because adolescents are seeking to establish their independence, their food choices sometimes are unwise and tend to be influenced by peer preference rather than parental advice. Teens frequently skip meals, especially breakfast, snack on foods that provide empty calories, and eat a lot of fast foods, which provides easy access to high-calorie, nutritionally unbalanced meals and nutritional deficiencies. Nutrients that are often deficient in the teen's diet include calcium, iron, zinc, vitamin A, vitamin D, vitamin B_6, and folic acid. Calcium needs increase during skeletal growth. Girls need additional iron because of losses during menstruation. Boys also need additional iron during this growth period.

In their quest for identity and independence, some adolescents experiment with food fads and diets. Adolescents often resist pressure from family members to eat balanced meals. Family caregivers can provide nutritious meals and snacks, regular mealtimes and a good example for the adolescents. A refrigerator stocked with ready-to-eat nutritious snacks can be a good weapon against snacking on empty calories.

Culture also influences adolescent food choices and habits. Be alert to cultural dietary influences on the adolescent; consider these when helping the adolescent and family devise an adequate food plan. Certain religions recommend a vegetarian diet; other persons follow a vegetarian diet for ecological or philosophical reasons. If planned with care, vegetarian diets can provide needed nutrients.

Health Education and Counseling

Before adolescents can take an active role in their own healthcare, they need information and guidance on the need for healthcare and how to meet that need most effectively. Education and counseling about sexuality, STIs, contraception, substance abuse, and mental health are a vital part of adolescent healthcare. Some of this teaching should and sometimes does come from family caregivers but often their lack of information or discomfort discussing these topics means that health professionals will have to do the job.

SEXUALITY. A good foundation in sex education can help adolescents take pride in having reached sexual maturity; otherwise, puberty can be a frightening, shameful experience. Girls who have not learned about menstruation until it occurs are understandably alarmed. Those who learned to regard it as "the curse" rather than an entrance into womanhood will not have positive feelings about this part of their sexuality.

Boys who are unprepared for nocturnal emissions may feel guilty, believing that they have caused these "wet dreams" by sexual fantasies or masturbation. They need to understand that this occurrence is normal and simply the body's method of getting rid of surplus semen.

Assuming that adolescents are prepared adequately for puberty, sex education during adolescence can deal with the important issues of responsible sexuality, contraception, and venereal disease. More adolescents today are sexually active than ever, resulting in an alarmingly rapid increase in teenage pregnancies and STIs. The incidence of HIV infection is particularly increasing among adolescents (CDC Fact Sheets, 2003). Girls need to learn the importance of regular pelvic examinations and Pap smears and the technique for the monthly self-care procedure of breast self-examination, Boys need to learn that testicular cancer is one of the most common cancers in young men between 15 and 34 years and must learn how and when to perform testicular self-examination.

Adolescents' growing awareness of their sexuality, sexually provocative material in the media, and lack of acceptable means to gratify sexual desires make masturbation a common practice during adolescence. Unlike young children's genital exploration, adolescent masturbation can produce orgasm in the female and ejaculation in the male. Generally, it is a private and solitary activity, but occasionally it occurs with other members of the peer group. Health professionals recognize masturbation as a positive way to release sexual tension and increase one's knowledge of body sensations. Reassure adolescents that masturbation is common in both males and females and is a normal outlet for sexual urges.

SEXUAL RESPONSIBILITY. Not all adolescents are sexually active, but the number of those who are increases with each year of age (CDC Fact Sheets, 2003). Although abstinence is the only completely successful protection, all adolescents need to have information concerning safe sex practices to be prepared for the occasion when they wish to be sexually intimate with someone. Adolescents do not have a good record of using contraceptives to prevent pregnancy. Many teens give excuses such as, "sex shouldn't be planned," because if it is planned, it is wrong or they feel guilty. They need to feel that it "just happened" in the heat of the moment, not because they really wanted or planned it. Many adolescents are beginning to realize that much more than pregnancy may be at risk, but their attitude of "it won't happen to me," which is typical of their developmental age, continues to contribute to their increasing sexual activity.

Some adults continue to resist providing contraceptive information to adolescents in school, believing that such information encourages teens to become sexually active. As HIV infection becomes a greater threat to every sexually active person, however, this argument becomes harder to defend. Adolescents need contraceptive information to prevent pregnancy, but more importantly they need straightforward information about using condoms to protect them against HIV infection. Other STIs that sexually active adolescents need to know about are syphilis, gonorrhea, genital herpes, genital warts, and chlamydial and trichomonal infections. Prevention of STIs is the primary aim of education for adolescents. If prevention proves ineffective, however, the most important factor is referral for treatment. Many adolescents are reluctant to seek treatment, fearing that their family caregivers will discover their activity. Crisis hotlines are valuable resources to assure adolescents that treatment is vital for them and their partners and that confidentiality is ensured.

Healthcare personnel who work with adolescents seeking treatment for an STI must be nonjudgmental, supportive, and understanding. The adolescents need treatment and information about preventing spread of the STI to others as well as how to prevent contracting another STI.

Many adolescents are not sexually active, but most spend time dating or socializing with peers. In recent years, the use of Rohypnol, also known as the "date rape drug," has become a concern for the adolescent as well as the young adult (see Chap. 10). Encourage adolescents to stay aware and alert to avoid becoming a victim of date rape. Teach them to avoid using alcohol and never to leave any drink unattended.

SUBSTANCE ABUSE. As adolescents search for identity and independence, they are susceptible to many pressures from society and their peers. Adolescents may experiment with substances that may be habit-forming or addictive and ultimately will harm them. This may be done "just for kicks," to "go along with the crowd" (peer group), or to rebel against the authority of family caregivers or other adults. Many adults also abuse some substances abused by adolescents; so to some adolescents, using these substances may appear sophisticated.

Alcohol is the mind-altering substance that teens most commonly abuse (Adger, 1999). Other substances that adolescents may abuse are tobacco (including smokeless tobacco), marijuana, cocaine or "crack," heroin, other street drugs, and prescription drugs (see Chap. 17).

MENTAL HEALTH. The turmoil that adolescents experience while searching for self-esteem and self-confidence can cause stress that may lead to depression, suicide, and conduct disorders. Academic and social pressures add to that stress. The family also may be under stress because of unemployment or economic difficulties, separation, divorce, or death of a caregiver. Healthcare personnel must be sensitive to signs that a teen is having problems. Adolescents need the opportunity to express their fears, concerns, and frustrations. The rapport between family caregivers and teens may not be such that adolescents can express these feelings to the family. Many schools have mental health personnel on staff that can provide counseling when needed. Mental health assessment is an important part of the adolescent's total health assessment. Mental health issues can stem from stressful situations, but often are related to chemical imbalances and problems in the brain (see Chap. 7). With the increased use of computers and Internet sites, Internet safety is an important aspect of adolescent mental health. Parents need to be aware of their adolescent's computer activities and the sites they access, especially communication sites such as chat rooms. Discussions with adolescents regarding safety concerns on Internet sites help to increase their awareness and decrease potential dangers. See Client and Family Teaching 6-4.

The Adolescent in the Healthcare Facility

When adolescents are hospitalized, it is usually because of a major health problem Adolescents must cope with the stress of hospitalization, possibly dramatic alterations in body image, partial or total inability to conform to peer group norms, and an interrupted search for identity. Adolescents fear loss of control and loss of privacy. Provide opportunities for the adolescent to make choices whenever possible. Protect the adolescent's privacy by providing screening and adequate covering during procedures.

Adolescents may react with anger and refuse to cooperate when their privacy or feelings of control are threatened. The admission interview for an adolescent may be more successful if the family caregiver and the adolescent are interviewed separately to provide the opportunity to gain information that the adolescent may not want to reveal in the presence of the family caregiver. Clear, hon-

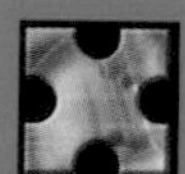

6-4 *Client and Family Teaching* Internet Safety

Signs that might indicate on-line risks in a child or adolescent:

- Spends large amounts of time on-line, especially at night
- Has pornography on computer
- Receives phone calls from adults you don't know
- Makes calls, especially long distance, to numbers you don't recognize
- Receives mail, gifts, or packages from someone you don't know
- Turns computer monitor off or changes screen when you enter room
- Becomes withdrawn from family

To minimize on-line concerns:

- Communicate and talk with child; openly discuss concerns and dangers.
- Spend time with child on-line.
- Use blocking software and devices.
- Use caller ID to determine who is calling your child.
- Maintain access to child's on-line account and monitor activity.

Adapted from FBI Publication, *A parent's guide to internet safety.* [On-line.]. Available: *http://www.fbi.gov/publications/pguide/pguidee.htm.*

est explanations about treatments and procedures are essential. Adolescents need to know what limits are set for their behavior while hospitalized. Many adolescents find it helpful to discuss their health problem with a peer who has had the same or a related problem. Adolescents need access to a telephone to contact peers and keep up social contacts. Recreation areas are important. Access to a computer and electronic mail might also help the teen stay connected to peers. Supervision is important to decrease misuse of computer privileges. The adolescent's health problem may require a lengthy hospitalization and intense rehabilitation efforts. Adequate preparation and guidance can help make that difficult experience easier and less damaging to normal growth and development.

Critical Thinking Exercises

1. *Tony brings 6-month-old Essie in for a routine checkup. Formulate a plan for the visit. Identify the characteristics to observe during the physical examination, nutritional factors to cover, and other age-appropriate teaching.*
2. *Four-year-olds sometimes are characterized as the "frustrating fours." After reviewing their growth and development characteristics, identify reasons you believe this may occur.*
3. *Delsey, the mother of 6-year-old Jasmine, is upset because Jasmine is a picky eater and often does not want to eat what Delsey has prepared. Discuss information you would share with this mother to advise her regarding nutrition in the school-age child.*

● NCLEX-STYLE REVIEW QUESTIONS 

1. The nurse is preparing to teach ninth grade students about reproduction and contraception. Which consideration is most important when preparing for the class?
   1. Examples of birth control methods are on open display for review.
   2. Pamphlets on sexually transmitted infections are sent home for further review.
   3. All information is appropriate for age, maturity level, and knowledge.
   4. All information is presented in current music and video format.
2. A parent confides in a nurse, "My toddler answers 'No' to every question." Which suggestion for handling this behavior is most appropriate to give the parent?
   1. Give the toddler choices to pick from.
   2. Give praise when "No" is not the response.
   3. Give a warning that this behavior must stop.
   4. Give a time-out for the negative behavior.
3. Which instruction to first-time mothers is crucial when starting their children on new foods?
   1. Offer a balanced group of meats and vegetables.
   2. Ensure that foods are thick in consistency.
   3. Give flavorful foods, which are best accepted.
   4. Offer one new food at a time.

connection

Visit the Connection site at **http://connection.lww.com/go/timbyEssentials** for links to chapter-related resources on the Internet.

References and Suggested Readings

Adger, H. (1999). Adolescent drug abuse. In *Oski's pediatrics: Principles and practice* (3rd ed.). Philadelphia: Lippincott Williams & Wilkins.

American Academy of Pediatrics. (2003). *Pediatric clinical practice guidelines & policies* (3rd ed.). Author.

Berger, K. S. (2001). *The developing person through the life span.* New York: Worth Publishers.

Brazelton, T. B., & Greenspan, S. (2001). *The irreducible needs of children: What every child must have to grow, learn, and flourish.* Cambridge, MA: Perseus Publishing.

Bufalini, M. (2001). Dental health life cycle. *Community Health Forum, 2*(6).

CDC Fact Sheets (2003). CDC Division of HIV/AIDS prevention. [On-line.] Available: http://www.cdc.gov/pubs/facts/htm. Accessed 2/21/04.

Deering, C. G., & Jennings, C. D. (2002). Communicating with children and adolescents. *American Journal of Nursing, 102*(3) 34–42.

Dudek, S. G. (2000). *Nutrition essentials for nursing practice* (4th ed.). Philadelphia: Lippincott Williams & Wilkins.

Gaylord, N. (2001). Parenting classes: From birth to 3 years. *Journal of Pediatric Health Care, 15*(4), 179.

Halsey, N. A., & Asturias, E. J. (1999). Immunization. In *Oski's pediatrics: Principles and practice* (3rd ed.). Philadelphia: Lippincott Williams & Wilkins.

Kula, K. S., & Wright, J. T. (1999). Oral problems. In *Oski's pediatrics: Principles and practice* (3rd ed.). Philadelphia: Lippincott Williams & Wilkins.

Mera, K., & Hackley, B. (2003). Childhood vaccines: How safe are they. *American Journal of Nursing, 103*(2), 79.

McClowry, S. G. (2002). The temperament profiles of school-age children. *Journal of Pediatric Nursing, 17*(1), 3–10.

Monsen, R. (2001). Giving children control and toilet training. *Journal of Pediatric Nursing, 16*(5), 375.

Nicoll, L. (2001). *Nurse's guide to the Internet* (3rd ed.). Philadelphia: Lippincott Williams & Wilkins.

Pillitteri, A. (2003). *Maternal and child health nursing* (4th ed.). Philadelphia: Lippincott Williams & Wilkins.

Spock, B., et. al. (1998). *Dr. Spock's baby and child care.* New York: Pocket Books.

Wong, D. L., Perry, S., & Hockenberry, M. (2002). *Maternal child nursing care* (2nd ed.). St. Louis: Mosby.

chapter 7

Caring for the Child or Adolescent With a Psychobiologic Disorder

Words to Know

brachycephaly
chelating agent
child neglect
dysfunctional family
echolalia
encephalopathy
fetal alcohol syndrome
incest
microcephaly
micrognathia
palpebral fissures
philtrum
pica
rumination
sexual abuse
sexual assault

Learning Objectives

On completion of this chapter, the reader will:

- Describe the characteristics and goals of treatment of autism.
- Explain why Down syndrome also is called trisomy 21.
- List 10 signs and symptoms of Down syndrome.
- Describe the characteristics of infants with fetal alcohol syndrome.
- List seven sources of lead that may cause chronic lead poisoning.
- Describe the symptoms, diagnosis, treatment, and prognosis of lead poisoning.
- List the prenatal, perinatal, and postnatal causes of mental retardation.
- Identify 10 possible characteristics seen in children with attention deficit-hyperactivity disorder.
- Identify how poor parenting skills may lead to child abuse.
- Identify the circumstances under which physical punishment can be classified as abusive.
- Describe the difference between accidental bruises to a child and those that have been inflicted abusively.
- Identify how a child may be emotionally abused.
- Describe the characteristics of the child with nonorganic failure to thrive.

This chapter offers a basic understanding of psychobiologic disorders seen in children. Care of children with developmental disorders is challenging for pediatric nurses as well as for family caregivers. Abuse and neglect have occurred throughout history; caring for and supporting children affected by abuse is a major role of the nurse.

DEVELOPMENTAL DISORDERS

• AUTISM

The American Psychiatric Association introduced the term *pervasive developmental disorder* in 1980. The main characteristic of pervasive developmental disorders is severe behavioral disturbance that affects the practical use of language as a means of communication, interpersonal interaction, attention, perception, and motor activity. One such disorder is autism. The word *autism* comes from the Greek word *auto* meaning "self" and was first used by Dr. Leo Kanner in 1943 to describe a group of behavioral symptoms in children.

Pathophysiology and Etiology

Although often called *infantile autism* because it is thought to be present from birth, autism usually is not diagnosed conclusively until after a child is 12 months old. Autistic children are totally self-centered and cannot relate to others; they often exhibit bizarre behaviors and are destructive to themselves and others.

Several theories exist about the cause of autism as well as its management. Autism appears to have organic and perhaps genetic causes. Researchers suggest that autism may result from a disturbance in language comprehension, a biochemical problem involving neurotransmitters, or abnormalities in the central nervous system and probably brain metabolism (Harris, 1999).

Because the cause of autism is not understood fully, treatment attempts have met with limited success. These children experience the normal health problems of childhood in addition to those that result from their behaviors.

Assessment Findings

The characteristics of autism are divided into three categories: inability to relate to others, inability to communicate with others, and obviously limited activities and interests. Children with autism do not develop a smiling response to others or an interest in being touched or cuddled. In fact, they can react violently at attempts to hold them. Their blank expressions and lack of response to verbal stimulation can suggest deafness. They do not show the normal fear of separation from parents that most toddlers exhibit. Often they seem not to notice family caregivers.

During their second year, children with autism become completely absorbed in strange repetitive behaviors such as spinning an object, flipping an electrical switch on and off, or walking around the room feeling the walls. Their bodily movements are bizarre: rocking, twirling, flapping arms and hands, walking on tiptoe, twisting and turning fingers. If others interrupt these movements or move objects in the environment, the child may throw a violent temper tantrum. Such tantrums may include self-destructive acts such as hand biting and head banging. Although infants and toddlers normally are self-centered, ritualistic, and prone to displays of temper, children with autism show these characteristics to an extreme degree coupled with an almost total lack of response to other people.

Children with autism are slow to develop speech, and any speech that develops is primitive and ineffective for communication. **Echolalia** ("parrot speech") is typical; children with autism echo words they have heard, such as on a television commercial, but offer no indication that they understand the words. Although these children are self-centered, their speech indicates that they seem to have no sense of self because they never use the pronouns "I" or "me."

Findings of standard intelligence tests that rely on verbal ability usually indicate that these children test in the mentally retarded range of intelligence (Harris, 1999). These children score poorly on intelligence tests but may have good memories and good intellectual potential.

To confirm a diagnosis of autism, at least eight of 16 identified characteristics must be present and all three categories must be represented. The symptoms of autism can suggest other disorders such as lead poisoning, phenylketonuria, congenital rubella, and measles encephalitis. Therefore, a complete physical and neurologic examination is necessary including vision and hearing testing, electroencephalography, radiographic studies of the skull, urine screening, and other laboratory studies. In addition, a complete prenatal, natal, and postnatal history including development, nutrition, and family dynamics is important.

Medical Management

The treatment of a child with autism is extremely challenging. Four goals toward which treatment is geared are as follows:

- Promotion of normal development
- Specific language development
- Social interaction
- Learning

Treatment using behavioral modification, pharmacotherapeutics, and other techniques must be planned individually and highly structured. Results are mixed, and no one technique has met with resounding success. The family needs therapy to help relieve guilt and understand this puzzling child. The overall long-term prognosis for children with autism is not optimistic; however, the outlook is better the earlier treatment begins. Facilitated communication involves working with the language development of children with autism by helping them express themselves through a computer keyboard. This method, however, is viewed as controversial and is not totally supported by the American Psychological Association.

Nursing Management

Nurses must recognize that autism places great stress on the entire family. The problems that cause family caregivers to seek diagnosis are difficult to live with; diagnosis itself is usually a lengthy and expensive process, and the hope for successful treatment is slight. Most caregivers of children with autism feel guilty despite the fact that current theories accept organic rather than psychological causes for the disorder. The possibility of genetic factors adds to this guilt. Often other children in the family who are not autistic suffer from a lack of attention because caregivers direct their energies almost totally to solving the problems of the youngster with autism.

Nurses who care for children with autism should consider the family caregivers as their most valuable source of information about the child's habits and communication skills. To gain the child's cooperation, the nurse must learn which techniques the caregivers use to communicate with the child. Establishing a relationship of trust between the child and the nurse is essential. To provide consistency, a constant primary nurse should care for this child.

In the hospital setting, a private or semiprivate room generally is preferred, with minimal visual and auditory stimulation. Familiar toys or other valued objects from home reduce the child's anxiety about the strange environment.

Stop, Think, and Respond ● BOX 7-1

What categories of characteristics are found in children with autism? What are some symptoms seen in the second year of life in these children? 

● DOWN SYNDROME

Down syndrome is the most common chromosomal anomaly, occurring in about 1 in 700 to 800 births (D'Alton and Stewart, 1999). Langdon Down first described the condition in 1866, but its cause was a mystery for many years. In 1932, it was suggested that a chromosomal anomaly might be the cause, but the anomaly was not demonstrated until 1959.

Pathophysiology and Etiology

Most people with Down syndrome have trisomy 21 (Fig. 7.1); a few have partial dislocation of chromosomes 15 and 21. When a child has trisomy 21, it means that three chromosomes are in the 21st position on a karyotype. Women older than 35 years are at increased risk of bearing a child with Down syndrome; however, children with Down syndrome are born to women of all ages (D'Alton & Stewart, 1999). Older women are more likely to choose to have an amniocentesis to determine if they are carrying a child with Down syndrome, which may lead to a decision about abortion. The growing trend toward routine screening of all pregnant women for an elevated maternal serum alpha-fetoprotein level may reduce the number of children born with Down syndrome, because parents will have the option to abort the pregnancy.

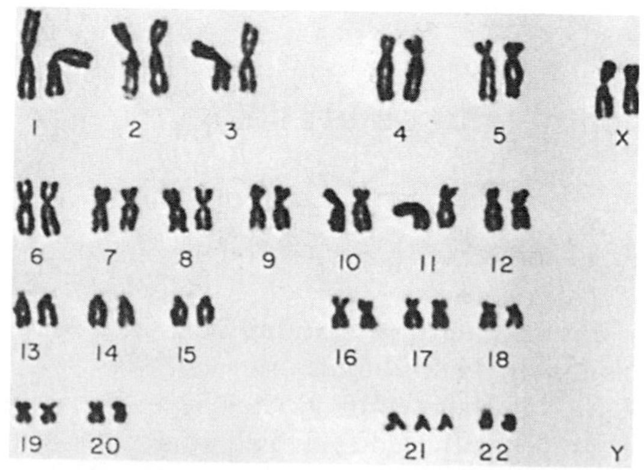

FIGURE 7.1 Karyotype showing trisomy 21. Note three chromosomes in the 21 position.

Assessment Findings

All forms of Down syndrome show a variety of abnormal characteristics. Mental status is usually within the moderate to severe range of retardation, with most children being moderately retarded. The most common anomalies include the following:

- **Brachycephaly** (shortness of head)
- Retarded body growth
- Upward and outward slanted eyes (almond-shaped) with an epicanthic fold at the inner angle
- Short, flattened bridge of the nose
- Thick, fissured tongue
- Dry, cracked, fissured skin that may be mottled
- Dry and coarse hair
- Short hands with an incurved fifth finger
- A single horizontal palm crease (simian line)
- Wide space between the first and second toes
- Lax muscle tone (often referred to as "double-jointed" by others)
- Heart and eye anomalies
- Greater susceptibility to leukemia than in the general population

Not all these physical signs are present in all people with Down syndrome. Some may have only one or two characteristics; others may show nearly all.

Medical and Nursing Management

The physical characteristics of the child with Down syndrome determine the medical and nursing management. Lax muscles, congenital heart defects, and dry skin contribute to many problems. Relaxed muscle tone may contribute to respiratory complications as a result of decreased respiratory expansion. Relaxed skeletal muscles contribute to late motor development. Gastric motility also is decreased, leading to problems with constipation. Congenital heart defects and vision or hearing problems add to the complexities of the child's care.

In infancy, the child's large tongue and poor muscle tone may contribute to difficulty breastfeeding or ingesting formula and can cause great problems when the time comes to introduce solid foods. Family caregivers need support during these trying times. As the child gets older, concern about excessive weight gain becomes a primary consideration.

Family caregivers of children with Down syndrome and other cognitive impairments need strong support and guidance from the birth of these children. Early intervention programs have yielded some encouraging results, but families must decide if they can manage the child at home. A child with cognitive impairment who is undisciplined or improperly supervised may threaten the safety of others in the home and the neighborhood. Caring for the child may demand so much sacrifice from other family members that the family eventually disintegrates.

Stop, Think, and Respond ● BOX 7-2

When a child with Down syndrome is said to have trisomy 21, what does this mean? What is the biggest concern regarding feeding the child with Down syndrome?

• FETAL ALCOHOL SYNDROME

Any ingestion of alcohol during pregnancy is considered unwise. Several factors related to maternal drinking may affect the fetus. The alcoholic mother may be malnourished. She may have an alcohol-induced illness such as gastric hemorrhage or cirrhosis of the liver. Alcohol crosses the placenta easily, directly affecting the fetus as well as being in the amniotic fluid that the fetus ingests. No safe range of maternal alcohol intake has been established, and any maternal drinking can cause infants to have poor intrauterine growth and congenital anomalies. Heavy maternal drinking produces even greater abnormalities (Bezold, 1999). The abnormalities characteristically seen in infants whose mothers consumed alcohol during pregnancy commonly are referred to as fetal alcohol effects (FAE) if the effects are mild or **fetal alcohol syndrome** (FAS) when the effects are severe.

Assessment Findings

Infants with FAS are shorter and weigh less than their peers and may have **microcephaly** (small head), facial deformities, hearing disorders, poor coordination, minor joint and limb abnormalities, heart defects, delayed development, and mental retardation. Facial deformities are characteristic and include short **palpebral fissures** (opening between the eyes); a flat **philtrum** (vertical groove in the middle of the upper lip); a thin upper lip; a short, upturned nose; and **micrognathia** (a small lower jaw). Infants may have a few or many of these abnormalities. These neonates are jittery and may show evidence of failure to thrive.

At birth, infants with FAS may be hypoglycemic from alcoholic effects. All infants at risk should be screened with a reagent strip in the nursery within the first few hours after birth. Symptoms of neonatal hypoglycemia for which the nurse should be alert include tremors, lethargy, seizures, irregular respirations, and apnea. These neonates also may have respiratory distress syndrome.

Many infants with FAE are not identified clearly. The effects of FAE include alcohol-related physical features, growth retardation, and various cognitive deficits. They are believed to be, at least in part, the result of the mother's consuming lower levels of alcohol as well as possible genetic differences in susceptibility.

Infants and toddlers with FAS often have difficulty with feedings. They also may be hyperactive or have attention deficit disorders, intellectual slowness, poor fine-motor control, and developmental delay of gross motor skills.

Medical and Nursing Management

Newborns with FAS need a quiet, nonstimulating environment. Intravenous fluids are administered as needed to avoid dehydration, and anticonvulsant drugs are administered if the infant is having seizures. Children with FAS and FAE need a supportive educational environment throughout their school years.

• LEAD POISONING (PLUMBISM)

Chronic lead poisoning has been a serious problem among children for many years. It is responsible for neurologic handicaps, including mental retardation, because of the effects of lead on the central nervous system. Infants and toddlers are potential victims because of their tendency to put any object within reach into their mouths. In some children, this habit leads to **pica** (the ingestion of nonfood substances such as laundry starch, clay, paper, and paint). Lead contamination also can affect the unborn fetus of a woman exposed to lead (such as lead dust from renovation of an older home). Screening for lead poisoning is part of a complete well-baby checkup between the ages 6 months and 6 years.

Pathophysiology and Etiology

The most common sources of lead poisoning are as follows:

- Lead-containing paint used on the outside or inside of older houses
- Furniture and toys painted with lead-containing paint; vinyl mini-blinds
- Drinking water contaminated by lead pipes or copper pipes with lead-soldered joints
- Dust containing lead salts from lead paint; emission from lead smelters

- Storage of fruit juices or other food in improperly glazed earthenware
- Inhalation of motor fumes containing lead or from burning of storage batteries
- Exposure to industrial areas with smelters or chemical plants
- Exposure to hobby materials containing lead (e.g., stained glass, solder, fishing sinkers, bullets)

The most common cause has been the lead in paint. Children tend to nibble on fallen plaster, painted wooden furniture (including cribs), and painted toys because they have a sweet taste. Fine dust that results from removing lead paint during remodeling also can harm young children in the household without parents being aware of exposure. In 1973, federal regulations banned the sale of paint containing more than 0.5% lead for interior residential use or use on toys. This legislation has not eliminated the problem, however, because many homes built before the 1960s in inner-city areas, small towns, and suburbs were painted with lead-based paint. Older mansions also may have lead paint because of the building's age. Only contractors experienced in lead-based paint removal should do renovation.

Assessment Findings

Acute episodes sometimes develop sporadically and early in the condition. The onset of chronic lead poisoning is insidious. Some early indications include irritability, hyperactivity, aggression, impulsiveness, or disinterest in play. Short attention span, lethargy, learning difficulties, and distractibility are other signs.

The condition may progress to **encephalopathy** (degenerative disease of the brain) because of intracranial pressure. Manifestations may include convulsions, mental retardation, blindness, paralysis, coma, and death.

The nonspecific nature of the presenting symptoms makes examination of the child's environmental history paramount. Testing blood lead levels is used as a screening method. Target screening is done in areas where the risk of lead poisoning is high. Finger sticks, or heel sticks for infants, can be used to collect samples for lead level screening.

Medical and Nursing Management

The most important aspect of treatment of a child with lead poisoning is to remove the lead from the child's system and environment. The use of a **chelating agent** (an agent that binds with metal) increases the urinary excretion of lead. Several chelating agents are available. Edetate calcium disodium, known as EDTA, is usually given intravenously because intramuscular administration is painful. Inappropriate dosage can result in renal failure. Dimercaptopropanol (dimercaprol), also known as BAL, causes excretion of lead through bile and urine; it may be administered intramuscularly. EDTA and BAL may be used together in children with extremely high levels of lead.

The oral drugs D-penicillamine (D-Penamine) and succimer (Chemet) may be used to treat children with lower blood lead levels. Both drugs come in capsules that can be opened and sprinkled on food or mixed in liquid for administration.

All the chelating drugs may have toxic side effects, and children being treated require careful monitoring with frequent urinalysis, blood cell counts, and renal function tests. Any child receiving chelation therapy should be under the care of an experienced healthcare team.

The prognosis after lead poisoning is uncertain. Early detection of the condition and removal of the child from the lead-containing surroundings offer the best hope. Follow-up should include routine examinations to prevent recurrence and to observe for signs of any residual brain damage not immediately apparent.

Although the incidence of lead poisoning has decreased, it is still prevalent. Measures to educate the public on the importance of preventing this disorder are essential to eliminate the problem. Education of family caregivers is an essential aspect of treatment (Client and Family Teaching 7-1).

Stop, Think, and Respond ● BOX 7-3

What is the most common cause of lead poisoning in children? What are the common sources of this material?

● MENTAL RETARDATION

The American Psychiatric Association (2000) defines mental retardation using two criteria: significantly subaverage general intellectual functioning—an intelligence quotient (IQ) of 70 or lower—and concurrent deficits in adaptive functioning. Adaptive functioning refers to how well a person can meet the standards of independence (activities of daily living) and social responsibility expected for his or her age and cultural group.

Mental retardation often occurs in combination with other physical disorders and has several potential causative factors. *Prenatal* causes include the following:

- Inborn errors of metabolism such as phenylketonuria, galactosemia, or congenital hypothyroidism. Early detection and treatment often can prevent damage.
- Prenatal infection such as toxoplasmosis or cytomegalovirus. Microcephaly, hydrocephalus, cerebral palsy, and other brain damage can result from intrauterine infections.

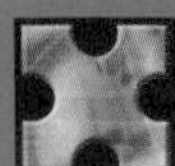

7-1 Client and Family Teaching
Preventing Lead Poisoning

- If you live in an older home, make sure your child does not have access to any chips of paint or chew any surface painted with lead-based paint. Look for paint dust on window sills, and clean with a high-phosphate sodium cleaner (the phosphate content of automatic dishwashing detergent is usually high enough).
- Wet-mop hard-surfaced floors and woodwork with cleaner at least once a week. Vacuuming hard surfaces scatters dust.
- Wash child's hands and face before eating.
- Wash toys and pacifiers frequently.
- Prevent child from playing in dust near an old lead-painted house.
- Prevent child from playing in soil or dust near a major highway.
- If your water supply has a high lead content, fully flush faucets before using for cooking, drinking, or making formula.
- Avoid contamination from hobbies or work.
- Make sure your child eats regular meals. Food slows absorption of lead.
- Encourage your child to eat foods high in iron and calcium.

From Centers for Disease Control and Prevention. (2002). Preventing lead poisoning in young children: a statement by The Centers for Disease Control. Atlanta, Author. [On-line.]. Available: *http://www.cdc.gov.*

- Teratogenic agents, such as drugs, radiation, and alcohol. These can have devastating effects on the central nervous system of a developing fetus.
- Genetic factors, or inborn variations of chromosomal patterns. These result in various deviations, the most common of which is Down syndrome (see earlier discussion).

Perinatal causes of mental retardation include the following:

- Birth trauma
- Anoxia from various causes
- Prematurity
- Difficult birth

In some instances, prenatal factors may have influenced the perinatal complications.

Postnatal causes include the following:

- Poisoning such as lead poisoning. Children who develop encephalopathy from chronic lead poisoning usually have significant brain damage.
- Infections and trauma, such as meningitis, convulsive disorders, and hydrocephalus
- Impoverished early environment such as inadequate nutrition and a lack of sensory stimulation. Emotional rejection in early life may irreparably damage a child's ability to respond to the environment.

Assessment Findings

The most common classification of mental retardation is based on IQ. Although controversy exists about the validity of tests that measure intelligence, this system is still the most useful for grouping these children.

The child with an IQ of 70 to 50 is considered mildly mentally retarded. He or she is a slow learner but can acquire basic skills. The child can learn to read, write, and do arithmetic to a fourth- or fifth-grade level but is slower than average in learning to walk, talk, and feed himself or herself. Retardation may not be obvious to casual acquaintances. With support and guidance, this child usually can develop social and vocational skills adequate for self-maintenance. Approximately 80% of retarded children are classified in this category (Accardo & Capute, 1999).

The moderately retarded child with an IQ of 55 to 35 has little, if any, ability to attain independence and academic skills and is referred to as *trainable.* Motor development and speech are noticeably delayed, but training in self-help activities is possible. This child may be able to learn repetitive skills in sheltered workshops. Some children may learn to travel alone, but few become capable of assuming complete self-maintenance. This category accounts for about 12% of retarded children (Accardo & Capute, 1999).

The child considered severely retarded tests in the IQ range of 40 to 20. This child's development is markedly delayed during the first year of life. He or she cannot learn academic skills but may be able to learn some self-care activities if sensorimotor stimulation begins early. Eventually this child probably will learn to walk and develop some speech; however, he or she always will need a sheltered environment and careful supervision.

The profoundly retarded child has an IQ lower than 20. This child has minimal capacity for functioning and needs continuing care. Eventually, the child may learn to walk and develop primitive speech but will never be able to perform self-care activities. Only about 1% of retarded children are in this category (Accardo & Capute, 1999).

Severe retardation usually is diagnosed at birth or during the first year. Children with milder retardation often are diagnosed when they begin school.

Medical Management

Knowledge about teaching children with cognitive impairment has increased dramatically, and new teaching methods have been yielding encouraging results (Accardo & Capute, 1999). Mildly and moderately retarded people can learn to perform tasks that enable them to achieve some degree of independence.

The child with cognitive impairment may not be identified until well into the preschool stage, because slow development often can be excused in one way or another. The family may be the best judge of the child's development, and healthcare personnel must listen carefully to any concerns or questions that caregivers express. When family members confront the fact that their child is retarded, they need to go through a grieving process, as do family members of any other child with a serious disorder. They need to mourn the loss of the normal child that they expected and resolve to give this child the best opportunities to develop his or her potential.

Early diagnosis and intervention are important tools to use in the care of the child with cognitive impairment. Early infant tests are difficult to administer and the results are inaccurate, but they may provide the family with some idea about the child's potential. The family must be aware that these are only predictions based on unreliable test data.

The child is usually kept at home in the family environment. The current philosophy of care for such a child is to approach teaching aggressively by encouraging learning in a supportive home environment where the child can relate closely to a few people whose role is to stimulate and encourage maximum development. The individual attention, security, and sense of belonging to a family are important factors in every child's growth and development.

NURSING PROCESS

● The Child With Cognitive Impairment

Assessment

The child with cognitive impairment is seen in the healthcare setting for diagnosis, treatment, and follow-up as well as routine health maintenance visits. During these visits, healthcare personnel may find communicating with the child difficult. A thorough interview with the child's caregiver can be helpful in learning about the child and family. Listen carefully to the caregiver, paying particular attention to any comments or concerns he or she has.

The interview and physical examination may be lengthy and detailed depending partially on the circumstances of the child's primary need for healthcare. Aside from the data collection needed as dictated by the current healthcare situation, also gather information about the child's habits, routines, and personal terminology (e.g., nicknames, toileting terms). Be careful to communicate at the child's level of understanding, and do not talk down to the child during the interview. Treat the child with respect. This approach helps gain cooperation from both family and child.

Diagnosis, Planning, and Interventions

Self-Care Deficit: Bathing/Hygiene, Dressing/Grooming, Feeding, Toileting related to cognitive or neuromuscular impairment (or both)

Expected Outcome: The child will develop skills to meet self-care needs within her or his ability.

- Design a teaching program that reflects the child's developmental level. Break each element of care into small segments and repeat those steps. *Consistency among all personnel who care for the child and any involved family members helps in teaching basic tasks. Learning takes place by habit formation and emphasizing the "three Rs:" routine, repetition, and relaxation.*
- Use praise generously and give small material rewards to aid in teaching. *Teaching this child can be time-consuming, frustrating, challenging, and rewarding. Praise and rewards give the child support and encouragement.*
- Challenge the child, but make the immediate small goals realistic and attainable. *Brushing teeth, brushing or combing hair, bathing, washing hands and face, feeding oneself, dressing independently, and basic safety are all self-care areas in which the child needs instruction and positive reinforcement.*
- Work at a level appropriate to the stage of the child's maturation, not the chronological age. *Physical disabilities in addition to retardation can affect the rate of physical development. These children often lack the ability to reason abstractly, which prevents transfer of learning or application of abstract principles to varied situations.*
- Watch for evidence of readiness for a new skill. *Most children with cognitive impairment increase in mental age, although slowly and to a limited level. Therefore, each child needs to be observed for readiness to learn new skills.*

Impaired Verbal Communication related to impaired receptive or expressive skills

Expected Outcome: The child's communication skills will improve, and the child will communicate needs and desires at his or her optimum level.

- Enlist the help of healthcare team members such as a speech therapist. *The child with cognitive impairment often has problems with language skills and forming various speech sounds because of an enlarged tongue or other physical deviations, including hearing impairment. A speech therapist can help develop a program specific to the child's needs.*
- Talk slowly and use pictures and articles when communicating with child. *Doing so gives the child time to process what is being said and reinforces what is being communicated.*
- Use a positive approach with examples and demonstrations. *This method achieves better results than does using a constant stream of "don't touch" or "stop that."*

- Be consistent in expectations and routines. *The child needs to know what to expect and finds security and support in routines and consistency.*

Delayed Growth and Development related to physical and mental disability

Expected Outcomes: (1) The child will attain the milestones of his or her stage of growth and development according to mental age. (2) Family caregivers will verbalize an understanding of the child's level of development.

- Provide environmental stimulation in a supervised setting. *Social interaction and activities are essential for development in all children, but the child with cognitive impairment needs much more environmental enrichment than the average child does. See Table 7.1 for suggested activities for providing this enrichment.*
- Teach and encourage family to reinforce socially acceptable behavior. *At home or in a healthcare facility, the child needs to know acceptable and unacceptable behaviors. Consistent discipline with instructions in simple, direct, concise language is important.*
- Teach family caregivers about the important landmarks of normal growth and development. *This information helps them understand the progressive nature of maturation and improves planning for the child.*

TABLE 7.1 EXAMPLES OF DEVELOPMENTAL STIMULATION AND SENSORIMOTOR TEACHING FOR RETARDED INFANTS AND YOUNG CHILDREN

DEVELOPMENTAL SEQUENCE	POSSIBLE ACTIVITIES TO ENCOURAGE DEVELOPMENT
Sitting	
1. Sit with support in caregiver's lap	Hold child in sitting position on lap, supporting under armpits. Do several times a day, gradually lessening the support.
2. Sit independently when propped	Place child in sitting position against firm surface with pillow behind the back and on either side. Leave the child alone several times a day.
3. Sit with increasingly less support	Allow child to sit on equipment that provides increasingly less support such as baby swing, feeder, walker, high chair.
4. Sit in chair without assistance	Place child in a chair with arms. Provide balance support at first, then gradually withdraw. Leave for 10 minutes at a time.
5. Sit without support	Place child on floor. Gradually withdraw assistance.
Self-Feeding	
1. Sucking	Encourage child to suck by putting food on pacifier, putting a drop on tongue, and so forth.
2. Drink from a cup	Put small amount of fluid in a baby cup. Raise cup to mouth by placing hands under child.
3. Grasp piece of food and place in mouth	Place bit of favorite food in child's hand. Guide hand and food to mouth. Gradually reduce support.
4. Transfer food from spoon to mouth	Move spoon to child's mouth with hand supporting baby's. Gradually withdraw support.
5. Scoop up food and transfer to mouth	Have child hold spoon by handle, scoop up food, and transfer to mouth. Do not allow child to use fingers. Progress from bowl to flat plate.
Stimulation of Touch	
1. Body sensation	Hold, cuddle, rock child.
2. Explore environment through touch	Brush skin with objects of various textures (feathers, silk, sandpaper). Place objects of different textures near child. Move hand to object.
3. Explore environment through mouth	Give child objects that can be chewed. Guide hand to mouth at first.
4. Explore tactile sensations	Expose child to hard, soft, warm, and cold objects.
5. Explore with water	Place hands or feet in water.

- Encourage the child to do activities within the limits of physical disabilities and cognitive functioning. *Abilities level off as these children reach the limits of their physical and mental capabilities. They proceed according to mental rather than chronological age.*

Compromised Family Coping related to emotional stress or grief

Expected Outcome: The family will cope effectively with the child's diagnosis.

- Support the family in working to accept the reality of the child's problem. *The family needs support to cope with the difficult task of helping the child develop his or her full potential. The family functions more effectively when caregivers accept the child as another member to help, love, and discipline.*
- Recognize the family's first reaction to learning that the child may have cognitive impairment is grief. *A parent may feel shame, assuming that he or she cannot produce a perfect child. Some rejection of the child is almost inevitable, at least initially, but the family must work through this to cope.*
- Encourage family caregivers to allow the child to acquire skills at his or her pace. *Some parents try to compensate for their feelings by overprotection or overconcern, making the child unnecessarily helpless.*

Risk for Social Isolation (family or child) related to fear of and embarrassment about the child's behavior or appearance

Expected Outcome: The family will interact with social groups and support networks.

- Encourage family members to talk with other families of impaired children. *Family members need to know that their feelings are normal. Others who have experienced similar feelings can offer support and guidance.*
- Offer information regarding support groups available. *One such group is the National Association of Retarded Citizens (http://www.thearc.org), a volunteer organization with chapters in many communities. The National Down Syndrome Society (http://www.ndss.org) is another excellent resource for the family of a child with Down syndrome.*
- Encourage participation in child and family activities such as Special Olympics. *Such organizations help the child to gain self-confidence and offer support to the family.*

Evaluation of Expected Outcomes

The child practices basic hygiene habits as well as dressing/grooming, feeding, and toileting skills within his or her abilities with support and supervision. The child can communicate basic needs to staff and family. Family caregivers identify the child's developmental level and set realistic goals; the child attains the highest level of functioning for his or her mental age. Family members verbalize feelings, mourn the loss of the "perfect child," and provide appropriate care to help the child reach optimum functioning. They make contact with support systems and establish relationships with other families who have children with cognitive impairment.

ATTENTION DEFICIT-HYPERACTIVITY DISORDER

Attention deficit–hyperactivity disorder (ADHD), or attention deficit disorder, is a syndrome characterized by degrees of inattention, impulsive behavior, and hyperactivity. Approximately 3% to 5% of all U.S. school-age children have ADHD; boys are more commonly affected than girls are (Mostofsky & Denckla, 1999). The cause is unclear: developmental lag, biochemical disorder, and food sensitivities are all theories under consideration.

Assessment Findings

The disorder affects every part of the child's life. The child with ADHD may have these characteristics:

- Is impulsive
- Is easily distracted
- Often fidgets or squirms
- Has difficulty sitting still
- Has problems following instructions despite being able to understand them
- Is inattentive when spoken to
- Often loses things
- Goes from one uncompleted activity to another
- Has difficulty taking turns
- Often talks excessively
- Often engages in dangerous activities without considering the consequences

These children also often demonstrate signs of clumsiness or poor coordination inappropriate for their age group, such as the inability to use a pencil or scissors in a child who is older than 3 or 4 years. No one child has all these symptoms. Although it was believed that these symptoms resolve by late adolescence, it now appears that they continue into adulthood at least for some people (retrieved October 18, 2003 from http://www.nimh.nih.gov/publicat/adhdcfm).

Although these children may have poor success in the classroom because of their inability to pay attention, they are not intellectually impaired. Poor impulse control also contributes to disciplinary problems at school. Some children with ADHD have learning disorders such as dyslexia and perceptual deficits. Self-confidence can suffer from feeling inferior to other children in the class. Special arrangements can be made to provide an educational atmosphere that is supportive for the child without the need for the child to leave the classroom.

Diagnosis can be made after the child is 3 years old, but often is not made until the child reaches school age and has trouble settling into the routine of the classroom setting. Diagnosis can be difficult and also may be controversial because many of the symptoms are subjective and rely on the assessment of caregivers and teachers. The symptoms may be a result of environmental factors that can include broken homes, stress, and nonsupportive caregivers. A careful, detailed history including school and social functioning, psychological testing, and physical and neurologic examinations can help make the diagnosis.

Medical Management

Treatment is multidisciplinary. Learning situations should be structured so that the child has minimal distractions and a supportive teacher. Home support is necessary and requires structured, consistent guidance from the caregivers. Medication is used for some children. Stimulant medications, such as methylphenidate (Ritalin) and dextroamphetamine (Dexedrine), often have been used. When given in large amounts, these medications may suppress the appetite and affect the child's growth. Using stimulants for a hyperactive child seems paradoxical, but these drugs apparently stimulate the area of the child's brain that aids in concentration, thus enabling the child to have better control.

Nursing Management

In the healthcare setting, maintain a calm, patient attitude toward the child with ADHD. Give only one simple instruction at a time. Limiting distractions, using consistency, and offering praise for accomplishments are invaluable methods of working with these children. The families of children with ADHD need a great deal of support. Primary family caregivers in particular can become frustrated and upset by the constant challenge of dealing with a child with ADHD. Building the child's self-esteem, confidence, and academic success must be the primary goals of all who work with these children.

> **Stop, Think, and Respond ● BOX 7-4**
>
> *Why do children with ADHD often have problems in school?*

CHILD ABUSE AND NEGLECT

Every family faces many types of stress at one time or another. Such stressful events include substance abuse, illness, job loss, economic crisis or poverty, relocation, birth, death, and trauma. How the family handles these stresses greatly affects each member's emotional, social, and physical health. A **dysfunctional family** is one that cannot resolve these stresses and work through them in a positive, socially acceptable manner. The atmosphere in such a family creates additional stress for all family members. Because of the lack of support within the family for individual members, these members respond negatively to real or perceived problems. Single-parent families often face multiple pressures at the same time; this dynamic creates additional stress and adds to the risk of dysfunctional coping. This may set the stage for child abuse or neglect. The term *child abuse* has come to mean any intentional act of physical, emotional, or sexual abuse, including acts of negligence committed by a person responsible for the care of the child.

Although child abuse has occurred throughout history, U.S. cultural practices evolved during the last few decades of the 20th century to emphasize the rights of children. Thus, society has come to regard any sort of mistreatment and abuse of children as unacceptable. Each year, increasing numbers of child abuse cases come to the attention of authorities. The actual number of abused children is not known, however, because many cases go undetected.

Child abuse is not limited to one age group and can be detected at any age. Surprisingly, adolescents have the greatest incidence of abuse. For children younger than 2 years, the rate is estimated at six per 1000; the rate for children 15 to 17 years escalates to more than 14 per 1000 (Wissow, 1999).

Child abuse has long-term as well as immediate effects. Abused children may be hyperactive or especially withdrawn; they may exhibit angry, antisocial behavior. Abusive parents often were abused themselves as children; thus, child abuse continues in a cyclical fashion across generations. Abusive parents can be found at all socioeconomic levels, but families with greater financial means may be able to evade detection more easily. Low-income families show greater evidence of violence, neglect, and sexual abuse according to some studies (Wissow, 1999). Commonly, abusive parents have inadequate parenting skills; therefore, they have unrealistic expectations of children and do not respond appropriately to their behavior.

State laws require healthcare personnel to report suspected child abuse. This requirement overrides concerns for confidentiality. Laws have been enacted that protect nurses who report suspected child abuse from reprisals by caregivers (e.g., being sued for slander) even if it is found that the child's situation is not a result of abuse. If the nurse does not report suspected child abuse, the penalty can be loss of the nursing license. Usually, the healthcare facility can hold a child for 72 hours after suspected abuse has been reported so that a caseworker can investigate the charge. After this 72-hour period, a hearing is held to determine if the charges are true and to decide placement of the child.

Types

Physical Abuse

Physical abuse often occurs when the caregiver is unfamiliar with normal child behavior. Inexperienced caregivers do not know what behaviors are normal for children and become frustrated when a child does not respond how they expect. For example, some young women become pregnant to have a child to love, and they expect the child to return that love in full measure. When the child resists the caregiver's control or seems to do the opposite of what is expected, the caregiver takes it as a personal affront and becomes angry, possibly responding with physical punishment. Some cultures support physical punishment for children, citing the old principle, "Spare the rod, spoil the child." Physical punishment that leaves marks, causes injury, or threatens the child's physical or emotional well-being, however, is considered abusive.

Young, active children often have several bruises that result from their usual activities. Most of these bruises occur over bony areas such as the knees, elbows, shins, and forehead. Bruises in areas of soft tissue, such as the abdomen, buttocks, genitalia, thighs, and mouth, may be suspicious. Bruises in the inner aspect of the upper arms may indicate that the child raised the arms to protect the face and head from blows. Bruises may be distinctive in outline, clearly indicating the instrument used; hangers, belt buckles, electrical cords, handprints, teeth (from biting), and sticks leave identifiable marks (Fig. 7.2). Bruises may be in varying stages of healing, which indicate that not all the injuries occurred during one episode.

Burns are another common injury seen in abused children. Although burns may be accidental in young children, certain types are highly suspicious. Cigarette

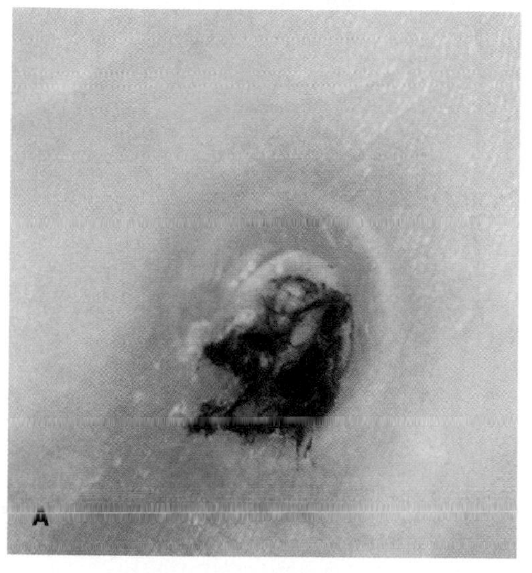

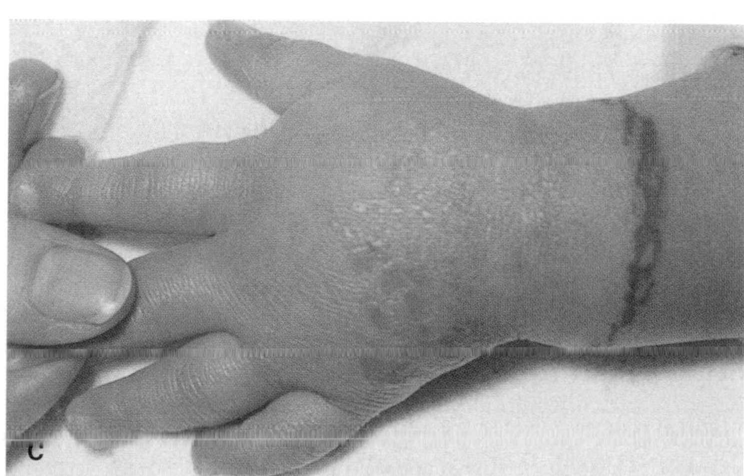

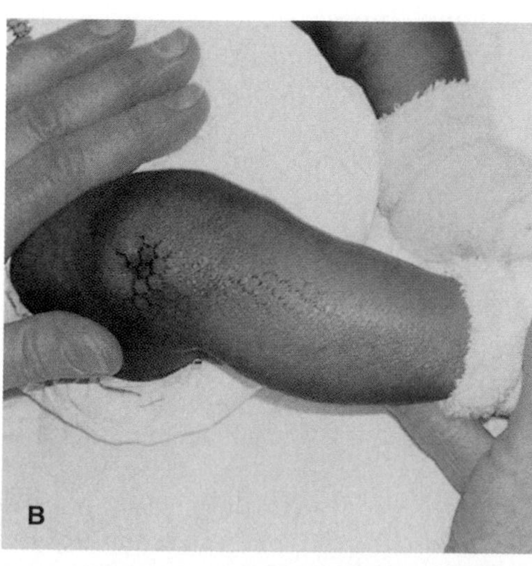

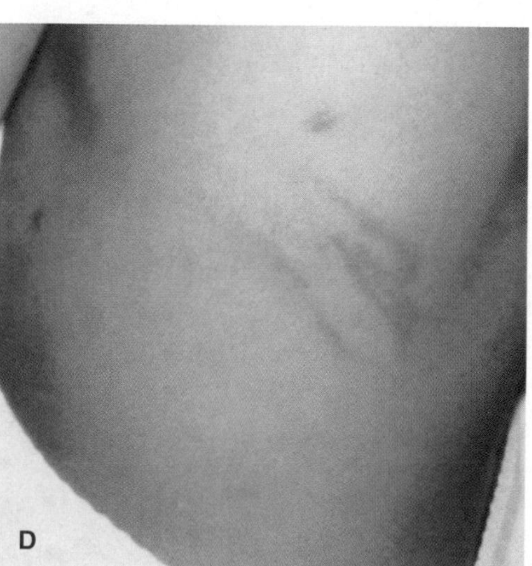

FIGURE 7.2 (**A**) Cigarette burn on child's foot. (**B**) Imprint from a radiator cover. (**C**) Rope burn from being tied to crib rail. (**D**) Imprint from a looped electrical cord.

burns, for example, are common abuse injuries. Burns from immersion of a hand in hot liquid, a hot register (as evidenced by the grid pattern), a steam iron, or a curling iron are not uncommon. Caregivers have been known to immerse the buttocks of a child in hot water if they thought the child was uncooperative in toilet training. Caregivers are often unaware of how quickly a child can be seriously burned. A burn that is neglected or not reported immediately must be considered suspicious until all the facts can be gathered and examined.

Use of technology can assist with the evaluation of signs or possible evidence of child abuse. A radiograph may reveal bone fractures in various stages of healing. Spiral fractures of the long bones of a young child are not common, and their presence might indicate possible abuse. Infants who have been harshly shaken may not show a clear picture of abuse, but computed tomography scanning may demonstrate cerebral edema or cerebral hemorrhage.

An important role of the healthcare team is to identify abusive or potentially abusive situations as early as possible. When a child comes to a physician's office or hospital because of physical injuries, family caregivers may attribute the injury to some action of the child's that is not in keeping with the child's age or level of development. The caregiver also may attribute the injury to an action of a sibling. Whenever the child's symptoms do not match the injury the caregiver describes, be alert for possible abuse. Do not accuse the caregiver before a complete investigation takes place, however.

Emotional Abuse and Neglect

Injury from emotional abuse can be just as serious and lasting as that from physical abuse, but it is much more difficult to identify. Several types of emotional abuse can occur:

- Verbal abuse such as humiliation, scapegoating, unrealistic expectations with belittling, and erratic discipline
- Emotional unavailability when caregivers are absorbed in their own problems
- Insufficient or poor nurturing or threatening to leave the child or otherwise end the relationship
- Role reversal in which the child must take on the role of parenting the parent and is blamed for the parent's problems

Children may show evidence of emotional abuse by appearing worried or fearful or having vague complaints of illness or nightmares. Caregivers may display signs of inappropriate expectations of the child when in the healthcare facility by sometimes mocking or belittling the child for age-appropriate behavior. In young children, failure to thrive may be a sign of emotional abuse. In older children, poor school performance and attendance, poor self-esteem, and poor peer relationships may be clues.

Child neglect is failure to provide adequate hygiene, healthcare, nutrition, love, nurturing, and supervision needed for growth and development. If a child is not given adequate care for a serious medical condition, the caregivers are considered neglectful. For example, if a child is seriously burned, even accidentally, and the caregivers do not take the child for evaluation and treatment until several days later, they may be judged to be neglectful. Often the child with failure to thrive as a result of being underfed, deprived of love, or constantly criticized can be classified as neglected; however, be careful not to make an unsubstantiated accusation.

Sexual Abuse

The Federal *Child Abuse Prevention and Treatment Act* defines **sexual abuse** as "the employment, use, persuasion, inducement, enticement, or coercion of any child to engage in, or assist any other person to engage in, any sexually explicit conduct" (from http://nccanch.acf.hhs.gov/pubs/factsheet/childmal.cfm). When a person has power or control over a child, that person, even if also a child, can be an abuser. For example, someone who is the same age but bigger or stronger could sexually abuse a child his or her own age.

As with other types of child abuse, sexual abuse knows no socioeconomic, racial, religious, or ethnic boundaries. Substance abuse, job loss, and poverty are contributing factors (Wissow, 1999). Like other forms of child abuse, sexual abuse is being recognized and reported more often.

Several terms commonly are used in discussions of sexual abuse. Legally, sexual contact between a child and another person in a caretaking position, such as a parent, babysitter, or teacher, is classified as sexual abuse. A sexual contact made by someone not functioning in a caretaker role is classified as **sexual assault.** Sexual abuse of children has existed in all ages and cultures, but it seldom has been admitted when perpetrated by parents or other relatives in the home. **Incest** (sexually arousing physical contact between family members not married to each other) is one form of sexual abuse. Incest includes fondling of breasts or genitalia, intercourse (vaginal or anal), oral-genital contact, exhibitionism, and voyeurism.

Regardless of the relationship of the perpetrator to the child, the outcome of the abuse is devastating. Episodes of sexual abuse that involve a person whom the child trusts seem to be the most damaging. Incest often goes unreported because the person committing the act uses intimidation by means of threats, appeals to the child's desire to be loved and to please, and convinces the child of the importance of keeping the act secret.

When a child is sexually assaulted by a stranger, the caregivers usually become aware of the incident, promptly report it, and take the child for a physical examination. In the case of incest, however, the child rarely tells another person what is happening. The child may exhibit physical complaints such as various aches and pains, gastrointestinal upsets, changes in bowel and bladder habits (including enuresis), nightmares, and acts of aggression or hostility. Some of these complaints or behaviors may be the presenting problem when a healthcare provider sees the child.

Nursing Management for the Abused or Neglected Child

When assessing a child who may have been abused or neglected, be thorough and complete in observation and documentation. The child should have a complete physical examination; carefully describe and accurately document all bruises, blemishes, lacerations, areas of redness and irritation, and marks of any kind on the child's body. It may be necessary to request that photographs be taken. Observe the interaction between the child and the caregiver, and carefully document observations using nonjudgmental terms. The child's body language may be revealing, so be alert for significant information. For example, if the child shrinks away from contact with the caregiver or healthcare practitioner or, on the other hand, is especially clinging to the caregiver, watch for other signs of inappropriate behavior. These assessments vary with the child's age (Table 7.2). Perhaps the most difficult part may be to maintain a nonjudgmental attitude throughout the interview and examination. Be calm and reassuring with the child; let the child lead the way when possible.

When possible, assign one nurse to care for the child so that the child can relate to one person consistently. Provide physical contact such as hugging, rocking, and caressing only if the child accepts it. Use play to help the child express feelings and fears in a safe atmosphere. Be careful not to do anything that might alarm or upset the child.

In some cases, one caregiver in the family may be an abuser while the other is not. The nonabusive caregiver is a victim as well as the child. Give the nonabusive caregiver an opportunity to express fears and anxieties. He or she may feel powerless in the situation.

While caring for the abused child when the caregiver is present, take the opportunity to observe how the caregiver relates to the child and how the child reacts to the caregiver. Give the caregiver the same courtesy extended to all caregivers. Offer a compliment when the caregiver does something well in caring for the child. Give the caregiver an opportunity to discuss in private any concerns—during this time you may be able to gain his or her confidence.

Often abuse occurs when a caregiver is unfamiliar with normal growth and development and the behaviors common to a particular stage. Help the caregiver develop realistic expectations. Discuss specific behaviors of the child that are upsetting to the caregiver and explain that these are common for the child's age.

The caregiver may be facing temporary or permanent placement of the child in another home. Help the caregiver and the child accept this change. Foster parents may need support from nursing staff to help ease the child's transition to the new home. Abused children must be followed carefully after discharge from the healthcare facility to protect their well-being.

NONORGANIC FAILURE TO THRIVE

Children who fail to gain weight and show signs of delayed development are classified as failure-to-thrive infants or children. Failure to thrive can be divided into two classifications: organic failure to thrive, which is a result of a disease condition, and nonorganic failure to thrive (NFTT), which has no apparent physical cause. It is important to differentiate these two classifications and to be careful not to make an unsubstantiated accusation of neglect in cases of organic failure to thrive. The section below discusses NFTT.

Assessment Findings

Children with NFTT are often listless and seriously below average weight and height, have poor muscle tone and a loss of subcutaneous fat, and are immobile for long periods. They may be unresponsive to (or actually try to avoid) cuddling and vocalization. Examination of the child is likely to reveal no organic cause for this condition. Examination of the family relationship, particularly the mother-child relationship, however, often provides important insights into the problem.

The family relationships of these children are often so disrupted that there is no warm, close relationship or attachment with a family caregiver. Often the father is absent or emotionally unavailable, adding to the mother's feelings of isolation and inadequacy and leading to an atmosphere of additional stress and conflict.

The problem is not with the caregiver alone or with the child but instead with their interaction and mutual lack of responsiveness. The caregiver does not stimulate the child; therefore, the child has no one to respond to and fails to do the "cute baby" things that would gain attention and stimulation. The child cannot accomplish the developmental task of establishing basic trust.

Children with NFTT often fall into the classification of "difficult" or irritable babies, but others may be listless and passive and do not seem to care about feedings. A common characteristic is **rumination** (voluntary regurgitation), perhaps as a means of self-satisfaction when these children do not receive the desired response from the caregiver. Rumination activates a chain of events that further strains the caregiver-child relationship. The child loses weight, sometimes becomes severely emaciated, grows increasingly listless and irritable, and smells "sour"

TABLE 7.2	SIGNS OF ABUSE IN CHILDREN
PHYSICAL SIGNS	**BEHAVIORAL SIGNS**
Physical Abuse	
Bruises and welts: may be on multiple body surfaces or soft tissue; may form regular pattern (e.g., belt buckle) Burns: cigar or cigarette, immersion (stocking/glovelike on extremities or doughnut-shaped on buttocks or genitals), or patterned as an electrical appliance (e.g., iron) Fractures: single or multiple; may be in various stages of healing Lacerations or abrasions: rope burns; tears in and around mouth, eyes, ears, genitalia Abdominal injuries: ruptured or injured internal organs Central nervous system injuries: subdural hematoma, retinal or subarachnoid hemorrhage	Less compliant than average Signs of negativism, unhappiness Anger, isolation Destructive Abusive toward others Difficulty developing relationships Either excessive or absent separation anxiety Inappropriate caretaking concern for parent Constantly in search of attention, favors, food, etc. Various developmental delays (cognitive, language, motor)
Physical Neglect	
Malnutrition Repeated episodes of pica Constant fatigue or listlessness Poor hygiene Inadequate clothing for circumstances Inadequate medical or dental care	Lack of appropriate adult supervision Repeated ingestions of harmful substances Poor school attendance Exploitation (forced to beg or steal; excessive household work) Role reversal with parent Drug or alcohol use
Sexual Abuse	
Difficulty walking or sitting Thickening or hyperpigmentation of labial skin Vaginal opening measures >4 mm horizontally in preadolescence Torn, stained, or bloody underclothing Bruises or bleeding of genitalia or perianal area Lax rectal tone Vaginal discharge Recurrent urinary tract infections Nonspecific vaginitis Venereal disease Sperm or acid phosphatase on body or clothes Pregnancy	Direct or indirect disclosure to relative, friend, or teacher Withdrawal with excessive dependency Poor peer relationships Poor self-esteem Frightened or phobic of adults Sudden decline in academic performance Pseudomature personality development Suicide attempts Regressive behavior Enuresis or encopresis Excessive masturbation Highly sexualized play Sexual promiscuity
Emotional Abuse	
Delays in physical development Failure to thrive	Distinct emotional symptoms or functional limitations Deteriorating conduct Increased anxiety Apathy or depression Developmental lags

because of frequent vomiting. None of this makes for an attractive baby to love, cuddle, and show off.

A physician must evaluate the child thoroughly to rule out a systemic or congenital disorder. Signs of deprivation are important elements in the diagnosis. When the child begins to improve in a nurturing atmosphere, the diagnosis is confirmed.

Medical and Nursing Management

Treatment initially depends almost entirely on good nursing care. By teaching child care skills, acting as a role model, and supporting caregiver-child interactions, the nurse can help reverse the child's growth failure and begin an improved caregiver-child relationship.

Prognosis is uncertain; much depends on the support and counseling the family receives. Long-term care is almost certainly necessary and may require several members of the healthcare team. A positive, nonjudgmental attitude on the part of the nurse can have a direct and lasting effect on the family's interaction with their child.

NURSING PROCESS

● The Child With Nonorganic Failure to Thrive

Assessment

Conduct a careful physical examination of the child including observing skin turgor, anterior fontanelle, signs of emaciation, weight, temperature, apical pulse, respirations, responsiveness, listlessness, and irritability. Observe for rumination or odor of vomitus.

When interviewing the family caregiver, carefully observe the interaction between the caregiver and the child and note the caregiver's responsiveness to the child's needs and the child's response to the caregiver. Listen carefully for underlying problems while talking with the family caregivers. Note if other supportive, involved people are present or if the caregiver is a single parent with no support system. Take a careful history of feeding and sleeping patterns or problems. Determine the caregiver's confidence in handling the child; note any apparent indication of feelings of stress or inadequacy.

Diagnosis, Planning, and Interventions

Imbalanced Nutrition: Less than Body Requirements related to inadequate intake of calories

Expected Outcome: The child's caloric intake will be adequate for child to have appropriate weight gain for age.

- Provide a diet adequate to meet child's daily requirements. *Initially, the child may not consume adequate calories; providing a diet to meet daily requirements will help the child maintain weight and continue growth.*
- Feed the child small, frequent feedings in a calm and quiet atmosphere. *Feeding the child every 2 or 3 hours may be necessary initially to reduce fatigue and improve appetite. Remaining quiet and relaxed decreases the child's anxiety.*
- Provide an environment without distractions and outside stimuli. *Even minor distractions easily divert attention. To decrease distractions and outside stimuli, the child may need to be closely snuggled and gently rocked. Feeding time should be pleasant and comforting.*
- Talk to child; encourage eating and offer direction to older child. *Children may need direction to prevent distraction and to enable them to focus on eating.*
- Encourage family caregiver to become involved in the child's feedings. *Promoting appropriate interaction between child and caregiver with guidance and support will help build their relationship.*
- Carefully document food and caloric intake. Keep strict intake and output records. *Doing so accurately monitors the child's intake and output to assess if daily needs are being met.*

Risk for Delayed Growth and Development related to physical or emotional neglect, lack of stimulation and insufficient nurturing

Expected Outcome: The child will grow and develop according to age-appropriate growth patterns and milestones.

- Hold, cuddle, and rock child when interacting and doing care. *These actions help meet the child's needs for human contact and tactile stimulation.*
- Provide sensory stimulation and age-appropriate activities. *Doing so promotes normal development of age-appropriate skills and milestones.*
- Use eye contact when working with the child. *Eye contact helps the child develop trust and stay engaged in activity or communication.*
- Offer explanations of treatments and situations to older children. *Fear and anxiety keep them from trying and participating in new activities.*

Impaired Parenting related to lack of knowledge and confidence in parenting skills

Expected Outcome: Family caregivers will demonstrate positive signs of good parenting.

- Point out to caregiver the child's development and responsiveness. *The caregiver who has not had a close, warm childhood relationship may not understand the child's needs for cuddling and stimulation.*
- Note and praise any positive parenting behaviors the caregiver displays. *Teaching must be done carefully and in a manner that doesn't further damage the caregiver's self-esteem. Many of these family caregivers are overly concerned about spoiling the child: it is important to dispel these fears.*
- Explain the need for the child to develop trust, and teach the caregiver about the developmental tasks appropriate for child. *Understanding of the child and age-appropriate behaviors increases the parent's comfort level.*

Evaluation of Expected Outcomes

The child's caloric intake increases to an appropriate daily intake; weight increases at a predetermined goal according to normal growth patterns. The child attains developmental milestones for stage of growth and development. The child has eye contact, visually follows the caregiver, and develops trust and security. Family caregivers exhibit appropriate response to the child, and their confidence and feelings of self-esteem increase.

Critical Thinking Exercises

1. *The third grade teacher at the school where you are the nurse complains that the new child in her classroom will just not sit still or listen. You suspect from her description of the child's behavior that the child may have ADHD. What signs and symptoms might indicate ADHD? What suggestions will you make regarding this child?*

2. *Your neighbor is a 17-year-old mother of an active 18-month-old. One day you overhear her yelling at the child, "Listen to me or I will beat you." Describe your feelings. What would you say and do in this situation?*

• NCLEX-STYLE REVIEW QUESTIONS

1. At a routine pediatric check-up, the nurse notes that a 10-month-old with Down syndrome has maintained the same weight for 3 months. When completing nutritional teaching with the family, which area of instruction is the highest priority?
   1. Types of nutritional snacks that are beneficial to eat between meals
   2. Feeding techniques to assist with a large tongue and poor muscle tone
   3. Recipes for spicy foods to combat undeveloped taste buds
   4. Food preparation techniques to aid in problems of malformed teeth
2. A nurse is answering the questions of a mother whose child has an IQ of 65. Which long-term instruction by the nurse is most appropriate?
   1. Families of such children frequently must consider long-term institutional care.
   2. Extended family members often shun children with mental retardation.
   3. Most children with mental retardation can develop social and vocational skills.
   4. Some children with mental retardation learn repetitive skills at sheltered workshops.
3. When establishing a plan of care for an elementary school child with attention deficit–hyperactivity disorder (ADHD), which consideration would the nurse identify as most likely to be a potential long-term problem?
   1. Intellectual impairment
   2. Poor social relationships
   3. Low self-confidence
   4. Explosive temper

connection

Visit the Connection site at **http://connection.lww.com/go/timbyEssentials** for links to chapter-related resources on the Internet.

References and Suggested Readings

Accardo, P. J., & Capute, A. J. (1999). Mental retardation. In *Oski's pediatrics: Principles and practice* (3rd ed.). Philadelphia: Lippincott Williams & Wilkins.

American Psychiatric Association. (2000). *Diagnostic and statistical manual of mental disorders text revision* (4th ed). Washington, DC: Author.

Bezold, L. I. (1999). Cardiovascular embryology. In *Oski's pediatrics: Principles and practice* (3rd ed.). Philadelphia: Lippincott Williams & Wilkins.

D'Alton, M. E., & Stewart, T. L. (1999). Fetal evaluation and prenatal diagnosis. In *Oski's pediatrics: Principles and practice* (3rd ed.). Philadelphia: Lippincott Williams & Wilkins.

Guevara, J., et al. (2001). Health care costs for children with attention deficit disorder. *Pediatrics, 108*(1), 71.

Harris, J. C. (1999). Pervasive developmental disorder and autistic disorder. In *Oski's pediatrics: Principles and practice* (3rd ed.). Philadelphia: Lippincott Williams & Wilkins.

Meaux, J. B. (2000). Stop, look, listen: The challenge for children with ADHD. *Issues in Comprehensive Pediatric Nursing, 23*(1), 1–13.

Mostofsky, S. H., & Denckla, M. B. (1999). School difficulties. In *Oski's pediatrics: Principles and practice* (3rd ed.). Philadelphia: Lippincott Williams & Wilkins.

Naslund, J. (2001). Modes of sensory stimulation. *Physiotherapy, 87*(8), 13–23.

Pillitteri, A. (2003). *Maternal and child health nursing* (4th ed.). Philadelphia: Lippincott Williams & Wilkins.

Sparks, S., & Taylor, C. (2001). *Nursing diagnosis reference manual* (5th ed.). Springhouse, PA: Springhouse Corporation.

VanRiper, M., & Cohen, W. (2001). Caring for children with Down's syndrome and their families. *Journal of Pediatric Health Care, 15*(3), 123.

Wissow, L. S. (1999). Child maltreatment. In *Oski's pediatrics: Principles and practice* (3rd ed.). Philadelphia: Lippincott Williams & Wilkins.

Wong, D. L., Perry, S., & Hockenberry, M. (2002). *Maternal child nursing care* (2nd ed). St. Louis: Mosby.

chapter 8

Caring for Children With Physical Disorders: Part 1

Words to Know

achylia
amblyopia
arthralgia
astigmatism
bilateral
binocular vision
carditis
cataract
chorea
circumoral pallor
clonus
conjunctivitis
coryza
croup
diplopia
ductus arteriosus
dysarthria
emetic
esotropia
exotropia
external hordeolum
foramen ovale
goniotomy
hemarthrosis
hirsutism
hyperopia
hypochylia
myopia
myringotomy
nuchal rigidity
opisthotonos
orthoptics
overriding aorta
polyarthritis
pulmonary stenosis
purpuric rash
refraction
right ventricular hypertrophy
spina bifida
strabismus
stridor
supernumerary
teratogenicity
unilateral
ventricular septal defect
ventriculoatrial shunting
ventriculoperitoneal shunting

Learning Objectives

On completion of this chapter, the reader will:

- Discuss acute laryngotracheobronchitis, including symptoms and treatment.
- State the major organs affected by cystic fibrosis.
- Describe the most common complication in cystic fibrosis and appropriate dietary and pulmonary treatment.
- List five common congenital heart defects and the blood flow associated with each.
- State the signs and symptoms of congestive heart failure in the child with congenital heart disease.
- Name the bacterium usually responsible for the infection that leads to rheumatic fever and accompanying major manifestations.
- State the most serious concern for the child with Kawasaki disease.
- Name the most common types of hemophilia and how each is inherited.
- Explain treatment for hemophilia.
- Differentiate between cleft lip and cleft palate.
- Differentiate the three types of spina bifida.
- State the most obvious symptoms of hydrocephalus.
- Describe two types of shunting performed for hydrocephalus.
- List five types of vision impairment.
- Differentiate between a child who is hard of hearing and one who is deaf.
- Describe the behavior of the infant with acute otitis media.
- List four complications of *Haemophilus influenzae* meningitis.
- Discuss the prenatal, perinatal, and postnatal causes of cerebral palsy.
- Differentiate between spastic and athetoid cerebral palsy.

Many disorders seen in infants and children affect the respiratory and cardiovascular systems. Nurses must understand how to care for children with respiratory and cardiovascular disorders as well as hematopoietic and lymphatic disorders. Neurologic and sensory disorders can be of great concern to family caregivers. Often the role of the nurse is one of support to children and families of children with these disorders.

RESPIRATORY DISORDERS

• ACUTE BRONCHIOLITIS/ RESPIRATORY SYNCYTIAL VIRUS

Acute bronchiolitis (acute interstitial pneumonia) is most common during the first 6 months of life and is seen rarely after the age of 2 years. Most cases occur in infants who have been in contact with older children or adults with upper respiratory viral infections. Acute bronchiolitis usually occurs in the winter and early spring. The causative agent is often respiratory syncytial virus (RSV).

Pathophysiology and Etiology

The bronchi and bronchioles become plugged with thick, viscid mucus, trapping air in the lungs. The infant can breathe in air but has difficulty expelling it. This hinders gas exchange, leading to cyanosis.

Assessment Findings

The onset of dyspnea is abrupt and sometimes preceded by a dry, persistent cough or nasal discharge. Shallow respirations, air hunger, cyanosis, and suprasternal and subcostal retractions are present. The chest becomes barrel-shaped from the trapped air; respirations are 60 to 80 breaths per minute. Dehydration may become a serious problem; the infant is often apprehensive, irritable, and restless. Diagnosis is based on clinical findings and confirmed by laboratory testing (enzyme-linked immunosorbent assay [ELISA]) of the mucus obtained by direct nasal aspiration or nasopharyngeal washing.

Medical and Nursing Management

The infant usually is hospitalized and treated with high humidity by mist tent, rest, and increased fluids. Oxygen also may be administered. Monitoring of oxygenation is done by pulse oximetry. Intravenous fluids are administered to ensure adequate intake. The infant is placed on contact transmission precautions to prevent the spread of infection. Antibiotics are not prescribed because the causative organism is a virus. Ribavirin (Virazole), an antiviral drug, may be used. It is administered as an inhalant by hood, mask, or tent. Ribavirin is classified as a category X drug, signifying a high risk for **teratogenicity** (causing damage to a fetus). Care must be taken to protect pregnant women when the drug is administered to a child with whom the pregnant woman might be in contact (Karch, 2003).

> **Stop, Think, and Respond ● BOX 8-1**
>
> *What is the most common cause of acute bronchiolitis? What precautions are necessary for people who are in contact with a child who has acute bronchiolitis and is receiving ribavirin?*

• CROUP SYNDROMES

Croup is not a disease but a group of disorders typically involving a barking cough, hoarseness, and inspiratory **stridor** (shrill, harsh respiratory sound). The disorders are named for the respiratory structures involved. For example, acute laryngotracheobronchitis affects the larynx, trachea, and major bronchi.

Spasmodic Laryngitis

Spasmodic laryngitis occurs between ages 1 and 3 years. The cause is undetermined; it may be of infectious or allergic origin. The attack may be preceded by **coryza** (runny nose) and hoarseness or by no apparent signs of respiratory irregularity during the evening. The child awakens after a few hours of sleep with a bark-like cough, increasing respiratory difficulty, and stridor. He or she becomes anxious, restless, and markedly hoarse. A low-grade fever and mild upper respiratory infection may be present.

This condition is not serious but is frightening both to the child and family. The episode subsides after a few hours; little evidence remains the next day. Attacks frequently occur two or three nights in succession.

Humidified air reduces laryngospasm. Taking the child into the bathroom and opening the hot water taps with the door closed is a quick method for providing moist air. An **emetic** (an agent that causes vomiting), such as syrup of ipecac, in a dosage less than that needed to produce vomiting, gives relief by helping reduce spasms of the larynx. Cool humidifiers may be used to provide high humidity. Sometimes exposure to cold air relieves the spasm—for instance, when parents take the child out into the night to go to the emergency department.

Acute Laryngotracheobronchitis

Acute laryngotracheobronchitis (bacterial tracheitis or laryngotracheobronchitis) may progress rapidly and become a serious problem within hours. Toddlers are affected most frequently. This condition is usually of viral origin, but bacterial invasion, usually staphylococcal, follows the original infection. It generally occurs after an upper respiratory infection with fairly mild rhinitis and pharyngitis.

The child develops hoarseness, a barking cough, and a fever that may reach 104°F to 105°F (40°C to 40.6°C). Laryngeal edema may occur and breathing becomes difficult; pulse is rapid and cyanosis may appear. Congestive heart failure and acute respiratory embarrassment can result.

Treatment is to maintain an airway and adequate air exchange followed by antimicrobial therapy. The child is placed in a croupette or mist tent that also can include the administration of oxygen. Racemic or nebulized epinephrine may be administered every 3 or 4 hours. Antibiotics are administered intravenously initially and continued after the temperature has normalized. Pulse oximetry is used to determine the degree of hypoxia.

NURSING PROCESS

● The Child With a Respiratory Disorder

Assessment

Conduct a thorough interview with caregivers. Include specific data such as when they first noticed the symptoms, the course of the fever thus far, a description of respiratory difficulties, signs of hoarseness, and the character of any cough. Collect data regarding how well the child has been taking nourishment and fluids. Ask about nausea, vomiting, urinary and bowel output, and history of exposure to other family members with respiratory infections.

Note measurement of temperature, apical pulse, respirations (rate, respiratory effort, retractions [costal, intercostal, sternal, suprasternal, substernal], and flaring of nares). Also note breath and lung sounds (crackles, wheezing), cough (dry, productive, hacking), irritability, restlessness, confusion, skin color (pallor, cyanosis), **circumoral pallor** (a white area around the mouth), cyanotic nail beds, skin turgor, anterior fontanelle (depressed or bulging), nasal passage congestion (color, consistency), mucous membranes (mouth dry, lips dry or cracked), and eyes (bright, glassy, sunken, moist, crusted).

Diagnosis, Planning, and Interventions

Maintaining adequate respiratory function is important with any respiratory condition or disorder. In addition, monitoring the child's intake and output helps prevent dehydration and related complications, which can ensue rapidly. Seeing a child in respiratory distress is upsetting to family caregivers; often nurses are responsible for supporting and teaching the family.

Ineffective Airway Clearance related to obstruction associated with edema, mucus secretions, nasal and chest congestion

Expected Outcome: Child's airway will remain clear and patent, with no evidence of retractions, stridor, hoarseness, or cyanosis.

- Provide an ice-cooled mist tent or cool vaporizer. *A moisturized atmosphere helps thin the mucus in the respiratory tract to ease respirations.*
- Suction or clear secretions when needed. *Clearing secretions helps keep the airway open.*
- Position the child to maximize ventilation; change position at least every 2 hours; use pillows and padding to maintain position. *Positioning provides for lung expansion and prevents slumping, which causes crowding of the diaphragm.*
- While client is in the mist tent, change bedding and clothing often. Stuffed toys are not recommended. *Bedding, clothes, and stuffed toys become saturated and are uncomfortable; they also contribute to an environment in which organisms flourish.*

Impaired Gas Exchange related to inflammatory process

Expected Outcome: Respiratory function will be within normal limits for age; respirations will be regular, breath sounds will be clear, and oxygen saturation levels will be within established limits.

- Monitor child at least every hour; uncover the child's chest and observe breathing efforts. Observe for tachypnea (rapid respirations); note the amount of chest movement, shallow breathing, and retractions. Listen with a stethoscope for breath sounds, particularly noting the amount of stridor. *Initial and ongoing assessment and monitoring indicate difficult breathing. Be continuously alert for warning signs of airway obstruction.*
- Observe for pallor, listlessness, circumoral cyanosis, cyanotic nail beds, and restlessness. *These indications of impaired oxygenation should be reported at once.*
- Administer oxygen by hood, mist tent, or nasal cannula as ordered. *Administration of oxygen increases the oxygen concentration in the blood.*
- Use oximetry to monitor oxygen saturation levels. *Changes in findings indicate respiratory decline.*
- Report increasing hoarseness. *This finding may indicate inflammation and edema in the respiratory tract.*

Risk for Deficient Fluid Volume related to respiratory fluid loss, fever, and difficulty swallowing

Expected Outcome: Fluid intake will be adequate for age and weight; child will exhibit good skin turgor and moist, pink mucous membranes. Urine output will be 1 to 3 mL/kg/hr.

- Clear the infant's nasal passages with a bulb syringe before feeding; feed slowly and without overtiring the child. *For hydration to be adequate, the infant must be able to take fluids without experiencing respiratory distress or exhaustion.*
- Offer small amounts of warm, clear fluids, juices, and water appropriate for age. *Small, frequent amounts of fluid help replace fluid losses and encourage the child to increase intake gradually.*
- Maintain accurate intake and output measurements; weigh the child daily. *Decreased intake or increased output will result in fluid deficit. Fluid needs are determined by the amount needed to maintain body weight with sufficient amounts added to replace additional losses.*
- Assess for dehydration: skin turgor, mucous membranes, and fontanelles. *Fluid loss or dehydration causes poor skin turgor, dry mucous membranes, and sunken fontanelles.*

Compromised Family Coping related to child's respiratory symptoms and illness
Expected Outcome: Family caregivers will verbalize an understanding of the child's condition and how to provide home care. They will ask appropriate questions and verbalize reduced anxiety.

- Teach and reassure family caregivers, encouraging them to discuss feelings of anxiety and helplessness. *Watching a child with severe respiratory symptoms is frightening; sharing feelings helps reduce emotional distress.*
- Use easily understood terminology; explain equipment, procedures, treatments, the illness, and the prognosis to the caregiver. *Understanding what is happening helps caregivers feel more in control of the situation.*
- Encourage caregivers to participate in child's care and to soothe and comfort child. *They may feel helpless. Verbalizing concerns and participating in the child's care will decrease these feelings, as well as support the child.*
- Actively listen to caregivers; use communication skills to respond to their worries and have them relate back specific facts. *Asking caregivers to verbalize their understanding of explanations, signs and symptoms to report, and effects of medications verifies that they comprehended the information accurately.*

Evaluation of Expected Outcomes

The child's airway is clear with no evidence of retractions, stridor, hoarseness, or cyanosis. Mucus secretions are thin and scant. Respiratory rate is within the normal range for the child's age; respirations are regular with clear breath sounds. The infant no longer uses respiratory accessory muscles to aid in breathing. Oxygen saturation levels are within established limits. The child exhibits good skin turgor and moist, pink mucous membranes. Urine output is 1 to 3 mL/kg/hr.

Caregivers cooperate with and participate in the child's care, appear more relaxed, verbalize feelings, and soothe the child. They accurately describe facts about the child's condition, ask appropriate questions, relate signs and symptoms to observe in the child, and name the effects, side effects, dosage, and administration of medications.

• CYSTIC FIBROSIS

Cystic fibrosis (CF) is a major dysfunction of all exocrine glands. The major organs affected are the lungs, pancreas, and liver.

Pathophysiology and Etiology

Cystic fibrosis is hereditary and transmitted as an autosomal recessive trait; thus, both parents must be carriers of the gene for CF to appear. The normal gene produces a protein, cystic fibrosis transmembrane conductance regulator, which serves as a channel through which chloride enters and leaves cells. The mutated gene blocks chloride movement, which brings on the apparent signs of CF. Blocking of chloride transport results in a change in sodium transport. This in turn results in abnormal secretions of the exocrine (mucus-producing) glands. They produce thick, tenacious mucus rather than the thin, free-flowing secretions normally produced. This abnormal mucus leads to obstruction of the secretory ducts of the pancreas, liver, and reproductive organs. Thick mucus obstructs the respiratory passages, causing trapped air and overinflation of the lungs. In addition, the sweat and salivary glands excrete excessive electrolytes, specifically sodium and chloride.

Assessment Findings

Signs and Symptoms

Meconium ileus is the presenting symptom in many newborns who later develop additional manifestations of CF. Depletion or absence of pancreatic enzymes before birth results in impaired digestive activity, and the meconium becomes viscid (thick) and mucilaginous (sticky). The thickened meconium fills the small intestine, causing complete obstruction. Clinical manifestations are bile-stained emesis, a distended abdomen, and no stool. Intestinal perforation with symptoms of shock may occur. These newborns taste salty when kissed because of the high sodium chloride concentration in their sweat.

A hard, nonproductive chronic cough and frequent bronchial infections occur. Development of a barrel chest and clubbing of fingers indicate chronic lack of oxygen. The abdomen becomes distended, and body muscles become flabby. Thick, tenacious mucus obstructs the pancreatic ducts, causing **hypochylia** (diminished flow of pancreatic enzymes) or **achylia** (no pancreatic enzymes), which leads to intestinal malabsorption and severe malnutrition. Malabsorption of fats causes frequent steatorrhea (see Chap. 9). Anemia or rectal prolapse is common if the pancreatic condition remains untreated. Frequently clients with CF develop diabetes.

Respiratory complications pose the greatest threat to children with CF. Abnormal amounts of thick, viscid mucus clog the bronchioles and provide an ideal medium for bacterial growth. Complications such as atelectasis and lung abscesses arise from severe respiratory infections. Bronchiectasis and emphysema may develop with pulmonary fibrosis and pneumonitis. In advanced disease, pneumothorax, right ventricular hypertrophy, and cor pulmonale are common complications. Cor pulmonale is a common cause of death.

The tears, saliva, and sweat of children with CF contain abnormally high concentrations of electrolytes; most clients have enlarged submaxillary salivary glands. In hot weather, the loss of sodium chloride and fluid through sweating produces frequent heat prostration. Males with CF who reach adulthood will most likely be sterile because of the blockage or absence of the vas deferens or other ducts. Females often have thick cervical secretions that prohibit the passage of sperm.

Diagnostic Findings

Diagnosis is based on family history, elevated sodium chloride levels in the sweat, analysis of duodenal secretions for trypsin content, a history of failure to thrive, chronic or recurrent respiratory infections, and radiologic findings of hyperinflation and bronchial wall thickening. Symptoms may be seen shortly after or months or years after birth. The principal diagnostic test to confirm CF is a sweat chloride test using the pilocarpine iontophoresis method, which induces sweating by using a small electric current that carries topically applied pilocarpine into a localized area of the skin.

Medical Management

In newborns, meconium ileus is treated nonoperatively with gentle hyperosmolar enemas. If they do not resolve the blockage of thick, gummy meconium, surgery is necessary. During surgery, a mucolytic such as Mucomyst may be used to liquefy the meconium. If this procedure is successful, resection may not be necessary.

In older children, treatment aims at correcting pancreatic deficiency, improving pulmonary function, and preventing respiratory infections. If bowel obstruction does occur (meconium ileus equivalent), the preferred management includes hyperosmolar enemas and increased fluids, dietary fiber, oral mucolytics, lactulose, and mineral oil.

The overall treatment goals are to improve the child's quality of life and to provide for long-term survival. Cooperation between the healthcare team and child and family is essential. With improved treatment, it is not unusual for a child with CF to grow into adulthood.

Dietary Treatment

Commercially prepared pancreatic enzymes given during meals and with snacks aid digestion and absorption of fat and protein. These enzymes come in capsules that can be swallowed or opened and sprinkled on the child's food. The child's diet should be high in carbohydrates and protein with no restriction of fats. The child may need 1.5 to 2 times the normal caloric intake to promote growth. These children have large appetites; however, they can receive little nourishment without a pancreatic supplement.

Because of the increased loss of sodium chloride, these children are allowed to use as much salt as they wish, even though onlookers may think it is too much. During hot weather, pretzels, salted bread sticks, and saltine crackers can provide additional salt.

Pulmonary Treatment

The treatment goal is to prevent and treat respiratory infections. Respiratory drainage is provided by thinning the secretions and through mechanical means, such as postural drainage and clapping. Antibacterial drugs for the treatment of infection are necessary as indicated. Some physicians prescribe a prophylactic antibiotic regimen when the child is diagnosed. Antibiotics may be administered orally or parenterally even in the home.

Immunization against childhood communicable diseases is extremely important for these chronically ill children. Physical activity, as the child can tolerate, is essential because it improves mucus secretion and helps the child feel better.

Respiratory modalities can be preventive or therapeutic. Handheld nebulizers are easy to use and convenient for ambulatory children. A bronchodilator such as theophylline or a beta adrenergic agonist such as albuterol may be administered either orally or through nebulization. Recombinant human DNA (DNase, Pulmozyme) breaks down DNA molecules in sputum, breaking up the thick mucus in the airways. A mucolytic such as Mucomyst may be prescribed during acute infection. Humidifiers can be useful. In summer, a room air conditioner can provide comfort and controlled humidity.

Chest physical therapy, a combination of postural drainage and chest percussion, is performed routinely at least every morning and evening, even if little drainage is apparent. Chest percussion (clapping and vibrating of the affected areas) helps loosen and move secretions from the lungs. Although time-consuming, chest physical therapy is part of the ongoing, long-term treatment, which the family must learn and continue at home.

Home Care

The home care for a child with CF places a tremendous burden on the family. Each day, family members spend much time performing treatments. They must learn to perform chest physical therapy, to operate respiratory equipment, and to administer IV antibiotics when necessary. They must plan the child's diet and regulate additional enzymes according to need. Family members must take great care to prevent exposing the child with CF to infections.

Family caregivers must guard against overprotection and undue limitation of the child's physical activity. Somehow, parents also must preserve a good family relationship, giving time and attention to other members of the family.

Physical activity is an important adjunct to the child's well-being and necessary to get rid of secretions. The family soon learns the child's capacity for exercise and can trust the child to become self-limiting as necessary.

Caring for a child with CF places great stress on financial resources. The expense of daily medications, frequent clinic or office visits, and sometimes lengthy hospitalizations can devastate an ordinary family budget even with medical insurance coverage. The Cystic Fibrosis Foundation (www.cff.org) is helpful in providing education and services.

Nursing Management

Conduct a parent interview that includes data concerning respiratory infections, the child's appetite and eating habits, stools, noticeable salty perspiration, history of bowel obstruction as an infant, and family history for CF. Also determine the caregiver's knowledge of the condition. Ask the child age-appropriate questions, involve the child in the interview process, and determine the child's perception of the disease and this current illness.

Include observation of respirations such as cough, breath sounds, and barrel chest; respiratory effort such as retractions and nasal flaring; clubbing of the fingers; and signs of pancreatic involvement such as failure to thrive and steatorrhea. Examine the skin around the rectum for irritation and breakdown from frequent foul stools.

Teach the child to cough effectively. Examine and document the mucus produced and increase fluid intake to help thin mucus secretions. Intravenous fluids and antibiotics may be necessary, especially when the child has an infection. Provide humidified air, either in the form of a cool mist humidifier or mist tent. Maintain the child in a semi-Fowler's or high Fowler's position to promote maximal lung expansion. Pulse oximetry is used to monitor oxygen saturation, and oxygen may be ordered. Give mouth care, perform chest physical therapy, and plan nursing care to conserve the child's energy and allow for rest time.

Help protect the child from any exposure to infectious organisms. Monitor vital signs to detect any indication of an infectious process, and restrict people with an infection from contact with the child. Increase the child's caloric intake to compensate for impaired absorption. Give high-calorie, high-protein snacks, pancreatic enzymes, and multiple vitamins and iron.

Evaluate the family's knowledge about CF to determine their teaching needs. Provide information for resources such as the Cystic Fibrosis Foundation, the American Lung Association (www.lungusa.org), and other local organizations. The family may have questions about genetic counseling and may need referrals.

Stop, Think, and Respond ● BOX 8-2

What causes cystic fibrosis? What organs does CF affect?

● SUDDEN INFANT DEATH SYNDROME

Sudden infant death syndrome (SIDS) is one of the leading causes of infant mortality worldwide (Carroll & Loughlin, 1999). Commonly called "crib death," SIDS is the sudden, unexpected death of an apparently healthy infant in whom the postmortem fails to reveal an adequate cause. The term SIDS is not a diagnosis, but rather a description of a syndrome. No single cause has been identified; SIDS can neither be prevented nor predicted.

The highest numbers of infants who die of SIDS are between 1 and 5 months, with the peak being 2 to 4 months (Carroll & Loughlin, 1999). SIDS is more often seen in low-birth weight infants, occurs more often in winter, and affects more male than female infants (Carroll & Loughlin, 1999). Because more infants with SIDS have been sleeping in a prone (face down) position than in a supine (lying on the back with face up) position, the American Academy of Pediatrics recommends that infants must be placed in a supine position to sleep.

Sudden infant death syndrome is rapid and silent. The history reveals that no cry has been heard, nor is there any evidence of a struggle.

The effects of SIDS on caregivers and families are devastating. Grief is coupled with guilt, even though SIDS cannot be predicted or prevented. Disbelief, hostility, and anger are common reactions. Prolonged depression usually follows the initial shock and anguish over the infant's death. The immediate response of emergency department staff should be to allow the family to express their grief, encouraging them to say goodbye to their baby and providing a quiet, private place for them to do so. Referrals should be made to the local chapter of the National SIDS Foundation. Many books and booklets have been written to help caregivers and siblings learn to cope with the feelings and emotions that occur when a child dies from SIDS. The best way to interact with caregivers is to actively listen and show compassionate concern.

CARDIOVASCULAR AND HEMATOPOIETIC DISORDERS ●

Cardiovascular system defects range from mild to severe. They may be detected immediately at birth or not for several months. Disorders involving the blood and blood-forming tissues are called hematopoietic disorders.

● CONGENITAL HEART DISEASE

When a newborn is suspected of having a heart abnormality, the family is understandably upset. Technological advances have progressed rapidly in this field, making earlier detection and successful repair much more likely.

Pathophysiology and Etiology

The heart begins beating early in intrauterine life. When first formed, the heart is a simple tube receiving blood from the placenta and pumping blood out into its developing body. During this period, the heart rapidly develops into its normal, but complex, four-chambered structure.

During fetal life the lungs are inactive, requiring only a small amount of blood to nourish their tissues. The umbilical arteries circulate blood to the placenta, where waste products and carbon dioxide are exchanged for oxygen and nutrients. The umbilical vein then returns blood to the fetus.

At birth, the umbilical cord is cut, and certain circulatory bypasses, such as the ductus arteriosus, foramen ovale, and ductus venosus, are no longer necessary. They close and atrophy during the first several weeks after birth. Rubella in the expectant mother during the first trimester is a common cause of cardiac malformation. Maternal alcoholism, maternal irradiation, ingestion of certain drugs during pregnancy, maternal diabetes, and advanced maternal age (older than 40 years) also increase the incidence. Maternal malnutrition and heredity are other contributing factors.

Assessment Findings

A cardiac murmur heard in infants may be functional and "innocent," disappearing as the child grows older. Conversely, it may be the chief manifestation of an abnormal heart or circulatory system. Infants with cardiac anomalies severe enough to cause circulatory difficulties have a history of being poor eaters, tiring easily from the effort to suck, and failing to grow or thrive normally.

Manifestations of congestive heart failure (CHF) may appear during the first year in infants with heart conditions. These infants tire easily, breathe hard, and refuse a bottle after 1 or 2 ounces, although they soon become hungry again. They are more comfortable if held upright. Other signs are failure to gain weight; a pale, mottled, or cyanotic color; a hoarse or weak cry; and tachycardia. Rapid respiration (with an expiratory grunt), flaring of the nares, and use of accessory respiratory muscles with retractions at the diaphragmatic and suprasternal levels are other clinical manifestations of CHF. Edema is a factor, and the heart generally shows enlargement. Anoxic attacks (fainting spells) are common. With some conditions, the young child may assume a squatting position, which reduces the return flow to the heart, thus temporarily reducing the workload of the heart. Clubbing of the fingers or toes, periods of cyanosis, and reduced exercise tolerance also may be seen.

The clinical symptoms of CHF are the primary basis for diagnosis of most congenital heart diseases. Chest radiographs that reveal an enlarged heart and electrocardiography indicate ventricular hypertrophy.

Medical Management

Treatment of CHF includes using digitalization to improve cardiac function; removing excess fluids with the use of diuretics, such as furosemide (Lasix); decreasing the workload on the heart by limiting physical activity; and improving oxygenation. Digoxin (Lanoxin) improves cardiac efficiency. ACE inhibitors (angiotensin-converting enzyme inhibitors) increase vasodilatation. Fluid restriction, elevating the head, bedrest, small, frequent feedings and oxygen help decrease the heart's workload. Advances in medical technology have enabled heart repairs to be performed on infants as young as 1 day.

Nursing Management

One of the nurse's roles is to help reduce anxiety in the child and family. Giving clear explanations of the defect, using understandable terms and diagrams, pictures, or models, is helpful. Cardiac catheterization may be performed before heart surgery. Closely observe the child, monitor the site used, and check the extremities for pulses, edema, skin temperature and color, and any other signs of poor circulation or infection. Monitor vital signs closely. When a child is admitted for cardiac surgery, conduct preoperative teaching for the family and child at an age-appropriate level. Describe the equipment to be used after surgery or show it using drawings and pictures. Teach the child how to cough and assist him or her to practice. At the end of surgery, specially trained personnel will take the child to the pediatric intensive care unit for skillful nursing.

Stop, Think, and Respond ● BOX 8-3

What symptoms would be most likely in a child who has congestive heart failure?

● CONGENITAL HEART DEFECTS

Congenital heart defects are described by a classification system based on blood flow characteristics:

- Increased pulmonary blood flow: ventricular septal, atrial septal, and patent ductus arteriosus
- Obstruction of blood flow out of the heart: coarctation of the aorta
- Decreased pulmonary blood flow: tetralogy of Fallot
- Mixed blood flow, in which saturated and desaturated blood mix in the heart, aorta, and pulmonary vessels: transposition of the great arteries

Types

Ventricular Septal Defect

Ventricular septal defect is the most common intracardiac defect (Fixler, 1999). It consists of an abnormal opening in the septum between the two ventricles, which allows blood to pass directly from the left to the right ventricle. No unoxygenated blood leaks into the left ventricle, so cyanosis does not occur.

A characteristic loud, harsh murmur associated with a systolic thrill occasionally is heard on examination. A history of frequent respiratory infections may occur during infancy, but growth and development are unaffected. Corrective surgery may be postponed until the child is 18 months to 2 years. The child may be placed on prophylactic antibiotics to prevent respiratory infections.

Atrial Septal Defects

In general, left-to-right shunting occurs in all true atrial septal defects. The atrial septum of many healthy people, however, houses a patent **foramen ovale** that normally causes no problems, because its valve is anatomically structured to withstand left chamber pressure, rendering it functionally closed. Atrial septal defects are amenable to surgery, and the opening is closed with sutures or a Dacron patch.

Patent Ductus Arteriosus

The **ductus arteriosus** is a vascular channel between the left main pulmonary artery and descending aorta. In fetal life, it allows blood to bypass the nonfunctioning lungs and go directly into the systemic circuit. After birth, the duct normally closes, eventually becoming obliterated and forming the ligamentum arteriosum. If the ductus arteriosus remains patent, however, the aorta continues to shunt blood into the pulmonary artery. This situation results in a flooding of the lungs and an overloading of the left heart chambers.

Symptoms of patent ductus arteriosus are often absent during childhood. Growth and development may be retarded in some children, with easy fatigability and dyspnea on exertion. The diagnosis may be based on a murmur over the pulmonary area, a wide pulse pressure, and a bounding pulse.

Surgical correction consists of closure of the defect by ligation or division of the ductus. The defect should be closed in childhood. Prognosis is good after a successful repair (Vick & Titus, 1999).

Coarctation of the Aorta

This anomaly consists of a constriction or narrowing of the aortic arch or the descending aorta, usually adjacent to the ligamentum arteriosum. Most children with this condition are asymptomatic until later childhood or young adulthood. A few infants have symptoms of dyspnea, tachycardia, and cyanosis, which are all signs of developing CHF.

In older children, the condition is diagnosed based on hypertension in the upper extremities and hypotension in the lower extremities. The radial pulse is readily palpable, but the femoral pulses are weak or even impalpable. Blood pressure is normal or elevated in the arms and low or undetectable in the legs. A high-pitched systolic murmur is usually present and heard over the base of the heart and over the interscapular area of the back.

Uncorrected coarctation may cause hypertension and cardiac failure later in life. Surgery consists of resection of the coarcted area with an end-to-end anastomosis of the proximal and distal ends of the aorta.

Tetralogy of Fallot

This consists of a grouping of heart defects (*tetralogy* denotes four abnormal conditions): (1) **pulmonary stenosis,** (2) **ventricular septal defect,** (3) **overriding aorta,** and (4) **right ventricular hypertrophy.** The child with tetralogy of Fallot may be precyanotic in early infancy, with the cyanotic phase starting at 4 to 6 months.

The infant presents with feeding difficulties, poor weight gain, dyspnea, and easy fatigability. Anoxic spells ("tet spells") are evidenced by sudden restlessness, gasping respiration, and increased cyanosis that lead to a loss of consciousness and possibly convulsions.

The preferred repair of these defects is total surgical correction. Successful total correction transforms a grossly abnormal heart into a functionally normal one. Most of these children, however, are left without a pulmonary valve.

Transposition of the Great Arteries

This severe defect was at one time almost always fatal. Advancements in diagnosis and treatment have increased the success rate in treatment of this disorder (Neches, Park, & Ettedgui, 1999). The aorta arises from the right ventricle instead of the left, and the pulmonary artery arises from the left ventricle instead of the right. These infants are usually cyanotic from birth and have a low rate of survival.

Nursing Management

The interview of the family caregiver must include information about the present illness and any previous episodes. Ask about problems during feeding; weight gain; episodes of rapid, difficult respirations or turning blue; and difficulty with lying flat. Note the quality and rhythm of the apical pulse. Observe respiratory status including any use of accessory muscles, retractions, breath sounds, rate, and type of cry. Examine the skin and extremities for color, skin temperature, and evidence of edema. Observe the infant closely for signs of easy fatigability or increased symptoms on exertion.

Monitor vital signs regularly to detect symptoms of decreased cardiac output. Watch for evidence of periorbital or peripheral edema, weigh the infant daily, and maintain intake and output measurements. Elevate the head of the crib mattress and administer oxygen as ordered. Give small, frequent feedings and gavage feedings as necessary.

Be understanding, empathetic, and nonjudgmental when communicating with and teaching the family. Following cardiac surgery, the child usually goes directly to a pediatric intensive care unit for care.

• RHEUMATIC FEVER

Rheumatic fever is a chronic disease affecting the connective tissue of the heart, joints, lungs, and brain. It is precipitated by a streptococcal infection such as strep throat, tonsillitis, scarlet fever, or pharyngitis, which may be undiagnosed or untreated. The resultant rheumatic fever may be the first indication of trouble.

Assessment Findings

Signs and Symptoms

A latent period of 1 to 5 weeks follows the initial infection. Onset is often slow and subtle. The child may be listless, anorectic, and pale. He or she may lose weight and complain of vague muscle, joint, or abdominal pain. Often there is a low-grade late afternoon fever.

Major manifestations of rheumatic fever are **carditis** (inflammation of the heart), **polyarthritis** (migratory arthritis), and **chorea** (disorder characterized by emotional instability, purposeless movements, and muscular weakness).

CARDITIS. Carditis is the major cause of permanent heart damage and disability. Presenting symptoms may be vague enough to be missed. The child may have a poor appetite, pallor, a low-grade fever, listlessness, or moderate anemia. Careful observation may reveal slight dyspnea on exertion. A soft systolic murmur over the apex of the heart may be present. Acute carditis may be the presenting symptom particularly in young children. An abrupt onset of high fever (perhaps as high as 104°F [40°C]), tachycardia, pallor, poor pulse quality, and a rapid decrease in hemoglobin are characteristic. Weakness, prostration, cyanosis, and intense precordial pain are common. Cardiac dilatation usually occurs. See Chapter 25.

POLYARTHRITIS. Polyarthritis moves from one major joint to another (ankles, knees, hips, wrists, elbows, shoulders). The joint becomes painful to either touch or movement (**arthralgia**) and hot and swollen. Body temperature is moderately elevated; the erythrocyte sedimentation rate (ESR) is increased.

CHOREA. The onset of chorea is gradual with increasing incoordination, facial grimaces, and repetitive involuntary movements. Movements may be mild and remain so, or they may become increasingly severe. Attacks tend to be recurrent and prolonged but are rare after puberty. The child may be sedated with phenobarbital, chlorpromazine (Thorazine), haloperidol (Haldol), or diazepam (Valium). Bed rest is necessary with protection such as padding the bedsides if the movements are severe.

Diagnostic Findings

Rheumatic fever is difficult to diagnose and sometimes impossible to differentiate from other diseases. The modified Jones criteria (Fig. 8.1) help in determining the

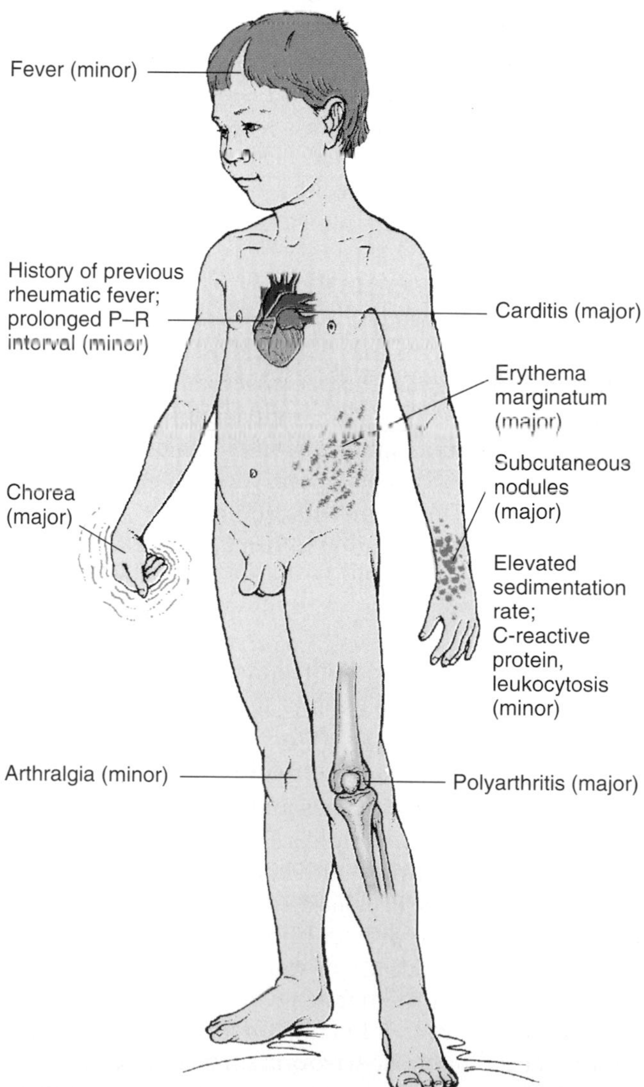

FIGURE 8.1 Major and minor manifestations of rheumatic fever.

diagnosis. Two major or one major and two minor criteria indicate a high probability if supported by evidence of a preceding streptococcal infection. Laboratory tests, although nonspecific, provide an evaluation of the disease activity to guide treatment. Two commonly used indicators are the erythrocyte sedimentation rate (ESR), which is elevated with an inflammatory process, and C-reactive protein, which remains elevated until clinical manifestations have ceased. C-reactive protein is not normally in the blood of healthy people, but it appears in the serum of people with rheumatic fever.

Medical Management

The chief concern is prevention of residual heart disease. As long as the rheumatic process is active, progressive heart damage is possible. Bedrest, which may last from 2 to several weeks, is essential to reduce the heart's workload. Residual heart disease is treated with digitalis, restricted activities, diuretics, and a low-sodium diet. Penicillin is administered to eliminate the hemolytic *streptococci.* If the child is allergic to penicillin, erythromycin is used. Acetylsalicylic acid (aspirin) is given to relieve pain, reduce inflammation, and decrease fever. For mild or severe carditis, corticosteroids may be used; diuretics are given in cases of severe carditis.

Nursing Management

Observe for any signs that may be classified as major or minor manifestations. Include observation for elevated temperature and pulse and careful examination for erythema marginatum, subcutaneous nodules, swollen or painful joints, or signs of chorea. A throat culture determines if there is an active infection. Obtain a complete, up-to-date history including information about a recent sore throat or upper respiratory infection, when the symptoms began, and what if any treatment was obtained. Position the child to relieve joint pain, carefully handle the joints when moving the child, and give warm baths and gentle range-of-motion exercises to alleviate joint discomfort. Monitor for side effects of corticosteroids such as **hirsutism** (abnormal hair growth) and "moon face." Quiet, age-appropriate games and rest periods between activities conserve the child's energy. The child with chorea may be frustrated with his or her inability to control the movements. Provide an opportunity for the child to express feelings; protect him or her from injury by keeping up and padding side rails.

The child with rheumatic fever must be maintained on prophylactic doses of penicillin for 5 years or longer. Whenever the child is to have oral surgery or dental work, he or she requires extra prophylactic precautions. Inform the family that a recurrence could have more serious effects, so a healthcare provider should investigate any upper respiratory infection.

• KAWASAKI DISEASE

Kawasaki disease (mucocutaneous lymph node syndrome) is an acute, febrile disease, most often seen in boys younger than 5 years. The cause appears to be an infectious agent. Following infection, the immune system becomes altered. Most cases occur in the late winter or early spring. The major complication of concern is cardiac involvement.

Assessment Findings

An elevated temperature (102°F to 104°F) is noted from the first day of the illness and may continue 1 to 3 weeks. Irritability; lethargy; inflammation in both conjunctiva; strawberry-colored tongue; dry, red, cracked lips; edema in the hands and feet; and red, swollen joints are visible. Skin on the fingers and toes peels in layers, and a rash covers the trunk and extremities. Cervical lymph nodes may be enlarged. The arteries, veins, and capillaries are inflamed, which can lead to serious cardiac concerns, including aneurysms and thrombus. The child may complain of abdominal pain.

The disease is seen in three stages:

- Acute—child has a high fever, does not respond to antibiotics or antipyretics, and is irritable.
- Subacute—The fever resolves, irritability continues, and the child is at greatest risk for aneurysms.
- Convalescent—Symptoms are gone; this phase continues until laboratory values are normal and the child's energy, appetite, and temperament have returned.

To be diagnosed with Kawasaki disease, the child must have an elevated temperature and four of the following symptoms: cervical lymphadenopathy; conjunctivitis; dry, swollen, cracked lips; strawberry tongue; aneurysm; abdominal pain; peeling of hands and feet; trunk rash; or red, swollen joints. The white blood cell count (WBC) and erythrocyte sedimentation rate (ESR) are elevated. During the subacute stage, the platelet count increases, which may lead to blood clotting and cardiac problems. Echocardiograms may show cardiac involvement.

Medical Management

A high dose of IV immunoglobulin (IVIG) therapy is given to relieve symptoms and prevent coronary artery abnormalities. Aspirin is used to control inflammation and fever and is continued for up to 1 year in lower doses as an antiplatelet.

Nursing Management

Nursing care for the child with Kawasaki disease focuses on relieving pain, discomfort, and itching. Monitor temperature, cardiac status, intake and output, and daily weight closely. Offer extra fluids and soft foods. Mouth and lip care help decrease the soreness. Passive range-of-motion exercises increase joint movement. Dealing with the irritability is sometimes difficult for both nurse and family. Rest and a quiet environment help decrease irritability. Encouraging the parents to have time away from the child is essential.

Discharge teaching includes information regarding the disease and symptoms, which may persist for some time. Most children recover without long-term effects, but cardiac involvement may not develop for some time after the child's recovery.

• HEMOPHILIA

Pathophysiology and Etiology

Hemophilia is one of the oldest known hereditary diseases. Defects in protein synthesis lead to deficiencies in any of the factors in the blood plasma needed for thromboplastic activity. These deficiencies result in delayed coagulation of blood. The principal factors involved are VIII, IX, and XI.

The mechanism of clot formation is complex. A simple description involves three stages:

1. Plasma-platelet interaction leads to the formation of prothrombin.
2. Prothrombin is converted to thrombin.
3. Thrombin converts fibrinogen into fibrin.

Fibrin then forms a mesh that traps red and white blood cells and platelets into a clot, closing defects in injured vessels. A deficiency in one of the thromboplastin precursors may lead to hemophilia.

Assessment Findings

Hemophilia is characterized by prolonged bleeding with frequent hemorrhages externally and into the skin, joint spaces, and intramuscular tissues. Bleeding from tooth extractions, brain hemorrhages, and crippling disabilities are serious complications. Death during infancy or early childhood is not unusual in severe hemophilia and results from a great loss of blood, intracranial bleeding, or respiratory obstruction caused by bleeding into the neck tissues. Serious hemorrhages may result from minor lacerations.

A careful examination of the family history and type of bleeding present is conducted. Abnormal bleeding beginning in infancy combined with a positive family history suggests hemophilia. A markedly prolonged clotting time is characteristic of severe factor VIII or IX deficiency, but mild conditions may have only a slightly prolonged clotting time. The partial prothrombin time is the test that most clearly demonstrates that factor VIII is low.

Common Types of Hemophilia

The two most common types of hemophilia are factor VIII deficiency and factor IX deficiency. These two types are briefly presented here.

Factor VIII Deficiency (Hemophilia A; Antihemophilic Globulin Deficiency; Classic Hemophilia)

Classic hemophilia is inherited as a sex-linked recessive Mendelian trait, with transmission to affected males by carrier females. Hemophilia A (classic hemophilia), the most common type, is also the most severe. The cause is a deficiency of antihemophilic globulin C, which is the factor VIII necessary for blood clotting.

Factor IX Deficiency (Hemophilia B; Plasma Thromboplastin Component Deficiency; Christmas Disease)

Christmas disease was named after a 5-year-old boy who was one of the first people diagnosed with a deficiency of factor IX. This sex-linked recessive trait appears in male offspring of carrier females and results from a deficiency of one of the necessary thromboplastin precursors: factor IX, the plasma thromboplastin component.

Medical Management

For many years, the only treatment for bleeding in hemophilia was the use of fresh blood or plasma. Commercial preparations now are available that supply factor VIII. These concentrates are supplied in dried form together with diluent for reconstitution and can be stored for a long time. A synthetic preparation, DDAVP (1-deamino-8-D-arginine vasopressin), is used in mild factor VIII deficiencies and von Willebrand disease, a Mendelian dominant trait present in both sexes, characterized by prolonged bleeding times, and classified with the hemophilias. One of the serious problems with using blood products of any kind has been the risk of exposure to hepatitis B and human immunodeficiency virus (HIV), the causative organism of acquired immunodeficiency syndrome (AIDS).

Nursing Management

Collect data by reviewing the child's history with the caregiver, including previous episodes of bleeding, usual treatment, medications the child takes, and current bleeding episode. Carefully observe the child for any signs of bleeding. Inspect the mucous membranes, examine the joints for tenderness and swelling, and check the skin for evidence of bruising. Ask about hematuria, hematemesis, headache, or black, tarry stools.

Bleeding into the joint cavities often occurs after some slight injury. The pressure of the confined fluid in the narrow joint spaces causes extreme pain. Promptly immobilize the extremity to prevent contractures (destruction of bone and joint tissues) to relieve pain and decrease bleeding. Ibuprofen is the only NSAID proven safe for these children. Use cold packs and elevate the extremity to decrease bleeding. Passive range-of-motion exercises help prevent joint contractures. Many clients who have had repeated episodes of **hemarthrosis** (bleeding into the joints) develop functional impairment of the joints. Physical therapy is helpful after the bleeding episode is under control.

Protect the child from trauma caused by limiting invasive procedures as much as possible. Avoid intramuscular injections. Apply cold compresses to the site of a procedure for 5 minutes or longer after it is finished. Pad crib sides, examine toys for sharp edges, emphasize the need to use a soft toothbrush, trim the nails to prevent scratching, and give adequate skin care to prevent irritation. Discuss safety measures for the home and child with family caregivers.

The family experiences anxiety over how much activity to allow the child, how to keep from overprotecting him or her, and how to help the child achieve a healthy mental attitude, all while preventing mishaps that may cause serious bleeding episodes. The financial strain on the family is considerable. The National Hemophilia Foundation is a resource for services and publications (http://www.hemophilia.org).

NEUROLOGIC DISORDERS

● CEREBRAL PALSY

Cerebral palsy (CP) is a group of disorders arising from a malfunction of motor centers and neural pathways in the brain. It is one of the most complex of the common permanent disabling conditions and often can be accompanied by seizures, mental retardation, sensory defects, and behavior disorders.

Pathophysiology and Etiology

Although the cause of CP cannot be identified in many cases, several causes are possible. It may result from damage to the parts of the brain that control movement; this damage generally occurs during the fetal or perinatal period, particularly in premature infants (Shapiro & Capute, 1999).

Prenatal causes of CP include any process that interferes with the oxygen supply to the brain, maternal infection, nutritional deficiencies, kernicterus (brain damage caused by jaundice) resulting from Rh incompatibility, and teratogenic factors such as drugs and radiation. *Perinatal* causes include anoxia immediately before, during, and after birth; intracranial bleeding; asphyxia; maternal analgesia; birth trauma; and prematurity. *Postnatal* causes include head trauma, infection, neoplasms, and cerebrovascular accident.

Prevention

Because brain damage in CP is irreversible, prevention is the most important aspect of care. Prevention focuses on prenatal care, perinatal monitoring, and postnatal prevention of infection and trauma.

Assessment Findings

Difficulty controlling voluntary muscle movements is one manifestation of damage to the central nervous system. Seizures, mental retardation, hearing and vision impairments, and behavior disorders often accompany the major problem. Delayed gross motor development, abnormal motor performance (e.g., poor sucking and feeding behaviors), abnormal postures, and persistence of primitive reflexes are other signs of CP. Diagnosis seldom occurs before 2 months of age and may be delayed until the 2nd or 3rd year, when the toddler attempts to walk and caretakers notice an obvious lag in motor development.

Several major types of CP occur, each of which has distinct clinical manifestations. *Spastic type,* the most common, is characterized by a hyperactive stretch reflex in associated muscle groups; increased activity of the deep tendon reflexes; **clonus** (rapid involuntary muscle contraction and relaxation); contractures affecting the extensor muscles, especially the heel cord; and scissoring caused by severe hip adduction. When scissoring is present, the child's legs are crossed and the toes point down. When standing, the child is on her or his toes. It is difficult for this child to walk on the heels or to run.

Athetoid type is marked by involuntary, uncoordinated motion with varying degrees of muscle tension. Children with this disorder are constantly in motion, and their entire bodies are in a state of slow, writhing muscle contractions whenever they attempt voluntary movement. Facial grimacing, poor swallowing, and tongue movements causing drooling; **dysarthria** (poor speech articulation); and hearing loss are also present.

Ataxia type is essentially a lack of coordination caused by disturbances in the kinesthetic and balance senses.

The least common type of CP, ataxia may not be diagnosed until the child starts to walk: the gait is awkward and wide-based.

Rigidity type is uncommon and characterized by rigid postures and lack of active movement.

Mixed type is seen when children have signs of more than one type of CP and usually are severely disabled. Postnatal injury may have caused the disorder.

Medical Management

Treatment of CP focuses on helping the child make the best use of residual abilities. Dental care is important because enamel hypoplasia is common, and children whose seizure disorders are controlled with phenytoin (Dilantin) are likely to develop gingival hypertrophy. Medications such as baclofen, diazepam, and dantrolene may be used to help decrease spasticity.

Physical therapists attempt to teach activities of daily living to children with CP by using methods based on principles of conditioning, relaxation, and residual patterns, and by stimulating contraction and relaxation of muscles. Braces are used to facilitate muscle training, reinforce weak or paralyzed muscles, or counteract the pull of antagonistic muscles. Orthopedic surgery sometimes is used to improve function and to correct deformities such as the release of contractures and the lengthening of tight heel cords.

Biomedical engineering has perfected devices that range from simple items, such as wheelchairs and specially constructed toilet seats, to completely electronic cottages. Feeding may be a challenge, so caregivers often need help finding a method that works for their child. Feeding aids include spoons with enlarged handles, plates with high rims and suction devices to prevent slipping, and covered cups.

Nursing Management

Interview and observe the child and family to determine the child's needs and level of development and the stage of family acceptance. Communicate with the family to learn as much as possible about the child's activities at home. Positioning to prevent contractures, providing modified feeding utensils, and suggesting appropriate educational play activities are all important aspects of the child's care.

• HYDROCEPHALUS

Hydrocephalus is characterized by excess cerebrospinal fluid (CSF) within the ventricular and subarachnoid spaces of the cranial cavity. Normally a delicate balance exists between the rate of formation and absorption of CSF: the entire volume is absorbed and replaced every 12 to 24 hours. In hydrocephalus, this balance is disturbed.

Pathophysiology and Etiology

Cerebrospinal fluid is formed mainly in the lateral ventricles by the choroid plexus and is absorbed into the venous system through the arachnoid villi. Cerebrospinal fluid circulates within the ventricles and the subarachnoid space. This colorless fluid consists of water with traces of protein, glucose, and lymphocytes.

In the *noncommunicating* type of congenital hydrocephalus, an obstruction occurs in the free circulation of CSF. This blockage causes increased pressure on the brain or spinal cord. In the *communicating* type of hydrocephalus, no obstruction of the free flow of CSF exists between the ventricles and spinal theca; rather, the condition results from defective absorption of CSF, leading to increased pressure on the brain or spinal cord. Congenital hydrocephalus is most often the obstructive or noncommunicating type.

Hydrocephalus may be recognized at birth, or it may not be evident until after a few weeks or months of life. The condition may not be congenital but instead may develop during later infancy or childhood as the result of a neoplasm, a head injury, or an infection such as meningitis.

When hydrocephalus occurs early in life before the skull sutures close, the soft, pliable bones separate to allow head expansion. This condition is manifested by a rapid increase in head circumference. The fact that the soft bones can yield to pressure in this manner may partially explain why many of these infants fail to show the usual symptoms of brain pressure and may exhibit little or no damage in mental function until later in life. Other infants show severe brain damage, which often has occurred before birth.

Assessment Findings

Signs and Symptoms

An excessively large head at birth is suggestive of hydrocephalus. Rapid head growth with widening cranial sutures is also strongly suggestive and may be the first manifestation of this condition. An apparently large head in itself is not necessarily significant. Normally every infant's head is measured at birth, and the rate of growth is checked at subsequent examinations. If an infant's head appears abnormally large or enlarging at birth, it should be measured frequently.

As the head enlarges, the suture lines separate and the spaces may be felt through the scalp. The anterior fontanelle becomes tense and bulging, the skull enlarges in all diameters, and the scalp becomes shiny with dilated veins. If pressure continues to increase without intervention, the eyes appear to be pushed downward slightly with the sclera visible above the iris (the so-called "setting sun" sign).

If the condition progresses without adequate drainage of excessive fluid, the head becomes increasingly heavy, the neck muscles fail to develop sufficiently, and the infant has difficulty raising or turning the head. Unless hydrocephalus is arrested, the infant becomes increasingly helpless and develops symptoms of increased intracranial pressure (IICP). These symptoms may include irritability, restlessness, personality change, high-pitched cry, ataxia, projectile vomiting, failure to thrive, seizures, severe headache, changes in level of consciousness, and papilledema.

Diagnostic Findings

Clinical manifestations, particularly an excessive increase in head circumference, are indications of hydrocephalus. Positive diagnosis is made with CT and MRI. Echoencephalography and ventriculography also may be performed to further define the condition.

Stop, Think, and Respond ● BOX 8-4

What signs and symptoms might indicate IICP? 

Medical Management

Surgical intervention is the only effective means of relieving brain pressure and preventing further damage to brain tissue. If brain damage is minimal, the child may be able to function within a normal mental range. Motor function usually is retarded. In some instances, surgical intervention may remove the cause of the obstruction, such as a neoplasm, cyst, or hematoma, but most children require placement of a shunting device that bypasses the point of obstruction, draining the excess CSF into a body cavity. This procedure arrests excessive head growth and prevents further brain damage.

Many shunt procedures use a silicone rubber catheter that is radiopaque so that its position may be checked through radiographic examination. The silicone rubber catheter reduces the problem of tissue reaction. A valve or regulator is an essential part of each catheter that prevents excessive build-up of fluid or too-rapid decompression of the ventricle.

The most common procedure, particularly for infants and small children, is **ventriculoperitoneal shunting** (VP shunt). This procedure drains the CSF from a lateral ventricle in the brain; the CSF runs through the subcutaneous catheter and empties into the peritoneal cavity. A VP shunt allows the insertion of some excess tubing to accommodate growth. As the child grows, the catheter needs to be revised and lengthened.

In **ventriculoatrial shunting,** CSF drains into the right atrium of the heart. This procedure cannot be used in children with pathologic changes in the heart. The bloodstream absorbs the CSF drained from the ventricle.

All types of shunts may have problems with kinking, blocking, moving, or shifting of tubing. The danger of infection in the tubing is a constant concern. Children with shunts require constant observation for signs of malfunction or infection.

The long-term outcome for a child with hydrocephalus depends on several factors. If untreated, prognosis is very poor, often leading to death. With shunting, prognosis depends on the initial cause of the increased fluid, its treatment, brain damage sustained before shunting, complications with the shunting system, and continued long-term follow-up. Some of these children can lead relatively normal lives if they have follow-up and revisions as they grow.

NURSING PROCESS

● Postoperative Care of a Child With a Shunt Placement

Assessment

Obtaining accurate vital and neurologic signs is necessary preoperatively and postoperatively. Measurement of the infant's head is essential. If the fontanelles are not closed, carefully observe them for any signs of bulging. Observe, report, and document all signs of IICP. If the child has returned for revision of an existing shunt, obtain a complete history preoperatively from the family caregiver to provide a baseline of the child's behavior.

Determine the level of knowledge family members have about the condition. For the family of the newborn or young infant, the diagnosis probably will be an emotional shock. Conduct the interview and examination of the infant with sensitivity and understanding.

Diagnosis, Planning, and Interventions

Following placement of a shunt in a child with hydrocephalus, closely monitor the child to be sure the shunt is functioning properly. Monitoring vital signs as well as neurologic status is a major nursing responsibility. Because the child frequently has an enlarged head, many nursing interventions relate to the accompanying problems and concerns. Activities to promote the growth and development of the child following the placement of a shunt must be planned according to the child's abilities and stage of development. Supporting and teaching family members helps decrease their anxiety and concern over their child.

Risk for Ineffective Cerebral Tissue Perfusion related to IICP

Expected Outcome: Child will be free from symptoms of excessive CSF.

- Monitor level of consciousness at least every 2 to 4 hours. Monitor neurologic status; check pupils for equality and reaction. *Change in level of consciousness or neurological status may indicate IICP or possible shunt malfunction.*
- Observe for a shrill cry, lethargy, or irritability. Measure and record head circumference daily. *Findings may indicate IICP or increased CSF, which might indicate malfunction of the shunt.*
- Keep child flat. *This position prevents a rapid decrease in ICP.*
- Keep suction and oxygen equipment convenient at the bedside. *IICP can cause respiratory concerns; therefore, emergency equipment should be accessible.*

Risk for Impaired Skin Integrity related to pressure from physical immobility

Expected Outcome: Child's skin will remain intact.

- Keep child's head turned away from the operative site; reposition at least every 2 hours as physician's orders permit. *These measures help increase circulation, prevent pressure on the shunt, and prevent pressure sores from forming on the side where the child rests.*
- Use a sheepskin pad or air or water mattress as ordered. *These devices help relieve pressure points and decrease skin breakdown.*
- Inspect the dressings over the shunt site immediately after the surgery, every hour for the first 3 to 4 hours, and then at least every 4 hours. *Dressings should be observed for any wetness or drainage from incision or shunt. A dry dressing reduces skin irritation.*

Risk for Infection related to the shunt

Expected Outcome: Child will remain free of infection

- Closely observe for and promptly report any redness, heat, or swelling. Monitor for elevated temperature and signs of lethargy. *These signs of infection should be monitored and reported.*
- Carry out appropriate procedures to care for the shunt; perform wound care meticulously as ordered. *Doing so decreases the likelihood of infectious bacteria entering the surgical site.*
- Administer antibiotics as prescribed. *They are given to prevent or treat infection.*

Risk for Delayed Growth and Development related to impaired ability to achieve developmental tasks

Expected Outcome: Child will have age-appropriate growth and development.

- Pick up, hold, cuddle, and comfort the child. *An uncomfortable or painful experience increases the need for emotional support. An infant perceives such support principally through physical contact made in a soothing, loving manner.*
- Talk to, play with, and provide age-appropriate activities. *Talking, laughing, and playing with the child are important aspects of care and stimulation.*
- Provide toys appropriate for the child's physical and mental capacity. *Age-appropriate toys and activities provide opportunities for essential development.*
- Place toys within easy reach and vision: a cradle gym, for example, may be tied close enough for the child to maneuver its parts. Turn crib so that vision is not obstructed. *Children need stimulation, contact, and social interaction for growth and development. An enlarged head is difficult to turn, so the child's position must promote contact with the environment.*

Anxiety related to family caregivers' fear of surgical outcome

Expected Outcome: Family caregivers will verbalize reduced anxiety.

- Explain to the family the condition and the anatomy of the surgical procedure in terms they can understand. *Accurate, nontechnical answers help reduce concerns.*
- Discuss the child's overall prognosis. Encourage family members to express anxieties and ask questions. *Supporting and listening to them helps decrease anxiety.*
- Give the family information about and encourage them to contact support groups such as the National Hydrocephalus Foundation (www.nhfonline.org). *Support from those who understand what the family is experiencing is helpful.*
- Demonstrate care of the shunt; have caregivers perform a return demonstration. Provide them with a list of signs and symptoms that they should report. *Knowing what to expect and report gives them specific guidelines and a feeling of control.*

Evaluation of Expected Outcomes

The child has no signs of IICP, such as lethargy, irritability, and seizure activity. Level of consciousness is stable. Vital signs are stable; there is no redness, drainage, or swelling at the surgical site; and the child shows no other signs of infection. The child's social and developmental needs are met, and the child interacts and plays appropriately with toys and surroundings. The family expresses fears and concerns, interacts appropriately, participates in the child's care, asks appropriate questions, and lists signs and symptoms to report.

• *HAEMOPHILUS INFLUENZAE* MENINGITIS

Pathophysiology and Etiology

Meningitis in infancy and childhood may result from various agents including meningococci, the tubercle bacillus, and the *Haemophilus influenzae* type B bacillus. The most common form is *H. influenzae* meningitis. Meningococcal meningitis is spread by droplets from an infected person; all other forms are contracted by invasion of the meninges via the bloodstream from an infection elsewhere.

The highest rates of *H. influenzae* meningitis are seen in children between 6 and 11 months (Kaplan, 1999).

Purulent meningitis is an infectious disease. In addition to standard precautions, droplet transmission precautions should be observed for 24 hours after the start of effective antimicrobial therapy or until pathogens can no longer be cultured from nasopharyngeal secretions. Current immunizations include the Hib, which is given at 2 months and repeated at 4, 6, and 12 months (see Table 5.1).

Assessment Findings

Onset may be either gradual or abrupt following an upper respiratory infection. Young infants with meningitis may have a characteristic high-pitched cry, fever, and irritability. Other symptoms include headache, **nuchal rigidity** (stiff neck) that may progress to **opisthotonos** (arching of the back), and delirium. Projectile vomiting may be present. Generalized convulsions are common in infants. Coma may occur early, particularly in older children. Meningococcal meningitis, which tends to occur as epidemics in older children, produces a **purpuric rash** (caused by bleeding under the skin) in addition to the other symptoms.

Early diagnosis and treatment are essential for uncomplicated recovery. A spinal tap is performed promptly whenever symptoms raise a suspicion of meningitis. For accurate results, the spinal tap is done before antibiotics are administered. Nurses assist by holding the infant during the spinal tap. Laboratory examination of the fluid reveals increased protein and decreased glucose content. Early in the disease, the spinal fluid may be clear but rapidly becomes purulent. The causative organism usually can be determined from stained smears of the spinal fluid, enabling specific medication to be started early without waiting for growths of organisms on culture media.

Medical Management

The child is initially isolated and treatment is started using IV administration of antibiotics. Third-generation cephalosporins, such as ceftriaxone (Rocephin), are commonly used, often in combination with other antibiotics. Antibiotics chosen for treatment depend on sensitivity studies. Later in the disease, medications may be given orally. Treatment continues as long as fever or signs of subdural effusion or otitis media persist. The administration of IV steroids early in the course has decreased the incidence of deafness as a complication. If seizures occur, anticonvulsants often are given.

Subdural effusion may complicate the condition. Fluid accumulates in the subdural space. Needle aspiration through the infant's open suture lines or bur holes (in the skull of the older child) is used to remove fluid. Repeated aspirations may be required.

Long-term complications of *H. influenzae* meningitis include hydrocephalus, nerve deafness, mental retardation, and paralysis. Early treatment with appropriate medications decreases the risk of complications.

Nursing Management

The infant or child with meningitis is obviously extremely sick, and the anxiety level of the family caregivers is high. Physical examination of the child includes using a neurologic evaluation tool to monitor neurologic status, including level of consciousness (see Chap. 5).

Closely monitor the child for signs of IICP: increased head size; headache; bulging fontanelle; decreased pulse; vomiting; seizures; high-pitched cry; increased blood pressure; change in eyes, level of consciousness, or pupil response; and irritability or other behavioral changes. Report an increase in blood pressure, decrease in pulse, change in neurologic signs, or signs of respiratory distress at once. Measure the infant's head circumference at least every 4 hours.

Place the child in a side-lying position with the neck supported and head elevated. Be sure to implement seizure precautions such as padding the crib sides and keeping sharp or hard items out of the crib.

The infectious process may increase secretion of the antidiuretic hormone produced by the posterior pituitary gland. As a result, the child may not excrete urine adequately, and body fluid volume excess will occur. Strictly measure intake and output, and monitor daily weight and electrolytes. Signs to report immediately are decreased urinary output, hyponatremia, increased weight, nausea, and irritability. The child may be placed on fluid restrictions.

• REYE SYNDROME

Reye (rhymes with "eye") syndrome is characterized by acute encephalopathy and fatty degeneration of the liver and other abdominal organs. It occurs in children of all ages but is seen more in young school-age children than in any other age group (Louis, 1999).

Pathophysiology and Etiology

Reye syndrome usually occurs after a viral illness, particularly an upper respiratory infection or varicella (chickenpox). Administration of aspirin during the viral illness has been implicated as a contributing factor. As a result, the American Academy of Pediatrics recommends not to give aspirin or aspirin compounds to children with viral infections (Louis, 1999).

Assessment Findings

Symptoms appear within 3 to 5 days after the initial illness. The child is recuperating unremarkably when he or she develops symptoms of severe vomiting, irritability, lethargy, and confusion. Immediate intervention is needed to prevent serious insult to the brain including respiratory arrest.

The history of a viral illness is an immediate clue. Liver function tests, including serum glutamic-oxaloacetic transaminase (SGOT), serum glutamic pyruvic transaminase (SGPT), lactic dehydrogenase (LDH), and serum ammonia levels, are elevated because of poor liver function. The child is hypoglycemic and has delayed prothrombin time.

Medical Management

The child with Reye syndrome often receives care in the intensive care unit because the disease may rapidly progress. Medical management focuses on supportive measures—improving respiratory function, reducing cerebral edema, and controlling hypoglycemia. Staging of the symptoms determines the specific treatment (Table 8.1).

Nursing Management

Carefully observe the child for overall physical status and any change in neurologic status. Accurate intake and output determinations are necessary to determine when fluids need to be adjusted to control cerebral edema and prevent dehydration. Administer osmotic diuretics (e.g., mannitol) as ordered to reduce cerebral edema. Monitor blood glucose level and bleeding time. Low blood glucose levels can lead to seizures; a prolonged bleeding time can indicate coagulation problems as a result of liver dysfunction.

Give the family opportunities to deal with their feelings; keep them informed about the child's care. Having a child in intensive care is a frightening experience, so make every effort to reassure the family with sincerity and honesty.

Since the American Academy of Pediatrics made its recommendation to avoid giving aspirin to children, especially during viral illnesses, the number of cases of Reye syndrome has steadily decreased (Louis, 1999). Teach families with young children to avoid the use of aspirin.

• SPINA BIFIDA

Spina bifida is a failure of the posterior laminae of the vertebrae to close as a result of a defect in the neural arch generally in the lumbosacral region. This leaves an opening through which the spinal meninges and spinal cord may protrude (Fig. 8.2).

Assessment Findings

A bony defect without soft-tissue involvement is called *spina bifida occulta.* In most instances, it is asymptomatic and presents no problems. A dimple in the skin or a tuft of hair over the site may cause one to suspect its presence, or it may be entirely overlooked.

When part of the spinal meninges protrudes through the bony defect and forms a cystic sac, the condition is termed *spina bifida with meningocele.* No nerve roots are involved, so no paralysis or sensory loss below the lesion appears. The sac may, however, rupture or perforate, introducing infection into the spinal fluid and causing meningitis. For this reason as well as for cosmetic purposes, surgical removal of the sac with closure of the skin is indicated.

In *spina bifida with myelomeningocele,* the spinal cord and the meninges protrude, with nerve roots embedded in the wall of the cyst. The effects of this defect vary in severity from sensory loss or partial paralysis below the lesion to complete flaccid paralysis of all muscles below

TABLE 8.1 STAGING OF REYE SYNDROME

STAGE	SYMPTOMS SEEN IN STAGE
Stage I	Lethargic, vomiting, follows verbal commands, normal posture
Stage II	Combative or stuporous, inappropriate verbalizing, normal posture
Stage III	Comatose, decorticate posture and response to pain
Stage IV	Comatose, decerebrate posture and response to pain
Stage V	Comatose, flaccid, seizures, no papillary response, no response to pain

Adapted from the National Institutes of Health Staging System, Louis, PT. (1999). Reye syndrome. In *Oski's pediatrics: Principles and practice* (3rd ed). Philadelphia: Lippincott Williams & Wilkins.

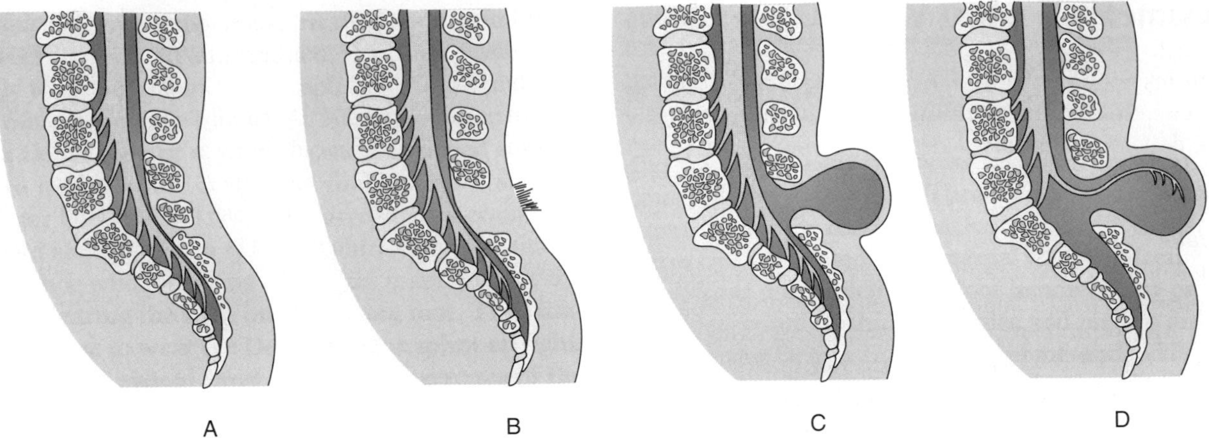

FIGURE 8.2 Degrees of spinal cord anomalies. (**A**) The normal spinal closure. (**B**) Occulta defect. (**C**) Meningocele defect. (**D**) Myelomeningocele defect clearly shows the spinal cord involvement.

the lesion. Complete paralysis involves the lower trunk and legs as well as bowel and bladder sphincters.

Making a clear-cut differentiation in diagnosis between a meningocele and a myelomeningocele on the basis of symptoms alone is not always possible. Myelomeningocele also may be termed *meningomyelocele;* the associated "spina bifida" always is implied but not necessarily named. *Spina bifida cystica* is the term used to designate either of these protrusions.

Elevated maternal alpha-fetoprotein (AFP) levels followed by ultrasonographic examination of the fetus may show an incomplete neural tube. An elevated AFP level in the maternal serum or amniotic fluid indicates the probability of central nervous system abnormalities. The best time to perform these tests is between 13 to 15 weeks' gestation when peak levels are reached. Most obstetricians perform AFP testing.

Diagnosis of the newborn with spina bifida is based on clinical observation and examination. Further evaluation of the defect may include magnetic resonance imaging (MRI), ultrasonography, computed tomography (CT) scanning, and myelography. The newborn requires careful examination for other associated defects, particularly hydrocephalus, genitourinary defects, and orthopedic anomalies.

Medical Management

Many specialists are involved in the treatment of these infants, including neurologists, neurosurgeons, orthopedic specialists, pediatricians, urologists, and physical therapists. After thoroughly evaluating the infant with spina bifida, they develop a plan of surgical repair and treatment.

The child requires years of ongoing follow-up and therapy. Surgery is required to close the open defect but may not be performed immediately, depending on the surgeon's decision.

Nursing Management

When collecting data during an examination, observe the child's movement and response to stimuli of the lower extremities. Carefully measure the head circumference and examine the fontanelles. Thoroughly document the observations made. When handling the infant, take great care to prevent injury to the sac. Monitor vital signs, neurologic signs, and behavior frequently to observe for any deviations from normal that may indicate an infection.

Until surgery is performed, the sac must be covered with a sterile dressing moistened in a warm sterile solution (often sterile saline), changed every 2 hours, and not allowed to dry because of the possible damage to the covering of the sac. Maintain the infant in a prone position so that no pressure is placed on the sac. After surgery, continue this positioning until the surgical site is well healed. Diapering is not advisable with a low defect, but the sac must be protected from contamination with fecal material. Placing a protective barrier between the anus and the sac may prevent this contamination. If the anal sphincter muscles are involved, the infant may have continual loose stools, which adds to the challenge of keeping the sac free from infection.

Perform range-of-motion exercises to prevent contractures. Position the infant so that the hips are abducted and the feet are in a neutral position. Massage the knees and other bony prominences with lotion regularly, then pad them, and protect them from irritation.

The family of an infant with such a major anomaly is in a state of shock on first learning of the problems. Be especially sensitive to their needs and emotions. Showing the family how to care for the infant, allowing them to participate in the care, and guiding them in performing return demonstrations are all methods to use. Refer the family to the Spina Bifida Association of America (http://www.sbaa.org). Although children with spina bifida have many long-term problems, their intelligence is not affected; many of these children grow into productive young adults who may live independently.

SENSORY DISORDERS

● CLEFT LIP AND CLEFT PALATE

Parents and family are naturally eager to see and hold their newborn and must be prepared for the shock of seeing the disfigurement of a cleft lip. They need encouragement and support as well as considerable instruction about the infant's feeding and care. The child born with a cleft palate but with an intact lip does not have the external disfigurement that may be so distressing to the new parent, but the problems are more serious.

Pathophysiology and Etiology

Although a cleft lip and a cleft palate often appear together, either defect may appear alone. In embryonic development, the palate closes later than the lip, and the failure to close occurs for different reasons.

The cleft lip and palate result from failure of the maxillary and premaxillary processes to fuse during the fifth to eighth week of intrauterine life. The cleft may be a simple notch in the vermilion line or may extend into the floor of the nose (Fig. 8.3). It may be either **unilateral** (one side of the lip) or **bilateral** (both sides). Cleft palate, which develops sometime between weeks 7 and 12 of gestation, is often accompanied by nasal deformity and dental disorders such as deformed, missing, or **supernumerary** (excessive in number) teeth.

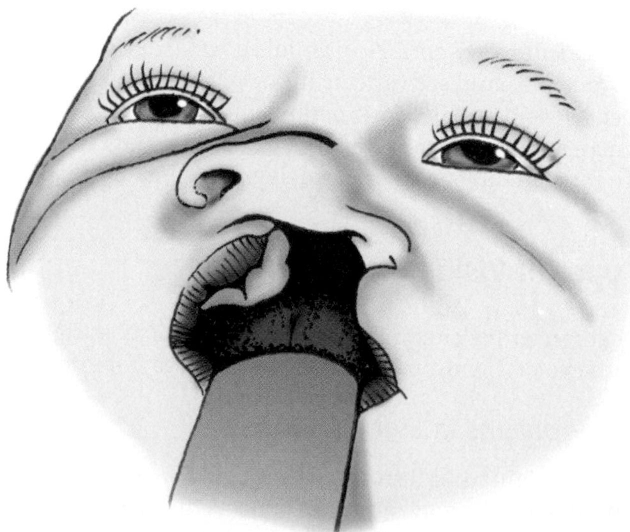

FIGURE 8.3 A cleft lip may extend up into the floor of the nose.

In an 8-week-old embryo, there is still no roof to the mouth; the tissues that are to become the palate are two shelves running from the front to the back of the mouth and projecting vertically downward on either side of the tongue. The shelves move from a vertical position to a horizontal position; their free edges meet and fuse in midline. Later bone forms within this tissue to compose the hard palate.

Normally, the palate is intact by the 10th week of fetal life. Exactly what happens to prevent this closure is not known for sure. Hereditary factors may play a part; the incidence of cleft palates is higher in the close relatives of people with the defect (Gorlin, 1999).

Assessment Findings

The physical appearance of the infant confirms the diagnosis of cleft lip. Diagnosis of cleft palate is made at birth with the close inspection of the newborn's palate. The examiner must insert a gloved finger into the newborn's mouth to feel the palate to determine that it is intact.

Medical Management

Surgery, usually performed by a plastic surgeon, is a major part of the treatment of a child with a cleft lip, palate, or both. Total care involves many specialists including pediatricians, nurses, orthodontists, prosthodontists, otolaryngologists, speech therapists, and occasionally psychiatrists.

Some plastic surgeons favor early repair, before the infant is discharged from the hospital; others prefer to wait until the infant is 1 or 2 months old, weighs about 10 pounds, and is gaining weight steadily. The goal in repairing the cleft palate is to give the child a union of the cleft parts to allow intelligible and pleasant speech and to avoid injury to the maxillary development. The timing of cleft palate repair is individualized according to the size, placement, and degree of deformity. The surgery may need to be done in stages over several years to achieve the best results. The optimal time for surgical repair of the cleft palate is considered to be between 6 months and 5 years of age. Because the child cannot make certain sounds when starting to talk, undesirable speech habits are formed that are difficult to correct. If surgery must be delayed beyond the 3rd year, a dental speech appliance may help the child develop intelligible speech.

Nursing Management

One primary concern in the nursing care of the infant with a cleft lip with or without a cleft palate is the emotional care of the family. Exploration of the family's acceptance of the infant is important.

Family caregivers who return to the hospital with the young infant for the repair of a cleft palate have already faced the challenges of feeding their baby. Ask questions about the feeding methods they found most effective. Feeding the infant with a cleft lip before repair may be time-consuming and tedious because the infant's ability to suck is inadequate. Breastfeeding may be successful because the breast tissue may mold to close the gap. A soft nipple with a crosscut made to promote easy flow of milk or formula may work well. Special cleft palate nipples molded to fit into the open palate area to close the gap may be used. Eyedroppers or Asepto syringes with a short piece of rubber tubing on the tip have been used with success. The person feeding the infant must be alert for signs of aspiration. See Client and Family Teaching 8-1.

To facilitate drainage of mucus and secretions, position the infant on the side, never on the abdomen, after a cleft lip or palate repair. Do not put anything in the infant's mouth to clear mucus because of the danger of damaging the surgical site, particularly with a palate repair.

Encourage sucking, which is important to the development of speech muscles. If the infant does not have a cleft lip or if the lip has had an early repair, he or she may learn sucking more easily, even though the suction generated is not as good as in the infant with an intact palate. A large nipple with holes that allow the milk to drip freely makes sucking easier.

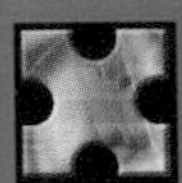

8-1 *Client and Family Teaching*
Cleft Lip/Cleft Palate

The nurse teaches as follows:

- Sucking is important to speech development.
- Holding the baby upright while feeding helps prevent choking.
- Burp the baby frequently, because he or she swallows a large amount of air during feeding.
- Don't tire the baby. Limit feeding times to 20 to 30 minutes maximum. If necessary, feed the baby more often.
- Feed strained foods slowly from the side of the spoon in small amounts.
- Don't be alarmed if food seeps through the cleft and out the nose.
- Have baby's ears checked any time he or she has a cold or upper respiratory infection.
- Talk normally to baby (no "baby talk"). Talk often; repeat baby's babbling and cooing. This helps in speech development.
- Try to understand early talking without trying to correct baby.
- Good mouth care is very important.
- Early dental care is essential to observe teething and prevent caries.

For an infant who has had a palate repair, no nipples, spoons, or straws are permitted; only a drinking glass or a cup is recommended. Do not place anything hard or sharp in the infant's mouth. Administer ordered analgesics to relieve pain, comfort the infant, and prevent crying, which is important to decrease the danger of disrupting the suture line.

For the first few postoperative hours, never leave the infant alone, because aspiration of mucus occurs quickly and easily. Because nothing is permitted in the infant's mouth, particularly the thumb or finger, elbow restraints are necessary. Be sure they are applied properly; check them frequently (see Fig. 5.4). Apply the restraint snugly but without hindering circulation. The older infant may need to be placed in a jacket restraint. Document the use of restraints. Remove them at least every 2 hours, but only one at a time, and control the released arm so that the thumb or fingers do not pop into the mouth.

Gentle mouth care with tepid water or clear liquid may be recommended to follow feeding. This care helps clean the suture area of any food or liquids to promote a cleaner incision for optimal healing.

The lip suture line is left uncovered after surgery. Keep it clean and dry to prevent infection and subsequent scarring. Apply a wire bow (Logan bar) or a butterfly closure across the upper lip and attach it to the cheeks with adhesive tape to prevent tension on the sutures caused by crying or other facial movement. Carefully clean the sutures after feeding with sterile cotton swabs and saline. Application of an ointment such as bacitracin may also be ordered.

The nurse and family caregivers must use every opportunity to provide sensory stimulation. Talking to the infant, cuddling and holding him or her, and responding to cries are important interventions.

• VISION IMPAIRMENT

Good vision is essential to a child's normal development. How well a child sees affects his or her learning process, social development, coordination, and safety. The sooner impairments are corrected, the better a child's chances are for normal or near-normal development.

Types of Vision Impairment

Children with vision impairments are classified as sighted with eye problems, partially sighted, or legally blind.

Eye Problems in Sighted Children

Among sighted children with eye problems, errors of **refraction** (the way light rays bend as they pass through the lens to the retina) are the most common. **Myopia** (nearsightedness) means that the child can see objects clearly at close range but not at a distance. When proper lenses are fitted, vision is corrected to normal. Myopia tends to be seen in families and often progresses into adolescence and then levels off.

Hyperopia (farsightedness) is a refractive condition in which the person can see objects better at a distance than close-up. It is common in young children and often persists into the first grade or even later. In most cases, correction is not needed in a preschooler. Teachers and parents should be aware of the considerable eye fatigue that may result from efforts at accommodation for close work.

Astigmatism may occur with or without myopia or hyperopia and is caused by unequal curvatures in the cornea that bend the light rays in different directions; this produces a blurred image. Slight astigmatism often does not require correction; moderate degrees usually require glasses for reading and watching television and movies; severe astigmatism requires glasses at all times.

Partial Sight

Children with partial sight have a visual acuity between 20/20 and 20/200 in the better eye after all necessary medical or surgical correction. These children also have a high incidence of refractive errors, particularly myopia. Eye injuries also cause loss of vision, as do conditions such as cataracts that can be improved by treatment but result in diminished sight.

Blindness

Blindness is legally defined as a corrected vision of 20/200 or less or peripheral vision of less than 20° in the better eye. Many causes of blindness have been reduced or eliminated such as retrolental fibroplasia (from excessive oxygen concentrations in newborns) and trachoma (a viral infection). Maternal infections are still a common cause of blindness.

Between 5 and 7 years, children begin to form and retain visual images; they have memory with pictures. Children who become blind before 5 years are missing this crucial element in their development. Blindness can seriously hamper the child's ability to form human attachments; learn coordination, balance, and locomotion; distinguish fantasy from reality; and interpret the surrounding world. How well the blind child learns to cope depends on the family's ability to communicate, teach, and foster a sense of independence.

Assessment Findings

Squinting and frowning while trying to read a blackboard or other material at a distance, tearing, red-rimmed eyes, holding work too close to the eyes while reading or writing, and rubbing the eyes are all signs of possible vision impairment. Although blindness is likely to be detected in early infancy, partial sight or correctable vision problems may go unrecognized until a child enters school unless vision screening is part of routine health maintenance.

A simple test kit for preschoolers is available for home use by family caregivers or visiting nurses. This kit is an adaptation of the Snellen E chart used for testing children who have not learned to read. The child covers one eye and then points the fingers in the same direction as the "fingers" on each E, beginning with the largest. Some examiners refer to these as "legs on a table."

With the Snellen chart, the letters on each line are smaller than those on the line above. If the child can read the 20-foot line standing 20 feet away from the chart, visual acuity is stated as 20/20. If the child can read only the line marked 100, acuity is stated as 20/100. The chart should be placed at eye level with good lighting and in a room free from distractions. One eye is tested at a time with the other eye covered.

Picture charts for identification also are used but are not considered as accurate. An intelligent child can memorize the pictures and guess from the general shape without seeing distinctly.

Medical Management

Significant medical and surgical advances have occurred in the treatment of cataracts, strabismus, and amblyopia. The earlier the child is treated, the better the child's chances of adequate vision for normal development and function. Errors of refraction are usually correctable. Corrective lenses for minor vision impairments should be prescribed early and checked regularly to be sure they still provide adequate correction.

Children who are partially sighted or totally blind benefit from association with normally sighted children. In most communities, education for these special children is provided within the regular school or in special classes that offer the child more specialized equipment and instruction.

Special equipment includes printed material with large print, pencils with large leads for darker lines, tape recordings, magnifying glasses, and typewriters. For children with a serious impairment whose participation in regular activities is sharply curtailed, talking books, raised maps, and Braille equipment are needed as well. These devices prevent isolation of the visually impaired child and minimize any differences from the other children.

Nursing Management

The child who is blind needs emotional comfort and sensory stimulation, much of which must be communicated by touch, sound, and smell. It is important for nurses to identify themselves when they enter or leave the room, explain sounds and other sensations that are new to the child, and let him or her touch the equipment that will be used in procedures. Explanations help reduce the child's fear and anxiety. A tactile tour of the room helps orient the child to the location of furniture and other facilities. The child with a visual impairment should be involved with as many peers and their activities as possible and be encouraged to be as independent as possible.

• CATARACTS

A **cataract** is a development of opacity in the crystalline lens that prevents light rays from entering the eye. Congenital cataracts may be hereditary or complications of maternal rubella during the first trimester of pregnancy. Cataracts also may develop later in infancy or childhood from eye injury or metabolic disturbances such as galactosemia and diabetes.

Surgical extraction of cataracts can be performed at an early age. With early removal, the prognosis for good vision improves. The infant or child is fitted with a contact lens. If only one eye is affected, the "good" eye is patched to prevent amblyopia (see strabismus). As the child gets older, he or she needs numerous lens changes.

• GLAUCOMA

Glaucoma may be of the congenital infantile type occurring in children younger than 3 years, of the juvenile type showing clinical manifestations after 3 years, or of the secondary type resulting from injury or disease. Increased intraocular pressure from overproduction of aqueous fluid causes the eyeball to enlarge and the cornea to become large, thin, and sometimes cloudy. Untreated, the disease slowly progresses to blindness. Pain may be present. **Goniotomy** (surgical opening into Schlemm's canal) provides drainage of the aqueous humor and is often effective in relieving intraocular pressure. Goniotomy may need to be performed multiple times to control intraocular pressure. Surgery is performed as early as possible to prevent permanent damage.

• STRABISMUS

Strabismus is the failure of the two eyes to direct their gaze at the same object simultaneously and is commonly called "squint" or "crossed" eyes. The muscular coordination of eye movements maintains **binocular** (normal) **vision** so that a single vision results. In strabismus, the visual axes are not parallel and **diplopia** (double vision) results. In an effort to avoid seeing two images, the central nervous system suppresses vision in the deviant eye causing **amblyopia** (dimness of vision from disuse of the eye), which is sometimes called "lazy eye."

A wide variation in the manifestation of strabismus exists; there are lateral, vertical, and mixed lateral and vertical types. In monocular strabismus one eye deviates while the other eye is used; in alternating strabismus, deviation alternates from one eye to the other. The term **esotropia** is used when the eye deviates toward the other eye; **exotropia** denotes a turning away from the other eye.

Treatment depends on the type of strabismus present. In monocular strabismus, occlusion of the better eye by patching to force the use of the deviating eye should be initiated at an early age. Patching continues for weeks or months. The younger the child is, the more rapid the improvement. The patching may be for set periods or continuous depending on the child's age. The older child needs continuous periods of patching, whereas the younger one may respond quickly to short periods of patching.

Glasses can correct a refractive error if amblyopia is not present. **Orthoptics** (therapeutic ocular muscle exercises) to improve the quality of vision may be prescribed to supplement the use of glasses or surgery.

Surgery on the eye muscle to correct the defect is necessary for children who do not respond to glasses and exercises. Many children need surgery after amblyopia has been corrected. Early detection and treatment of strabismus are essential for a successful outcome. The correction is believed to be necessary before the child reaches 6 years or the visual damage may be permanent; however, some authorities believe that correction can be successful up to 10 years.

• EYE INJURY AND FOREIGN OBJECTS IN THE EYE

Eye injuries are fairly common, particularly in older children. Ecchymosis of the eye (black eye) is of no great importance unless the eyeball is involved. A penetrating wound of the eyeball is potentially serious—BB shots, in particular, are dangerous—and requires an ophthalmologist's attention. With any history of an injury, a thorough examination of the entire eye is necessary. See Chapter 43 for more discussion.

• EYE INFECTIONS

External hordeolum, known commonly as a stye, is a purulent infection of the follicle of an eyelash generally caused by *Staphylococcus aureus.* Localized swelling, tenderness, pain, and a reddened lid edge are present. The maximal tenderness is over the infected site. The lesion progresses to suppuration with eventual discharge of the purulent material. Warm saline compresses applied for about 15 minutes three or four times daily give some relief and hasten resolution, but recurrence is common.

The stye should never be squeezed. Antibiotic ointment may help prevent accompanying conjunctivitis and recurrence.

Conjunctivitis is an acute inflammation of the conjunctiva. In children, a virus, bacteria, allergy, or foreign body may be the cause. Bacterial conjunctivitis is most common. The purulent drainage, a common characteristic, can be cultured to determine the causative organism. Because of the danger of spreading infection, bacterial conjunctivitis is treated with ophthalmic antibacterial agents such as erythromycin, bacitracin, sulfacetamide, and polymyxin. Because ointments blur vision, eye drops are used during the day and ointments at night. Before applying medication, warm moist compresses can be used to remove the crusts that form on the eyes. The child with bacterial conjunctivitis should be kept separate from other children until the condition has been treated. The use of separate washcloths and towels and disposable tissues is important to prevent spread of infection among family members.

● NURSING CARE FOR THE CHILD UNDERGOING EYE SURGERY

Anyone experiencing sensory deprivation finds it difficult to stay in touch with reality. A child whose eyes are covered is particularly vulnerable. A child who wakens from surgery to total darkness may panic, as evidenced by trembling and nervousness. The child needs a family caregiver or loved one to stay during the time when vision is restricted.

The child should be as well prepared for the event as possible, but the small child has no experience to help in understanding what actually will happen. One preoperative preparation might be to play a game with a blindfold to help the child become used to having his or her eyes covered.

Restraints should not be used indiscriminately, but most small children need some reminder to keep their hands away from the sore eye unless someone is beside them to prevent them from rubbing it or from removing eye dressings. Elbow restraints are useful, although they do not prevent rubbing the eye with the arm. Flannel strips applied to the wrists in clove-hitch fashion can be tied to the bedsides in such a manner as to allow freedom of arm movement but to prevent the child from damaging the operative site.

● HEARING IMPAIRMENT

Hearing loss is one of the most common disabilities in the United States, with as many as 33 children born each day with a hearing impairment (Ansel, Landa, & Luethke, 1999). Depending on the degree of loss and age at detection, the problem can moderately to severely impair a child's development. Development of speech, human relationships, and understanding of the environment all depend on hearing. Infants at high risk for hearing loss should be screened during the first year of life (Scott & Tyson, 1999).

Types of Hearing Impairment

Hearing loss ranges from mild (hard of hearing) to profound (deaf). A child who is hard of hearing has a loss of hearing acuity but can learn speech and language by imitating sounds. A deaf child has no hearing ability.

Conductive Hearing Loss

In this type of impairment, middle ear structures fail to carry sound waves to the inner ear. Conductive hearing loss most often results from chronic serous otitis media or other infection and can make hearing levels fluctuate. Chronic middle ear infection can destroy part of the eardrum or the ossicles, which leads to conductive deafness. This type of deafness is seldom complete and responds well to treatment.

Sensorineural (Perceptive) Hearing Loss

Damage to the nerve endings in the cochlea or to the nerve pathways leading to the brain causes this type of hearing loss, which is generally severe and unresponsive to medical treatment. Diseases such as meningitis and encephalitis, hereditary or congenital factors, and toxic reactions to certain drugs (such as streptomycin) may be responsible. Maternal rubella is believed to be one of the common causes of sensorineural deafness in children (Sanchez & Siegel, 1999).

Mixed Hearing Loss

Some children have both conductive and sensorineural hearing impairments. In these instances, the conduction level determines how well the child can hear.

Central Auditory Dysfunction

Although this child may have normal hearing, damage to or faulty development of the proper brain centers makes the child unable to use the auditory information received.

Assessment Findings

Mild to moderate hearing loss often remains undetected until the child moves outside the family circle into nursery school or kindergarten. The hearing loss may have been gradual, and the child may have become such a skilled lip reader that neither the child nor the family is aware of the partial deafness.

The child should be observed for an apparent inability to locate a sound and a turning of the head to one side when listening. The child who fails to comprehend when spoken to, who gives inappropriate answers to questions, who consistently turns up the volume on the television or radio, or who cannot whisper or talk softly may have hearing loss.

Children who are profoundly deaf are more likely to be diagnosed before 1 year of age than are children with mild to moderate hearing loss. The child who is suspected of having a hearing loss should be referred for a complete audiologic assessment including pure-tone audiometric, speech reception, and speech discrimination tests. Children with sensorineural impairment generally have a greater loss of hearing acuity in the high-pitched tones. The loss may vary from slight to complete. Children with a conductive loss are more likely to have equal losses over a wide range of frequencies.

A child's hearing should be tested at all frequencies by a pure-tone audiometer in a soundproof room. Speech reception and speech discrimination tests measure the amount of hearing impairment for both speech and communication. Accurate measurements usually can be made in children as young as 3 years if the test is introduced as a game.

Deafness, mental retardation, and autism sometimes are diagnosed incorrectly because the symptoms can be similar. Deaf children may fail to respond to sound or develop speech because they cannot hear. Mentally retarded or autistic children may show the same lack of response and development even though they do not have a hearing loss.

Medical Management

When the type and degree of hearing loss have been established, the child or even infant may be fitted with a hearing aid. Hearing aids are helpful only in conductive deafness. These devices only amplify sound; they do not localize or clarify it.

It is believed that deaf children can best learn to communicate by a combination of lip reading, sign language, and oral speech. Family members are the child's first teachers; they must be aware of all phases of development—physical, emotional, social, intellectual, and language—and seek to facilitate it.

A deaf child depends on sight to interpret the environment and to communicate. Thus, it is important to be sure that the child's vision is normal and if it is not, to correct that problem. Training in the use of all the other senses—sight, smell, taste, and touch—makes the child better able to use any available hearing.

The John Tracy Clinic in Los Angeles is dedicated to young children (birth through age 5) born with severe hearing loss or who have lost hearing through illness before acquiring speech and language. The clinic's purpose is "to find, encourage, guide, and train the parents of deaf and hard-of-hearing children, first in order to reach and help the children, and second to help the parents themselves." Information about the clinic can be obtained by calling toll-free (800) 522-4582 or visiting http://www.johntracyclinic.org.

Nursing Management

When the deaf child is in a healthcare facility, the child's primary caregiver should be present during the stay to help the child communicate needs and feelings. When speaking to the deaf child, stand or sit face to face on the child's level. Be certain that a deaf child can see you before you touch him or her. Demonstrate each procedure before it is performed, showing the child the equipment or pictures of the equipment to be used. Follow demonstrations with explanations to be sure the child understands. Keep a night-light in the child's room; sight is a critical sense to the deaf child. Put the hearing aid in a safe place when the child is not wearing it.

• OTITIS MEDIA

Otitis media is one of the most common infectious diseases of childhood. The eustachian tube of infants is shorter and wider than in older children and adults (Fig. 8.4). The tube is also straighter, thereby allowing nasopharyngeal secretions to enter the middle ear more easily. *Haemophilus influenzae* is an important causative agent of childhood otitis media.

Assessment Findings

A restless infant who repeatedly shakes the head and rubs or pulls at one ear should be checked for an ear infection. These behaviors often indicate that the infant is having ear pain. Symptoms include fever, irritability, and hearing impairment. Vomiting or diarrhea may occur.

Examination of the ear with an otoscope is done in the infant by pulling the ear down and back to straighten the ear canal. In the older child the ear is pulled up and back. The examination reveals a bright-red, bulging eardrum in otitis media. Spontaneous rupture of the eardrum may occur, in which case drainage will be purulent, and the pain caused by the pressure build-up in the ear will be relieved. If present, purulent drainage is cultured to determine the causative organism and appropriate antibiotic.

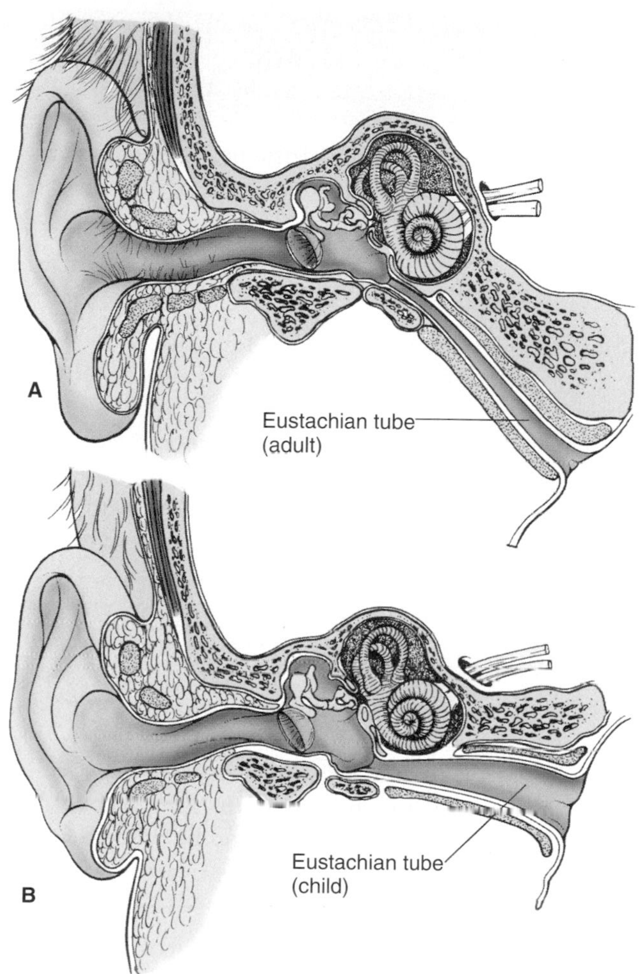

FIGURE 8.4 Comparison of the eustachian tube in the adult (**A**) and the infant (**B**).

Medical Management

Antibiotics are used during the period of infection and for several days following to prevent mastoiditis or chronic infection. A 10-day course of amoxicillin is a common treatment. Most infants respond well to antibiotics.

Some infants and young children have repeated episodes of otitis media. Children with chronic otitis media may be put on a prophylactic course of an oral penicillin or sulfonamide. **Myringotomy** (incision of the eardrum) may be performed to establish drainage and to insert tiny tubes into the tympanic membrane to facilitate drainage. In most cases, the tubes eventually fall out spontaneously. Attention to chronic otitis media is essential because permanent hearing loss can result from frequent occurrences.

Mastoiditis (infection of the mastoid sinus), a possible complication of untreated acute otitis media, was much more common before the advent of antibiotics. Currently it is seen only in children who have an untreated ruptured eardrum or inadequate treatment (through noncompliance of caregivers or improper care) of an acute episode.

Nursing Management

Most infants and young children with otitis media receive care at home; therefore, a primary nursing responsibility is to teach family caregivers about prevention and treatment. See Client and Family Teaching 8-2.

Stop, Think, and Respond ● BOX 8-5

Why are infants more likely than adults to get otitis media? What bacterium often causes otitis media?

Critical Thinking Exercises

1. *The mother of a 2-year-old, who is upset because her child has awakened with a bark-like cough and a high-pitched harsh sound when taking a breath, calls the pediatric triage nurse at 10:00 PM. What questions should the nurse ask this mother? What should the mother do to try to relieve the child's symptoms? What further instructions should the nurse give this mother?*
2. *How would you respond to the family of a child who died from SIDS when they ask, "What caused our baby to die? What are the risk factors for SIDS?"*
3. *The family of Scott, a 6-year-old with hemophilia, is concerned that Scott might get AIDS from his treatments. What is the likelihood of Scott being HIV-positive or of contracting AIDS from his treatments? What explanation will you give this family to reassure them?*
4. *Diane's baby was born with a bilateral cleft lip and cleft palate. When you bring the baby to Diane for feeding, she breaks down and sobs uncontrollably. What would your immediate response be? How would you support and reassure this mother? What treatments and procedures might be done for this child?*

● NCLEX-STYLE REVIEW QUESTIONS 

1. A 3-year-old arrives in the emergency department with a dry and nonproductive cough, digital clubbing, steatorrhea, malnutrition, and a blood glucose level of 128. Laboratory results reveal abnormally high sodium chloride in the sweat. Based on these symptoms, the nurse gathers teaching information related to which condition?
   1. AIDS
   2. Reye syndrome
   3. Kawasaki disease
   4. Cystic fibrosis
2. An obstetric nurse is instructing expectant mothers on sudden infant death syndrome (SIDS). Which of the following would the nurse stress as a risk factor for SIDS?
   1. Prone position for sleep
   2. Post-term delivery
   3. Age range of 6 to 9 months
   4. Respiratory infections

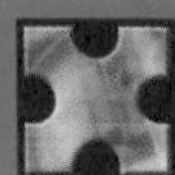

8-2 *Client and Family Teaching* Otitis Media

The eustachian tube is a connection between the nasal passages and the middle ear. The eustachian tube is wider, shorter, and straighter in the infant, allowing organisms from respiratory infections to travel into the middle ear to cause infection (otitis media).

PREVENTION

- Hold infant in an upright position or with head slightly elevated while feeding to prevent formula from draining into the middle ear through the wide eustachian tube.
- Never prop a bottle.
- Do not give infant a bottle in bed. This allows fluid to pool in the middle ear, encouraging organisms to grow.
- Protect infant from exposure to others with upper respiratory infections.
- Protect infant from passive smoke; do not permit smoking in baby's presence.
- Remove sources of allergies from home.
- Observe for clues to ear infection: shaking head, rubbing or pulling at ears, and fever, combined with restlessness or screaming and crying.
- Be alert to signs of hearing difficulty in toddlers and preschoolers. This may be the first sign of an ear infection.
- Teach toddler or preschooler gentle nose blowing.

CARE OF CHILD WITH OTITIS MEDIA

- Have child with upper respiratory infection who shows symptoms of ear discomfort checked by a healthcare professional.
- Complete the entire amount of antibiotic prescribed, even though the child seems better.
- Heat (such as a heating pad on low setting) may provide comfort, but an adult must stay with the child.
- Soothe, rock, and comfort child to help relieve discomfort. The child is more comfortable sleeping on side of infected ear.
- Give pain medications (such as acetaminophen) as directed. Never give aspirin.
- Provide liquid or soft foods; chewing causes pain.
- Hearing loss may last up to 6 months after infection.
- Follow-up with hearing test should be scheduled as advised.

3. Which assessment finding by the nurse would indicate that a client had ataxic cerebral palsy?
  1. Slow, writhing movements
  2. Voluntary, jerky movements
  3. Lack of coordination and balance
  4. Muscle tremors and rigidity

connection

Visit the Connection site at **http://connection.lww.com/go/timbyEssentials** for links to chapter-related resources on the Internet.

References and Suggested Readings

Ansel, B. M., Landa, R. M., & Luethke L. E. (1999). Development and disorders of speech, language and hearing. In *Oski's pediatrics: Principles and practice* (3rd ed.). Philadelphia: Lippincott Williams & Wilkins.

Carroll, J. L., & Loughlin, G. M. (1999). Sudden infant death syndrome. In *Oski's pediatrics: Principles and practice* (3rd ed.). Philadelphia: Lippincott Williams & Wilkins.

Cooper, K. E. (2001). The effectiveness of ribavirin in the treatment of RSV. *Pediatric Nursing, 27*(1).

England, A. C., Dalheim Rydstrom, I., & Astrid, N. (2001). Being the parent of a child with asthma. *Pediatric Nursing, 27*(4), 365.

Fixler, D. E. (1999). Epidemiology of congenital heart disease. In *Oski's pediatrics: Principles and practices* (3rd ed.). Philadelphia: Lippincott Williams & Wilkins.

Gorlin, R. J. (1999). Craniofacial defects. In *Oski's pediatrics: Principles and practices* (3rd ed.). Philadelphia: Lippincott Williams & Wilkins.

Hagerman, R. J. (1999). *Neurodevelopmental disorders: Diagnosis and treatment.* New York: Oxford University Press.

Kaplan, S. L. (1999). Haemophilus influenzae. In *Oski's pediatrics: Principles and practices* (3rd ed.). Philadelphia: Lippincott Williams & Wilkins.

Karch, A. M. (2003). *2003 Lippincott's Nursing Drug Guide.* Philadelphia: Lippincott Williams & Wilkins.

Kline, M. K. (1999). Otitis media. In *Oski's pediatrics: Principles and practices* (3rd ed.). Philadelphia: Lippincott Williams & Wilkins.

Louis, P. T. (1999). Reye syndrome. In *Oski's pediatrics: Principles and practices* (3rd ed.). Philadelphia: Lippincott Williams & Wilkins.

Malhotra, A., & Krilow, L. (2001). Viral croup. *Pediatrics in Review, 22*(1), 5.

Naslund, J. (2001). Modes of sensory stimulation. *Physiotherapy, 87*(8), 13–23.

Neches, W. H., Park, S. C., Ettedgui, J. A. (1999). Transposition of the great arteries. In *Oski's pediatrics: Principles and practices* (3rd ed.). Philadelphia: Lippincott Williams & Wilkins.

North American Nursing Diagnosis Association. (2003). *NANDA nursing diagnoses: Definitions and classification 2003–2004.* Philadelphia: Author.

Parini, S. (2001). Eight faces of meningitis. *Nursing 2001, 31*(8), 51.

Pillitteri, A. (2003). *Maternal and child health nursing* (4th ed.). Philadelphia: Lippincott Williams & Wilkins.

Sanchez, P. J., & Siegel, J. D. (1999). Rubella. In *Oski's pediatrics: Principles and practices* (3rd ed.). Philadelphia: Lippincott Williams & Wilkins.

Scott, D. T., & Tyson, J. E. (1999). Follow-up of infants discharged from newborn intensive care. In *Oski's pediatrics: Principles and practices* (3rd ed.). Philadelphia: Lippincott Williams & Wilkins.

Shapiro, B. K., & Capute, A. J. (1999). Cerebral palsy. In *Oski's pediatrics: Principles and practices* (3rd ed.). Philadelphia: Lippincott Williams & Wilkins.

Skoner, D. P. (2002). Balancing safety and efficacy in pediatric asthma management. *Pediatrics, 109*(2), 381.

Sparks, S., & Taylor, C. (2001). *Nursing diagnosis reference manual* (5th ed.). Springhouse, PA: Springhouse Corporation.

Vick, W. G., III, & Titus, J. L. (1999). Defects of the atrial septum, including the atrioventricular canal. In *Oski's pediatrics: Principles and practices* (3rd ed.). Philadelphia: Lippincott Williams & Wilkins.

Wong, D. L., Perry, S., & Hockenberry, M. (2002). *Maternal child nursing care* (2nd ed.). St. Louis: Mosby.

chapter 9

Caring for Children With Physical Disorders: Part 2

Words to Know 

ankylosis
ascites
celiac syndrome
chordee
colic
currant jelly stools
diabetic ketoacidosis
encopresis
enuresis
gastroenteritis
halo traction
hernia
insulin reaction
intercurrent infections
intussusception
Kussmaul breathing
kyphosis
leukopenia
lordosis
orchiopexy
polydipsia
polyphagia
polyuria
scoliosis
steatorrhea
striae
synovitis
tinea

Learning Objectives

On completion of this chapter, the reader will:

- Explain the diagnosis of celiac disease.
- Differentiate between mild diarrhea and severe diarrhea.
- Describe the five types of hernias that infants may have.
- State another name for congenital megacolon and its common symptoms.
- Describe the diagnosis and treatment of intussusception.
- Identify the symptoms of pyloric stenosis.
- Describe what to include in an age-appropriate teaching plan for children with type 1 diabetes mellitus.
- Discuss the importance of good skin care, correct insulin administration, and exercise for children with diabetes.
- Describe the symptoms of nephrotic syndrome.
- Name the drugs of choice and their primary purpose in the treatment of juvenile rheumatoid arthritis.
- List three signs and symptoms of congenital dislocation of the hip.
- Describe the treatment for congenital dislocation of the hip.
- State the two most common skeletal deformities in the newborn.
- Identify the most common form of muscular dystrophy and its characteristics.
- Discuss the importance of early treatment for clubfoot.
- Identify the causative organism of thrush.
- Describe the treatment for pediculosis of the scalp, explaining the protection the nurse must use when treating a child with this condition in the hospital.
- Discuss communicable diseases for which children are immunized.
- Describe infectious mononucleosis.

Disorders dealing with the gastrointestinal system of infants and children range from mild to serious in nature. Many children are affected by these disorders and it is important for the nurse to be aware of the speed at which complications can arise. Endocrine, urinary, and renal disorders also have a wide range of severity. Because of the active nature of children, musculoskeletal disorders are common during childhood.

GASTROINTESTINAL DISORDERS

• CELIAC SYNDROME/GLUTEN-INDUCED ENTEROPATHY

Intestinal malabsorption with **steatorrhea** (fatty stools) is a condition with various causes, the most common being cystic fibrosis and gluten-induced enteropathy (the so-called idiopathic celiac disease). The term **celiac syndrome** is used to designate malabsorptive disorders in general.

Pathophysiology and Etiology

Idiopathic celiac disease is a basic defect of metabolism precipitated by the ingestion of wheat gluten or rye gluten, which leads to impaired fat absorption. The exact cause is not known. The most widely accepted theory is an inborn error of metabolism, with an allergic reaction to the gliadin fraction of gluten (a protein factor in wheat) as a contributing, or possibly the sole, factor.

Assessment Findings

Signs generally do not appear before 6 months of age and may be delayed until 1 year or later. Manifestations include chronic diarrhea with foul, bulky, greasy stools and progressive malnutrition. Anorexia and a fretful, unhappy disposition are typical. The onset is generally insidious with failure to thrive, bouts of diarrhea, and frequent respiratory infections. If the condition becomes severe, the effects of malnutrition are prominent. Retarded growth and development, a distended abdomen, and thin, wasted buttocks and legs are characteristic signs.

Celiac crisis, an emergency, may interrupt the chronic course of this disease. Frequently, the trigger is an upper respiratory infection. The child vomits copiously; has large, watery stools, and becomes severely dehydrated. As the child becomes drowsy and prostrate, an acute medical emergency develops. Parenteral fluid therapy is essential to combat acidosis and to achieve normal fluid balance.

One way to determine if the cause of a small child's failure to thrive is celiac disease is to initiate a trial gluten-free diet and observe the results. Improvement in the nature of the stools and general well-being with weight gain should follow, although several weeks may elapse before confirmation of clear-cut manifestations. Conclusive diagnosis can be made by a biopsy of the jejunum through endoscopy that shows changes in the villi. Serum screening of IgG and IgA antigliadin antibodies shows the condition and also aids in monitoring progress of therapy.

Medical Management

Response to a diet that excludes rye, wheat, and oats is generally good, although respiratory infections may bring relapses. The omission of wheat products in particular should continue through adolescence, because ingestion of wheat appears to inhibit growth in these children.

The young child usually is started on a starch-free, low-fat diet. If the condition is severe, this diet consists of skim milk, glucose, and banana flakes. Bananas contain invert sugar and are usually well tolerated. Lean meats, puréed vegetables, and fruits are added gradually to the diet. Eventually fats may be added, and the child can be maintained on a regular diet with the exception of all wheat, rye, and oat products.

Commercially canned creamed soups, cold cuts, frankfurters, and pudding mixes generally contain wheat products. The forbidden list also includes malted milk drinks, some candies, many baby foods, and breads, cakes, pastries, and biscuits unless they are made from corn flour or cornmeal. The child needs double amounts of vitamins A and D to supplement the deficient diet.

Nursing Management

The primary focus of nursing care is to help caregivers maintain a restrictive diet for the child. Family teaching should include information regarding the disease and the need for long-term management as well as guidelines for a gluten-free diet. Caregivers must learn to carefully read the list of ingredients on packaged foods before purchasing anything. The diet of the young child may be monitored fairly easily, but when the child goes to school, monitoring becomes a much greater challenge. As the child grows, caregivers and children might need additional nursing support to help them make dietary modifications.

Stop, Think, and Respond ● BOX 9-1

What are the common symptoms of celiac disease? What is usually removed from the diet of a child with celiac disease?

● COLIC

Pathophysiology and Etiology

Colic consists of recurrent paroxysmal bouts of abdominal pain and is fairly common in young infants. It often disappears at approximately 3 months of age, but this is small comfort to caregivers vainly trying to soothe a colicky infant. Although many theories have been proposed, none has been accepted as the causative factor.

Assessment Findings

Attacks occur suddenly, usually late in the day or evening. The infant cries loudly and continuously and appears to be in considerable pain, but otherwise seems healthy, nurses or takes formula well, and gains weight as expected.

The baby may be momentarily soothed only by rocking or holding but eventually falls asleep, exhausted from crying. Differential diagnosis should be made to rule out an allergic reaction to milk or certain foods. Changing to a nonallergenic formula helps determine if there is an allergic factor or lactose intolerance. If the baby is breastfed, the mother's diet should be studied to determine if anything she is eating might be affecting the baby. Intestinal obstruction or infection also must be ruled out.

Medical and Nursing Management

No single treatment is consistently successful. Medications such as sedatives, antispasmodics, and antiflatulents are sometimes prescribed, but their effectiveness is inconsistent. The family must remember that the condition will pass, even though at the time it seems it will last forever. Reassure family caregivers that their parenting skills are not inadequate. Support the family and promote coping skills by providing family teaching (Client and Family Teaching 9-1).

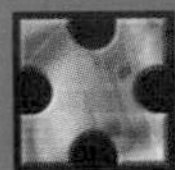

9-1 *Client and Family Teaching* Colic

The nurse teaches the family as follows:

- Rock the baby in a rocker. Alternatively, pick up the baby and, with baby's abdomen down across your knees, swing your legs side to side. (Be sure to support the baby's head.)
- Walk around the room while rocking the baby in your arms or a front carrier. Hum or sing to the child.
- Try a bottle, but do not overfeed. Give a pacifier if baby has eaten well within 2 hours.
- Baby may like the rhythmic movements of a baby swing.
- Try taking baby outside or for a car ride.
- When feeding the baby, try methods to decrease gas formation (i.e., frequent burping, giving smaller feedings more frequently); position baby in infant seat after eating.
- Try doing something to entertain but not overexcite baby.
- Gently rub baby's abdomen if it is rigid.
- Sit with baby resting on your lap with legs toward you; gently move baby's legs in pumping motion.
- Try putting baby down to sleep in a darkened room.
- Keep remembering that it is temporary. Stay as calm and relaxed as possible.

● DIARRHEA AND GASTROENTERITIS

Diarrhea in infants is a fairly common symptom of several conditions. It may be mild with slight dehydration or extremely severe, requiring prompt and effective treatment. Infectious diarrhea commonly is referred to as **gastroenteritis.**

Pathophysiology and Etiology

Simple diarrhea that does not respond to treatment can quickly progress to severe, life-threatening diarrhea. Some conditions that cause diarrhea require readjustment of the infant's diet. Elimination of the offending food can control allergic reactions. Overfeeding as well as underfeeding or an unbalanced diet also may be the cause of diarrhea in an infant.

Contact with contaminated food or human or animal fecal waste through the oral-fecal route causes many diarrheal disturbances in infants. The infectious organisms may be salmonella, *Escherichia coli,* dysentery bacilli, and various viruses, most notably rotaviruses. Determining the causative factor is difficult in many instances. Because of the seriousness of infectious diarrhea and the danger of its spread, the child with moderate or severe diarrhea often is isolated until the causative factor has been proved to be noninfectious.

Assessment Findings

Mild diarrhea may present as little more than loose stools; the frequency of defecation may be two to 12 per day. The infant may be irritable and have a loss of appetite. Vomiting and gastric distention are not significant factors, and dehydration is minimal.

Mild or moderate diarrhea can rather quickly become severe diarrhea in an infant. Vomiting usually accompanies the diarrhea; together, they cause large losses of body water and electrolytes. The infant becomes severely dehydrated and is gravely ill. The skin becomes extremely dry and loses its turgor. The fontanelle becomes sunken, and the pulse is weak and rapid. The stools become greenish liquid and may be blood-tinged.

Stool specimens may be collected for culture and sensitivity testing to determine the causative infectious organism, if there is one. Subsequently, effective antibiotics can be prescribed as indicated.

Medical Management

Treatment to stop the diarrhea must be initiated immediately. Establishing normal fluid and electrolyte balance is the primary concern in treating gastroenteritis. The infant with acute dehydration may be given oral feedings of commercial electrolyte solutions, such as Pedialyte or Rehydralyte. This treatment is called *oral rehydration therapy*. After the diarrhea has stopped, feedings are restarted gradually. Once commonly used, the BRAT diet (ripe *b*anana, *r*ice cereal, *a*pplesauce, and *t*oast) has become somewhat controversial because it is high in calories, low in energy and protein, and does not provide adequate nutrition. Salty broths should be avoided. After the infant has been rehydrated, he or she can return to breastfeeding or formula-feeding. Foods can be added slowly as the infant's condition improves, returning to a regular diet.

In severe diarrhea with shock and severe dehydration, oral feedings are discontinued completely. Fluids to be given intravenously must be calculated carefully to replace the lost electrolytes. Frequent laboratory determinations of the infant's blood chemistries are necessary to guide the physician in this replacement therapy. For the infant who has had a serious bout of diarrhea, soybean formula may be given for a few weeks to avoid a possible reaction to milk proteins.

Nursing Management

The interview with the family caregiver must include specific information about the history of bowel patterns and the onset of diarrheal stools with details on number and type of stools per day. Suggest terms to describe the color and odor of stools to assist the caregiver with descriptions. Inquire about recent feeding patterns, nausea, and vomiting. Ask the caregiver about fever and other signs of illness in the infant and signs of illness in any other family members.

Physical examination of the infant includes observation of skin turgor and condition including excoriated diaper area, temperature, anterior fontanelle (depressed, normal, or bulging), apical pulse rate (observing for weak pulse), stools (character, frequency, amount, and color of any blood), irritability, lethargy, vomiting, urine (amount and concentration), lips and mucous membranes of the mouth (dry, cracked), eyes (bright, glassy, sunken, dark circles), and any other notable physical signs.

To prevent the spread of possibly infectious organisms to other pediatric clients, follow standard precautions issued by the Centers for Disease Control and Prevention. Wear gowns and gloves when handling articles contaminated with feces. Limit visitors to family only. Carry out good handwashing and also teach it to family caregivers.

To reduce irritation and excoriation of the buttocks and genital area, cleanse those areas frequently and apply a soothing protective preparation such as lanolin or A and D Ointment. Change diapers as quickly as possible after soiling. Leaving the diaper off and exposing the buttocks and genital area to the air is often helpful.

An infant can dehydrate quickly and face serious problems after less than 3 days of diarrhea. Carefully count diapers and weigh them to determine the infant's output accurately. Closely observe all stools. Document the number and character of the stools, as well as the amount and character of any vomitus. Weigh the infant daily on the same scale, early in the morning before the morning feeding. Monitor intake and output strictly. IV fluids may be given to rest the GI tract, restore hydration, and maintain nutritional requirements.

When starting oral fluids, begin with electrolyte solutions and progress to half-strength and then full-strength formula. The breastfed infant can continue breastfeeding. The infant who is NPO needs to have his or her sucking needs fulfilled by offering a pacifier.

Monitor vital signs at least every 2 hours if there is fever. Do *not* take the temperature rectally, as insertion of a thermometer into the rectum can stimulate stools as well as cause trauma and tissue injury to sensitive mucosa. Follow appropriate procedures for fever reduction.

Being the family caregiver of an infant who has become so ill in such a short time is frightening. Suggest to the caregiver ways to console the infant by soothing, gentle stroking of the head, and speaking softly. Explain to family caregivers the importance of GI rest for the infant. They (especially if young or poorly educated) may not understand the necessity for NPO status. Increased understanding on their part can improve cooperation. See Client and Family Teaching 9-2.

Stop, Think, and Respond ● BOX 9-2

What is the most serious concern for the infant with diarrhea? What symptoms would be noted in the infant?

● HERNIAS

A **hernia** is the abnormal protrusion of part of an organ through a weak spot or other abnormal opening in a body wall. Complications occur depending on the amount of circulatory impairment involved and how much the herniated organ impairs the functioning of another organ. Most hernias can be repaired surgically.

Diaphragmatic Hernia

In a congenital hernia of the diaphragm, some of the abdominal organs are displaced into the left chest through an opening in the diaphragm. The heart is pushed toward the right, and the left lung is compressed. Rapid, labored respirations and cyanosis are present on the first day of life, and breathing becomes increasingly difficult.

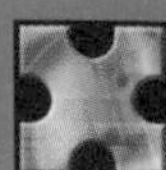

9-2 *Client and Family Teaching* Diarrhea and Vomiting

The nurse teaches the family as follows:

DIARRHEA

The danger in diarrhea is dehydration (drying out). Children who become dehydrated can become very sick. Increasing liquids is helpful. Solid foods may need to be decreased so the child will drink more.

Suggestions

- Give liquids in small amounts (3 or 4 tbsp) approximately every 30 minutes. If this goes well, slightly increase the amount each time. Do not force the child to drink—he or she may vomit. Liquids recommended for vomiting also may be given for diarrhea.
- Give solid foods in small amounts. Do not give milk for 1 or 2 days, because this can make diarrhea worse.
- Give only nonsalty soups or broths.
- Soft foods to give in small amounts include applesauce, fine chopped or scraped apple without peel, bananas, toast, rice cereal, plain unsalted crackers or cookies, and any meats.

Call the physician if:

- Child develops sudden high fever
- Stomach pain becomes severe
- Diarrhea becomes bloody (more than a streak of blood), more frequent, or severe
- Child becomes dehydrated (dried out)

Signs of dehydration

- Child has not urinated for 6 hours or more.
- Child has no tears when crying.
- Child's mouth is dry or sticky to touch.
- Child's eyes are sunken.
- Child is less active than usual.
- Child has dark circles under eyes.

Warning: Do not use medicines to stop diarrhea for children younger than 6 years unless specifically directed by the physician. These medicines can be dangerous if not used properly.

VOMITING

Vomiting usually will stop in a few days and can be treated at home as long as the child is getting some fluids.

Warning: Some medications used to stop vomiting in older children or adults are dangerous in infants or young children. DO NOT use any medicine unless your physician has told you to do so for *this child.* Give child clear liquids to drink in small amounts.

Suggestions

- Pedialyte, Lytren, Rehydralyte, Infalyte
- Flat soda (no fizz) (use caffeine-free type; do not use diet soda)
- Jello water—double the amount of water, let stand to room temperature
- Ice popsicles
- Gatorade
- Tea
- Solid Jell-O
- Broth (not salty)

How to give: Give small amounts often. One tbsp every 20 minutes for the first few hours is a good rule of thumb. If the child keeps this down without vomiting, increase to 2 tbsp every 20 minutes for the next few hours. If there is no vomiting, increase the amount the child may have. If the child vomits, wait for 1 hour before offering more liquids.

Surgery is essential and may be performed as an emergency procedure. During surgery, the abdominal viscera are withdrawn from the chest and the diaphragmatic defect is closed. This defect may be minimal and easily repaired or so extensive that pulmonary tissue has failed to develop normally. The outcome of surgical repair depends on the degree of pulmonary development. The prognosis in severe cases is guarded.

Omphalocele

Omphalocele is a relatively rare congenital anomaly. Some of the abdominal contents protrude through into the root of the umbilical cord and form a sac lying on the abdomen. This sac may be small with only a loop of bowel or large and containing much of the intestine and the liver. Peritoneal membrane instead of skin covers the sac. These defects may be detected during prenatal ultrasonography so that prompt repair may be anticipated.

At birth, the defect should be covered immediately with gauze moistened in sterile saline; it then may be covered with plastic wrap to prevent heat loss. Surgical replacement of the organs into the abdomen may be difficult with a large omphalocele because there may not be enough space in the abdominal cavity. Other congenital defects are often present. With large omphaloceles, surgery may be postponed and the surgeon will suture skin over the defect, creating a large hernia. As the child grows, the abdomen may enlarge enough to allow replacement.

Umbilical Hernia

Normally the ring that encircled the fetal end of the umbilical cord closes gradually and spontaneously after birth. When this closure is incomplete, portions of omentum and intestine protrude through the opening. More common in preterm and African American infants, umbilical hernia is largely a cosmetic problem. While upsetting to parents, it is associated with little or no morbidity. In rare instances, the bowel may strangulate in the sac and require immediate surgery. Almost all these hernias close spontaneously by 3 years; hernias that do not close should be surgically corrected before the child enters school.

Inguinal Hernia

Primarily common in males, inguinal hernias occur when the small sac of peritoneum surrounding the testes fails to close off after the testes descend from the abdominal sac into the scrotum. This failure allows the intestine to slip into the inguinal canal, with resultant swelling. If the intestine becomes trapped (incarcerated) and circulation to the trapped intestine is impaired (strangulated), surgery is necessary to prevent intestinal obstruction and gangrene of the bowel. As a preventive measure, inguinal hernias normally are repaired as soon as they are diagnosed.

• CONGENITAL AGANGLIONIC MEGACOLON

Pathophysiology and Etiology

Congenital aganglionic megacolon, also called Hirschsprung's disease, is characterized by persistent constipation resulting from partial or complete intestinal obstruction of mechanical origin. In some cases, the condition may be severe enough to be recognized during the neonatal period; in other cases the blockage is not diagnosed until later infancy or early childhood.

Parasympathetic nerve cells regulate peristalsis in the intestine. The name *aganglionic megacolon* actually describes the condition because no parasympathetic ganglion cells are found within the muscular wall of the distal colon and rectum. As a result, the affected portion of the lower bowel has no peristaltic action. Thus, it narrows, and the portion directly proximal to (above) the affected area becomes greatly dilated and filled with feces and gas.

Assessment Findings

Failure of the newborn to have a stool in the first 24 hours may indicate several conditions, one of which is megacolon. Other neonatal symptoms suggestive of complete or partial intestinal obstruction include bile-stained emesis and generalized abdominal distention. Gastroenteritis with diarrheal stools may be present, and ulceration of the colon may occur.

The affected older infant or young child has severe constipation dating back to early infancy. Stools are ribbon-like or consist of hard pellets. Formed bowel movements do not occur except with the use of enemas, and soiling does not occur. The rectum is usually empty because the impaction occurs above the aganglionic segment.

As the child grows older, the abdomen becomes progressively enlarged and hard. General debilitation and chronic anemia are usually present. Differentiation must be made between this condition and psychogenic megacolon from coercive toileting or other emotional problems. The child with aganglionic megacolon does not withhold stools or defecate in inappropriate places, and no soiling occurs. Definitive diagnosis is made through barium studies and must be confirmed by rectal biopsy.

Surgical Management

Treatment involves surgery with resection of the aganglionic portion of the bowel. A colostomy often is performed to relieve the obstruction. This allows the infant to regain any weight lost and also gives the bowel a period of rest to return to a more normal state. Resection is deferred until later in infancy.

Nursing Management

Ask family caregivers about the onset of constipation, the character and odor of stools, the frequency of bowel movements, and any poor feeding habits, anorexia, and irritability. Observe the child for a distended abdomen and signs of poor nutrition. Record weight and vital signs.

Give enemas as ordered to achieve bowel elimination and also before any diagnostic and surgical procedures. Administer colonic irrigations with saline solutions. Never administer soapsuds or tap water enemas, because the lack of peristaltic action causes the enemas to be retained and absorbed into the tissues, leading to water intoxication. This could cause syncope, shock, or even death after only one or two irrigations.

Parenteral nutrition may be needed to improve nutritional status because the constipation and distended abdomen cause loss of appetite.

Children need careful explanations to reduce fears. Encourage family caregivers to stay with the young child if possible to increase feelings of security.

Following surgery, skin integrity, especially around the colostomy stoma, is very important. Give careful attention to the area around the colostomy. Record and report redness, irritation, and rashy appearances of the skin around the stoma. Observe for signs of pain such as crying, increased pulse and respiratory rate, restlessness, guarding of the abdomen, or drawing up the legs. Administer analgesics promptly as ordered.

If an NG tube is left in place after surgery, accurate intake and output determinations and reporting the character, amount, and consistency of stools help determine when the child may have oral feedings. Record and report the drainage from the NG tube every 8 hours; immediately report any unusual drainage such as bright-red bleeding.

Show the family caregiver how to care for the colostomy at home. Discuss topics such as devices and their use, daily irrigation, and skin care.

● INTUSSUSCEPTION

Pathophysiology and Etiology

Intussusception is the invagination, or telescoping, of one portion of the bowel into a distal portion. It occurs most commonly at the juncture of the ileum and colon, although it can appear elsewhere in the intestinal tract. The invagination is from above downward, the upper portion slipping over the lower portion and pulling the mesentery along with it.

This condition occurs more often in boys than in girls and is the most common cause of intestinal obstruction in childhood. The highest incidence occurs in infants between 4 and 10 months. The condition usually appears in healthy babies without any demonstrable cause. Possible contributing factors may be the hyperperistalsis and unusual mobility of the cecum and ileum normally present in early life. Occasionally, a lesion such as Meckel's diverticulum or a polyp is present.

Assessment Findings

The infant who previously appeared healthy and happy suddenly becomes pale, cries out sharply, and draws up the legs in a severe colicky spasm of pain. This spasm may last for several minutes after which the infant relaxes and appears well until the next episode, which may occur 5, 10, or 20 minutes later.

Most of these infants start vomiting early. Vomiting becomes progressively more severe and eventually is bile-stained. The infant strains with each paroxysm, emptying the bowels of fecal contents. The stools consist of blood and mucus, thereby earning the name **currant jelly stools.** Signs of shock appear including a rapid, weak pulse; increased temperature; shallow, grunting respirations; pallor; and marked sweating. Because these signs coupled with the paroxysmal pain are quite severe, professional healthcare often is initiated early.

The physician usually can make a diagnosis from the clinical symptoms, rectal examination, and palpation of the abdomen during a calm interval when it is soft. A baby is often unwilling to tolerate this palpation, and sedation may be ordered. A sausage-shaped mass can often be felt through the abdominal wall.

Medical and Surgical Management

This condition is an emergency; prolonged delays in treatment are dangerous. The telescoped bowel rapidly becomes gangrenous, but adequate treatment during the first 12 to 24 hours should have a good outcome with complete recovery. The outcome becomes more uncertain as the bowel deteriorates, making resection necessary.

Immediate treatment consists of IV fluids, NPO status, and a diagnostic barium enema. The barium enema often can reduce the invagination simply by the pressure of the barium fluid pushing against the telescoped portion. The barium enema should not be done if signs of bowel perforation or peritonitis are evident. Abdominal surgery is performed if the barium enema does not correct the problem. Surgery may consist of manual reduction of the invagination, resection with anastomosis, or possible colostomy if the intestine is gangrenous.

If the invagination was reduced, the infant is returned to normal feedings within 24 hours and discharged in about 48 hours. Carefully observance for recurrence during this period is necessary.

● PYLORIC STENOSIS

The *pylorus* is the muscle that controls the flow of food from the stomach to the duodenum. Pyloric stenosis is characterized by hypertrophy of the circular muscle fibers of the pylorus, with a severe narrowing of its lumen.

Pathophysiology and Etiology

Pyloric stenosis is classified as a congenital defect, even though symptoms are rare during the first days of life. Its cause is unknown, but it occurs more frequently in white males and has a familial tendency (McEvoy, 1999). The pylorus becomes thickened to as much as twice its size, is elongated, and has a consistency resembling cartilage. As a result of obstruction at its distal end, the stomach becomes dilated.

Assessment Findings

The infant with pyloric stenosis usually does not show symptoms until the third week of life. Symptoms rarely appear after the second month. During the first weeks of life, the infant often eats well and gains weight, then starts vomiting occasionally after meals. Within a few days, vomiting increases in frequency and force, becoming projectile. The vomited material is sour, undigested food; it may contain mucus but never bile, because it has not progressed beyond the stomach.

Because the obstruction is mechanical, the baby does not feel ill, is ravenously hungry, and is eager to try again and again, but the food invariably comes back. As the condition progresses, the baby becomes irritable, loses weight rapidly, and becomes dehydrated. Alkalosis develops from the loss of potassium and hydrochloric acid, and the baby becomes seriously ill.

Constipation becomes progressive because little food gets into the intestine, and urine is scanty. Gastric peristaltic waves passing from left to right across the abdomen usually can be seen during or after feedings.

Diagnosis usually is based on the clinical evidence. The nature, type, and times of vomiting are documented. When the infant drinks, gastric peristaltic waves are observed. An experienced physician often can feel the olive-sized pyloric mass through deep palpation. Ultrasonographic or radiographic studies with barium swallow show an abnormal retention of barium in the stomach and increased peristalsis.

Medical Management

A surgical procedure called a pyloromyotomy (also known as Fredet-Ramstedt operation) is the treatment of choice. This procedure simply splits the hypertrophic pyloric muscle down to the submucosa, allowing the pylorus to expand so that food may pass. Prognosis is excellent if surgery is performed before the infant is severely dehydrated.

Nursing Management

When interviewing family caregivers, ask when the vomiting started and determine its character (undigested formula with no bile, vomitus progressively more projectile). Also ask about constipation and scanty urine. Obtain the infant's weight and observe skin turgor and condition (including excoriated diaper area), anterior fontanelle (depressed, normal, or bulging), temperature, apical pulse rate (observing for weak pulse and tachycardia), irritability, lethargy, urine (amount and concentration), lips and mucous membranes of the mouth (dry, cracked), and eyes (bright, glassy, sunken, dark circles). Observe for visible gastric peristalsis when the infant is eating.

If the infant is severely dehydrated and malnourished, IV fluids and electrolytes are necessary for rehydration to prepare for surgery and to correct hypokalemia and alkalosis. Carefully monitor the IV site for redness and induration. Feedings of formula thickened with infant cereal and fed through a large-holed nipple may be given to improve nutrition before surgery. A smooth muscle relaxant may be ordered before feedings. Feed the infant slowly while he or she is sitting in an infant seat or being held upright. Burp the infant frequently to avoid gastric distention. Document the feeding given, approximate amount retained, and frequency and type of emesis.

The family caregivers are anxious because their infant is obviously seriously ill and will have to undergo surgery. Include the caregivers in the preparation for surgery and offer explanations and support.

Postoperatively, position the infant on the side to prevent aspiration of mucus or vomitus. Observe the infant's behavior to evaluate discomfort and pain. Excessive crying, restlessness, listlessness, resistance to being held and cuddled, rigidity, and increased pulse and respiratory rates can indicate pain. Administer analgesics as ordered. The first feeding, given 4 to 6 hours postoperatively, is usually an electrolyte replacement. Accurate intake and output and daily weight determinations are required.

Stop, Think, and Respond ● BOX 9-3

What symptom is seen in the infant with pyloric stenosis? What causes this symptom?

TYPE 1 DIABETES MELLITUS

Type 1 diabetes mellitus affects many children between 5 and 15 years of years of age; incidence of this condition continues to increase (Plotnick, 1999). Diabetes often is considered an adult disease (see Chap. 52); management of diabetes in children differs from that in adults and will be discussed here, including important aspects geared to the child's developmental stage.

Pathophysiology and Etiology

An acute infection during childhood may trigger a mechanism in genetically susceptible children, activating beta-cell dysfunction and disrupting insulin secretion. In children, diabetes causes an abrupt, pronounced decrease in insulin production, resulting in a decreased ability to derive energy from food eaten. The body uses large amounts of protein and fat to supply the child's energy needs, causing loss of weight and slowed growth. This combination of failure to gain weight and lack of energy may be the initial reason the child comes to the healthcare provider's attention. A healthcare provider may not see the child, however, until symptoms of ketoacidosis are evident.

Assessment Findings

In children, symptoms of diabetes often have an abrupt onset. Classic symptoms of type 1 diabetes mellitus are **polyuria** (dramatic increase in urinary output, probably with enuresis), **polydipsia** (increased thirst), and **polyphagia** (increased hunger and food consumption). Weight loss or failure to gain weight and lack of energy usually accompany these symptoms, even though the child has increased food consumption.

If the child's symptoms are not noted and referred for diagnosis, the disorder is likely to progress to **diabetic ketoacidosis,** which is characterized by drowsiness, dry skin, flushed cheeks and cherry-red lips, acetone breath with a fruity smell, and **Kussmaul breathing** (abnormal increase in the depth and rate of respiratory movements). Nausea and vomiting may occur. If untreated, the child lapses into coma and exhibits dehydration, electrolyte imbalance, rapid pulse, and subnormal temperature and blood pressure. Treatment for ketoacidosis includes correction of fluid depletion; IV regular insulin is given along with IV electrolyte fluids.

Early detection and control are critical in minimizing later complications of diabetes. At each visit to a healthcare provider, children with a family history of diabetes should be monitored for glucose using a finger stick glucose test and for ketones in the urine using a urine dipstick test. If the blood glucose level is elevated or ketonuria is present, a fasting blood sugar (FBS) is performed.

Medical Management

Management of diabetes in children includes insulin therapy as well as a meal and exercise plan. Treatment of the child with diabetes involves the family, child, and several healthcare team members. After diabetes is diagnosed, the child may be hospitalized for a period to be stabilized. The child's teacher, the school nurse, and others who supervise the child during daily activities must be informed of the diagnosis.

Insulin therapy is an essential part of the treatment of diabetes in children. The dosage of insulin is adjusted according to blood glucose levels so that the levels are maintained near normal. Two kinds of insulin are often combined for the best results (see Chap. 52 for a discussion of insulin types). The introduction of the rapid-acting insulin Lispro or Humalog has greatly changed insulin administration in children. This insulin can be administered immediately after the child has eaten so the amount of food eaten can be considered when determining the dosage. Many children are controlled on an insulin regimen in which a dose containing a short-acting insulin and an intermediate-acting insulin are given at two times during the day: the first before breakfast and the second before the evening meal. Children's insulin doses have to be regulated individually to keep their blood glucose levels as close to normal as possible.

Insulin overload leads to an **insulin reaction** (insulin shock, hypoglycemia), resulting in too-rapid metabolism of the body's glucose. Contributing factors include a change in the body's requirement, carelessness in diet (such as failure to eat proper amounts of food), an error in insulin measurement, or excessive exercise. Because diabetes in children is very unstable and fluctuating, the child is subject to insulin reactions. Some symptoms of impending insulin shock in children are any type of odd, unusual, or antisocial behavior; weakness; nervousness; lethargy; headache; blurred vision and dizziness; and undue fatigue or hunger. Other symptoms might include pallor, sweating, convulsions, and coma. Children often have hypoglycemic reactions in the early morning. As they become regulated and observe a careful diet at home, parents need not watch so closely but should thoroughly understand all aspects of this condition.

Treatment of an insulin reaction should be *immediate.* Parents should give the child sugar, candy, orange juice, or a commercial product designed for this emergency. Repeated or impending reactions require consultation with the physician.

If the child cannot take a sugar source orally, glucagon should be administered subcutaneously to promptly increase the blood glucose level. Every adult responsible for a child with diabetes should clearly understand the procedure for administering this drug and have easy access to it. Glucagon is available as a pharmaceutical product and packaged in prefilled syringes for immediate use. It is administered in the same manner as insulin.

Glucagon acts within minutes to restore consciousness, after which the child can take candy or sugar. This treatment prevents the long delay while waiting for a physician to administer IV glucose or an ambulance to reach the child. It is, however, not a substitute for proper medical supervision.

The need for insulin continues to increase until the child reaches full growth. Family caregivers need to know that this is normal and that the child's condition is not worsening.

The child may not be able to take over management of the insulin dose as early as blood glucose monitoring, but he or she can watch the preparation of the syringe and learn the technique for drawing up the dosage. It may be helpful to encourage the child to watch the process until it becomes routine. By the time the child is 8 or 9 years old, caregivers should encourage him or her to talk with them about the dose and to practice working with the syringe. The child also may draw up the dose and prepare for self-administration. The age at which this is possible varies. No two children mature at the same rate; some may be able to do this much earlier than others. Automatic injection devices can help the child self-administer insulin at a younger age. Caregivers should encourages the child to take over the management of the therapy when ready. If included in decision-making, the child can learn the importance of the routine and accept the restrictions the disease imposes.

An insulin pump is a method of continuous insulin administration useful for some children with diabetes. The child can use the pump to release extra insulin at meals and other times when needed by pressing a button. The pump does not sense the blood glucose level; therefore, careful blood glucose monitoring at least four times a day is necessary to adjust the dosage as needed. The child must remove the pump to bathe, swim, or shower. He or she may want to wear loose clothing that will hide the pump.

Adolescence is an extremely trying period for many with diabetes. Clients with diabetes, like other adolescents, must work from dependence to independence. Even when an adolescent has accepted responsibility for self-care, it is not unusual for him or her to rebel against the control that this condition demands, become impatient, and appear to ignore future health. The teen may skip meals, drop diet controls, or neglect glucose monitoring. Going barefoot and neglecting proper foot care also can cause problems. Caregivers naturally become concerned and are apt to give the adolescent more controls to rebel against. Family, teachers, nurses, and physicians should take special care to see that these young people find enough maturing satisfaction in other areas and do not need to rebel in this vital area.

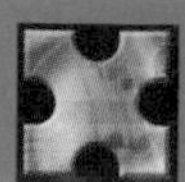

9-3 *Client and Family Teaching*
Diabetic Food Plan for Children

The nurse teaches the family as follows:

- Plan well-balanced meals that appeal to the child.
- Be positive when talking with the child about foods he or she can eat; downplay negatives.
- Space three meals and three snacks throughout the day. Divide daily caloric intake to provide 20% at breakfast, 20% at lunch, 30% at dinner, and 10% at each snack. Calories should be made up of 50% to 60% carbohydrates, 15% to 20% protein, and no more than 30% fat.
- Avoid concentrated sweets such as jelly, syrup, pie, candy bars, and soda pop.
- The child may use artificial sweeteners.
- The child must not skip meals. Make every effort to plan meals with foods the child likes.
- Include foods that contain dietary fiber such as whole grains, cereals, fruits and vegetables, nuts, seeds, and legumes. Fiber helps prevent hyperglycemia.
- Dietetic food is expensive and unnecessary.
- Keep complex carbohydrates available for the child to eat before exercise and sports activities to provide sustained carbohydrate energy sources.
- Teach child day by day about the food plan to encourage independence in food selections when at school or away from home.

Nursing Management

The child with diabetes needs a sound nutritional program that provides adequate nutrition for normal growth while it maintains blood glucose levels close to normal. The food plan should be well balanced with foods that consider the child's preferences, cultural customs, and lifestyle (Client and Family Teaching 9-3). Help the child and caregiver to understand the importance of eating regularly scheduled meals. Assist them to plan special occasions so that the child does not feel left out of celebrations. Include children in meal planning when possible so that they learn what is permissible and what is not.

Skin breakdowns, such as blisters and minor cuts, can become major problems for the child with diabetes. Teach the caregiver and child to inspect the skin daily and promptly treat even small breaks. Teach them to dry the skin well after bathing. Emphasize good foot care, including wearing well-fitting shoes, inspecting between toes for cracks, trimming nails straight across, wearing clean socks, and not going barefoot.

Children with diabetes may be more susceptible to urinary tract and upper respiratory infections. Teach children and caregivers to be alert for signs of urinary tract infection and instruct them to report signs promptly. These children are more susceptible to long-term complications of an infection. They should never skip insulin during illness; they should check blood glucose levels every 2 to 4 hours during this time. They need to increase fluids. Instruct caregivers to contact the care provider when the child becomes ill, especially if the child is vomiting, cannot eat, or has diarrhea, so that close supervision can be maintained. It is extremely important for the child to wear a Medic Alert identification medal or a bracelet with information about diabetic status.

On initial diagnosis of diabetes, check the blood glucose level as often as every 4 hours until the child achieves some stability. Teach the child and caregiver how to perform monitoring. Because this procedure involves a finger stick, the child may object and resist it. Consider the child's developmental stage when performing the testing. School-age children can be involved in much of the process.

Monitor the child closely for signs of hypoglycemia or hyperglycemia. Teach the child and family the signs of both hypoglycemia and hyperglycemia (Box 9-1). Instruct the child to get help immediately when signs of hypoglycemia occur. If there is any doubt as to whether the child is having a hypoglycemic or a hyperglycemic reaction, treat it like hypoglycemia.

BOX 9-1 ● Signs of Hypoglycemia and Hyperglycemia

HYPOGLYCEMIA
- Shaking
- Irritability
- Hunger
- Diaphoresis
- Dizziness
- Drowsiness
- Pallor
- Changed level of consciousness
- Feeling "strange"

HYPERGLYCEMIA
- Polyphagia (excessive hunger)
- Polyuria (excessive urination)
- Dry mucous membranes
- Poor skin turgor
- Lethargy
- Change in level of consciousness

Teach the family caregiver and child the correct way to give insulin. A doll may be used to practice the actual administration until the caregiver (and child, if old enough) is comfortable and confident. This part of the treatment is probably the most threatening aspect of the illness. The child and family need a great deal of empathy and warm support.

When the diagnosis of diabetes is confirmed, the family caregiver may feel devastated. A young child will not understand the implications, but the school-age or adolescent child will experience great fear and anxiety. The caregiver may have feelings of guilt, resentment, or denial. All these feelings and concerns must be recognized and resolved to work successfully with the child who has diabetes.

The school-age or older child may experience some strong feelings of inadequacy or being "sick" and must express and handle these feelings. Encourage the child to become active in helping with self-care. Summer camps for children with diabetes available in many areas can help develop the child's self-assurance.

URINARY AND RENAL DISORDERS

● CRYPTORCHIDISM

Pathophysiology and Etiology

Shortly before or soon after birth, the male gonads (testes) descend from the abdominal cavity into their normal position in the scrotum. Occasionally, one or both of the testes do not descend, a condition called cryptorchidism. The testes are usually normal in size; the cause for failure to descend is not clearly understood.

Assessment Findings

In most infants with cryptorchidism, the testes descend by the time the infant is 1 year old. If one or both testes have not descended by this age, treatment is recommended. If both testes remain undescended, the male will be sterile.

Medical and Surgical Management

A surgical procedure called **orchiopexy** is used to bring the testes down into the scrotum and anchor them there. Some physicians prefer to try medical treatment—injections of human chorionic gonadotropic hormone—before surgery. If injections are unsuccessful, orchiopexy is performed, usually when the child is 1 to 2 years old. Prognosis for a normal functioning testicle is good when the surgery is performed at this young age and no degenerative action has occurred before treatment.

● HYDROCELE

Hydrocele is peritoneal fluid that accumulates in the scrotum through a small passage called the processus vaginalis, a fingerlike projection in the inguinal canal through which the testes descend. Usually the processus closes soon after birth; if the processus does not close, fluid from the peritoneal cavity passes through causing hydrocele. This is the same passage through which intestines may slip, causing an inguinal hernia. If the hydrocele remains by the end of the first year, corrective surgery is performed.

● ENURESIS

Pathophysiology and Etiology

Enuresis, or bedwetting, is involuntary urination beyond the age when children commonly acquire control of urination. Many children do not acquire complete nighttime control before 5 to 7 years of age, and occasional bedwetting may be seen in children as late as 9 or 10 years. Boys have more difficulty than girls do; in some instances enuresis may persist into adulthood. Enuresis may have a physiologic or psychological cause and may indicate a need for further exploration and treatment. Physiologic causes may include a small bladder capacity, urinary tract infection, and lack of awareness of the signal to empty the bladder because of sleeping too soundly. Persistent bedwetting in a 5-year-old or 6-year-old may be the result of rigorous toilet training before the child was physically or psychologically ready. Enuresis in the older child may be a way to express resentment toward family caregivers or a desire to regress to an earlier level of development to receive more care and attention. Emotional stress can be a precipitating factor. The healthcare team also needs to consider the possibility that enuresis can be a symptom of sexual abuse.

Medical and Nursing Management

If a physiologic cause has been ruled out, efforts to discover possible causes, including emotional stress, are essential. If the child is interested in achieving control—for instance, to go to camp or visit friends overnight—waking the child during the night to go to the toilet or limiting fluids before retiring may be helpful. Nevertheless, these measures should not replace searching for the cause. The family caregiver may become extremely frustrated about having to deal with smelly, wet bedding every morning. The child may go to great efforts to hide the fact that the bed is wet. Help from a pediatric mental health professional may be warranted. Healthcare personnel must take a supportive, understanding attitude toward the problems of the caregiver and child, providing each of them the freedom and an environment to express feelings.

• ENCOPRESIS

Encopresis is chronic involuntary fecal soiling beyond the age when control is expected (approximately 3 years of age). Speech and learning disabilities may accompany this problem. If no organic causes (e.g., worms, megacolon) exist, encopresis indicates a serious emotional problem and a need for counseling for the child and family caregivers. Some experts believe that overcontrol or undercontrol by a caregiver can cause encopresis. Recommendations for treatment differ; the most important goal, however, is recognition of the problem and referral for treatment and counseling.

• EXSTROPHY OF THE BLADDER

Pathophysiology and Etiology

This urinary tract malformation usually is accompanied by other anomalies such as epispadias, cleft scrotum, cryptorchidism (undescended testes), a shortened penis, and cleft clitoris. It also is associated with malformed pelvic musculature, resulting in a prolapsed rectum and inguinal hernias. Children with this defect have a widely split symphysis pubis and posterolaterally rotated hip sockets, causing a waddling gait.

In this condition, the anterior surface of the urinary bladder lies open on the lower abdomen. The exposed mucosa is red and sensitive to touch and allows direct passage of urine to the outside. This condition makes the area vulnerable to infection and trauma.

Surgical Management

Surgical closure of the bladder is preferred within the first 48 hours of life. Final surgical correction is completed before the child goes to school. If bladder repair is not done early in the child's life, the family caregivers must learn how to care for this condition and how to deal with their feelings toward this less-than-perfect child. Their emotional reaction may be further complicated if the malformation is so severe that the sex of the child may be determined only by a chromosome test.

Nursing Management

Direct nursing care of the infant with exstrophy of the bladder toward preventing infection, preventing skin irritation around the seeping mucosa, meeting the infant's need for touch and cuddling, and educating and supporting the family during this crisis.

• HYPOSPADIAS AND EPISPADIAS

Pathophysiology and Etiology

Hypospadias is a congenital condition in which the urethra terminates on the ventral (underside) surface of the penis instead of at the tip. A cordlike anomaly (a **chordee**) extends from the scrotum to the penis, pulling the penis downward in an arc. Urination is not affected, but the boy cannot void while standing in the normal male fashion. In epispadias, the opening is on the dorsal (top) surface of the penis.

Surgical Management

Surgical repair is desirable between ages 6 and 18 months, before body image and castration anxiety become problems. Microscopic surgery makes early repair possible. Surgical repair is often accomplished in one stage as outpatient surgery. These infants should not be circumcised, because the foreskin is used in the repair. Severe hypospadias may require additional surgical procedures. Surgical repair is indicated in cases of epispadias.

• NEPHROTIC SYNDROME

Pathophysiology and Etiology

Several different types of nephrosis have been identified in nephrotic syndrome. The most common type in children is called lipoid nephrosis, idiopathic nephrotic syndrome, or minimal change nephrotic syndrome (MCNS).

All forms of nephrosis have early characteristics of edema and proteinuria; therefore, definite clinical differentiation cannot be made early in the disease.

Nephrotic syndrome has a course of remissions and exacerbations that usually lasts for months. The recovery rate is generally good with the use of intensive steroid therapy and protection against infection. The cause of MCNS is unknown. In rare cases, it is associated with other specific diseases. Most cases occur between 2 and 6 years of age.

Assessment Findings

Edema is usually the presenting symptom, appearing first around the eyes and ankles. As the swelling advances, the edema becomes generalized with a pendulous abdomen full of fluid. Respiratory embarrassment may be severe, and edema of the scrotum on the male is characteristic. The edema shifts when the child changes position while lying quietly or walking. Anorexia, irritability, and loss of appetite develop. Malnutrition may become severe; however, the generalized edema masks the loss of body tissue, causing the child to present a chubby appearance and to double his or her weight. After diuresis, the malnutrition becomes quite apparent. These children are usually susceptible to infection, and repeated acute respiratory conditions are the usual pattern. This is intensified by the immunosuppression caused by the administration of prednisone.

Laboratory findings include marked proteinuria, especially albumin, with large numbers of hyaline and granular casts in the urine. Hematuria is not usually present, although a few red blood cells may appear in the urine. The blood serum protein level is reduced, and the level of cholesterol in the blood (hyperlipidemia) is increased.

Medical Management

The management of nephrotic syndrome is a long process with remissions and, commonly, recurrence of symptoms. The use of corticosteroids has induced remissions in most cases and has reduced recurrences. Corticosteroid therapy usually produces diuresis in about 7 to 14 days, but the drug is continued until a remission occurs. Prednisone is the drug most commonly used. After the diuresis occurs, intermittent therapy is continued every other day or for 3 days a week. Daily urine testing for protein is continued whether the child is at home or in the hospital.

Diuretics have not been effective in reducing the edema of nephrotic syndrome, although a loop diuretic (furosemide) may be administered if the edema causes respiratory embarrassment. Immunosuppressant therapy may be used to reduce symptoms and prevent further relapses in children who do not respond adequately to corticosteroids. Cyclophosphamide (Cytoxan) is the drug most commonly used. Cyclophosphamide has serious side effects such as **leukopenia** (leukocyte count less than 5,000/mm^3), gastrointestinal symptoms, hematuria, and alopecia. The length of therapy is usually 2 or 3 months. Family caregivers need encouragement and support for the long months of treatment.

NURSING PROCESS

● The Child With Nephrotic Syndrome

Assessment

Observe for edema when performing the physical examination. Weigh the child and record the abdominal measurements to serve as a baseline. Obtain vital signs including blood pressure. Note any swelling around the eyes, ankles, and other dependent parts; record the degree of pitting. Inspect the skin for pallor, irritation, or breakdown. Examine the scrotal area of the young boy for swelling, redness, and irritation. Question the caregiver about the onset of symptoms, the child's appetite, urine output, and signs of fatigue or irritability.

Diagnosis, Planning, and Interventions

Children with nephrotic syndrome usually are hospitalized for diagnosis, thorough evaluation of their general health and specific condition, and institution of therapy. The child with nephrotic syndrome is especially at risk for respiratory infections because the edema and the corticosteroid therapy lower the body's defenses. If the child has an infection, a course of antibiotic therapy may be given. Unless unforeseen complications develop, the child is discharged with complete instructions for management. The nurse's role in caring for the child with nephrotic syndrome includes, but is not limited to, the following.

Excess Fluid Volume related to fluid accumulation in tissues and third spaces.

Expected Outcome: The child's intake and output will be within normal limits, edema will be decreased, and skin turgor will be normal.

- Accurately measure and document intake and output. *Imbalances may indicate fluid retention. Accurate measurement gives a baseline for evaluating fluid balance.*
- Weigh the child at the same time every day on the same scale in the same clothing. *Consistent measurement of the child's weight will reflect fluid accumulations and volume changes accurately.*
- Measure the child's abdomen daily at the level of the umbilicus; make certain that all staff personnel measure at the same level. Note the desired location for measuring on the nursing care plan. *The abdomen may be enlarged greatly with **ascites** (edema in the peritoneal cavity). The abdomen can even become marked with **striae** (stretch marks). Measuring the abdomen consistently gives a baseline for monitoring fluid excess.*

- Test the urine regularly for albumin and specific gravity. *Protein lost in the urine of the child with nephrotic syndrome is usually albumin. A high specific gravity indicates fluid retention.*

Risk for Imbalanced Nutrition: Less than Body Requirements related to anorexia

Expected Outcome: Nutritional intake will be adequate to meet normal growth needs.

- Monitor and record the child's dietary intake. *Doing so will reveal nutrients the child is consuming. Although the child may look plump, underneath the edema is a thin, possibly malnourished child.*
- Offer a visually appealing and nutritious diet. *Ascites diminishes the appetite because of a full feeling in the abdomen. Appetite is poor for several reasons: the child may be lethargic, apathetic, and simply not interested in eating; a no-added-salt diet may be unappealing to the child; corticosteroid therapy may decrease the appetite.*
- Consult the child and family to learn which foods are appealing. *Cater to the child's wishes as much as possible to perk up a lagging appetite. A dietitian can help plan appealing meals.*
- Serve six small meals a day. *Doing so may help increase the child's total intake better than the customary three meals a day.*

Risk for Impaired Skin Integrity related to edema

Expected Outcome: The child's skin integrity will be maintained.

- Inspect all skin surfaces regularly for breakdown. *Doing so helps detect concerns and prevent skin breakdown. Edematous tissue does not heal well; breaks in the skin can easily become infected, causing further concerns.*
- Turn and position the child every 2 hours. *Lethargic children may not turn themselves. Position changes help increase circulation, decrease pressure, and promote skin integrity.*
- Protect skin surfaces from pressure by means of pillows and padding. Protect overlapping skin surfaces from rubbing. *Doing so avoids skin breakdown caused by pressure areas and rubbing.*
- Bathe the child regularly, being careful to wash the skin surfaces and dry them completely. *These steps promote comfort and increase circulation.*
- If the scrotum is edematous, use a soft cotton support to provide comfort. *Doing so reduces skin irritation and breakdown.*

Fatigue related to edema and disease process

Expected Outcome: The child's energy will be conserved.

- Bed rest is common during the edema stage of the condition. *The child rarely protests because of fatigue. The sheer bulk of the edema makes movement difficult.*
- Gradually increase activity as tolerated, but balance with rest periods and encourage the child to rest when fatigued. *When diuresis occurs several days after beginning prednisone, the child may feel less fatigued and be allowed more activity. Rest helps the child conserve energy.*
- Plan quiet, age-appropriate activities that interest the child. *Most children love having someone read to them. Coloring books, dominoes, puzzles, and some computer and board games are quiet activities that many children enjoy and require less energy.*
- Involve the family in providing some of these activities. *Many children are cared for at home; family involvement throughout the illness is a comfort to the child.*

Risk for Infection related to immunosuppression

Expected Outcome: The child will be free from signs and symptoms of infection.

- Protect the child from anyone with an infection: staff, family, visitors, and other children. *The child with nephrotic syndrome is prone to respiratory infections; contact with infected people increases the likelihood of the child being infected.*
- Perform and teach handwashing and strict medical asepsis. *Handwashing is the single best way to avoid exposure to pathogens, which may cause infection.*
- Monitor vital signs every 4 hours; observe for any early signs of infection. *Elevation of temperature and changes in vital signs might be indicators of infection.*

Deficient Caregiver Knowledge related to disease process, treatment, and home care

Expected Outcome: Family caregivers will verbalize an understanding of the disease process, treatment, and the child's home care needs.

- Provide a written plan to help family caregivers follow the treatment program successfully. *The family must keep a careful record of home treatment for the healthcare provider to review at regular intervals.*
- Teach family caregivers about possible reactions with the use of steroids and the adverse effects of abruptly discontinuing these drugs. *Understanding these aspects well may help reduce or eliminate forgetting to give the medication or neglecting to refill the prescription.*
- Encourage family caregivers to report promptly any symptoms they think that the medication is causing. *Knowledge of symptoms to watch for helps increase prompt reporting.*
- Teach the family that the necessary special care is important to keep the child in optimum health, and to report promptly any **intercurrent infections** (those occurring at the same time as an already existing disease). *Prompt reporting of any infection leads to earlier initiation of treatment.*
- Teach family that exacerbations are common and probable. Stress the information that they should report including rapidly increasing weight, increased proteinuria, or signs of infections. *Any of these may be a reason to alter the therapeutic regimen or change the specific antibiotic agents used.*
- Encourage family to relate back information taught. *Having the family verbalize information learned can assist with clarifications and reinforcements.*

- Encourage family to express feelings of concern. *The prolonged course of the disorder and characteristic relapses can upset the family. Encouraging verbalization of feelings helps them feel supported.*

Evaluation of Expected Outcomes

The child has appropriate weight loss and decreased abdominal girth and eats 80% or more of his or her meals. Skin remains free of breakdown with no redness or irritation. The child rests as needed and engages in quiet diversional activities. He or she has normal vital signs with no respiratory or gastrointestinal symptoms. The family can explain nephrotic syndrome and describe aspects of medications given. They state signs and symptoms of infection, discuss home care, and ask and answer appropriate questions. The family verbalizes feelings and concerns related to caring for a child with a chronic illness; the family receives adequate support.

● URINARY TRACT INFECTIONS

Pathophysiology and Etiology

Infections of the urinary tract are fairly common in the "diaper age," in infancy, and again between 2 and 6 years. The condition is more common in girls than in boys except in the first 4 months, when it is more common in boys. Although many different bacteria may infect the urinary tract, intestinal bacteria, particularly *Escherichia coli,* are often the cause of acute episodes. The female urethra is shorter and straighter than the male urethra, so it is more easily contaminated with feces. Inflammation may extend into the bladder, ureters, and kidney.

Assessment Findings

In infants, symptoms may be fever, nausea, vomiting, foul-smelling urine, weight loss, and increased urination. Occasionally there is little or no fever. Vomiting is common, and diarrhea may occur. The infant is irritable. In acute pyelonephritis (inflammation of the kidney and renal pelvis), onset is abrupt with a high fever for 1 or 2 days. Convulsions may occur during the period of high fever. In preschool children, bedwetting may be a symptom.

Diagnosis is based on the finding of pus in the urine under microscopic examination. The urine specimen must be fresh and uncontaminated. A "clean catch" voided urine, properly performed, is essential for microscopic examination. If a culture is needed, the infant may be catheterized, but this usually is avoided if possible. A suprapubic aspiration also may be done to obtain a sterile specimen. In the cooperative, toilet-trained child, a clean midstream urine sample may be obtained successfully.

Medical Management

Simple UTIs may be treated with antibiotics (usually sulfisoxazole or ampicillin) at home. The child with acute pyelonephritis is hospitalized. Fluids are given freely. Symptoms usually subside within a few days after antibiotic therapy has been initiated, but this is not an indication that the infection is completely cleared. Medication must be continued after symptoms disappear. An IV pyelogram or ultrasonographic study may be performed to assess the possibility of structural defects if the child has recurring infections.

Nursing Management

During the interview with the family caregiver, gather information about the present illness: when the fever started and its course thus far, signs of pain or discomfort on voiding, recent change in feeding pattern, any vomiting or diarrhea, irritability, lethargy, abdominal pain, unusual odor to urine, chronic diaper rash, and signs of febrile convulsions. If the child is toilet-trained, ask caregivers about toileting habits (How does the child wipe? Does the child wash the hands when toileting?). Also ask about the use of bubble baths and the type of soap used, especially for girls.

Collecting data regarding the child includes temperature, observation of a wet diaper or urine in an older child, inspection of the perineal area for rash, and any irritability and lethargy. A urine specimen is needed on admission. A midstream urine collection method is desirable, and catheterization is avoided if possible. Record and report any indications of urinary burning, frequency, urgency, or pain.

In the child who has repeated UTIs, observe his or her interactions with family caregivers to detect any indications that sexual abuse may have caused the infection. Look for possible indications of sexual abuse, such as bruising, bleeding, and lacerations of the external genitalia, especially in the child who is extremely shy and frightened.

Monitor the infant's temperature frequently, at least every 2 hours if it is higher than 101.3° F (38.5° C). If the infant has a fever, follow the procedures to reduce elevated temperatures. Administer antibiotics and antipyretic medications as ordered.

Encourage the child to void every 3 or 4 hours to prevent recurrent infection. Monitor and measure urine output. Weigh an infant's diaper for accuracy.

Increasing the child's fluid intake is necessary to help dilute the urine and flush the bladder, as well as to reduce body temperature. An increase in fluid intake also helps decrease the pain experienced on urination.

Family caregivers are the key people in helping prevent recurring infections. See Client and Family Teaching 9-4.

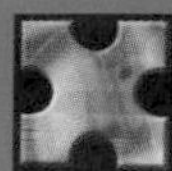

9-4 *Client and Family Teaching* Urinary Tract Infection

The nurse teaches the family as follows:

- Change infant's diaper when soiled; clean baby with mild soap and water and dry completely.
- Teach girls to wipe from front to back.
- Teach child to wash hands before and after going to the toilet.
- Bubble baths create a climate that encourages bacteria to grow, especially in young girls.
- Teach young girls to take showers. Avoid using water softeners in tub baths.
- Encourage child to try to urinate every 3 or 4 hours and to empty the bladder.
- Girls should wear cotton underpants to provide air circulation to perineal area.
- Encourage child to drink fluids, especially cranberry juice.
- Older girls should avoid whirlpools or hot tubs.

● WILMS' TUMOR (NEPHROBLASTOMA)

Pathophysiology and Etiology

Wilms' tumor, an adenosarcoma in the kidney region, is one of the most common abdominal neoplasms of early childhood. The tumor arises from bits of embryonic tissue that remain after birth. This tissue can spark rapid cancerous growth in the area of the kidney. The tumor is rarely discovered until it is large enough to be palpated through the abdominal wall. As the tumor grows, it invades the kidney or renal vein and disseminates to other parts of the body.

Medical and Surgical Management

When the child is being evaluated and treated, a sign must be visibly posted stating that abdominal palpation should be avoided because cells may break loose and spread the tumor. Treatment consists of surgical removal as soon as possible after the growth is discovered, combined with radiation and chemotherapy.

Prognosis is best for the child younger than 2 years but has improved markedly for others with improved chemotherapy. Follow-up consists of regular evaluation for metastasis to the lungs or other sites. All long-term implications for chemotherapy apply to this child (see Chap. 19).

MUSCULOSKELETAL DISORDERS

● JUVENILE RHEUMATOID ARTHRITIS

Connective tissues such as the musculoskeletal system and skin and mucous membranes provide a supportive framework and protective covering for the body. Juvenile rheumatoid arthritis (JRA) is the most common connective tissue disease of childhood.

Pathophysiology and Etiology

In JRA, joint inflammation occurs first; if untreated, inflammation leads to irreversible changes in joint cartilage, ligaments, and menisci (the crescent-shaped fibrocartilage in the knee joints), eventually causing complete immobility. Occurrence of JRA appears to peak at two age levels: 1 to 3 years and 8 to 12 years. It can be subdivided into three different types: systemic; polyarticular, involving five or more joints; and oligoarthritis (pauciarticular), involving four or fewer joints, most often the knees and ankles.

Medical and Nursing Management

The treatment goal is to maintain mobility and preserve joint function. Treatment can include drugs, physical therapy, and surgery. Early diagnosis and drug therapy to control inflammation and other systemic changes can reduce the need for other types of treatment.

Enteric-coated aspirin was long the drug of choice for JRA; however, because of the concern of aspirin therapy and Reye syndrome (see Chap. 8), nonsteroidal anti-inflammatory drugs (NSAIDs) are frequently replacing aspirin in treatment of JRA. Aspirin may still be used because it is effective, inexpensive, and easily administered, and has few side effects when carefully regulated. Acetaminophen is not appropriate because it lacks anti-inflammatory properties. Teach family caregivers the importance of regular administration of medications even when the child is not experiencing pain. The primary purpose of aspirin or NSAIDs is not to relieve pain but to decrease joint inflammation. When aspirin or NSAIDs are no longer effective, gold preparations, steroids, D-penicillamine, or immunosuppressives may be used. All these are toxic and must be closely monitored.

Physical therapy includes exercise, application of splints, and heat. Joints must be immobilized by splinting during active disease, but gentle daily exercise is necessary to prevent **ankylosis** (immobility of a joint).

Stress to caregivers the importance of encouraging the child to perform independent activities of daily living to maintain function and independence. Depending on the degree of disease, activity, range-of-motion exercises, isometric exercises, swimming, and riding a tricycle or bicycle may be part of the treatment plan. Inform caregivers that these exercises should not increase pain; if exercise does trigger increased pain, the amount of exercise should be decreased.

● HIP DYSPLASIA

Pathophysiology and Etiology

Hip dysplasia results from defective development of the acetabulum with or without dislocation. The malformed acetabulum permits dislocation with the head of the femur becoming displaced upward and backward. The condition is difficult to recognize during early infancy. A family history of the defect indicates increased observation of the young infant. The condition is often bilateral and more common in girls than in boys.

Assessment Findings

Early recognition and treatment before an infant starts to stand or walk are important for successful correction. The first examination should be part of the newborn assessment. Experienced examiners may detect an audible click when examining the newborn using the Bartow and Ortolani tests. These tests, used together on one hip at a time, involve dislocating and relocating the acetabulum in adduction and abduction; only an experienced practitioner should conduct them. The tests are effective only for the first month; after that, the clicks disappear. Signs that are useful after this include:

- Asymmetry of the gluteal skin folds (higher on the affected side) (Fig. 9.1A)
- Limited abduction of the affected hip (Fig. 9.1B). This is tested by placing the infant in a dorsal recumbent position with the knees flexed, then abducting both knees passively until they reach the examination table without resistance. If dislocation is present, the affected side cannot be abducted more than 45 degrees.
- Apparent shortening of the femur (Fig. 9.1C)

After the child has started walking, later signs include lordosis, swayback, protruding abdomen, shortened extremity, duck-waddle gait, and a positive Trendelenburg sign. To elicit this sign, the child stands on the affected leg and raises the normal leg. The pelvis tilts down rather than up toward the unaffected side.

X-ray studies usually are made to confirm the diagnosis in the older infant. Uncorrected dislocation causes limping, easy fatigue, hip and low back discomfort, and postural deformities.

Medical Management

When the dislocation is discovered during the first few months, treatment consists of manipulation of the femur into position and the application of a brace. The most common type of brace used is the Pavlik harness (Fig. 9.2). The physician assesses the infant weekly while the infant is in the harness and adjusts the harness to align the femur gradually. Sometimes no further treatment is needed. If treatment is delayed until after the child has started to walk or if earlier treatment is ineffective, open reduction followed by application of a spica cast usually is needed. A spica cast, or spica hip cast as it is often called, covers the lower part of the body from the waist down and either one or both legs, usually leaving the feet open. The cast maintains the legs in a froglike position, with the hips abducted. There may be a bar placed be-

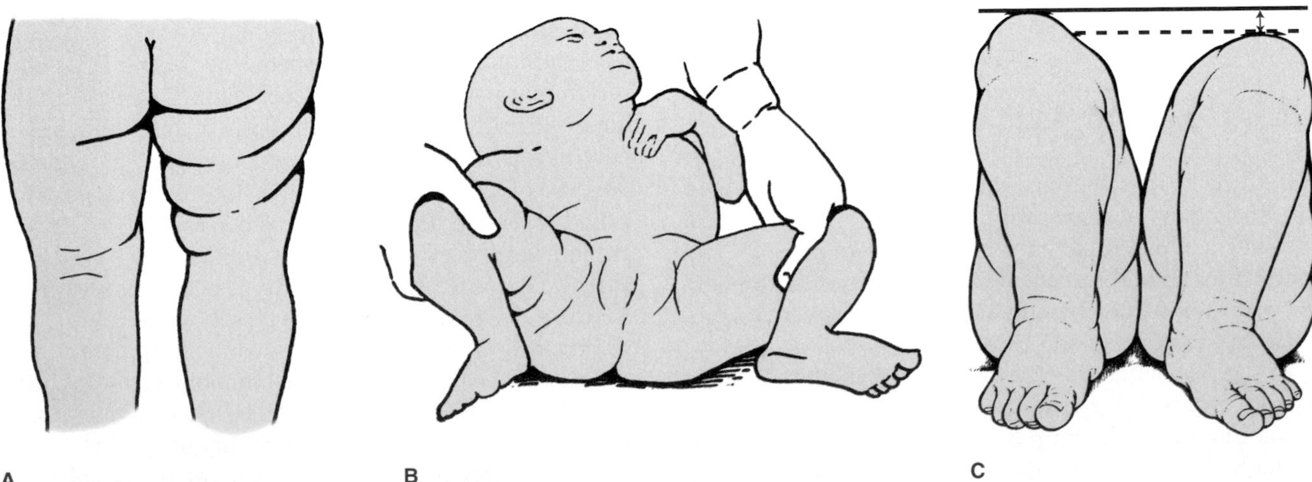

FIGURE 9.1 Congenital hip dislocation. (**A**) Asymmetry of the gluteal folds of the thighs. (**B**) Limited abduction of the affected hip. (**C**) Apparent shortening of the femur.

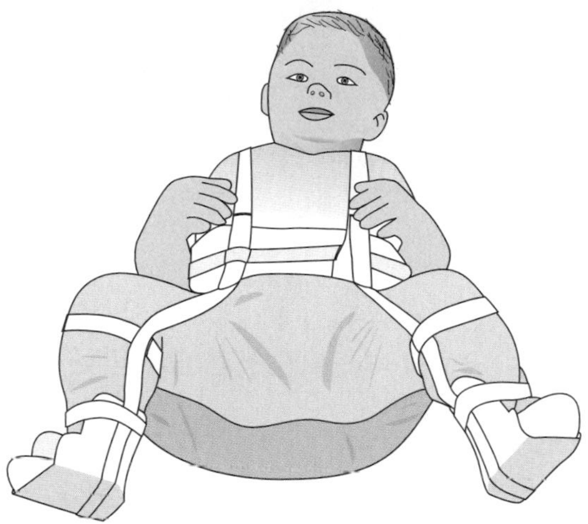

FIGURE 9.2 Proper positioning of an infant in a Pavlik harness. The harness is composed of shoulder straps, stirrups, and a chest strap. It is placed on both legs, even if only one hip is dislocated.

tween the legs to help support the cast. After the cast is removed, a metal or plastic brace is applied to keep the legs in wide abduction.

> **Stop, Think, and Respond ● BOX 9-4**
>
> *What are the three diagnostic findings in the child who has hip dysplasia?*

NURSING PROCESS

The Child in an Orthopedic Device or Cast

Assessment

Although the actual hospitalization of the child may be relatively short (if no other abnormalities require hospitalization), the nurse must teach the family about cast care or care of the child in an orthopedic device such as a Pavlik harness. Determine the family caregiver's ability to understand and cooperate. Emotional support of the family is important. Observation of the child varies depending on the orthopedic device or cast used. Immediately after application, observe for signs that the cast is drying evenly. Check the toes for circulation and movement. Check the skin at the edges of the cast for signs of pressure or irritation. If an open reduction has been performed, observe the child for signs of shock and bleeding in the immediate postoperative period.

Diagnosis, Planning, and Interventions

Acute Pain related to discomfort of orthopedic device or cast

Expected Outcome: The child will show signs of being comfortable.

- Administer analgesics as ordered and document effectiveness. *Analgesics may need to be given depending on the injury or situation to keep the child comfortable.*
- Offer the infant nonnutritive sucking, stroking, cuddling, and talking. *The infant may be irritable and fussy because of the restricted movement caused by the device or cast. Useful methods of soothing help infant feel secure and comfortable.*
- Spend time with the older child and provide diversional activities, such as books, toys, and arts and crafts. *Diversional activities help keep the child from focusing on pain and on the restricted movement caused by the cast or device.*
- Check the child for signs of skin irritation from the device or cast. *Irritation can lead to discomfort and pain, as well as skin breakdown.*
- The child in a cast may be held after the cast is completely dry. Do not remove the harness or orthopedic device unless the provider grants specific permission for bathing. *Offering comfort to the child by holding and caressing helps decrease discomfort and anxiety.*

Risk for Impaired Skin Integrity related to pressure of the cast on the skin surface

Expected Outcome: The child's skin will remain intact.

- When handling the cast, use the palms of the hands to avoid excessive pressure on the cast. *Pressure on a wet cast can cause indentations, which can create areas of pressure on skin under the cast.*
- Carefully inspect the skin around the cast edges for signs of irritation, redness, or edema. *Rough edges can cause irritation and skin breakdown.*
- Petal the edges of the cast around the waist and toes. *Doing so will protect the skin around the edges of the cast as well as help prevent the edges of the cast from crumbling and falling into the cast.*
- Protect the cast with plastic covering around the perineal area. *This measure helps keep the cast from being soiled and getting moist. If the covering becomes soiled, remove it, wash and dry thoroughly, then reapply or replace it.*
- Monitor the skin under the straps or parts of an orthopedic device frequently; massage the skin gently. *Doing so relieves pressure under the shoulder straps or device and increases circulation. Extra padding may be placed to prevent pressure areas.*
- Avoid using powders and lotions. *Caking of them can cause areas of irritation.*
- Daily sponge baths are important. *They increase comfort and keep skin clean and dry.*
- Observe carefully for any restriction of breathing caused by tightness over the abdomen and lower chest area. *If the cast is too tight, the child cannot breathe deeply and have adequate oxygenation. Vomiting after a feeding may indicate that the cast is too tight over the stomach. It may have to be removed and reapplied.*
- Prevent the child from pushing any small particles of food or toys down into the cast. *Teach the older child*

that anything pushed inside the cast can cause irritation and skin injury.

- Blow cool air using the cool setting on a hair dryer or fan or use Asepto syringe to decrease itching under the cast. *Cool air will not cause skin irritation or injury.*
- Use disposable diapers for the infant in a cast. *Diapering can be a challenge. Disposable diapers are usually the most effective way to protect the cast and prevent leakage.*

Risk for Delayed Growth and Development related to restricted mobility secondary to orthopedic device or cast
Expected Outcome: The child will attain appropriate developmental milestones.

- Provide infant with stimulation of a tactile nature, such as mobiles, musical toys, and stuffed toys. Hold the infant if possible and encourage interaction. Provide a pacifier if the infant desires it. *Sensory stimulation and touch promote development in the infant.*
- Provide the older child with age-appropriate activities, games, and toys. *Activities should be geared so the child can use existing skills to help develop and master higher-level skills.*
- Do not permit the child to cry for long periods. Keep feeding times relaxed. *Responding to needs in a consistent, relaxed manner helps develop security in the pediatric client.*
- Promote activities that encourage the child to use the free hand, interact with siblings and other children, and allow the child to see and experience new things in the environment. *Diversionary activities should include transporting the child to other areas in the home or car. Strollers and car seats may be adapted to allow safe transportation. For toddlers, a wagon or large skateboard may provide a movable base to explore the environment and encourage independence.*

Deficient Knowledge of family caregivers related to home care of the child in the orthopedic device or cast
Expected Outcome: The family caregivers will learn home care of the child.

- Determine family caregivers' knowledge; design a thorough teaching plan. *Because the child will receive care at home most of the time, family caregivers must understand needed care.*
- Use complete explanations, written guidelines, demonstrations, and return demonstrations. *These measures give family members information they can use as a guideline, especially at home. Return demonstration allows for evaluation of understanding of what has been taught.*
- Provide the family with a resource person whom they may call when a question arises and encourage them to feel free to call that person. *This measure provides family support and decreases anxiety and concerns of not knowing how to care for the child.*

Evaluation of Expected Outcomes

The child is alert and content with no long periods of fussiness. The infant interacts with caregivers with cooing, smiling, and eye contact. Skin around the edges of the cast shows no signs of redness or irritation. The diaper area is clean, dry, intact, and protected from soiling. The child responds positively to audio, visual, and diversionary activities and shows age-appropriate development. The family demonstrates care of the child in the orthopedic device or cast, asks pertinent questions, and identifies a resource person to call.

● LEGG-CALVÉ-PERTHES DISEASE (COXA PLANA)

Pathophysiology and Etiology

Legg-Calvé-Perthes disease is an aseptic necrosis of the head of the femur. It occurs four to five times more often in boys than in girls (Sponseller, 1999). It can be caused by trauma to the hip, but generally the cause is unknown.

Assessment Findings

Symptoms first noticed are pain in the hip or groin and a limp accompanied by muscle spasms and limitation of motion. These symptoms mimic **synovitis** (inflammation of a joint, which is most commonly the hip in children), which makes immediate diagnosis difficult. For a definitive diagnosis, radiographic examination may need to be repeated several weeks after the initial visit to demonstrate vascular necrosis.

The disease has three stages; each lasts 9 months to 1 year. In the first stage, radiographic studies show opacity of the epiphysis. In the second stage, the epiphysis becomes mottled and fragmented. During the third stage, reossification occurs.

Medical Management

In the past, immobilization of the hip through the use of braces and crutches and bed rest with traction or casting was considered essential for recovery without deformity. Restricting a child's activity for 2 years or more, however, was extremely difficult. Current treatment focuses on containing the femoral head within the acetabulum during the revascularization process so that the new femoral head will form to make a smoothly functioning joint. The method of containment varies with the portion of the head affected. Use of a brace that holds the necrotic portions of the head in place during healing is considered an effective method of containment. Reconstructive surgery is now possible, enabling the child to return to normal activities within 3 to 4 months. Prognosis for complete recovery without difficulty later in life depends on the child's age at the time of onset, the amount of involvement, and the cooperation of the child and family caregivers.

Nursing Management

Nursing care focuses on helping the child and caregivers to manage the corrective device and the importance of compliance to promote healing and avoid long-term disability.

● MUSCULAR DYSTROPHY

Pathophysiology and Etiology

Muscular dystrophy is a hereditary, progressive, degenerative disease of the muscles. The most common form is Duchenne (pseudohypertrophic) muscular dystrophy. This X-linked recessive hereditary disease occurs almost exclusively in males and is carried by females. When muscular dystrophy has been diagnosed in a child, the mother and the siblings should be tested to see if they have the disease or are carriers.

Assessment Findings

The first signs are noted in infancy or childhood, usually within the first 3 to 4 years of life. The child may have delayed walking, develop a waddling gait, and be unable to climb stairs. Later, trunk muscle weakness develops. Mild mental retardation often accompanies this disease. The child cannot rise easily to an upright position from a sitting position on the floor; instead he or she rises by climbing up the lower extremities with the hands (Fig. 9.3). Weakness of leg, arm, and shoulder muscles progresses gradually. Increasing abnormalities in gait and posture appear by school age with **lordosis** (forward curvature of the lumbar spine, or swayback), pelvic waddling, and frequent falling. The child becomes progressively weaker, usually becoming wheelchair-bound by 10 to 12 years (middle school or junior high school age). The disease continues into adolescence and young adulthood, when the client usually succumbs to respiratory or heart failure.

In addition to symptoms in the first 2 years of life, highly increased serum creatinine phosphokinase levels as well as a decrease in muscle fibers seen in a muscle biopsy can confirm the diagnosis.

Medical and Nursing Management

No effective treatment for the disease has been found, but research is rapidly closing in on genetic identification, which promises changes in treatment in the future (DeVivo & DiMauro, 1999). Encourage the child to be as active as possible to delay muscle atrophy and contrac-

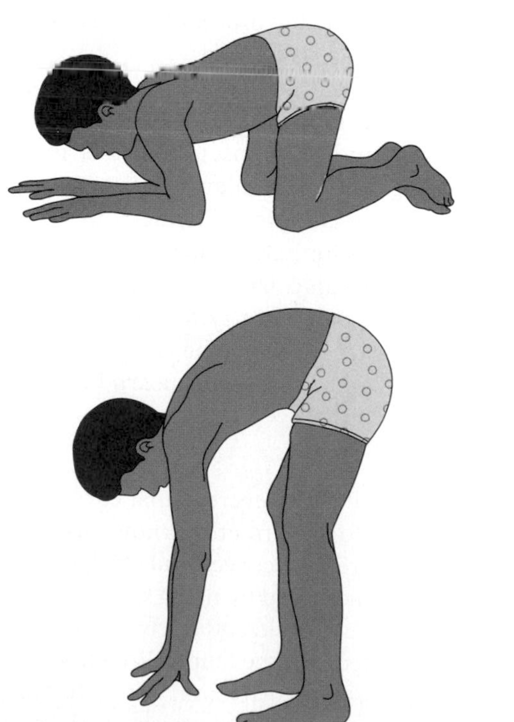

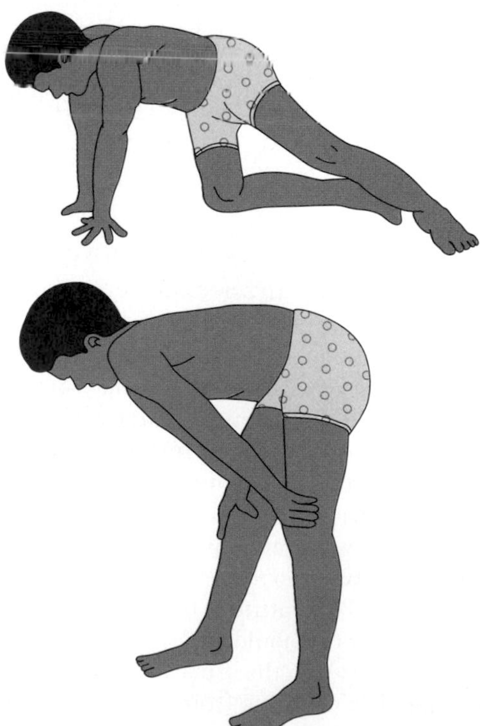

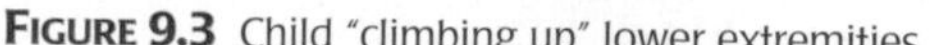

FIGURE 9.3 Child "climbing up" lower extremities.

tures. To help keep the child active, physiotherapy, diet to avoid obesity, and parental encouragement are important.

When a child becomes wheelchair-bound, **kyphosis** (humpback) develops and causes decreased respiratory function and increased incidence of infections. Breathing exercises are a daily necessity for these children.

Advise the family to keep the child's life as normal as possible, which may be difficult. This disease can drain the family's emotional and financial reserves. Suggest assistance through the Muscular Dystrophy Association—USA (National Headquarters, 3300 E. Sunrise Drive, Tucson, AZ 85718, 800-572-1717, http://www.mdausa.org), through local chapters of this organization, and by talking with other parents who face the same problem.

● SCOLIOSIS

Scoliosis, a lateral curvature of the spine, occurs in two forms: structural and functional (postural). Functional scoliosis is more common.

Pathophysiology and Etiology

Most cases of structural scoliosis are idiopathic (no cause is known). Congenital deformities or infection cause a few, and rotated and malformed vertebrae are seen in others. Idiopathic scoliosis is seen in school-age children 10 years or older. Although mild curves occur as often in boys as in girls, idiopathic scoliosis requiring treatment occurs more frequently in girls (Sponseller, 1999).

Functional scoliosis can have several causes: poor posture, muscle spasm from trauma, or unequal length of legs. Correction of the primary problem leads to the elimination of functional scoliosis.

Assessment Findings

Nurses play an important role in screening for scoliosis. Many states require regular examination of students for scoliosis, beginning in the fifth or sixth grade. Scoliosis screening should last through at least eighth grade. School nurses often do the initial screening; nurses in other healthcare settings are responsible for further screening during regular well-child visits. All nurses who work in healthcare settings with children 10 years and older should conduct or assist with screening programs.

During examination, observe the undressed child from the back. Note any lateral curvature of the spinal column; asymmetry of the shoulders, shoulder blades, or hips; and any unequal distance between the arms and waist. Then ask the child to bend at the hips (touch the toes) and observe for prominence of the scapula on one side and curvature of the spinal column.

Medical Management

Treatment is either nonsurgical or surgical. Curvatures less than 25 degrees are observed closely but not treated. Curvatures between 25 degrees and 40 degrees usually are corrected with a brace. Curvatures more than 40 degrees usually are corrected surgically. Treatment is long term and often lasts through the rest of the child's growth cycle.

Electrical stimulation may be used for mild curvatures, but its effectiveness is unclear. Other nonsurgical treatments include the use of braces and traction.

Braces

The Milwaukee brace was the first type of brace used for scoliosis but is now used more commonly to treat **kyphosis,** an abnormal rounded-out curvature of the spine also called "humpback." Either the Boston or the thoracic-lumbar-sacral orthotic (TLSO) brace is used to treat scoliosis. The Boston brace and the TLSO brace are made of plastic and customized to fit the child.

To achieve the greatest benefit, the child should wear the brace constantly except during bathing or swimming. He or she wears the brace over a T-shirt or undershirt to protect the skin. The healthcare provider monitors the fit of the device closely and teaches the child and caregiver to notify the provider if there is any rubbing. During the first few weeks of wearing the brace, the child can be given a mild analgesic for discomfort and aching. The provider also may prescribe certain exercises to be done several times a day. He or she teaches the child these exercises before applying the brace; however, the child does them while the brace is in place.

Wearing a brace creates a distinct change in body image, especially in older school-age children or adolescents, when body consciousness is at an all-time high. Wearing clothing similar to that of peers helps the child to feel more accepted. The need to wear the brace and deal with its limitations may cause anger; the change in body image can cause grief. It is important for the child to have an opportunity to discuss his or her feelings. Sometimes it helps for the client in a brace to talk with others who had scoliosis to learn how they coped.

Traction

When a child has severe spinal curvature or cervical instability, a form of traction known as **halo traction** may be used to reduce curves and straighten the spine. Halo traction is achieved by using stainless steel pins inserted into the skull while countertraction is applied by using pins inserted into the femur. Weights are increased gradually to promote correction. When the curvature has been corrected, spinal fusion is performed. In some cases, halo traction might be used following surgery if there is cervical instability.

Surgical Treatment

Surgical treatment includes the use of various instruments, such as rods, screws, and hooks placed along the spinal column to realign the spine, followed by spinal fusion to maintain the corrected position. This major surgery is done in cases of severe curvatures, and the child and family must be well prepared for it. The child can expect postoperative pain and must endure days of remaining flat in bed, being turned only in a log-rolling fashion.

Postoperatively the neurovascular status of the extremities is monitored closely. The child may use a patient-controlled analgesia pump to control pain. A Foley catheter usually is inserted because of the need to remain flat. The rods remain in place permanently. In some cases the child may be placed in a body cast for some time to ensure spinal fusion. Approximately 6 months after surgery, the child will be able to participate in most activities except contact sports (e.g., tackle football, gymnastics, wrestling). Because the bones are fused and rods are implanted, this procedure arrests the child's growth in height, which contributes to emotional adjustments that the child and family must make.

Nursing Management

The child with scoliosis must be reassessed every 4 to 6 months. Document the degree of curvature and related impairments. Provide privacy and protect the child's modesty. The child must practice and perform prescribed exercises as directed. Encourage and support the child during these exercises.

When a brace is applied, the child may need to be in traction for 1 or 2 weeks before the procedure. This can be emotionally traumatic. Be sensitive to the child's emotional state.

After the brace is first applied, check the child regularly to confirm proper fit. Observe for any areas of rubbing, discomfort, or skin irritation; adjust the brace as necessary. Instruct the child and caregiver to report reddened areas to the care provider for appropriate adjustments. Advise them to massage skin under the pads daily and that daily bathing and wearing clean cotton underwear or a T-shirt protects the skin.

Evaluate the child's environment after application of the brace; take precautions to prevent injury. Help the child practice moving safely: going up and down stairs; getting in and out of vehicles, chairs, and desks; and getting out of bed. Teach the child to avoid hazardous surfaces. Advise family caregivers to contact school personnel to ensure that the child has comfortable, supportive seating at school and that adjustments are made in the physical education program.

Self-image and the need to be like others are very important at this age. Learning to be confident enough to handle the comments of peers can be difficult for the child. Give the child frequent opportunities to express feelings about being different. Encourage the child to find extracurricular activities with which the brace will not interfere.

Family caregivers also may be concerned about the diagnosis. Be certain that the child and caregivers completely understand the importance of wearing the brace continually. To encourage compliance, teach them about possible complications of spinal instability and possible further deformity if correction is unsuccessful.

● TALIPES EQUINOVARUS

In talipes equinovarus (congenital clubfoot), the entire foot is inverted, the heel is drawn up, and the forefoot is adducted. The equinovarus foot has a clublike appearance, hence the term clubfoot. The Latin *talus,* meaning ankle, and *pes,* meaning foot, make up the word *talipes,* which is used in connection with many foot deformities. *Equinus,* or plantar flexion, and *varus,* or inversion, denote the kind of foot deformity in this condition.

Assessment Findings

Talipes equinovarus is the most common congenital foot deformity. It appears as a single anomaly or in connection with other defects such as myelomeningocele. It may be bilateral (both feet) or unilateral (one foot). The cause is unclear, though a hereditary factor occasionally is observed (Sponseller, 1999). A hypothesis that has received some acceptance proposes an arrested embryonic growth of the foot during the first trimester of pregnancy (Sponseller, 1999).

Talipes equinovarus is detected easily in newborns but must be differentiated from a persisting "position of comfort" assumed in utero. Use of passive exercise may correct the positional deformity easily; a true clubfoot deformity is fixed. The positional deformity should be explained to parents at once to prevent anxiety.

Medical and Surgical Management

Correction that begins during the neonatal period usually includes manipulation and bandaging or application of a cast. The cast often is applied while the infant is still in the neonatal nursery. The foot is first gently moved into as nearly normal a position as possible. Force should not be used. The cast is applied over the foot and ankle (and usually to mid-thigh) to hold the knee in right-angle flexion. Casts are changed frequently to provide gradual, atraumatic correction—every few days for the first several weeks, then every week or two. Treatment continues, usually for months until radiograph and clinical observation confirm complete correction. After correction with a cast, a Denis Browne splint with shoes attached may be used to maintain the correction for another 6 months or longer (Fig. 9.4). After overcorrection is complete, the child should wear a special clubfoot shoe, which is a laced shoe whose turning out makes it appear that the child is wearing the shoe on the wrong foot. The child may continue to wear the Denis Browne splint at night, and caregivers should carry out passive exercises of the child's foot.

Children who do not respond to nonsurgical measures, especially older children, need surgical correction. This approach involves several procedures depending on the age of the child and the degree of the deformity. It may involve lengthening the Achilles tendon, capsulotomy of the ankle joint, release of medial strictures, and operating on the bony structure for the child older than 10 years. Prolonged observation after correction by any means should be carried out at least until adolescence; any recurrence is treated promptly.

Nursing Management

When a plaster of Paris cast is used, there should be some type of waterproof material protecting the skin from the cast's sharp plaster edges. One method is to apply strips of adhesive vertically around the edges of the cast in a manner called *petaling.* To petal a cast, strips of adhesive are cut 2 or 3 inches long and 1 inch wide. One end is notched and the other end is cut pointed to aid in smooth application.

Teach family caregivers appropriate cast care. The older infant may resist wearing the Denis Browne splint, so educate family caregivers about the importance of gentle, but firm, insistence that the child must wear the splint.

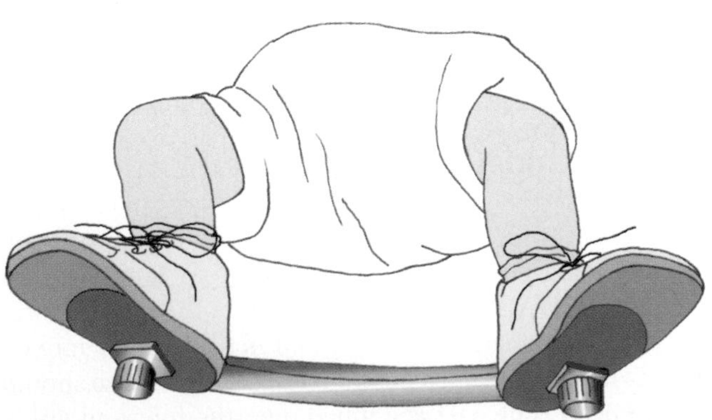

FIGURE 9.4 A Denis Browne splint with shoes attached is used to correct clubfoot.

INTEGUMENTARY DISORDERS

● CANDIDIASIS

Candida albicans is the causative agent for thrush and some cases of diaper rash. Thrush appears in the infant's mouth as a white coating that looks like milk curds. Newborns can be exposed to a maternal vaginal infection with *C. albicans* during delivery. Poor handwashing practices and inadequate washing of bottles and nipples are other contributing factors. In addition, infants and toddlers may experience episodes of thrush or diaper rash after antibiotic therapy, which may upset the balance of normal intestinal flora, leading to candidal overgrowth.

Application of nystatin (Mycostatin, Nilstat) to the oral lesions every 6 hours is an effective treatment for thrush. Treatment for diaper rash caused by *C. albicans* is the application of nystatin ointment or cream to the affected area. In all cases, good hygiene practices should be reinforced.

● DIAPER RASH

Pathophysiology and Etiology

Diaper rash is common in infancy, causing the baby discomfort and fretfulness. Bacterial decomposition of urine produces ammonia, which is irritating to an infant's tender skin. Diarrheal stools also produce a burning erythematous area in the anal region. Some infants seem more susceptible than others, possibly because of inherited sensitive skin. Prolonged exposure to wet or soiled diapers, use of plastic or rubber pants, inadequate cleansing of the diaper area (especially after bowel movements), sensitivity to some soaps or disposable diaper perfumes, and the use of strong laundry detergents without thorough rinsing are common causes. Yeast infections, notably candidiasis, are also causative factors (see earlier discussion).

Nursing Management

Teach caregivers that the primary treatment is prevention. Instruct them to change diapers frequently without waiting for obvious leaking. Manufacturers of disposable diapers constantly are trying to improve the ability of disposable diapers to wick wetness away from the infant's skin. Diapers washed at commercial laundries are sterilized, preventing the growth of ammonia-forming bacteria. Diapers washed at home should be presoaked (good commercial products are available), washed in hot water with a mild soap, and rinsed thoroughly with an antiseptic added to the final rinse. Drying diapers in the sun or in a dryer also helps destroy bacteria.

Exposing the diaper area to the air helps clear up dermatitis. Discourage the use of baby powder when diapering, because caked powder contributes to an environment in which organisms thrive. Cleaning the diaper area from front to back with warm water and drying thoroughly with each diaper change helps improve or prevent the condition. If soap is necessary when cleaning stool from the infant's buttocks and rectal area, remind caregivers to be certain that they have rinsed the soap completely before diapering. Use of commercial wet wipes may aggravate the condition. If the area becomes excoriated and sore, the healthcare provider may prescribe an ointment. See Client and Family Teaching 9-5.

● ACUTE INFANTILE ECZEMA

Infantile eczema is an atopic dermatitis considered at least partly an allergic reaction to an irritant. It is fairly common in infants older than 3 months. It is uncommon in breastfed babies before they start additional foods.

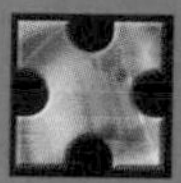

9-5 *Client and Family Teaching* Diaper Rash

The nurse teaches the family as follows:

- Rinse all the baby's clothes thoroughly to eliminate soap or detergent residue that may irritate skin.
- Rinse cloth diapers in clear water. Do not use fabric softeners; they can cause a skin reaction.
- Use plastic or rubber diaper covers only when necessary. They hold moisture, which worsens the rash.
- Change diapers as soon as wet or soiled. Disposable diapers hold moisture the same as plastic or rubber covers.
- Avoid fastening diaper too tightly, which irritates baby's skin.
- Expose baby's bottom to air without diapers as much as possible to help rash heal.
- Do not overdress or overcover baby. Sweating makes rash worse.
- Wash baby's bottom with lukewarm water only, using wet cotton balls or pouring over bath basin or sink. Pat dry with soft cloth. Do not use commercial baby wipes. Do not rub rash.
- A cool, wet cloth placed over red diaper rash is very soothing. Try this for 5 minutes three or four times a day.
- Use ointment only as recommended by healthcare provider. Apply very thin layer only. Wash off at each diaper change.
- Dry diaper area thoroughly before rediapering. A hair dryer on low warm setting used after patting dry may help.

Pathophysiology and Etiology

Three factors characterize infantile eczema:

- Hereditary predisposition
- Hypersensitivity of the deeper layers of the skin to protein or protein-like allergens
- Allergens to which the child is sensitive that may be inhaled, ingested, or absorbed through direct contact such as house dust, egg white, and wool

Infants who have eczema tend to have allergic rhinitis or asthma later in life (Tunnessen & Krowchuk, 1999).

Assessment Findings

Eczema usually starts on the cheeks and spreads to the extensor surfaces of the arms and legs. Eventually it may affect the entire trunk. Initial reddening of the skin is followed quickly by papule and vesicle formation. Itching is intense, and the infant's scratching makes the skin weep and crust. Hemolytic *streptococci* or *staphylococci* easily infect the areas.

The most common allergens involved in eczema are as follows:

- Foods: egg white, cow's milk, wheat products, orange juice, tomato juice
- Inhalants: house dust, pollens, animal dander
- Materials: wool, nylon, plastic

Diagnosis, however, is not simple. Often trial by elimination is as effective as any other diagnostic tool. Skin testing on a young infant generally is not considered valid, so it is discouraged as a means of diagnosis.

Medical Management

An elimination diet may help rule out offending foods. A hypoallergenic diet consisting of a milk substitute such as soy formula, vitamin supplement, and other known hypoallergenic foods is given. If the skin condition improves, other foods are added one at a time at an interval of approximately 1 week; the provider and caregiver note the effects and eliminate any foods that cause a reaction. The protein of egg white is such a common offender that most pediatricians advise against feeding whole eggs to infants until late in the first year.

Caregivers must take great measures to prevent the child from becoming undernourished. They always must conduct an elimination program under the supervision of a competent pediatric nurse practitioner, dietitian, or physician.

Caregivers must keep children with eczema away from anyone who has recently been vaccinated for smallpox (e.g., someone vaccinated in preparation for travel). Protecting the child from anyone with a herpes simplex infection (cold sore) also is important. Lesions that become infected with herpes simplex may lead to a generalized reaction. In the child with severe eczema and many lesions, body fluid loss from oozing through the lesions can be serious. The infant may have severe pain and be gravely ill with this complication.

Oral antibiotics may be ordered for a coexistent staphylococcal or streptococcal infection. Oral antihistamines and sedatives may help relieve itching and allow rest. If no infection exists, topical hydrocortisone ointments may be used to relieve inflammation. Wet soaks or colloidal baths also may be prescribed for their soothing effects. The water should be tepid for further soothing, and soap may not be used because of its drying effect. Lubrication is essential to retain moisture and prevent evaporation after the bath. Emollients containing lanolin or petrolatum, such as Eucerin, may be prescribed.

Caregivers should help protect the child against inhalant and contact allergens as much as possible. In the infant's bedroom, they should remove window drapes or curtains, dresser scarves, and rugs or ensure that these articles are made of washable fabric that can be laundered frequently. The crib mattress should have a nonallergenic covering and be washed frequently. Feather pillows, carpets, and area rugs may need to be eliminated; stuffed toys should be washable. It may be necessary to provide new homes for household pets. A home, especially an older one with a damp basement, may harbor molds that shed allergenic spores. Bathrooms arc also places for molds and mildews to hide, especially in warm, humid climates.

Nursing Management

Data collection about the infant with eczema includes obtaining vital signs, observing general nutritional state, and completely examining all body parts. Carefully document the eruptions and their location and size. Note unaffected as well as weeping and crusted areas.

Advise caregivers to cover the lesions with light clothing, especially materials that help keep the child from scratching. Remind them to cut the child's nails closely and to use mitten-like hand coverings. Use restraints only if necessary. If ointments or wet dressings must remain in place on the infant's face, caregivers can make a mask by cutting holes into a cotton stockinette-type material to correspond to eyes, nose, and mouth. They can keep wet dressings in place on the rest of the body by wrapping the infant "mummy" fashion.

Instruct caregivers to plan soothing baths, such as a colloidal bath (Aveeno), just before the baby's naps or bedtime. They should time medications such as sedatives or antihistamines so that they will be effective immediately after the bath when the infant is most relaxed.

If an elimination diet is being used, ensure that the diet is carefully balanced within the framework of foods permitted and supplemented with vitamin and mineral preparations as needed.

When possible, these children should stay out of the healthcare facility because of concerns about contracting an infection. If placement is necessary, these infants should be put in a room alone or where no other child has any type of infection.

Help family caregivers understand the condition and possible food, contact, or inhalant allergens. They should avoid overdressing and overheating the infant, because perspiration causes itching. Advise them to use mild detergent to launder the infant's clothing and bedding.

Children with eczema are frequently active and "behaviorally itchy." Assist caregivers in handling challenging behavior.

Stop, Think, and Respond ● BOX 9-5

What are the most common allergens that cause infantile eczema?

● FUNGAL INFECTIONS

Fungi that live in the outer (dead) layers of the skin, hair, and nails can develop into superficial infections. **Tinea** (ringworm) is the term commonly applied to these infections, which are further differentiated according to the body part infected.

Tinea Capitis (Ringworm of the Scalp)

Ringworm of the scalp is called *tinea capitis* or *tinea tonsurans.* The most common cause is *Microsporum audouinii,* which is transmitted from person to person through combs, towels, hats, barber scissors, or direct contact. A less common type, *Microsporum canis,* is transmitted from animal to child.

Tinea capitis begins as a small papule on the scalp and spreads, leaving scaly patches of baldness. The hairs become brittle and break off easily. Griseofulvin, an oral antifungal, is the treatment of choice. Because treatment may be prolonged (3 months or more), compliance must be reinforced. Children who are being properly treated may attend school. Hair loss is not permanent.

Tinea Corporis (Ringworm of the Body)

Tinea corporis, ringworm of the body, affects the epidermis and may appear on any body part. Lesions appear as scaly rings with clearing in the center, resembling those of scalp ringworm. The child usually contracts tinea corporis from contact with an infected dog or cat. Topical antifungal agents, such as clotrimazole, econazole nitrate, tolnaftate, and miconazole, are effective. Griseofulvin also is used.

Tinea Pedis (Ringworm of the Feet; Athlete's Foot)

Tinea pedis (athlete's foot) is scaling or cracking of the skin between the toes. Microscopic examination of scrapings from the lesions is necessary for definite diagnosis. Transmission is direct or indirect contact with skin lesions from infected people. Contaminated sidewalks, floors, pool decks, and shower stalls spread the condition to those who walk barefoot. Tinea pedis is usually found in adolescents and adults (Tunnessen & Krowchuk, 1999).

Care includes washing the feet with soap and water, then gently removing scabs and crusts and applying a topical agent such as tolnaftate. Griseofulvin by mouth is also useful. During the chronic phase, the use of ointment, scrupulous foot hygiene, frequent changing of white cotton socks, and avoidance of plastic footwear are helpful. Continuing application of a topical agent for up to 6 weeks is recommended.

Tinea Cruris (Ringworm of the Inner Thighs and Inguinal Area)

Tinea cruris (jock itch) results from the same organisms that cause tinea corporis. It is more common in athletes and uncommon in preadolescents. It is pruritic and localized to the area. Treatment is the same as for tinea corporis. Sitz baths also may be soothing.

• IMPETIGO

Impetigo is a superficial bacterial skin infection. In newborns, the primary causative organism is *Staphylococcus aureus*. In older children, the most common causative organism is group A beta-hemolytic streptococci. Impetigo lesions in newborns are usually bullous (blister-like); in older children, lesions are nonbullous.

Impetigo in the newborn nursery is cause for immediate concern, because the condition is highly contagious and can spread through a nursery quickly. Nurses caring for infants with impetigo must follow contact (skin and wound) precautions, including wearing cover gowns and gloves. They should segregate these infants from other infants in the nursery to deter spread of the disease. Nurses can soak off crusts with warm water followed by application of topical antibiotics such as Bacitracin and Neosporin. They must cover the infant's hands or apply elbow restraints to prevent scratching of lesions. Careful handwashing by nursing personnel and family members is essential.

Older children with impetigo receive treatment at home. Family caregivers must learn and implement hygiene practices to prevent spreading impetigo to other children in the household and day care center, nursery school, or elementary school. Lesions occur primarily on the face but may spread to any part of the body. The crusts and drainage are contagious. Because the lesions are pruritic (itchy), the child must learn to keep his or her fingers and hands away from the lesions. Caregivers should trim the child's nails to prevent scratching of lesions. Family members should not share towels or washcloths. Medical treatment includes oral penicillin or erythromycin for 10 days. Daily washing of the crusts helps speed healing. Mupirocin (Bactroban) ointment may be used.

Because this infection is commonly streptococcal in older children, rheumatic fever or acute glomerulonephritis may follow. Alert family caregivers to this rare possibility.

• PARASITIC INFECTIONS

Parasites are organisms that live on or within another living organism from which they obtain their food supply. Lice and scabies mites live by sucking the blood of a host.

Pediculosis

The causes of pediculosis (lice infestation) are *Pediculus humanus capitis* (head lice), *Pediculus humanus corporis* (body lice), and *Phthirus pubis* (pubic lice). Head lice are the most common infestation in children. Animal lice are not transferred to humans.

Children exchange head lice through direct contact or indirectly through combs, headgear, or bed linen. Lice, which are rarely visible, lay their eggs (called *nits*) on the head where they attach to hair strands. The nits can be seen as tiny, pearly white flecks attached to the hair shafts. They look much like dandruff, but dandruff flakes can be flicked off easily, whereas nits are tightly attached and not easily removed. They hatch in approximately 1 week, and lice become sexually mature in approximately 2 weeks. Severe itching of the scalp is the most obvious symptom.

Use of lindane (Kwell) shampoo, which is prescribed by a physician, is suggested if over-the-counter medications are not effective in treating the condition. After wetting the hair with warm water, the Kwell is applied like any ordinary shampoo; about 1 ounce is used. The head should be lathered for 4 minutes, then rinsed thoroughly and dried. After the hair is dry, it should be combed with a fine-toothed comb dipped in warm white vinegar to remove remaining nits and nit shells. Shampooing may be repeated in 2 weeks to remove any lice that may have been missed as nits and since hatched. Avoid getting Kwell into the eyes or on mucous membranes. When treating a child in the hospital for pediculosis, wear a disposable gown, gloves, and head cover for protection.

Family caregivers often are embarrassed when a school nurse sends word that their child has head lice. Reassure them that lice infestation is common and can happen to any child; it is not a reflection on housekeeping. Inspect all family members and treat them as needed. See Client and Family Teaching 9-6 for other useful information.

Scabies

Scabies is a skin infestation caused by the mite *Sarcoptes scabiei.* The female mite burrows in areas between the fingers and toes and in warm folds of the body, such as the axilla and groin, to lay eggs. Burrows are visible as dark lines, and the mite is seen as a black dot at the end of the burrow. Itching is severe, leading to scratching with resulting secondary infection.

The areas are treated with lindane lotion or crotamiton (Eurax). The body is first scrubbed with soap and water; lotion is then applied on all areas of the body except the face. With lindane, a second coat can be applied, then all washed off in 24 hours. For crotamiton, a second coat is applied in 24 hours; the client waits an additional 48 hours to wash it off. Caregivers should follow the tips recommended for pediculosis. All who had close contact with the child within 30 to 60 days should be treated. The rash and itch may continue for several weeks even though the mites have been eliminated successfully.

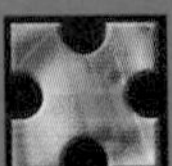

9-6 *Client and Family Teaching* Eliminating Pediculi Infestation

- Wash all bedding and clothing of the child in hot water; dry in a hot dryer.
- Vacuum carpets, car seats, mattresses, and upholstered furniture very thoroughly. Discard vacuum dust bag.
- Wash pillows, stuffed animals, and other washable items the same way you wash clothing.
- Dry-clean nonwashable items.
- If items cannot be washed or dry-cleaned, seal in plastic bag for 2 weeks to break reproductive cycle of lice.
- Wash combs, brushes, and other hair items (e.g., rollers, curlers, barrettes) in shampoo and soak for 1 hour.
- If you discover the infestation, report to child's school or day care.
- Schools should disinfect headphones.

IMMUNE DISORDERS

• COMMUNICABLE DISEASES

Understanding various communicable diseases and their prevention, symptoms, and treatment requires knowledge of the terms in Box 9-2. Some communicable diseases require specific precautions to prevent their spread. Specific transmission precaution procedures can be found in the procedure manuals of individual institutions.

Explain to the child and caregivers the reason for transmission precautions, which are to protect the child from

BOX 9-2 ● Common Terms in Communicable Disease Nursing

Active immunity: stimulates development of antibodies to destroy infective agent, without causing disease. Occurs when vaccine is given
Antibody: a protective substance the body produces in response to the introduction of an antigen
Antigen: a foreign protein that stimulates the formation of antibodies
Antitoxin: an antibody that unites with and neutralizes a specific toxin
Carrier: a person in apparently good health whose body harbors the specific organisms of a disease
Causative agent: pathogen that causes disease
Enanthem: an eruption on a mucous surface
Endemic: habitual presence of a disease within a given area
Epidemic: an outbreak in a community of a group of illnesses of similar nature in excess of the normal expectancy
Erythema: redness of the skin produced by congestion of the capillaries
Exanthem: an eruption appearing on the skin during an eruptive disease
Host: a human, animal, or plant that harbors or nourishes another organism
Immunity: passive: immunity acquired by administration of an antibody. *Active:* immunity acquired by an individual as the result of his or her own reactions to pathogens. Natural: resistance of the normal animal to infection
Incubation period: the time interval between the infection and the appearance of the first symptoms of the disease
Macule: a discolored skin spot not elevated above the surface
Mode of transmission: mechanism by which infectious agent is spread or transferred to humans
Natural immunity: resistance to a pathogen or infection; genetically determined
Pandemic: a worldwide epidemic
Papule: a small, circumscribed, solid elevation of the skin
Passive immunity: antibodies obtained from an immune person, given to someone exposed to disease to prevent him or her from getting disease
Period of communicability: time which infectious agent can be transmitted or passed from an infected person or animal to another person
Pustule: a small elevation of epidermis filled with pus
Toxin: a poisonous substance produced by certain organisms, such as bacteria
Toxoid: a toxin that has been treated to destroy its toxicity but that retains its antigenic properties
Vaccine: a suspension of attenuated or killed microorganisms administered for the prevention of a specific infection

the threat of infection and others from the infection the child has. Otherwise, the child may think that the precautions are a form of punishment. Families are more likely to follow correct procedures if they understand the need for them. Transmission precautions may intensify the normal loneliness of being ill, so the child needs extra attention and stimulation during this time.

The recommended schedule of childhood immunization is found in Chapter 5. Urge caregivers of children with incomplete immunizations to bring the immunizations up to date. For families of limited means, free immunizations are available at clinics.

● INFECTIOUS MONONUCLEOSIS

Pathophysiology and Etiology

The cause of infectious mononucleosis ("mono"), sometimes called the "kissing disease," is the Epstein-Barr virus, one of the herpes virus groups. Saliva transmits the organism. No immunization is available, and treatment is symptomatic. Adolescents and young adults seem most susceptible to this disorder, although sometimes it also is seen in younger children.

Assessment Findings

Infectious mononucleosis can present various symptoms ranging from mild to severe and that mimic hepatitis. Symptoms include fever; sore throat with enlarged tonsils; thick, white membrane covering the tonsils; palatine petechiae (red spots on the soft palate); swollen lymph nodes; and enlargement of the spleen accompanied by extreme fatigue and lack of energy. In some instances, headache, abdominal pain, and epistaxis are also present.

Diagnosis of infectious mononucleosis is based on clinical symptoms, laboratory evidence of lymphocytes in the peripheral blood (with 10% or more abnormal lymphocytes present in a peripheral blood smear), and a positive heterophil agglutination test. Monospot is a valuable diagnostic test—rapid, sensitive, inexpensive, and simple to perform. Monospot can detect significant agglutinins at lower levels, thus allowing earlier diagnosis. Infectious mononucleosis often is confused with streptococcal infections because of the fever and the appearance of the throat and tonsils.

Medical and Nursing Management

No cure exists for infectious mononucleosis; treatment is based on symptoms. An analgesic-antipyretic, such as acetaminophen, usually is recommended for the fever and headaches. Encourage fluids and a soft, bland diet to reduce throat irritation. Corticosteroids sometimes are prescribed to relieve the severe sore throat and fever. Bed rest is suggested to relieve fatigue but is not imposed for a specific time. If the spleen is enlarged, the adolescent is cautioned to avoid contact sports that might cause a ruptured spleen. Because the immune system is weakened, the adolescent must take precautions to avoid secondary infections.

The course of infectious mononucleosis is usually uncomplicated. Fever and sore throat may last from 1 week to 10 days. Fatigue generally disappears 2 to 4 weeks after the appearance of acute symptoms but may last as long as 1 year. The limitations that this disorder imposes on the teenager's school and social life may cause depression. In most instances, however, the adolescent can resume normal activities within 1 month after symptoms present.

Nursing care includes encouraging the adolescent to express feelings about the interruptions the illness is causing in school, social, and work plans. Long-term effects are rare.

Critical Thinking Exercises

1. *Ten-month-old Hayden has severe diarrhea. What symptoms and physical signs would you look for in this child? What documentation would be especially important?*
2. *You are caring for 3-year-old Cassie who has had several urinary tract infections. Her mother asks you what causes them. What will you tell this mother? What specific things will you teach regarding prevention and treatment?*
3. *Jillian, 12 years old, has scoliosis and must wear a TLSO brace. She says she thinks it is really ugly. What feelings do you think Jillian might have? How will you respond?*
4. *The caregiver of a 5 year old who has just started kindergarten calls you upset because her child has been sent home from school with a note advising her that there has been an outbreak of head lice. Three other children between the ages of 2 and 10 years are in the home. Explain to this caregiver what to do in this situation.*

● NCLEX-STYLE REVIEW QUESTIONS 

1. When assessing a child diagnosed with nephrotic syndrome, which of the following nursing considerations is most important?
   1. Consistent measurements of weight and abdominal girth
   2. Output of bowel and bladder elimination
   3. Pain scale use and pain management regimen
   4. Assessment of skin turgor and skin integrity
2. The nurse is educating a 13-year-old newly diagnosed with diabetes mellitus. Which statement by the child indicates that nutritional instructions have been effective?
   1. "The more that I eat, the higher my blood sugar will be."
   2. "I will eat a complex carbohydrate snack after my soccer game."

3. "If I feel shaky, I will take my blood sugar and drink some orange juice."
4. "I will never be able to have any sweets or anything that I really like again."

3. A school nurse is conducting routine scoliosis screenings for the eighth grade. During the assessment, she finds that one student has scoliosis of 30°. The student tearfully asks, "What will they do for this?" Which of the following is the nurse most correct to advise?
1. "Surgical intervention will be likely to straighten the spine."
2. "A molded brace will likely be used to stop curvature progression."
3. "Skeletal traction will likely be used to realign the vertebrae in the spine."
4. "Range-of-motion exercises will likely be taught to strengthen the back muscles."

connection

Visit the Connection site at **http://connection.lww.com/go/timbyEssentials** for links to chapter-related resources on the Internet.

References and Suggested Readings

Azar, R., & Solomon, C. R. (2001). Coping strategies of parents facing child diabetes mellitus. *Journal of Pediatric Nursing, 16*(6), 418.

Chin, K. R., et al. (2001). A guide to early detection of scoliosis. *Contemporary Pediatrics, 18*(9) 77.

DeVivo, D. C., & DiMauro, S. (1999). Hereditary and acquired types of myopathy. In *Oski's pediatrics: Principles and practice* (3rd ed.). Philadelphia: Lippincott Williams & Wilkins.

Goldberg, M. J. (2001). Early detection of developmental hip dysplasia. *Pediatrics in Review, 22*(4), 131–34.

Hockenberry, M. J., Wilson, D., Winkelstein, M. L., & Kline, N. E. (2003). *Wong's nursing care of infants and children* (7th ed.). St. Louis: Mosby.

Katz, D. R. (2001). Adolescent idiopathic scoliosis: The effect of brace treatment on the incidence of surgery. *Physical Therapy, 81*(9), 1591.

Kelekman, J., et al. (1999). Diabetes update in the pediatric population. *Pediatric Nursing, 25*(6), 666.

Lawless, M. R., & McElderry, D. H. (2001). Nocturnal enuresis: Current concepts. *Pediatrics in Review, 22*(12), 399–407.

Lifschitz, C. H. (1999). Celiac disease. In *Oski's pediatrics: Principles and practice* (3rd ed.). Philadelphia: Lippincott Williams & Wilkins.

Maniatis, A. K., et al. (2001). Continuous subcutaneous insulin infusion therapy for children and adolescents: An option for routine diabetes care. *Pediatrics, 107*(2), 351.

McEvoy, C. F. (1999). Developmental disorders of gastrointestinal function. In *Oski's pediatrics: Principles and practice* (3rd ed.). Philadelphia: Lippincott Williams & Wilkins.

Pillitteri, A. (2003). *Maternal and child health nursing* (4th ed.). Philadelphia: Lippincott Williams & Wilkins.

Plotnick, L. P. (1999). Type 1 (insulin-dependent) diabetes mellitus. In *Oski's pediatrics: Principles and practice* (3rd ed.). Philadelphia: Lippincott Williams & Wilkins.

Questions and answers about scoliosis in children and adolescents. (2001). National Institute of Arthritis and Musculoskeletal and Skin Diseases, National Institutes of Health [On-line.] Available: www.niams.nih.gov/hi/index.htm.

Splete, H. (2001). Catch curves like scoliosis in time for bracing. *Pediatric News, 35*(11), 42.

Sponseller, P. D. (1999). In *Oski's pediatrics: Principles and practice* (3rd ed.). Philadelphia: Lippincott Williams & Wilkins.

Tunnessen, Jr., W. W., & Krowchuk, D. P. (1999). Pediatric dermatology. In *Oski's pediatrics: Principles and practice* (3rd ed.). Philadelphia: Lippincott Williams & Wilkins.

Wedge, J. H., et al. (2001). Congenital clubfoot. *Current Pediatrics, 11*(5), 332–340.

chapter 10

Biopsychosocial Aspects of Caring for Young and Middle Adults

Words to Know 

adolescent moratorium
androgeny
basal metabolic rate (BMR)
blended family
climacteric
domestic violence
extended family
gender role
Generation X
Generation Y
generativity
intimacy
isolation
keratotic lesion
menopause
mid-life crisis
nuclear family
osteoporosis
personal protection order
presbycusis
presbyopia
rape
sandwich generation
single-parent family
stagnation
temporary restraining order
traditional family

Learning Objectives

On completion of this chapter, the reader will:

- Describe the attributes associated with psychosocial development in young and middle adulthood.
- Give three components that are used to determine if a person meets or exceeds a safe weight.
- Give examples of drugs used to facilitate smoking cessation.
- Name two growing practices among young adults that affect the integrity and safety of the integument.
- List examples of life events that mark the transition from adolescence to young adulthood.
- Cite at least one benefit of androgeny.
- Describe the current status of sexuality among young adults.
- Name four types of family structures in which young adults may be members.
- Name two consequences young adults experience in relation to unemployment and downsizing.
- Name three types of rape.
- List three drugs that potentiate the commission of rape.
- Identify two principles that are followed when caring for rape victims.
- List six aspects of nursing care when treating a rape victim.
- Identify the most dangerous period for victims of domestic violence.
- Discuss at least three areas for health teaching when caring for young adults.
- Discuss unique problems that nurses deal with when caring for middle-aged adults.

Nurses provide care to individuals from birth to old age. An important nursing intervention is preparing clients for physical changes and common life experiences that occur at various life stages. Nurses must be knowledgeable about how aging affects health and familiar with social changes that are characteristic of each period in the life cycle.

The first part of this chapter discusses physical and psychosocial development of the young adult, exploring common societal problems that first appear or are especially prevalent in young adulthood. The second part discusses physical and psychosocial development of the middle adult, exploring common societal problems that first appear or are especially prevalent in middle adulthood.

YOUNG ADULTHOOD

Young adults who graduated from college in 1998 are described as belonging to **Generation Y.** They may also be called Echo Boomers to differentiate them from older young adults labeled as **Generation X.** Age, alphabetical designations of X and Y, and euphemistic labels fail to fully explain today's young adults.

Developmental Stage and Task: Intimacy Versus Isolation

Erikson observed that developmental tasks during young adulthood, 18 to 35 years, involve leaving home, forming lasting relationships with nonrelatives, and committing to a career. If young adults form friendships with others and have significant, intimate relationships with one person, a basis for closeness with others results. Young adults then acquire the positive attribute of **intimacy,** the ability to enter into personal relationships that reaffirm one's identity. Acquiring intimacy during this period enhances young adults' ability to become productive and happy members of society. Inability to form close relationships with others results in loneliness and **isolation.**

Physical Characteristics

Most people are healthiest and attain peak physical performance as young adults. Physical condition begins to decline after 20 years (Vander Zanden, 2000). Chronic diseases are very rare among young adults. This age group is more likely to experience acute infectious illnesses and trauma from injuries. Success in treating victims of major trauma increases the numbers of survivors with varying degrees of disability. The following is a brief overview of typical physical characteristics of young adults.

Weight

Weight fluctuates in relation to activity. Young adults consume more calories in relation to energy expenditures they once had as adolescents. Consequently, overweight and obesity become new problems for many young adults. The National Institutes of Health (NIH) (1998) report that about 55% of adults in the United States are overweight. The NIH released federal obesity clinical guidelines that recommend three components for determining if a person meets or exceeds a safe weight. They include (1) body mass index (BMI), (2) waist circumference, and (3) risk factors for diseases and conditions associated with obesity. One method for calculating BMI is to multiply 703 times the weight in pounds and then divide by height in inches, squared. According to the NIH guidelines, a BMI of 25 to 29.9 is considered overweight; a person is considered obese if the BMI is 30 or greater. A waist circumference that measures more than 40 inches in men and more than 35 inches in women increases health risks. When the first two measurements exceed desirable limits and the person has a personal or family history of hypertension, diabetes, high cholesterol, heart disease, and respiratory disorders, the probability for premature death increases.

DIETS. An obvious technique used to control or reduce weight is dieting. Around 40% of young adult women and 24% of young adult men diet (Vander Zanden, 2000). Young adults are prone to fad diets rather than making low-calorie selections. Characteristics of fad diets include prolonged periods of fasting, severe restrictions of amounts of food, restrictions of particular food groups, and claims for fast and easy weight loss.

Strict dieting can cause nutritional deficits and a "yo-yo" effect of weight loss followed by weight gain. Some young adults develop eating disorders (see Chap. 16). The healthiest way to lose weight is to exercise, limit calories, and consume a variety of foods. These measures help to suppress the appetite, enhance loss of body fat, increase lean body mass, improve self-image, reduce anxiety and depression, and facilitate stress management.

EXERCISE. Many people begin to exercise because aerobic exercise can prevent cardiovascular diseases. Young adults use indoor fitness centers and outside settings for walking, jogging, cycling, swimming, and roller-blading. The number of adults who exercise, however, is still below the national goals set in *Healthy People 2010.* By 2010, the goal is to increase from the current 15% to 30% the proportion of adults who engage in regular, preferably daily, moderate physical activity for at least 30 minutes (U.S. Department of Health and Human Services, 2000). Moderate activity includes walking at approximately 3 to 4 miles per hour, easy cycling, leisurely swimming, golfing without a cart, playing table tennis, canoeing at 2 to 4 miles per hour, and mowing the yard with a power mower (Vander Zanden, 2000).

Respiratory System

With the exceptions of upper or lower respiratory tract infections, the lungs remain highly functional throughout young adulthood among nonsmokers and persons who are not chronically exposed to significant levels of air pollution. Young adults with scoliosis, a lateral curvature of the spine, may have diminished respiratory volumes.

Smokers and those who inhale smoke passively (i.e., those who inhale air emitted from exhaled smoke or smoke from a burning cigarette, pipe, or cigar) are exposed to harmful chemicals such as nicotine, tar, carbon monoxide, and hydrogen cyanide. Chronic exposure increases the rate of respiratory infections, pulmonary and cardiovascular diseases, and lung cancer. The number and severity of asthma attacks is higher among smokers and those who inhale smoke passively. Maternal smoking lowers infant birth weight. A link exists between low birth weight and the incidence of sudden infant death syndrome (SIDS). Although many smokers continue to perpetuate their habit into later years of adulthood, various drugs can assist with smoking cessation (Drug Therapy Table 10.1).

Cardiovascular System

Minor changes occur in the heart and vascular system. One percent of myocardial strength is lost with each year of adulthood. Blood pressure gradually increases after age 20. Early narrowing of the coronary arteries and other vascular changes begin as well. A diet high in saturated fat contributes to the building of plaque on the walls of the coronary arteries, beginning the pathologic process of atherosclerosis (see Chap. 27). Effects of this process, however, are not evident for many years.

Drug Therapy Table 10.1 DRUGS FOR SMOKING CESSATION

DRUG CLASS AND EXAMPLES	SIDE EFFECTS	NURSING CONSIDERATIONS
Antidepressants		
bupropion (Zyban)	Weight loss, insomnia, restlessness, agitation, dry mouth, headache, tremors, excessive sweating, seizures, hypertension	Dose is different when used to treat depression. Begin drug therapy 1 week before cessation of smoking. Drug is contraindicated for pregnant or breast-feeding women. Use with alcohol increases seizure potential. Blood pressure increases when used with smoking or nicotine products for smoking cessation. This drug can induce psychotic behavior when combined with marijuana.
Nicotine Products		
Nicotine patch *(Nicoderm, Nicotrol, Habitrol)*	Itching, burning, or tingling at site of patch when first applied; tachycardia; increased blood pressure, redness at site when patch is removed Nicotine overdose: headaches, dizziness, upset stomach, vomiting, diarrhea, mental confusion, weakness, or fainting	Consult the physician if application site becomes swollen or very red. Caution client against wearing the patch and smoking or using tobacco products. Avoid if client is allergic to adhesive tape. Monitor blood pressure and heart rate. Keep away from children.
Nicotine gum *(Nicorette)*	Tachycardia, elevated blood pressure	Advise client to chew the gum slowly until a slight tingling occurs or a peppery taste is noted, then place it between the cheek and gum until the taste or tingling is almost gone. Explain that 9 to 12 pieces of gum per day usually control the urge to smoke, but up to 20 to 30 pieces of gum are safe depending on the strength of the gum. Use an alternate product if there is evidence of temporomandibular joint disease or the person has dentures or vulnerable dental work. Monitor blood pressure and heart rate. Keep away from children.
Nicotine inhaler	Cough and throat irritation, cardiac and central nervous system stimulation	Nicotine is delivered to the mouth and throat, where it is absorbed through the mucous membranes; the inhaler does not deliver nicotine to the lungs. Caution is necessary for people who have bronchospastic disease; drugs for asthma may need to be adjusted. Monitor blood pressure and heart rate. Keep away from children.
Nicotine nasal spray *(Nicotrol)*	Nasal and sinus irritation, cardiac and central nervous system stimulation	Instruct client to inhale when compressing the nasal pump to distribute nicotine to nasal mucosa. This is not to be used longer than 6 months. Monitor blood pressure and heart rate. Drug-seeking people may abuse this system. Keep away from children.

Cognition and Sensory Perception

The young adult's brain is totally developed although it continues to change in structure and complexity. Additional life experiences refine a person's ability to problem-solve. According to Vander Zanden (2000, p. 633), young adults become more adaptive and knowledgeable about themselves, form values, and develop increased depth in thinking, logical reasoning, and using imagination. As a result, they acquire characteristics of adult maturity (Box 10-1).

Sensory organs undergo slight changes. Hearing, which is most acute at about age 14, gradually declines. Significant hearing loss, if identified at this time, is more likely associated with a history of childhood middle ear infections or exposure to loud music during adolescence.

Musculoskeletal System

Young adults are generally physically strong and resilient. They enjoy remarkable agility and stamina because the musculoskeletal system is functioning optimally. Proprioception, the ability to sense and coordinate body movements, and speed of reaction time reach their peak between ages 20 and 30. By about age 20, changes in general appearance are no longer as rapid as during adolescence. Growth for nonpregnant women and most men is complete. Some men grow a few more inches between ages 18 and 20.

Upper body strength is greater among men than women because of their higher percentage of muscle fibers. Men also have athletic and fitness advantages because the greater size of their heart, lungs, and blood volume facilitates greater aerobic capacity. Because women have more subcutaneous fat than men, they have an advantage in using fat stores when necessary for additional energy (Murray & Zentner, 2001).

Integumentary System

Skin blemishes, a problem during puberty and adolescence, tend to resolve. Facial hair for young men is more widely distributed and requires daily shaving. Wisdom teeth or third molars, if present, erupt during early young adulthood. Men who inherit male pattern baldness may note early thinning or loss of hair at the hairline.

TATTOOS. Micropigmentation, the application of pigment to the skin, is used medically as an adjunct to procedures such as breast reconstruction surgery (see Chap. 54). It has also been used to recreate the appearance of eyebrows on persons who have lost their facial hair (see Chap. 63). A growing trend among young adults is to have a tattoo, a graphic design using permanently colored pigments, applied to their skin. The pigments in tattoo inks pose several health risks. Allergies to the pigments can occur; once applied, the pigments are difficult or impossible to remove. The pigments can also interfere with the quality of magnetic resonance imaging (MRI) when the metallic components of the procedure interact within the pigment, causing swelling or burning in the area of the tattoo.

Infection is another potential complication. Unless the equipment, including components that hold needles, is sterilized, the potential exists for transmitting blood-borne infectious diseases, such as hepatitis (see Chap. 49) and AIDS (see Chap. 37). The American Association of Blood Banks rejects potential blood donors who have received a tattoo in the past year.

Other consequences of tattooing are related to traumatized skin. A granuloma, an inflammatory nodular lesion, may form. Body cells, sensing the pigment particles as foreign, attack the particles (see Chap. 35). Some persons, especially those with darkly pigmented skin, have a tendency to form keloids, an overgrowth of scar tissue.

A common problem is that the person regrets having a tattoo or is dissatisfied with its appearance. Tattoos can be removed, but the skin rarely returns to its pretattoo appearance. Techniques for changing the skin's appearance include the following:

- Laser treatments, which tend only to lighten tattoos
- Dermabrasion, which mechanically rubs away the skin layers, sometimes leaving scar tissue in its place
- Salabrasion, which uses a salt solution rather than a sanding disc or wire brush to abrade the skin
- Scarification of the skin with an acid solution
- Plastic surgery, in which fluid-filled balloons are inserted under the skin to stretch it so that once the tattooed skin is removed, the wound edges can be approximated
- Retattooing to camouflage the existing tattoo

BODY PIERCING. Body piercing, the act of inserting a metal ring, barbell, or other device through the lips, cheeks, nose, tongue, eyebrow, or other areas, is a growing trend among young adults. Infection, allergic reactions, and bleeding are potential complications. The airway may be obstructed from swelling when the tongue is pierced. Oral devices can damage teeth, interfere with speaking and swallowing, and cause respiratory complications if devices are inhaled.

BOX 10-1 ● Characteristics of Adult Maturity

- Developing personal self-reliance
- Learning from past experiences
- Communicating feelings
- Respecting others
- Coping with stressors
- Restraining impulses
- Being accountable
- Accepting consequences of decisions

Social Characteristics

The young adult's social network undergoes major changes: relationships with high school classmates dwindle after graduation; peer conformity loses its importance; and new acquaintances at college, work, or in the community replace former close friendships. Eventually, young persons establish their independence; develop their own lifestyles; form new relationships with friends, coworkers, and a significant other; and take on increasing responsibilities, such as working full-time and raising children. Education after high school and employment offer the means for achieving greater independence.

Marking the Transition

In the United States, identifying the end of adolescence and the beginning of young adulthood is difficult. The transition is less clear than it is in other less industrialized cultures, where rituals provide formal rites of passage. For example, in aboriginal Australia 16-year-old boys leave home for a *walkabout,* which tests survival skills and cunning to stay alive in country outback areas for approximately 6 months. Upon return, the village accepts the adolescent as a mature adult.

In the United States, the traditional mark of adulthood was a person's ability to live independently of parental support. Prior to World War II, most adolescents assumed adult roles very quickly. That trend has changed. Sociologists observe that an immediate need for adolescents to become independent members of society no longer exists. Instead, there is an **adolescent moratorium,** during which persons aged 18 to 27 years may continue to live at home with parental support while working or going to school.

Society encourages individuals to prove readiness for adulthood by participating in activities outside the home and school. Examples include youth ministry and community service. Other life events help demonstrate passage into maturity.

> **Stop, Think, and Respond ● BOX 10-1**
>
> *How is initiation into a gang or fraternity similar to a rite of passage like a walkabout?*

Gender Roles

Developing qualities that transform adolescents into mature adults is a gradual process, such as development of gender roles. **Gender role,** behaviors ascribed by society as either feminine or masculine, continues to be refined during young adulthood. Young adults may cling to or reject society's stereotypical notions about gender differences such as men must make more money than women and women are primary nurturers. Some may experience extreme conflict when circumstances, such as a traumatic injury or chronic disease, interfere with their perception of gender role. The best outcome occurs when young adults develop a perspective of androgeny. **Androgeny** is the belief that it is acceptable to perform roles traditionally ascribed to men or women regardless of gender.

The feminist movement raised America's consciousness of social and gender inequities. It liberated women from being homemakers to working full-time or part-time outside the home. Both sexes now feel more comfortable seeking employment in previous gender-specific occupations and professions. Men are accepted in nursing and women are accepted as physicians. Financial inequities still exist among women in male-dominated positions, however, and fewer women are heads of businesses and corporations.

Sexuality

Young adults are very sexually active and abortion is more common (Daccy & Travers, 1996). By age 22, 90% of young adults have had a sexual relationship with one or more partners (Vander Zanden, 2000). Although AIDS is the leading cause of death among 25- to 44-year-old African-American men and the fifth leading cause of death among all races and both sexes in this age group (see Chap. 37), AIDS has had little effect on whether couples have unprotected sex. Many unmarried and non-monogamous young adults use condoms only to prevent pregnancy. Consequently, if a woman is using a reliable contraceptive (e.g, taking an oral contraceptive), neither she nor her male partner is likely to use a condom during intercourse. The result is that many young adults are acquiring and spreading sexually transmitted diseases (STDs).

On a positive note, sexual promiscuity has decreased, meaning that when sexual intercourse occurs, it is generally between individuals who are involved in an ongoing social relationship. And, although young adults have multiple sex partners before marriage, the number of sexual contacts they have is fewer than those of previous generations. A small number of young adults are vowing to remain sexually abstinent until married.

Although heterosexuality is the norm, homosexuality does not carry the stigma it once did. Many gay men and lesbians have committed monogamous relationships.

Family Structures

Although some cohabitating adults choose to remain childless, most young adults marry and have children. More young adults, however, are marrying later in life than age mates of previous generations. The average age for marriage is now 25 to 26 years old (Vander Zanden, 2000). Later age at marriage contributes to smaller family sizes. Many women wait until their 30s and even 40s to have their first child. Reproductive technology is facilitating pregnancies for women who previously would have been childless such as perimenopausal women, single women, and lesbians. Some infertile couples may feel unfulfilled. Nurses can refer childless couples to local and international agencies providing adoptive services.

A **nuclear family,** or **traditional family,** consists of a married man and woman with biologic offspring. Other family variations are common. A **single-parent family** is one in which one biologic parent provides for the well-being of one or more children. A **blended family** refers to a married couple who are caretakers of children from each spouse's previous marriage(s). An **extended family** is multigenerational.

Prevalent Psychosocial Problems

Young adults face many crises, including job insecurity, unemployment, and sexual harassment. Crime and violence are national problems involving young adults. The highest rates of violent crime (i.e., murder, forcible rape, aggravated assault, robbery) occur among those aged 15 to 25 years (Butts, 1999). The leading cause of death among 18 to 35 year olds is homicide, supporting the validity of crime statistics (Fig. 10.1). In 1995, 77% of murder victims were males, and 88% were 18 years of age or older (U.S. Department of Justice, 1996). Crime also includes such problems as rape, domestic violence, and stalking, the victims of which are primarily women.

Unemployment and Downsizing

Close to 2 million Americans lose their jobs each year; more than 20% of adults who lose their jobs are out of work for at least 6 months (Carson & Arnold, 1999). To remain profitable and competitive, employers are reducing their numbers of full-time workers. Thus, many young adults are part-time, temporary, and subcontracted workers. Consequently, many working young adults do not receive health insurance and other full-time benefits.

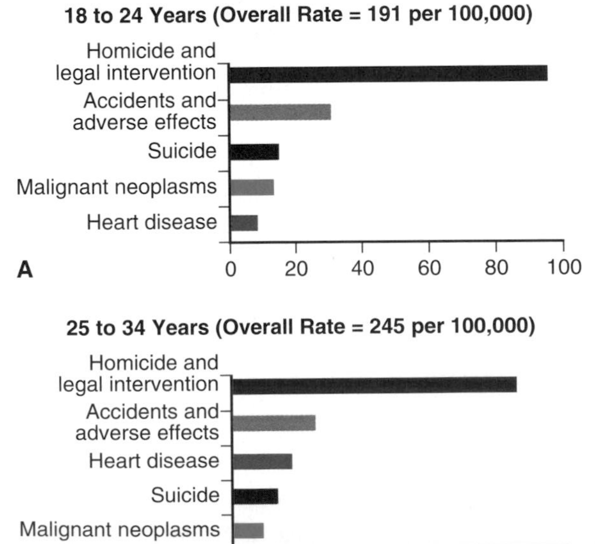

FIGURE 10.1 Note that death by homicide far surpasses the other leading causes of death in adults aged (**A**) 18 to 24 and (**B**) 25 to 34. (Source: www.iihe.org/information/Databook1996/T17_DeathCausesLeadingAge.htm)

Rape

Rape is any forced sexual act in which there is vaginal, oral, or anal penetration, including that which is performed with an inserted object. Rape occurs even if the victim consents out of fear of violence or death. Rape is a crime. It is not motivated by a desire for sex. Rather, it is a manifestation of a need for dominance and control using sex as a weapon.

Although women are the usual victims and men are the usual perpetrators, rape can occur regardless of gender. Rape even occurs among gays and lesbians. Rape statistics are unreliable because an estimated 84% of cases are unreported. Researchers believe that one out of every three women will be raped in her lifetime (District of Columbia Rape Crisis Center, 1998).

TYPES OF RAPE. There are three types of rape: (1) *stranger rape,* in which the victim does not know the perpetrator, (2) *marital rape,* which involves spouses, and (3) *date rape,* also called acquaintance rape, in which the victim knows the assailant. Date rapes account for more than 60% of all rapes (Cooperation Extension, 2001). Gang rape, which is less common, involves several perpetrators (Fontaine and Fletcher, 2003). Box 10-2 gives information on methods of preventing rape.

Stop, Think, and Respond ● BOX 10-2

A student returns to her apartment from the library. Her boyfriend accuses her of being out with another man. He pulls her into the bedroom and insists on having sex. She resists, but her boyfriend says, "If you love me, prove it." They have sex. Has a rape occurred?

DATE-RAPE DRUGS. There is an increased use of drugs that lead to date rape. Three common methods are involved:

- Alcohol (the most common)—the majority of rapes occur when one or both people are drinking and experience disinhibition and impaired judgement
- Combination of alcohol and flunitrazepam (Rohypnol)—known as the *date rape drug,* called "Rophie" for short—potentiates alcohol and interferes with memory
  - Drug is tasteless, colorless, odorless, and dissolves quickly in drinks
  - Sedation occurs in 15 to 20 minutes—lasts 6 hours
  - Causes temporary paralysis, inability to speak, and unconsciousness

BOX 10-2 ● Advice for Rape Prevention

- Install deadbolt locks on doors.
- Keep ground floor windows and patio doors secured.
- Use a door viewer to identify visitors.
- Do not let a stranger into your home or apartment.
- Avoid going alone to a basement laundry room in an apartment building.
- Use your first initial and last name on your mailbox and phone listing.
- Ask a friend to accompany you on walks; some colleges and universities have volunteers that will escort students to and from their dormitory to other places on campus such as the library.
- Carry a whistle and keys in your hand while walking alone.
- Yell, "Call 911. I'm being attacked" rather than "Help," to which few people respond.
- Avoid listening to tapes, compact discs, or radios with earphones while walking; it may distract your attention.
- Park in well-lit areas.
- Stay in your locked car when there is a mechanical problem and put on flashing hazard lights.
- Ask someone to call the police rather than leave your car.
- Keep your distance if someone asks for information from a car.

    - Most rapes are not reported—victim has little or no recall
    - If rape is suspected, drug is not detected in blood after 4 hours and not in urine after 72 hours
- Gamma hydroxy-butyrate (GHB)—central nervous system depressant that produces drowsiness, dizziness, unconsciousness, seizures, respiratory depression, and coma

See Client and Family Teaching 10-1.

RAPE AVOIDANCE TECHNIQUES. Predicting rape is difficult. Rapists, however, are often controlling men who exhibit loss of temper, jealousy, physical or verbal abuse, and intolerance of differences of opinion. What may seem to be minimal faults early in a relationship can escalate into something more serious later.

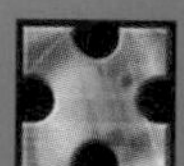

10-1 *Client and Family Teaching* Avoiding Rape Drugs

To avoid being drugged and subsequently raped, the nurse can teach clients the following:

- Do not accept alcoholic beverages from strangers.
- Report seeing someone dropping any substance into a drink.
- Open all cans or bottles of beverages yourself.
- Avoid mixed drinks served in glasses.
- Never leave a drink unattended while dancing or using the rest room.
- Watch as any mixed drink is being prepared.
- Seek medical attention if you think you have been drugged.

Trusting one's instincts is always best. If a person has the slightest premonition that a situation may become dangerous, it is important to leave. The longer a possible victim remains in the immediate environment, the greater the potential for rape. If there is no avenue for escape, the person should say "No!" with conviction. Potential victims of rape should avoid smiling when saying "No" because it sends a mixed message. They should say the word "rape" to emphasize the seriousness of what may happen. Emotionally charged words often cause a potential rapist to reconsider the consequences of persisting. If aborting an attack is impossible, the victim should resist if it is safe to do so. Resisting is foolhardy, however, if the rapist has a weapon.

CARING FOR RAPE VICTIMS. Rape victims need treatment as soon as possible following the assault. Feelings of shame, fear, and disbelief often interfere with obtaining appropriate care. Those who seek medical attention often display one of the following responses: an *expressive style* of response in which the victim cries or sobs and is restless, hyperalert, and tense or a *controlled style* of response in which the victim is calm, composed, and subdued (Carson & Arnold, 1996). Victims with a controlled response contradict the stereotypical expectation and are less likely to be believed than those who are intensely emotional. Nurses should not assume that a person who remains controlled is any less traumatized by the rape than one who is expressive. Above all, healthcare workers and law enforcement officers must believe all victims who say they were raped and convey that the rape was not the victim's fault.

The rape victim must not bathe or shower, douche, or destroy clothing. Initial treatment involves attending to injuries, providing prophylaxis against pregnancy and STDs, giving emotional support, and collecting legal evidence. Nursing Care Plan 10-1 provides extensive information on nursing care and management of rape.

Rape victims sometimes experience long-term consequences of their attack, especially those who refuse counseling or are not referred for counseling. Clients who have been raped are at risk for the development of posttraumatic stress disorder (see Chap. 14).

Domestic Violence

The notion that all couples and families "live happily ever after" is false. Unfortunately, some loving relationships turn violent. **Domestic violence** is a pattern of physical, sexual, and psychological attacks that adults use to control their intimate relationships (Gerard, 2000). Domestic violence involves:

- Couples who are or were formerly married, living together, or dating
- People related by blood, marriage, or adoption
- Couples who have one or more minor children in common

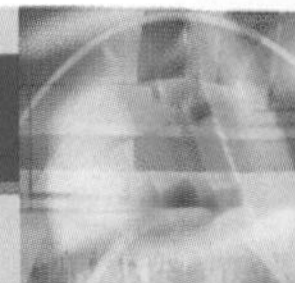

Nursing Care Plan 10-1

THE CLIENT WHO HAS BEEN RAPED

Assessment

- Ask the client:
  - Time, location, and circumstances of the attack
  - Identity of perpetrator, if known
  - Description of perpetrator, if unknown
  - Type of sexual assault: oral, vaginal, anal
  - For female client, date of last menstrual period
  - Current use of condom or other contraceptive by victim or perpetrator
  - Date of last consensual intercourse
  - Current or recent treatment for STD
  - Who to call for emotional support and safety after treatment
  - If a rape crisis advocate can be contacted
  - If the client needs temporary shelter upon discharge
- Examine the client for physical injuries.

Nursing Diagnosis: **Rape Trauma Syndrome**

Expected Outcome: Client will work through feelings associated with rape and recover from the experience.

Interventions	*Rationales*
Ensure privacy but remain with client at all times.	Privacy ensures client's dignity. Staying with client reduces fear and anxiety.
Convey that the rape was not the client's fault.	Many rape victims blame themselves; dispel this false belief.
Remain nonjudgmental.	Clients often feel unjustifiably shameful and guilty.
Ask permission to photograph client and areas of injury.	Giving the opportunity to decide restores a sense of control for client; photographs demonstrate the magnitude of rape and physical assault to a jury.
Identify each person involved in client's care and treatment and purpose for his or her involvement.	Client may feel revictimized when approached by strangers. Information reduces anxiety.
Explain the process of collecting evidence.	Evidence is necessary for future legal prosecution. Even if the client does not want to prosecute the perpetrator, he or she may change that decision in the future.
Assist client to remove clothes—place them in evidence bag. Assist physician to collect head and pubic hair, swabs from vagina, penis, mouth, and anus. Collect saliva and blood samples. Scrape or clip fingernails—deposit specimens in evidence kit. Perform tests for STDs. Assure that specimens are sealed and accurately marked.	Accurate collection of physical evidence helps to successfully prosecute perpetrator, match for DNA evidence, and diagnose and treat STDs.
Offer and explain the purpose of postcoital contraception.	Postcoital contraception prevents implantation of a fertilized ovum and avoids pregnancy.

(continued)

Nursing Care Plan 10-1 (Continued)

THE CLIENT WHO HAS BEEN RAPED

Interventions	*Rationales*
Notify a support person, rape crisis counselor, or both.	The support of a significant other and encouragement to process the rape verbally help reduce the potential for post-traumatic stress disorder.
Offer client an opportunity to shower after physical evidence has been obtained.	Meeting hygiene needs helps to eliminate the physical and emotional trauma of being sexually violated.
Provide disposable underwear and a scrub suit until client has access to personal clothing.	Clean clothing restores dignity.
Arrange for temporary shelter in a safe house if client fears returning home.	Client may have flashbacks of the rape if he or she returns to the place of the assault before feeling a measure of safety.
Arrange a referral for long-term counseling.	Individual and group therapies help clients recover from psychological trauma.
Schedule a date for medical follow-up.	Postdischarge assessment will verify prevention of pregnancy and prevention or appropriate management of STDs.

Evaluation of Expected Outcome: Client returns to a similar level of functioning as before the rape.

Statistics on domestic violence are staggering. Although men are battered, in about 95% of cases, men are the batterers. One woman in four is physically abused by her partner (Gerard, 2000), resulting in 2 to 3 million severe assaults every year. A woman is beaten every 15 seconds, and 2000 to 4000 women are murdered every year by their husbands or live-in boyfriends (Fontaine & Fletcher, 2003). Abusive partners often lived with and observed their own parents' violent relationships, which conditions them to believe that violence within a relationship is normal. Other reasons that cause a person to become violent include feelings of inadequacy, depression, and substance abuse.

Physical abuse is obvious by the resulting injuries. If physical abuse is occurring, generally other types of abuse are too. Psychological abuse includes verbal insults, threats that create fear for one's life (especially if the victim reveals the abuse to others), isolation, and control over daily activities. Batterers of spouses or partners commonly abuse children as well.

PATTERN OF DOMESTIC VIOLENCE. Most cases of domestic violence follow a three-stage pattern: tension-building, acute battering, and a honeymoon period. During the *tension-building phase,* which may last several years, there is verbal abuse and minor forms of physical abuse such as slapping and shoving. The *acute battering phase* is manifested by overt violence like choking, breaking bones, or using a weapon. This phase generally lasts for 24 hours or less. During the *honeymoon phase,* which shortly follows the acute battering phase, the batterer appears remorseful and behaves in ways to convince the victim that he or she will be nonviolent. The batterer may send flowers or give some other token of affection. Most victims want to believe that the relationship will improve, and they may even blame themselves for triggering the violent episode. As tension returns, however, the cycle of violence is repeated.

CARING FOR VICTIMS OF DOMESTIC VIOLENCE. Nurses are likely to see female victims of domestic violence in Emergency Departments (EDs). These women often come alone and present with repeated injuries (particularly to the head, upper body, and breasts) or stress-related disorders. Previous hospital records may be linked to repeated abuse; in fact, acts of violence and subsequent injuries tend to escalate in severity over time. During the history, the client's explanation for the injury may be incompatible with the extent of the trauma.

Unlike cases of child abuse, nurses are not obligated to report their suspicions of abuse between partners to legal authorities. But nurses can intervene in other ways, as discussed in Nursing Guidelines 10-1.

Nursing Implications

When caring for young adults, nurses must be aware of common patterns of behavior affecting health and well-being of individuals within this age group. Clients in this

NURSING GUIDELINES 10-1

Interventions In Cases Of Domestic Violence

- Ask the client if the injuries are the result of physical abuse.
- Assess if the client wants help in leaving the batterer. A woman may choose to remain in an abusive relationship for several reasons (Table 10.1), and nurses must respect her choice. Danger is greatest when a woman attempts to terminate the relationship with the batterer. According to Gerard (2000, p. 56), "About 70% of intimate partner violence victims who are murdered die either as they're trying to leave or after they've moved."
- Discuss safe places for the person to retreat when there is potential for future violence. If escape is impossible, rooms to avoid include the bathroom (where no exit is possible) and rooms where weapons may be kept (kitchen or bedroom).
- Tell the victim to memorize phone numbers of people who can help during an altercation. The victim should develop a "code word" with phone contacts to alert them to need for assistance.
- Provide the address and phone number of one or more domestic assault shelters; shelters house victims and their children for 4 to 6 weeks while providing food, counseling, and help with finding employment, alternative housing, and financial assistance.
- Explain the process of obtaining an emergency **personal protection order,** a document that forbids contact between the batterer and victim for a specified period, or a **temporary restraining order,** a court-ordered directive requiring that the batterer avoid all contact with the victim.
- Advise the client to call the police if her physical safety is threatened. Police are more likely to arrest a person who violates a court-ordered directive.
- Recommend that the client insist that responding police officers complete an official report and write down the number of the report before leaving so it can be accessed in the future.
- Encourage clients to press charges against the batterer. Prosecuting attorneys make the final decisions about whether to prosecute a batterer based on if evidence is sufficient to win the case.
- Tell the victim to contact the Legal Aid Office or Friend of the Court for legal assistance. A batterer may be tried in a civil court more successfully than in a criminal court.
- Suggest that police or a friend photograph any evidence of physical injury which may be used in court if the victim brings criminal charges against the batterer.
- Offer the phone number of the community mental health association where therapists are available for crisis intervention and group and family therapy.
- Recommend discussing personal safety with an employer and the employer's security officer; provide a photo of the abuser.

age group have minimal knowledge of community healthcare resources. Nurses are likely to find that young adults tend to seek healthcare only when they experience an emergency. In many cases, young adults delay seeking medical care because they cannot pay for treatment.

Health Promotion

Young adults perceive themselves as perpetually healthy and invincible. Consequently, many disregard early warning signs of diseases. They often do not consider preventive health measures a priority and disregard healthy behaviors such as obtaining early prenatal care, performing breast or testicular self-examinations, or scheduling regular health and dental examinations. Nurses can distribute educational materials about important health promotion measures at local community health fairs. They may also speak to members of service organizations like the Rotary Club, Big Brothers and Big Sisters, and 4-H leaders.

Illness and Hospitalization

Young adults continue to adjust to their physical characteristics and work through feelings about sexuality. They are apt to be anxious when faced with a medical examination or need for surgery. Careful explanations are essential, as is providing privacy. Such measures convey the nurse's concern about their welfare, understanding of their feelings, and respect for their need for dignity. During database interviews, nurses often find that young adult clients have no knowledge about their family's health history nor their personal history of childhood diseases. Nurses need to collaborate with a family member or rely on past medical records to obtain a comprehensive health history.

During hospitalization, young adults are as frightened as younger clients but show their fear in less obvious ways. Nurses must realize that young adults also require reassurance. It is important to allow young adults to express ideas and ask questions about matters that interest or concern them, and by conveying respect for them as individuals. The nurse also helps young adults cope with their illness, whether temporary or permanent, and teaches them preventive healthcare measures.

Human Immunodeficiency Virus

Nurses who work in public health agencies, acute care settings, and long-term healthcare facilities are likely to see an increase in young adults diagnosed with HIV. Individuals infected with HIV can remain asymptomatic for 10 years or more, yet they are capable of transmitting the virus to others. This information indicates a need for nurses to educate teenagers and adults about the advantages of sexual abstinence, maintaining monogamous relationships with uninfected partners, or using other safer sex practices. Unfortunately, when HIV becomes

TABLE 10.1 REASONS PEOPLE REMAIN IN ABUSIVE RELATIONSHIPS

EMOTIONAL	FINANCIAL	SOCIAL
Fear for life Hope that the batterer will change Belief that batterer is basically a good person Belief that batterer has more good qualities than bad	Lack of employment No access to cash or bank assets	Lack of support from friends and family Acceptance of responsibility for saving the relationship Blame of batterer's behavior on substance abuse, finances, or job-related stressors Correlation of ending the relationship with failure Protection of public image of family Belief that it is better for children to be raised by two people rather than one Lack of knowledge about a means to end the relationship Desire to protect children from greater harm

active, infected adults succumb to and need treatment for opportunistic infections and eventually require terminal care (see Chap. 37).

MIDDLE ADULTHOOD

Middle age, generally from ages 35 to 65 years, is characterized as the "established years." During this period, the person may actualize earlier struggles of youth, adolescence, and young adulthood to establish a home and career. Middle-aged adults can analyze their assets and channel their energies into accomplishing life goals that remain unfulfilled. The middle years are characterized by pursuit of activities that provide self-satisfaction and community responsibility.

Demographics

Middle-aged Americans compose about one-fifth of the U.S. population. Many of them entered the job market and made their way in the labor force during the late 1960s and 1970s. Now, one American turns 50 years old every 7.6 seconds. Each middle adult is experiencing life stresses and major changes. Many are feeling the psychological pressures associated with the shift from the industrial age to the information age.

Developmental Stage and Task: Generativity Versus Stagnation

The task of terminating early adulthood involves reviewing the past, considering how one's life is going, and deciding the future. Many begin to experience the gap between earlier life aspirations and current achievements. They may wonder about continuing with earlier life choices. During this period, a person may choose a different career path or redefine his or her current roles. This is a time when people take "stock" of current life situations, analyze, and make necessary adjustments.

Triggered by the realization that life is rapidly advancing, the middle years are a time when adults take inventory of their lives. As young adults, these people focused on setting goals. As middle adults, they evaluate if, and how well, they are achieving their goals.

Middle-aged adults are more likely to ponder the purpose for and value of their existence. Knowing that their remaining years are limited, they want to survey their achievements and pursue opportunities for self-fulfillment, a characteristic referred to as **generativity.** Middle-aged adults become more caring, giving, and productive. Many spend time comforting, advising, and listening to younger family members or close friends and volunteering in civic activities.

On self-examination, some middle-aged adults are disappointed to find that they have not invested their energies wisely. The feeling that they have accomplished nothing of true significance along with a lack of commitment to future endeavors is referred to as **stagnation.** Box 10-3 summarizes the major developmental tasks of the middle-aged adult.

Physical Characteristics

The middle years are productive years, yet the pace of living changes subtly. Evidence of declining physical abilities becomes apparent. The incidence of various health problems increases with age. About 35 million Americans (1 in 7) have disabilities ranging from arthritis, diabetes, and emphysema to mental disorders. People can maximize their chances for a healthy long life by altering their

BOX 10-3 ● Major Developmental Tasks of the Middle-Aged Adult

- Reassessing life accomplishments and goals
- Adjusting to role changes
- Accepting physical, emotional, and social changes associated with middle age
- Planning for retirement
- Strengthening relationships with spouse, family, friends, or companions
- Adjusting to responsibilities for aging parents
- Developing skills, hobbies, or activities that provide satisfaction

lifestyles to include various health conscious practices such as exercising regularly and eating a healthy diet.

The human body, which has been functioning optimally for several decades, tends to work less efficiently. Early signs of aging appear, which can be traumatic, especially in the U.S. culture, which emphasizes youth and glamour.

Weight

As a person moves into middle adulthood, weight becomes a concern. About 50% of the adult population weighs above the upper limit of normal. About 40% become overweight as a result of genetics. Others become overweight from changes in the **basal metabolic rate** (BMR), the minimum energy a person uses in a resting state. Sex and age affect BMR, which drops quickly during adolescence and then more slowly during adulthood. Decreased BMR is caused by a drop in the ratio of lean body mass to fat. Thus, if a person continues to eat the same foods, he or she will tend to gain weight.

Adults tend not to exercise routinely, which compounds weight gain. Added weight is responsible for many health problems. Adults with weight problems need to work closely with their physicians and a nutritionist who can assist with meal planning. Adults should avoid fad diets and crash diets, as they do more harm than good. Eating properly and following a routine exercise program can ward off unwanted pounds.

Respiratory System

The lungs begin to change. The extent of such changes depends on lifestyle, predisposition to illnesses such as asthma, and environmental hazards. Staying active and either walking or engaging in some form of aerobic exercise will maintain lung function.

Smoking is a serious problem in the United States and leads to many health deficits such as emphysema, lung cancer, and chronic lung changes and conditions. Smoking is the number one controllable cause of cancer, responsible for at least 30% of cancer deaths. Various smoke reduction programs are available to those who wish to make this lifestyle change.

Cardiovascular System

Cardiovascular disease is the leading killer of adults today. Genetics and lifestyle play important roles. Men are at higher risk in comparison to premenopausal women; however, the risks equalize for men and women after menopause. African-American men are at a higher risk of heart disease than are white men.

Arteries continue to fill with deposits of fat, while calcium infiltrates the fatty plaque making the arteries hard and inelastic. Mild hypertension (high blood pressure) is a common sign of early heart disease and can also affect the kidneys and brain. Medications can help reduce high blood pressure. Regular blood pressure screenings several times a year are recommended during the middle years.

Cholesterol, a white, waxy fat that occurs naturally in the body, has become the "buzz word" in health since the 1990s. The National Cholesterol Education Program suggests regular testing of cholesterol levels starting at age 20 years. Dietary changes to reduce consumption of saturated fats and increasing activity level through regular exercise can raise the beneficial high-density lipoprotein (HDL) cholesterol and lower the damaging low-density lipoprotein (LDL) cholesterol. Educating adults about maintaining a healthy lifestyle by watching their weight, decreasing salt intake, decreasing cholesterol and fats, decreasing alcohol intake, decreasing or stopping smoking, learning stress management techniques, and increasing exercise can reduce the risk of hypertension and cardiac problems.

Neurologic System

Intellectual and stimulating hobbies, such as reading, working with computer programs, and solving crossword puzzles, can slow the process of brain cell loss. Other factors affect brain activity, such as alcohol intake or diseases such as cerebrovascular accident (stroke), Parkinson's disease, or Alzheimer's disease. A cerebrovascular accident occurs when blood circulation to the brain fails. Brain cells die from decreased blood flow and the resulting lack of oxygen. Both blockage and bleeding can be involved. Stroke is the third leading killer of Americans and the most common cause of disability. Each year more than 500,000 Americans have a stroke, with about 145,000 dying. Strokes occur in all age groups, both sexes, and all races of every country.

Cognition and Sensory Perception

Visual accommodation, the ability to focus an image on the retina, gradually declines. Between age 40 to 50 years, many people notice difficulty in reading small print or performing other tasks that require close vision. This condition, called **presbyopia,** results from a loss of elasticity in the lens of the eye. Because the lens tends to be more rigid, middle adults need more time to adjust to rapid changes in light and darkness. Changes in the lens, such as thickening, decreased flexibility, and increased opacity, cause glare sensitivity. Other eye conditions, such as glaucoma, dry eye, or floaters, can appear. Another condition called *macular degeneration* may become apparent, which can fade, distort, or blur vision. Annual eye examinations may prevent many of these eye conditions (see Chap. 43).

Presbycusis is hearing loss associated with aging. High-pitched sounds diminish first. Some people, particularly those in their later middle years, find that the decrease interferes with hearing and communicating with others.

Teeth strength may begin to decline, which could cause teeth to fall out. Dental examinations every 6 months are recommended.

Taste buds are replaced at a slower rate, which may account for changes in food-related tastes. Smell receptors begin to deteriorate, also affecting the sense of taste.

Reproductive System

Couples have a variety of contraceptive measures available to limit family size during their reproductive years. The use of oral contraceptives, however, especially among middle-aged women who smoke, increases the risk for blood clot formation.

Climacteric refers to abrupt changes in the body caused by alterations in the secretion and balance of hormones. Women between ages 40 and 55 years experience a dramatic physiologic change in the reproductive system known as **menopause** (see Chap. 53). Ovulation becomes irregular toward late mid-life and eventually ceases. Reduced estrogen also causes changes in secondary sex characteristics (Box 10-4).

As men age, the ability to achieve and sustain an erection slightly diminishes, and the prostate gland enlarges. Male fertility extends long past that of women.

Mid-life men and women remain at risk for HIV/AIDS. The number of cases among middle and older women has been steadily increasing, mainly among postmenopausal women who no longer use birth control. Because of their age or monogamous marital status, these women do not see themselves as being at risk for HIV/AIDS or other sexually transmitted diseases (STDs). Health providers also do not regularly ask for sexual histories or test for HIV/AIDS/STDs in this population. Anyone who is sexually active, however, is at risk for HIV/AIDS (see Chap. 37).

BOX 10-4 ● Secondary Sex Changes With Decreased Estrogen

- Breasts begin to droop and sag.
- Vaginal mucous membranes become dry and easily irritated.
- Pubic hair becomes sparse and gray.
- Vaginal lubrication decreases.
- Mood swings are common.
- Hot flashes and headaches occur.
- Bones become more brittle as a result of loss of calcium.
- Vascular changes are accelerated.

Urinary System

Men older than age 50 years begin to notice slight changes in urinary patterns, such as hesitancy, reduced force of urinary stream, or fullness in the bladder. These signs are indicators of prostatic hypertrophy (see Chap. 55). Women who have had several children often experience stress incontinence from a relaxation of the pelvic floor muscles. Coughing, sneezing, or laughing may cause leakage of urine.

Musculoskeletal System

Height remains constant until the late stages of middle adulthood when there is a slight decline. Adipose and connective tissues gradually replace muscle mass, which compromises strength. Muscles can begin to atrophy, although this development is less noticeable in men. Regular exercise combining both cardiovascular exercise and strength training can prevent most muscle aging.

Range of joint motion diminishes from a sedentary lifestyle or damage to joints from hard work. Bone mass becomes increasingly porous, particularly in women after menopause, leading to **osteoporosis.** Women should take calcium supplements or drugs that prevent bone resorption as recommended by their physician. These debilitating processes can go unnoticed until a simple injury has serious consequences, such as a fracture or delayed healing.

Rheumatoid arthritis (RA), an inflammatory disease that causes pain, swelling, and loss of joint function, can occur in middle age (see Chap. 61). Some have mild forms of RA; others live with serious disability. Physicians classify RA as an autoimmune disease, which means that the person's own immune system is attacking his or her own body tissue (see Chap. 36). Although no single test for RA is available, especially in its early stages, laboratory and radiographic tests can determine the extent of bone damage and monitor the progression of this disease. See Chapter 61 for more detail about treatment and nursing management of RA.

Integumentary System

Subcutaneous fat disappears toward the end of the middle-age period, giving the face a bony appearance. Age lines or wrinkles are evident at the forehead, corners of the eyes, and mouth. The skin appears wrinkled and dry from chronic exposure to the sun.

Keratotic lesions, elevated, darkly pigmented skin plaques, appear as moles on the scalp, face, neck, or trunk (Fig 10.2). The hair loses texture and color. Baldness becomes more evident among men. Change in the balance of estrogen and testosterone causes facial hair or

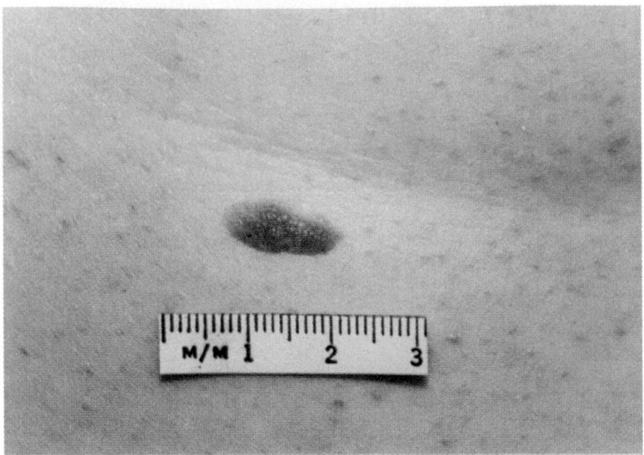

FIGURE 10.2 Keratotic lesion.

hair growth about the nipples and chest area in postmenopausal women.

> **Stop, Think, and Respond ● BOX 10-3**
>
> *What advice would you give to "sun worshippers"?* 

Social Characteristics

During middle age, most adults remain socially involved with relatives and friends. As their children marry, the social network of middle adults expands to include sons- and daughters-in-law. When children leave home, middle-aged couples have more time to spend with each other. For many couples, this strengthens the relationship. Others find that the relationship has changed since the years of childrearing, causing them to feel distant and estranged from each other. Irreconcilable differences may lead to separation or divorce.

Couples who remain together tend to be more financially secure than they were during early adulthood. Many start to focus on ensuring that their savings will be adequate during their retirement years.

Adults in this age group are often described as the **sandwich generation,** because many are raising children while assuming increasing responsibility for aging parents. As a result, they are "sandwiched" between two generations. Some middle adults also care for their grandchildren. These added responsibilities can thwart the middle-aged adult's independence and create a crisis. Well-adjusted middle adults view the added responsibilities of aging parents and children as part of life.

> **Stop, Think, and Respond ● BOX 10-4**
>
> *Middle adulthood is also labeled as the "empty nest years," symbolizing the departure of children from the parental home. What are some potential problems that may result from the "empty nest"?*

Prevalent Psychosocial Issues and Problems

Personality is viewed as the combination of particular dynamic traits that continue to develop and change throughout adulthood. For many middle-aged adults, new events and challenges influence their personality.

Aging tends to be emotionally difficult in the U.S. culture. Many Americans value youth and energy more than the experience and wisdom that accompany passing years. Many people associate mid-life with change and loss. Depression in mid-life is common but often unrecognized and untreated. Suicide risk increases with age, especially for adult men.

Some middle-aged clients develop a **mid-life crisis,** in which they view themselves as less likely to accomplish the goals of their youth. Even those who have accomplished their goals and seem successful have feelings of dissatisfaction. To relieve feelings of insecurity and unhappiness over the loss of their youth, some have cosmetic surgery, wear clothing styles more characteristic of younger adults, have extramarital affairs, or abandon their current lifestyle to seek a more meaningful existence.

Financial insecurity also stresses middle-aged adults. Unemployment jeopardizes pension plans, retirement packages, and health insurance benefits. Without insurance coverage, serious illness or injury can mean financial ruin. Caring for elderly parents can be a financial burden as well. Some middle-aged adults feel guilty for not providing the care that aging parents require and worry about finding adequate care or nursing home.

Nursing Implications

Many middle-aged clients are concerned about their physical condition after the illness or death of a friend. They recognize the negative effects of neglecting their health and seek to reform poor health habits. Nurses must identify health risks and teach clients ways to modify or refrain from behaviors that contribute to preventable diseases. Health teaching includes smoking cessation, refraining from excessive alcohol, eating a low-fat diet, exercising regularly, and obtaining regular screening for colorectal, prostate, breast, and cervical cancer. Monthly breast self-examination is important for women in this age group to aid in early detection of breast cancer. Nurses also stress the importance of routine annual examinations, blood work, and other tests to assist in the early detection of many diseases, which is key to treatment and recovery.

Nutrition

Weight tends to increase in middle age, related to excessive calories, decreased metabolic rate, and less activity. A person's diet should include all nutrients he or she needs to maintain and repair body tissue; however, decreased caloric intake is necessary to compensate for decreased activity levels and metabolism.

Because calcium in the bone is constantly being broken down and replenished, calcium requirements remain high. A regular exercise program helps to prevent weight gain, maintains bone mass, and compensates for lowered metabolism.

As adults age, poor dentition may affect the ability to chew food. If the diet is deficient in whole grains, fresh fruits, and uncooked vegetables to compensate for the inability to chew, stool volume and moisture are reduced, which contributes to bowel irregularity and constipation. Nurses should assess for such problems and help the client address them as necessary.

Sleep

Many middle-aged adults fill every hour of the day with activity; consequently, many are also sleep-deprived. Several factors can affect the quality of sleep, including use of caffeine, stimulants, or other medications. Changes in circadian rhythms can also affect sleep patterns. Many middle adults commonly go to sleep, waking a few hours later and unable to return to sleep. Another factor that may disrupt sleep during these years is parents who are waiting for teenagers to come home.

Nurses should assess all clients for sleep disturbances. A few simple techniques such as limiting or eliminating caffeine, engaging in stress reduction techniques (see Chap. 12), attending to stressful issues earlier in the day, cooling the room temperature, taking a warm bath or reading before bed, or listening to soft music may help.

Sexuality

Although sexuality exists throughout the life span, the frequency and vigor of intercourse are likely to decrease during middle adulthood. Sexual effectiveness does not automatically disappear as humans age. Healthy men and women often enjoy sexual functioning well into their 80s. Unfortunately, many clients accept social definitions of themselves as sexless. Believing that they will naturally lose their sexual effectiveness becomes a self-fulfilling prophecy, even though their bodies have not lost the capacity for sex.

Nurses should address issues related to sexuality for all adults. They need to answer questions honestly and provide information and referrals to help clients continue to enjoy this part of life for as long as they desire. For more information on particular issues, treatments, and teaching, see Unit 14.

Critical Thinking Exercises

1. *What data would suggest that a person has positively adjusted to young adulthood?*
2. *When planning a health promotion program for a group of young adults, what topics are most important to include?*
3. *A middle-aged client is admitted for observation after experiencing chest pain. Based on what you know about the physical, emotional, and social characteristics of a person in this age group, what assessments are important to make? Why?*

● NCLEX-STYLE REVIEW QUESTIONS 

1. The nurse is providing client teaching to a middle-aged woman diagnosed with osteoporosis. The nurse is confident that the client has understood the instructions when the client states that to preserve bone mass, she should:
   1. Establish a regular exercise program.
   2. Drink four quarts of milk per day.
   3. Explore use of herbal supplements.
   4. Increase daily intake of caffeine.
2. A nurse is working on a college campus advising young adult women about methods to prevent rape. Which of the following would the nurse teach to be the best method?
   1. Carry a flashlight when going out after dark.
   2. When at the bar, limit drinking to two alcoholic beverages.
   3. After dark, call security to escort the student to the dorm.
   4. Turn the volume down on headsets when walking or jogging.
3. A postmenopausal woman comes to the clinic for a routine annual examination. The client reports that she experiences vaginal dryness during intercourse. Which response by the nurse is most appropriate?
   1. "How long have you had this problem?"
   2. "We better tell the doctor."
   3. "Is your partner upset about your problem?"
   4. "Such dryness is normal from decreased estrogen levels."

connection

Visit the Connection site at **http://connection.lww.com/go/timbyEssentials** for links to chapter-related resources on the Internet.

References and Suggested Readings

Arslanian-Engoren, C. (2000). Gender and age bias in triage decisions. *Journal of Emergency Nursing, 26*(2), 117–124.

Benetos, A., Thomas, F., Safar, M. E., et al. (2001). Should diastolic and systolic blood pressure be considered for cardiovascular risk evaluation: A study in middle-aged men and women. *Journal of the American College of Cardiology, 37*(1), 163–168.

Butts, J. (1999). Youth violence: Perception versus reality. [Online.] Available: http://www.urban.org/crime/module/butts/youth_violence.html.

Carson, V. B., & Arnold, E. N. (1999). *Mental health nursing.* Philadelphia: W. B. Saunders.

Chisholm, J. F. (1999). The sandwich generation. *Journal of Social Distress & the Homeless, 8*(3), 177–191.

Dacey, J., & Travers, J. F. (1996). *Human development across the lifespan.* Madison: Brown & Benchmark.

Davis, N. B., et al. (1999). Motor vehicle crashes and positive toxicology screens in adolescents and young adults. *Journal of Trauma Nursing, 6*(1), 15–18.

DeLaune, S. C., & Ladner, P. K. (1998). *Fundamentals of nursing: Standards and practice.* Albany, NY: Delmar.

District of Columbia Rape Crisis Center. [On-line.] Available: http://www.dcrcc.org.

Dudek, S. (2000). *Nutrition essentials for nursing practice* (4th ed.). Philadelphia: Lippincott Williams & Wilkins.

Edelman, C. L. (2002). *Health promotion throughout the lifespan* (5th ed.). St. Louis: Mosby–Year Book.

Equal Employment Opportunity Commission. (2001). Laws enforced by the EEOC. [On-line.] Available: http://www.eeoc.gov.laws.html.

Fontaine, K. L., & Fletcher, J. S. (2003). *Mental health nursing* (5th ed.). Upper Saddle River, NJ: Pearson Education, Inc.

Fournier, R. A. (1999). The sandwich generation: A continuing education offering. *DNA Reporter, 23*(4), 16–19.

Gerard, M. (2000). Domestic violence, how to screen and intervene. *RN, 63*(12), 52–56.

Kenney, J. W. (2000). Women's 'inner-balance': A comparison of stressors, personality traits, and health problems by age groups. *Journal of Advanced Nursing, 31*(3), 639–650.

Lauer, J. C., & Lauer, R. H. (1999). *How to survive and thrive in an empty nest.* Oakland, CA: New Harbinger Publications.

Martin, M., Grünendahl, M., & Martin, P. (2001). Age differences in stress, social resources, and well-being in middle and older age. *Journals of Gerontology. Series B: Psychological Sciences and Social Sciences, 56B*(4), 214–222.

Murray, R. B., & Zentner, J. P. (2001). *Health promotion strategies through the life span* (7th ed.). Upper Saddle River, NJ: Prentice Hall.

National Commission Against Drunk Driving. (2001). 21–34 Year old young adults, the commission communities project. [On-line.] Available: http://ncadd.com/21_34/index.cfm.

National Institutes of Health. (1998). First federal obesity clinical guidelines released. [On-line.] Available: http://www.nih.gov/news/pr/jun98/nhlbi-17.htm.

Peacock, J. M., Folsom, A. R., Knopman, D. S., et al. (2000). Dietary antioxidant intake and cognitive performance in middle-aged adults. *Public Health Nutrition, 3*(3), 337–343.

Rosdahl, C. B. (2003). *Textbook of basic nursing* (8th ed.). Philadelphia: Lippincott Williams & Wilkins.

Schott-Baer, D., & Kotal, B. (2000). Frequency and effectiveness of self-care actions and menopause symptoms of middle-aged working women. *MEDSURG Nursing, 9*(6), 302–307.

University of Nebraska Cooperation Extension. (2001). [On-line.] Available: http://www.ianr.unl.edu/pubs/family/nf244.htm.

U.S. Department of Health and Human Series, Office of Disease Prevention and Health Promotion. (2000). *Healthy people 2010.* [On-line.] Available: http://www.health.gov.healthypeople.

U.S. Department of Justice, Office of Attorney General. (1999). 1999 Report on cyberstalking: A new challenge for law enforcement and industry. [On-line.] Available: http://www.cybercrime.gov/cyberstalking.htm.

U.S. Department of Justice, Federal Bureau of Investigation. (1996). Uniform crime reporting program press release. [On-line.] Available: http://www.fbi.gov/ucr.

U.S. Department of Justice, Drug Enforcement Agency. (2001). Gamma hydroxybutyrate (GHB). [On-line.] Available: http://usdoj.gov/dea/concern/ghb.htm.

U.S. Food and Drug Administration. (2000). Tattoos and permanent makeup. [On-line.] Available: http://vm.cfsan.fda.gov/~dms.

Vander Zanden, J. W. (2000). *Human development* (7th ed.). Boston: McGraw Hill.

chapter 11

Biopsychosocial Aspects of Caring for Older Adults

Words to Know 

ageism
antioxidants
autophagocytosis
despair
ego integrity
elder abuse
free radicals
gerontology
kyphosis
life review
pet therapy
reality orientation
reminiscence therapy
senescence
validation therapy

Learning Objectives

On completion of this chapter, the reader will:

- List five trends for which society should prepare in view of the growing population of aging adults.
- Identify developmental tasks for older adults.
- Contrast the developmental characteristics of ego integrity and despair.
- Define gerontology.
- Discuss three theories of aging.
- Discuss physical and social characteristics that are unique to adults older than 65 years.
- Discuss factors that affect the emotional health of older adults.
- Define ageism and how it affects older adults.
- Discuss ways that a nurse's attitude concerning the aged can affect their care.
- List approaches the nurse can use when teaching older adults.
- Identify nursing care measures that are especially important when providing physical care for an older adult.
- Describe pet therapy, reality orientation, and reminiscence therapy.

Older adults play a vital role in society, the home, the workplace, and the community. They offer others with less maturity the wisdom of life experiences. Healthcare workers help older adults to maintain their independence, health, and productivity.

OLDER ADULTHOOD

Senescence is the last stage in the life cycle. During senescence, body processes gradually deteriorate. Diet, exercise, stress reduction, and health promotion activities can slow the rate of senescence. This developmental period is subdivided into three categories: the young-old, ages 65 to 74; the middle-old, ages 75 to 84; and the old-old, older than age 85.

Demographics

The number of people older than age 65 is increasing rapidly. Life expectancy has extended for both sexes. Males can expect to live an average of 73 years, and females an average of 79 years (National Institute on Aging, 2001). By 2050, the population of Americans who live to be 85 will represent almost 5% of the U.S. population (Federal Interagency Forum on Aging Related Statistics, 2000). By 2000, centenarians (those age 100 years or older) increased

35% above the number in 1990 (Administration on Aging, 2001).

Developmental Stage and Task: Ego Integrity Versus Despair

During late adulthood, older adults have developmental tasks to complete (Box 11-1). They must discover activities to fill the time previously spent at work and raising families. These activities must sustain a sense of usefulness and self-worth. Older adults must also adjust to losses such as loss of friends or a spouse, loss of income, loss of health and agility, and loss of independence. Aging adults must face their own death.

As aging adults deal with life's remaining challenges, they acknowledge the permanency of past decisions and actions. They develop either a sense of ego integrity or despair as they reflect on their lives. **Ego integrity** is a feeling of personal satisfaction that life has been happy and fulfilling. **Despair** results when a person views life as disappointing and unfulfilling and anguishes over what might have been.

Most older adults engage in **life review,** a process of looking back at one's life and reviewing decisions, choices, conflicts, and resolutions. For integrity to emerge in the older adult, a life review results in belief that life has been meaningful and well spent. If, after a life review, the older adult sees life as ineffective, with poor decisions and unresolved conflict, he or she will feel despair.

Theories of Aging

Gerontology is the study of aging, including physiologic, psychological, and social aspects. It is a young science, as most significant advances in this field have been made since 1950. Research findings enhance understanding of the nature of aging and function. Scientists conduct research to determine actual causes of the aging processes. The goal is to find ways to extend both the quantity and the quality of life.

BOX 11-1 ● Developmental Tasks of the Older Adult

- Adjust to the physical limitations brought about by aging.
- Find satisfaction in retirement.
- Secure acceptable living arrangements.
- Develop meaningful social relationships.
- Adjust to losses accompanying aging (e.g., loss of friends, family, or spouse through death, reduced income, or functional loss).
- Recognize meaning in one's life.
- Accept and prepare for one's own death.

Physical characteristics change throughout the life cycle—hair turns gray, skin wrinkles, bones demineralize, and blood vessels become hard and inelastic. It is not clear what biologic mechanisms trigger these changes. Several theories attempt to explain the aging process. These include:

- **Autophagocytosis** (literally means "to eat self")—Portions of cells are consumed to reduce their size. This occurs when cells sense adverse conditions. Smaller cells decrease energy needs and increase potential for survival. A brown-colored residue called *lipofuscin* forms during this process. This cellular pigment accumulates in older people. Cell shrinkage contributes to decreased weight and height and atrophy of tissues and organs.
- Stress response—Hans Selye, an early 20th century physician, defined the *general adaptation syndrome,* which stated that physiologic responses to physical, psychological, and social changes (which produce biologic stress) are always the same. Gerontologists believe that defense mechanisms associated with stress responses eventually weaken and lead to death.
- Immune system decline—As people age, the immune system becomes impaired, weakening the body's defenses, and leaving it vulnerable to infection and cancer. Others theorize that with immune system decline the body identifies normal cells as foreign, causing the body's defenses to attack healthy cells, advancing the aging process (autoimmune theory of aging).
- Faulty DNA replication—Deoxyribonucleic acid (DNA) molecules in each cell program cellular reproduction. DNA is susceptible to damaging agents (such as free radicals—see below) that are locked onto DNA molecules, interfering with cell reproduction. Aging cells cannot resist cell damage. As a result, tissue disorganization and organ failure occur.
- **Free radicals**—Unstable atoms with excessive energy cause harm to DNA molecules and may be responsible for age-related changes. Chronic exposure to toxins such as radiation contributes to cellular changes. Healthy cells use **antioxidants** to block chemical reactions that create free radicals. Investigations are in process to learn more about the antioxidant effects of vitamins C and E, and provitamin A, also known as *beta carotene.*

Physical Characteristics

In older adults, functional decline will occur without any specific illness. In caring for older clients, nurses must recognize normal physiologic variations that accompany aging. In addition, older adults often manifest diseases with milder or atypical symptoms. Many physical changes seen in older adults are a progression of the changes that occur during middle age (see Chap. 10). Since aging is not a uniform process, organ systems age at different rates, producing alterations in functions. Norms for health and illness are not established for older adults as they are in younger age groups. Landmarks of normal aging are not thoroughly understood. Nurses can compare the older person's patterns of health and illness with current ability, using the client as the standard. The nurse also considers capabilities, social support, and the environment as to effects on overall functioning. Knowledge about the client's particular situation provides an approach to care and helps ensure accurate assessment, interpretation of data, interventions, and evaluations.

Respiratory System

The lungs of the older adult are exposed for many years to smoke, bacteria, and multiple environmental irritants. Age-related changes that do affect the respiratory system are so gradual that most older adults compensate for their effects. Normal aging includes a reduced alveolar surface area, loss of elastic recoil, a decrease in vital capacity and oxygen saturation, decline in host defense and intolerance for exercise.

The rib cage becomes rigid as cartilage calcifies. The thoracic spine shortens and osteoporosis may cause stooped posture, decreasing available lung space, and limiting ability to take deep breaths. Abdominal muscles become weaker, causing decreased inspiratory and expiratory effort. The alveoli enlarge and become thin although numbers remain constant in the absence of chronic pulmonary disease.

Cardiovascular System

Cardiovascular changes associated with aging include decreased cardiac output (volume of blood pumped by the heart), stiffened aorta and arteries, and decreased circulatory system response to demands of activity and exercise. Vital signs changes include increased blood pressure, irregular pulse, and shortness of breath on exertion. Older adults experience postural hypotension (rapid drop in blood pressure when rising or standing from a lying or sitting position). Impaired arterial circulation causes skin to feel cool and the feet to appear purplish or bluish when in a dependent position. Varicose veins (bulging, twisted veins in the legs) cause lower extremities to swell and fatigue easily.

Classic symptoms of cardiovascular diseases in older adults are altered or absent in older adults, so it is important to thoroughly assess clients. Nursing interventions should focus on preventing further disease by helping older people minimize risk factors. Ways to reduce risks are stopping smoking, lowering cholesterol, eating well-balanced meals, limiting salt intake, performing stress reduction techniques, and exercising regularly.

Neurologic System

Many adults worry whether they are thinking, remembering, and making decisions with the same acuity as when they were younger. As early as age 40, adults notice occasional mental lapses. A decline in cognition may accompany normal aging. There is less decline or no decline for people with favorable lifestyles and good health.

The incidence of serious cognitive deficits, like Alzheimer's disease (see Chap. 18), increases with age. Most older adults have better long-term memory than short-term memory. They respond less quickly to questions in an interview. Nurses should not assume, however, that clients are cognitively impaired. Diminished hearing or anxiety slows a client's responses.

Clinical depression, common among older adults, may be mistaken for dementia. Age-related changes in the nervous system are from disease states. Normal changes that occur have little effect on thinking and cognition. Structural changes that accompany aging include loss of neurons and brain weight, accumulations of lipofuscin in the neuronal cytoplasm, slowed synaptic transmissions, and loss of peripheral nerve function. Functional changes include slowed reaction time, impaired thermoregulation, and changes in sleep wave patterns.

Stop, Think, and Respond ● BOX 11-1

Do you think learning stops or changes as a person ages?

Sensory Perception

Most older adults wear glasses. The *presbyopia* (age-related loss of visual acuity for near vision) that began in the middle years becomes more pronounced. Visual acuity declines at an accelerated rate as eye structures degenerate. Most people older than age 70 have some degree of cataract formation. Many avoid driving at night because of difficulty in adjusting to the glare of oncoming headlights.

Hearing loss becomes more pronounced. *Presbycusis* (age-related hearing loss) that began in the middle years progresses. Presbycusis is gradual with initial loss of ability to hear high-pitched sound, followed by decreased ability to hear middle- and low-pitched sounds. Nurses must look for signs of hearing loss because older adults do not always report hearing difficulties.

Position sense and reaction time decline gradually until about age 70, when the rate of decline becomes rapid. Deterioration of these two faculties, together with diminished vision, is a common cause of accidents. Consequently, many older adults are injured in falls.

Stop, Think, and Respond ● BOX 11-2

What are the signs of hearing loss that an older adult may display?

Gastrointestinal System

Changes in the gastrointestinal system are usually not life-threatening, but they may cause the greatest concern and are the source of many complaints for older adults. Gastrointestinal (GI) problems such as constipation, indigestion, diarrhea, nausea, vomiting, weight gain or loss, or increased flatulence (gas) are bothersome and increase even without organic disease. Gallbladder disease and cancers of the GI tract increase with age. Poor nutrition, medications, emotions, inactivity, and various health factors influence the status of the gastrointestinal system.

Age affects virtually every area of the GI tract. In the oral cavity, taste buds decrease in number and saliva production diminishes. Poor dental hygiene can cause problems with chewing. Older adults are at increased risk for aspiration because food remains in the esophagus for a longer time and the gag reflex is weaker. Decreased gastric acid secretions impair absorption of iron, vitamin B_{12}, and proteins. Colon cells atrophy and peristalsis slows, resulting in constipation and flatulence.

Older adults use various measures to treat their GI complaints. Self-treatment delays assessment and diagnosis of GI problems. Good health habits can prevent some GI problems. Dental hygiene and regular dental visits can prevent many disorders that threaten nutritional intake. Proper quantity and quality of food enhances general health and minimizes risk of indigestion and constipation. Nurses should educate older adults on the relationship between medications and gastrointestinal health.

Reproductive Changes

Changes in sexual response may alter genitourinary function and contribute to embarrassment and general discomfort for older adults. Breasts of older women lose their suppleness and hang flat against the chest wall. Men appear to have more prominent breasts related to slightly decreased testosterone. Clients remain sexually active, but need more stimulation to become aroused. In men, the penis and testes shrink, whereas the prostate gland enlarges. Erections are briefer. In women, the vagina becomes shorter and narrower, and the walls become thin and less elastic. The vulva may atrophy. Vaginal secretions diminish, causing discomfort and bleeding during intercourse.

Urinary System

Both men and women develop urinary problems as they age. Bladder capacity decreases in both sexes. The bladder also loses muscle tone; emptying may be incomplete. Men awaken at night to void because the enlarged prostate gland blocks complete emptying of urine, making it necessary to urinate more frequently. For women, ligaments and muscles stretched during pregnancy fail to keep the bladder suspended. As elastic tissue and pelvic floor muscles weaken, stress incontinence, leakage of urine with increased abdominal pressure during coughing, sneezing, laughing, or lifting, occurs. Another type of chronic incontinence is urge incontinence, leakage of urine because of an inability to delay voiding. Decreased renal blood flow occurs because of decreased cardiac output and reduced glomerular filtration rate.

Musculoskeletal System

Older adults continue to experience decreases in height that began in middle adulthood as a result of compression of disks between the vertebrae. This, combined with weakened chest muscles, causes the spine to have a thoracic curve known as **kyphosis** or humpback. With a change in the center of gravity, older adults assume a wider stance when standing and walking. The hips and the knees tend to be flexed. There may be stiffness in the weight-bearing joints and limited range of motion. Muscles atrophy, but are more clearly defined because of loss of subcutaneous fat. There is general, progressive loss of muscle fibers leading to flabby, thin muscles, particularly of the arms and legs.

Physical limitations seen in older adults are the result of inactivity, not degenerative changes. Remaining as active as possible helps slow the loss of physical ability. Arthritis is the leading chronic condition affecting the musculoskeletal system among people older than age 65. Arthritis results in joint stiffness, limited movement, and deformity. Osteoporosis causes bone mass loss, particularly in older women, and places older adults at increased risk for spontaneous fractures (see Chap. 61).

Integumentary System

Aging contributes to gradual changes in older clients' integument and their ability to adjust to heat and cold. These changes include:

- Skin:
  - Dry, thin, flaky, and easily irritated
  - *Lentigines* or *liver spots* form on exposed areas of the body (Fig. 11.1)
  - Increased capillary fragility causing easy bruising
  - Poor healing related to diabetes and vascular disease
  - Loss of subcutaneous tissue contributing to wrinkles and sagging tissue

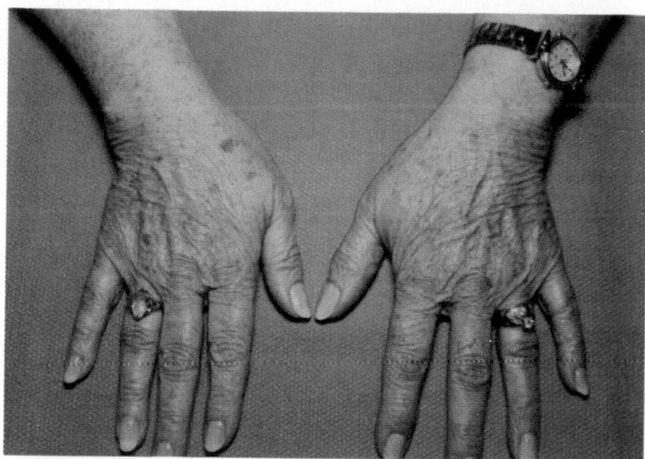

FIGURE 11.1 Senile lentigines. (Courtesy of Ken Timby)

- Hair:
  - Thinner and drier
  - Graying of hair related to loss of melanin production
  - Slower hair growth
  - Hairline recession in both men and women
  - Men experience longer, coarser hair growth in eyebrows, ears, and nose
- Nails:
  - Thicken and are brittle related to poor circulation—especially toenails (Fig. 11.2)
  - Diminished nail growth
  - Longitudinal striations in nails that cause splitting of nail surface
- Oral condition—gums recede and teeth loosen as jaw bones shrink; clients may lose teeth, especially if they do not practice good oral hygiene
- Loss of ability to adjust to temperature extremes:
  - Lowered metabolism makes it difficult to keep warm
  - Slowed dilation of blood vessels in the skin contributes to ineffective sweating and lowered ability to lose heat

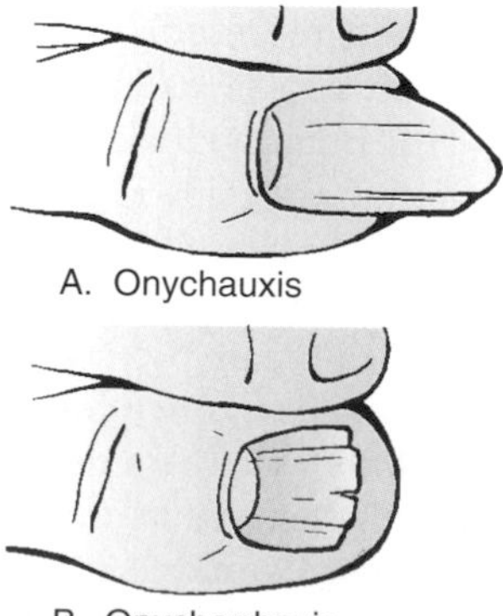

FIGURE 11.2 (**A**) Onychauxis is characterized by nail hypertrophy, which may be a consequence of aging. (**B**) Onychorrhexis, associated with aging, results in brittle, fragile, uneven nail edges.

Chapter 63 discusses many of the skin disorders that older adults experience. Pathologic skin changes are related to sun exposure. Older adults also have benign skin disorders that are worrisome and unattractive. They also are prone to minor trauma that causes bruising and tearing.

Social Characteristics

Healthy older adults usually maintain fairly active lives. Some become more active, learning new hobbies and socializing with new friends, because they have more time. For many, old age involves continued learning and emotional growth. Working and raising a family previously provided many social contacts for the older adult. Some older adults feel bored and lonely when they retire, with a loss of self-esteem because former activities and contacts are curtailed. Outcomes of this time period are linked to a person's overall attitude about life. There is growing evidence that staying active and maintaining social contacts or acquiring new acquaintances is a way to stay health both mentally and physically.

Prominent Psychosocial Issues and Problems

Although personality continues to evolve throughout life, basic temperament is stable into old age. If a client's temperament was cheerful and optimistic during youth, he or she will usually keep that demeanor in old age. A bitter, complaining young person will often carry that attitude into old age.

The ability to cope with crises of diminished health, dependence, leisure time, fixed income, and alternative housing depends on coping skills established earlier in life. Many older adults experience loss. Effective coping skills acquired throughout life will assist older adults to overcome grief and accept losses. This is also a time to plan for life-end decisions, such as burial arrangements, living wills and advance directives.

Older adults experience difficult transitions and concerns. The first is **ageism,** behaviors and beliefs that depict older adults in negative, inaccurate, or stereotypical ways. Older adults are characterized as sick, feeble, rigid, disagreeable, opinionated, or demented people living in the past. In reality, older adults are remarkably healthy and productive until the extremes of old age. Some Americans believe that the significant part of life is over after middle age. This view undermines the dignity of older people who sense that they are not expected to remain physically or mentally healthy. Ageism prevents older adults from obtaining new jobs or forces them into early retirement. In some situations, older adults are avoided, treated disrespectfully, or ignored.

In 1998 about 67% of older persons lived alone or in a family setting (American Association of Retired Persons, 1999). Others lived with a companion or in supervised living arrangements. Many older adults find dependence on others difficult to accept, even when they recognize the need for it. Some deny that they need assisted living and insist on remaining at home even when it jeopardizes their safety. Finding safe and affordable living accommodations is difficult for many older people. Retirement communities combine smaller residences with conveniences such as an infirmary, shopping services, and recreational facilities. Older adults must part with treasured objects to accommodate a smaller dwelling. Familiar objects and mementos are extremely comforting to older adults.

For many, retirement is a time of freedom and to experience many activities, depending on how well the person planned financially. Working after retirement should be a choice but some people experience financial problems and continued work is necessary. Older adults face economic concerns related to decreased income. Compulsory retirement or serious and chronic illnesses are major factors contributing to financial worries. Although studies show that older workers are conscientious, careful, accurate, and dependable, many employers are reluctant to hire them. There are more older adults engaged in part-time employment, and employers are recognizing their value because trends show more retired people re-entering the work force.

Medical expenses increase for older adults, adding to economic concerns. The enactment of Medicare, federal legislation providing health benefits to the aged, was an important advance in helping older adults meet health-care costs.

Older adults also need others to do tasks they can no longer perform, such as lawn care, painting, and cleaning. Most older adults rely on Social Security, a fixed income that does not increase at the same rate as the cost of living. As older adults live longer, their money does not stretch as far.

All people have emotional needs for love, companionship, and acceptance. Hobbies or other special interests and social contacts help older adults cope. Some are involved in community volunteer work or activities and meeting places specifically for older adults. The problem of loneliness is acute for many older people. Older adults also face separation from family and friends and the death of a spouse. Community meal sites and senior centers try to meet the older adult's need for companionship by providing opportunities for socialization.

Pets also fill the void (Fig. 11.3). They serve as family substitutes, provide comfort, and decrease feelings of loneliness. Many extended care facilities use **pet therapy** and have a resident cat or dog. The activity and playfulness of animals stimulate aged persons who are uncommunicative. Pets decrease anxiety and depression and provide older adults with the feeling of being needed and loved.

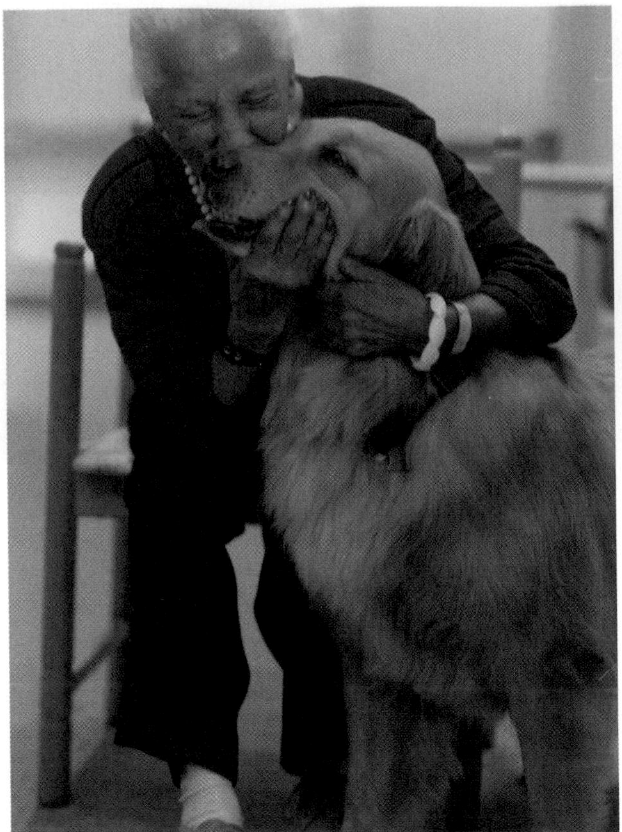

FIGURE 11.3 Pets provide companionship to many older adults.

Many older adults experience depression. Symptoms such as fatigue, irritability, loss of interest in surroundings, decreased ability to concentrate, or feelings of worthlessness are often viewed as natural consequences of aging. Many older adults with depression receive no treatment. This is unfortunate because older adults respond well to antidepressants such as amitriptyline (Elavil), nortriptyline (Aventyl, Pamelor), trazodone (Desyrel, Trazon), and fluoxetine (Prozac).

Although older adults represent only 13% of the population, they account for 20% of all suicide attempts. More suicide attempts occur in individuals age 65 or older than in any age group. Risk for suicide is greater among those who live alone, have health problems, or abuse alcohol. Death of a spouse is also associated with an increased risk of suicide. Nurses or healthcare providers investigate any expressions of hopelessness or helplessness. It is appropriate to ask older adults who seem depressed if they are considering harming themselves or ending their life.

Many older adults who live alone, particularly those living in urban settings, are vulnerable to crimes against their property and person. Some cope with these fears by becoming isolated prisoners in their own homes. Older adults are also the victims of fraud or con games. Older adults may become victims of **elder abuse** when they depend on others for care and support. Abuse may be physical, in the form of beatings; psychological, in the form of threats; social, in the form of abandonment or unreasonable confinement; and material, in the form of theft or mismanagement of money. The abuser is often a caretaker or family member. Older adults at risk for abuse are frail, dependent, and cognitively or physically impaired. Adult Protective Services, a division of each state's Department of Social Services, investigates and safeguards older adults who are suspected victims of abuse.

Nursing Implications

Caring for older adults occurs in a variety of healthcare settings, and requires accurate assessments, interventions, restorative care to promote independence, and referrals to appropriate community resources. Older clients need time to learn new information and respond to changes in their routines. Nurses adapt their approach if the client has a visual or hearing deficit. Older clients have experience in many things—teaching the client should build on past experiences and knowledge. The following information outlines several overall aspects of care for the older adult.

Psychosocial Issues

Nurses must recognize the high incidence of depression and suicide potential in older adults in all settings. Changes in behavior such as increased alcohol consumption, decreased social interests, or complaints of fatigue, anger, or hopelessness should alert nurses to ask the client about suicidal thoughts or intentions. If the client does have such thoughts, report them to your supervisor and the primary care physician. It is important to make the environment safe (remove weapons, sharps, and medications). Stay with the client until other arrangements are made to keep the client safe (see Chap. 15 for more information on depression and suicide).

Nutrition and Diet Modification

Nutritional deficiencies are serious problems for older adults. Dietary insufficiencies are related to loss of or changes in teeth, boredom at eating alone, fatigue, or lack of money. The diet of older adults tends to be high in carbohydrates, which are more affordable on a fixed income. Also, many shop irregularly, and depend on a stockpile of processed foods that have an extended shelf life. Older adults benefit from a diet lower in calories but high in nutrients because absorption of the nutrients is diminished.

Some older clients require a soft diet and foods that are easy to digest. Chewing is difficult for some because of diminished production of saliva or improperly fitted dentures. Many benefit from supplemental vitamins and minerals or nourishing between-meal snacks. Tracking body weight is a good assessment tool for evaluating the nutritional status of older adults. Report a weight gain or loss of 5% in a 4-week period to the primary care provider for analysis.

Physical Care

Promoting hygiene and grooming helps older adults maintain dignity and self-respect. Physical limitations may alter how clients care for themselves, but nurses need to encourage self-care. Older adults can quickly lose their ability for self-care if someone does everything for them, because they feel inept or incapable. Clients may be slower in movements and responses, but are easily confused or anxious or prone to accidents if rushed. It is best for nurses to provide clients with all that is needed for self-care and allow clients to proceed at their own pace.

Daily partial baths or a biweekly tub bath/shower are adequate for older adults. Frequent bathing can be too drying. Clients will need assistance to get in and out of the tub, a stall shower, and/or a shower chair if weak or unsteady. Showers provide the most thorough rinsing of soap and minimize skin irritations.

Some older women may require cleansing douches or medication related to vaginal discharge or urinary incontinence. The vaginal mucosa is thin and subject to infection. Careful perineal care and use of disposable pads can keep the client clean and comfortable.

Pay close attention to the client's integument. Applying cream or lotion to dry extremities after a client bathes promotes circulation and prevents skin breakdown. Before trimming a client's toenails, the client should soak feet in water. Older adults with very thick nails, diabetes, or peripheral vascular disease should have professional nail care.

Elimination

Bowel and urinary elimination may pose problems for older adults. Urinary frequency is common. Take care to prevent falls when the client gets up to use the toilet, ensuring that the call button is nearby so that the client can obtain assistance. Leave a commode, bedpan, or urinal in easy reach for those unable to wait for assistance.

Constipation is more likely in those who are immobile, fail to drink sufficient fluids, or lack sufficient dietary bulk. Helping clients maintain adequate fiber and fluid intake and have a regular time for evacuation helps restore regularity. Physicians can order enemas, mild laxatives, or stool softeners if other methods of relieving constipation are ineffective.

Mobility

Confinement in bed causes adverse effects among older people. Older adults expand their chests less fully. Confinement in bed accentuates this problem, leading to the development of hypostatic pneumonia (pneumonia that occurs as a result of shallow breathing).

Pressure ulcers (bed sores) are common among older adults because of diminished subcutaneous fat. Frequent position changes and pressure-relieving devices are necessary for inactive clients. Muscle tone is readily lost during prolonged bed rest, resulting in extreme weakness. Promote alternative activity such as active or passive exercises.

Safety

Nurses ensure that the environment is safe for the older client. Beds left in a high position are a potential danger because older adults misjudge the distance to the floor and fall when getting out of bed. The bed is left in the low position except when giving direct nursing care. A dim nightlight helps older people become oriented to the surroundings and prevents falling or tripping over objects when the client gets out of bed.

Nighttime agitation and confusion are common among older adults, particularly when they are moved from familiar surroundings to a hospital or nursing home. This problem is commonly mismanaged. Physical restraints increase the client's frustration and distress. It is better for the nurse to determine the cause of the confusion and then attempt to reduce or eliminate it. Causes of agitation include the need to urinate, discomfort of constipation, being too hot or cold, fatigue, pain, fear, or loneliness. Meeting physical or emotional needs may quiet a restless client.

Sleep

Older adults usually require less sleep. Keeping older clients awake and active during the day facilitates sleep at night. Sedatives and hypnotics, even in low doses, can result in wakefulness, excitement, and confusion. Nurses can provide a warm, caffeine-free beverage, extra blanket, or soft music to promote restful sleep.

Reality Orientation

Measures to help older clients maintain contact with reality can prevent episodes of confusion. The older adult benefits from **reality orientation** (Nursing Guidelines 11-1). Reality orientation involves using various techniques that reinforce the client's awareness of the date, time, place, names or roles of individuals involved in their care, and current events.

Communication

Encouraging communication involves stimulating older adults to talk about past experiences and events. This is referred to as **reminiscence therapy.** Older adults have a need to talk about past events, achievements, and losses. Asking them to recall their personal history encourages communication between older adults, healthcare personnel, and family.

NURSING GUIDELINES 11-1

Reality Orientation

- Prominently display the date.
- Identify yourself and address the client by name each time you interact with him or her.
- Reinforce the time of day during routine activities (e.g., "Mrs. Green, it's 2 PM and time for your pill.")
- Give the client a few pages of the newspaper to read.
- Discuss current events.
- Compare events from day to day.
- Routinely tune in radio or television news programs.
- Encourage social interaction with other clients.

Validation therapy, developed by Naomi Feil (1992), is a method of communicating with the confused and disoriented elderly persons who act out in inappropriate ways because of permanent and progressive loss of cognitive ability. Feil believes these individuals are seeking to communicate feelings through their behavior. In validation therapy, nurses reassure clients and gain understanding of their behavior or words spoken. For example, the woman who cares for and nurtures a doll may need validation of her role as a mother or the assurance of the love of her children. In this case, the nurse says, "I know you love your children" or "You are such a good mother." To say, "That is not a baby, but a doll," is presenting reality, but would cause emotional pain or agitation in many older adults. By seeking to validate feelings, the nurse provides comfort and affirms feelings.

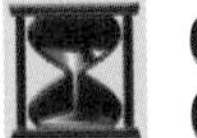

GENERAL GERONTOLOGIC CONSIDERATIONS

Older clients with arthritis or other conditions that cause loss of strength or coordination may request that prescriptions be filled without using childproof caps.

Nurses caring for older adults must dispel stereotypical thinking and view their clients as individuals with unique qualities and characteristics.

Critical Thinking Exercises

1. *An 82-year-old client sits alone all day in the nursing home. He spends his time staring at the television without interest. When nurses try to involve him in various activities, he is irri-*

tated or says that he is too tired. What are some reasons for the client's behavior? What actions(s) could you take to help him?

2. *The nursing home asks you to help organize a reality orientation program for the older residents. Many nursing assistants are unaware of the intervention. How would you explain reality orientation to the nurse assistants? What are some suggestions you could make to reinforce reality for the elderly clients in the nursing home?*

● NCLEX-STYLE REVIEW QUESTIONS 

1. A 75-year-old man gets up twice per night to urinate. Based on knowledge of normal sensory changes in older adults, which advice would be most appropriate for the nurse to give the client to prevent falls and injury during the night?
    1. Put on slippers before getting out of bed.
    2. Use a flashlight to show the way to the bathroom
    3. Place a urinal at the bedside.
    4. Leave a nightlight on in the bathroom.
2. When working with the following clients at a health clinic, the nurse correctly identifies that the client at greatest risk for elder abuse is:
    1. A 72-year-old man with diabetes who lives in a retirement village
    2. A 75-year-old woman with dementia who lives with her daughter
    3. An 80-year-old man with alcoholism who lives alone
    4. An 85-year-old woman with hypertension who lives with her husband
3. A 75-year-old hospitalized client is supposed to be discharged from the hospital in the morning. Prior to discharge, the nurse provides instructions about new medications. Considering age-related physical changes in older adults, which modification to teaching would be most appropriate for the nurse to implement?
    1. Provide a well-lit, quiet environment for teaching.
    2. Write out the instructions on the discharge summary form.
    3. Repeatedly ask the client if he has any questions.
    4. Ask the pharmacist to explain the side effects.

connection—

Visit the Connection site at **http://connection.lww.com/go/timbyEssentials** for links to chapter-related resources on the Internet.

References and Suggested Readings

Administration on Aging. (2001). A profile of older Americans. Department of Health and Human Services. [On-line.] Available: http://www.aoa.dhhs.gov.

American Association of Retired Persons. (1999). A profile of older Americans. [On-line.] Available: http://www.research.aarp.org.

Courts, N. F., Barba, B. E., & Tesh, A. (2001). Family caregivers' attitudes toward aging, caregiving, and nursing home placement. *Journal of Gerontological Nursing, 27*(8), 44–52.

Dudek, S. G. (2001). *Nutrition handbook for nursing practice* (5th ed.). Philadelphia: Lippincott Williams & Wilkins.

Eliopoulos, C. (2001). *Gerontological nursing* (5th ed.). Philadelphia: Lippincott Williams & Wilkins.

Federal Interagency Forum on Aging-Related Statistics. (2000). Older Americans 2000: Key indicators of well-being. Administration on Aging, Agency for Healthcare Research and Quality, Bureau of Labor Statistics. [On-line.] Available: http://www.agingstats.gov.

Feil, N. (1992). *Validation: The Feil method.* Cleveland, OH: Edward Feil Productions.

Feldt, K. S., & Oh, H. L. (2000). Pain and hip fracture outcomes for older adults. *Orthopaedic Nursing, 19*(6), 35–44.

Gomez, R. G., & Madey, S. F. (2001). Coping with hearing loss model for older adults. *Journals Of Gerontology. Series B: Psychological Sciences and Social Sciences, 56B*(4), 233–235.

Hirst, S. P., & Raffin, S. (2001). "I hated those darn chickens . . ." The power in stories for older adults and nurses. *Journal of Gerontological Nursing, 27*(9), 24–29, 55–56.

McBean, L. D., Groziak, S. M., Miller, G. D., et al. (2001). Healthy eating in later years. *Nutrition Today, 36*(4), 192–201.

National Institute on Aging. (2001). Aging America poses unprecedented challenge. [On-line.] Available: http://www.nia.nih.gov.

Van Wynen, E. A. (2001). Healthy people 2010. A key to successful aging: learning-style patterns of older adults. *Journal of Gerontological Nursing, 27*(9), 6–15.

chapter 12

Interaction of Body and Mind

Words to Know 

alternative medical systems
alternative therapy
biological-based therapies
body-based therapies
brain mapping
complementary therapy
coping mechanisms
distress
energy therapies
eustress
general adaptation syndrome
hardiness
immunopeptides
limbic system
mental status examination
mind-body interventions
neuropeptides
neurotransmitters
placebo effect
psychobiologic disorders
psychobiology
psychoneuro-endocrinology
psychoneuro-immunology
psychosomatic diseases
receptor
soma
spiritual healing
stress
stress management
stress-related disorder

Learning Objectives

On completion of this chapter, the reader will:

- Explain why mental illnesses are now considered psychobiologic disorders.
- Discuss two new areas of neuroscience being studied to learn more about psychobiologic disorders.
- Name two chemical substances transmitted between neurons, giving examples of each.
- List examples of techniques used to assess clients with psychobiologic disorders.
- Distinguish between stress, eustress, and distress.
- Describe the general adaptation syndrome, and name its three stages.
- Explain the purpose of coping mechanisms and the outcomes that may result from their use.
- List the defining features of hardiness.
- Discuss methods that are sometimes used to predict a person's vulnerability for acquiring stress-related disorders.
- Discuss techniques that the nurse can suggest for helping clients cope with stressors.
- Discuss the rationale for a mind–immune system connection.
- Discuss explanations for the development of psychosomatic diseases.
- Differentiate between the terms *complementary therapy* and *alternative therapy*.
- List five categories of psychobiologic interventions that the National Center for Complementary and Alternative Medicine investigates.

The mind, central nervous system (CNS), and body, once thought of as completely separate structures, are now viewed as a single communicating entity. Research has uncovered anatomic and chemical links between body and mind. New fields of science examine these linkages and their effects on health.

Psychobiology is the study of the biochemical basis of thought, behavior, affect, and mood. **Psychobiologic disorders** are conditions of biologic abnormalities in the brain and altered cognition, perception, emotion, behavior, and socialization. **Psychoneuroendocrinology** is the study of how fluctuations in pituitary, adrenal, thyroid, and reproductive hormones alter cognition, perception, behavior, and mood. **Psychoneuroimmunology** studies the connections among the emotions, CNS, neuroendocrine system, and immunologic system. Research in psychoneuroimmunology field studies how stress predisposes a person to health problems. All these overlapping fields study the anatomy, physiology, and pathology of the brain.

THE BRAIN AND PSYCHOBIOLOGIC FUNCTION

The brain is made up of the cerebrum, brain stem, and cerebellum (Fig. 12.1). The *cerebrum,* the brain's largest component, controls sensory perception, voluntary movement, personality, intelligence, language, thoughts, judg-

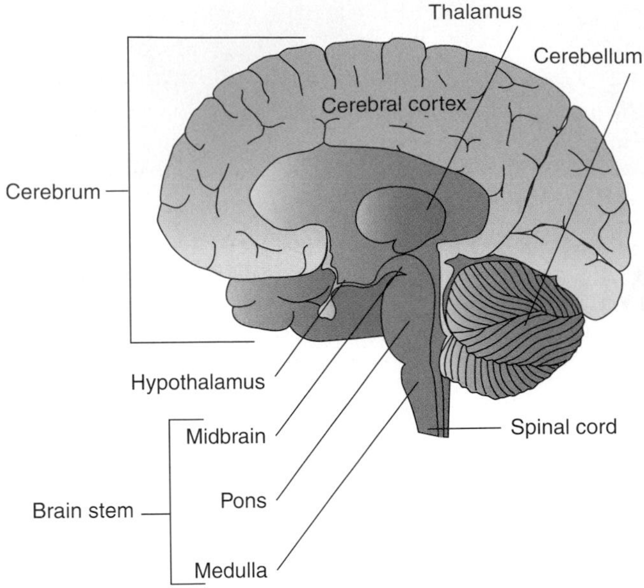

FIGURE 12.1 Brain structures.

ment, emotions, memory, creativity, and motivation. The outer layer of the cerebrum processes information for appropriate functional areas of the brain. The *cerebral cortex* is the major pathway of physiologic intercommunication. The **limbic system** is a network within the brain that contains structures involved in emotions and related physiologic functions. It includes the *thalamus,* which connects many brain centers and modulates movement, sensation, behavior, and emotions. The limbic system also includes the *hypothalamus,* which controls the autonomic nervous system and coordinates the endocrine and immune systems via pituitary-adrenocortical connections (Porth, 2002). Because of its neuroendocrine and neuroimmunologic roles, the limbic system affects and determines many psychobiologic activities.

Stop, Think, and Respond ● BOX 12-1

Which two structures in the brain play the greatest role in connecting the mind with physiologic functions?

Receptors are structures found on the surface of cells throughout the body and brain. Each cell has millions of different receptors. These receptors sense and pick up chemical messengers that arrive in the extracellular fluid. A chemical messenger is like a specific key that fits into and binds with a specific receptor. Only those messengers that have molecules in exactly the right shape can bind with specific receptors. For example, opiate receptors can bind only with chemicals in the opiate group such as heroin, morphine, or endorphins. Once binding occurs, the message is received and the cell begins to respond.

Chemical messengers, or **neurotransmitters,** may be natural or man-made, and the message may cause the cell to perform any number of activities. Neurotransmitters (Table 12.1) communicate information that affects thinking, behavior, and bodily functions. The chemicals are synthesized in the neurons and stored in vesicles in the axons. They are released and attach themselves (bind) momentarily to receptors on postsynaptic neurons. After the chemicals transmit their information, they either

TABLE 12.1 SELECTED NEUROTRANSMITTERS

NEUROTRANSMITTER	ABBREVIATION	EXAMPLES OF FUNCTIONS
Serotonin (5-hydroxytryptamine)	5-HT	Stabilizes mood Induces sleep Regulates temperature Controls appetite
Dopamine	DA	Integrates thoughts Promotes movement in concert with ACH Stimulates hypothalamic endocrine activity Enhances judgment
Norepinephrine	NE	Affects attention and concentration Raises energy level Heightens arousal
Acetylcholine	ACH	Assists memory storage Promotes movement in concert with DA Prepares for action
Gamma-aminobutyric acid	GABA	Reduces arousal and aggression Inhibits excitatory neurotransmitters like NE and DA Decreases seizure potential

become inactive or weakened, or are recaptured by releasing neuron for future use, a process called reuptake.

Neurons are classified by the type of neurotransmitter they release; for example, cholinergic neurons release acetylcholine, and dopaminergic neurons release dopamine.

Neuropeptides are a separate type of neurotransmitter. They include chemicals such as:

- Substance P, which transmits the sensation of pain
- Endorphins and enkephalins, morphine-like neuropeptides that interrupt transmission of substance P and promote a feeling of well-being
- Neurohormones released by interactions among the hypothalamus, pituitary, and the endocrine glands they stimulate

Different areas of the brain contain different types of neurons with specific neurotransmitters. Each neurotransmitter has either a stimulating or inhibiting effect on neurons. All brain function, including thoughts, emotions, or messages to organs and muscles, depends on these neurotransmitters (Barry, 1996).

Receptors for neurotransmitters and neuropeptides are located throughout the CNS and in the endocrine and immune systems. This finding suggests that these systems communicate with each other through chemical messages. This concept has tremendous implications for how the mind and emotions can affect physical well-being and how physical status can affect the mind (Barry, 1996).

PSYCHOBIOLOGIC ILLNESS

Many still believe that mental illness results from character defects, demonic possession, or punishment by God. This explains why individuals with mental illness are sometimes feared and stigmatized. The study of brain structure, chemistry, and genetics is providing scientific information about mental illness. Brain pathology is seen as the major factor contributing to mental illnesses, or psychobiologic disorders. Three major types of psychobiologic disorders are somatoform and anxiety disorders (see Chaps. 13 and 14), mood disorders (see Chap. 15), and thought disorders (see Chap. 18). Other conditions with a biologic basis include eating disorders (see Chap. 16) and chemical dependency (see Chap. 17).

Pathophysiology and Etiology

The neurotransmitters dopamine, norepinephrine, epinephrine, serotonin, and acetylcholine are often implicated in the psychobiology of mental illness. Neurotransmitters are concentrated in different areas of the brain. Disruption of a neurotransmitter system results in specific symptoms associated with that area of the brain. For example, serotonin is found in areas that regulate sleep, appetite, sexual behavior, and mood. Imbalances in serotonin may be responsible for depression, eating disorders, sleep disturbances, and obsessive-compulsive disorder.

Other insights into brain physiology came from observing effects of medications on behavior and symptoms (psychopharmacology). An example is antianxiety medications, such as the benzodiazepines (see Chap. 14), which activate gamma-aminobutyric acid (GABA) receptors that inhibit arousal, excitement, and aggression.

Psychological factors (forces that shape behavior) also influence psychological equilibrium and may be tied to brain chemistry as well. Some researchers believe that the neurotransmitter network links emotion, memory, and learned behavior (Pert & Chopra, 1999). Sigmund Freud proposed that disordered behavior results from intrapersonal (within oneself) conflicts that arise during specific stages of development. For example, he correlated compulsive neatness and stinginess with rigid toilet-training. Erik Erikson and Harry Stack Sullivan theorized that mental health or illness depends on social relationships and interpersonal interactions. Other theorists suggest that mental stability is affected by significant others and social systems, such as neighborhood, city, and country. B. F. Skinner proposed that adaptive and maladaptive behaviors are learned and repeated because of rewarding reinforcement. This perspective is applied in various circumstances, such as when young children are offered candy to induce toilet training.

Stop, Think, and Respond ● BOX 12 2

What do you think may be the physiologic and psychological consequences if an infant is not held very much, is not talked to affectionately, or is ignored when hungry?

Assessment Findings

Signs and Symptoms

Brain dysfunction can cause a mix of psychobiologic signs and symptoms. The American Psychiatric Association (2000) has established symptoms for each specific mental disorder in the *Diagnostic and Statistical Manual of Mental Disorders,* 4th edition, text revision (DSM-IV-TR). The DSM-IV-TR is a book that classifies psychiatric disorders. Commonly seen symptoms include anxiety, mood changes, abnormal eating patterns, chemical dependence, or thought disturbances. Ultimately, the client's signs and symptoms affect relationships with others and interfere with age-related role responsibilities.

Mental Status Examination

A **mental status examination** is one component of a thorough neurologic examination. The examiner observes the client and asks questions about cognition and mental state. Areas covered in an extensive mental status examination include physical appearance, orientation, attention and concentration, short- and long-term memory, movement and coordination, speech patterns, mood, intellectual performance, perception, insight, judgment, and thought content.

Psychological Tests

Psychological tests are used to detect personality characteristics, interpersonal conflicts, and self-concept (Table 12.2).

Diagnostic Findings

Measuring levels of neurotransmitters and neuropeptides is difficult, expensive, and sometimes impossible. A definitive diagnosis for many psychobiologic disorders is usually achieved by ruling out other diseases with similar symptoms. The reader is referred to Chapter 38 for a description of tests such as electroencephalography (EEG), computed tomography (CT) scan, magnetic resonance imaging (MRI), and positron emission tomography (PET).

Brain mapping, a new diagnostic tool, compares a client's brain activity patterns (from an EEG or other electronic image) with a computerized database of electrophysiologic abnormalities. A growing database of distinctive patterns for seizure disorders, schizophrenia, depression, dementia, anxiety disorders, attention deficit/hyperactivity disorder, and others now exists for comparison.

TABLE 12.2 PSYCHOLOGICAL TESTS

TEST	DESCRIPTION
Minnesota Multiphasic Personality Inventory (MMPI)	This true-or-false test of 550 questions is used to analyze which of nine clinical personality traits are manifested by the client's responses.
Beck Depression Inventory	Client rates self according to statements that concern mood.
Draw-a-Person (tree, house, family) Test	Client's drawing is analyzed for symbolism about his or her self-perception or other emotional data.
Word Association Test	Client is asked to quickly provide a response to words, such as "mother . . . work . . .", etc. Responses are analyzed for psychological significance.
Thematic Apperception Test (TAT)	Client is asked to look at pictures and then tell a story about them. Recurring themes in the stories suggest the underlying basis of emotional problems.
Rorschach Test	The client is asked to indicate what he or she sees in each of 10 separate inkblots.

Medical and Nursing Management

Treatment of psychobiologic disorders depends on the specific diagnosis. Modalities include drug therapy, psychotherapy, cognitive therapy, and behavior modification (see Chaps. 13 through 18). The goal of drug therapy is to correct the biochemical abnormality. Best results occur with mood disorders (see Chap. 15), anxiety disorders (see Chaps. 13 and 14), and schizophrenia (see Chap. 18). Psychotherapy, cognitive therapy, and behavior modification attempt to uncover repressed thoughts and emotions and identify healthier coping mechanisms. Nurses play an active role in all aspects of treatment, including administering and monitoring response to drug therapy, implementing behavior modification plans, and providing individual and group counseling.

THE BRAIN AND PSYCHOSOMATIC FUNCTION

Brain chemistry and its effects on physical health are currently being widely researched as well. Emotions, which originate in brain structures and chemicals, can powerfully influence an individual's health and sense of well-being.

According to Selye's theory (1956), **stress** is a physiologic response to biologic stressors like surgical trauma, psychological stressors such as fear, or sociologic stressors like increased family responsibilities. Stress is implicated in the development or exacerbation of autoimmune diseases, anorexia nervosa, obsessive-compulsive disorder, panic attacks, thyroid conditions, heart disease, functional and inflammatory disorders of the gastrointestinal tract, chronic pain conditions, and diabetes. Stress is not an entirely negative concept. Just the right amount of stress, called **eustress,** maintains a healthy balance in life. Eustress helps individuals to pursue goals, solve problems, or manage life's predictable and unpredictable crises. Excessive, ill-timed, or unrelieved stress is called **distress.** It triggers the **general adaptation syndrome,** a nonspecific physiologic response (Box 12-1). This response, which can cycle many times through the alarm and resistance stages before reaching the exhaustion stage, occurs through the neuroendocrine and autonomic nervous systems.

Stop, Think, and Respond ● BOX 12-3

How might failing one test be considered eustress but failing several tests be considered distress?

BOX 12-1 ● General Adaptation Syndrome

Stressor
↓
ALARM
↓
Autonomic nervous system

↓ Sympathetic division (norepinephrine)
↓
- Increased heart rate
- Increased force of heart contraction
- Increased rate and depth of respirations
- Vasoconstriction
- Increased blood pressure
- Increased muscle tension

↓ Parasympathetic division (acetylcholine)
↓
- Decreased gastric motility
- Increased intestinal peristalsis
- Contraction of urinary bladder muscles

RESISTANCE
↓
Hypothalamus/pituitary/adrenal axis
↓
Adrenocorticotropic hormone (ACTH)
↓
Adrenal cortex
Glucocorticoids (cortisol)
–Increased serum glucose level
–Altered fat and protein metabolism
–Decreased capillary permeability
–Decreased inflammatory response
Mineralocorticoids (aldosterone)
–Conservation of sodium
–Excretion of potassium
–Reduced urine output
|
EXHAUSTION
↓
Cardiac failure
Renal failure
Inadequate immune response

Physiologic Stress Response

The autonomic nervous system consists of the sympathetic and parasympathetic divisions. The most common pathway for the stress response is through the sympathetic division, which uses norepinephrine to stimulate body systems, arousal, and anxiety in response to stress. This response overrides control of the parasympathetic nervous system, which slows many metabolic processes. Some people respond to stressors through the parasympathetic pathway. Instead of being stimulated to fight or flee, parasympathetic responders become "frozen by fear." Becoming motionless is beneficial among various animals. For example, possums "play dead" when a predator is nearby, causing the predator to lose interest. Some theorists argue that taking a similarly less aggressive stance could help humans to avoid confrontation.

Psychological Stress Response

Just as the body responds to stressors, the *psyche,* or mind, also reacts to stress. **Coping mechanisms** are unconscious tactics humans use for protection from feeling inadequate or threatened. These mechanisms function like "psychological first-aid" by helping temporarily to avoid the emotional effects of a stressful situation. When used appropriately and in moderation, coping mechanisms allow maintenance of psychological equilibrium and lead to psychological growth. If a person overuses coping mechanisms, he or she becomes dysfunctional. Some individuals develop maladaptive coping mechanisms such as abusing alcohol or other substances.

A particularly effective coping style is called **hardiness** (Kobasa, 1979). Characteristics of hardiness are:

- A commitment to something meaningful versus a sense of alienation
- A sense of having control over sources of stress versus a feeling of helplessness
- The perception of life events as a challenge rather than a threat

Refer to Nursing Guidelines 12-1 for interventions that can foster effective coping skills and a sense of hardiness.

PSYCHOSOMATIC ILLNESSES

Psyche refers to the mind, and **soma** refers to the body. The term "psychosomatic" means pertaining to the mind–body relationship, and psychosomatic illness refers to illnesses influenced by the mind. The term psychosomatic illness is often used interchangeably with **stress-related disorder.** In the past, psychosomatic had a negative con notation, suggesting that a client's illness was not legitimate. Psychoneuroimmunologic research has given the term a more holistic meaning, reflecting the concept that the mind and body are not separate. **Psychosomatic diseases** (Box 12-2) are legitimate medical conditions associated with or aggravated by stress. Many healthcare providers now believe that all illnesses, if not psychosomatic in origin, have psychosomatic components.

Pathophysiology and Etiology

Biologic Factors

In addition to known effects of stress on the autonomic nervous system, studies show that stressful events, such as preparing for tests or undergoing job strain, also affect the immune system. The immune system defends the body against cancer and invading microorganisms. Stress can lower the numbers of white blood cells, the immune system's disease fighters. Research shows that chronic stress or very intense stress, such as the death of a spouse,

NURSING GUIDELINES 12-1

Fostering Effective Coping Skills

- Explore the coping strategies the client has found helpful in the past and encourage their continued use.
- Encourage clients to re-establish priorities and to strike a healthy balance between work and play.
- Suggest cultivating relationships with family and friends who are supportive.
- Teach the client assertiveness skills by role-playing how to (1) clearly state feelings, and (2) say "no" to unreasonable requests.
- Discuss time management techniques like (1) getting up earlier, (2) avoiding procrastination, (3) performing stressful tasks when the client has maximum energy, and (4) eliminating or delegating unwanted tasks.
- Recommend a daily exercise program to reduce stimulating neurotransmitters and release endorphins and enkephalins such as (1) beginning with a 5- to 10-minute workout, (2) increasing the duration by 5 minutes each day, and (3) building up to a 30- to 45-minute period of exercise.
- Tell the client to avoid using alcohol or other nonprescribed sedative drugs as forms of self-treatment.
- Suggest writing about feelings in a diary if verbalizing traumatic or angry thoughts is difficult.
- Suggest stress management education and joining a support group.

has a greater effect on health than temporary stressors. This finding is particularly true when a person lacks supporting relationships. A connection seems to exist between poorer immune function and loneliness; when individuals share emotions with others, immune functions improve.

Research supports a biologic connection between the mind and the immune system in that that the immune system and brain communicate with each other through the chemical messenger system using neurotransmitters and immunopeptides. **Immunopeptides** (or immunotransmitters) are called *cytokines* (see Chap. 35) and function in the same way as neurotransmitters; they relay messages throughout the immune system and the brain (Pert & Chopra, 1999). Immune cells can also secrete small quantities of neurochemicals. Nerve cells connecting organs of the immune system (thymus, spleen, and lymph nodes) to the brain have been identified. This ability to communicate through chemicals implies that the immune system can make the brain aware of processes at distant sites in the body and that the brain can send messages directing the immune system's actions. The powerful actions of neurotransmitters, especially in states of excess or depletion, suggest that the psychological state can significantly affect immune function.

Many psychosomatic or stress-related diseases involve allergic, inflammatory, or altered immune responses (see Chap. 36). They are characterized by physical symptoms that cycle through periods of *remission,* or absence, and *exacerbation,* or recurrence, with symptomatic episodes often occurring when the client is under stress. The brain–immune connection suggests that changes in body chemistry during periods of stress trigger an autoimmune (self-attacking) response or result in immunosuppression. Invasion of the body by cancer cells or disease-causing microorganisms, however, is not sufficient cause for disease; disease occurs when defenses are compromised or cannot recognize unnatural cells or pathogens. For this reason, psychological variables that influence immunity have the potential to influence the onset and progression of immune system-mediated diseases.

BOX 12-2 ● Stress-Related Diseases and Disorders

Allergic and hypersensitivity disorders	Hypertension
Anovulation	Infertility
Bronchial asthma	Irritable bowel syndrome
Bruxism	Low back pain
Cancer	Multiple sclerosis
Cardiac dysrhythmias	Psoriasis
Connective tissue disorders	Rheumatoid arthritis
Eczema	Temporomandibular joint disorder
Hair loss	Tension headaches
Herpes simplex infection	Tic disorders
	Ulcerative colitis

Psychological Factors

There is an association of certain psychological characteristics with an increased incidence of illness. Research suggests that there may be a generic, disease-prone personality with character traits that include anger and hostility, depression, anxiety, and other features (Pelletier, 1977). The type of disease that develops is related to an individual's health habits, environmental exposure, family history, and other socioeconomic factors.

Assessment Findings

Many stress-prone individuals seek medical attention when they experience symptoms in one or more organs affected by the autonomic nervous system. Clients may present with heart palpitations, pounding headaches, breathlessness, tightness in the chest, chest pain, chronic pain, irritability, epigastric pain, abdominal discomfort and bloating, or constipation alternating with diarrhea. Other illnesses, including cancer and heart disease, are not so obviously related to stress but are thought to have a psychosomatic component. Biopsychosocial effects of stress and mental state should be considered in evaluating and treating illness.

Diagnostic tests are done to determine the extent of the disease and physical causes for the client's symptoms. Such things as excessive caffeine intake, cocaine use, mitral valve prolapse, hyperthyroidism, hypoglycemia, and lactose intolerance can mimic signs and symptoms of some stress-related diseases. Thus, it is important to conduct tests before assuming that the disorder is stress induced.

Medical and Nursing Management

Treatment involves standard medical care pertinent to the diagnosis, control of the physical symptoms, and implementation of methods effective in managing stress and supporting the immune system. Nurses have an important role in the treatment and education of clients regarding these methods. Stress management and other techniques have gained acceptance based on studies that suggest psychological factors can reduce the effects of stress on the immune system and facilitate healing. **Stress management** programs offer instruction in relaxation techniques and effective coping strategies including assertiveness training and developing a network of social support.

PSYCHOBIOLOGIC INTERVENTIONS

Psychobiologic interventions use the mind and body to alter disease. The placebo effect is an example of how the mind and body are connected. Traditional medicine is now investigating and integrating broader approaches, known as complementary and alternative therapies, to manage and treat various disorders.

The Placebo Effect

A *placebo* is an inactive substance that cannot alter physiology, yet does in a significant number of people. The **placebo effect** refers to healing or improvements that occur because the individual believes a treatment will be effective.

The placebo effect was first observed during drug research. In most clinical drug trials, half of the research volunteers receives the drug being studied, while the other half receives a placebo. None of the volunteers or researchers know which subjects are receiving the actual drug. When results of the studies are analyzed, researchers find that 30% or more of those who receive a placebo experience improvement. A person's belief system can positively influence health and may show that a purely psychological basis for recovery exists. When clients believe in the treatment regimen or have faith in the prescriber, it potentiates a positive outcome.

Stop, Think, and Respond ● BOX 12-4

What response would you expect if you gave 100 people a red-colored candy that you said would increase their desire for sex?

Complementary and Alternative Therapies

The National Institutes of Health established the National Center for Complementary and Alternative Medicine (NCCAM) in 1998. NCCAM defines a **complementary therapy** as one used *in addition to* conventional medical treatment. In contrast, an **alternative therapy** is one used *instead of* conventional medical treatment. The NCCAM studies complementary and alternative therapies, educates scientists and healthcare providers on the nature and principles of complementary and alternative therapies, and provides the results of research findings.

The NCCAM subdivides complementary and alternative therapies, which approximately 42% of Americans use (Fontanarosa & Lundberg, 1998), into five general groups: (1) alternative medical systems, (2) mind-body interventions, (3) biological-based therapies, (4) body-based therapies, and (5) energy therapies.

Alternative Medical Systems

Alternative medical systems evolved from non-Western cultures and existed before the beginning of modern medicine. Table 12.3 compares differences between alternative and conventional medical systems.

CHINESE MEDICINE. Although the term *Chinese medicine* is used, this medical system also includes contributions from Japan, Korea, and other Southeast Asian countries. Chinese medicine believes that health is the outcome of balancing *yin* and *yang,* opposite forces that must remain equalized to maintain *qi,* life's energy force. Forces that alter *qi,* either by depleting or obstructing it, cause illness. Correcting an imbalance between two attributes like motion and stillness or hot and cold restores harmony and health. Treatment measures such as acupuncture, herbal remedies, diet, exercise, and massage are used to restore *qi.*

AYURVEDIC MEDICINE. *Ayurvedic medicine* has its roots in India and is the oldest system of medicine in the world. It is based on spiritual practices of Tibetan monks. Ayurvedic medicine helps individuals become unified with nature to develop a strong body, clear mind, and tranquil spirit. One belief is that *prana,* or the life force (similar to the *qi* in Chinese medicine), moves through various centers in the body called *chakras.* The Ayurvedic doctor prescribes modalities such as yoga, herbal medicine, fasting and eating cleansing foods, meditation, and massage to maintain or restore the dynamic flow of the *prana.*

TABLE 12.3 DIFFERENCES BETWEEN ALTERNATIVE AND CONVENTIONAL MEDICAL SYSTEMS

ALTERNATIVE MEDICAL SYSTEMS	CONVENTIONAL MEDICAL SYSTEMS
Originated approximately 1500 BC or earlier	Originated with Hippocrates in approximately 5 BC
Believe that health results from harmony among the person, his or her environment (nature, universe), and energy force	Believe that health results from normal physiologic function
Focus on maintaining a healthy state	Focus on treating illness or injury
Do not correlate symptoms of disease with any specific organ or anatomic location	Correlate symptoms with the organ or location of the person's disorder
Identify with and are sensitive to cultural traditions	Recognize cultural differences but may not incorporate the client's beliefs into the treatment regimen
Incorporate religious principles	Do not reject spirituality, but do not apply any religious significance to a person's illness or recovery
Rely heavily on medicinal plants	Rely on manufactured pharmaceuticals
Accept the efficacy of treatment approaches based not on specific scientific explanation but rather traditional use	Demand scientific evidence for the mechanisms of treatment and replication of results through unbiased research
Do not have established educational standards for practitioners	Require practitioners to have formal education beyond college
Do not regulate practice	Require formal licensure for practice

NATIVE AMERICAN MEDICINE. Native Americans perceive disease as a result of disharmony with Mother Earth, possession by an evil spirit, or violation of a taboo. They rely on a *shaman,* a person within the tribal community who is both a medicine man (or woman) and a spiritual figure with the extraordinary ability to heal. The shaman has power to achieve an altered state of consciousness to journey to the spirit world or assume the persona of another life form, such as an eagle or mountain lion.

Native Americans believe that the shaman obtains knowledge from a higher power during a trance-like state, accompanied by chanting, drumming, dancing, or by consuming psychoactive botanicals. The shaman is able to determine the cause and remedies for sick individuals. Remedies may include herbs, meditation, fasting, and sweating. The shaman may fashion a talisman, a symbolic figure that the sick individual wears to ward off evil spirits or exorcise bad spirits.

Mind-Body Interventions

Mind-body interventions are techniques that rely on the power of the mind to alter body functions or symptoms.

BIOFEEDBACK. *Biofeedback* enables clients to voluntarily control body temperature, heart rate, blood pressure, and brain waves. Initially, clients are monitored for physiologic activity, such as heart rate. A machine provides feedback and clients try to alter a particular function (e.g., decrease heart rate). If the machine's signal changes, it helps them determine if they are successful. Eventually, clients do not need the machine; they can alter their physiology at will. Biofeedback is used to reduce hypertension and rapid heart rates, manage pain, abort seizures, relieve migraines, and dilate peripheral blood vessels.

IMAGERY. *Imagery* uses the mind to visualize a positive physiologic effect. Clients conjure up mental images of their body waging and winning a battle with a disease. For example, clients might visualize their body producing white blood cells in large numbers. They then imagine the white cells destroying cancer cells. Laboratory values of white cell counts taken before and after such imagery sessions often show that numbers of white blood cells dramatically increase.

HUMOR. *Humor* can be used therapeutically. Laughter stimulates the immune system by increasing the number of white blood cells and lowering cortisol, which suppresses immune function. Laughter can cause the release of neuropeptides (endorphins and enkephalins).

HYPNOSIS. *Hypnosis* is a therapeutic intervention that facilitates a physiologic change through the power of suggestion. Hypnotism may help individuals overcome habits like smoking, relieve chronic pain, and extinguish irrational fears.

SPIRITUAL HEALING. *Spiritual healing* restores health through a higher power (God or some other metaphysical force). An intermediary person may channel the healing force, acting strictly as a facilitator. Healing may occur through the sick person's prayers or those said by others on his or her behalf. The medical community has not yet entirely accepted spiritual healing as legitimately therapeutic.

Biological-Based Therapies

Biological-based therapies use natural products such as herbs, aromas, and even bee venom.

HERBAL THERAPY. The use of plants as *herbal therapy,* a technique for treating disease and disorders, has been mostly handed down orally from generation to generation in various world locales. Their use is commonly referred to as "folk medicine" because their benefits are largely anecdotal rather than based on scientific investigation.

Approximately 25% of prescription drugs are derived from plants. Drugs manufactured from plant sources generally contain one or more extracts from the plant or a synthesized, molecularly similar structure. Herbalists argue that using only parts of a plant changes the effects that are achieved from using the whole plant. Consequently, interest in self-treatment using herbs has been renewed (Table 12.4). Clients use herbs in juices, teas, powders, salves, and many other forms.

Presently, herbal therapy is not regulated like pharmaceutical drugs are in the United States. In 1994 Congress passed the Dietary Supplement Health and Education Act, which defines a "dietary supplement" as supplying one or more essential nutrients missing from the diet and including vitamins, minerals, amino acids, herbs, and other botanicals. As such, herbs are classified as nutritional supplements and are not held to the same standards of unified dosages, safety, and efficacy as drugs. Manufacturers of herbal preparations, however, cannot claim that the herbal product prevents or treats a disease because that automatically places the substance in the category of a drug, which is highly regulated.

To avoid federal regulation, labels on herbal products can suggest medicinal use as long as they also contain a disclaimer that the Food and Drug Administration has not evaluated the product. More information will be

TABLE 12.4 POPULAR HERBS USED IN THE UNITED STATES

HERB	BOTANICAL NAME	CLAIM FOR USE	PRECAUTIONS
Chamomile	*Chamomilla recutita*	Relieves digestive disorders	Avoid if allergic to ragweed, asters, chrysanthemums, or members of the daisy family.
Echinacea	*Echinacea augstifolia*	Boosts immune function and speeds healing	Avoid if allergic to plants in the daisy family; prolonged use may reduce effects.
Ephedra	*Ephedra vulgaris*	Relieves asthma, stimulates the central nervous system, promotes weight loss, increases energy	Action is similar to that of amphetamine; ephedra can cause tachycardia, headache, hypertension, seizures, insomnia, chest pain, decreased intestinal motility, and death from stroke or heart attack.
Garlic	*Allium sativum*	Lowers blood pressure, thins the blood	Possible side effects include intestinal gas; combining garlic with aspirin or other anticoagulants can prolong bleeding.
Ginkgo	*Ginkgo biloba*	Improves memory	Possible side effects include gastrointestinal distress, headaches, and allergic reactions; use with caution if taking aspirin or other blood-thinning drugs.
Ginseng	*Panax gensema*	Increases energy and helps in dealing with stress	Use may raise blood pressure and serum glucose level and can increase the growth of estrogen-dependent cancer.
Kava	*Piper methysticum*	Reduces stress and anxiety	Large doses can produce an intoxicating effect; long-term use can lead to dry, scaly skin.
St. John's Wort	*Hypericum perforatum*	Treats mild depression	Use may cause sensitivity to light; interactions with other drugs can be dangerous.
Saw palmetto	*Serenoa repens*	Relieves enlargement of the prostate gland	Avoid tea versions because the herb dissolves poorly; nausea and gastrointestinal distress are possible.
Valerian	*Valerian officinalis*	Relieves anxiety and insomnia	Possible side effects include blurred vision, excitability, and changes in heartbeat if taken in large doses or for more than 2 weeks.

available as the NCCAM studies herbs more scientifically. Clients who use herbs need to (1) find out what they are, (2) not use a product without information, (3) use the lowest dose initially, (4) increase the dose gradually, and (5) never exceed the maximum dose. Even herbs have possibly lethal side effects. Consulting with a physician before using herbs and disclosing that information before any medication is prescribed is best. Use of herbs is not recommended for pregnant or lactating women, infants, and children younger than age 6 years.

AROMATHERAPY. Most people have a positive or negative association of odors of certain substances with various people, places, or feelings. *Aromatherapy* uses scents to alter emotions and biologic processes. For therapeutic uses, scents from botanical oils of lavender, peppermint, and the like are released by adding them to bath water, permeating the air where they are inhaled, or rubbing them on the skin. Olfactory nerves carry the scented molecules to the limbic system. As discussed earlier, the limbic system is the brain area used for learning, memory, and emotions. Once the limbic system is stimulated, it triggers physiologic and psychological responses via neurotransmitters like serotonin, endorphins, or norepinephrine, released by the hypothalamus. The neurotransmitters can, in turn, affect nervous, endocrine, and immune system functions. Some believe that aromatherapy helps control blood pressure and hormone secretions; relieve pain, depression, and anxiety; or promote higher states of alertness. More research is needed to validate the physiologic actions of various scents, evaluate how best to use them, and determine why one type of aroma affects people differently.

APITHERAPY. *Apitherapy,* the medicinal use of bee venom, to date has been used to treat various inflammatory joint conditions (e.g., rheumatoid arthritis). It is also used to treat multiple sclerosis. Bee venom contains various enzymes that may stimulate the adrenal glands and induce the release of cortisol, an anti-inflammatory and immunosuppressant hormone. Physicians currently consider apitherapy an unconventional treatment and do not recommend its use nor support a client's request for it. Nevertheless, experiments have demonstrated relief of symptoms among research volunteers (Kuthan, 2000).

Body-Based Therapy

Body-based therapies are healing methods that use manipulation and movement to improve health and restore biologic functions.

MASSAGE THERAPY, REFLEXOLOGY, AND SHIATSU. *Massage therapy* involves applying pressure and movement to stretch and knead soft body tissues. Massage therapists use the warmth of their hands, elbows, and forearms and lubricating oils to stimulate circulation and relieve physical and psychologic tension. Benefits of massage include relief from discomfort and improved mobility or functional use of affected parts of the body.

Reflexology is a complementary health practice in which manual pressure is applied to the feet and hands. Those who practice reflexology claim that locations in the extremities contain reflex centers composed of more than 7000 nerve endings linked to body organs and tissues. When pressure is applied to a reflex area, the impulse travels from peripheral nerves to the spinal cord and brain. As a result, reflexologists believe that reconditioning or reprogramming the neural reflex improves the body's ability to facilitate natural healing.

Shiatsu is a Japanese word that means "finger pressure." Shiatsu has many similarities to acupressure and acupuncture because practitioners apply pressure to acupoints within various body meridians (energy channels). Each meridian correlates with an organ or its function. Acupoints are locations along the meridians where Asians believe the body's life force, *qi* or *chi,* moves. Unblocking and strengthening qi rebalances the body's energy and restores health.

CHIROPRACTIC. *Chiropractic* theory proposes that subluxation (malalignment) of the spinal vertebrae alters nerve activities that regulate body functions in distant organs. To treat various disorders, chiropractors, the single largest group of U.S. alternative-complementary practitioners, perform spinal manipulation as a generic method for curing neuromuscular disorders and a host of other diseases. Millions of people seek chiropractic treatment with some improvement in their symptoms. Chiropractic treatment is further legitimized because (1) many health insurance policies cover it, (2) the federal government provides Medicare and Medicaid reimbursement for it, and (3) the costs are an approved income tax deduction (Jarvis, 2001).

YOGA AND TAI CHI. *Yoga* developed in India, and *tai chi* has its origins in China. Both incorporate techniques that combine mental and physical exercises for the purpose of integrating body and mind. There are several branches of yoga; *hatha yoga* is most commonly practiced in the United States. Advocates of *hatha yoga* attribute the following benefits to its practice:

- Relaxation and centeredness
- Relief of headaches, insomnia, anxiety, and pain
- Increased musculoskeletal flexibility
- Improved breathing
- Overall contentment

The Chinese believe that tai chi exercises restore *qi* or *chi.* The exercises require standing and shifting body weight from one foot to another while performing a series of slow, choreographed arm movements. It is accompanied by slow, controlled breathing and visualization of energy circulating throughout the body. It is believed that tai chi exercises tone the whole body without exertion and cardiac risks associated with other aerobic forms of physical exercise, restore health, and prevent disease.

Energy Therapies

Energy therapies are techniques that claim to manipulate electromagnetic fields within the body.

REIKI. *Reiki* (pronounced "ray-key") shares many features with what Westerners may call "therapeutic touch" and spiritual healing. Reiki is a Japanese method of healing introduced to the Western world in the 1800s. *Rei* means "spirit" and *ki* is translated like *qi* or *chi*. Basically, those who use Reiki believe that *ki* promotes health and healing. They further believe that when *ki* is blocked and a person is ill, a Reiki practitioner can channel energy—not from his or her own body, but from the universe—to the sick person's body. Once *ki* is restored, healing occurs.

The practitioner transfers energy within the universe by laying-on of hands. Direct contact between the practitioner and client is the usual method of healing. Healing can also occur from a distance because the Japanese believe that the spirit is not confined by time or space. In other words, the practitioner and ill person can be geographically separate. The practitioner then moves his or her hands on an object that symbolically represents the sick person while visualizing the transmission of energy. The belief is that the recipient draws in the energy, which goes where it is needed.

ACUPUNCTURE. *Acupuncture* is a healing therapy in which a needle is placed in one or more acupoints to unblock *qi*. Acupuncture is considered a form of energy therapy because its ultimate goal is to restore the balance and free flow of energy within the body. Some acupuncturists take the technique one step further by manipulating the needles with an electric current. When used in this manner, it is referred to as electroacupuncture.

ELECTROMAGNETIC THERAPY. *Electromagnetic therapy* promotes healing using either electricity, magnets, or both. Microcurrent therapy, using low-intensity electrical currents to alter cellular physiology, is currently used to treat nonhealing fractures and to relieve pain. Magnetism is used diagnostically at present with MRI.

The theory concerning electromagnetism is based on the physiologic principle that cellular membranes emit electrical currents, verified by recording electrical energy as in electrocardiograms. Science confirms that nerve stimulation causes the resting membrane potentials of cells to change to action potentials. A magnet changes the direction of an electrical current by separating charged ions. Theoretically, electromagnetic therapy (1) affects the cell membrane by changing the ion exchange of electrolytes like calcium, sodium, and potassium, (2) stimulates the release of endorphins, naturally produced morphine-like chemicals, or other neurotransmitters through the cell's membrane, or (3) rebalances the electromagnetic field within the body.

Although many questions remain about electromagnetic theory, it now includes static magnet therapy and pulsed magnetic field therapy. Static magnet therapy refers to wearing stationary magnets, which are stronger than everyday refrigerator type magnets, directly on the body. The static magnets are incorporated in bracelets, necklaces, belts, wraps, and even mattress pads. Pulsed magnetic field therapy uses devices that apply very low frequency electricity (50 Hz) to body areas at intervals of 25 pulses per second for 600 seconds (10 minutes) followed by an interval of rest. Supposedly, the pulsing effect produces rising and falling levels in the body's magnetic field.

Electromagnetic therapeutic devices are used haphazardly for many unrelated conditions such as fibromyalgia, post-polio syndrome, peripheral neuropathy, multiple sclerosis, depression, epilepsy, and urinary incontinence. More research is needed to determine if there really are beneficial results.

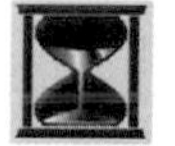

GENERAL GERONTOLOGIC CONSIDERATIONS

The function of the immune system diminishes with age, resulting in increased incidences of infection, cancer, and autoimmune disease.

Elderly clients who have developed positive coping skills continue to cope well as they age.

Some older adults feel helpless and cannot cope when released from a healthcare facility without adequate discharge planning.

Emotional distress and impaired self-care abilities have been identified as major contributors to rehospitalization of older adults.

Loss of a network for support increases an older adult's vulnerability and reaction to stressors.

Adults who have chronic psychosomatic diseases are likely to manifest debilitating effects in late adulthood.

Critical Thinking Exercises

1. *What would you say to someone who characterizes mental illness as the manifestation of a poor or weak character?*
2. *What suggestions would you offer to someone who has developed a stress-related (psychosomatic) disorder?*

• NCLEX-STYLE REVIEW QUESTIONS 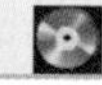

1. When the student health nurse assesses a college freshman, which of the following is the best example that the student is experiencing eustress?
   1. The student says she is achieving a 3.0 grade point average in her classes.
   2. The student says she has frequent respiratory infections.

3. The student says she feels tired and overwhelmed.
4. The student says she needs to find a part-time job.

2. A 60-year-old woman recently lost her husband to a sudden heart attack. She is assuming all the responsibilities that her husband normally completed. Which statement made by the widow is typical of normal grieving following such an experience?
1. "I have had a bad cold three times this winter. Normally, I am never sick."
2. "I am experiencing difficulty falling asleep at night and require a sleeping pill."
3. "I have been having chest pain and frequent panic attacks at night."
4. "I have lost all desire to live since my husband's passing."

3. A client in the physician's office states that she has been having frequent headaches, insomnia, anxiety, and pain and asks the nurse for an alternative therapy suggestion. Following an asymptomatic physical examination, which alternative therapy would benefit the wide range of symptoms expressed?
1. Chiropractic
2. Aromatherapy
3. Yoga
4. Apitherapy

connection

Visit the Connection site at **http://connection.lww.com/go/timbyEssentials** for links to chapter-related resources on the Internet.

References and Suggested Readings

American Psychiatric Association. (2000). *Diagnostic and statistical manual of mental disorders* (4th ed., text revision). Washington, DC: Author.

Barrett, S. (2001). How the dietary supplement health and education act of 1994 weakened the FDA. [On-line.] Available: http://www.quackwatch.com/02ConsumerProtection/dshea.html.

Barry, P. (1996). *Psychosocial nursing: Care of physically ill patients and their families* (3rd ed.). Philadelphia: Lippincott Williams & Wilkins.

Bensing, K. (March 18, 2002). Spotlight on mental illness. *Advance for Nurses,* 39.

Benson, H. (2000). *The relaxation response.* New York: Avon Books.

Dossey, L. (1996). *Prayer is good medicine: How to reap the healing benefits of prayer.* San Francisco: Harper.

Dossey, L. (1999). *Reinventing medicine: Beyond mind-body to a new era of healing.* San Francisco: Harper.

Fisher, M. J. (2000). Better living through the placebo effect—self-delusion as a form of wellness. *The Atlantic, 286*(4), 16–20.

Fontanarosa, P. B., & Lundberg, G. D. (1998). Alternative medicine meets science. *Journal of the American Medical Association, 280*(18), 1618–1619.

Fox, S., et al. (1999). Neurologic mechanisms in psychoneuroimmunology. *Journal of the American Association of Neuroscience Nurses, 31*(2), 87–97.

Hatler, C. W. (1998). Using guided imagery in the emergency department. *Journal of Emergency Nursing, 24*(6), 518–523.

International Academy of Advanced Reflexology. (2001). Reflexology accurately defined. [On-line.] Available: http://www.reflexology.net.

Jarvis, W. T. (2001). Why chiropractic is controversial (1990). [On-line.] Available: http://www.chirobase.org/01General/controversy.html.

Kaye, J., et al. (2000). Stress, depression, and psychoneuroimmunology. *Journal of the American Association of Neuroscience Nurses, 32*(2), 93–101.

Kobasa, S. (1979). Stressful life events, personality and health: An inquiry into hardiness. *Journal of Personality and Social Psychology,* 42(1), 1–11.

Kuthan, F. (2000). Bee venom treatment of rheumatic disorders. [On-line.] Available: http://www.apitherapy.org/aas/kuthan.html and http://www.apitherapy.org.

Pelletier, K. (1977). *Mind as healer, mind as slayer.* New York: Dell.

Pert, C., & Chopra, D. (1999). *Molecules of emotions: Why you feel the way you feel.* New York: Scribner.

Porth, C. M. (2002). *Pathophysiology: Concepts of altered states* (6th ed.). Philadelphia: Lippincott Williams & Wilkins.

Selye, H. (1956). *The stress of life.* New York: McGraw-Hill.

Townsend, M. C. (2000). *Psychiatric mental health nursing: Concepts of care* (3rd ed.). Philadelphia: F. A. Davis.

chapter 13

Caring for Clients With Somatoform Disorders

Words to Know 

body dysmorphic disorder
conversion disorder
factitious disorders
histrionic
hypochondriasis
insight-oriented therapy
la belle indifference
malingering
Munchausen's syndrome
Munchausen's syndrome by proxy
pain disorder
secondary gain
somatization
somatization disorder
somatoform disorders

Learning Objectives

On completion of this chapter, the reader will:

- Describe the coping mechanism referred to as somatization.
- Describe somatoform disorders.
- Explain why malingering and syndromes classified as factitious disorders are not somatoform disorders.
- Discuss three explanations for the development of somatoform disorders.
- Explain the meaning of insight-oriented therapy.
- Name two nursing diagnoses common to clients with somatoform disorders.

The care of clients who suffer from somatoform disorders is challenging because the symptoms, which are very real and distressing, do not result from any specific pathology. By understanding the psychological origins of these disorders, nurses can provide better care for clients who suffer physically from underlying emotional factors.

SOMATOFORM DISORDERS

Somatoform disorders are conditions with a basis in the coping mechanism of somatization. Approximately 2% to 15% of the U.S. population have various types of somatoform disorders (Videbeck, 2004). Sometimes somatoform disorders are misdiagnosed as medical diseases, so the incidence could be higher. **Somatization** is the manifestation of unconscious emotional distress through physical symptoms. Although many people have physical illnesses made worse by stress and emotional conflict (see Chap. 12), somatizers (people with somatoform disorders) have no physiologic basis for their symptoms and often go from doctor to doctor seeking relief. The psychological origin of the somatizer's symptoms is unknown to the client, and the illnesses seem very real. All somatoform disorders share three characteristics:

1. Physical symptoms resemble a medical illness, but cannot be objectively identified.
2. Psychological factors promote and maintain the symptoms or cause their periodic recurrence.
3. Unconscious motivators influence the course of the disorder; the client does not consciously control the symptoms (Videbeck, 2004).

Somatoform disorders are not to be confused with **malingering,** deliberate faking of an illness to acquire financial compensation, obtain drugs, or be relieved of responsibilities from work or school. Nor are they **factitious disorders,** in which people purposefully cause illness-like symptoms. One example of a factitious disorder is **Munchausen's syndrome,** in which a person self-induces an illness (e.g., by taking nonlethal amounts of poison) to acquire medical treatment. A second example is **Munchausen's syndrome by proxy,** in which a person makes another person—usually his or her own child—sick. The person creates a life-threatening situation to gain attention from medical personnel and notoriety for saving the child's life. For example, a mother may revive a child with cardiopulmonary resuscitation (CPR) after first smothering the child.

Types

Somatization Disorder

A person with **somatization disorder** has combinations of multiple unexplained somatic complaints (Box 13-1) with no medical explanation. Chronic symptoms cause the person to seek medical attention, sometimes from more than one physician simultaneously. More women than men develop somatization disorder, which explains why it was formerly referred to as hysteria ("hyster" referring to uterus). The term *hysteria* has a connotation of high states of emotion, also characteristic of affected individuals.

Hypochondriasis

Hypochondriais is a somatoform disorder in which a person is preoccupied with minor symptoms and develops an exaggerated belief that they signify a life-threatening illness. When medical diagnostic workups show normal findings, clients with hypochondriasis may be convinced that their illness is so complex that it eludes diagnosis. As symptoms continue and frustration mounts, these individuals become increasingly anxious and invest time, energy, and money to discover a cause for their concerns.

Conversion Disorder

Conversion disorder is characterized by a sudden loss of motor or sensory function, such as paralysis or deafness, following a stressful event or experience. Often the manifestation of the symptom holds some symbolic meaning. For example, people may become blind after witnessing a traumatic event. Although the anatomic structures in their visual tracts and centers for vision in the brain are normal, they cannot see. Theorists believe that the blindness is a defense mechanism to prevent them from ever having to see a similar event. Because the physical malady is a protective mechanism, affected persons appear unconcerned that it exists, referred to as ***la belle indifference.***

Pain Disorder

Persons with **pain disorder,** formerly known as somatic pain disorder, experience pain in one or more anatomic sites without any identifiable medical condition. As in conversion disorder, the onset, severity, continuation, or recurrence of the pain is related to psychological factors. The person generally experiences perverted beneficial effects because the pain provides an excuse from unwanted responsibilities or garners sympathetic attention from family and social acquaintances. Pain disorder can lead to abuse of analgesic medications and unnecessary surgery when physicians deal with the condition on a physical rather than a psychological level.

Body Dysmorphic Disorder

People who develop **body dysmorphic disorder** are convinced that some feature of their bodies is flawed. Although most people believe that their appearance could be improved in some way, those with body dysmorphic disorder exaggerate the significance of what others would describe as a minor characteristic. People with body dysmorphic disorder may glance frequently in reflective surfaces, touch or pick at their skin, measure or repeatedly palpate the defect, continually request reassurance about the defect, performing elaborate grooming rituals, use various means to disguise the defect, avoid social situations in which others could observe the defect, or become anxious around other people (Watkins, 2001). Those with body dysmorphic disorder may become socially isolated, unable to concentrate, desirous of cosmetic surgery, depressed, or suicidal.

BOX 13-1 ● Examples of Somatic Complaints

GASTROINTESTINAL SYMPTOMS
Nausea, bloating, vomiting, diarrhea, food intolerance

PAIN SYMPTOMS
Headache; abdominal discomfort; pain in the back, extremities, chest, or rectum; pain during urination, menstruation, or sexual intercourse

SEXUAL SYMPTOMS
Disinterest in sex, erectile or ejaculatory dysfunction, irregular menses, excessive menstrual bleeding, vomiting throughout pregnancy

PSEUDONEUROLOGIC SYMPTOMS
Impaired coordination or balance, paralysis or localized weakness, difficulty swallowing or lump in the throat, inability to speak, urinary retention, hallucinations, loss of touch or pain sensation, double vision, blindness, deafness, seizures, amnesia, loss of consciousness other than fainting

Pathophysiology and Etiology

Several theories exist to explain somatoform disorders. One is that the chronic release of neurotransmitters and neuroendocrine hormones in response to stress exhaust or deplete regions in the brain that facilitate adaptation and coping behaviors. Another theory suggests that physical symptoms provide relief from psychological tension when the person cannot deal with it consciously. Yet another explanation is that the conversion of emotional pain into a physical disorder serves as a justifiable way to obtain attention and compassion from others—an outcome referred to as **secondary gain.** Regardless of cause, clients with somatoform disorders experience physical distress that interferes with the quality of their lives. The disorder may impair social interactions and affect the ability to perform activities of daily living (ADLs) and role responsibilities.

Assessment Findings

Clients seek diagnosis and treatment for symptoms that generally involve a variety of body systems, pain, or a unique body characteristic. Some may have illnesses that are highly symbolic in nature (e.g., imagined heart ailments after termination of a romance). Some somatizers appear **histrionic,** a term that derives from the word hysteria, when describing their symptoms. They are animated, dramatic, and prone to exaggeration. Others, like those with conversion disorder, appear apathetic. They often have multiple symptoms, and many provide a history of extensive medical consultations, diagnostic procedures, and surgical interventions. Symptoms still persist or others replace them. The physical examination usually reveals symptoms that do not fit with known patterns of disease or injury. Often, these symptoms become more distressing during emotional crises, although most somatizers do not acknowledge such a relationship. Symptoms often provide some secondary gain: they distract from dealing with emotional problems, provide a means for gaining attention, or relieve the client from performing unwanted responsibilities.

Stop, Think, and Respond ● BOX 13-1

A middle manager must make monthly verbal presentations to his company's board of directors. A day or two before the board meetings, he develops severe diarrhea. At times, he asked the board to postpone his report or allow him to submit a written report. He has seen his physician about the diarrhea many times. Results of diagnostic tests were unremarkable. He asked for a referral to a gastroenterologist, but had the same results. Based on information about somatoform disorders, explain what may be involved. 

Despite comprehensive laboratory and diagnostic tests, no etiology or pathology is identified. Current medications may be temporarily discontinued to determine if a drug–drug or drug–food interaction or an interaction with some other environmental substance explains the client's symptoms. When investigative approaches prove negative, it is presumed that the symptoms are the result of a psychobiologic process.

Medical Management

Differentiating the somatizer from a client with a medical illness is important. The physician attempts to find the pathologic basis while treating the symptoms. Clients with pain disorder are referred to specialty pain clinics to learn nonpharmacologic interventions for the relief of their discomfort.

Repeated diagnostic testing with negative results reinforces the client's belief that the physician is inept. Although many clients with somatoform disorders resist it, they may be referred to psychiatrists or psychologists for insight-oriented psychotherapy.

Insight-oriented psychotherapy helps clients understand the cause and relationship between their emotional distress and physical symptoms. Goals of treatment include avoiding further unnecessary procedures and diagnostic testing, minimizing disability, and helping the client find other coping mechanisms that prevent translating emotional stress into bodily symptoms. Therapy may be brief and followed by one or two sessions as needed. Antianxiety medications such as Xanax and Valium are avoided or prescribed for only a brief period because of their abuse and addiction potential. Antidepressant drugs are used if the client becomes despondent (see Chap. 15).

Nursing Management

Inform the client about the preparation for diagnostic procedures, how each test is conducted, and care that will be provided afterward. Administer prescribed medications according to medical orders. Emotional support is essential; avoid conveying that you think that the symptoms are unreal or that the client can consciously control them. Planned nursing interventions help the client learn alternatives, other than somatization, for dealing with life events. If psychological counseling becomes part of the medical treatment plan, reinforce the idea that the mind influences the body and that both may need treatment occasionally. See the teaching tips provided in Client and Family Teaching 13-1.

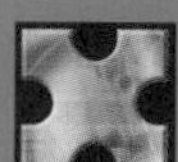

13-1 *Client and Family Teaching* Somatoform Disorders

The nurse teaches the client and family as follows:

- Expressing emotions and feelings is important.
- When an illness develops, explore the possibility that emotional conflicts coexist.
- Consult with a physician who can validate whether the present symptoms are disease-related or a recurrence of a somatoform disorder.
- Focus attention on behaviors that are unrelated to the expression of physical symptoms.
- Treat the time during an illness "matter-of-factly"; avoid special favors or attention that rewards the sick role.

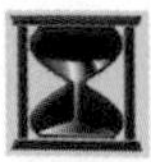

GENERAL GERONTOLOGIC CONSIDERATIONS

Loss of a support network increases an older adult's vulnerability and reaction to stressors.

Socially isolated older adults may focus on themselves and be preoccupied with bodily illness.

By focusing on somatoform disorders, older adults may obtain more attention and care from family members than they would otherwise.

Incidence of somatoform disorders increases in older adults. Healthcare providers must evaluate all physical symptoms before treating older adults for a somatoform disorder.

Critical Thinking Exercises

1. *Discuss the physical, emotional, social, and financial implications that can result from having a somatoform disorder.*
2. *What behaviors might be therapeutic to avoid the development of somatoform disorders?*

• NCLEX-STYLE REVIEW QUESTIONS 

1. When a nurse reviews a client's health record, which of the following is a common finding for someone who suffers from a somatoform disorder?
   1. Laboratory test results outside normal limits
   2. Multiple physician referrals
   3. Family history of cancer
   4. History of drug abuse
2. An 18-year-old client has been diagnosed with a somatoform disorder. Her mother is trying to understand why she would want to get attention and compassion in this way from others. The best explanation the nurse can provide is that acquiring attention for health-related problems is a form of:
   1. *La belle indifference*
   2. Secondary gain
   3. Histrionics
   4. Conversion disorder
3. When a nursing assistant asks if hypochondriasis means that the client is not really sick, the most accurate response from the nurse is that a client with this type of illness:
   1. Thinks minor symptoms are a life-threatening disorder
   2. Thinks he is sick, but the test results are all negative
   3. Would rather be hospitalized than have to go to work
   4. Has an illness that has influenced his emotions

connection

Visit the Connection site at **http://connection.lww.com/go/timbyEssentials** for links to chapter-related resources on the Internet.

References and Suggested Readings

Fortinash, K. M., & Holoday-Worret, P. A. (2000). *Psychiatric mental health nursing* (2nd ed.). St. Louis: Mosby.

Mind matters. Fear of being sick can become an illness. (1999). *Health News, 17*(2), 10.

Schatz, D., et al. (2000). The relationship of maternal personality characteristics to birth outcomes and infant development. *Birth: Issues in Perinatal Care and Education, 27*(1), 25–32.

Townsend, M. C. (2000). *Psychiatric mental health nursing: Concepts of care* (3rd ed.). Philadelphia: F. A. Davis.

Videbeck, S. L. (2004). *Psychiatric mental health nursing* (2nd ed.). Philadelphia: Lippincott Williams & Wilkins.

Watkins, C. E. (2001). Body dysmorphic disorder. [On-line.] Available: http://www.baltimorepsych.com/body_dysmorphic_disorder.htm.

chapter 14

Caring for Clients With Anxiety Disorders

Words to Know 

agoraphobia
anxiety
anxiety disorders
anxiolytics
behavioral therapy
cognitive therapy
compulsion
desensitization
fear
flashbacks
generalized anxiety disorder
limbic system
obsession
obsessive-compulsive disorder
panic disorder
phobic disorders
post-traumatic stress disorder
psychic numbing
psychotherapy
social phobia

Learning Objectives

On completion of this chapter, the reader will:

- Differentiate anxiety from fear.
- Name four levels of anxiety, explaining the differences among each level.
- Give six areas of nursing management that apply to the care of anxious clients.
- Give three examples of anxiety disorders.
- List categories of drugs used to treat anxiety disorders.
- Name and discuss two types of psychotherapy used to treat anxiety disorders.
- List six nursing interventions that are helpful for reducing anxiety.
- Discuss areas of teaching for clients with anxiety disorders.

Although anxiety and fear are normal human responses, anxiety disorders are not. Anxiety disorders may be strictly biologic, learned, the result of unconscious emotional conflicts, or a combination of all three. This chapter explores anxiety and fear and discusses how to intervene for an anxious client. It also explores anxiety disorders and nursing care of those who have them.

ANXIETY AND FEAR

Anxiety differs from fear, but these terms are often used interchangeably. **Anxiety** is a vague uneasy feeling, without an identifiable cause. It occurs when a person anticipates nonspecific danger. **Fear** is a feeling of terror in response to someone or something specific perceived as dangerous or threatening. Fear and anxiety are common reactions of patients in healthcare facilities. Recognizing signs of escalating anxiety, understanding its consequences, and intervening appropriately are important interventions.

Levels of Anxiety

Anxiety ranges from mild, which is constructive, to moderate, severe, and panic (Table 14.1). Mild anxiety prepares an individual to take action in appropriate situations. For example, mild anxiety before a test causes most people to study. Moderate, severe, and panic levels of anxiety are counterproductive; they provoke responses that interfere with well-being.

Stop, Think, and Respond ● BOX 14-1

Give examples of situations that provoke mild anxiety and the appropriate outcomes that generally result. Discuss situations that may trigger more extreme levels of anxiety and their potential consequences. 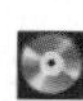

Nursing Management

Assist the anxious client by implementing interventions that maintain or restore a sense of calm and control.

TABLE 14.1 LEVELS OF ANXIETY

LEVEL	BEHAVIORAL MANIFESTATIONS	PHYSICAL MANIFESTATIONS
Mild	Attention is heightened. Sensory perception is expanded. Focus is on stimuli. Reality is intact. Information processing is accurate. Person feels in control.	Muscle tone increases. Heart rate, blood pressure, and breathing slightly increase. Perspiration is noticeable.
Moderate	Person is more easily distracted. Concentration is slightly impaired. Person can redirect attention. Learning takes more effort. Perception narrows. Problem-solving becomes difficult. Person is irritable and feels inadequate.	Muscles are tense. Slight leg or hand tremors may occur. Rate, pitch, and volume of speech change. Respiratory depth and vital signs increase. Sleep is disturbed.
Severe	Attention span decreases. Person cannot concentrate or remain focused. Perception is reduced. Ability to learn is impaired. Information processing is inaccurate or incomplete. Person is aware of extreme discomfort. Effort is needed to control emotions. Person feels incompetent.	Symptoms include hyperventilation, dizziness, tachycardia, heart palpitations, and hypertension. Fine motor movement is impaired. Communication is limited.
Panic	Person exaggerates details. Perception is distorted. Learning is disabled. Thoughts are fragmented. Person cannot control emotions and feels helpless.	Speech is incoherent. Movements are haphazard, usually in an effort to escape. Symptoms include dyspnea, fainting, tremors, and diaphoresis.

Building Trust

Building trust is especially critical to developing a therapeutic relationship with an anxious client. Being available and attentive to the client's needs contributes to this trust. Do not leave an anxious client alone, especially during a new or potentially frightening experience.

Restoring Comfort

Nurses' interventions are guided by what brings relief to a person. Ask the client what would be comforting. Some clients find it helpful for the nurse to support them in nonverbal ways, like remaining with them without talking or holding a hand. Others prefer to talk about how they feel, but are more relaxed if the nurse remains physically distant.

Modifying Communication

Do not interrupt anxious clients when they talk. Verbalizing does not relieve anxiety, but it can be beneficial, helping to process information and explore methods for dealing with problems. Some clients prefer not to discuss their anxiety and fears with the nurse. Respect the client's right to privacy, but offer a referral to a health professional with counseling expertise.

Adjusting Teaching

Because an anxious client's attention and concentration are limited, directions or explanations must be simple, brief, and repeated frequently. To determine a client's level of comprehension, asking the person to paraphrase what he or she has been taught is helpful. Reducing sensory stimulation, such as dimming the lights and eliminating noise, is beneficial. Do not expect the client to show a great deal of self-reliance or independence until he or she feels more relaxed and secure.

Helping Problem-Solve

Anxiety impairs problem-solving ability, and clients seek advice in decision-making. Instead of influencing their clients' choices, nurses help clients follow a step-by-step problem-solving process to formulate decisions:

1. Identify problems
2. Determine their causes
3. Explore possible solutions
4. Examine pros and cons of each option
5. Select the choice most compatible with personal values

Once the client makes a decision, advocate on the client's behalf—even if it is not one you would personally choose. Also respect the client's right to change his or her mind at any time.

Ensuring Safety

Persons experiencing panic-level anxiety can act impulsively and endanger their safety (e.g., jumping out of a window, running into the street). Remain calm to help such individuals reduce anxiety to a more manageable level. Having only one nurse interact with the client is better, because multiple sources of stimulation add to a client's agitation. If the client is very unstable, it is wise to avoid touching or getting physically close to him or her. Intruding within the client's personal space is likely to increase anxiety.

ANXIETY DISORDERS

Anxiety disorders are psychobiologic illnesses resulting from activation of the autonomic nervous system, chiefly the sympathetic division. They tend to be chronic and sometimes appear without any logical explanation.

Types

Generalized Anxiety Disorder

Generalized anxiety disorder (GAD) is characterized by chronic worrying on a daily basis for 6 or more months. There is generally more than one focus of worry. For example, a person may be worried about finances, job performance, and personal health. Often, worrying in out of proportion with reality. At least six other signs and symptoms of anxiety accompany the client's distress. When the client seeks medical attention, test results fail to reveal physical disorders (Box 14-1).

Panic Disorder

Panic disorder is the most extreme manifestation of anxiety. Those who are affected experience abrupt onset of physical symptoms and terror that include intense apprehension; tachycardia; palpitations; chest pain; smothering or choking sensations; hyperventilation; lightheadedness; feeling of impending doom; and fear of fainting, dying, losing control, or going insane.

Panic episodes may last minutes to less than 1 hour and then spontaneously subside. The first instinct during a panic attack is to escape to a safer place. When a client suddenly leaves without explanation, others will see this behavior as strange.

A person experiencing a panic attack cannot identify its cause but associates the location or concurrent activity as the precipitating event. These individuals cope by avoiding situations or places where attacks occurred. As attacks recur in a variety of circumstances, however, people with panic disorder often develop agoraphobia. **Agoraphobia** is a fear of experiencing panic attacks in public, causing public humiliation. Consequently, many of those with panic disorder permanently confine themselves to their homes.

BOX 14-1 ● Examples of Conditions That Resemble Generalized Anxiety Disorder

- Mitral valve prolapse
- Hypoglycemia
- Hyperthyroidism
- Premenstrual syndrome
- Menopause
- Dementia
- Abuse of psychostimulants (cocaine, caffeine, weight loss drugs)
- Sedative (alcohol, opioids, barbiturates) withdrawal

Phobic Disorders

Phobic disorders are conditions in which a person develops an exaggerated fear, such as irrational fear of insects, animals, or various life experiences, some of which are potentially dangerous. When a person with a phobic disorder is exposed to the phobic stimulus, he or she develops symptoms of anxiety that may reach severe or panic levels. He or she generally goes to extremes to avoid the object of the phobia or painfully endures the phobic stimulus despite the fact that it causes severe distress. Most people with phobic disorders are aware of how illogical the phobia is and how unrealistic their disabling response has become.

One common phobic disorder is social phobia. Persons who develop **social phobia,** also known as *social anxiety,* fear situations that point attention to themselves. Examples include speaking publicly or attending a party. The greatest worry for those with social phobia is that they will be embarrassed or criticized for failing to meet acceptable standards.

Post-traumatic Stress Disorder

Post-traumatic stress disorder (PTSD) is a condition involving a delayed anxiety response 3 or more months after an emotionally traumatic experience, such as witnessing or being the victim of a violent crime or being in a natural disaster. Although traumatic experiences are somewhat relative, they must be extraordinarily severe to cause PTSD. Circumstances of the traumatic event involve actual or threatened death or injury to self or others and produce fear, helplessness, or horror. Some feel guilty for having survived such an event when others just as deserving of life died.

Initially, the affected person avoids dealing with the tragedy and detaches from others using a technique referred to as **psychic numbing.** Eventually, however, the person can no longer stifle his or her memories.

Months or years later, memories may resurface in recurrent nightmares or **flashbacks,** in which the person feels as if he or she is reliving the precipitating event. This feeling may also occur when the person is exposed to a situation that resembles the original trauma, like associating the explosive sound of fireworks with military gunfire.

To relieve symptoms of guilt, grief, anger, or sadness, some clients with PTSD abuse substances like alcohol or other mind-altering and mood-altering drugs. When such coping strategies prove ineffective, they may act out aggressively. They may respond violently if startled from sleep. Those who suspect that they may have PTSD should consult a mental health professional for a definitive diagnosis.

Stop, Think, and Respond ● BOX 14-2

Discuss how nurses who care for seriously burned victims may develop PTSD.

Obsessive-Compulsive Disorder

Obsessive-compulsive disorder (OCD) is manifested by performance of an anxiety-relieving ritual (**compulsion**) to terminate a disturbing, persistent thought (**obsession**). Obsessions may involve concerns about potential danger or being contaminated with germs. They are intrusive, and cannot be dismissed from these clients' consciousness. To relieve anxiety, clients with OCD repetitively perform a tension-relieving compulsion that generally falls into one or more of the following categories:

- Cleaning, such as repetitious scrubbing
- Washing, such as repeated bathing or handwashing
- Checking, such as repeatedly verifying that doors are locked
- Counting, such as a bank teller repeatedly making sure that the money count is accurate
- Touching, such as having to touch the door frame before entering a room

Clients with OCD may feel compelled to perform the same act repeatedly for a specific number of times or in a prescribed sequence. The more the person resists performing the compulsive act, the more the anxiety escalates. The same is true if another person interrupts, alters, or forbids the ritual. Because rituals are often excessive and time-consuming, they may lead to problems in social relationships, failure in school, or loss of employment. Most clients with OCD recognize that their thoughts and behaviors border on ridiculous but cannot stop independently.

Pathophysiology and Etiology

Genetic studies suggest that many anxiety disorders have familial patterns. This finding implies an inherited faulty physiology, maladaptive learning, or acquisition of personality traits modeled after those displayed by significant others.

Symptoms occur because the neurotransmitter norepinephrine floods the limbic system. A minority of individuals respond to stress via the parasympathetic route, in which the neurotransmitter acetylcholine causes symptoms. The **limbic system,** which surrounds the brain stem, is a ring of structures made up of lobes of the cerebrum, thalamus, hypothalamus, and others. This complex neural tissue is a physiologic network for emotions, survival and behavioral responses, motivation, and learning. Biochemical changes brought on by the autonomic nervous system trigger physical arousal in the cortex and the neuroendocrine pathways involving the hypothalamus, pituitary, and adrenal glands.

Other biochemical mechanisms also may contribute to development of anxiety disorders. A dysregulation of gamma-aminobutyric acid (GABA), a neurotransmitter that should buffer or extinguish activity of norepinephrine, is one possibility. The second possibility is depletion of serotonin (5-HT), which would explain why some clients with anxiety disorders develop depression or improve when receiving treatment with antidepressant drugs (see Chap. 15).

Assessment Findings

Although anxiety causes behavioral, cognitive, and emotional effects, most clients seek treatment for physical signs and symptoms (cardiovascular, respiratory, neuromuscular, gastrointestinal, integumentary problems) (Table 14.2). For example, clients may be concerned about palpitations, breathlessness, chronic fatigue, tension headaches, and sleep disturbances. In many clients, blood pressure is elevated and heart rate increased. Some clients report having unrealistic worries or fears or exaggerated startle reactions, experiencing flashbacks of previously traumatic events, avoiding situations that provoke symptoms, or performing ritualistic behaviors.

Findings from laboratory blood tests and diagnostic tests like electrocardiography are essentially normal. Positron emission tomography (PET) and computed tomography (CT) scans have shown abnormal brain use of glucose in clients with anxiety disorders. Magnetic resonance imaging (MRI) has demonstrated atrophy in some brain areas in selected anxiety disorders. Diagnosis of most clients with anxiety disorders, however, is based on symptomatology and history.

Medical Management

Medical management of anxiety disorders includes drug therapy combined with cognitive and behavioral psychotherapy. Drug therapy relieves symptoms associated with anxiety, but does not eliminate causative factors. Once drug therapy is implemented, however, clients

TABLE 14.2 COMMON SIGNS AND SYMPTOMS OF ANXIETY

RESPONSES	SIGNS AND SYMPTOMS
Physical	
Cardiovascular	Hypertension, tachycardia, palpitations, fainting*
Respiratory	Dyspnea, rapid breathing, hyperventilation, choking sensation, tightness in the chest
Neuromuscular	Tremors, restlessness, insomnia, muscle tension, excessive sleep,* generalized weakness, dizziness
Gastrointestinal	Anorexia, nausea, diarrhea,* constipation, feeling of fullness
Urinary	Frequency and urgency of urination*
Integumentary	Diaphoresis, sweaty palms, pallor, blushing,* dry mouth
Behavioral	Crying, rapid speech or mutism, hypervigilance, being easily startled or accident-prone, social isolation, physical escape, avoidance, loss of interest in sexual activity, pacing, fidgeting, nail-biting, picking at skin, seeking comfort in food or alcohol, absenteeism, failure to complete or poor performance of tasks
Cognitive	Forgetfulness, poor judgment, lack of motivation, confusion, nightmares, intrusive thoughts, preoccupation, decreased attention and concentration, inability to recall information
Emotional	Unrealistic fears, mood swings, easily angered, impatient, intolerant, nervous

*Indicates a parasympathetic rather than a sympathetic nervous system response.

are more capable of dealing with issues affecting their daily lives.

Drug Therapy

Drugs that (1) reduce or block levels of norepinephrine or (2) normalize levels of serotonin are most commonly prescribed for anxiety disorders. They include anxiolytics, beta-adrenergic blockers, central-acting sympatholytics, and occasionally antidepressants (Drug Therapy Table 14.1). Clients must be aware that it may take several weeks to feel the beneficial effects of drug therapy.

ANXIOLYTICS. **Anxiolytics**, sometimes referred to as minor tranquilizers, are drugs that relieve symptoms of anxiety. They include benzodiazepines like alprazolam (Xanax), lorazepam (Ativan), and diazepam (Valium) and nonbenzodiazepine drugs like buspirone (BuSpar). Clients should not take alcohol or other sedating drugs when taking anxiolytics. They should consult a physician before discontinuing drug therapy. Abrupt discontinuation can cause withdrawal symptoms that mimic anxiety. Clients should also avoid caffeine, nicotine, or stimulating drugs like diet pills that interfere with desired effects of anxiolytic drug therapy.

Stop, Think, and Respond ● BOX 14-3

What health teaching is appropriate when a client will begin taking an anxiolytic drug?

BETA-ADRENERGIC BLOCKERS. Receptors for norepinephrine are referred to as alpha-adrenergic and beta-adrenergic receptors. When norepinephrine stimulates beta-adrenergic receptors in the heart and lungs, heart rate, forcefulness of heart contraction, and dilation of bronchi all increase. The body is prepared for "fight or flight." In anxiety disorders, norepinephrine prepares the body for a similar response. Blocking the beta-adrenergic receptors with drugs like propranolol (Inderal), atenolol (Tenormin), or metoprolol (Lopressor) reduces this sympathetic nervous system stimulation that causes some symptoms associated with anxiety.

Beta-adrenergic blocking agents do not cause sedation, tolerance, or addiction. They do lower blood pressure and subsequently can cause episodes of dizziness or fainting when rising quickly from a lying or sitting position. Other major side effects include bradycardia and reduced blood glucose level. Those taking a nonselective beta-adrenergic blocker—one that interferes with bronchodilation—may experience fatigue, dyspnea, and wheezing.

CENTRAL-ACTING SYMPATHOLYTICS. Central-acting sympatholytics block alpha-2 receptors for norepinephrine in the brainstem. Consequently, they reduce heart rate and blood pressure. Examples include clonidine (Catapres), methyldopa (Aldomet), and guanabenz (Wytensin). Although these drugs are prescribed more often to control primary hypertension, they potentially have beneficial effects among anxious individuals with elevated blood pressure. Clonidine is also used to control hypertension among individuals who experience withdrawal symptoms when abruptly abstaining from alcohol or anxiolytic therapy.

ANTIDEPRESSANTS. OCD seems to respond to administration of some antidepressants, including selective serotonin reuptake inhibitors (SSRIs) and tricyclic antidepressants (TCAs). Sertraline (Zoloft) is also approved for treatment

DRUG THERAPY TABLE 14.1 DRUGS USED TO TREAT ANXIETY

DRUG CATEGORY AND EXAMPLES	MECHANISM OF ACTION	SIDE EFFECTS	NURSING CONSIDERATIONS
Benzodiazepines *alprazolam (Xanax)*	Exact mechanism of action not understood, but is thought to increase the inhibitory effects of GABA, making the cells less responsive to norepinephrine	Transient mild drowsiness, sedation, fatigue, lightheadedness, constipation, diarrhea, nausea, dry mouth, drug dependence	Instruct client to avoid alcohol and other CNS depressants. Warn client that cimetidine, disulfiram, omeprazole, valproic acid, and oral contraceptives increase the effects of these drugs. Tell client to avoid operating machinery, report all side effects, and avoid stopping the drug abruptly.
Nonbenzodiazepine anxiolytics *buspirone (BuSpar)*	Exact mechanism unknown but does bind with serotonin and dopamine receptors	Dizziness, nervousness, insomnia, headache, lightheadedness, dry mouth, abdominal distress, vomiting, palpitations, chest pain, hyperventilation	Instruct client to avoid alcohol and other CNS depressants and operating machinery, and to report side effects. Inform client that frequent small meals and sucking on ice chips will alleviate gastrointestinal disturbances and dry mouth.
Beta-adrenergic blockers *propranolol hydrochloride (Inderal)*	Decrease the effects of the sympathetic nervous system by reducing CNS sympathetic outflow and blocking beta-adrenergic receptors	Fatigue, nausea, vomiting, diarrhea, flatulence, constipation, bradycardia, hypotension, congestive heart failure, dysrhythmias, erectile dysfunction, decreased libido, decreased activity tolerance	Monitor heart rate, blood pressure, and postural changes. Instruct client to avoid alcohol, to report all side effects, and not to discontinue the drug abruptly. Review all medications because propranolol can interact with many other drugs. Administer with food. Warn clients with diabetes that propranolol may obscure signs and symptoms of hypoglycemia and thus to manage serum glucose carefully.
Central-acting sympatholytics *clonidine hydrochloride (Catapres)*	Decrease the sympathetic outflow from the CNS and inhibit sympathetic nervous system effects	Drowsiness, sedation, dizziness, constipation, dry mouth, anorexia, erectile dysfunction, weight gain, weakness, nightmares	Monitor blood pressure and postural changes. Instruct client to avoid alcohol. Inform client to take drug as prescribed and not to miss doses or abruptly discontinue use. Tell client to report any side effects and that side effects will disappear once the drug is discontinued.

CNS = central nervous system; GABA = gamma-aminobutyric acid.

of social phobia. The symptoms of PTSD are somewhat relieved by some SSRIs and TCAs. Antidepressants are discussed in more detail in Chapter 15.

Psychotherapy

Psychotherapy involves talking with a psychiatrist, psychologist, or mental health counselor. Some clients respond better when therapy sessions are conducted one on one; others, such as those with PTSD, respond better to group interactions.

In **cognitive therapy,** the therapist helps clients alter irrational thinking, correct faulty belief systems, and replace negative self-statements with positive ones based on the theory that it is not events that provoke anxiety, but the person's interpretation of events. **Behavioral therapy** attempts to extinguish undesirable responses by learning other adaptive techniques. One example sometimes used with clients who have phobic disorders or OCD is **desensitization,** which involves providing emotional support while gradually exposing a person to whatever it is that provokes anxiety.

NURSING PROCESS

● The Client With Anxiety

Assessment

Observe for evidence of various levels of anxiety: pacing, talking excessively, complaining, crying, being withdrawn, or trying to run away. Encourage the client to express anxiety by asking open-ended questions such as, "How are you feeling now?" Having the client rate his or her anxiety level using a scale from 0 to 10 is helpful. The client should indicate the level at which anxiety is tolerable. Ask if the client has an effective method for controlling anxiety. Observe the client's mood for signs of concurrent depression and assess the client's use of and knowledge about medications to treat the disorder.

Diagnosis, Planning, and Interventions

Anxiety related to faulty perception of danger
Expected Outcome: The client's anxiety will return to a tolerable level.

- Reduce as much external stimuli, such as noise, bright lights, and activity, as possible. *Numerous stimuli escalate anxiety because they interfere with attention and concentration. Dealing simultaneously with multiple stimuli can tax the client's energy.*
- Maintain a calm manner when interacting with the client. *An anxious nurse can increase anxiety in a client. Modeling a controlled state promotes a similar response in the client.*
- Take a position at least an arm's length away from the client. *Invading an anxious client's personal space may increase his or her discomfort.*
- Avoid touching the client without first asking permission. *An anxious client may misinterpret unexpected touching as a threatening gesture.*
- Establish trust by being available to the client and keeping promises. *Insecurity can be relieved if the client knows he or she can depend on assistance from the nurse.*
- Advise client to seek out the nurse or another supportive person when feeling the effects of anxiety. *The earlier that anxiety is de-escalated, the sooner the client will experience relief of symptoms.*
- Stay with client during periods of severe anxiety. *The nurse's presence can help the client stay in control or restore control to a more comfortable level.*
- Follow a consistent schedule for routine activities. *Unpredictability heightens anxiety; consistency helps a client manage time and cope with personal demands.*
- Encourage the client to identify what he or she perceives to be a threat to emotional equilibrium. *Processing situations verbally may give the client perspective on perceived threats so that they are more realistic and less exaggerated.*
- Use a soft voice, short sentences, clear messages, and specific directions when exchanging information. Assist the client who becomes agitated. *Anxious clients have a short attention span and reduced ability to concentrate, so they may be unable to follow lengthy or complicated information. Assistance relieves unnecessary distress.*
- Instruct and help the client with moderate or severe anxiety to perform one or more of the following until anxiety is within a tolerable level:
    - Count slowly backward from 100. *Distraction redirects the client's attention from distressing physiologic symptoms to the task at hand.*
    - Breathe slowly and deeply in through the nose and out through the mouth. *Slowing respirations aborts hyperventilation and subsequent potential for fainting, peripheral tingling, and numbness from respiratory alkalosis.*
    - Offer a warm bath or back rub. *Warm running water promotes relaxation; massage relaxes muscles and possibly releases endorphins, natural chemicals that promote a sense of well-being.*
    - Progressively relax groups of muscles from the toes to the head. *Consciously relaxing muscles relieves tension and fatigue.*
    - Repeat positive statements such as, "I am in control," "I am safe," "I am relaxed." *Positive self-talk can be transformed into reality.*
    - Visualize a pleasant, relaxing place. *Imagery can transform a person's aroused state to one that is more relaxed.*
    - Listen to a relaxation tape or soothing music. *Distraction helps to refocus attention to less anxiety-provoking stimuli.*
    - Engage in a large-muscle activity such as riding an exercise bicycle or going for a brisk walk. *Activity uses norepinephrine and can reduce it to a more manageable amount.*
- Administer antianxiety medication prescribed on an as-needed (prn) basis if nonpharmacologic approaches are ineffective. *Medication may be necessary to ensure the client's or others' safety if there is a potential for loss of control or violent acting out.*

Evaluation of Expected Outcomes

Following successful nursing interventions, the client deals with anxiety-provoking stimuli realistically and implements measures to decrease anxiety. He or she has extended periods during which anxiety is at a tolerable level and participates in normal activities without becoming incapacitated by anxiety. The client develops more self-confidence, becomes more self-reliant in managing symptoms of anxiety, and manages day-to-day stressors without becoming incapacitated.

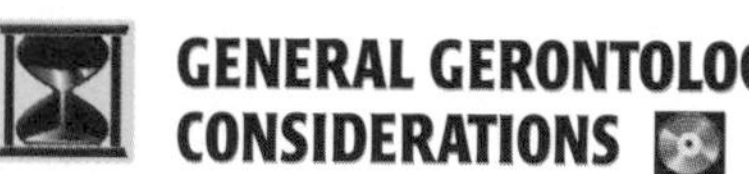

GENERAL GERONTOLOGIC CONSIDERATIONS

Feelings of vulnerability and limitations associated with age may contribute to anxiety in older adults.

Because the kidneys excrete most antianxiety agents, older adults with impaired kidney function are at increased risk for toxicity when taking these medications.

Anxiety may be manifested in the older adult as confusion, behavior changes, or withdrawal.

Many older adults on fixed incomes experience financial problems related to housing and medical expenses that can produce anxiety.

Antianxiety drugs may cause short periods of memory impairment that can aggravate an already existing cognitive disorder.

Before administering a benzodiazepine to an older adult, assess for sleep problems, especially snoring. These drugs have the potential to exacerbate sleep apnea.

Short-acting benzodiazepines such as alprazolam (Xanax) are preferred in older adults because they are less likely than longer-acting benzodiazepines to cause toxicity, leading to excessive sedation and depression.

Buspirone is commonly used to treat anxiety in older adults. The drug does not produce dependence or interact with benzodiazepines or alcohol. A decrease in anxiety may occur in about 1 week; however, the drug may take up to 4 weeks before a full therapeutic response occurs.

The drugs used to treat anxiety may cause dizziness or lightheadedness, increasing the risk of falling in older adults.

Critical Thinking Exercises

1. *Discuss nursing interventions that would be appropriate when a client tells you that he or she feels anxious about her upcoming surgery.*
2. *What interventions should a nurse implement if a client suddenly experiences a panic attack?*

• NCLEX-STYLE REVIEW QUESTIONS 

1. When a client arrives at an outpatient clinic, the nurse is correct in concluding that the client is anxious when the nurse observes the client
   1. Pacing around the waiting room
   2. Sitting in the corner of the room
   3. Flipping through the pages of a magazine
   4. Talking to others who are waiting
2. What information is most important for the nurse to provide a 52-year-old client with a history of panic disorder who is given a prescription for alprazolam (Xanax)?
   1. Avoid consuming alcohol while taking this drug.
   2. Long-term use will not cause drug dependency.
   3. This drug has a side effect of insomnia.
   4. Benefits of drug therapy will be seen immediately.

connection

Visit the Connection site at **http://connection.lww.com/go/timbyEssentials** for links to chapter-related resources on the Internet.

References and Suggested Readings

Anxiety disorders lead mental ills in United States. (1996). *Public Health Reports, 111*(July/August), 293–294.

Barstow, D. G. (2000). Post-traumatic stress disorder: A student nurse's personal experience of terror. *Journal of Psychosocial Nursing and Mental Health Services, 38*(4), 29–33.

Fortinash, K. M., & Holoday-Worret, P. A. (2000). *Psychiatric mental health nursing* (2nd ed.). St. Louis: Mosby.

Giger, J. N., Davidhizar, R., Poole, V. L., et al. (2000). Breakthrough in psychiatric care: Pharmacological treatment of obsessive-compulsive disorders with implications for nursing care. *Journal of Practical Nursing, 50*(1), 23, 25–29, 31.

Laidlow, T. M., Falloon, I. R. H., Barnfather, D., et al. (1999). The stress of caring for people with obsessive compulsive disorders. *Community Mental Health Journal, 35*(5), 443–450.

Tan, W., & Tsai, T. W. (2000). Antidepressants and cognitive-behavioral therapy effective in panic disorder. *Patient Care, 34*(16), 13, 67.

VanderZyl, S. K. (1999). Anxious? You're not alone. *Nursingmatters, 10*(11), 4.

Videbeck, S. L. (2004). *Psychiatric mental health nursing* (2nd ed.). Philadelphia: Lippincott Williams & Wilkins.

chapter 15

Caring for Clients With Mood Disorders

Words to Know 

affect
bipolar disorder
delusions
dopamine
electroconvulsive therapy
euthymic
gamma aminobutyric acid
hallucinations
hypertensive crisis
major (unipolar) depression
mania
melatonin
monoamine hypothesis
mood
mood disorders
norepinephrine
photoperiods
phototherapy
psychomotor agitation
psychomotor retardation
psychotherapy
psychotic depression
reactive (secondary) depression
reuptake
seasonal affective disorder
serotonin
serotonin syndrome

Learning Objectives

On completion of this chapter, the reader will:

- Discuss signs and symptoms of mood disorders.
- Describe neurotransmitters that, when imbalanced, affect mood.
- Identify types of drugs that are used to treat mood disorders and nursing considerations related to their administration.
- Give criteria that indicate a high risk for suicide.
- Discuss nursing measures that are useful in preventing suicide.
- Discuss the nursing management of clients with common mood disorders.

Mood refers to a person's overall feeling state occurring as a continuum, with extremes of emotion existing at both ends or poles (Figure 15.1). Mood is displayed in a person's **affect,** the verbal and nonverbal behavior that communicates feelings.

People with normal moods are referred to as **euthymic**—capable of experiencing a variety of feelings, all of which are situationally appropriate. Individuals with **mood disorders** experience an extreme persistent mood or severe mood swings interfering with social relationships. Primary mood disturbances include major (unipolar) depression and bipolar disorder, formerly called manic-depressive syndrome.

Dysthymia, a feeling of unremitting sadness, is less severe than major depression. In **psychotic depression,** an extreme form of depressive disorder, some individuals experience **hallucinations,** sensory phenomena like hearing voices or seeing images, and **delusions,** fixed false beliefs that are often persecutory in nature. Cyclothymia, alternating sad and elated moods, resembles bipolar disorder, but extremes of mood are less pronounced. **Mania** is the frenzied state of euphoria exhibited by persons during the manic phase of bipolar disorder. **Seasonal affective disorder** (SAD) is a mood disorder characterized by depressive feelings developing during darker winter months and disappearing in the spring.

MAJOR DEPRESSION

Depression, a common experience, can be a normal reaction to loss, disappointment, or overwhelming events. A sad feeling that can be directly attributed to a situation or cause is referred to as **reactive** or **secondary depression.** Generally, reactive depression is self-limiting; when circumstances change or supportive others provide help, depression is relieved. Many people experience **major** or **unipolar depression,** a sad mood with no obvious relationship to situational events. Depression is also a comorbid (coexisting) condition among people with anxiety disorders and substance abuse (see Chaps. 14 and 17).

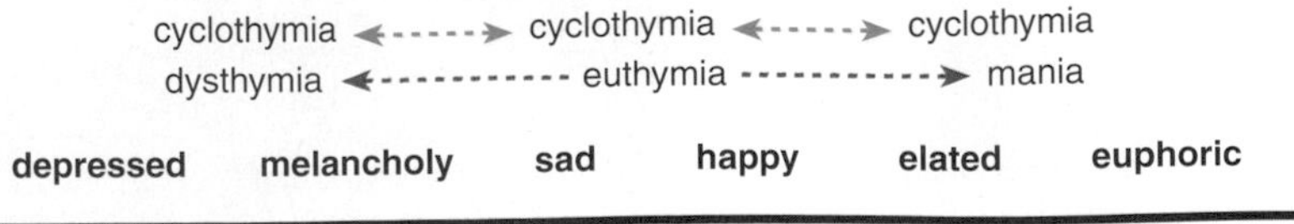

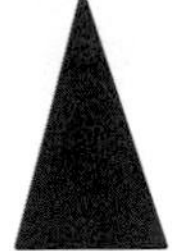

FIGURE 15.1 Mood continuum.

Pathophysiology and Etiology

Brain function, and consequently mood, depends on the dynamic interplay of neurotransmitters. Moods are likely generated by the limbic system, which is the center for emotions. Possible biologic mechanisms that may trigger major depressive symptoms include those related to genetics, dysregulation of neurotransmitters, and neuroendocrine imbalance. Psychological and social theories suggest that infantile rejection or neglect, learned feelings of helplessness, chronic exposure to discrimination, or distorted or false perceptions about oneself contribute to depression. Although these latter factors should not be dismissed, research in brain chemistry gives more support to biologic explanations.

Genetics

Mood disorders tend to be prevalent among close blood relatives, suggesting a genetic link. Even when raised separately, identical twins have a higher incidence of depressive episodes when one is affected (Kelsoe, 2000). Researchers are studying the DNA of fairly homogenous groups (e.g., the Amish) for variations in chromosome patterns among relatives who have mood disorders and those who do not. Preliminary evidence shows that differences exist in at least two chromosomes, but more research is needed (Videbeck, 2004).

Stop, Think, and Respond ● BOX 15-1

What other reason might explain why people who are related manifest similar disturbances in mood? 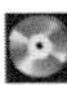

Neurotransmitter Dysregulation

A widely accepted psychobiologic theory for depression is the **monoamine hypothesis,** which proposes imbalances in one or more monoamine neurotransmitters, serotonin, norepinephrine, and dopamine, cause depression. The hypothesis rests on evidence of lowered levels of a metabolite of **serotonin,** 5-HIAA, in depressed people. Second, **norepinephrine** levels may be low or high among people affected by depression. Low levels of norepinephrine may explain why some depressed people develop **psychomotor retardation,** characterized by lack of energy, increased sleep, and little interest in daily events or responsibilities. On the other hand, some depressed people may have excessive norepinephrine, and are more likely to experience **psychomotor agitation** with such stimulating manifestations as insomnia, pacing, and distractability, rather than lethargy. Third, symptoms of some depressed clients suggest excess **dopamine,** associated with distortion of thoughts. In moderate to severe depression, this may be evidenced as overreactive guilt, self-blame, self-pity, and low self-worth.

Neuroendocrine Imbalance

Interactions of the pituitary, adrenal cortex, thyroid gland, and ovaries may also play a role in producing depression by altering levels of hormones. These endocrine glands are stimulated and suppressed via the hypothalamus, a structure within the limbic system. Abnormal levels of cortisol, a hormone produced by the adrenal cortex, and variations in thyroid hormones are accompanied by changes in mood and motor activity. The hypothalamus also influences the pituitary gland's stimulation of reproductive hormones. The latter hormonal relationships help to explain the altered mood states associated with premenstrual syndrome (PMS) (also known as late luteal phase dysphoric syndrome), menopause, and postpartum depression.

Assessment Findings

The predominant feature of major depression is a persistent sad mood accompanied by multiple physiologic and cognitive (thought) changes. Because symptoms of depression may be similar to other conditions (Box 15-1), a tentative diagnosis is made while investigating and eliminating alternative reasons for clinical findings.

BOX 15-1 ● Signs and Symptoms of Major Depression

Sad mood
Appetite change (increased or decreased)
Disturbed sleep (insomnia or hypersomnia)
Inability to concentrate
Marked decrease in pleasure
Apathy, including lack of interest in sex
Guilty feelings
Energy changes (restlessness or inactivity)
Suicidal thoughts

Studies that identify 5-HIAA in cerebrospinal fluid and the metabolite of norepinephrine (MPHG) in urine are financially prohibitive except for research purposes. Blood levels of serotonin can be measured more easily, but some question if the level in blood correlates with the level necessary for normal mood in the brain. Furthermore, some managed care groups consider diagnostic laboratory tests of neurotransmitter levels unnecessary. Third-party payers often maintain that a diagnosis of depression can be confirmed or ruled out by the client's clinical presentation and by performing other standard tests for disorders that mimic depression. Findings that indicate alternative diagnoses to depression include low thyroid function test results suggesting hypothyroidism (see Chap. 51), abnormal blood glucose levels suggesting diabetes mellitus (see Chap. 52), low hemoglobin level indicative of anemia (see Chap. 33), and detection of drug abuse in a urine drug screen (see Chap. 17).

Neurologic imaging tests like computed axial tomography (CAT) scans or magnetic resonance imaging (MRI) may be performed to eliminate diagnoses such as brain tumor or cerebrovascular accident as causes for a client's altered mood. A positron emission tomography (PET) scan may show a change in activity within the prefrontal cortex suggestive of a mood disorder. The physician may omit imaging tests if he or she thinks the clinical evidence strongly supports the diagnosis of depression.

Medical Management

Drug Therapy

The three main categories of drugs that relieve the symptoms of depression are tricyclic antidepressants (TCAs), monoamine oxidase inhibitors (MAOIs), and selective serotonin reuptake inhibitors (SSRIs) (Drug Therapy Table 15.1). A fourth group of medications is called atypical antidepressants because they that do not fall in any of the three major chemical families.

All antidepressants increase or potentiate levels of serotonin. **Serotonin syndrome** is a potentially life-threatening condition that results from elevated levels of serotonin in the blood. Manifestations include fever, sweating, shivering, feelings of intoxication, confusion, restlessness, anxiety, disorientation, ataxia, tachycardia, hypertension, tremors, and muscular spasms and rigidity. The following factors place a client at risk for serotonin syndrome:

DRUG THERAPY TABLE 15.1 ANTIDEPRESSANTS

DRUG CATEGORY AND EXAMPLES	MECHANISM OF ACTION	SIDE EFFECTS	NURSING CONSIDERATIONS
Tricyclic antidepressants (TCAs) *amitriptyline (Elavil), nortriptyline (Pamelor), imipramine (Tofranil)*	Block the reuptake of serotonin and norepinephrine	Orthostatic hypotension, sedation, dry mouth, blurred vision, weight gain, constipation, urinary retention, cardiac dysrhythmias	Inform client that symptomatic relief may not occur for 2 to 4 weeks or longer. Caution client to rise slowly from a lying or sitting position. Inform client that blurred vision and dry mouth will decrease over time. Discuss the increased potential for suicide as energy increases before depression resolves. Discontinue the drug gradually.
Monoamine oxidase inhibitors (MAOIs) *phenelzine (Nardil), tranylcypromine (Parnate)*	Block the enzyme that breaks down monoamines	Headache, insomnia, severe hypertension with certain foods and drugs, orthostatic hypotension, transient erectile dysfunction, constipation or diarrhea, dry mouth, blurred vision	Provide information on diet and drug restrictions to avoid hypertensive crisis. Advise client to wear a MedicAlert bracelet. Educate client about potentially lethal interaction with meperidine (Demerol) Explain that there may be a 2- to 6-week delay before symptoms improve. Advise client to take last dose before bedtime to avoid sleep disturbances. Allow at least a 14-day interval between discontinuing a TCA and initiating an MAOI.
Selective serotonin reuptake inhibitors *fluoxetine (Prozac), sertraline (Zoloft), paroxetine (Paxil)*	Block the reuptake of serotonin but not norepinephrine	Weight loss, insomnia, tremor, nervousness, headache, decreased libido, erectile dysfunction, interference with liver enzymes that potentiates the risk for altered metabolism of other drugs	Instruct client to avoid caffeine and other foods or drugs that are cardiac stimulants. Monitor blood pressure and heart rate. Allow at least 14 days before switching to an MAOI. Monitor for serotonin syndrome, which can result from a drug–drug interaction.

- Antidepressants from different classes such as MAOIs and SSRIs are coprescribed.
- The time between weaning from one antidepressant drug to initiating another is inadequate.
- Other serotonergic agonists, drugs that stimulate serotonin receptors, are combined with antidepressant therapy. Serotonergic agonists include dextromethorphan (Benylin, Pertussin, Delsym), meperidine (Demerol), and lithium (Eskalith, Lithane).

Temporarily withholding the antidepressant is recommended initially. In severe cases, symptoms can be managed with anxiolytic drugs like diazepam (Valium), beta-adrenergic blockers like propranolol (Inderol), or skeletal muscle relaxants like dantrolene (Dantrium), while supporting breathing with mechanical ventilation.

TRICYCLIC ANTIDEPRESSANTS. Tricyclic antidepressants (TCAs) were the first group of drugs used to treat depression; they occasionally are prescribed for clients with chronic pain. TCAs were named because they have three chemical attachments in their organic molecular structure. Many variations of drugs in this category have been developed since the first tricyclics. The subsequent modifications are referred to as bicyclics and even heterocyclics according to the changes in their molecules. Collectively, they may be called "cyclic" antidepressants.

Cyclic antidepressants block the **reuptake** of serotonin and norepinephrine interfering with reabsorption of these neurotransmitters by the releasing presynaptic neuron. This creates a sustained effect.

One disadvantage of cyclic antidepressants is the lag time between initiation of drug therapy and relief of depressive symptoms. It may take from 10 to 28 days or longer, depending on the specific cyclic drug, before a client notes any change in mood. Another disadvantage is that cyclics are highly lethal if taken in an overdose. Because suicide is not uncommon among depressed clients, the physician must consider limiting the number of cyclics that are filled in any one prescription. Regardless of the prescribed class of antidepressant, clients with psychomotor retardation may attempt suicide once their level of energy increases. Nurses should not be lulled into thinking that a depressed client is necessarily nonsuicidal just because he or she is more active. In fact, close observation is even more important at this time.

MONOAMINE OXIDASE INHIBITORS. Monoamine oxidase is an enzyme that breaks down monoamine neurotransmitters. Inhibiting this enzyme allows neurotransmitters to continue stimulating receptor sites for norepinephrine, serotonin, and, to some extent, dopamine. Monoamine oxidase inhibitors (MAOIs) are the least prescribed category of antidepressants because they have a high potential for food–drug interactions and drug–drug interactions (Box 15-2). When an MAOI is combined with foods containing tyramine, another monoamine, clients are likely to develop a potentially fatal **hypertensive crisis** with symptoms such as elevated blood pressure, headache, nausea, vomiting, sweating, palpitations, visual changes, neck stiffness, sensitivity to light, and tachycardia. The nurse must teach clients about dietary and drug restrictions, which continue for at least 2 weeks after stopping the drug.

BOX 15-2 ● Food, Beverage, and Drug Restrictions During Monoamine Oxidase Inhibitor Drug Therapy

FOOD AND BEVERAGES TO AVOID

Aged, hard cheese	Pepperoni, sausage
Chocolate	Sour cream
Pickled herring	Broad beans (fava beans)
Overripe bananas	Monosodium glutamate
Chicken liver	Beer
Dried fish	Soy sauce
Fermented meat (salami)	Red wine
Yogurt	Meat tenderizer

DRUGS TO AVOID

Cold and allergy medications	Meperidine (Demerol)
Appetite suppressants	Antidepressants in other categories
Antiasthmatics	Local anesthetics with epinephrine
Antihypertensives	

Stop, Think, and Respond ● BOX 15-2

What information would you offer to a person who has just started MAOI therapy and plans to go out for pizza and beer?

SELECTIVE SEROTONIN REUPTAKE INHIBITORS. Selective serotonin reuptake inhibitors (SSRIs) interfere primarily with the reabsorption of serotonin. They have lesser effects on other neurotransmitter levels. The accumulated serotonin prolongs stimulation of neuroreceptor sites. SSRIs are the newest and most prescribed group of drugs for treatment of depression. They are used for several reasons: (1) they have milder side effects, (2) they are unlikely to cause death in cases of overdose, (3) dosages do not need much adjustment after initiation of therapy, and (4) the lag time is short, perhaps 3 to 10 days.

Although SSRIs cause side effects, these problems tend to dissipate within weeks of starting drug therapy. If side effects do not resolve, they can be managed with additional medications like a mild hypnotic for sleep. Unfortunately, sexual dysfunction is a frequent and undesirable side effect. Alterations in sexual activity are a leading cause of noncompliance. Lowering the dose of SSRIs can reduce sexual side effects.

ATYPICAL ANTIDEPRESSANTS. Several additional drugs relieve depression but do not belong to the major categories of antidepressants. Some examples include nefazodone (Serzone), venlafaxine (Effexor), and maprotiline (Ludiomil). The atypical drugs are used as alternatives for clients who do not respond to trials with other standard classes of antidepressants.

Stop, Think, and Respond ● BOX 15-3

How would you respond to a client who reports feeling just as depressed as when he or she began antidepressant drug therapy 4 days earlier?

Psychotherapy

Psychotherapy, talking with a psychiatrist, psychologist, or mental health counselor, promotes coping with emotional problems, gaining insight into behaviors, and learning techniques that can improve well-being. Various types of psychotherapy are available:

- *Psychodynamic psychotherapy* is patterned after a Freudian model. Clients discuss early life experiences to raise repressed feelings to a conscious level.
- *Interpersonal psychotherapy* is facilitated by a bond that develops between the therapist and client. The empathy and trust help clients gain understanding of their condition and the courage and support to overcome it.
- *Supportive psychotherapy* helps clients learn about their disorder and treatment techniques, improve or develop new social skills, obtain positive reinforcement for progress, and give encouragement to persevere.
- *Cognitive therapy* helps clients replace negative, and often illogical, ways of thinking with more positive outlooks (see Chap. 14).
- *Behavioral therapy* endeavors to change unhealthy ways of behaving. Clients are rewarded verbally or in some other way when they alter their behavior positively (see Chap. 14).

Psychotherapy is often more productive after depressed clients respond to antidepressant drug therapy. Clients should be advised that if they feel uncomfortable or dissatisfied with a particular practitioner or style of therapy, they can be referred elsewhere.

Electroconvulsive Therapy

Electroconvulsive therapy (ECT) uses the application of an electric stimulus to one or both temporal regions of the head to produce a brief, generalized seizure. Although the exact mechanism of action is unknown, the belief is that ECT achieves its effect by either increasing circulating levels of monoamine neurotransmitters or by improving transmission to the receptor site. ECT is generally reserved for depressed clients who:

- Have not responded to drug therapy
- Are intolerant of the side effects of antidepressant medications
- Are so seriously suicidal that waiting for antidepressants to become effective jeopardizes their safety

Except for clients who are extremely suicidal, ECT can be administered on an ambulatory, outpatient basis. Many clients experience aftereffects including headache, soreness of skeletal muscles, temporary confusion, short-term patchy memory loss, and brief learning disability. ECT is usually contraindicated for clients with cardiac or neurovascular pathologies.

NURSING PROCESS

● The Depressed or Suicidal Client

Assessment

Besides assessing the client physically and monitoring mood and affect, nurses can use various assessment questionnaires as a database for quantifying a person's mood state and tracking changes that occur during treatment. Examples include the Beck Depression Inventory, a self-assessment tool, and the Hamilton Rating Scale for Depression (HAMD), which is administered by a mental health worker. If a client is depressed, the nurse must assume that he or she may also be suicidal. Suicide is the third leading cause of death among 15 to 24 year olds. Older adults commit almost 20% of all suicides, with the greatest incidence among men aged 80 to 84 years (Centers for Disease Control, 2002). One of the most reliable suicide assessment techniques is to bluntly ask, "Do you feel like killing yourself?" Unfortunately, some depressed clients conceal their suicidal thoughts, provide only vague verbal or behavior clues (Box 15-3), or

BOX 15-3 ● Clues of Suicidal Intentions

CLEAR VERBAL CLUES
"I'm planning to kill myself."
"I wish I were dead."

VAGUE VERBAL CLUES
"I just can't stand it any longer."
"Nobody needs me anymore."
"Life has lost its meaning for me."
"You won't be seeing me anymore."
"I'm getting out."
"Everybody would be better off without me."

BEHAVIORAL CLUES
Giving away a valued possession
Donating large sums of money to charity
Putting personal affairs in order
Writing poetry with morbid themes
Composing a suicide note
Making funeral arrangements
Buying a gun; stockpiling pills
Lifting of depressed mood (may indicate a plan and energy to carry it out)

assume that others are aware of their despair but have chosen to ignore it.

If a client admits to being suicidal, determine if the client has a suicide plan, which increases the seriousness of the risk. Assess if the plan is feasible and of high or low lethality. High-lethality methods are those from which possibility of rescue is remote, including shooting or hanging oneself or jumping from a bridge or building. Low-lethality methods allow a window of time for the suicidal person to be found and rescued; examples include overdosing on medications or cutting the wrists.

Determine the level at which the depressed client can carry out activities of daily living. Depressed clients may not eat, bathe, shave, or shampoo or style their hair. In some cases, they neglect self-care because they lack energy. They may also ignore cleanliness and grooming because of low self-esteem or little concern for social acceptance.

Diagnosis, Planning, and Interventions

Risk for Suicide related to feelings of hopelessness
Expected Outcomes: (1) The client will not harm self. (2) The client will identify a reason for living.

- If hospitalized, move client close to nursing station. *Facilitates close and frequent observation.*
- Encourage a client who is not hospitalized to contact a friend or relative rather than remain alone. *Presence of a supportive person can deter a suicide attempt.*
- Talk to a nonhospitalized client on the phone as long as possible while contacting a 911 operator. *Delays a potential suicide attempt or provides time to obtain assistance from emergency personnel who can intervene.*
- Make a verbal or written contract with the client that he or she will not attempt suicide. *Clients often honor such commitments.*
- Confiscate any objects the client may use for self-harm, such as belts, shoelaces, safety razors, sharp combs, keys, or knives. *Reduces resources he or she has for attempting suicide.*
- Inspect client's mouth, looking under the tongue and within the buccal cavity, after administering medications. *Suicidal clients may conceal and hoard medications until they stockpile sufficient numbers for an overdose.*
- Observe client's whereabouts at least every 15 minutes, and spend time interacting with him or her. *Reduces client's potential time for attempting or completing suicide and increases the response time available to resuscitate a person who has attempted suicide.*
- Keep client busy and involved in activities. *Shifts client's attention away from his or her emotional pain and hopelessness.*

Ineffective Coping related to feelings of helplessness and worthlessness
Expected Outcome: The client will identify one or more alternatives to suicide.

- Acknowledge client's feeling of despair. *Demonstrates that the nurse notices the person and is perceptive.*
- Indicate that you want to help. *Offering assistance is characterized as a therapeutic use of self. Reassures client that you will not abandon him or her and that he or she is worthy of help.*
- Emphasize hope, previous positive experiences, and outcomes. *Reinforces that client has potential to overcome current difficulties based on past success.*
- Explore other courses of action rather than suicide. *Alternatives help client consider options for dealing with current situation.*
- Appeal to client's ambivalence by indicating that current feelings are likely to change given additional time. *Most suicidal clients will delay or dismiss suicidal activities if they believe that they will feel better eventually.*
- Discuss previous coping strategies and encourage using some that were effective in the past. *Offers the possibility that similar actions can achieve a positive result.*
- Develop a plan for maintaining future safety such as talking with a trusted friend or calling a crisis hotline. *If a plan is developed, there is a possibility that the client will implement it.*

Evaluation of Expected Outcomes

The client implements new or previously successful coping strategies to manage emotional problems. He or she eats sufficiently to maintain adequate nutrition and his or her weight before illness.

SEASONAL AFFECTIVE DISORDER

Seasonal affective disorder (SAD) develops during darker winter months and spontaneously disappears in the spring. It is more prevalent among people living in northern states, such as Washington, Michigan, and the New England states. Native Alaskans do not manifest the disorder as much as those who move there.

Pathophysiology and Etiology

The best explanation for SAD is that it is a primitive biologic response triggered by **photoperiods,** daytime hours that are short because of fewer hours of sunlight. The condition actually resembles characteristics of hibernating animals. Theorists believe that light rays follow a visual pathway to the hypothalamus, the center for regulating sleep, hunger, libido, and mood. The hypothalamus relays the light-sensing data to the pineal gland, which regulates production of a hormone called melatonin. **Melatonin,** which also affects regulation of serotonin, induces sleep during dark hours and is suppressed by daylight. When hours of daylight become fewer, production of melatonin is extended. In northern latitudes, melatonin secretion is sustained until spring, when days become brighter and longer.

Assessment Findings

Clients with SAD use the terms *sleepy, fatigued,* and *lethargic* to describe themselves in the winter. Lack of energy turns into feeling irritable, unable to concentrate, worthless, guilty, depressed—even suicidal. Some report cravings for carbohydrates, leading to weight gain, much like an animal preparing to sleep through the winter. As clients with SAD become more depressed and irritable, they are less inclined to interact socially. Many tend to stay indoors and dread leaving home.

The depression is bimodal; it cycles with the seasons. After prolonged winter depression, most report a lifting of spirits in the spring. Some also describe feeling energetic, more motivated, hyperactive, and even euphoric until late fall, when the depressive pattern repeats itself.

At this time no diagnostic tests can confirm SAD. Physicians rely on clients' reports of cycling moods that correlate with the ratio of sunlight.

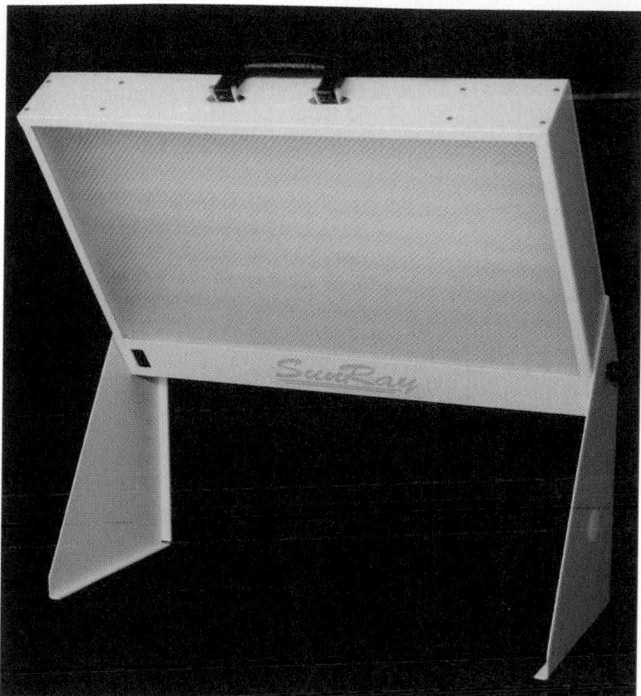

FIGURE 15.2 Phototherapy products such as a light box relieve the symptoms of seasonal affective disorder. (Courtesy of Light Therapy Products.)

Medical Management

For those who cannot move to a sunnier location, phototherapy is the best alternative for treating SAD. **Phototherapy** is a technique using artificial light to simulate the intensity of sunlight. The artificial light is produced by fluorescent bulbs at 2500 to 10,000 lux, the international measurement of illumination. Ten thousand lux is about 10 to 20 times as bright as ordinary indoor light.

The frequency and duration for phototherapy can vary, but a common prescription is to sit by the light source from 30 minutes to 2 hours per day, preferably in the early morning hours (Figure 15.2). The client should not look directly at the light, but instead glance periodically at it to relieve symptoms in 1 to 2 weeks. Other models are available as well. A head-mounted light that shines on the face during daytime activities facilitates mobility. Bedroom phototherapy lights can be set with an automatic timer to come on at a predawn schedule. Even though the sleeper's eyes are closed, it is believed that the light penetrates the eyelids, which triggers a decline in melatonin—much like daybreak naturally activates arousal from sleep.

Nursing Management

Most clients with SAD are treated as outpatients. The nurse provides information on how to implement phototherapy and supplement its beneficial effects. The most important principle to stress is that natural sunlight is brighter and better than any artificial substitute. The nurse also should teach measures found in Client and Family Teaching 15-1.

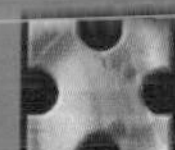

15-1 *Client and Family Teaching* Seasonal Affective Disorder (SAD)

The nurse must teach the client who experiences SAD and his or her family the following:

- Avoid the use of eyeglasses or contact lenses that are coated to shield ultraviolet radiation because the coating interferes with light transmission to the pineal gland.
- Add more lamps and bright fixtures at home and work.
- Install skylights.
- Trim shrubs and trees from around windows.
- Use translucent curtains or shades rather than heavy drapes.
- Sleep and work in an east-facing room.
- Take brief walks outside around noon without sunglasses.
- Jog after sun-up and before sundown.
- Take up an outdoor winter sport.

BIPOLAR DISORDER

Bipolar disorder is characterized by cycling between depression, euthymia, and euphoria. Each dysfunctional mood is likely to last several months, although depressive phases tend to be longer than manic phases. Some individuals experience a mild manic phase, referred to as *hypomania;* others, known as *rapid cyclers,* experience at least four episodes of mania and depression per year.

Pathophysiology and Etiology

Extremes in levels of monoamines—excessive in mania and inadequate during depression—seem to be responsible for the symptoms of bipolar disorder. In severe cases, excess dopamine may cause distorted thinking and hallucinations. Insufficient **gamma aminobutyric acid** (GABA), an inhibitory neurotransmitter, may counteract the effects of monoamines. Altered blood calcium levels may also contribute to development of bipolar disorder because calcium is required for exciting neurons. Genetic predisposition is also implicated.

Assessment Findings

Signs and symptoms of the depressive phase of bipolar disorder are the same as those for major depression. During the manic phase, clients are hyperactive and often display an exaggerated sense of their own importance. They can quickly become angry and aggressive with those who attempt to restrain their burst of energy and wild ideas. Because judgment is impaired, reckless and impulsive behavior like sexual promiscuity, criminal activity, spending sprees, gambling, and risky business transactions can occur. The surge of norepinephrine allows clients experiencing the manic phase to go without sleep for long periods. It also causes rapid thinking accompanied by racing speech. When extremely ill, some individuals experience psychotic features such as hallucinations. Combined with delusions (illogically false beliefs), the client with bipolar disorder can become homicidal or suicidal.

It may eventually be possible to predict who will develop bipolar disorder with the use of gene mapping. At present, however, no objective tests are available, and the diagnosis is based on the client's history.

Medical Management

Bipolar disorder is managed by the administration of one or more mood-stabilizing medications (Drug Therapy Table 15.2). Lithium (Eskalith, Lithane, Lithobid), a chemical element, is usually the initial drug of choice. It controls both depressive and manic symptoms in clients who respond to lithium monotherapy (single-drug treatment). The American Psychiatric Association's Practice Guideline for the Treatment of Bipolar Disorder (1994) now recommends anticonvulsants such as valproic acid derivatives (Depakote, Depakene, Valproate) and others such as carbamazepine (Tegretol), alone or in combination with lithium, for controlling mood swings. Antipsychotics such as haloperidol (Haldol) (see Chap. 18) may also be prescribed for a brief period to induce sedation and control hallucinations and delusions. Some propose using calcium-channel blockers, but there is little research to support this.

Lithium

Lithium is a naturally occurring element found in stone and spring water that flows from underground sources. Pharmaceutical preparations are available for those who are lithium-deficient. When ingested, lithium carries on functions like other electrolytes. It moves easily through cell membranes, but it is less easily removed. Some believe that this feature may stabilize cell membranes, leading to the equalization of moods. Another possibility is that lithium regulates the activity between neurotransmitters like serotonin, norepinephrine, dopamine, and their receptor sites. However, lithium:

- May be ineffective for some
- Has a delay of 5 to 14 days in achieving therapeutic benefits
- Has a narrow range of safety between a therapeutic serum level (0.8 to 1.2 mEq) and toxic level (1.5 mEq)
- May be nontherapeutic or dangerously elevated when taken in combination with other drugs, such as tetracycline, haloperidol, theophylline, and carbamazepine
- Causes side effects that challenge compliance
- Requires periodic laboratory tests to monitor serum blood levels

Lithium crosses the placental barrier, so its use is contraindicated in pregnant women. Lithium is water-soluble and present in all body fluids, including breast milk; lithium in breast milk is toxic to infants. Loss of body fluid from diarrhea, diuretics, and excessive perspiration can lead to concentrated blood levels and lithium toxicity. Since the body always attempts to balance cations with anions, lithium may be retained if sodium levels are low. Providers must stress the importance of maintaining an adequate ingestion of salt to all clients who rely on lithium to control their disorder.

Anticonvulsants

Anticonvulsants may achieve therapeutic effects by enhancing the action of GABA in much the same way that benzodiazepines reduce anxiety (see Chap. 14). One of the first anticonvulsants used to treat bipolar disorder

DRUG THERAPY TABLE 15.2 MOOD-STABILIZING MEDICATIONS

DRUG EXAMPLES	MECHANISM OF ACTION	SIDE EFFECTS	NURSING CONSIDERATIONS
lithium carbonate (Eskalith, Lithane, Lithobid)	Alters sodium transport in nerve and muscle cells; increases intraneural stores and inhibits release of norepinephrine and dopamine	Hand tremors, nausea, vomiting, diarrhea, thirst, polyuria, sedation, thyroid dysfunction, wrist and ankle edema at therapeutic level	Administer with meals. Withhold if serum level is >1.5 mEq. Female clients should use contraception and avoid breast-feeding.
valproic acid (Depakote)	May increase levels of GABA	Drowsiness, mild tremor, ataxia, nausea, vomiting, diarrhea, blood dyscrasias, liver toxicity	Administer with meals. Caution client to avoid activities that require alertness and coordination. Monitor blood for therapeutic level.
carbamazepine (Tegretol)	Decreases rate of neuronal impulse transmission	Dizziness, drowsiness, unsteady gait, nausea, vomiting, fluid retention, edema, blood dyscrasias, skin rash, liver toxicity	Administer with meals. Caution client to avoid activities that require alertness and coordination. Risk of central nervous system toxicity increases when given with lithium. Risk of liver toxicity increases when given with a monoamine oxidase inhibitor. Monitor blood for therapeutic levels. Female clients should use contraceptives.
clonazepam (Klonopin)	May increase brain levels of GABA	Drowsiness, dizziness, unsteady gait, nausea, vomiting, constipation, blood dyscrasias, dry mouth, liver toxicity	Collaborate with the physician on baseline blood tests before initiating therapy. Administer drug with food or milk. Drowsiness may be potentiated if combined with alcohol or other sedative drugs. Monitor laboratory findings during therapy and withhold drug if there is bone marrow suppression or serious elevation in liver enzymes. Advise sucking on hard candy or more frequent oral hygiene to relieve dry mouth. Advise women that incidence of birth defects increases if drug is taken during pregnancy, and to use a reliable contraceptive while taking this drug. Never discontinue the drug abruptly.

GABA = gamma-aminobutyric acid.

was carbamazepine (Tegretol). It is still used to manage the symptoms of clients at the onset of acute mania. In addition, it is effective in decreasing the incidence and frequency of mood swings among rapid cyclers. Carbamazepine stimulates drug metabolism by the liver, so maintaining consistent therapeutic drug levels is difficult. Clients who take carbamazepine are at risk for infection because the drug impairs white blood cell formation. Serum drug levels and leukocyte counts must be monitored periodically.

Valproic acid derivatives like Depakote are usually preferred to carbamazepine. These derivatives also enhance GABA activity. Clients who take valproic acid tend to experience gastrointestinal symptoms like nausea, vomiting, and diarrhea. Some develop sedation and ataxia, putting them at risk for injury. There must be periodic assessment of liver function and blood cell counts. Although it can be combined with lithium and used for long-term management of bipolar disorder, valproic acid is unsafe during pregnancy.

Nursing Management

Nursing Care Plan 15-1 provides a detailed discussion of care for the client with bipolar disorder. Before discharge, educate the client and his or her significant others on the disease process, how prescribed drugs help in symptom management, drug effects and side effects, signs of drug toxicity and actions to take, frequency of blood tests, and the advantages of wearing a MedicAlert bracelet.

In addition to arranging outpatient therapy, inform the client and others of support groups that can continue the educational and therapeutic processes. Both the client and those who live in the same environment need to understand the signs of relapse, such as an inability to

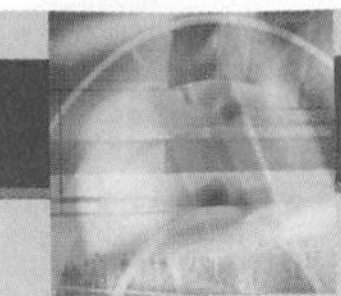

Nursing Care Plan 15-1

THE CLIENT WITH BIPOLAR DISORDER/ACUTE MANIC PHASE

Assessment

- It may be necessary to perform the initial assessment and physical examination in brief increments. Bipolar clients have short attention spans and poor concentration and are easily frustrated if their activity is curtailed. Use the family as a more objective resource for necessary information, which is valuable since the client's symptoms usually create multiple crises.
- Determine types of prescribed medications the client takes and if he or she is compliant with the medication regimen. Sometimes antidepressants trigger manic symptoms because they raise monoamine neurotransmitter levels.
- Ask about the client's use of alcohol or other controlled substances since many clients with bipolar disorder attempt to self-medicate to control their moods or use drugs recreationally because of their poor judgment.
- Obtain information about the client's recent sleep patterns, hydration, and dietary intake.
- Observe the client's attention to hygiene and manner of dress. Check the female client's last date of menstruation and if she has consistently used contraception.
- Prepare the client for laboratory and diagnostic tests that will likely include an electrocardiogram (ECG), thyroid function studies, and blood chemistry tests. Note if the client is voiding in sufficient quantities and inquire as to the client's bowel elimination patterns including the date of the last bowel movement.
- Record baseline vital signs.
- Listen to the client's thought content during verbal interactions. The client is likely to speak loudly and rapidly. At the very least, bipolar clients express expansive and elaborate ideas or schemes. Some may have paranoid ideas or inflate their own importance. They may experience hallucinations.

Nursing Diagnosis: **Disturbed Thought Processes** related to excessive levels of monoamines

Expected Outcome: Client will be oriented to time, place, and person.

Interventions	*Rationales*
Orient client to person, place, time, and events.	Racing thoughts often interfere with comprehension.
Provide information in small amounts, using brief sentences.	Brief discussions accommodate for short attention span.
Reduce distracting stimuli such as noise and stimulation.	External stimuli potentiate client's internal activity.
Present reality when client is delusional; do not press the issue if it causes agitation.	Failing to present reality reinforces that client's delusions are real. Persistence may create conflict or cause client to act out violently.
Monitor client's whereabouts to ensure that he or she does not wander from unit or healthcare agency.	Bipolar clients are impulsive and resist being confined. Healthcare personnel are responsible for safety at all times.

Evaluation of Expected Outcome:

- Client becomes oriented.
- Client interacts appropriately for the situation.

Nursing Diagnoses: **Risk for Other-Directed Violence** and **Risk for Self-Directed Violence**

Expected Outcome: Client will not injure self or others.

(continued)

Nursing Care Plan 15-1 (Continued)

THE CLIENT WITH BIPOLAR DISORDER/ACUTE MANIC PHASE

Interventions	Rationales
Take client to a room or other secluded area when he or she shows signs of aggression.	Decreased stimulation may restore self-control.
Set firm limits for behavioral expectations using a modulated and controlled tone of voice.	Client remains informed of the kinds of behavior that will not be tolerated. A modulated, controlled voice is less likely to provoke a confrontation.
Offer client a large-muscle activity like playing basketball or riding an exercise bicycle.	Exercise releases energy and reduces the potential for an angry outburst.
Administer a prescribed short-acting sedative if aggressive behavior escalates and endangers others.	A sedate client is more responsive to directions from others and less likely to become physically violent.
Obtain an order to seclude or restrain if client becomes violent.	Legally, restraints must be avoided unless absolutely necessary to protect others because clients have the right to the least restrictive treatment.
Initiate suicidal precautions if data suggest vulnerability for self-harm.	The client's safety is a priority of care.

Evaluation of Expected Outcome:

- Client has no angry outbursts.
- Client demonstrates self-control.

Nursing Diagnosis: **Bathing/Hygiene Self-Care Deficit** related to decreased attention and concentration

Expected Outcome: Client will be clean and groomed each day.

Interventions	Rationales
Prepare necessities for bathing, grooming, and hygiene for client. Supervise hygiene and provide assistance if needed.	Distractability may interfere with client's ability to organize hygiene items. Client may be less thorough without nurse's supervision.
Spread uncompleted hygiene tasks throughout remainder of the day.	All hygiene needs may not be met at one time.
Help client to dress appropriately and remain dressed.	Bipolar clients may dress flamboyantly or seductively unless supervised. Poor judgment may result in episodes of nudity.

Evaluation of Expected Outcome: Client resumes independent responsibility for self-care and activities of daily living.

sleep for several days in a row or increasingly impulsive behavior such as making unnecessary purchases. Also review the signs of cycling into a depressed mood so that indications for reinitiating medical care are clear.

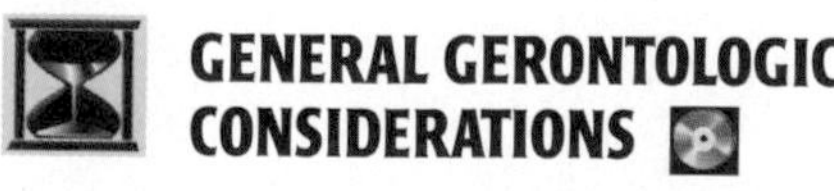

GENERAL GERONTOLOGIC CONSIDERATIONS

Impaired regulation of neurotransmitters in older adults suggests that they may be biologically predisposed to depression and thought disorders.

Cognitive impairment in the depressed older adult can be easily confused with dementia. It is important to distinguish between the two because depression in the elderly can usually be treated successfully.

In older adults, psychotropic drugs are prescribed at the lowest possible dosage that will produce a therapeutic effect because of the potential for increased adverse reactions and possible toxicity.

Risk for orthostatic hypotension from psychotropic drugs is increased in older adults because of decreased functioning of the blood pressure-regulating mechanism.

Older adults may require longer administration (up to 8 weeks) than other clients to obtain a therapeutic effect when taking antidepressants.

Antidepressants must be used cautiously in older adults with cardiovascular disease. Older men with prostatic enlargement are more susceptible to urinary retention.
Older adults who seek treatment for subacute physical symptoms, such as loss of appetite, trouble sleeping, lack of energy, and weight loss, may actually be depressed.
The losses that accompany aging and chronic or terminal illness may trigger feelings of hopelessness, which increase the risk for suicide.
Older adults who are depressed often use a lethal means to ensure successful suicide. The highest suicide rate is seen in older adults between ages 75 to 80 years.
As individuals with bipolar disorder age, their depressive episodes may increase in frequency and last longer.
Older adults who are prescribed lithium to treat bipolar disorder require careful monitoring. Because the kidneys eliminate lithium, age-related changes in the elderly may reduce renal clearance, predisposing these clients to lithium toxicity.

Critical Thinking Exercises

1. *Two depressed clients are in a psychiatric hospital. One feels suicidal, but has no plan for carrying it out. The other indicates that he would kill himself with a gun, but has none. Describe the similarities and differences in their nursing care.*
2. *What physical consequences might occur for the client in a manic episode?*
3. *What problems might family members experience as a result of living with a person with a mood disorder?*

• NCLEX-STYLE REVIEW QUESTIONS 

1. The nurse provides client teaching about dietary restrictions while taking monoamine oxidase inhibitors (MAOIs). Which is the best evidence that the client has understood the nurse's instructions?
    1. The client says it is okay to eat pepperoni pizza.
    2. The client says it is okay to eat a salami sandwich.
    3. The client says it is okay to eat a carton of yogurt.
    4. The client says it is okay to eat a turkey sandwich.

2. After gathering the following data on a client with depression, which statement indicates the highest risk for suicide?
    1. "I feel hopeless about the future."
    2. "I plan to use my mother's gun."
    3. "I would be better off dead."
    4. "I cannot stand the stress anymore."

connection

Visit the Connection site at **http://connection.lww.com/go/timbyEssentials** for links to chapter-related resources on the Internet.

References and Suggested Readings

Abrams, A. C. (2000). *Clinical drug therapy* (6th ed.). Philadelphia: Lippincott Williams & Wilkins.

American Psychiatric Association. (1994). Practice guideline for the treatment of patients with bipolar disorder. *American Journal of Psychiatry, 151*(12s), iii–36.

Centers for Disease Control and Prevention. (2002). Suicide in the United States. [On-line 6/19/03.] Available: http://www.cdc.gov/ncipc/factsheets/suifacts.htm.

Cole, M. R. (1999). Bridging the great divide: Management of the patient with bipolar disorder. *Nursing Spectrum, 11A*(3), 8–9.

Fortinash, K. M., & Holoday-Worret, P. A. (2000). *Psychiatric mental health nursing* (2nd ed.). St. Louis: Mosby.

Hass, S. S. (August 5, 2002). More than blue. *Advance for Nurses,* 26–28.

Heffern, W. A. (2000). Psychopharmacological and electroconvulsive treatment of anxiety and depression in the elderly. *Journal of Psychiatric and Mental Health Nursing* 7(3), 199–204.

Kaye, J., Morton, J., Bowcutt, M., et al. (2000). Stress, depression, and psychoneuroimmunology. *Journal of Neuroscience Nursing, 32*(2), 93–100.

Kelsoe, J. R. (2000). Mood disorders: Genetics. In B. J. Sadock & V. A. Sadock (Eds.), *Comprehensive textbook of psychiatry* (Vol. 1) (7th ed., pp. 1308–1328). Philadelphia: Lippincott Williams & Wilkins.

Miller, S. M. (2000). One nurse's story of bipolar disease. *Nursing Spectrum, 12A*(15), 21–22.

Patient suicide: Court faults nurse's referral of patient to chemical dependency program. (2000). *Legal Eagle Eye Newsletter for the Nursing Profession, 8*(9), 3.

Pollack, L. E., & Cramer, R. D. (2000). Perceptions of problems in people hospitalized for bipolar disorder: Implications for patient education. *Issues in Mental Health Nursing, 21*(8), 765–778.

Reviewing anxiety and mood disorders. (2002). *Nursing 2002, 32*(6), 76–77.

Tredgett, J. (2000). Lithium clinic update. *Mental Health Nursing, 20*(5), 13–15.

U.S. Preventive Services Task Force. (2002). Screening for depression: Recommendations and rationale. *American Journal of Nursing, 102*(7), 77–80.

Videbeck, S. (2004). *Psychiatric mental health nursing* (2nd ed.). Philadelphia: Lippincott Williams & Wilkins.

chapter 16

Caring for Clients With Eating Disorders

Words to Know 

anorexia nervosa
binge-eating disorder
body mass index
bulimarexia
bulimia nervosa
compulsive overeating
eating disorders
endocannabinoids
food binges
lanugo
leptin
melanin-concentrating hormone
normal eating
orexin A
orexin B
purge
satiety
water loading

Learning Objectives

On completion of this chapter, the reader will:

- Differentiate normal eating from eating disorders.
- Discuss types of eating disorders.
- Name neurotransmitters, neurohormones, and other chemicals that affect the appetite and satiety center in the brain.
- Discuss reasons why most clients with anorexia induce self-starvation.
- Give the healthy adult range for body mass index.
- List components of treatment for clients with anorexia nervosa.
- Name problems that are the focus of nursing management when caring for clients with anorexia nervosa.
- Discuss the nurse's role in managing the nutrition of a client with anorexia nervosa.
- Give examples of how clients with bulimia compensate for binging.
- Name problems, besides nutrition, that nurses focus on when caring for clients with bulimia nervosa.
- Discuss psychosocial problems that may accompany overeating syndromes.

A rich variety of foods, sufficient for energy needs, growth and repair of cells, and maintenance of a healthy weight, is required to preserve health. Depending on variables such as age, sex, physical condition, activity level, and height, **normal eating** involves consuming approximately 1500 to 2500 calories per day, usually spread over three meals and two to three snacks. Normal eating occurs in response to hunger and ceases when **satiety** (a feeling of comfortable fullness) is attained. This chapter deals with conditions characterized by disordered eating.

Collectively, **eating disorders** are those in which eating

- Is consistently less than the client's caloric needs to maintain a healthy weight
- Occurs without hunger or fails to bring about satiety
- Is accompanied by anxiety and guilt
- Results in physiologic imbalances or medical complications

Eating disorders affect 500,000 people in the United States at any given time. They are most prevalent among middle to upper middle class young women between ages 12 to 25 years. Clients with eating disorders may try to keep their illness secret. Family and friends may become aware of the problem only after repeatedly noting emotional and behavioral symptoms (Table 16.1) or when serious health consequences ensue. Anorexia nervosa, bulimia nervosa, binge-eating disorder, and compulsive overeating are eating disorders. Obesity is a consequence of overeating; therefore, some obese clients also have eating disorders.

ANOREXIA NERVOSA

Anorexia nervosa is characterized by an obsession with thinness that is achieved through self-starvation. It occurs more often in women than in men; 1 in 200 girls aged 12 to 18 years develops anorexia nervosa. Although men also develop eating disorders, they are less likely to disclose such problems to a health professional. Even

TABLE 16.1 SIGNS AND SYMPTOMS OF EATING DISORDERS

EATING DISORDER	PHYSICAL	EMOTIONAL	BEHAVIORAL
Anorexia nervosa	Decrease of 25% in body weight; weight is 85% or less of normal; lanugo; alopecia; cold intolerance; amenorrhea; constipation; abdominal pain	Distorted body image; hatred of a particular body part; low self-esteem; depression; isolation; perfectionism	Restriction of food choices and intake; ritualistic handling of food (cutting into tiny pieces, arranging food a certain way, using certain plates and utensils only); weighing oneself frequently; denial of hunger
Bulimia nervosa	Inability to accurately interpret hunger and fullness signals; swelling of parotid glands ("chipmunk cheeks"); frequent weight fluctuations; irregular menses	Feeling unable to control eating; depressive mood and frequent mood swings; black-and-white thinking; exaggerated concern about weight	Excessive exercise, use of diuretics, and laxatives; secret eating of high-calorie, high-carbohydrate foods; alternately binging and fasting
Binge eating and compulsive overeating	Obesity; discomfort after eating	Preoccupation with weight, eating, and dieting; attributes professional and social success and failure to weight; feels disgust or guilt after eating; feels lack of control over eating	Frequent dieting, restricts activities because of embarrassment about weight; eating when not hungry; rapid eating; eating alone

when they do, the information is often dismissed, untreated, and unreported.

There are two subtypes of clients with anorexia: those who lose weight by exclusively restricting their intake of calories, and those who manifest **bulimarexia,** a pattern of both food restriction and purging discussed later in this chapter, to avoid absorbing the food that is consumed.

Pathophysiology and Etiology

The exact cause of anorexia nervosa is unknown. Many authorities believe that anorexia and other eating disorders result from a combination of cultural, social, physiologic, and psychological factors. Increasing evidence connects genetics and altered physiology.

Culturally and socially, extremely skinny role models in the media suggest to young women and men that thinness is linked with attractiveness and success. The image, portrayed as ideal, is unhealthy and unrealistic for most people. Self-starvation, rigorous physical activity, or both is sometimes the only way to achieve a similar appearance. Some athletes like gymnasts or ballet dancers restrict food intake believing that low body weight improves performance.

Physiologic influences play a key role in eating disorders. Neurotransmitters and neurohormones may influence eating by binding with receptors in the appetite center of the hypothalamus. Clients with anorexia may experience a down-regulation or insensitivity to norepinephrine and have increased serotonin levels, which fool the brain into believing satiety has occurred despite minimal intake (Kaye & Weltzin, 1991). Weight loss is a side effect of drugs that increase serotonin level, such as the selective serotonin reuptake inhibitors (see Chap. 15). Variations in the gene for serotonin receptors have been found in clients with anorexia. In 1999, researchers located receptors in the human brain for **melanin-concentrating hormone** (Saito, Nothacker, et al., 1999). In animal studies, low levels of this hormone caused weight loss, while high levels promoted obesity. Finally, **leptin,** a substance manufactured in human fat cells, acts on receptors in the hypothalamus, where it inhibits food intake. Clients with anorexia may have excessive leptin.

In terms of psychological influences, theorists have noted that persons with anorexia nervosa are often perfectionists, have low self-esteem, and possess an intense desire to please others. Some consider the refusal to eat a form of self-control that clients with anorexia use to cope with stressful life experiences or dysfunctional family relationships.

Assessment Findings

Signs and Symptoms

Persons with anorexia do experience hunger, but they control the urge to eat because of a morbid fear of becoming fat. Clients with anorexia consume an average of 600 to 900 calories or less per day. Their weight eventually is 85% or less than others of similar build, age, and height. Most consider themselves obese despite appearing emaciated.

Most anorexic clients deny that they are in jeopardy of dying. They may appear skeleton-like and develop a growth of fine body hair called **lanugo** that, in the absence of subcutaneous fat, helps maintain body temperature by reducing heat loss. These clients tend to be hypotensive and may have irregular, low pulse rates, making them prone to fainting. Severe malnutrition causes anorexic clients to be constipated, feel cold most of the time, have frequent chronic infections, and cease menstruating. Many conceal their starvation by hiding or disposing of food and dressing in bulky clothing.

Complications

Failure to consume adequate nourishment eventually deprives body systems of the nutritional elements required for homeostasis, growth, and cellular repair. Low serum estrogen levels lead to osteopenia (low bone mass) and premature osteoporosis (severe demineralization of bones), both of which lead to stress fractures, particularly of the spine and hips (Thrash et al., 2000). Starvation can cause vitamin deficiencies, fluid and electrolyte imbalances, and death from cardiac failure or dysrhythmia.

Diagnostic Findings

Body mass index (BMI), a mathematical computation based on height and weight (Box 16-1), is used to evaluate a person's size in relation to norms within the adult population. Clients with anorexia typically have a BMI of 16 or less. Anemia is usually present, and electrolyte levels, especially potassium and sometimes sodium, are often dangerously low. Deficiencies in serum proteins are reflected in low albumin, transferrin, and ferritin levels. Cardiac irregularities are identified by electrocardiography. Bone densiometry studies are used to determine the presence and severity of osteopenia.

BOX 16-1 ● Body Mass Index Formula, Calculation, and Interpretation

FORMULA

$$BMI = \frac{\text{weight in kg}}{\text{height m}^2}$$

CALCULATION

1. Divide pounds by 2.2 = kilograms.
2. Divide height (inches) by 39.4 = meters.
3. Square the answer in step 2 by multiplying the number times itself.
4. Divide weight in kg by m^2.

INTERPRETATION

Anorectic	BMI = ≤16
Underweight	BMI = 16–<18.5
Healthy	BMI = 18.5–24.9
Overweight	BMI = 25–29.9
Obese	BMI = 30–34.9
Severely obese	BMI = 35–39.9
Extremely obese	BMI = ≥40

Stop, Think, and Respond ● BOX 16-1

Besides weighing less that normal for one's height, what other findings suggest that an underweight person has anorexia nervosa?

Medical Management

Treatment involves four aspects: nutritional therapy, psychotherapy, drug therapy, and family counseling. Nutritional therapy includes providing nourishing meals, supplemental vitamins and minerals, intravenous fluids and electrolytes, tube feedings, or total parenteral nutrition. Once the client's weight improves or stabilizes, outpatient treatment begins.

To promote compliance with the weight-gain regimen, behavioral therapy (see Chap. 14) is instituted. By eating, the client earns privileges, such as having visitors and participating in social and physical activities. The privileges are rewards used to reinforce desired behavior. Individual and group psychotherapies are used to help clients gain insight into distorted perceptions of thinness and the motivations for continuing with dangerous weight-loss behaviors. Counseling and involvement in self-help groups for several years are often indicated.

Antidepressant medications such as amitriptyline (Elavil) are administered (see Chap. 15). Bulimarexic clients have responded to drug therapy with the antihistamine cyproheptadine (Periactin), which has antiseritonergic activity. Supplemental vitamins and minerals containing iron, potassium, and calcium may be included to compensate for natural sources that the client is not consuming. Stool softeners or laxatives may be necessary to counteract constipation resulting from deficient dietary fiber. Family counseling aims at relieving power struggles between those who try to convince the client to eat and the client who refuses. It also focuses on learning skills for undoing *enmeshment,* the habit of family members being so involved with one another that personal identities are lost and contact with others outside the family is excluded.

NURSING PROCESS

● The Client With Anorexia Nervosa

Assessment

Perform a physical assessment, noting signs of malnutrition such as absence of body fat; dry skin, scalp, and hair; fine hair covering the body; edema from hypoproteinemia; and cold hands and feet. Monitor vital signs regularly to detect hypothermia, bradycardia, or hypotension. Cardiac monitoring can detect dysrhythmias caused by hypokalemia. The client is weighed as accurately as possible with minimal clothing, and BMI is calculated.

Obtain a nutritional history and identify the date of the client's last menstrual period. Question as to whether the client restricts food intake or combines it with purging. Noting the form of purging is important. Keep in mind that excessive exercise is a form of purging. Observe the client's mood and anxiety level and asks about family dynamics or other stressors.

Diagnosis, Planning, and Interventions

Imbalanced Nutrition: Less than Body Requirements related to fear of gaining weight

Expected Outcomes: (1) The client will consume an established amount of calories each day and gain 2 to 5 pounds by a mutually agreed upon target date. (2) The client will attain and maintain a BMI of at least 18.5.

- Assign the same few nurses to the client's care. *Promotes a therapeutic alliance, and reduces potential for manipulation.*
- Establish a contract for expected weight restoration and target date; include rewards for reaching goals and consequences of failure to achieve goals. *Promotes self-involvement and a sense of ownership in the plan. Makes the client aware of the management of outcomes in the therapeutic plan.*
- Weigh the client regularly, but randomly. *Random weights are generally more accurate. Client cannot falsify weight by* ***water loading,*** *a technique in which clients with anorexia attempt to demonstrate weight gain by consuming a large volume of water and avoiding urination before being weighed.*
- Work with the dietitian to provide at least six to eight meals each day with a total caloric value between 1500 to 2000 calories; gradually increase total calories to between 2500 to 4000 calories/day. *The client is much more likely to work toward weight gain if food is offered frequently and is not heavily calorie loaded. To gain 1 pound of weight, a person must consume 3500 calories that are not used for basic metabolism and activities.*
- Set a limit of 30 minutes to consume the meal. *Clients with anorexia practice various rituals such as cutting food into small pieces and rearranging food on the plate without actually eating. Informing clients of the time limit may provide an incentive to consume food.*
- Observe or sit with the client during meals. *Prevents the client from hiding rather than eating food.*
- Remove the dietary tray after 30 minutes without commenting on food that has not been eaten. *Removal of food at designated time avoids a power struggle. Negative comments reinforce that the client was victorious in resisting the urge to eat. Withholding any comments avoids an adversarial image.*
- Record the type and amount of food consumed. *Provides information to evaluate the client's progress and calculate caloric intake.*
- Restrict the client's use of the bathroom for 2 hours after meals or accompany the client to the bathroom. *Allows time for consumed food to enter the small intestine for absorption rather than being vomited.*
- Give the client a liquid nutritional supplement to replace the uneaten calories at meals. *Clients may consume liquids that are calorie-loaded rather than solid food.*
- Implement behavioral rewards or consequences consistently and fairly. *Deviation from or inconsistent application of guidelines reduces the effectiveness of the plan of care.*
- Administer prescribed drug, vitamin, and mineral therapy, and ensure that the client attends group and individual psychotherapy. *Resistance to the therapeutic regimen is common. Anorexia requires management with medical, nutritional, and psychological modalities.*

Disturbed Body Image related to unresolved psychosocial conflicts

Expected Outcome: The client will develop a realistic perception of self and insight into motivation for thinness.

- Encourage the client to talk about perceptions of body image, but avoid opposing the client's views. *Disagreeing tends to further entrench the client's beliefs.*
- Offer the observation that fixation with weight control diverts attention and energy needed to deal with real issues surrounding psychosocial conflicts. *Offering alternative views can raise awareness.*
- Help client clarify issues underlying the need to control weight gain and promote weight loss. *Helps develop insight.*
- Suggest that perfection is impossible and that no body image is worth dying for. *Calling attention to the seriousness of the health problem may promote modifications in the client's behavior.*

Evaluation of Expected Outcomes

The client consumes nutritious food, resulting in gradual weight gain and a BMI greater than 18.5. The person no longer perceives himself or herself as fat. Evidence of enhanced insight is based on the client's self-disclosure that withholding consumption of food created a sense of power and provided a way to achieve an unrealistic image of perfection.

Client and Family Teaching 16-1 presents education points for families of clients with anorexia nervosa.

BULIMIA NERVOSA

Bulimia nervosa is characterized by two episodes of secret **food binges** (rapid consumption of many calories) per week followed by behaviors intended to prevent weight gain. The abnormal eating pattern persists for at least 6 months. There are two types of clients with bulimia: (1) those who **purge** (eliminate nutrients) after

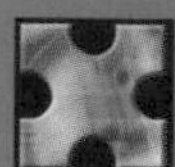

16-1 *Client and Family Teaching* Anorexia Nervosa

The nurse counsels and educates family members by offering the following suggestions:

- Focus on the person rather than the eating disorder.
- Provide unconditional love.
- Avoid inflicting guilt for the family distress that the disorder causes in daily living.
- Give the client the power to make decisions and facilitate changes in matters other than eating.
- Avoid being manipulated by the person with anorexia nervosa.
- Explain that it is common for clients with anorexia nervosa to discredit the staff of the eating disorder team, the facility, and the treatment approaches.
- Demonstrate united support for one another and the plan for the client's treatment.
- Prepare for rehospitalization if the client becomes medically unstable or experiences a relapse.

binging, with self-induced vomiting, laxatives, enemas, or diuretics; (2) those who do not purge but compensate by fasting, using diet pills, or engaging in excessive exercise (see binge-eating disorder later in this chapter).

In contrast to clients with anorexia nervosa, persons with bulimia nervosa are generally older at the onset of the disorder and are overweight or normal weight. They usually admit that their eating behavior is abnormal and are ashamed of habitually binging and purging.

Pathophysiology and Etiology

Researchers believe that the hypothalamus is the center for appetite regulation. Stimulation of the lateral area of the hypothalamus promotes eating; stimulation of the ventromedial area causes individuals to feel satiated (full), and thus eating behavior ceases. Neurotransmitters turn on and off these two areas of the hypothalamus. Clients with bulimia may have a biochemically induced compulsion to eat created by increased sensitivity to norepinephrine within the hypothalamus and reduced levels of serotonin, which disguises the point of satiety. Since serotonin is synthesized from the essential amino acid tryptophan, binge eating may act as a mechanism to supply tryptophan so as to increase serotonin levels, similar to how drinking water relieves thirst.

In 1998, researchers found two hormones that they named **orexin A** and **orexin B** after the Greek word, *orexis,* which means appetite (Leutwyler, 1998). When laboratory animals were injected with orexin hormones, which attach to receptors in the lateral hypothalamus, the animals consumed 8 to 10 times the normal amount of food. Researchers hypothesized that orexins A and B contribute to binge eating and obesity in humans. Leptin, a substance manufactured in human fat cells, is believed to suppress orexigenic (appetite-stimulating) chemicals (DiMarzo, et al., 2001). Therefore, binge eating may occur in the absence of leptin or when receptors for leptin are reduced.

Whatever the cause, once a binge begins, it is difficult to control. Eating is terminated by abdominal pain, interruption (discovery) by others, or sleeping. After the eating frenzy, clients with bulimia feel so guilty that they purge, fast (abstain from food for a longer than usual time—not days on end like someone with bulimarexia), or exercise.

Assessment Findings

Signs and Symptoms

During a binge, clients consume 3000 to 11,500 calories in 2 hours or less. Self-induced vomiting results in hoarseness, inflammation of the esophagus and oral pharynx, calluses on the back of the hand and fingers from repeatedly stimulating the gag reflex, erosion of tooth enamel, and swollen parotid glands. Clients tend to be of normal weight or slightly overweight. Their weight can fluctuate as much as 10 pounds in 1 week.

Complications

Self-induced vomiting and use of emetics like ipecac damage teeth; abuse of laxatives and enemas contributes to constipation. The nonprescribed use of diuretics and diet pills predisposes the clients to fluid, electrolyte, and cardiac problems. Some clients with bulimia also compulsively abuse drugs or alcohol. Shame and guilt may trigger suicidal thoughts or attempts.

Diagnostic Findings

Diagnosis is based on clinical findings and history of persistent binging and purging. Serum electrolyte levels may be altered. An x-ray of the upper gastrointestinal tract shows an overstretched or stenotic esophagus from frequent regurgitation and inflammation followed by scarring.

Medical Management

Treatment includes drug therapy with antidepressants (see Chap. 15), individual and group psychotherapy, and behavior modification techniques (see Chap. 15). Treatment of most clients with bulimia nervosa is managed on an outpatient basis.

NURSING PROCESS

● The Client With Bulimia Nervosa

Assessment

Weigh the client and calculate the BMI. Examine teeth to detect dental damage and examine conjunctiva for ruptured blood vessels caused by forced vomiting. Ask questions concerning (1) the frequency of binging and purging episodes, (2) the client's state of mind prior to a binge, (3) the types and amounts of food that the client consumes during a binge, and (4) the nature of the purge. Inventory medications, such as emetics, diuretics, and laxatives, that the client uses for purging. If exercise is the technique the client uses to purge, the type of activity and average duration of exercise are essential to note.

Collect the history and current health information, explain the medical therapy regimen, and refer the client to the dietitian for a safe weight loss program (if necessary). Provide emotional support. Some important areas to reinforce during health teaching include the following:

- Follow a dietary plan compatible with the food pyramid (Fig. 16.1).
- Eat at a slow pace.
- Eat only in the presence of others.

Diagnosis, Planning, and Interventions

Imbalanced Nutrition: More than Body Requirements related to compulsion to binge

Expected Outcomes: (1) The client will delay urge to binge or purge. (2) The client will consume no more than 2000 to 3000 calories per day divided among three meals plus or minus snacks. (3) The client will maintain a stable weight.

- Help client identify feelings, situations, or foods that trigger binging episodes. *Raising awareness of triggering events can break the cycle of binging and purging.*
- Explore alternative coping strategies for dealing with triggering stimuli. *Techniques for controlling impulses can abort a binging episode.*
- Explain that starving leads to binging and that excessive restriction is a major contributor to this disorder. *Eating regularly, but in controlled amounts, reduces hunger.*
- Tell the client to restrict eating to the kitchen or dining room at only specific times. *Restricting location and time for eating interferes with usual patterns of binge eating. Private binges often occur in other locations, such as in the living room while watching television.*
- Instruct client to wait at least 1 hour after a meal before succumbing to a binge. *Delaying a binge helps client separate normal from abnormal eating and from turning a normal meal into a binge.*
- Discuss alternatives for aborting or interrupting eating binges, such as eating with a family member or friend, calling a friend for support, leaving the binging location, and stocking low-calorie food. *Binging takes place when the client is alone and with a low potential for being discovered. Consuming low-calorie foods may minimize anxiety and reduce potential for purging.*
- Suggest that the client adulterate binge food like dropping it in dirt or soaking it in vinegar if all else fails. *Making food unpalatable is a behavior modification technique, called negative reinforcement.*

Situational Low Self-Esteem related to poor impulse control and ineffective methods to control weight

Expected Outcome: The client will report increased self-esteem.

- Discuss keeping a diary or journal where entries describe incidents when client overcame the urge to

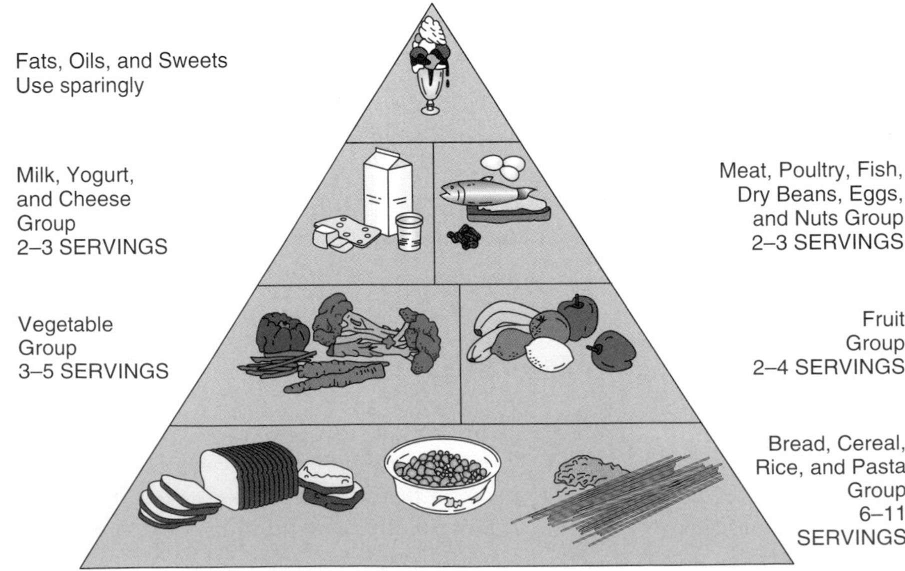

FIGURE 16.1 Food pyramid.

binge or purge. *Provides an objective resource for self-evaluation of progress.*

- Encourage client to read previous diary or journal entries whenever negative thoughts intrude. *Provides self-affirming evidence that he or she is making progress.*
- Help dispel faulty perception that losing control over binging and purging means the client is a total failure. *Clients overlook positive attributes and condemn themselves because of a single weakness.*
- Refer the client to a dietitian. *Loss of weight without purging increases self-esteem. A dietitian can develop a personalized plan for meeting nutritional needs while facilitating gradual weight loss if needed.*

Evaluation of Expected Outcomes

The client's caloric intake is in accordance with her or his metabolic needs. Binging and purging are reduced or eliminated. The client successfully implements alternative strategies for managing compulsive behaviors and has positive self-regard.

Stop, Think, and Respond • BOX 16-2

Where is the appetite center, and what substances stimulate or suppress it?

BINGE-EATING DISORDER AND COMPULSIVE OVEREATING

Binge-eating disorder is characterized as inability to control overeating, feeling guilty, but not engaging in compensating behaviors to prevent weight gain. **Compulsive overeating** is characterized as eating when not hungry or regardless of feeling full. Some individuals have both problems simultaneously. Either may result in obesity.

Pathophysiology and Etiology

The cause of overeating syndromes is still unknown. People with eating disorders suffer from anxiety, depression, and compulsive behavior. Biochemical factors may be involved in binge eating and compulsive overeating. Similarly to anorexia and bulimia nervosa, it is likely that an imbalance of neurotransmitters involving norepinephrine and serotonin, or neurohormones like orexin A and B or leptin, affects the appetite center in the brain. Additional neuroendocrine disequilibrium may involve cortisol, a hormone that the adrenal cortex releases in response to stress (see Chap. 12); reduced cholecystokinin, a hormone secreted by the mucosa of the upper small intestine that causes laboratory animals to stop eating when feeling full; and imbalances in neuropeptides Y and YY, psychoactive chemicals that stimulate eating behavior in research animals. Scientists recently located brain receptors for **endocannabinoids,** natural chemicals with marijuana-like properties, which activate the appetite center (DiMarzo, et al., 2001; Mechoulam & Fride, 2001). The existence of endocannabinoids helps explain why marijuana users develop ravenous hunger, called "the munchies," and why dronabinol (Marinol), synthetic tetrahydrocannabinol (THC)—the active ingredient in marijuana—helps those with cancer and AIDS gain weight. Increased amounts of or increased sensitivity to endocannabinoids may explain some syndromes characterized by overeating. Also, the fact that many overeaters state they use food as a way of coping with stress should not be overlooked.

Assessment Findings

Signs and Symptoms

Overeaters are typically overweight with a history of unsuccessful dieting attempts. Clients tend to eat without being hungry. They prefer high-sugar and high-fat foods to nibble over several hours or gorge on until they feel uncomfortably full. Some report they overeat or binge when angry, sad, bored, or anxious. They often have a history of other compulsive behaviors such as alcohol or drug abuse. Some reveal they have considered suicide or have performed self-mutilation, such as cutting and burning themselves, pulling their hair, and interfering with wound healing to cope with their intense feelings, to punish themselves, or to experience physical pain to counteract the consequences of feeling emotionally numb.

Complications

Overeating leads to many physical and emotional problems. Many individuals develop hyperlipidemia (elevated blood fat levels), hypertension, type 2 diabetes mellitus, degenerative arthritis, and sleep apnea. They are at increased risk for gallbladder disease, heart disease, and some types of cancer. Many feel unhappy, ashamed, and disgusted with themselves. They tend to become socially isolated to avoid being noticed and possibly rejected.

Diagnostic Findings

People with overeating syndromes generally have a BMI of 30 or above. Other laboratory and diagnostic tests reflect secondary complications from obesity such as elevated blood sugar, cholesterol, and serum lipid levels.

Medical Management

A comprehensive approach to treating overeating syndromes involves weight reduction, psychotherapy, and self-help support groups. The first step is a sensible weight-loss regimen prescribed by a dietitian. Strict dieting is discouraged because it tends to worsen binge eating. To help clients lose weight and remain compliant, short-term drug therapy may be used. Prescribed medications include antidepressants such as selective serotonin reuptake inhibitors (e.g., fluoxetine [Prozac]) that promote weight loss (see Chap. 15).

Support groups, like Overeaters Anonymous, or group therapy in eating disorder clinics are helpful adjuncts to individual psychotherapy. In some cases, surgery is an option for severely obese clients with medical complications.

Nursing Management

When interviewing the client, it is important to show sensitivity to the individual's self-consciousness about weight and emotional problems. During a comprehensive physical assessment, ensure privacy when measuring weight and height. Education points are presented in Client and Family Teaching 16-2.

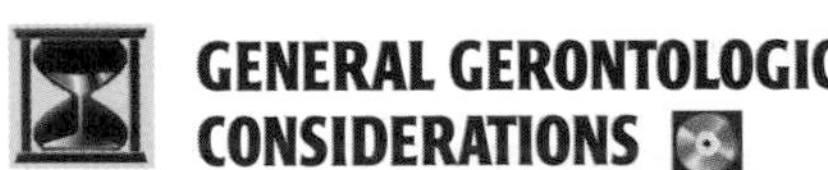

Older adults may experience severe weight loss as the result of major depression, but it is extremely rare for older adults to have an excessive fear of gaining weight or an excessive desire for weight loss. Assess any adult with significant weight loss for depression.

In addition to depression, weight loss in older adults can be related to bereavement, confusion, ill-fitting dentures, diminished sensations of taste and smell, or inability to self-feed. Consider these factors when assessing any older adult with significant weight loss.

At times, older adults may simply refuse to eat, resulting in self-starvation. Self-starvation over the loss of health, diagnosis of a terminal disease, or inability to cope with life's losses is related to major depression or faulty coping skills and is not classified as an eating disorder.

Critical Thinking Exercises

1. *Based on the food pyramid, explain the components of a healthy daily diet.*
2. *Calculate the BMI of a person who weighs 175 pounds and is 63 inches tall. What conclusion is appropriate based on your calculation?*
3. *What weight loss strategies are appropriate to recommend and discourage for an obese client who is a compulsive overeater?*

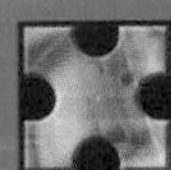

16-2 *Client and Family Teaching* Overeating Syndromes

The nurse counsels clients with overeating syndromes as follows:

- Get treatment from professionals who are experienced in treating eating disorders.
- Follow directions for taking prescribed medications; report any untoward effects.
- Avoid popular nonprescription diet pills. They generally contain central nervous system stimulants, which can increase heart rate and blood pressure and cause dizziness, irritability, insomnia, and dry mouth.
- Strict dieting or fasting is the leading cause of binging.
- Exercise according to the advice of a physician to reduce appetite and increase weight loss.
- Avoid nutritional and weight loss centers because they generally do not offer comprehensive services most clients need to keep from gaining weight once reaching the target weight.
- Read food labels and understand that those that say "sugar free" or "contains no cholesterol" do not mean that ingredients are calorie free or low calorie.
- Talk to a close friend or support person about feelings.
- Attend an Overeaters Anonymous meeting. This free self-help group is modeled after the 12-step program of Alcoholics Anonymous.
- Remember that recovery is a day-by-day process; it is self-defeating to dwell on the lack of previous success or relapses that may occur.

● NCLEX-STYLE REVIEW QUESTIONS 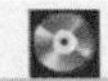

1. The nurse has been working with a college-aged client who has bulimia on measures to control her eating disorder. In reviewing the following nursing measures, which one is most effective for a client with bulimia?
    1. Restricting the use of the bathroom after meals
    2. Keeping a daily consumption food inventory
    3. Avoiding meals in fast-food establishments
    4. Keeping a daily calorie count
2. When gathering data on a client suffering from anorexia nervosa, which of the following requires immediate nursing intervention?
    1. Formation of lanugo
    2. Stress fractures
    3. Cardiac dysrhythmias
    4. Amenorrhea
3. To obtain accurate data for determining the progress of a client with anorexia nervosa, which of the following is most important for the nurse to control just prior to weighing the client?
    1. The number of calories the client consumes
    2. The volume of water the client drinks
    3. The amount of exercise the client performs
    4. The time of day the client is weighed

connection

Visit the Connection site at **http://connection.lww.com/go/timbyEssentials** for links to chapter-related resources on the Internet.

References and Suggested Readings

DiMarzo, V., Goparaju, S., Wang, L., et al. (2001). Leptin-regulated endocannabinoids are involved in maintaining food intake. *Nature, 410,* 822–825.

Kaye, W. H., & Weltzin, T. E. (1991). Serotonin activity in anorexia and bulimia nervosa: Relationship to the modulation of feeding and mood. *Journal of Clinical Psychiatry, 52,* 41–48.

Leutwyler, K. (1998). The discovery of two new hormones gives researchers food for thought. *Scientific American.* [On-line.] Available: http://www.sciam.com.

Mechoulam, R., & Fride, E. (2001). Physiology: A hunger for cannabinoids. *Nature, 410,* 763–765.

Orbanic, S. (2001). Understanding bulimia: Signs, symptoms, and the human experience. *American Journal of Nursing, 101*(3), 35–42.

Ricca, V., Mannucci, E., Zucchi, T., et al. (2000). Cognitive-behavioral therapy for bulimia nervosa and binge eating disorder. *Psychotherapy and Psychosomatics, 69*(6), 287–295.

Schmidt, U. (2001). Treating eating disorders—ethical, legal and personal issues. *Behavior Research and Therapy, 39*(3), 369.

Saito, Y., Nothacker, H. P., Wang, Z., et al. (1999). Molecular characterization of the melanin-concentrating-hormone receptor. *Nature, 400,* 265–269.

Thrash, L. E., & Anderson, J. (2000). The female athlete triad: Nutrition, menstrual disturbances, and low bone mass. *Nutrition Today, 35*(5), 168–174.

chapter 17

Caring for Chemically Dependent Clients

Words to Know 

alcoholism
aversion therapy
blackouts
chemical dependence
cross-tolerance
detoxification
environmental tobacco smoke
methadone maintenance therapy
opiate dependence
polydrug abuse
relapse
rule of one hundreds
substance abuse
tolerance
withdrawal

Learning Objectives

On completion of this chapter, the reader will:

- Discuss health and social consequences of substance abuse.
- Describe commonly abused addictive substances and at least three other categories of abused drugs.
- Discuss the meaning of withdrawal.
- Explain mechanisms by which tolerance occurs.
- List steps in the progression toward chemical dependence.
- Explain physiologic and psychosocial factors for the development of chemical dependence.
- Explain ways abused drugs produce their effects.
- Define alcoholism and accompanying symptoms.
- Name components of treatment for alcoholism.
- List potential health consequences of tobacco use.
- Discuss the components of a successful smoking cessation program.
- Name drugs commonly abused by persons who use cocaine.
- Give reasons for methadone maintenance therapy.

Substance abuse and chemical dependence are serious public health and social problems. They contribute significantly to *morbidity* (incidence of disease) and *mortality* (deaths) from liver damage, cardiopulmonary disease, and infectious diseases such as hepatitis and acquired immunodeficiency syndrome (AIDS). Alcohol and drug abuse also are major contributors to domestic violence and child abuse, crime, traffic and boating fatalities, assaults, and murders.

SUBSTANCE ABUSE AND CHEMICAL DEPENDENCE

Substance abuse is the use of a drug that is different from its accepted purpose. Generally, it is the consequences of inappropriately taking drugs—primarily mind-altering and mood-altering substances—that are of major concern. Commonly abused drugs include alcohol, cocaine, heroin, hallucinogens, amphetamines, marijuana, barbiturates, volatile hydrocarbons such as those found in glue, and nicotine. Because of their widespread use, alcohol and nicotine contribute most to morbidity and mortality, and thus are the most harmful substances. Tobacco use is so widely accepted and its psychoactive properties are so subtle that its negative social and occupational effects seem minor. Yet tobacco is an addictive substance that contributes annually to the deaths of 430,000 people—as many as are caused by alcohol, cocaine, heroin, suicide, homicide, motor vehicle accidents, fire, and AIDS combined (National Center for Chronic Disease Prevention and Health Promotion, 2000).

Withdrawal refers to physical symptoms and craving for a drug that occur when a person abruptly stops using an abused substance (Table 17.1). **Chemical dependence** means that a person must take a drug to avoid withdrawal symptoms. Addiction is sometimes used interchangeably with dependence, but addiction more accurately refers to the drug-seeking behaviors that interfere with work,

TABLE 17.1 COMMONLY ABUSED SUBSTANCES

DRUG	EFFECTS	SIGNS AND SYMPTOMS OF TOXICITY	SIGNS AND SYMPTOMS OF WITHDRAWAL
Alcohol	Central nervous system depressant • Lethargy • Slurred speech • Slowed motor reaction • Impaired judgment • Decreased social inhibition	Nausea and vomiting, loss of coordination, belligerence, stupor, coma	Anxiety, agitation, elevated vital signs, hyperactive reflexes, tremors, diaphoresis, insomnia, hallucinations, seizures
Cocaine	Central nervous system stimulant • Tachycardia • Hypertension • Increased energy • Feeling of well-being • Insensitivity to pain and fatigue • Weight loss	Restlessness, paranoia, irritability, auditory hallucinations, convulsions, respiratory or cardiac arrest	Depressed mood, lethargy, impaired concentration, craving for drug
Heroin	Central nervous system depressant • Initial brief rush of euphoria • Sedation • Reduced motivation, attention, and concentration • Altered sensitivity to stressors • Pain relief • Lowered vital signs, especially respiratory rate • Slowed peristalsis • Constricted pupils • Decreased interest in sex	Respiratory depression, hypothermia, pinpoint pupils, coma	Yawning, runny nose, perspiration, goose bumps, anorexia, vomiting, diarrhea, dilated pupils, insomnia, elevated vital signs, drug craving

relationships, and normal activities (Box 17-1). **Tolerance** refers to reduction in a drug's effect that follows persistent use. It results because the body develops mechanisms for using the drug more effectively or inactivating the drug more efficiently. A person must take increasing amounts of the substance to obtain the desired effect.

Pathophysiology and Etiology

Causes of chemical dependence are complex and involve many psychobiologic factors. Substance abuse often begins with curious experimentation and progresses to habituation, psychological and physical dependence, and finally addiction (Table 17.2). One factor that explains substance abuse is the self-reinforcing pleasurable effects that some substances produce in the limbic system of the brain. Stimulant drugs such as cocaine and amphetamines affect levels of norepinephrine, dopamine, and acetylcholine. Depressant drugs such as alcohol, heroin, and barbiturates cause effects similar to those of gamma-aminobutyric acid (GABA), endorphins, and enkephalins. These drugs either mimic the neurotransmitters by attaching to their receptor sites or block their reuptake.

Psychosocial dynamics also play a part in substance use and abuse. Family members, peers, and role models who use alcohol, tobacco, and other drugs influence impressionable teenagers and youngsters. Promotion of alcohol in U.S. culture also fosters its use and abuse. Many people abuse drugs in a dysfunctional effort to cope with psychosocial stressors.

BOX 17-1 ● Signs of Alcohol or Drug Addiction

- Regularly drinking or taking more than was originally planned
- Unsuccessfully attempting to reduce or regulate use
- Spending excessive time obtaining, consuming, or recovering from the effects of the drug
- Continuing use despite negative consequences
- Drinking or consuming drugs alone
- Failing to fulfill major role obligations at work, school, or home
- Exhibiting tolerance to alcohol and sedative drugs
- Displaying withdrawal symptoms when drug is not consumed

Treatment

Initiating treatment is a difficult hurdle in treating chemical dependence. Clients deny their addiction, rationalize substance use, or blame life situations for their drug and drinking habits. Often, dependent individuals must "hit bottom" before they seek help. Once they seek treatment and withdrawal is managed, recovering individuals must

TABLE 17.2 PATTERNS OF SUBSTANCE ABUSE

EXPERIMENTATION	HABITUATION	DEPENDENCE	ADDICTION
Initial use	Repeated use	Frequent use	Unremitting use
Low dose	Uniform doses	Doses increase	High doses
Finds experience pleasurable	Seeks to re-experience pleasure	Craves ongoing pleasure from drug	Needs drug to feel "normal"
No discomfort from abstinence	No discomfort from abstinence	Experiences minor physical discomfort if drug is not used	Experiences severe withdrawal symptoms if drug is not used

learn new methods of coping with stressors, repair relationships damaged by addiction, and develop new interests and activities to fill the time once devoted to using drugs or alcohol.

Although some individuals quit taking abused substances unassisted, most people benefit from chemical detoxification and a treatment plan that involves abstinence, counseling, and support of peers through a 12-step program. Twelve-step programs are free and provide specific guidelines (steps) for becoming and staying drug or alcohol free. Frequent (daily, if necessary) attendance at meetings is encouraged. During meetings, members share their experiences and discuss the 12 steps and other topics related to recovery.

• ALCOHOL DEPENDENCE

Alcoholism is a chronic, progressive multisystem disease characterized by an inability to control the consumption of alcohol. Unchecked, alcoholism is fatal. Serious medical consequences of alcoholism are dose-related. On a drink-by-drink comparison, women are more likely to develop health problems earlier than men because they generally weigh less than men. The same amount of alcohol will be more concentrated and more toxic to women than to men.

Pathophysiology and Etiology

In alcoholism, evidence suggests that a genetic component alters metabolism of alcohol in those with the disease (Li, 2000). Instead of acetaldehyde converting to acetic acid, some acetaldehyde combines with dopamine to form an addictive substance called tetrahydroisoquinoline (TIQ). TIQ is formed only in the brains of alcoholics. Other research has identified a variant gene for dopamine among alcoholics that locks onto receptors, triggering sensations of pleasure and reward (Hill, et al., 1999).

Assessment Findings

Signs and Symptoms

Although the client may deny problem drinking, he or she typically has a history of increasing alcohol consumption. The person may hide containers of alcohol and drink privately at any time during the day. Many clients manifest a great tolerance for alcohol and a **cross-tolerance** (reduced effect) when taking sedative-hypnotic drugs. **Blackouts,** periods of amnesia involving events and activities during drinking, occur even in early stages. Family and friends note alcoholic behaviors, and social or legal repercussions occur. A history of social, financial, civic, and occupational problems reflects the individual's inability to control drinking despite negative consequences.

Acutely intoxicated alcoholics may enter a tertiary care hospital with altered mental status, acute gastric bleeding, or as victims of trauma or violence. When hospitalization occurs, management of alcohol withdrawal is very important. Withdrawal from alcohol results in nervous system stimulation manifested by tremors, sweating, hypertension, tachycardia, heart palpitations, craving for alcohol, seizures, and hallucinations.

Stop, Think, and Respond ● BOX 17-1

What assessment findings suggest that a person who consumes alcohol is an alcoholic rather than a social drinker?

Complications

Alcohol-related physical symptoms may accompany persistent drinking. Esophagitis, gastritis, enlarged liver, esophageal and rectal bleeding, and pancreatitis are common. Memory is impaired, and clients may experience erectile dysfunction or decreased libido. Studies implicate alcohol in liver cancer, cerebrovascular accident, metabolic deficiencies, aspiration pneumonia, cardiomyopathy, blood dyscrasias, and neurologic disorders. Infants born to women who drank alcohol during pregnancy may have fetal alcohol syndrome (FAS), which causes physical and intellectual deficits.

Diagnostic Findings

A blood alcohol level (BAL) measures the percentage of alcohol in the blood, indicating the extent of alcohol toxicity (Table 17.3). Elevated levels of glutamyltransferase (GTT), aspartate transferase (AST), and alanine transferase (ALT) reflect alcohol-induced liver disease. Levels of pancreatic enzymes (amylase and lipase) may also be elevated.

Medical Management and Rehabilitation

To break progression of alcoholism, clients undergo detoxification, nutritional therapy, psychotherapy, and drug therapy. They are encouraged to continue rehabilitation by joining a support group such as Alcoholics Anonymous.

Detoxification

Alcohol withdrawal without detoxification is a potentially fatal process. **Detoxification** (detox) involves stabilizing the client with a sedative drug while the alcohol is metabolized from his or her system. Withdrawal symptoms are controlled until they subside. Drugs used in detoxification are lorazepam (Ativan), diazepam (Valium), and chlordiazepoxide (Librium) (Drug Therapy Table 17.1). Initially, high doses and frequent drug administration compensate for the client's cross-tolerance. These drugs are gradually tapered and discontinued. A beta-adrenergic blocker such as propranolol (Inderal) is given to reduce dangerously elevated heart rates and blood pressures that can occur. Alcoholism is related to thiamine deficiency, which can lead to dementia. Because thiamine is necessary for the metabolism of glucose, glucose solutions must be avoided until thiamine is administered. Once thiamine is administered, intravenous (IV) hydration with glucose and additional vitamins, such as folic acid, support the client metabolically until the condition stabilizes.

Nutritional Therapy

Alcoholics often are undernourished and deficient of B vitamins. Injections of thiamine for 3 days followed by oral administration and folic acid supplements are often prescribed. Vitamin therapy prevents neurologic complications known as Wernicke's encephalopathy and Korsakoff's psychosis.

Psychotherapy

Individual or group psychotherapy helps the client to gain greater insight into emotional problems that led to or resulted from alcohol dependence. Family therapy with spouse and children includes sharing how alcoholism affected each person so that healing may begin.

Drug Therapy

Disulfiram (Antabuse) is a drug given to recovering alcoholics who cannot control the compulsion to drink. It is a form of **aversion therapy** because it deters drinking by causing unpleasant physical reactions when alcohol is consumed or absorbed through the skin (see Drug Therapy Table 17.1). Health teaching includes a list of products that contain alcohol such as liquid cough suppressants (Box 17-2). The client must be informed that life-threatening cardiopulmonary complications and even death can occur when disulfiram and alcohol are combined. Naltrexone (Trexan, ReVia), a narcotic antagonist, is also used as an adjunct for recovering alcoholics. It decreases the effects of alcohol should the person **relapse** (return to drinking).

Support Groups

Alcoholics Anonymous was the first 12 step self-help program. Founded in 1926 by an alcoholic physician, AA is composed of and run by recovering alcoholics to help people who are dependent on alcohol get and stay sober. AA emphasizes personal accountability, spirituality, and powerlessness over alcohol. Family members of clients with alcoholism may benefit from attending meetings of Al Anon, Alateen, or Adult Children of Alcoholics (ACOA) to learn more about how alcoholism has affected them.

TABLE 17.3 BLOOD ALCOHOL LEVEL AND ASSOCIATED IMPAIRMENT

BLOOD ALCOHOL LEVEL	PERCENTAGE OF BLOOD ALCOHOL	PHYSICAL AND BEHAVIORAL EFFECTS
50 mg/dL	0.05%	Mood changes, loosening of inhibition, decreased judgment, slight euphoria
80–100 mg/dL	0.08–0.1%	Reduced muscle coordination, decreased reaction time, impaired vision
200 mg/dL	0.2%	Staggering, poor control of emotions, easily angered
300 mg/dL	0.3%	Mental confusion, stupor
400 mg/dL	0.4%	Coma
500 mg/dL	0.5%	Respiratory depression, death

DRUG THERAPY TABLE 17.1 DRUGS USED IN THE RECOVERY FROM CHEMICAL DEPENDENCE

DRUG CATEGORY AND EXAMPLES	SIDE EFFECTS	NURSING CONSIDERATIONS
Benzodiazepine		
chlordiazepoxide hydrochloride (Librium)—management of acute alcohol withdrawal	Sedation, confusion, restlessness, bradycardia, tachycardia, urinary retention or incontinence, drug dependence	If giving intravenously, use a large vein and monitor vital signs carefully. Intramuscular injection can be quite painful; reconstitute with special diluent only, monitor injection sites, administer slowly. Observe client for excessive sedation, and use cautiously in clients with impaired kidney or liver function.
Antialcoholic Agent		
disulfiram (Antabuse)—blocks oxidation of alcohol, resulting in the accumulation of acetaldehyde	*If alcohol is used:* flushing, throbbing headaches, dyspnea, vomiting, tachycardia, hypotension, blurred vision; severe reactions can result in convulsions, myocardial infarction, death. *Disulfiram alone:* drowsiness, headache, dermatitis	Do not administer until at least 12 hours have elapsed since last exposure to alcohol. Inform client to avoid all sources of alcohol and to wear a medical identification bracelet. Arrange for follow-up liver and blood studies. Inform client of potential side effects and to report them to a healthcare provider.
Smoking Deterrent		
nicotine transdermal (Nicotrol)—binds to nicotinic receptors in central and peripheral nervous system	Headache, insomnia, diarrhea, constipation, pharyngitis, burning and itching at site, backache, chest pain, dysmenorrhea	Explain application, site rotation, and disposal of used patches so that pets or children do not come in contact with product. Inform client of side effects and to report any that occur.
Narcotic Antagonist		
naltrexone hydrochloride (Trexan, ReVia)—blocks the effects of opioids and aids in the abstinence from alcohol	Insomnia, anxiety, nervousness, low energy, abdominal pain, nausea, vomiting, decreased sexual potency, delayed ejaculation, rash, joint and muscle pain, increased thirst	Induces sudden withdrawal so do not use until 7 to 14 days have elapsed since last exposure to opioids. Inform client that small doses of opioids will have no effect. Larger doses may overcome the inhibiting effect, but coma or death may occur. Tell the client to report any side effects.
Narcotic Agonist Analgesic		
methadone (Dolophine)—binds with opioid receptors in the CNS and produces euphoria, analgesia, and sedation	Light-headedness, dizziness, sedation, nausea, vomiting, respiratory depression, circulatory depression, shock, cardiac arrest	A single liquid oral dose is used for maintenance. Constipation may be severe; ensure that client is taking a stool softener. Use with caution in clients receiving sedatives, hypnotics, tranquilizers, tricyclic antidepressants, and monoamine oxidase inhibitors—respiratory depression, hypotension, and coma can occur.

Stop, Think, and Respond ● BOX 17-2

Explain why the first of AA's 12 steps leading to recovery from alcoholism is "We admitted we were powerless over alcohol—and that our lives had become unmanageable."

BOX 17-2 ● Obscure Sources of Alcohol

- Liquid cough and cold medications
- Liquid sleep medications
- Flavoring extracts
- Mouthwash
- Rubbing alcohol
- Aftershave lotions
- Fruitcake with alcohol

NURSING PROCESS

● The Client With Alcohol Dependence

Assessment

Examine the client from head to toe, noting any signs of injuries, abdominal enlargement, jaundiced skin or sclera, and blood in body fluids or stool indicating complications from liver damage or portal hypertension (see Chap. 49). Include questions about the use of alcohol when establishing the client's database. The CAGE Screening Test is helpful in detecting alcoholic behaviors (Box 17-3). If the client admits to consuming alcohol, determine the type, how much, and when the last drink was consumed. The latter information is important because withdrawal symptoms occur within 3 to 72 hours after a client's last drink. Administer a breath alcohol concentration test as soon as

BOX 17-3 ● CAGE Questionnaire for Alcoholism

1. Have you ever felt that you ought to **C**ut down on your drinking?
2. Have people **A**nnoyed you by criticizing your drinking?
3. Have you ever felt **G**uilty about your drinking?
4. Have you ever had a drink first thing in the morning to steady your nerves or get rid of a hangover (**E**ye-opener)?

From Ewing, J. A. (1984). Detecting alcoholism: The CAGE questionnaire. *Journal of the American Medical Association, 252,* 1905–1907.

possible upon contact with the client to obtain an approximation of the client's current alcohol level. A history of seizures or other severe symptoms in previous withdrawals merits close observation for a similar reaction.

Monitor the client for signs and symptoms of withdrawal. Nurses often use the **Rule of One Hundreds** as an indicator of escalating withdrawal. It refers to a body temperature greater than or equal to 100°F, pulse rate greater than or equal to 100 beats/min, or diastolic blood pressure greater than or equal to 100 mm Hg. The rise in any one of these three vital signs suggests the need for sedative medication, because physiologic consequences of withdrawal may be extremely difficult to counteract once they have begun.

Diagnosis, Planning, and Interventions

PC: Alcohol Withdrawal

Expected Outcome: The nurse will manage and minimize alcohol withdrawal.

- Assess the client's vital signs and other data, such as hand tremors, hyperactive tendon reflexes, diaphoresis, anxiety, insomnia, and disorientation, that suggest physiologic stimulation. *As the body metabolizes alcohol, it releases norepinephrine, causing autonomic nervous system stimulation.*
- Consult with physician regarding need for a detoxification drug. *The physician is responsible for prescribing a drug for detoxification based on assessment data.*
- Administer prescribed detoxification medication. *Prevents rapid and dangerous withdrawal.*
- Repeat assessments for withdrawal at least every 2 hours. *Client may require more medication if physiologic stimulation is not controlled.*
- Monitor for seizure activity, hallucinations, extreme tremors, and agitation. *If early and minor symptoms of alcohol withdrawal are not managed effectively, the client's withdrawal will progress in severity because of dopamine stimulation.*

Imbalanced Nutrition: Less than Body Requirements related to inadequate dietary intake

Expected Outcome: The client's will consume at least 75% of food that is served.

- Obtain weight. *Provides a baseline to evaluate subsequent nutritional intake.*
- Determine the client's food preferences. *A person is more likely to consume food that he or she likes.*
- Collaborate with the dietary department to provide six small meals each day and an ample variety of snacks. *The client is likely to consume more food if the quantity is distributed throughout the day.*
- Monitor dietary intake and record data in the medical record. *Provides an objective means to evaluate client's progress.*

Health-Seeking Behavior: Abstinence from Alcohol related to a desire to manage a chronic, fatal disease

Expected Outcomes: (1) The client will verbalize that alcohol abuse is an illness that requires ongoing treatment and support. (2) The client will understand the connection between alcohol and its associated activities and develop nonalcohol-related interests and contacts. (3) The client will formulate a plan for attaining and maintaining sobriety.

- Let the client express feelings concerning potential losses. *Discussing effects of abstinence is the first step in working through grief.*
- Explore alternatives that may substitute for potential losses. *Identifying activities and other people with whom to socialize may substitute for void caused by abstaining from alcohol.*
- Encourage the family or significant others to support one another. *Physical and emotional burdens associated with life-altering changes can be lightened if shared among many people who are meaningful to the client.*
- Promote sharing of experiences between the client and others who are further ahead in their recovery. *Role models who are dealing with similar issues can motivate and encourage the client.*
- Provide the locations of AA meetings. *Knowing the locations and times of meetings allows the client to make personal choices in pursuing his or her recovery.*
- Explain that a sponsor may be selected from among those who attend AA meetings. *A sponsor provides social and emotional support throughout recovery.*
- Recommend that the client begin reading the "Big Book" of AA. *This book describes the traditional 12 steps that lead to recovery.*

Evaluation of Expected Outcomes

Vital signs are stable, and symptoms of withdrawal are controlled. The client eats a well-balanced diet and sleeps an adequate number of hours per night. The client demonstrates a willingness to cope with losses associated with overcoming dependence on alcohol. He or she also moves forward with measures to remain sober, such as participating in AA.

● NICOTINE DEPENDENCE

Nicotine, the stimulant drug in tobacco, is the most heavily used addictive, mood-altering substance in the United States. It is absorbed by inhaling tobacco in cigarettes, cigars, and pipes, or through the mucous membranes of the mouth from loose tobacco. Smoking raises blood carbon monoxide levels and causes constriction of peripheral blood vessels. It disrupts the structure of alveoli, causing them to become overstretched and inelastic. It is implicated in the development and recurrence of gastric ulcers. Smokeless tobacco (chewing tobacco) exposes the oral cavity to carcinogens, inhaled tobacco targets the lungs and distant organs, and cigars or pipes repeatedly expose the oral cavity and esophagus to harmful substances.

U.S. society condones and even endorses tobacco use. While smoking and tobacco use have decreased in recent decades, approximately 25% of adults use tobacco. Estimates of associated medical costs are $53 billion annually. Passive absorption of smoke can also cause disease in nonsmokers.

Nicotine produces tolerance, resulting in increased use over time and withdrawal symptoms when use is discontinued. Users light up or chew to maintain blood and brain levels; nicotine is then distributed throughout the body, metabolized in the liver, and excreted by the kidneys. Tobacco use is a conditioned, learned response, meaning that past patterns of use reinforce the habit of smoking. Smoking cessation strategies must target both physical dependence and conditioned related behaviors.

Consequences

Smoking is responsible for most deaths from lung cancer and chronic obstructive lung disease. Other cancer deaths and deaths from coronary artery disease are also related to smoking. Tobacco contains more than 40 carcinogenic chemicals. It is the major cause of oropharyngeal cancers and contributes to cerebrovascular disease, peripheral vascular disease, and cancers of the urinary tract, esophagus, and pancreas.

Breathing **environmental tobacco smoke** (also called secondhand smoke or passive smoke), the smoke given off by the burning end of a cigarette, pipe, or cigar and the exhaled smoke from the lungs of a smoker, is potentially injurious to others. Breathing secondhand smoke can cause headaches and eye, nose, and throat irritation. Nonsmokers exposed to environmental tobacco smoke have increased rates of heart disease, lung and other types of cancer, and lower respiratory infections. Risk of sudden infant death syndrome (SIDS) is increased among infants whose mothers smoked throughout the pregnancy and after delivery. Asthma in children is increased in frequency and severity when these children are exposed to an environment with passive smoke.

Medical Management

Healthcare providers encourage smokers and tobacco users to quit and provide materials that inform them of methods to do so. Various levels of intervention are available, including counseling and follow-up or enrollment in behavior modification programs. These programs help clients manage temptation and extinguish preconditioned cues to smoke. They also provide rewards for goal achievement. Pharmacologic therapy using nicotine substitutes (gum, patch, inhaler) (see Drug Therapy Table 17.1), which are gradually tapered and stopped, help clients avoid withdrawal symptoms.

Relapse is common, and only 10% to 15% of smokers who quit remain tobacco-free for 1 year. Attempts to quit, however, are a predictor for eventual success; 60% of those who try and fail do ultimately succeed.

Nursing Management

Nurses help clients who smoke by counseling them to quit and providing them with information on various smoking-cessation programs. Nurturing a client's belief that he or she can be successful is an important supportive measure. Many clients fear gaining weight after smoking cessation. Typical weight gain in the year after cessation is 9 to 10 pounds. Help clients plan strategies to offset weight gain, such as walking programs, substituting fruits for high-calorie desserts, and reducing dietary fat. Sugarless hard candy or chewing gum may keep the client's mouth busy without adding calories. If clients are unwilling to quit, inform them of passive smoke's danger to others and encourage abstinence from smoking in the presence of nonsmokers, especially children. Also actively promote individual and community health by learning smoking cessation techniques and attending seminars.

Advise nonsmokers on techniques for reducing inhalation of passive smoke:

- Do not permit others to smoke within one's home or workplace.
- If smoking takes place within the home, increase ventilation by opening windows or using exhaust fans.
- Avoid riding in a car with someone who smokes; the small area contributes to a high concentration of toxic smoke, which increases exposure.

• COCAINE DEPENDENCE

Cocaine is a central nervous system (CNS) stimulant obtained from the leaves of the coca plant. The powder form of cocaine is snorted (inhaled through the nose) or dissolved and injected intravenously. Crack, a purified form of cocaine with a crystalline or rocklike appearance, is smoked either by placing it in a pipe or by sprinkling it onto or mixing it with tobacco or marijuana. Cocaine may be freebased, which reduces the drug to its purest form. The person then smokes freebased cocaine by sprinkling it onto a cigarette or inhaling it through a pipe. Freebased cocaine provides an intense physical experience as the drug is absorbed, more so than when it is taken by other routes. It also increases the risk of toxic effects and overdose reactions. Metabolism of cocaine, which is rapid, is generally followed by an intense craving to use the drug again. Cravings can recur months or years after abstinence.

Assessment Findings

Signs and Symptoms

Signs and symptoms of the drug's effect may be brief (see Table 17.1) because cocaine is fully metabolized in several minutes. Signs correlate with its route of administration and consequences of chronic use, such as ulceration of the nasal mucosa and perforation of the nasal septum in those who snort cocaine; needle marks along the pathways of veins in those who inject cocaine intravenously; burns on faces, fingertips, or eyebrows in those who may also use or lean over a lighted pipe. Smoking cocaine can cause a chronic cough and pulmonary congestion.

Clients who are addicted to cocaine often have a problem with **polydrug abuse,** abuse of more than one substance. Often they take sedative drugs such as alcohol, minor tranquilizers, barbiturates, and marijuana to offset their agitation and irritability.

Complications

Long-term abusers of cocaine experience anorexia, weight loss, memory impairment, personality and behavioral changes, paranoia, psychosis, and hallucinations. Stimulant abuse can cause rapid and severe hypertension, cardiac dysrhythmias, seizures, cerebral hemorrhage (stroke), myocardial infarction (heart attack), and respiratory arrest. Some people who use cocaine experience bizarre skin sensations referred to as "cocaine bugs," which lead to scratching and scarring. Newborns can also experience withdrawal symptoms if their mothers have recently used cocaine.

Diagnostic Findings

Drug toxicology tests are done on blood and urine. Metabolites of cocaine can be found in urine up to 36 hours after its use. Other abused substances are also identified.

Medical Management and Rehabilitation

Cocaine toxicity (see Table 17.1) requires immediate treatment because the condition is life-threatening. Referral to Cocaine Anonymous, based on the same principles as AA, provides ongoing support to those addicted to cocaine. Participation in individual and group psychotherapy and Cocaine Anonymous is encouraged to help the client eliminate all forms of drug abuse. The recreational use of other drugs can lead to relapse.

To help persons addicted to cocaine with recovery, medications like bromocriptine (Parlodel) and amantadine (Symmetrel) are used temporarily. They increase or mimic effects of dopamine, the neurotransmitter most likely responsible for the rewarding and reinforcing effects of cocaine. Antidepressants relieve the dysphoria (depression) that occurs during withdrawal. Amino-acid precursors such as phenylalanine and tyrosine, substances from which the neurotransmitters norepinephrine and dopamine are made, are included in drug therapy to replace levels depleted by chronic use.

Nursing Management

Assess the client's history of drug use and current physical condition, including signs of toxicity and withdrawal. If needed, implement medical treatment during a life-threatening emergency. Later, explain effects of drug abuse and risks for continuing drug-taking behaviors. Monitoring the client for suicidal ideation (see Chap. 15) and administering medications that provide support during withdrawal are essential nursing interventions.

• OPIATE DEPENDENCE

Opiate dependence is an addiction to CNS depressant drugs, narcotics, either derived from or chemically similar to opium. Opioid is a term for synthetic narcotics. Some examples of opiate drugs include heroin (diacetylmorphine), codeine, morphine, meperidine (Demerol), methadone, hydromorphone (Dilaudid), oxycodone, and opium as in tincture of paregoric. Opiates produce sedation after initial euphoria. The rate of tolerance and chemical dependence is related to drug, dose, and frequency of use.

Assessment Findings

Refer to heroin in Table 17.1 for effects of opiates. The pupils are generally pinpoint in size. Constipation is associated with slowed peristalsis. Chronic use is evidenced by anorexia, weight loss, constipation, malnutrition, needle marks, and scarring (tracks) along the paths of veins.

Respiratory depression can lead to unconsciousness and death. Sharing needles during IV administration of any abused substance can lead to AIDS, hepatitis, and septicemia. Abscesses may develop in punctured skin and veins. General debilitation increases susceptibility to tuberculosis and anemia. Neonates in withdrawal are observed to have a high-pitched cry, tremors, insomnia, increased respirations, vomiting, diarrhea, dehydration, and convulsions.

A urine drug screen reveals evidence of opiate use. Rapid recovery (within 2 to 5 minutes) from lethargy, hypotension, and respiratory depression after IV administration of a narcotic antagonist such as naloxone (Narcan) supports the diagnosis of narcotic overdose.

Medical Management and Rehabilitation

Withdrawal symptoms are treated with the alpha-adrenergic blocker clonidine (Catapres) to inhibit the release of norepinephrine. Methadone (Dolophine), a synthetic narcotic, may be used to eliminate or control withdrawal symptoms.

One method for helping those addicted to heroin stay off IV or street-supplied narcotics is methadone maintenance therapy. **Methadone maintenance therapy** involves substituting one addicting drug for another. The advantage is that because methadone is a synthetic drug prepared by a pharmaceutical company, the drug is untainted and the dose is reliable. The rationale behind methadone maintenance therapy is that it forestalls withdrawal, avoids a toxic overdose, reduces the potential for bloodborne infections, and theoretically reduces crime because the drug is provided legally. Some addicts, however, may combine methadone with a depressant drug of choice, increasing the potential for overdose and death. The practice of testing the urine before providing methadone is one way of screening and eliminating those who are abusing the system.

Naltrexone (Trexan, ReVia) is also used for opiate addiction. If clients return to opiate abuse while taking naltrexone, they do not experience the previous level of opiate effects.

Psychotherapy is an important aspect of rehabilitation. It involves treating the complex web of social problems that accompanies the addiction. Clients also are referred to Narcotics Anonymous, a self-help organization modeled after AA.

Nursing Management

The nurse's role is similar to that discussed for other types of chemical dependence, with a few exceptions that apply to administering drug therapy. If naltrexone is prescribed, the client must be opiate-free for at least 7 days before administration begins. Advise the client who takes methadone to tell healthcare providers or wear a Medic-Alert tag in case the client needs a narcotic, tranquilizer, or barbiturate. Because methadone is a narcotic, lower doses of other sedative drugs are necessary because the combination can potentiate their depressant action.

OTHER ABUSED SUBSTANCES

Various other substances are abused and addictive. Some examples include hallucinogens, amphetamines, marijuana, barbiturates, tranquilizers, and volatile hydrocarbons. Signs and symptoms follow the same pattern as with previously discussed substances: experimental use progresses through stages of increased use until dependence and addiction occur; there is failure to meet social, familial, or occupational obligations with increased defensive mechanisms to explain behavior; disturbances in mood and physical function occur as the result of drug abuse. Treatment and recovery include withdrawal, abstinence, and ongoing enrollment in a support group.

GENERAL GERONTOLOGIC CONSIDERATIONS

Alcoholism may be difficult to identify in the older adult because symptoms such as tremors, unsteady gait, or memory loss mimic changes associated with aging.

Alcohol abuse diminishes significantly after age 70.

Older adults who drink alcohol exhibit greater impairment than younger adults and recover more slowly.

Prolonged use of alcohol can result in neurologic deficits such as confusion, ataxia, and loss of cognitive ability.

Older adults may abuse over-the-counter and prescription drugs rather than illicit drugs.

Acute alcohol withdrawal in older adults is serious and may be life-threatening.

Administration of disulfiram to older adults requires caution. This drug interferes with the actions of several drugs (e.g., warfarin, nitroglycerin) that are often a part of the older adult's medication regimen.

Critical Thinking Exercises

1. *What information would you offer to a smoker who claims that "smoke-free environments" violate his or her right to smoke?*
2. *From which type of substance could a person be withdrawing if the following assessments are made? The person has a runny nose and tearing eyes. Frequent yawning is observed. The pilomotor muscles around hair follicles produce the appearance of "goose bumps." The person is experiencing nausea, vomiting, abdominal cramps, and diarrhea.*

NCLEX-STYLE REVIEW QUESTIONS 

1. A 46-year-old client with alcoholism is brought to the emergency department with cardiopulmonary symptoms. She states that she is taking disulfiram (Antabuse) but has not had any alcoholic beverages. Which question by the nurse is a priority?
   1. "How long have you been an alcoholic?"
   2. "What time was your last dose of disulfiram?"
   3. "Have you eaten any foods containing tyramine?"
   4. "Have you taken any other medications?"

2. Approximately 24 hours after admission, the client who abuses alcohol becomes very restless and yells that he must kill all the bugs in his room. In this situation, it is essential for the nurse to:
   1. Place the client in restraints.
   2. Close the door to seclude the client.
   3. Reassure the client that he is not seeing bugs.
   4. Remain at the client's bedside.

3. Which set of vital signs indicates the potential need for sedative medication during a period of acute alcohol withdrawal?
   1. T-97.2, P-88, R-24, BP-124/80
   2. T-99, P-68, R-20, BP-90/60
   3. T-100.6, P-120, R-28, BP-180/110
   4. T-99.2, P-80, R-16, BP-160/90

connection

Visit the Connection site at **http://connection.lww.com/go/timbyEssentials** for links to chapter-related resources on the Internet.

References and Suggested Readings

Compton, P., & McCaffery, M. (2001). Controlling pain. Treating acute pain in addicted patients. *Nursing, 31*(1), 17.

Henderson-Martin, B. (2000). No more surprises: Screening patients for alcohol abuse. *American Journal of Nursing, 100*(9), 26–33.

Hill, S. Y., Zezza, N., Wipprecht, G., et al. (1999). Linkage studies of D2 and D4 receptor genes and alcoholism. *American Journal of Medical Genetics, 88,* 676–685.

Li, T. (2000). Pharmacogenetics of responses to alcohol and genes that influence alcohol drinking. *Journal of Studies on Alcohol, 61*(1), 5–12.

McGee, E. M. (2000). Alcoholics anonymous and nursing: lessons in holism and spiritual care. *Journal of Holistic Nursing, 18*(1), 6–26.

National Center for Chronic Disease Prevention and Health Promotion. Office on Smoking and Health. (2000). Reducing tobacco use. A report of the Surgeon General-2000. [On-line.] Available: http://www.cdc.gov/tobacco.

Olms, D. (1983). *The disease concept of alcoholism.* Bellville: Gary Whiteaker Company.

Ryan, L. A., & Ottlinger, A. (1999). Implementation of alcohol withdrawal program in a medical-surgical setting: improving patient outcomes. *Journal of Addictions Nursing, 11*(3), 102–106.

Sachse, D. S., & Kearney, K. (2000). Emergency. Delirium tremens. *American Journal of Nursing, 100*(5), 41–42.

Schmidt, J., & Williams, E. (1999). When all else fails, try harm reduction. *American Journal of Nursing, 99*(10), 67–70.

Stewart, K. B., & Richards, A. B. (2000). Recognizing and managing your patient's alcohol abuse. *Nursing, 30*(2), 56–59.

chapter 18

Caring for Clients With Dementia and Thought Disorders

Words to Know 

acalculia
acetylcholine
agnosia
agraphia
alexia
Alzheimer's disease
aphasia
apraxia
ataxia
cognitive functions
conservatorship
delirium
delusions
dementia
depot injections
durable power of attorney
extrapyramidal symptoms
guardianship
hallucinations
incompetent
mentation
negative symptoms
neuritic plaques
neurofibrillary tangles
positive symptoms
prions
respite care
restraint alternatives
schizophrenia
voice dismissal

Learning Objectives

On completion of this chapter, the reader will:

- Differentiate delirium from dementia.
- Describe etiologic factors and pathologic changes associated with Alzheimer's disease.
- Name the first symptom of Alzheimer's disease.
- Identify methods for diagnosing Alzheimer's disease.
- Explain the mechanism of drug therapy in Alzheimer's disease.
- Describe the focus of nursing management when caring for clients with Alzheimer's disease.
- Discuss characteristics of schizophrenia.
- Describe psychobiologic explanations for schizophrenia.
- Differentiate positive from negative symptoms of schizophrenia.
- Discuss common medical management of schizophrenia.
- Name examples of antipsychotic drugs and their mechanisms of action.
- Explain the term *extrapyramidal symptoms,* and list examples.
- Describe techniques to prevent noncompliance with drug therapy in clients with schizophrenia.
- Summarize the nursing management of clients with schizophrenia.

Changes in **mentation,** mental activity, can occur anytime during life. **Cognitive functions,** such as short-term memory and learning ability, change gradually as people age, but many acute, chronic, reversible, and irreversible conditions that impair thinking processes can occur any time. Although older adults are at greatest risk for cognitive impairment, such impairment is not necessarily a normal consequence of aging, and may be treatable. Depression and other medical disorders, such as hypothyroidism, can manifest as mental dysfunction. Mental changes require investigation to determine if anything can reverse the symptoms.

DELIRIUM

Delirium is a sudden, transient state of confusion. The period of confusion depends on the cause of the delirium. Clients with delirium may have difficulty processing information, and be disoriented as to the date, time of day, and location. They may experience impaired judgement or inability to perform intellectually. Some clients with delirium may be suspicious or frightened or behave inappropriately.

Delirium can result from high fever, head trauma, brain tumor, drug intoxication or withdrawal, metabolic disorders (e.g., liver or renal failure), or inflammatory disorders of the central nervous system (CNS) such as meningitis or encephalitis. Treating the underlying medical condition usually restores mental functions.

DEMENTIA

Dementia more commonly affects older adults. There is a decline in memory and other mental functions which are severe enough to affect an alert person's daily life (Small, Rabins, Barry, et al., 1997). Various disorders are characterized by dementia, including Alzheimer's disease, cerebrovascular disorders (see Chap. 40), and Parkinson's disease (see Chap. 39). In contrast to delirium, dementia is manifested by a gradual, irreversible loss of intellectual abilities.

Stop, Think, and Respond ● BOX 18-1

A client is 60 years old. He developed a headache and high fever 24 hours ago. When he is aroused, he thinks he is in the city in which he spent his boyhood. He calls for his mother who has been dead for more than 10 years. Is this client manifesting delirium or dementia?

ALZHEIMER'S DISEASE

Alzheimer's disease is a progressive, deteriorating brain disorder. The two types are early onset (before 60 years) and late onset (after 60 years), with late onset being more common.

Pathophysiology and Etiology

Having a first-degree relative with Alzheimer's disease nearly doubles the risk for acquiring this form of dementia. Inherited genetic abnormalities on chromosomes 14, 19, and 21 are associated with early-onset Alzheimer's disease. Research about Alzheimer's disease suggests other abnormalities, defects in neurotransmitters, and elevated levels of specific amino acids. Other suggestions related to cause include aluminum toxicity leached from cooking utensils and metal food containers; mercury absorption from the metal amalgam used in dental fillings (Kranhold, 2001); and infection by **prions,** small proteins that cause neurologic diseases like bovine spongiform encephalopathy (mad cow disease) in animals and Creutzfeldt-Jakob disease, a form of dementia, in humans (Prusiner, 1998).

In dementia of the Alzheimer's type, four pathologic changes occur in the brain:

1. The size of the cortex decreases.
2. The neurotransmitter **acetylcholine** (critical for memory and cognition) is deficient, especially in the cortex and hippocampus.
3. **Neuritic plaques,** deposits of beta amyloid (starchy component) and degenerating nerve cells, are found.
4. **Neurofibrillary tangles,** twisted bundles of nerve fibers (Fig. 18.1), appear.

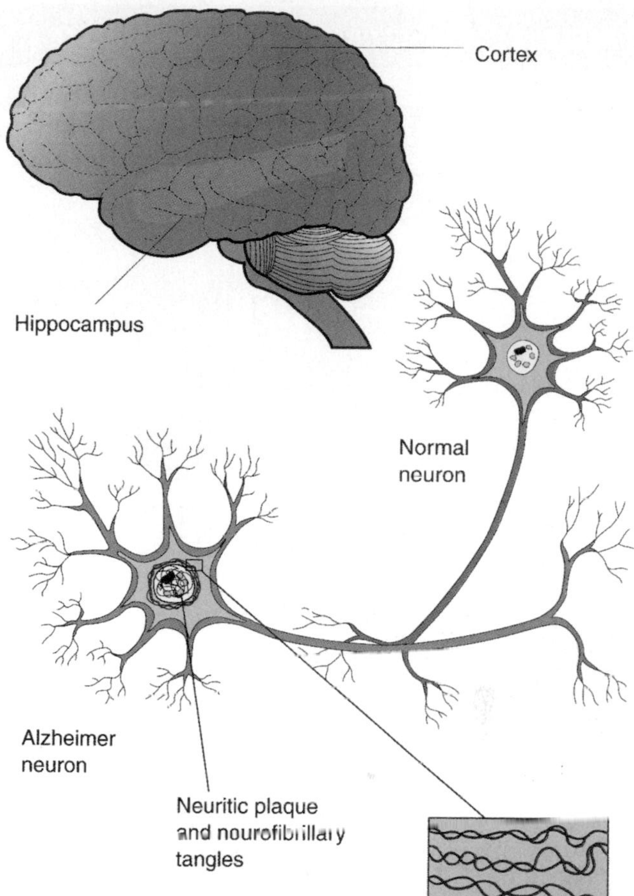

FIGURE 18.1 Neurofibrillary tangling and neuritic plaques in Alzheimer's disease.

The decreased size of the cerebral cortex along with acetylcholine deficiency explain cognitive deficits and alterations in emotions that accompany the disease. The degree to which plaque and tangles are present is directly related to the severity of disease manifestations.

Assessment Findings

Signs and Symptoms

Alzheimer's disease progresses through seven distinct stages corresponding with those identified in the Global Deterioration Scale (Table 18.1). Progression from one stage to another occurs at different rates among affected individuals. Early stages may last 2 to 4 years or longer; it may take as long as 5 to 10 years before a person needs constant care.

Onset is usually insidious. Symptoms may develop slowly over years. Memory loss, the classic symptom, is confined at first to recent information. Long-term memory and ability to make appropriate judgments and problem-solve become impaired as well. Disturbances in behavior, personality changes, and depression also occur. As the dis-

TABLE 18.1 GLOBAL DETERIORATION SCALE

STAGE	CHARACTERISTIC	MANIFESTATIONS
1	Normal mentation	None
2	Forgetfulness	Concern for self-identified memory changes such as forgetting location of items, forgetting familiar names No objective demonstration of memory deficit No social consequences for minor memory loss
3	Early confusion	One or more of the following: getting lost in an unfamiliar location decline in work performance noticed by others deficit in word and name finding little retention of what has been read difficulty remembering names of new acquaintances loss or misplacement of valuable objects impaired ability to concentrate Objective demonstration of memory deficit Denial of memory and cognitive deficits Mild to moderate anxiety
4	Late confusion	Deficits in the following areas: current and recent events personal history counting backward in series of numbers traveling and handling finances Inability to perform complex tasks such as preparing dinner for guests Strong denial of impairment Blunted affect Retreat from challenges
5	Early dementia	Assistance of others needed Memory loss for important information like address and telephone number Some disorientation to time or place Difficulty counting backward by 4s or 2s May have difficulty choosing proper clothing
6	Middle dementia	May forget name of spouse or significant others Unaware of recent events and experiences Memory of past sketchy Unaware of date and surroundings Difficulty counting backward and sometimes forward in 10s Requires assistance with activities of daily living May be incontinent Needs assistance to travel Confuses day and night Personality and emotional changes such as: delusional thinking repetition of cleaning anxiety, agitation, violence cannot keep a thought long enough to carry it out
7	Late dementia	Loss of verbal ability Grunting may be evident Incontinent; requires help with toileting and feeding Loss of motor skills for walking, sitting, head control, and smiling

Adapted from Reisberg, B., Ferris, S. H., Leon, J. J., & Crook, T. (1982). The global deterioration scale (GDS): An instrument for the assessment of primary degenerative dementia. *American Journal of Psychiatry, 139,* 1136–1139.

ease advances, memory, cognition, awareness, and ability to care for self deteriorate markedly. Clients may wander and become lost. Periodic incidences of violent behavior are possible. Problems with speaking (**aphasia**), reading (**alexia**), writing (**agraphia**), and calculating (**acalculia**) develop. Inability to recognize objects and sounds (visual, tactile, and auditory **agnosia**), difficulty walking (**ataxia**), and tremors occur. In the final stage of the disease, an inability to accomplish activities of daily living (ADLs; **apraxia**), such as grooming, toileting, and eating, despite intact motor function, makes the client totally dependent on others.

Diagnostic Findings

Ruling out Alzheimer's disease in clients who are experiencing similar signs and symptoms can spare them emotional agony, as well as saving time and money spent on nonspecific tests. The diagnosis of Alzheimer's is usually made by excluding other causes for the client's symptoms. A computed tomography (CT) scan shows shrinking of the cerebral cortex, but this is not apparent in the early stages of the disease. Photon emission tomography (PET) and magnetic resonance imaging (MRI) provide structural and metabolic information about the brain. Electroencephalography (EEG) detects slower than normal brain waves. None of these diagnostic tests is specific for Alzheimer's disease, which until recently could only be confirmed during a postmortem examination of the brain. A new diagnostic test called Nymox AD7C detects evidence of beta-amyloid protein in cerebrospinal fluid.

Medical Management

No cure exists for Alzheimer's disease. Treatment is mainly supportive using one of various drugs currently available. Although maintaining a client's independence in a familiar environment for as long as possible is best, the physician continues to assess the client's safety and burden on caregivers. Eventually, clients may go to an extended care facility, many of which have a unit dedicated to care of clients suffering from Alzheimer's or other forms of dementia.

Current drugs approved for treatment of Alzheimer's disease include cholinesterase inhibitors like tacrine (Cognex), donepezil (Aricept), and galantamine hydrobromide (Reminyl) (Drug Therapy Table 18.1). These drugs increase acetylcholine by inhibiting cholinesterase, the enzyme that degrades it. When administered in the early to middle stages of Alzheimer's disease, some clients improve, some stay the same, some progress more slowly, and some fail to respond. All clients eventually get worse over time.

One new drug, memantine, was recently approved in the U.S. Memantine's mechanism of action is different from the cholinesterase inhibitors. Memantine is a neuroprotective drug classified as an *N*-methyl-D-aspartate (NMDA) antagonist. By blocking NMDA receptors, the drug protects neurons from excessive stimulation by glutamate, an excitatory neurotransmitter responsible for neuronal death. Clients in advanced stages of Alzheimer's disease experienced less deterioration when taking

DRUG THERAPY TABLE 18.1 ALZHEIMER'S DISEASE

DRUG CATEGORY AND EXAMPLES	MECHANISM OF ACTION	SIDE EFFECTS	NURSING CONSIDERATIONS
Cholinesterase Inhibitor			
tacrine (Cognex)	Provides for increased levels of acetylcholine in the cortex by inhibiting cholinesterase, the enzyme that breaks down acetylcholine	Headache, fatigue, confusion, seizures, dizziness, nausea, vomiting, diarrhea, gastrointestinal upset, abdominal pain, loss of appetite, skin rashes, hepatotoxicity	Administer on an empty stomach on an around-the-clock schedule. Do not abruptly discontinue. Arrange for regular blood tests to determine aminotransferase levels. Inform client and family of side effects and to report any that occur. Tell client to exercise caution if performing tasks that require alertness.
donepezil (Aricept)	Inhibits the breakdown of acetylcholine	Nausea, vomiting, diarrhea, bradycardia, possible exacerbations of asthma and chronic obstructive pulmonary disease, muscle cramps, loss of appetite	Tell client that frequent small meals may minimize gastrointestinal upset. Monitor heart rate, and report bradycardia (heart rate <60 beats per minute).
galantamine hydrobromide (Reminyl)	Increases concentration of acetylcholine by blocking action of acetylcholinesterase	Nausea, vomiting, anorexia, diarrhea, weight loss	Tell client to take drug at morning and evening meals.
N-Methyl-D-Aspartate (NMDA) Antagonist			
memantine	Blocks NMDA receptors		

memantine than others who were given a placebo (Merz Pharmaceuticals, 2002).

Working from the premise that high homocysteine (an amino acid created during protein metabolism) levels interfere with memory, some physicians are also prescribing folic acid (folate) supplements. Folate lowers homocysteine levels.

Antidepressants or tranquilizers may help agitated or depressed clients.

Nursing Management

The major focus of nursing management is to help the client and caregiver maintain the highest possible quality of life by supporting mental and physical functions and ensuring safety. Most clients initially receive care in their homes, and home health nurses instruct the family about physical care, disease process, and treatment. They also will provide emotional support and intervene if family caregivers become overburdened. When transfer of the client from the home to an extended care facility becomes necessary, the nurse meets the client's physical needs on a full-time basis and helps the family cope during the client's deterioration. See Client and Family Teaching 18-1 and Nursing Care Plan 18-1.

SCHIZOPHRENIA

Schizophrenia is a thought disorder characterized by deterioration in mental functioning, disturbances in sensory perception, and changes in affect (emotion). Clients with schizophrenia improve with drug therapy but never fully recover. Because the condition is lifelong and appears in young adulthood, it causes anguish for families who must deal with the burden of healthcare costs and responsibility for caring for a loved one with this illness.

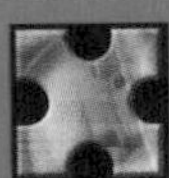

18-1 *Client and Family Teaching* Cognitive Disorders

The nurse helps the family cope by teaching about the client's illness, the treatment plan, and prognosis:

- Encourage the family to be supportive and involved, while allowing the client to remain as independent as possible.
- Give the family a referral to a social worker and crisis telephone numbers.
- Direct the family to local community mental health associations and support groups.

Pathophysiology and Etiology

Schizophrenia, historically attributed to emotional dysfunction, is now categorized as a psychobiologic disease because of recent findings in brain and neurotransmitter chemistry. Many neurotransmitter imbalances are involved in schizophrenia. Dopamine excess is believed to be the major cause of the symptoms, with imbalances of norepinephrine, serotonin (5-HT), and gamma-aminobutyric acid (GABA) (see Chap. 12) also playing a role. The disease has a familial or genetic component. Other theories suggest anatomic and physiologic changes associated with schizophrenia result from a viral infection experienced by the affected individual's mother during pregnancy. The neurochemical imbalance produces a variety of manifestations characterized by disturbed thinking, with themes that may include suspiciousness; persecution; being controlled; grandiosity (belief in one's importance); religious fixation; or preoccupation with sex, a love interest, illness, or a body part.

Assessment Findings

Symptoms generally begin during late adolescence to early adulthood. Clients manifest a range of symptoms categorized as positive or negative. **Positive symptoms** include delusions, hallucinations, and fluent but disorganized speech. **Negative symptoms,** sometimes called defect symptoms, are marked by impoverished speech and inability to enjoy relationships or express emotions (Box 18-1). Positive symptoms are more easily managed than negative symptoms. Classic symptoms are inexplainable sensory experiences such as hearing voices or seeing apparitions of people who are not really there. These occur in combination with peculiar patterns of speaking and odd motor behaviors. The client also tends to abandon relationships and interactions with others and loses motivation for working, going to school, or engaging in other goal-driven behaviors. Hygiene and appearance tend to lose their previous importance.

Diagnosis is made primarily on the symptomatology and by ruling out other possible causes. CT and PET scans, MRIs, and brain mapping (see Chap. 12) may show decreased brain size and activity, especially in the frontal and temporal lobes.

Medical Management

Clients with schizophrenia are referred to care of psychiatrists. Once the client is within the mental health system, every effort is made to avoid institutionalization. The exception is when the client is dangerous to self or others. Community mental health services are selected to meet the client's needs for psychotherapy, drug adminis-

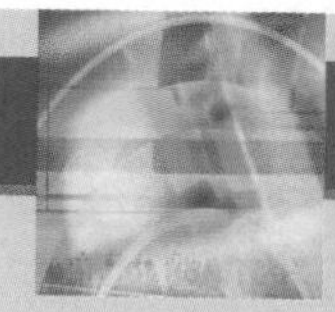

Nursing Care Plan 18-1

THE CLIENT WITH ALZHEIMER'S DISEASE

Assessment

- Interview both client and family, because the client may be unable to give a complete or objective history regarding memory, sleep patterns, moods, and self-care activities. Assess caregiver's strengths, limitations, and ability to manage caretaking activities.
- Perform a complete head-to-toe physical examination. Be especially attentive to muscular strength, balance, and gait.
- Determine client's mental status. Identify level of orientation, short-term and long-term memory, social behavior, emotional status, cognitive and motor skills, and ability to perform ADLs.

Nursing Diagnosis: **Caregiver Role Strain** related to being overwhelmed by responsibilities, fatigue, and depression

Expected Outcome: Caregiver will experience less anxiety as knowledge about implementing plans that will provide needed relief increases.

Interventions	*Rationales*
Assess caregiver's strengths, limitations, and ability to manage caretaking activities.	The caregiver may experience sleep deprivation, physical injury, and social isolation if no one else is available to assist with client care.
Suggest scheduling **respite care,** brief relief from caretaking responsibilities, with family and friends on a regular rotating basis.	Dividing caretaking responsibilities promotes physical endurance and emotional stability.
Provide a list of agencies that offer social services such as the county's commission on aging and Social Security and Medicare agencies.	Clients may be unaware of services available for assistance or how to contact them.
Develop a list of people to contact in an emergency, including a 24 hour hotline for the home health nursing agency.	Having a plan helps clients obtain assistance in a crisis
Recommend that caregiver and client take care of legal matters such as wills, transferring titles, and preparing an advance directive.	Attending to legal matters before severe cognitive changes occur is best.
Suggest establishing **durable power of attorney,** designating who may make decisions regarding finances or healthcare when the client becomes **incompetent,** the legal term for the inability to understand the risks or benefits of decisions.	Such measures ensure that a person selected by the client has access to unencumbered funds and follows the client's wishes regarding healthcare decisions.
Advise caregiver to obtain **guardianship** or **conservatorship,** court-appointed responsibility, for managing the client's care and assets if the client is already incompetent.	The client's financial assets may be frozen unless the court stipulates that another person can have access to private accounts.
Encourage the caregiver to temporarily place the client in a long-term nursing facility to take a well-deserved vacation.	Giving the caregiver a temporary option for a vacation may help to sustain his or her ability to continue caring for the client.

Evaluation of Expected Outcome:

- Caregiver seeks relief from responsibilities at least 1 or 2 days a week.
- Caregiver and client take care of legal issues.

Nursing Diagnosis: **Risk for Interrupted Family Processes** related to guilt over placing the client in a care facility

Expected Outcome: Family will remain united and supportive over the decision to transfer the client's care to others.

(continued)

Nursing Care Plan 18-1 (Continued)

THE CLIENT WITH ALZHEIMER'S DISEASE

Interventions	*Rationales*
Acknowledge and empathize with the family's ambivalent feelings.	Family is more likely to accept transfer of the client's care if the nurse demonstrates empathy.
Emphasize skills and services that the facility provides.	Knowledge that the facility offers many services to promote and maintain the client's well-being enhances acceptance of the decision.
Let the family participate in developing and revising the plan of care.	Family participation promotes a team approach to managing the client's care.
Keep the family informed of the client's progress or lack thereof.	Communication is often the key to good interpersonal relationships.
Encourage the family to visit and participate in the client's care as much as they want.	Promoting continued interactions conveys a sense that family is included rather than excluded from the client's life.
Allow the family privacy during interactions with the client, and make an area available to them for special occasions like birthdays.	Making special accommodations for family activities individualizes care.
Keep a current list of family phone numbers, listing the relationships of members to the client and indications for which they prefer to be called.	Accurate information is important when communication is necessary.
Prepare the family for the likely deterioration.	Realistic preparation for the progression of the disease promotes anticipatory grieving and acceptance of the client's potentially terminal condition.

Evaluation of Expected Outcome:

- Family members reconcile themselves to the difficult decision to transfer the care of the client to a nursing care facility.
- They remain involved in the client's care and understand the changes that accompany the disease process.

Nursing Diagnosis: **Impaired Memory** related to global cognitive deficits

Expected Outcome: Client will be reoriented and participate in life experiences to his or her potential.

Interventions	*Rationales*
Orient client frequently to person, place, and time.	Frequent reminders accommodate for impairment in memory.
Place a large-faced clock and calendars at multiple places within the client's environment.	External clues help the client maintain orientation or become oriented with minimal effort.
Assign consistent caregivers and maintain a structured daily routine.	Repetition and consistency reduce episodes of confusion.
Attach something the client can recognize to the door of his or her room.	The client is more likely to find his or her room by looking for a familiar clue like his or her name printed in large letters or a brightly colored bow.
Make sure the client wears an identification bracelet with an address and telephone number. Maintain a current photograph in the medical record.	Clients with Alzheimer's disease are known to wander and not recall their current residence. Having the means to identify the client aids in search-and-rescue efforts.

Evaluation of Expected Outcome: Client becomes reoriented with techniques such as verbal reminders and environmental clues like a large-faced clock and calendar and can participate in activities that occur at consistent times throughout the day.

(continued)

Nursing Care Plan 18-1 (Continued)

THE CLIENT WITH ALZHEIMER'S DISEASE

Nursing Diagnosis: **Risk for Trauma** related to ataxia and propensity for wandering

Expected Outcome: Client will move about freely and safely within the healthcare facility but will not leave the facility unsupervised.

Interventions	*Rationales*
Help the client don supportive walking shoes when out of bed.	Supportive shoes promote a stable gait and posture.
Provide assistance with ambulation. Remove hazards, such as foot stools, small tables, or liquid spills, from the ambulatory area.	Assistance reduces the potential for falls. Removing obstacles and slippery surfaces promotes safer ambulation.
Keep the environment well lighted.	The ability to see helps the client avoid environmental hazards.
Maintain the bed in low position.	Should a fall occur, the bed in low position reduces the potential for serious injury.
Use **restraint alternatives,** protective or adaptive devices for fall protection and postural support.	Physical restraints increase the potential for injury; clients have the right to the least restrictive intervention.
Place a bed monitor under the client's mattress.	Bed monitors alert caregivers when a client gets out of bed without signalling for assistance.
Install alarms on exit doors, and respond immediately when one sounds.	An alarm alerts caregivers when someone leaves who is unauthorized to do so.

Evaluation of Expected Outcome:

- No injuries occur.
- The client's whereabouts are known at all times.

Nursing Diagnosis: **Impaired Verbal Communication** related to expressive or receptive aphasia

Expected Outcome: Client will communicate with healthcare professional at whatever level is possible.

Interventions	*Rationales*
Approach from the front, make eye contact, and look for a response to your voice.	Obtaining the client's attention promotes verbal interaction.
Get the client's attention by using the name to which he or she is most likely to respond.	Using a client's name increases cognitive awareness and potential for social interaction.
Keep explanations or directions short and simple.	Being succinct makes it easier for the client to process information and respond appropriately.
Give gentle reminders or model the desired response.	Reminding and modeling compensate for failing memory or loss of language skills.
Involve client in one idea or task at a time.	Keeping ideas and tasks to a minimum promotes attention and concentration.
Reduce environmental stimuli like noise and activity.	Excess stimulation interferes with attention and concentration and may agitate the client.
Promote interactions that tap into the client's long-term memory such as reminiscing; offer client verbal cues such as, "I understand you were . . . (a school teacher)."	Long-term memory is retained more than short-term memory; recalling information promotes social interaction and elevates self-esteem.

(continued)

Nursing Care Plan 18-1 (Continued)

THE CLIENT WITH ALZHEIMER'S DISEASE

Interventions	*Rationales*
Give client plenty of time to respond to questions. Try to understand what client wants to convey.	Impaired language skills make communication more difficult.
Repeat information that you believe the client is trying to communicate.	Rephrasing or paraphrasing helps ensure accurate interpretation of the client's thoughts.
Include client in small group activities, even if there is little or no socialization.	Despite the appearance of being uninvolved, participation may stimulate the client's awareness.
Change activities or distract the client if he or she becomes angry, hostile, or uncooperative.	The nurse is responsible for ensuring the safety of the client, other clients, and staff.

Evaluation of Expected Outcome: Client understands spoken works and responds verbally.

tration, and social needs, such as housing, job assistance, and money management, in an outpatient setting.

Antipsychotic drugs are the mainstay of treatment. These drugs, also called major tranquilizers or neuroleptics, belong to several different chemical families, but all block receptors for dopamine. Some examples of antipsychotic drugs are haloperidol (Haldol), fluphenazine (Prolixin), risperidone (Risperdal), clozapine (Clozaril), and olanzapine (Zyprexa) (Drug Therapy Table 18.2).

BOX 18-1 ● Positive and Negative Symptoms of Schizophrenia

POSITIVE

Delusions, false beliefs that cannot be changed by logical reasoning
Hallucinations, sensory experiences that others do not perceive; can be auditory, visual, tactile, olfactory, or gustatory (involving taste)
Loose associations, a sequence of ideas that are slightly connected
Inappropriate affect, a display of emotional feeling inconsistent with the situation
Peculiarities in speech like *echolalia,* repeating what others say; *rhyming; word salad,* using unrelated words in a sentence; or *neologisms,* inventing new words
Bizarre behavior such as *stereotopy* (repetitious movement) and *echopraxia* (mimicking the movements of others)

NEGATIVE

Concrete thinking, an inability to explain abstract ideas
Thought blocking, an inability to recall information for a time
Symbolism, attaching significance to an insignificant object or idea
Blunted or *flat affect,* little or no display of feeling
Anhedonia, inability to experience pleasure
Catatonia, immobility
Posturing, assuming statuesque positions
Autism, social withdrawal
Self-neglect of hygiene, eating, work, finances, and the like
Poverty of thought, lacking any opinions or ideas

Risperidone, clozapine, and olanzapine, newer drugs called *atypical antipsychotics,* produce their effects with reduced incidence of **extrapyramidal symptoms** (EPS), movement disorders associated with traditional drugs (Box 18-2). But clozapine has the potential adverse effect of dangerously depressing bone marrow function, and clients who take clozapine must undergo a weekly blood count. If the client's white blood cell count drops too low, the drug is discontinued. Anticholinergic drugs such as trihexyphenidyl (Artane) and benztropine (Cogentin) are given to prevent or relieve EPS. Antipsychotics are sometimes combined with anticonvulsant drugs such as clonazepam (Klonopin) and carbamazepine (Tegretol).

Noncompliance with drug therapy is the leading cause for the return of disease symptoms and the need for short-term hospitalization. For this reason, some nonhospitalized clients are given **depot injections,** intramuscular injections of antipsychotic drugs in an oil suspension that are gradually absorbed over 2 to 4 weeks.

Nursing Management

When caring for clients with schizophrenia in acute care or community mental health settings, nurses perform a mini mental status examination during the initial contact and periodically thereafter to monitor for changes. They assess the client for delusions, bizarre speech patterns, hallucinations, agitation, stupor, and social withdrawal. They also assess the client's physical status including hygiene and nutritional condition.

Administer antipsychotic drugs as prescribed. Do not argue with the client about the validity of any delusions, because clients may become more fixated on their delusions, defensive, or hostile if others challenge them. Instead, try to shift the client's focus to what is real and direct the client to a quiet place during periods of agitation.

DRUG THERAPY TABLE 18.2 TREATMENT OF SCHIZOPHRENIA

DRUG CATEGORY AND EXAMPLES/ MECHANISM OF ACTION	SIDE EFFECTS	NURSING CONSIDERATIONS
Antipsychotics		
haloperidol (Haldol) Blocks postsynaptic dopamine receptors	Drowsiness, pseudoparkinsonism, dystonia, akathisia, neuroleptic malignant syndrome, dysrhythmias, suppression of cough reflex, anaphylactoid reactions, anemia, dry mouth, constipation, urinary retention	Monitor older clients for dehydration and aspiration potential. Withdraw drug gradually. Tell client to avoid driving. Instruct client to drink fluids and report any side effects.
fluphenazine (Prolixin) Blocks postsynaptic dopamine receptors	Drowsiness, extrapyramidal syndromes, dysrhythmias, suppression of cough reflex, dry mouth, constipation, urinary retention	Tell client to avoid alcohol. Do not mix oral concentrate with caffeine-containing beverages, teas, or apple juice. Monitor older clients for signs of dehydration. Tell client to drink plenty of fluids and to report any side effects.
risperidone (Risperdal) Blocks dopamine and serotonin receptors in the brain	Insomnia, agitation, headache, anxiety, drowsiness, nausea, vomiting, constipation, tardive dyskinesias, neuroleptic malignant syndrome, seizures	Monitor client for seizures when initiating therapy or increasing dose. Increase dose gradually until therapeutic effect is achieved. Tell client not to stop taking drug abruptly or to make up missed doses, but to contact the healthcare provider. Instruct client not to take this drug during pregnancy and to report any side effects.
olazapine (Zyprexa) Blocks dopamine and serotonin receptors	Dizziness, drowsiness, headache, weight gain, orthostatic hypotension, extrapyramidal symptoms	Instruct clients in measures to offset orthostatic hypotension, such as rising slowly and doing ankle pumps before standing. Monitor for extrapyramidal symptoms. Initiate anticholinergic drugs. Decrease, discontinue, or switch medications as directed.

If a client is experiencing a hallucination, state that you do not hear or see anyone, but acknowledge that the experience must seem real and frightening to the client. Staying with the client throughout the hallucination also is essential. Healthcare personnel should not touch clients without warning. Other methods of dealing with hallucinations include calling auditory hallucinations "the voices" rather than using a personal pronoun like "they" or "them"; asking the client to share the content of the hallucination; distracting the client from attending to the hallucination; and teaching the technique of **voice dismissal,** which refers to saying "stop" or "be gone."

To assist with social skills, accompany the client to group meetings and activities. Such support may help the client participate in situations perceived as threatening or causing social discomfort. Do not pressure the client to participate, but share time with the client after the group interaction, using open-ended questions to explore the client's perception of the experience. Verbal compliments when the client speaks voluntarily with others or acts appropriately in social situations can empower the client to make further attempts at interaction. Also give suggestions for improvements and act as a mentor.

BOX 18-2 ● Extrapyramidal Side Effects (EPS)

Movement Disorder	Explanation
Akinesia (pseudoparkinsonism)	The client appears to have symptoms of Parkinson's disease (see Chap. 39) such as hand tremors, stooped posture, stiff shuffling gait.
Akathisia	The client cannot sit or stand still.
Dystonia	Sudden severe muscle spasm occurs, usually in the neck, tongue, or eyes.
Tardive dyskinesia	Client makes involuntary muscle movements, usually in the face, such as tongue thrusting, continuous chewing, grimacing, lip smacking, blinking; irreversible once manifested.

Stop, Think, and Respond ● BOX 18-2

Discuss appropriate nursing interventions when a client with schizophrenia expresses a delusional belief or experiences a hallucination.

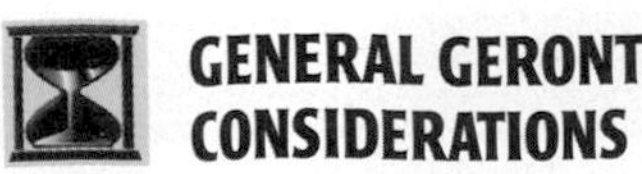

GENERAL GERONTOLOGIC CONSIDERATIONS

Alzheimer's disease affects approximately 30% of individuals older than age 85.

Tacrine can be dissolved in orange juice or other liquid if the older adult has difficulty swallowing.

Older adult clients require lower dosages of antipsychotic drugs.

The older adult taking haloperidol (Haldol) is at risk for dehydration. Report lethargy, decreased thirst, weakness, and dry mucous membranes.

Older adults are particularly susceptible to tardive dyskinesia while taking antipsychotic drugs. Report symptoms immediately because the drug must be discontinued.

Critical Thinking Exercises

1. *Discuss similarities and differences between Alzheimer's disease and schizophrenia.*
2. *In what ways are interventions for altered mentation different for a client with Alzheimer's disease and schizophrenia?*

• NCLEX-STYLE REVIEW QUESTIONS

1. A 76-year-old woman in a personal care home has been recently diagnosed with late-onset Alzheimer's disease. When the nurse's aide asks if there is a deficiency in a neurotransmitter, the correct answer by the nurse is that clients with Alzheimer's disease have a deficiency in:
   1. Acetylcholine
   2. Epinephrine
   3. Norepinephrine
   4. Serotonin
2. The most therapeutic technique for helping clients with dementia remain oriented is to:
   1. Call each client by his or her first name.
   2. Ask the clients to identify a goal for the day.
   3. Assign clients to small jobs each day.
   4. Post large calendars with the current date.
3. The activities coordinator at a skilled nursing facility is creating a schedule for activities. The best technique for reducing confusion among clients with dementia is to:
   1. Wear a name tag when caring for the clients.
   2. Adhere to a consistent routine of unit activities.
   3. Provide diversional activities like field trips.
   4. Distribute a list of the day's scheduled events.

connection

Visit the Connection site at **http://connection.lww.com/go/timbyEssentials** for links to chapter-related resources on the Internet.

References and Suggested Readings

Armstrong, M. (2001). The pressures felt by informal carers of people with dementia. *Nursing Standard, 15*(17), 47–55.

Brooker, D., & Duce, L. (2000). Well-being and activity in dementia: A comparison of group reminiscence therapy, structured goal-directed group activity and unstructured time. *Aging & Mental Health, 4*(4), 354–358.

Froelich, T. F., Robinson, J. T., & Inouye, S. K. (1998). Screening for dementia in the outpatient setting: The time and change test. *Journal of the American Geriatric Society, 46*(12), 1506–1511.

Gray, R., & Gournay, K. (2000). What can we do about acute extrapyramidal symptoms? *Journal of Psychiatric and Mental Health Nursing, 7*(3), 205–211.

Kranhold, K. (2001; May 10). Dentists battle "gag" on warning about mercury. *Wall Street Journal,* Eastern edition 327 (92), Section B:1.

Lo, R., & Brown, R. (2000). Caring for family carers and people with dementia. *International Journal of Psychiatric Nursing Research, 6*(2), 684–694.

Lynch, M., & Wagstaff, C. (1999). Managing care of the patient with schizophrenia—before and after surgery. *Journal of Practical Nursing, 49*(4), 12–15.

Merz Pharmaceuticals. (2002). Memantine. [On-line.] Available at: http://www.memantine.com. NIMH funds study of drugs for schizophrenia and Alzheimer's. *Journal of Psychosocial Nursing and Mental Health Services, 37*(12), 7.

Petersen, R. C. (2000). Aging, mild cognitive impairment, and Alzheimer's disease. *Neurologic Clinics, 18*(4), 789–805.

Prusiner, S. B. (1998). The prion diseases. *Brain Pathology, 8*(3), 499–513.

Rempusheski, V. F., & Hurley, A. C. (2000). Advance directives and dementia. *Journal of Gerontological Nursing, 26*(10), 27–34.

Schafer, C., Sodoma, C., Gonzalez, S., et al. (2000). Your turn. How do you structure the day for individuals with dementia? *Journal of Gerontological Nursing, 26*(10), 52–53.

Small, G. W., Rabins, P. V., Barry, P. B., et al. (1997). Consensus statement of the American Association for Geriatric Psychiatry, the Alzheimer's Association, and the American Geriatrics Society. *Journal of the American Medical Association, 278,* 1363–1371.

Solomon, P. R., & Pendlebury, W. W. (1998). Recognition of Alzheimer's disease: The 7 minute screen. *Family Medicine, 30*(4), 265–271.

Webster, J. (2001). Unraveling Alzheimer's disease and other dementias. *Home Health Care Consultant, 8*(1), 10–18.

Weitzel, C. (2000). Could you spot this psych emergency? *RN, 63*(9), 35–38.

Yeaworth, R. (2000). Coalition to change assisted living regulations governing special units for dementia patients. *Nursing Outlook, 48*(6), 314–315.

chapter 19

Caring for Clients With Cancer

Words to Know 

alopecia
antineoplastic
apheresis
benign
brachytherapy
cancer
carcinogens
chemotherapy
engraftment
extravasation
gene therapy
immunotherapy
leukopenia
malignant
metastasis
myelosuppression
neoplasms
neutropenia
oncology nursing
radiation therapy
stomatitis
thrombocytopenia
vesicants

Learning Objectives

On completion of this chapter, the reader will:

- Discuss the pathophysiology and etiology of cancer.
- Compare benign and malignant tumors.
- Name factors that contribute to the development of cancer.
- Identify the warning signs of cancer.
- Describe ways to reduce the risks of cancer.
- Explain methods for diagnosing cancer.
- Describe systems for staging and grading malignant tumors.
- Differentiate various treatments and methods for managing cancer.
- Discuss various adverse effects that occur with cancer treatments and methods used to treat those effects.
- Describe emotions associated with the diagnosis of cancer.
- Use the nursing process as a framework for caring for clients with cancer.

Cancer is characterized by abnormal, unrelated cell proliferation. Cancerous tumors invade healthy tissues and compete with normal cells for oxygen, nutrients, and space. Nurses in all settings care for clients of all ages with cancer. The nursing specialty related to care of clients with cancer is **oncology nursing.** A diagnosis of cancer is frightening to most people, although reactions depend on the particular diagnosis, location, stage, treatment, effects on bodily functions, and prognosis.

CANCER

Pathophysiology

The cell is the basic structural unit in plants and animals. Differentiated cells work together to perform specific functions. Cell regeneration occurs through cell division and reproduction. Abnormal changes in cells develop for many reasons. These abnormal cells reproduce in the same way as normal cells, but do not have regulatory mechanisms to control growth. Abnormal cell growth proliferates in an uncontrolled and unrestricted way.

New growths of abnormal tissue are called **neoplasms** or tumors. The first part of the tumor's name indicates the particular cell or tissue. The suffix *-oma* indicates it is a tumor. Four main tumor classifications according to tissue type are *carcinomas* (cancers originating from epithelial cells), *lymphomas* (cancers originating from organs that fight infection), *leukemias* (cancers originating from organs that form blood), and *sarcomas* (cancers originating from connective tissue, such as bone or muscle). Tumors also are classified according to cell of origin and whether growth is **benign,** not invasive or spreading, or **malignant,** invasive and capable of spreading (Table 19.1).

Benign tumors remain at their site of development. They may grow large, but their growth rate is slower than that of malignant tumors. They do not usually cause death unless their location impairs the function of a vital organ, such as the brain. Malignant tumors grow rapidly and are likely to cause **metastasis** (spreading), unless removed. Cancer metastasizes by direct extension to adjacent tissues, from lymph vessels into tissues adjacent to lymphatic vessels, by transport from blood or lymph systems, or by diffusion within a body cavity. The *primary*

TABLE 19.1 CLASSIFICATION OF TUMOR CELLS

ORIGIN	MALIGNANT	BENIGN
Skin	Basal cell carcinoma	
	Squamous cell carcinoma	Papilloma
	Malignant melanoma	Nevus (mole)
Epithelium	Adenocarcinoma	Adenoma
Muscle	Myosarcoma	Myoma
Connective tissue		
Fibrous tissue	Fibrosarcoma	Fibroma
Adipose (fatty) tissue	Liposarcoma	Lipoma
Cartilage	Chondrosarcoma	Chondroma
Bone	Osteosarcoma	Osteoma
Nerve tissue	Neurogenic sarcoma	Neuroma
	Neuroblastoma	Ganglioneuroma
	Glioblastoma	Glioma
Bone marrow	Multiple myeloma	
	Leukemia	

site is the area where malignant cells first form. The *secondary* or metastatic sites are regions to which cancer cells have spread. Metastasis is a discouraging characteristic of cancer because even one malignant cell can give rise to a metastatic lesion in a distant part of the body. Metastatic tumors are treated aggressively when possible to improve quality of life and lengthen survival time. Cancer is known to spread to lymph nodes that drain the tumor area. When a malignant tumor is removed, generally lymph node dissection is also done, along with a wide excision of the tumor.

Etiology

Cancer is the second leading cause of death in the United States, where half of all men and one-third of all women will develop cancer during their lives (American Cancer Society, 2001). Lung cancers are the most deadly for both men and women. Common cancers in men include prostate, lung, and colon. Breast, lung, and colon cancer most commonly affect women.

Damage to cellular DNA causes cancer cells to develop. Inherited cancers occur when damaged DNA passes to the next generation. Certain factors and agents also contribute to the development of cancer. These factors are called **carcinogens** and include chemical agents, environmental factors, dietary substances, viruses, defective genes, and medically prescribed interventions.

Assessment

Signs and Symptoms

Cancer is slow growing. At first there may be no or vague symptoms or signs. It is important to educate clients about prevention and self-examination so that cancer can be diagnosed as early as possible. Seven warning signals of cancer include:

1. A change in bowel habits or bladder function
2. Sores that do not heal
3. Unusual bleeding or discharge
4. Thickening or lump in breast or other body parts
5. Indigestion or difficulty swallowing
6. A recent change in a wart or mole
7. A nagging cough or hoarseness

Better education has improved awareness of warning signals and factors that may influence cancer development. Public education focuses on periodic physical examinations and cancer screening programs. Box 19-1 lists healthy habits that reduce cancer risk.

Diagnostic Findings

A client's history, physical examination, and diagnostic studies contribute to the diagnosis of cancer. The physical examination may be unremarkable, but the client's history is suspicious. The client also is evaluated for risk factors. Many diagnostic studies are used to establish a diagnosis of cancer.

LABORATORY TESTS. Specific cancers alter the chemical composition of blood and other body fluids. There are specialized tests for *tumor markers,* specific proteins, antigens, hormones, genes, or enzymes that cancer cells release. Tumor markers are not normally present in or not found in large quantities in the blood. Examples of

BOX 19-1 ● Healthy Lifestyle Habits That Reduce the Risk of Cancer

- Learn and regularly practice self-examination techniques.
- See physician or nurse practitioner regularly.
- Include periodic colon examinations, mammograms, Pap smears, testicular examinations, and prostate-specific antigen testing as indicated.
- Eat a healthy diet.
- Abstain from smoking or using tobacco products.
- Avoid overexposure to the sun; use sunscreen with SPF of 15 or greater.
- Maintain weight within suggested limits.
- Exercise regularly.
- Practice safety in the workplace to avoid exposure to chemicals and radiation.
- Limit alcohol intake.

tumor markers include alpha-fetoprotein, carcioembryonic antigen, and prostate-specific antigen.

Other laboratory tests may be useful in establishing a diagnosis. Although abnormal values do not directly indicate a malignant process, they provide a total clinical picture. For example, a complete blood count (CBC) may indicate anemia in a client with possible colon cancer. Occult blood in the stool may indicate colorectal cancer.

RADIOLOGIC AND IMAGING TESTS. Several radiologic and imaging tests are used to diagnose cancer. X-ray studies with plain films or contrast media and specialized equipment detect tumors in specific organs. Computed tomography (CT) scan provides three-dimensional cross-sectional views of tissues to determine tumor density, size, and location. Magnetic resonance imaging (MRI) uses magnetic fields for sectional images and helps visualize tumors hidden by bones. Positron emission tomography (PET) scan uses computed cross-sectional images with increased concentration of radioisotopes in malignant cells. It provides information about the biologic activity of the cells and assists in differentiating benign and malignant processes and responses to treatment. Ultrasound uses high frequency sound waves to detect abnormalities of a body organ or structure.

OTHER STUDIES. Biopsy means the excision of tissue samples from the body for direct microscopic examination for malignant or premalignant processes. In a frozen section study, a tumor or node is removed during surgery and taken to the pathologist for immediate examination. The specimen is quickly frozen and then sliced into very thin pieces to be examined under a microscope. With endoscopy, fiberoptic instruments enable light to travel straight or at various angles and illuminate the area being examined. Through cytology, microscopic examination of cells from various body areas is used to diagnose malignant or premalignant disorders.

Staging of Tumors

Before a client is treated for cancer, tumors are staged and graded based on how they grow and the cell type. The American Joint Commission on Cancer developed a grading system referred to as the TNM classification: *T* indicates size of the tumor, *N* stands for involvement of regional lymph nodes, and *M* refers to presence of metastasis (Table 19.2). Once the TNM descriptions are established, they are grouped together in a simpler set of stages that include tumor size, evidence of metastasis, and lymph node involvement.

- *Stage I:* Malignant cells are confined to the tissue of origin, with no signs of metastasis.
- *Stage II:* Spread of cancer is limited to the local area, generally to area lymph nodes.

TABLE 19.2 TNM STAGING SYSTEM AND CLASSIFICATION

SYMBOL	MEANING
T	Tumor
TX	Primary tumor cannot be assessed
T0	No evidence of primary tumor
T1s	Carcinoma in situ
T1, T2, T3, T4	Progressive increase in tumor size and extension
N	Regional lymph nodes
NX	Regional lymph nodes cannot be assessed clinically
N0	No regional lymph node involvement
N1, N2, N3	Increase in regional lymph node involvement
M	Distant metastasis
MX	Cannot be assessed
M0	No distant metastasis
M1	Distant metastasis present
Example: T2, N1, M0	Indicates the primary tumor has grown and spread to regional lymph nodes but is not metastasized
G1	Well-differentiated grade
G2	Moderately well-differentiated grade
G3, G4	Poorly to very poorly differentiated grade

- *Stage III:* Tumor is larger, probably has invaded surrounding tissues, or both.
- *Stage IV:* Cancer has invaded or metastasized to other parts of the body.

Grading of tumors involves differentiation of the malignant cells. Basically there are two classifications: differentiated and undifferentiated. Cancer cells are evaluated in comparison to normal cells. *Well-differentiated* cells are those that most closely resemble the tissue of origin. *Undifferentiated cells* bear little resemblance to the tissue of origin. Cell differentiation is graded from I to IV. The higher the number, the less differentiated is the cell type. Tumors with poorly differentiated cells are graded IV. These tumors are very aggressive and unpredictable, and prognosis is usually poor.

Medical and Surgical Management

Surgery

Surgery ranges from tumor excision alone to extensive excision, including removal of the tumor and adjacent structures such as bone, muscle, and lymph nodes. The type and extent of surgery depends on the extent of disease, actual pathology, client's age and physical condition, and anticipated results. When tumors are confined and have not invaded vital organs, surgery is more likely to be curative and is referred to as the *primary treatment.* In some cases, the entire tumor cannot be removed but as much of it as possible is removed, referred to as *debulking.* Two types of excisions are done. The first is *local excision,* in which the tumor is removed along with a small margin of healthy tissue. The other type is *wide* or *radical excision,* which removes the primary tumor, lymph nodes, any involved adjacent structures, and surrounding tissues that pose a risk for metastasis.

Salvage surgery is done when there is a local recurrence of cancer. It is generally more extensive. For example, a cancerous tumor may be removed from the breast (lumpectomy). If a tumor reappears, a mastectomy will most likely be done.

Prophylactic surgery may be done if the client is at considerable risk for cancer. According to Smeltzer and Bare (2004), prophylactic surgery may be done when there is a family history or genetic predisposition, ability to detect cancer at an early stage, and client's acceptance of the postoperative outcome. Examples of prophylactic surgery include mastectomy and hysterectomy. Clients need careful preoperative counseling and teaching to be fully aware of the consequences following surgery.

Surgery for relief of uncomfortable symptoms or prolonging life is considered *palliative.* Examples include removal of excess fluid to increase comfort, such as *paracentesis* (removal of fluid from the abdominal cavity) and *thoracentesis* (removal of fluid from the chest). Surgical procedures that relieve pain include nerve blocks, placement of epidural catheters for administration of epidural analgesics, and placement of venous access devices for administration of parenteral analgesics.

Reconstructive or *plastic surgery* may be done after extensive surgery to correct defects. Some surgeries are disfiguring or so profound that clients have difficulty adjusting to body changes. In these cases, radiation therapy may be a better option.

Radiation Therapy

Radiation therapy uses high-energy ionizing radiation, such as high-energy x-rays, gamma rays, and radioactive particles (alpha and beta particles, neutrons, and protons) to destroy cancer cells. Cells are destroyed from disrupted cell function and division and alteration of DNA molecules. Cell death can occur immediately or when the cell can no longer reproduce.

The goal of radiation therapy is to destroy malignant, rapidly dividing cells without permanently damaging surrounding healthy tissues. Radiation therapy may destroy both normal and malignant cells, but the more rapidly reproducing malignant cells are more sensitive to radiation because it affects cells undergoing mitosis (cancer cells) more than cells in slower growth cycles (normal cells). Radiation therapy may be applied externally or internally, both with curative and palliative intent. Nearly 60% of all clients with cancer will receive some form of radiation; about 60% of those clients will be cured (Washington & Leaver, 1997).

EXTERNAL RADIATION THERAPY. External radiation therapy or external beam radiation uses high-energy x-rays aimed at a specific body location. A treatment plan, using beams from multiple directions, is developed and customized for each client. Linear accelerators are machines that deliver external beam radiation.

External radiation therapy enables treatment of large body areas, targeting the tumor and nearby lymph nodes. Clients usually have daily radiation treatments over several weeks as outpatients. Their skin is marked with a marker or tattoo to identify reference points for the treatment plan. Clients are instructed not to wash off these markings until therapy is complete. Clients are not radioactive when receiving external beam radiation therapy.

INTERNAL RADIATION THERAPY. Internal radiation therapy (**brachytherapy**) refers to short-distance therapy. It involves direct application of a radioactive source on or within a tumor and delivers a high dose of radiation to a small area. Common methods include interstitial implants, intracavitary implants, and systemic therapy. It delivers a high dose of radiation to a specific tumor, applying less radiation to adjacent normal tissues. Brachytherapy is used alone or combined with surgery, chemotherapy, and external radiation therapy.

Sealed brachytherapy sources include interstitial and intracavitary implants. Needles, seeds, wires, or catheters contain the radioactive source and are implanted directly into the tumor. For intracavitary implants, the radioactive source is placed directly in the body cavity and an applicator holds it in place. When the implants are removed, no radioactivity is left in the body. In some cases seeds are left in permanently, such as with prostate or brain cancer (Nevidjon & Sowers, 2000). The radioactivity of the seeds decays over several weeks or months, depending on the radioactive element's half-life. Clients generally go home if they have permanent implants. Clients must stay away from other people for a few days while the radiation is most active. They must restrict close contact with children or pregnant women to 5 minutes and no closer than 6 feet for 2 months after the implant.

Clients must be hospitalized when receiving sealed brachytherapy because they will emit radiation during therapy. Specific orders for treatment and precautions to be taken, as well as the type and dosage of the radioactive substance, time and area of insertion, type of applicator used, and when to remove the material are noted in the client's chart. Box 19-2 lists safety measures when a client is receiving radiation therapy. Everyone involved

BOX 19-2 ● Safety Measures for Protecting Healthcare Personnel and Visitors From Excessive Exposure to Radiation

Client is placed in private room; some rooms have walls that are lined with lead.
Standardized sign is placed on door to designate the room as a radiation room.
Anyone entering the room must have knowledge of the precautions required. Children younger than age 18 and pregnant women are never permitted in the room.
Healthcare personnel limit time spent in the room and limit distance from source of radiation by working as far from the source of radiation as possible.
The physician and radiation safety personnel are notified if the sealed sources become dislodged.
When the client has unsealed sources, gloves must be worn at all times. Policies regarding disposal of body fluids and contaminated articles such as dressings must be adhered to.

in the client's care must recognize the necessity for limitations to radiation exposure.

Unsealed radiation sources (radiation in a suspension or solution or radiopharmaceutical therapy), such as iodine 131, may be administered orally, intravenously, or into a body cavity. Various body parts take up these sources in doses sufficient to treat cancer or, if received in small amounts, to diagnose cancer. This type of radiation has systemic effects and is excreted primarily in urine, but also through saliva, sweat, and feces. To reduce exposure, clients are asked to:

- Wash hands carefully after going to the bathroom.
- Flush toilet several times after each use.
- Use separate eating utensils and towels.
- Wash laundry separately.
- Drink plenty of fluids to help flush radioactive substances away.
- Avoid kissing and sexual contact.

Nursing Guidelines 19-1 provide standard interventions for clients receiving radiation therapy. When providing information, clients need to know the type and duration of treatment, what is required of the client, possible side effects, skin and mouth care, nutritional and dietary concerns, and precautions needed.

Expected side effects may result from destruction of normal cells in the area being irradiated and are specific to the anatomic site treated. They include the following:

- **Alopecia** (hair loss)
- Erythema (local redness and inflammation of the skin)
- Desquamation (shedding of epidermis, which can be dry or moist)
- Alterations in oral mucosa, including **stomatitis** (inflammation of the mouth), xerostomia (dryness of the mouth), change or loss in taste, and decreased salivation
- Anorexia (loss of appetite)
- Nausea and vomiting
- Diarrhea
- Cystitis (inflammation of the bladder)
- Pneumonitis (inflammation of the lungs)
- Fatigue
- **Myelosuppression** (depression of bone marrow function) if marrow-producing sites are irradiated,

NURSING GUIDELINES 19-1

Managing Clients Receiving Radiation Therapy

- Provide information regarding the safety of radiation: effects on others, effects on tumor, and side effects related to radiation.
- Teach client about the actual procedure of external or internal radiation therapy.
- Explain the need for optimal nutritional intake.
- Protect the skin from irritation.
- Assess skin and mucous membranes for changes, particularly the areas being treated.
- Advise client that effects of radiation on skin include redness, tanning, peeling, itching, hair loss, and decreased perspiration.
- Cleanse with mild soap (be careful not to wash radiation marks) and tepid water. Advise the client to shave with electric razors.
- Moisturize with mild, water-based lubricant lotions.
- Advise client to wear loose cotton clothing and to protect skin from sun exposure, chlorine, and wind. He or she must avoid heat lamps and heating pads and report any blistering (use prescribed creams or ointments).
- Maintain intact oral mucous membranes.
- Teach client to:
  - Report oral burning, pain, open lesions, or problems with swallowing; use nonalcoholic mouthwash.
  - Brush with soft toothbrush and avoid electric toothbrushes.
  - Floss gently; use WaterPik cautiously.
  - Keep lips moist with lip balm.
  - Avoid alcoholic beverages, very hot drinks and foods, highly seasoned foods, acidic foods, and tobacco products.
  - Assess lesions—culture as necessary.
- Monitor client for signs of bone marrow suppression: decreased leukocyte, erythrocyte, and platelet counts.
- Assess for signs of bleeding; assess lesions and culture as necessary.
- Monitor for signs and symptoms related to area of irradiation: cerebral edema, malabsorption, pleural effusion, pneumonitis, esophagitis, cystitis, and urethritis.
- Encourage client to share fears and anxieties related to radiation therapy.
- Inform client that fatigue is a common effect of radiation therapy.

resulting in anemia (decreased red blood cells, hemoglobin, or volume of packed red blood cells), **leukopenia** (decreased white blood cell count), and **thrombocytopenia** (decreased platelet count)

Effects of radiation are cumulative. Often clients experience chronic or long-term side effects after completing therapy. These effects result from decreased blood supply and normal tissue destruction. Changes are irreversible. Possible effects include fibrosis (abnormal formation of scar tissue) in the small intestine, lungs, and bladder; cataracts; disturbances in blood cell formation; sterility; and new cancers.

When radioisotopes are used to treat cancer, three safety principles must always be kept in mind: time, distance, and shielding (where applicable).

Time. *Time* refers to the length of exposure. The less time spent in the vicinity of a radioactive substance, the less radiation is received. Healthcare personnel must plan carefully and work quickly and efficiently to spend minimal time at the bedside. Careful psychological preparation helps the client accept the limited amount of nursing time.

Distance. *Distance* refers to length in feet between the person entering the room and the radioactive source (client). The inverse square law applies to radiation exposure. Rate of exposure varies inversely to the square of the distance from the source (client). For example, nurses standing 4 feet from the source of radiation receive 25% of the radiation they would receive if they stood 2 feet from the source.

Shielding. *Shielding* is the use of any type of material to decrease radiation that reaches an area. The material usually used is lead, such as lead-lined gloves and lead aprons. Other materials, such as concrete walls, are capable of shielding. See Client and Family Teaching 19-1.

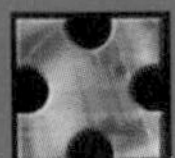

19-1 *Client and Family Teaching* Radiation Therapy

The nurse instructs clients who receive radiation therapy on an outpatient basis as follows:

- Avoid using ointments or creams on the area receiving radiation therapy unless prescribed or instructed to by a physician or radiation therapist.
- Avoid extremes of heat or cold, including heating pads, ultraviolet light, diathermy, whirlpool, sauna, steam baths, or direct sunlight.
- If receiving radiation to the head or scalp, avoid shampooing with harsh shampoos (baby or mild shampoo is acceptable), tinting, permanent waving, hair dryers, curling irons, and any hair products or treatments unless approved by the physician or radiation therapist.
- Bathe carefully. Avoid using soap and friction over the irradiated area. Do *not* wash off skin markings because they serve as guides for setting and adjusting the treatment machine over the area to be radiated.
- Wear loose clothing to avoid irritating the irradiated areas.

Chemotherapy

Chemotherapy uses **antineoplastic** agents to treat cancer cells locally and systemically. These agents may be used alone or combined with other therapies to cure cancer, prevent it from metastasizing, slow its growth, destroy tumor cells that have metastasized, or relieve symptoms. Antineoplastic agents work by interfering with cellular function and reproduction. They are classified according to their relationship to cell division and reproduction.

CELL CYCLE-SPECIFIC DRUGS. Antineoplastic drugs are most effective during cell division. Cell cycle-specific drugs are used to treat rapidly growing tumors because they attack cancer cells when they enter a specific phase of cell reproduction. Chemotherapy is administered in multiple repeated doses to produce a greater cell kill and to halt the growth of tumor cells. Examples of cell cycle-specific agents are topoisomerase I inhibitors, antimetabolites, mitotic spindle poisons, and miscellaneous agents (Drug Therapy Table 19-1).

CELL CYCLE-NONSPECIFIC DRUGS. Cell cycle-nonspecific drugs are effective during any phase of the cell cycle, whether reproducing or resting. They are used for large, slow-growing tumors. The amount of drug given is more important than the frequency. Cell cycle-nonspecific drugs have more prolonged effects on cells, which result in cell damage and destruction. They are often given in combination with cell cycle-specific drugs and may also be combined with or follow radiation therapy. Examples of cell cycle-nonspecific agents are alkylating agents, antitumor antibiotics, nitrosureas, hormones, and miscellaneous agents (see Drug Therapy Table 19-1).

ROUTES AND DEVICES FOR ADMINISTRATION OF CHEMOTHERAPY. Chemotherapeutic drugs are administered by several routes. The most common are the oral and intravenous (IV) routes, but they also may be given intramuscularly, intraperitoneally, intra-arterially, intrapleurally, topically, intrathecally, or directly into a cavity. IV administration is monitored closely to prevent the drug from leaking into surrounding tissues, referred to as **extravasation.** Most agents can be very irritating. Blistering and tissue necrosis are possible effects of extravasation. If a client complains of burning or pain

DRUG THERAPY TABLE 19.1 ANTINEOPLASTIC AGENTS

DRUG CATEGORY AND EXAMPLES	MECHANISM OF ACTION	CELL CYCLE SPECIFICITY	SIDE EFFECTS
Alkylating Agents			
busulfan, carboplatin, chlorambucil, cisplatin, cyclophosphamide, dacarbazine, hexamethyl ifosfamide, melamine, melphalan, nitrogen mustard, thiotepa	Alters DNA structure by misreading DNA code, initiating breaks in the DNA molecule, cross-linking DNA strands	Cell cycle–nonspecific	Bone marrow suppression, nausea, vomiting, cystitis (cyclophosphamide, ifosfamide), stomatitis, alopecia, gonadal suppression, renal toxicity (cisplatin)
Nitrosoureas			
carmustine (BCNU), lomustine (CCNU), semustine (methyl CCNU), streptozocin	Similar to the alkylating agents; cross the blood–brain barrier	Cell cycle–nonspecific	Delayed and cumulative myelosuppression, especially thrombocytopenia; nausea, vomiting
Topoisomerase I Inhibitors			
irinotecan, topotecan	Induces breaks in the DNA strand by binding to enzyme topoisomerase I, preventing cells from dividing	Cell cycle–specific	Bone marrow suppression, diarrhea, nausea, vomiting, hepatotoxicity
Antimetabolites			
5-azacytadine, cytarabine, edatrexate fludarabine, 5-fluorouracil (5-FU), FUDR, gemcitabine, hydroxyurea, leustatin, 6-mercaptopurine, methotrexate, pentostatin, 6-thioguanine	Interferes with the biosynthesis of metabolites or nucleic acids necessary for RNA and DNA synthesis	Cell cycle–specific (S phase)	Nausea, vomiting, diarrhea, bone marrow suppression, proctitis, stomatitis, renal toxicity (methotrexate), hepatotoxicity
Antitumor Antibiotics			
bleomycin, dactinomycin, daunorubicin, doxorubicin (Adriamycin), idarubicin, mitomycin, mitoxantrone, plicamycin	Interferes with DNA synthesis by binding DNA; prevent RNA synthesis	Cell cycle–nonspecific	Bone marrow suppression, nausea, vomiting, alopecia, anorexia, cardiac toxicity (daunorubicin, doxorubicin)
Mitotic Spindle Poisons			
Plant alkaloids: etoposide, teniposide, vinblastine, vincristine (VCR), vindesine, vinorelbine	Arrests metaphase by inhibiting mitotic tubular formation (spindle); inhibit DNA and protein synthesis	Cell cycle–specific (M phase)	Bone marrow suppression (mild with VCR), neuropathies (VCR), stomatitis
Taxanes: paclitaxel, docetaxel	Arrests metaphase by inhibiting tubulin depolymerization	Cell cycle–specific (M phase)	Bradycardia, hypersensitivity reactions, bone marrow suppression, alopecia, neuropathies
Hormonal Agents			
androgens and antiandrogens, estrogens and antiestrogens, progestins and anti-progestins, aromatase inhibitors, luteinizing hormone–releasing hormone analogs, steroids	Binds to hormone receptor sites that alter cellular growth; block binding of estrogens to receptor sites (antiestrogens); inhibit RNA synthesis; suppress aromatase of P450 system, which decreases estrogen level	Cell cycle–nonspecific	Hypercalcemia, jaundice, increased appetite, masculinization, feminization, sodium and fluid retention, nausea, vomiting, hot flashes, vaginal dryness
Miscellaneous Agents			
asparaginase, procarbazine	Unknown or too complex to categorize	Varies	Anorexia, nausea, vomiting, bone marrow suppression, hepatotoxicity, anaphylaxis, hypotension, altered glucose metabolism

during the chemotherapy infusion, the drug must be discontinued. **Vesicants** are particularly damaging antineoplastics, in that they cause tissue necrosis affecting underlying tendons, nerves, and blood vessels. Sloughing and ulceration of the skin may be so severe that the client will need skin grafts. If vesicants are being administered, there are protocols for treating the extravasation. General measures include stopping administration of the drug, leaving the needle in place, gently aspirating the residual drug and blood into the tubing or needle, and injecting a neutralizing solution.

Various vascular devices are used to administer chemotherapy and are particularly beneficial for long-term chemotherapy. Clients do not have to endure repeated venipunctures. Venous access devices are special catheters inserted into a peripheral or central vein so that the catheter tip is located in the superior vena cava or right atrium. Examples include peripheral indwelling catheters (PIC lines), peripherally inserted central catheters (PICC lines), and external catheters (Hickman catheters, Broviac catheters). Another type is the implanted vascular access device (IVAC), also referred to as a port. A metal or plastic port encloses a self-sealing silicone rubber septum. The port is surgically implanted subcutaneously. A silicone catheter attached to the port is threaded subcutaneously to the right atrium. To access the port, a needle is inserted in the self-sealing septum of the port.

Chemotherapy infusion pumps are used for some cancers. They provide constant infusion of an antineoplastic drug directly into the cancerous organ. A small pump (similar in size to a hockey puck) is surgically implanted subcutaneously in the abdomen or applied externally.

ADVERSE EFFECTS OF CHEMOTHERAPY. Nursing management of the client receiving chemotherapy varies depending on the drug, dose administered, and route used (Nursing Guidelines 19-2). Some clients experience little discomfort or few adverse effects. Others have a wide range of symptoms. Tissues most susceptible to chemotherapy are those with rapidly growing cells, such as epithelial tissue, hair follicles, and bone marrow. Chemotherapy can potentially harm all body systems. Common adverse effects associated with chemotherapy are as follows:

- Nausea and vomiting during the first 24 hours following chemotherapy administration; use of concurrent antiemetics helps to reduce incidence and severity.
- Stomatitis and mouth soreness or ulceration
- Alopecia
- Myelosuppression results from inhibition of the manufacture of red and white blood cells and platelets. Severe anemia, bleeding tendencies, leukopenia, **neutropenia** (decreased neutrophils), and thrombocytopenia are possible if bone marrow depression is profound. Blood transfusions may be necessary, as well as protection of the client from infections.
- Fatigue related to the above effects, chemotherapy, and increased metabolic rate that accompanies cell destruction.

See Client and Family Teaching 19-2.

NURSING GUIDELINES 19-2

Managing Clients Receiving Chemotherapy

- Monitor client for symptoms of anaphylactic reaction: urticaria (hives), pruritus (itching), sensation of lump in throat, shortness of breath, wheezing.
- Assess for electrolyte imbalances.
- Teach client and family to report excessive fluid loss or gain, change in level of consciousness, increased weakness or ataxia (lack of muscle coordination), paresthesia (numbness, prickling, or tingling), seizures, persistent headache, muscle cramps or twitching, nausea and vomiting, or diarrhea.
- Prevent extravasation of vesicant drugs. Implement measures to treat extravasation of vesicant medications if it occurs.
- Teach client to increase fluid intake to 2500 to 3000 mL/day unless contraindicated.
- Assess for signs of bone marrow depression: decreased white and red blood cell, granulocyte, and platelet counts.
- Assess for signs of bleeding and infection.
- Monitor for signs of renal insufficiency:
  - Elevated urine specific gravity
  - Abnormal electrolyte values
  - Insufficient urine output (<30 mL/hour)
  - Elevated blood pressure, BUN (blood urea nitrogen), and serum creatinine
- Inform client about the reasons for nausea and vomiting.
- Administer antiemetics before and during administration of chemotherapy, or as indicated.
- Encourage the following dietary modifications:
  - Eat small, frequent meals.
  - Eat slowly.
  - Eat cool, bland foods and liquids.
  - Suck on hard candy during chemotherapy if taste alterations occur.
  - Avoid hot or very cold liquids, food with fat and fiber, spicy foods, and caffeine.
- Assess oral mucosa for dryness, redness, swelling, lesions, ulcerations, viscous (sticky) saliva, or white patches.

Stop, Think, and Respond ● BOX 19-1

You are assigned to a client recently diagnosed with lung cancer. Surgery is planned, followed by chemotherapy. Your client says that he has heard that large doses of vitamin C would contribute to postoperative healing and enhance chemotherapy. He asks if he should begin megadoses of vitamin C. How should you respond?

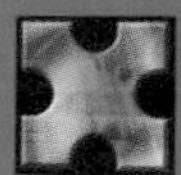

19-2 *Client and Family Teaching* Chemotherapy

The nurse instructs clients receiving chemotherapy on an outpatient basis to:

- Keep all appointments for chemotherapy treatments.
- Follow recommendations of the physician or healthcare personnel regarding diet, oral fluids, and adverse effects to report.
- Purchase a wig, cap, or scarf before therapy begins, if hair loss is anticipated. Hair usually begins to grow again within 4 to 6 months after therapy; new growth may have a slightly different color and texture.
- Have periodic evaluations and examinations as recommended.

Bone Marrow Transplantation

Cancers sensitive to high doses of chemotherapy and radiation therapy may be treated with bone marrow transplantation (BMT). Survival rate after BMT for malignant disease is about 50%. There are four possible sources for BMT: autologous, allogeneic, syngeneic, or stem cell transplant.

AUTOLOGOUS BONE MARROW TRANSPLANTATION. *Autologous BMT* involves harvesting the client's own bone marrow and storing it in a frozen state. The client then receives intensive chemotherapy (ablative chemotherapy) and radiation therapy to eliminate any remaining tumor. The client's own bone marrow is then reinfused. Harvested bone marrow may be treated with chemotherapy to kill malignant cells. Until bone marrow is established (referred to as **engraftment**), the client is at high risk for infections and bleeding. This type of BMT is done for clients who have cancer affecting the bone marrow but do not have a matched donor or for clients who have aggressive cancer that has not affected the bone marrow (Smeltzer & Bare, 2004). Clients having autologous BMT do not require immunosuppressant drugs. A risk persists that tumor cells remain in the bone marrow.

ALLOGENIC BONE MARROW TRANSPLANTATION. *Allogeneic BMT* is done for clients with cancer affecting the bone marrow. A compatible donor, one with the same leukocyte antigen as the client, donates bone marrow. The client receives ablative chemotherapy and often also has total body irradiation to destroy cancer cells and bone marrow. The client then receives the donor bone marrow. It takes 2 to 4 weeks for transplanted marrow to establish itself and begin producing blood cells. Clients receive immunosuppressant drugs, which may include cyclosporine and azathioprine (Imuran), to prevent rejection of the bone marrow, referred to as *graft-versus-host disease* (GVHD). GVHD occurs with allogenic BMT because the T lymphocytes in the donor's marrow view the recipient's tissues as "foreign," causing an immune reaction. The first 3 months following allogenic BMT are the most critical for the client in terms of rejection, infection, hemorrhage, nausea, vomiting, and fatigue.

SYNGENEIC BONE MARROW TRANSPLANTATION. *Syngeneic BMT* is possible only if the client has an identical twin. The process is the same as for allogeneic BMT. Because the donor is an identical tissue match, however, the recipient needs fewer immunosuppressant drugs, as there is no issue with bone marrow rejection.

STEM CELL TRANSPLANT. The most recent innovation in BMTs is peripheral *stem cell transplant.* Clients having this type of BMT receive chemotherapy and hematopoietic growth factors that stimulate production of hematopoietic stem cells. The stem cells are collected by **apheresis** (process of separating blood into components) for later reinfusion. Stem cells are essentially bone marrow because of their role in engraftment and repopulation of hematopoietic tissue (Smeltzer & Bare, 2004). Following collection of stem cells, clients have ablative chemotherapy and possibly radiation therapy. Stem cells are then reinfused. Recovery tends to be faster than with other BMTs.

NURSING MANAGEMENT. Nursing management for the client receiving any form of BMT is crucial. Before the procedure, the nurse evaluates the client's physical condition, organ function, nutritional status, complete blood studies (including assessment for past antigen exposure such as HIV, hepatitis, or cytomegalovirus), and psychosocial status.

When clients are ready to receive a BMT, they undergo intensive chemotherapy and possibly whole body radiation. Because a large amount of tissue is treated, nausea, vomiting, diarrhea, and stomatitis are common. Until transplanted bone marrow begins to produce blood cells, clients have no physiologic means to fight infection, making them very prone to infection. They are at high risk for dying from sepsis and bleeding before engraftment. Nurses *must* monitor clients closely and take measures to prevent infection. Clients are also at risk for bleeding, renal complications, and liver damage.

Following a BMT, the client is closely monitored for at least 3 months because of possible complications related to the transplant. Infections are common, as is GVHD. The client's immune system is deficient because of the chemotherapy and radiation therapy. Throughout the entire BMT, the nurse assesses the client's psychological status. Clients experience many mood swings and need support and assistance throughout this process.

Their families and significant others also require support. See Nursing Guidelines 19-3.

Immunotherapy

Immunotherapy uses biologic response modifiers (BRMs) to stimulate the body's natural immune system to restrict and destroy cancer cells. Many of these treatments are new and in trial phases. Research demonstrates that the body's natural immunity, a process of surveillance, recognition, and attack of foreign cells, is a defense against cancer (see Chap. 35). Use of BRMs attempts to manipulate the natural immune response by restoring, modifying, stimulating, or augmenting natural defenses (Smeltzer & Bare, 2004).

Results of immunotherapy vary. Some clients respond well; others have little or no response. Generally, immunotherapy is not instituted until surgery, radiation therapy, and chemotherapy have failed. The three categories of immunotherapy are nonspecific, monoclonal antibody, and cytokines.

Hyperthermia

Hyperthermia or thermal therapy uses temperatures greater than 41.5°C (106.7°F) to destroy tumor cells. Heat is in the form of radiowaves, ultrasound, microwaves, magnetic waves, hot water baths, or immersion in hot wax. Methods of delivery include extracorporeal circulators, probes, or infusion of heated chemotherapeutic agents into the blood or directly into a cancerous organ. A client may also be immersed in heated water or paraffin. Tumor cells are more sensitive to the harmful effects of high temperatures.

> **NURSING GUIDELINES 19-3**
>
> ***Managing Clients Receiving a Bone Marrow Transplant***
>
> - Assess client's nutritional status.
> - Monitor for signs and symptoms of infection and renal insufficiency (see Nursing Guidelines 19-2).
> - Assess for signs and symptoms of graft-versus-host disease (GVHD): irritability, pulmonary infiltration, hepatitis, enlarged spleen, enlarged lymph nodes, anemia, sepsis, diarrhea, maculopapular rash, and skin desquamation.
> - Implement Standard Precautions and use protective isolation as needed.
> - Assist with thorough hygiene.
> - Review information related to prevention of infection, signs of rejection, importance of adherence to medical regimens and follow-up, medication instructions, and dietary needs.
> - Encourage client to discuss anxieties and fears.
> - Provide ongoing information about recovery phase and status of recuperation.

Hyperthermia is combined with other therapies. When used with radiation therapy, tumor cells are more sensitive to radiation and cannot repair themselves at all. Hyperthermia alters cell membrane permeability so that uptake of chemotherapy is increased. It enhances the function of immunotherapeutic agents. Clients receiving hyperthermia may experience local burns and tissue damage, electrolyte imbalances, fatigue, GI disturbances, and neuropathies.

Gene Therapy

Scientists theorize that many cancers result from gene alterations. Strategies to confront this problem include **gene therapy,** which involves replacing altered genes with correct genes, inhibiting defective genes, and introducing substances that destroy genes or cancer cells (Smeltzer & Bare, 2004). Scientists predict that gene therapy will play a significant role in the future prediction, diagnosis, and treatment of cancer. It is currently being investigated in the treatment of brain tumors, melanoma, and renal, breast, and colon cancers.

Clinical Trials

Clinical trials provide methods to test new treatments for specific cancers. Trials may involve a new drug, a new combination of existing drugs, or new therapies. The process for new treatments to become accepted practice is lengthy. Before testing on humans, testing is done on laboratory animals. Following animal testing, there are four phases:

1. Phase I—Treatment is given to a small group of people to determine dosing, schedule for treatment, and toxicity. Participants are generally clients for whom standard treatment has been ineffective. Clients are fully aware of the trial's experimental nature.
2. Phase II—Treatment is given to a larger group of clients to further determine effectiveness with specific cancers and to get better information about dosing, side effects, and toxicity. Clients are similar to clients selected for Phase I.
3. Phase III—If treatment appears effective in Phase II, then a larger number of clients are selected and compared with clients receiving accepted treatments for a particular type of cancer. At this point, the new treatment has had significant testing and review.
4. Phase IV—In this phase there is further testing of newly accepted treatments for other uses, dosing, and toxicity.

Complementary and Alternative Therapy

Complementary and alternative therapy includes imagery, medicinal therapy, special diets, and mystical and spiritual approaches. Alternative therapy refers to treatments not proven to be effective in treating a particular disease, but used instead of conventional treatments. Examples include hydrogen peroxide therapy, hydrazine sulfate, and essiac tea (American Cancer Society, 2001). Table 19.3 briefly describes some methods used to treat cancer. It is difficult for healthcare professionals to condone unconventional therapies because many methods do not have a scientific foundation. There are legal and ethical implications if healthcare personnel participate in unaccepted treatments. Information provided to clients must be factual and understandable. Although some alternative methods have successfully augmented conventional treatments, many methods have no positive effects, and some are actually harmful.

Nursing Management

Managing the care of clients with cancer is challenging. The diagnosis itself implies multiple problems, and the treatments result in many secondary problems. This care requires a comprehensive plan designed to meet or assist the client and family's needs. In addition to the discussion below, see Nursing Care Plan 19-1.

Pain is a major problem for clients with cancer. Sources of pain include bone metastasis; nerve compression; obstructed blood vessels, lymph systems, or organs; inflammation; ulceration; infection; or necrosis. Pain ranges from dull aching to sharp unrelenting throbbing.

Clients with cancer also experience fatigue, a frequent side effect of cancer treatments that rest fails to relieve. Fatigued clients are constantly weary, lack energy, and often feel too weak to carry out normal activities. The nurse must assess clients for other stressors that contribute to fatigue, such as pain, nausea, fear, and lack of adequate support. The nurse works with other healthcare team members to treat the client's fatigue.

Another major problem for clients with cancer is infection. Many factors predispose clients with cancer to infection: impaired skin and mucous membranes, chemotherapy, radiation therapy and other therapies, the malignancy itself, malnutrition, medications, invasive catheters and IV lines, contaminated equipment, age, chronic illness, and prolonged hospitalization (Smeltzer & Bare, 2004). Nurses must provide scrupulous care to clients with cancer and monitor for signs and symptoms of infection, including fever, elevated WBC counts, pain, redness, swelling, and drainage.

Psychological Support

The diagnosis of cancer is frightening and overwhelming. Psychological support is as important as medical treatments and physical care. Clients have many reactions ranging from anxiety, fear, and depression to feelings of guilt related to viewing cancer as a punishment for past actions or failure to practice a healthy lifestyle. They may express anger related to the diagnosis and their inability to be in control. Clients have the right to know their diagnosis, treatment plan, and prognosis so they can make informed decisions. A client may never accept a cancer diagnosis. When provided with adequate information and supported psychologically, clients are more likely to face their diagnosis and be involved with their care and treatment. Families and significant others also require support.

Client and Family Teaching

Clients and their families or significant others require education to understand diagnostic procedures, make treatment choices, participate in preventing complications, and recognize side effects and other adverse signs. Teaching focuses on medications, treatments, procedures, adverse effects associated with treatment, possible changes in body image or function, resources for support, and follow-up needed after discharge from the hospital.

TABLE 19.3 ALTERNATIVE METHODS OF CANCER TREATMENT

METHOD	DESCRIPTION
Imagery, relaxation techniques, stress reduction exercises, yoga, biofeedback, massage, and music therapy	These methods are used to reduce pain, promote relaxation, and enhance conventional treatment methods based on beliefs that there is a link between the immune system and cancer and that these methods boost the immune system's ability to fight the cancer cells.
Medicinal agents	Many "cures" for cancer have been concocted from plants, herbs, flowers, and fluids of humans and animals. Although a few merit scientific investigation, many are considered quackery. The use of vitamins, minerals, proteins, and other ingredients is advocated for treatment of many cancers and prevention of treatment side effects.
Special diets	Many diet regimens are advocated as treatment for certain cancers or as adjuncts to treatment. Examples include organic foods, macrobiotic diets, and particular foods that reportedly kill cancer cells.
Spiritual methods	These methods are derived from powers of faith that people believe will help them to overcome cancer. Examples include faith healing, laying on of hands, and prayer.

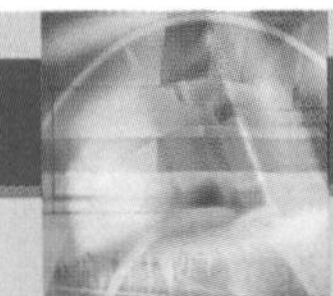

Nursing Care Plan 19-1

THE CLIENT WITH CANCER

Assessment

- Assess client's level of understanding about the diagnosis, treatment, and follow-up care.
- Determine the client's strengths, coping mechanisms, response to diagnosis, and emotional and physical support systems.
- Evaluate the family's response to illness.
- Check client's overall physical condition, energy and pain levels, and nutritional and fluid status.

Nursing Diagnosis: **Anxiety** related to diagnosis, prognosis, treatments, changes in health status

Expected Outcome: Client demonstrates decreased anxiety. Refer to Chapter 14 for nursing interventions.

Evaluation of Expected Outcome: Client and family share anxieties about diagnosis and care.

Nursing Diagnosis: **Fatigue** related to side effects of treatments, weakness from cancer, and physical and psychological stress

Expected Outcomes: (1) Client will participate in daily care as much as possible. (2) Client will identify measures to conserve and improve energy.

Interventions	*Rationales*
Identify energy level by asking client to evaluate it on a scale of 0 (not tired) to 10 (totally exhausted).	Establishes current level of fatigue.
Plan care around energy level and include rest periods.	Reduces physical stress and conserves energy.
Encourage adequate protein and calorie intake.	Increases activity tolerance.
Encourage use of relaxation techniques and mental imagery.	Promotes relaxation and reduces psychological stress.

Evaluation of Expected Outcomes:

- Client can participate in care without becoming exhausted.
- Client can identify need for rest.

Nursing Diagnosis: **Disturbed Body Image** related to side effects of treatments, weight loss, and changes in appearance

Expected Outcomes: Client will verbalize understanding of changes in appearance. Client will demonstrate coping methods and adaptation to changes he or she is experiencing.

Interventions	*Rationales*
Explore strengths and resources with client.	Promotes a positive self-image.
Discuss possible changes in weight and hair loss. Suggest that the client select a wig before hair loss occurs.	Decreases anxiety associated with a change in appearance.
Acknowledge client's anger, sadness, or depression.	Assists client to cope.
Refer client to a support group or counseling.	Allows client to share feelings and recognize that he or she is not alone.

Evaluation of Expected Outcomes: Client states acceptance of change or loss and demonstrates ability to adjust.

(continued)

Nursing Care Plan 19-1 (Continued)

THE CLIENT WITH CANCER

***Nursing Diagnosis: Imbalanced Nutrition:* Less than Body Requirements** related to loss of appetite, difficulty swallowing, side effects of chemotherapy, or obstruction by tumor

Expected Outcomes: Client will increase dietary intake. Client will demonstrate understanding of the need for adequate intake of nutrients and fluids.

Interventions	*Rationales*
Monitor daily food intake.	Provides baseline data.
Encourage intake of sufficient calories, nutrients, and fluids (see Nursing Guidelines 19-2), offering small frequent meals and fluids.	Reduces sensation of fullness and decreases stimulus to vomit.
Administer antiemetics as ordered prior to meals.	They are more effective when given before nausea.
Monitor laboratory studies for signs of dehydration, biochemical imbalances, and malnutrition.	Reveals evidence of imbalances and assists in making needed interventions.

Evaluation of Expected Outcomes: Client demonstrates minimal weight loss and verbalizes necessity to have adequate intake.

When developing a plan for client and family teaching, consider facts such as the type of malignancy, treatment given, proposed treatments, client's condition, and effectiveness of the family support system. These facts will determine the areas to discuss in more detail. Be aware of any explanations or information that other healthcare providers give to the client and family. Allow time for clients to express their feelings or discuss home care. Doing so also helps identify issues the client or family does not understand.

The Terminally Ill Client

Nursing management of terminally ill clients can be both physically and emotionally difficult. It must include both client and family. Nurses must carry out tasks gently to reduce the possibility of pain and discomfort and to keep the client as comfortable as possible. Pay attention to controlling pain, providing adequate fluid and nutrition, keeping the client warm and dry, and controlling odors (when present). An important part of nursing care is to help the client maintain dignity, despite an illness that often requires dependence on others for activities of daily living.

GENERAL GERONTOLOGIC CONSIDERATIONS

Older adults with cancer may have additional problems with nutrition, adequate fluid intake, skin care, and complications related to inactivity.

Older adults often have decreased resistance to infection, which may pose problems if they receive antineoplastic agents that have a depressant effect on bone marrow.

Because of concurrent disease and the effects of aging on the body's tissues and organs, older adults may not receive the same treatments for cancer that younger clients do.

Older adults, faced with long and sometimes rigorous cancer treatment, may refuse treatment. Those who have undergone extensive surgery for cancer require detailed home care planning before discharge from the hospital.

Arthritis, as well as general muscular stiffness, may make lying supine on an x-ray table difficult for older adults. It may be necessary to pad bony prominences and provide support to the back or legs during radiation therapy.

The skin of older adults is often dry. They may experience intense itching and dryness during and after radiation therapy; therefore, additional treatment of skin problems may be necessary. Inspect the skin frequently for signs of breakdown, excessive scratching, and infection.

Older adults are more prone to electrolyte imbalance. Excessive vomiting during or after treatments may result in a serious electrolyte imbalance.

Older adults who receive internal radiation therapy may experience difficulty in lying still until the end of the treatment. Check these clients more frequently for displacement of the applicator.

Critical Thinking Exercise

1. *A client with endometrial cancer has been told that she will be treated with internal radiation therapy. Discuss what information to include in her teaching plan.*

• NCLEX-STYLE REVIEW QUESTIONS

1. A client diagnosed with cancer comes to the clinic after receiving a combination of radiation and chemotherapies. She complains of nausea, vomiting, and diarrhea.

The nurse should initially assess for signs and symptoms related to:

1. Fatigue
2. Dehydration
3. Infection
4. Anemia

2. At a routine clinic visit, the nurse weighs a client who has cancer and finds that he has lost 25 pounds since undergoing cancer treatment. The best suggestion the nurse can make to increase the client's caloric intake is to eat:

1. Red meat
2. Larger portions
3. Foods high in fat
4. Small, frequent meals

3. A nurse instructs a group of young adults at a community center about behaviors that can decrease the risk of cancer. Which information is most applicable for this age group?

1. Avoid smoking and prolonged sun exposure.
2. Schedule yearly mammograms or prostate examinations.
3. Perform self-examination techniques four times per year.
4. Eat a diet low in salt and fat.

connection

Visit the Connection site at **http://connection.lww.com/go/timbyEssentials** for links to chapter-related resources on the Internet.

References and Suggested Readings

American Cancer Society. (2001). *Cancer reference information.* Available: http://www.cancer.org.

Bullock, B. L., & Henze, R. L. (2000). *Focus on pathophysiology.* Philadelphia: Lippincott Williams & Wilkins.

Cerrato, P. L. (2000). Preventing cancer. *RN, 63*(11), 38–44.

Eremita, D. (2001). Dolasetron for chemo nausea. *RN, 64*(3), 38–40.

Giarelli, E., Pisano, R., & McCorkle, R. (2000). Stable and able. *American Journal of Nursing, 100*(12), 26–31.

Haylock, P. J. (2000). The universal specialty. *American Journal of Nursing, 100*(4), 9.

Houldin, A. D. (2000). *Patients with cancer: Understanding the psychological pain.* Philadelphia: Lippincott Williams & Wilkins.

Jaquette, S. G. (2000). The octopus and me. *American Journal of Nursing, 100*(4), 23–4.

Mayer, D. K. (2000). Cancer overview. *American Journal of Nursing, 100*(4), 24D–H.

Myers, J. M. (2000). Chemotherapy-induced hypersensitivity reaction. *American Journal of Nursing, 100*(4), 53–54.

Nevidjon, B. M., & Sowers, K. W. (2000). *A nurse's guide to cancer care.* Philadelphia: Lippincott Williams & Wilkins.

Perin, M. L., & Pasero, C. (2000). Corticosteroids for cancer pain. *American Journal of Nursing, 100*(4), 15–16.

Sinopli, T. (September 21, 2002). Highly curable cancer. *Advance for Nurses,* 25–27.

Smeltzer, S. C., & Bare, B. G. (2004). *Brunner & Suddarth's textbook of medical-surgical nursing* (10th ed.). Philadelphia: Lippincott Williams & Wilkins.

Starr, J. H. (2000). Radiation is lonely. *RN, 63*(8), 40–42.

Thayler-DeMers, D. (2000). The cancer survival toolbox. *American Journal of Nursing, 100*(4), 87.

Washington, C. M., & Leaver, D. T. (1997). *Principles and practice of radiation therapy: Practical applications.* St. Louis: Mosby.

Worthington, K. (2000a). Chemotherapy on the unit. *American Journal of Nursing, 100*(4), 88.

Worthington, K. (2000b). Guarding against radiation exposure. *American Journal of Nursing, 100*(5), 104.

Zu-Kei Lin, R. (April 29, 2002). Hodgkin's disease. *Advance for Nurses.* 33–34.

chapter 20

Caring for Clients in Shock

Words to Know 

adrenocorticotropic hormone
anaerobic metabolism
anaphylactic shock
antidiuretic hormone
cardiac output
cardiogenic shock
catecholamines
colloid solutions
compensation stage
corticosteroid hormones
crystalloid solutions
decompensation stage
distributive shock
endotoxins
hypovolemic shock
hypoxia
irreversible stage
ischemia
neurogenic shock
obstructive shock
oliguria
positive inotropic agents
renin-angiotensin-aldosterone system
septic shock
shock
vasopressors

Learning Objectives

On completion of this chapter, the reader will:

- Define shock.
- Name general categories of shock.
- Identify subcategories of distributive shock.
- List pathophysiologic consequences of shock.
- Name the stages of shock.
- Describe physiologic mechanisms that attempt to compensate for shock.
- Discuss signs and symptoms manifested by clients in shock.
- Name diagnostic measurements used when monitoring clients in shock.
- Give medical approaches for treating shock.
- List complications of shock.
- Discuss the nursing management of clients with shock.

This chapter discusses shock and its various types, pathophysiologic consequences, and assessment findings, which may vary according to type. It also presents the medical and nursing management of clients in shock.

SHOCK

Shock is a life-threatening condition that occurs when arterial blood flow and oxygen delivery to tissues and cells are inadequate. It develops as a consequence of one of three events: (1) blood volume decreases, (2) the heart fails as an effective pump, or (3) peripheral blood vessels massively dilate (Collins, 2000). In some cases, the body implements compensatory mechanisms to counteract the effects of shock. In other cases, shock progresses until therapeutic measures are implemented. If physiologic and therapeutic measures are inadequate, organs are damaged and death may follow.

Types

The four main categories of shock are hypovolemic, distributive, obstructive, and cardiogenic, depending on the cause (Smeltzer & Bare, 2004) (Table 20.1). More than one type of shock can develop simultaneously. Hypovolemic shock is most common, but cardiogenic shock is most lethal (Mower-Wade et al., 2001).

Hypovolemic Shock

In **hypovolemic shock,** extracellular fluid volume is significantly reduced, primarily due to lost or reduced blood or plasma (water component). Intravascular, interstitial, and intracellular fluid volumes are interdependent. Loss from one location results in a similar loss in the others. Thus, a deficit of intravascular volume (plasma) reduces the net circulating volume.

Hypovolemic shock can develop when overall fluid volume is depleted from significant bleeding, such as during surgery, after trauma, or after delivery of an infant. It also may result from significant fluid loss, as with burns,

TABLE 20.1 TYPES OF SHOCK

TYPE	CAUSE	EXAMPLES
Hypovolemic shock	Decreased blood volume	Hemorrhage (frank and internal) Extreme diuresis Severe diarrhea or vomiting Dehydration Third-spacing
Distributive shock	Redistribution of intravascular fluid from arterial circulation to venous or capillary areas	
Neurogenic		Spinal cord injury
Septic		Toxic reaction to gram-negative bacterial infection
Anaphylactic		Severe allergic reaction
Obstructive shock	Impaired filling of heart with blood	Cardiac tamponade (see Chap. 24) Dissecting aneurysm Tension pneumothorax (see Chap. 23)
Cardiogenic shock	Decreased force of ventricular contraction	Myocardial infarction Cardiac dysrhythmia (see Chaps. 26 and 27)

large draining wounds, reduced fluid intake, suctioning, or disorders in which fluid losses exceed fluid intake, such as diabetes insipidus (see Chap. 51).

Distributive Shock

In **distributive shock,** or *normovolemic shock,* the amount of fluid in the circulatory system is not reduced, yet fluid circulation does not permit effective tissue perfusion. Vasodilatation, a prominent characteristic of distributive shock, increases the space in the vascular bed. Central blood flow is reduced because peripheral vascular or interstitial areas exceed their usual capacity. Three types of distributive shock are neurogenic, septic, and anaphylactic shock.

NEUROGENIC SHOCK. **Neurogenic shock** results from an insult to the vasomotor center in the medulla of the brain or to peripheral nerves that extend from the spinal cord to the blood vessels. Spinal cord or head injury or overdoses of opioids, opiates, tranquilizers, or general anesthetics can cause neurogenic shock. Sympathetic nervous system tone is impaired, resulting in decreased arterial vascular resistance, vasodilatation, and hypotension. Blood remains distributed in the periphery, so that the heart does not fill adequately, cardiac output is reduced, tissue perfusion is compromised, cells are deprived of oxygen and switch to anaerobic metabolism, and metabolic acidosis develops.

SEPTIC SHOCK. **Septic shock,** or *toxic shock,* is associated with overwhelming bacterial infections. It occurs most commonly with gram-negative bacteremia (bacteria in the blood) caused by such pathogens as *Escherichia coli,* species of *Pseudomonas,* and gram-positive drug-resistant *Staphylococcus aureus* and *Streptococcus.* **Endotoxins,** harmful chemicals released by bacterial cells, are probably the major cause of septic shock. They trigger an immune response in which vasoactive chemicals, such as cytokines (see Chap. 35), dilate blood vessels and increase capillary permeability, causing vascular fluid to shift to the interstitium. Clients with septic shock have an elevated leukocyte count and initially manifest a fever accompanied by warm, flushed skin and a rapid, bounding pulse. As septic shock progresses, clients eventually develop cold, pale or mottled skin and hypotensive symptoms, findings common with other forms of shock.

ANAPHYLACTIC SHOCK. **Anaphylactic shock** (see Chap. 36) is a severe allergic reaction that follows exposure to a substance to which a person is extremely sensitive. Common allergic substances include bee venom, latex, fish, nuts, and penicillin. The body's immune response to the allergic substance causes mast cells in the connective tissues, bronchi, and gastrointestinal tract to release histamine and other chemicals. Vasodilatation, increased capillary permeability with swelling of the airway and subcutaneous tissues, hypotension, and hives or an itchy rash result (Fig. 20.1).

Obstructive Shock

Obstructive shock occurs when the heart or great vessels are compressed. The compression reduces space available for blood in the heart, compromising the volume of blood that enters and leaves the heart en route to the lungs and tissues. Any condition that fills the thoracic cavity with fluid, air, or tissue can lead to obstructive shock. Examples include increased fluid or blood in the pericardial sac (cardiac tamponade, see Chap. 25); air that accumulates between the layers of pleura (tension pneumothorax, see Chap. 23); or abdominal tissue, fluid,

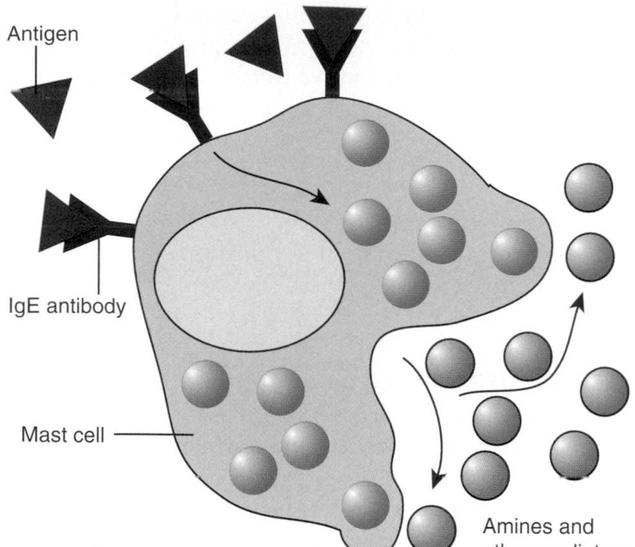

FIGURE 20.1 Vasodilation, increased capillary permeability, smooth muscle contraction, and eosinophilia characterize an anaphylactic reaction. Systemic reactions may involve laryngeal stridor, angioedema, hypotension, and bronchial, gastrointestinal, or uterine spasm. Local reactions are characterized by hives.

or air that crowds the diaphragm, as in an enlarged liver and ascites (see Chap. 49).

Cardiogenic Shock

In **cardiogenic shock,** heart contraction is ineffective, reducing **cardiac output,** the volume of blood ejected from the left ventricle per minute. A myocardial infarction (MI) with subsequent heart failure (see Chaps. 27 and 30) is a leading cause of cardiogenic shock.

> **Stop, Think, and Respond ● BOX 20-1**
>
> *Indicate the type of shock each client is most likely experiencing:*
>
> - *Client A has had an MI and cardiac arrest; paramedics resuscitated him. He is now having difficulty breathing, a rapid heart rate, and chest pain. Urine output is 50 mL in the last 4 hours.*
> - *Client B was involved in a motor vehicle collision. Paramedics note a substantial bruise on his right upper thigh, which is much larger than his left upper thigh. Based on assessment findings and a distorted alignment of the right leg, they suspect a fractured pelvis or femur. They also suspect a ruptured spleen because the client has abdominal tenderness. He is hypotensive with pale and cool skin.*
> - *Client C was pruning roses when a bee stung her. Within minutes she had difficulty breathing and lost consciousness. Her neighbor called 911. Paramedics note that the client is hypotensive, tachycardic, and barely able to breathe.*

Pathophysiology

Regardless of the type, many complex events accompany shock, which usually progresses through three stages: (1) compensation, (2) decompensation, and (3) irreversible (Fig. 20.2).

Compensation Stage

The **compensation stage** is the first stage of shock, in which several physiologic mechanisms attempt to achieve stability. If natural or medical means can reverse shock, chances of uncomplicated recovery are greatly improved. If shock progresses, positive outcomes are less predictable. Compensatory mechanisms include release of catecholamines; activation of the renin-angiotensin-aldosterone system; and production of antidiuretic and **corticosteroid hormones,** chemicals that promote fluid retention and reabsorption.

CATECHOLAMINES. **Catecholamines** are neurotransmitters that stimulate responses by the sympathetic nervous

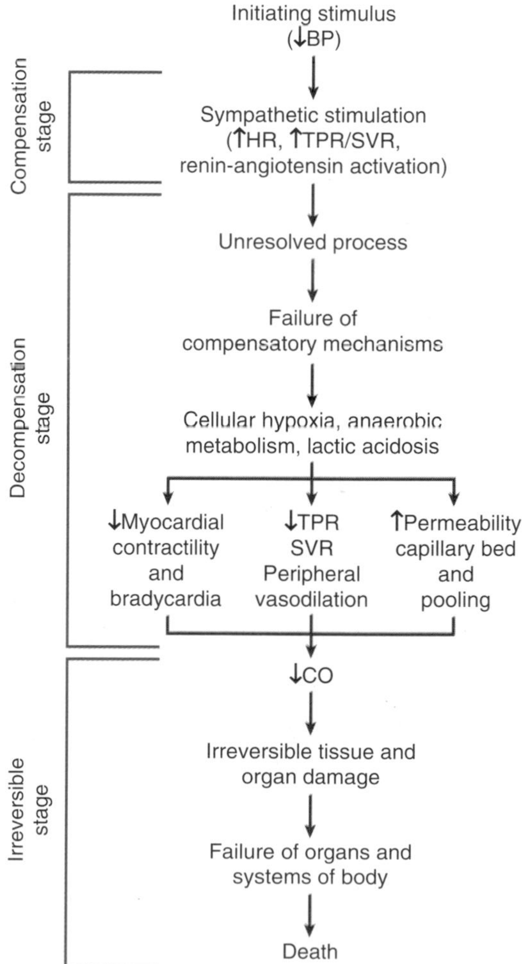

FIGURE 20.2 Stages of shock. *BP,* blood pressure; *CO,* cardiac output; *HR,* heart rate; *SVR,* systemic vascular resistance; *TPR,* total peripheral resistance.

system. To compensate shock, the sympathetic nervous system releases endogenous catecholamines, epinephrine and norepinephrine into the circulation. They increase heart rate and the contractile ability of the myocardium. Venous return to the right atrium subsequently increases, as does blood sent to the lungs. Bronchial dilatation increases the amount of oxygenated air entering the lungs, followed by a more efficient exchange of oxygen and carbon dioxide (CO_2).

RENIN-ANGIOTENSIN-ALDOSTERONE SYSTEM. The **renin-angiotensin-aldosterone system** is a mechanism that restores blood pressure (BP) when circulating volume is diminished. In response to low renal (kidney) blood perfusion, the juxtaglomerular cells release renin, an enzymatic hormone in nephrons of the kidneys. Release of renin causes chemical reactions that eventually produce angiotensin II, a potent vasoconstrictor that raises BP. Angiotensin II stimulates the hypothalamus to signal the adrenal cortex to release aldosterone, a mineralocorticoid promoting reabsorption of sodium and water by the kidney, which increases blood volume.

ANTIDIURETIC HORMONE AND CORTICOSTEROID HORMONES. Low blood volume also stimulates the pituitary to secrete **antidiuretic hormone** (ADH), also known as *vasopressin,* and **adrenocorticotropic hormone** (ACTH). ADH promotes reabsorption of water that the kidneys would ordinarily excrete. ACTH stimulates the adrenal glands to secrete *glucocorticoids,* which help the body respond to stress, and *mineralocorticoids,* such as aldosterone, that conserve sodium and promote potassium excretion. They play an active role in controlling sodium and water balance.

Decompensation Stage

The **decompensation stage** occurs as compensatory mechanisms fail. The client's condition spirals into cellular hypoxia, coagulation defects, and cardiovascular changes.

CELLULAR HYPOXIA. **Hypoxia** refers to decreased oxygen reaching the cells. Hypoxic cells switch from aerobic metabolism to **anaerobic metabolism,** a less efficient mechanism for meeting energy requirements. When energy supply falls below demand, pyruvic and lactic acids increase, causing metabolic acidosis. Cellular structural integrity is impaired because without sufficient adenosine triphosphate (ATP), the energy source for operating the sodium and potassium pumps, sodium and water enter the cell and potassium exits into the extracellular fluid (Fig. 20.3). Eventually, cells swell and rupture, making them unable to carry out electrochemical processes. Lysosomes, the cellular structure for breaking down cellular waste, leak enzymatic fluid and cause further cellular destruction.

COAGULATION DEFECTS. Cellular damage causes an inflammatory response. Platelets become sticky and accu-

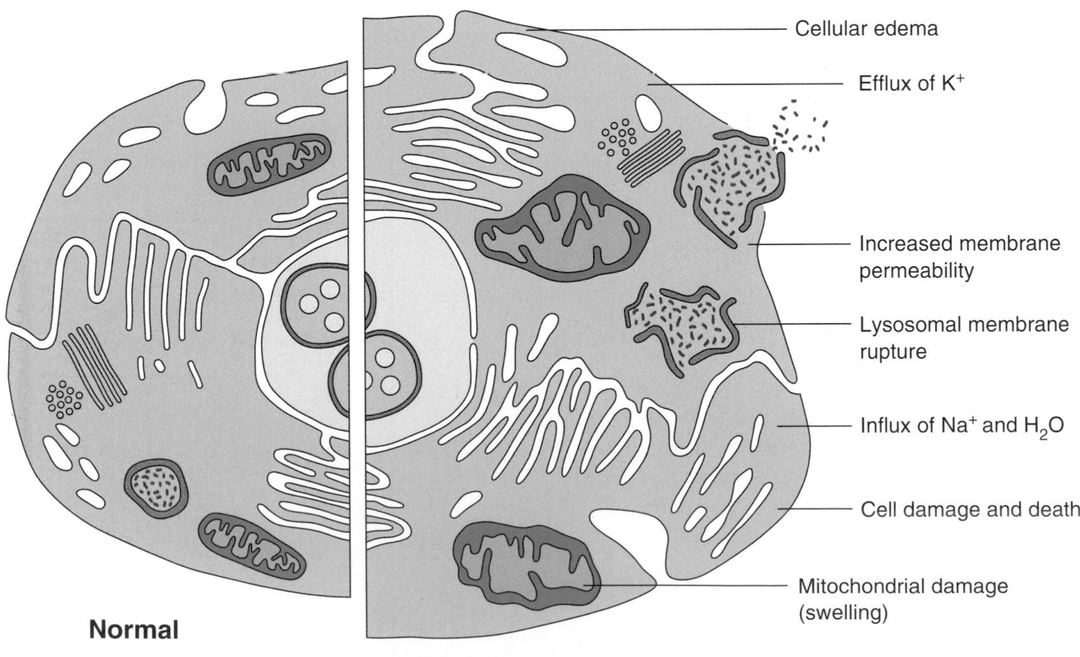

FIGURE 20.3 Cellular effects of shock. The cell swells, the cell membrane becomes more permeable, and fluids and electrolytes seep from and into the cell. Mitochondria and lysosomes are damaged, and the cell dies. (From Smeltzer, S. C., & Bare, B. G. [2004]. *Brunner & Suddarth's textbook of medical–surgical nursing* [10th ed., p. 246.]. Philadelphia: Lippincott Williams & Wilkins.)

mulate in the blood vessels of the volume-depleted client, predisposing him or her to microemboli formation. Clots compromise the ability of the red blood cells (RBCs) to deliver oxygen throughout the body, leading to cell and organ death.

CARDIOVASCULAR CHANGES. Impaired myocardial cells cannot maintain sufficient heart rate and force of contraction to circulate blood efficiently. Brain cells in the medulla cannot sustain the stimulus for vasoconstriction. Blood vessels dilate, blood pools in the periphery or leaks into the interstitium, cardiac output decreases, and BP falls. Clinical signs include bradycardia, hypotension, confusion, lethargy, decreased urine production, cold, pale skin, and reduced peristalsis. Aggressive interventions are necessary to prevent the irreversible stage of shock and ensure the client's survival.

Irreversible Stage

The **irreversible stage** occurs when significant cells and organs are damaged. The client's condition reaches a "point of no return" despite medical interventions. Multiple systems fail. When the kidneys, heart, lungs, liver, and brain cease to function, death is imminent.

Assessment Findings

Signs and Symptoms

The nurse monitors for evidence that blood volume or circulation is becoming compromised. Although shock develops quickly, early signs and symptoms are evident during the decompensation stage. Critical assessments include vital signs, characteristics of peripheral pulses, and changes in mentation, skin, and urine output (Table 20.2).

ARTERIAL BLOOD PRESSURE. In shock, both systolic and diastolic arterial BPs fall because cardiac output decreases or the vascular bed size increases. Hypotension may be rapid and sudden or slow and insidious. For the normotensive (normal BP) adult, average systolic BP is 120 mm Hg. A systolic BP of 90 to 100 mm Hg indicates impending shock, whereas 80 mm Hg or below indicates shock. If it is difficult to auscultate BP but a peripheral pulse can be palpated, the BP is at least 80 mm Hg (Collins, 2000).

Knowing a client's previous BP is useful. Regardless of the numeric figure, a progressive fall in BP is serious. A BP of 120/82 mm Hg usually is considered normal. If an individual with an original BP of 190/112 mm Hg has a BP of 120/82 mm Hg, shock may be developing. The nurse must inform the physician of any fall in systolic BP below 100 mm Hg, any fall of 20 mm Hg or more below the client's usual systolic BP, or any trend in progressively decreasing BP.

PULSE PRESSURE. *Pulse pressure* is the numeric difference between systolic and diastolic BP. If a client has a BP of 120/80 mm Hg, the pulse pressure is 40 mm Hg. A pulse pressure between 30 and 50 mm Hg is considered normal, with 40 mm Hg being a healthy average. In shock, the pulse pressure tends to narrow (decrease) as the falling systolic pressure nears the diastolic pressure.

PULSE RATE, VOLUME, AND RHYTHM. In hypovolemic shock, the pulse rate and other assessment data identify the severity of shock and provide an approximate reduction in blood volume. As cardiac output decreases, compensatory tachycardia initially develops to increase cardiac output. Pulse volume becomes weak and thready as circulating volume diminishes. In the later stages, the pulse may be slow and imperceptible. Pulse rhythm may change from regular to irregular. Hypoxia, if it affects heart tissue, is a leading cause of dangerous cardiac dysrhythmias (see Chap. 28).

RESPIRATIONS. In shock, tissues receive less oxygen. In response, the body tries to obtain more oxygen by breath-

TABLE 20.2 SHOCK CLASSIFICATION AND ESTIMATED BLOOD LOSS

ASSESSMENT DATA	CLASS I	CLASS II	CLASS III	CLASS IV
Pulse rate	<100	>100	>120	>140
Pulse pressure	Normal or increased	Decreased	Decreased	Decreased
Blood pressure	Normal	Normal	Decreased	Decreased
Respirations	14–20	20–30	30–40	>35
Urine output/hr	≥30 mL	20–30 mL	5–15 mL	Negligible
Mental status	Slightly anxious	Mildly anxious	Anxious and confused	Confused and lethargic
Blood loss	≤750 mL	750–1000 mL	1500–2000 mL	≥2000 mL
Percentage of total blood volume lost*	≤15%	15%–30%	30%–40%	≥40%

*Estimates are based on an adult male weighing 70 kg.
(Adapted from American College of Surgeons. [1993]. *Advanced trauma life support for physicians.* Chicago: Author.)

ing faster. Rapid respirations help move blood in the large veins toward the heart. Respirations are shallow, and the client may be heard grunting. In early stages, the client is hungry for air, but in profound shock as death nears, the respiratory rate decreases.

TEMPERATURE. Heat-regulating mechanisms are depressed in shock. Diaphoresis increases heat loss. With the possible exception of septic shock, subnormal body temperature is characteristic.

MENTATION. Altered cerebral function often is the first sign of inadequate oxygen delivery to the tissues. Mild anxiety, increasing restlessness, agitation, or confusion accompany shock. As the condition worsens, the client becomes listless and stuporous, ultimately losing consciousness.

SKIN. In all but the early stages of septic and neurogenic shock, the skin is cold and clammy. As peripheral blood vessels constrict to direct blood from the skin to more vital organs (heart, kidneys, brain), the skin becomes paler. Eventually the skin may appear mottled (i.e., a mix of pale and cyanotic areas lacking any uniform consistency). Capillary filling longer than 3 seconds and cyanosis of the nailbeds, lips, and earlobes indicate oxygen deficiency. In clients with highly pigmented skin (such as African-American clients), cyanosis is detected by inspecting the conjunctiva and oral mucous membranes. Lack of cyanosis does not prove absence of hypoxia because cyanosis is one of the last signs to appear.

URINE OUTPUT. Reduced cardiac output decreases renal blood flow, leading to decreased urine output. Vasoconstriction, the physiologic response to shock, also contributes to markedly reduced renal blood flow. The rate of urine formation is often an important indicator of the status of a client in shock. When shock is quickly reversed, urine output usually returns to normal. Continued **oliguria** (decreased urine formation) indicates renal damage, caused by reduced blood flow to the kidney.

Stop, Think, and Respond ● 20-2

Which stage of shock is characterized by the following physiologic changes?

1. *Client is unconscious, with a slow pulse, systolic BP of 85 mm Hg, and mottled skin color.*
2. *Client is alert and oriented, with tachycardia but normal BP and skin color.*
3. *Client is somewhat disoriented, with BP lower than earlier assessment and pale skin.*

Diagnostic Findings

Arterial blood gas (ABG), central venous pressure, and pulmonary artery pressure measurements support a diagnosis of shock. They also are used to monitor response to treatment.

ARTERIAL BLOOD GAS (ABG) MEASUREMENTS. ABG specimens are drawn from a direct arterial puncture or indwelling arterial catheter (see Chap. 24). In shock, partial pressure of oxygen in arterial blood (PaO_2, normally 80 to 100 mm Hg) falls below 60 mm Hg. The partial pressure of CO_2 in arterial blood ($PaCO_2$) may be normal or decreased. A pulse oximeter measures the amount of oxygen bound to hemoglobin, or the saturated oxygen (SpO_2) level, which normally is 95% to 100%. If the SpO_2 level is above 90%, it is assumed that the PaO_2 is 60 mm Hg or above.

CENTRAL VENOUS PRESSURE. *Central venous pressure* (CVP) is the pressure of blood in the right atrium or venae cavae. CVP measures hemodynamic variables in shock: venous return, quality of right ventricular function, and vascular tone. Trends in CVP measurements are useful in managing a client in shock (see Chap. 24). Normal CVP is 4 to 10 cm H_2O. In hypovolemic shock, CVP is lower than normal; in cardiogenic shock, it usually is above normal.

PULMONARY ARTERY PRESSURE. CVP measurements indicate the status of right ventricular function, but do not provide information about left ventricular function, which is more pertinent to circulation than right. Knowing fluid pressures on the left side of the heart is more meaningful. To assess left ventricular function, a special catheter is inserted into the vena cava and advanced through the right atrium and right ventricle into the pulmonary artery. The catheter, connected to a monitor, measures *pulmonary artery pressure* (PAP) or *pulmonary capillary wedge pressure* (PCWP) (see Chap. 24). Normal PAP ranges from 20 to 30 mm Hg systolic and from 8 to 12 mm Hg diastolic. Normal PCWP ranges from 4 to 12 mm Hg. In shock, PAP measurements usually are low, reflecting the low volume of blood in the arterial system.

Medical Management

Aggressive treatment of conditions that predispose to shock may prevent it. Once shock develops, treatment depends on its type and level and usually includes one or more of the following: intravenous (IV) fluid therapy, vasopressor drug therapy, and mechanical devices that restore blood circulation to cells.

Intravenous Fluid Therapy

IV fluids are prescribed to restore intravascular volume. The total volume, type of solution(s), and rate of administration vary according to the etiology of shock. Usually, a ratio of 3:1 is followed; that is, 3 L of fluid is administered for every 1 L of fluid lost. This amount stabilizes the client, replaces the deficit, and provides a reserve to prevent shock from recurring. Initially, as much as 250 to 500 mL may be infused in 1 hour. Solutions may include **crystalloid solutions,** which contain dissolved substances such as sodium, other electrolytes, or glucose in water; **colloid solutions,** which contain proteins (such as albumin) to increase osmotic pressure; and blood and blood products if blood loss has been major.

To ensure oxygenation of tissues, especially in cases of hemorrhage or if the hemoglobin level is 70 g/L or less, administering whole blood or packed RBCs is best. One unit of RBCs can increase an adult's hemoglobin by 10 g/L (Gilcreast et al., 2001). Clients who are alert and capable of making informed decisions but refuse blood transfusions on the basis of religious beliefs (e.g., Jehovah's Witnesses) require bloodless alternatives and measures that conserve blood and its oxygen-carrying capacity. Such measures include the following:

- Drawing the minimum volume of blood for laboratory analysis
- Restricting movement and activity to only that which is essential
- Reinfusing the client's own blood that has been collected in a closed-circuit cell saver
- Using lasers and electrocautery devices to minimize bleeding during surgery
- Administering pharmacologic agents like erythropoietin to stimulate the bone marrow to manufacture RBCs
- Administering cryoprecipitate, factor VIII, and thrombin to promote *hemostasis,* control of bleeding using substances in the body's natural coagulation process

Drug Therapy

Medical management of shock is extremely complex; drugs are carefully titrated and used alone or in combination to improve cardiovascular status (Drug Therapy Table 20.1). Adrenergic drugs are primarily used to treat

DRUG THERAPY TABLE 20.1 AGENTS TO TREAT SHOCK

DRUG CATEGORY AND EXAMPLES	MECHANISM OF ACTION	SIDE EFFECTS	NURSING CONSIDERATIONS
Vasopressor Agents (Alpha-Adrenergic Activity) *norepinephrine (Levophed), metaraminol (Aramine), phenylephrine (Neo-Synephrine)*	Increase peripheral vascular resistance and raise BP	Headaches, restlessness, palpitations, tremors, nausea, vomiting, anxiety, dizziness	Protect from light. Monitor BP closely during administration. Monitor intake and output. Avoid abrupt withdrawal of these medications.
Positive Inotropic Agents (Beta-Adrenergic Activity) *dobutamine (Dobutrex), isoproterenol (Isuprel), milrinone (Primacor), inamrinone (Inocor)*	Strengthen cardiac contraction and increase cardiac output	Headache, tremors, nervousness, fatigue, palpitations, nausea, vomiting, anxiety, flushing	Inform client to report anginal pain. Observe for dysrhythmias. Monitor BP, pulse, respirations, intake, output, and weight.
digoxin (Lanoxin)		Visual disturbances, diaphoresis, confusion	Take apical pulse for 1 full minute before giving. Note rate and rhythm. Withhold if pulse is below 60 or above 110 beats/min. Do not administer with an antacid. Monitor serum levels for possible toxicity.
Combined Alpha- and Beta-Adrenergic Activity *epinephrine (Adrenalin), dopamine (Intropin)*	Strengthen myocardial contraction, increase cardiac rate and output	Nervousness, anxiety, tremors, headache, weakness, nausea, vomiting, palpitations	Protect from light. Do not use discolored solutions. Monitor BP, pulse, respirations, intake, and output. Check blood glucose levels, which may increase.

shock. **Vasopressors,** drugs with alpha-adrenergic activity, increase peripheral vascular resistance and raise BP. They are administered after fluid therapy increases intravascular fluid volume. If not, vasoconstrictive qualities further impair cellular circulation.

Drugs with beta-adrenergic activity that increase heart rate and improve the force of heart contraction are **positive inotropic agents** (*inotropic* means affecting the force of muscular contraction).

Many drugs, such as epinephrine and dopamine, have combined alpha- and beta-adrenergic effects. Epinephrine is the drug of choice in anaphylactic shock. Anaphylactic shock is also treated with an antihistamine, ACTH, or adrenal corticosteroids to counter the allergen. Antidysrhythmics and drugs that reduce peripheral vascular resistance, like calcium channel blockers, angiotensin-converting enzyme inhibitors, and vasodilators like the nitrates, are appropriate for cardiogenic shock.

Mechanical Devices

Mechanical devices help improve cardiac output or redistribute blood. Those used in the treatment of cardiogenic shock include the intra-aortic balloon pump (IABP) and ventricular assist device (VAD; see Chap. 31). First responders (paramedics) may use a pneumatic antishock garment (PASG), also called *military antishock trousers* (MAST), which redistributes blood from the lower extremities to the central circulation. PASGs and MAST must be used following strict guidelines.

A new type of antishock garment known as Dyna Med Anti-Shock Trousers (DMAST) has been developed. In contrast to PASGs, the DMAST is noninflatable, uses lower pressures to promote central circulation, and can be applied in less than 60 seconds (Fig. 20.4).

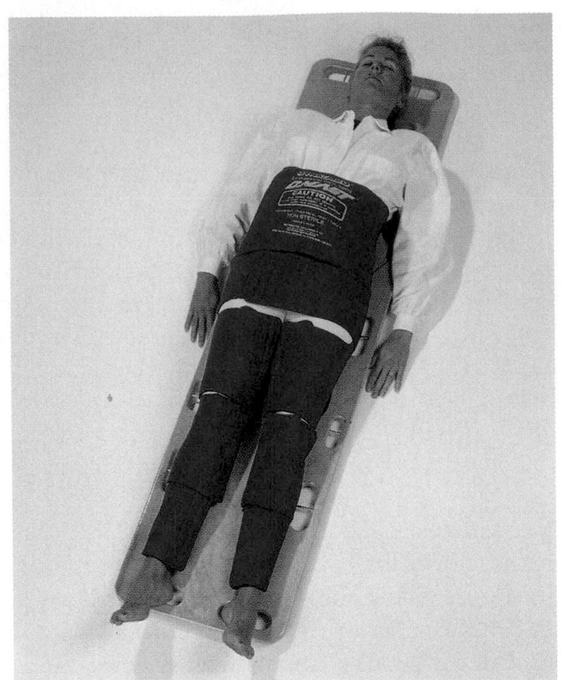

FIGURE 20.4 Dyna Med Anti-Shock Trousers (DMAST).

Prognosis and Complications

When shock is treated adequately and promptly, the client usually recovers. Recovery may be tenuous because of secondary complications, which almost always result from tissue hypoxia and organ **ischemia,** reduced oxygenation. Life-threatening complications include kidney failure, neurologic deficits, bleeding disorders, acute respiratory distress syndrome (see Chap. 23), stress ulcers, and sepsis that can lead to multiple organ dysfunction.

NURSING PROCESS

● The Client in Shock

Regardless of the cause, prolonged shock is incompatible with life. In few instances is the careful attention to nursing practices and principles more important than in the management of a client in impending or actual shock.

Assessment

Assess for early signs of shock and report such findings to the physician immediately. Check vital signs on initial contact and frequently thereafter. Observe skin color and temperature and assess the rate and quality of radial and peripheral pulses. Monitor urine output and determine respiratory rate and effort to detect evidence of dyspnea or airway obstruction resulting from edema, which accompanies anaphylactic shock. Inspect for bleeding or other causes that may explain the developing symptoms of shock. Determine level of consciousness and orientation status regularly to detect changes. In cases of suspected cardiogenic shock, auscultate the chest for abnormal lung and heart sounds. Check laboratory test results for evidence of low RBCs and hemoglobin, findings that correlate with hypovolemic shock. An elevated white blood cell count supports septic shock. Analysis of ABG findings is essential for evidence of hypoxemia and metabolic acidosis. Apply a pulse oximeter to monitor SpO_2. Monitor the results of coagulation tests such as platelet counts, the international normalized ratio, prothrombin time, and partial thromboplastin time.

Diagnosis, Planning, and Interventions

Implement measures to control bleeding, other fluid losses, or fluid maldistribution, and to promote blood circulation to the brain and vital organs. Support of breathing is necessary to ensure adequate blood oxygenation. Use measures to maintain normal body temperature and implement medical therapy as directed. Other care includes, but is not limited to, the following:

Decreased Cardiac Output related to (specify) blood loss, impaired fluid distribution, impaired circulation, inadequate heart contraction, massive vasodilatation

Expected Outcome: Cardiac output will be of adequate volume, as evidenced by heart rate between 60 and 120 beats/minute, systolic BP between 90 and 139 mm Hg, urine output greater than 35 to 50 mL/hour, alert mental status, and warm, dry skin.

- Restrict activity to total rest. *Decreases cellular oxygen requirements. Reduces heart rate, allowing heart to fill with more blood between contractions.*
- Administer IV fluids or blood products at the prescribed rate, ensuring patency of the IV catheter(s). *IV fluids replace fluid lost or trapped in the interstitial space. Administration of whole blood or packed cells increases tissue and cellular oxygenation.*
- Administer prescribed vasopressor or inotropic drugs. *They can raise BP, increase the force of heart contraction, and promote blood circulation to the kidneys to ensure waste excretion.*
- Measure fluid intake and compare with voided urine output; obtain a medical order for insertion of an indwelling catheter if hourly urine output measurements are necessary. *Urine output above 35 to 50 mL/hour or 500 mL/day indicates kidney perfusion is sufficient for excretion of toxic wastes. Urine output aids in evaluating the effectiveness of therapeutic interventions.*

Impaired Tissue Perfusion related to reduced cardiac output secondary to blood loss, heart failure, altered body fluid distribution, vasodilatation, and bradycardia secondary to neurologic trauma or adverse effects from central nervous system depressants

Expected Outcomes: (1) Systolic BP will be at least 90 mm Hg, with hourly urine output 50 mL or greater. (2) Peripheral pulses will be strong. (3) Capillary refill time will be between 2 and 3 seconds. (4) Skin will be warm. (5) Client will be alert and oriented.

- Control frank bleeding by applying direct pressure to the site. *Compresses the area and slows blood loss from the vascular system.*
- Maintain client in a supine position with legs elevated 12 inches (higher than the heart) unless there is head injury, heart failure, increased intracranial pressure, possible spinal cord injury, or dyspnea. *Elevating the legs promotes blood perfusion to heart, lungs, and brain.*
- Administer oxygen as ordered. *Higher percentage of oxygen increases the oxygen bound to hemoglobin and dissolved in blood so that cells can maintain aerobic metabolism.*
- Implement measures to reduce the work of the heart in cardiogenic heart failure, such as administering diuretics, vasodilators, and antidysrhythmics. *A heart in failure is best supported by reducing the volume it must circulate, decreasing the arterial resistance that it must overcome to eject blood, and slowing the heart to reduce its oxygen requirements.*
- Prepare the client in cardiogenic shock for insertion of an IABP or VAD. *Mechanically supporting or enhancing natural heart contractions improves cardiac output and tissue perfusion (see Chap. 31).*
- Immobilize possible spinal injuries and splint fractures. *Reducing complications from trauma can minimize the potential for neurogenic and hypovolemic shock.*

Impaired Gas Exchange related to edema of the airway secondary to a severe allergic reaction leading to anaphylactic shock

Expected Outcomes: (1) SpO2 level will be at least 90%, PaO2 will be 80 to 100 mm Hg, and PaCO2 will be 35 to 45 mm Hg. (2) Airway will be patent, respiratory rate will be no more than 24 breaths/minute at rest, and breathing will be quiet and effortless.

- Assist with the insertion of an artificial airway and ventilatory support (see Chap. 22). *Facilitates maintenance of a patent airway; artificial ventilation ensures that respiratory gases enter and leave the lungs.*
- Suction airway when secretions compromise gas exchange. *Removes fluid that occupies space in the airways needed for the movement and exchange of gases.*
- Administer prescribed adrenergic, bronchodilating, anti-inflammatory, and antihistamine medications. *Improves the potential for gas exchange.*

Hypothermia related to hemorrhage

Expected Outcome: Body temperature will be restored to normal range.

- Keep client dry and covered. *Measures that prevent evaporation and heat loss from radiation interfere with the loss of body heat.*
- Raise the room temperature to approximately 80°F. *Raises body temperature by convection.*
- Place client on a warming blanket or direct warming lights to the client's body. *Conduction and radiation transfer heat.*
- Keep client's head covered with a turban made of stockinette or other material. *Reduces heat loss, which can be significant from the head.*
- Warm IV solutions and blood products. *Raises the temperature of tissues where they are circulated.*
- Warm humidified air that is mixed with oxygen during mechanical ventilation. *Increases core body temperature.*

Hyperthermia related to altered temperature regulation secondary to sepsis

Expected Outcome: Body temperature will be reduced to normal range.

- Administer prescribed antipyretics. *They block the production of prostaglandins, which elevate the temperature set point within the hypothalamus.*
- Place client on a cooling mattress. *Contact with a cool surface lowers body temperature.*
- Control shivering. *Shivering increases body heat through contraction of skeletal and pilomotor muscles in the skin.*

- Administer a tepid sponge bath. *Body temperature is lowered when the heat of the skin vaporizes water.*
- Administer prescribed antibiotics. *They reduce or destroy pathogens responsible for sepsis.*

Evaluation of Expected Outcomes

Vital signs are stable. Tissue perfusion is satisfactory, as evidenced by adequate urine output; strong, palpable peripheral pulses; warm, dry skin; and intact sensorium. Capillary refill is immediate. ABGs are within normal range. Blood pH is between 7.35 and 7.45. The client is normothermic.

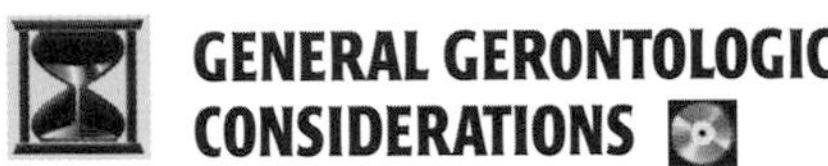

GENERAL GERONTOLOGIC CONSIDERATIONS

Older adults, particularly those with cardiac disease, are prone to cardiogenic shock. They also have a decreased percentage of body water and are more likely to develop hypovolemic shock.

Critical Thinking Exercises

1. *Which types of shock usually are accompanied by warm skin rather than cool skin?*
2. *In which type of shock does the client manifest a slow rather than a rapid heart rate?*

• NCLEX-STYLE REVIEW QUESTIONS 

1. A nurse stops to assist at a severe car accident and notes a large pool of blood under the body of a victim. The nurse immediately assesses for signs and symptoms related to:
    1. Hypovolemic shock
    2. Anaphylactic shock
    3. Septic shock
    4. Distributive shock
2. Postoperatively, a client exhibits signs and symptoms of hypovolemic shock. After reviewing the physician's orders, which nursing action should receive priority?
    1. Administer 3 liters oxygen via nasal cannula.
    2. Send a request for blood to the blood bank.
    3. Infuse normal saline IV fluid at 150 cc/hour.
    4. Give a dose of epinephrine (Adrenalin).
3. A nursing home resident is admitted to the hospital with a diagnosis of septic shock. If the physician ordered all the following, the nurse is most correct in reviewing which laboratory test result because it is most indicative of septic shock?
    1. Red blood cell count
    2. White blood cell count
    3. Arterial blood gas results
    4. Prothrombin time

connection

Visit the Connection site at **http://connection.lww.com/go/timbyEssentials** for links to chapter-related resources on the Internet.

References and Suggested Readings

Atassi, K. A., & Harris, M. L. (2001). Disseminated intravascular coagulation. *Nursing, 31*(3), 64.

Bullock, B. L., & Henze, R. L. (2000). *Focus on pathophysiology.* Philadelphia: Lippincott Williams & Wilkins.

Carroll, P. (2001). Anaphylaxis. *RN, 64*(12), 45–49.

Collins, T. (2000). Understanding shock. *Nursing Standard, 14*(49), 35–39.

Edwards, S. (2001). Shock: Types, classifications and explorations of their physiological effects. *Emergency Nurse, 9*(2), 29–38.

Frank, L. R. (2000). Is MAST in the past? The pros and cons of MAST usage in the field. *Journal of Emergency Medical Services, 25*(2), 38–41, 44–45.

Gilcreast, D. M., Avella, P., Camarillo, E., et al. (2001). Trauma: Treating severe anemia in a trauma patient who is a Jehovah's witness. *Critical Care Nurse, 21*(2), 69–81.

Mower-Wade, D. M., Bartley, M. K., & Chiari-Allwein, J. L. (2001). How to respond to shock. *Dimensions of Critical Care Nursing, 20*(2), 22–27.

Putman, H., & May, K. R. (2001). Relief for patients with severe allergies. *RN, 64*(6), 26–31.

Rembacz, J. M., & Abel, C. J. (2000). Pericardial tamponade. *American Journal of Nursing, 100*(9, Suppl.), 10–14, 24–26.

Smeltzer, S. C., & Bare, B. G. (2004). *Brunner & Suddarth's textbook of medical-surgical nursing* (10th ed.). Philadelphia: Lippincott Williams & Wilkins.

Stoll, E. H. (2001). Sepsis and septic shock. *Clinical Journal of Oncology Nursing, 5*(2), 71–72.

chapter 21

Introduction to the Respiratory System

Words to Know 

adenoids
alveoli (sing. alveolus)
bronchioles
bronchi (sing. bronchus)
carina
cilia
diaphragm
diffusion
epiglottis
ethmoidal sinuses
frontal sinuses
glottis
hilus
interstitium
larynx
lungs
maxillary sinuses
mediastinum
nasal septum
nasopharynx
oropharynx
paranasal sinuses
parietal pleura
perfusion
pharynx
pleura
pleural space
respiration
sphenoidal sinuses
thoracentesis
tonsils
trachea
turbinates (conchae)
ventilation
visceral pleura
vocal cords

Learning Objectives

On completion of this chapter, the reader will:

- Describe structures of the upper and lower airways.
- Explain the normal physiology of the respiratory system.
- Differentiate respiration, ventilation, diffusion, and perfusion.
- Describe oxygen transport.
- Define forces that interfere with breathing, including airway resistance and lung compliance.
- Identify elements of a respiratory assessment.
- List diagnostic tests that may be performed on the respiratory tract.
- Discuss preparation and care of clients having respiratory diagnostic procedures.

The respiratory system provides oxygen for cellular metabolic needs and removes carbon dioxide (CO_2), a waste product of cellular metabolism. Respiratory disorders and diseases are common, ranging from mild to life-threatening. Disorders that interfere with breathing or the ability to obtain sufficient oxygen greatly affect respiratory and overall health status.

RESPIRATORY ANATOMY

The respiratory system is divided into the upper airway (Fig. 21.1) and lower airway. The following sections briefly describe the anatomic structures of both divisions.

Upper Airway

Nose

Nasal bones and cartilage support the external nose. The nares are the external openings of the nose. The internal nose is divided into two cavities separated by the **nasal septum.** Each nasal cavity has three passages created by the projection of turbinates or conchae from the lateral walls. The vascular and ciliated mucous lining of the nasal cavities warms and humidifies inspired air. Mucus secreted from the nasal mucosa traps small particles (e.g., dust, pollen). **Cilia** (fine hairs) move mucus to the back of the throat. This movement helps prevent irritation to and contamination of the lower airway. The nasal mucosa also contains olfactory sensory cells that are responsible for the sense of smell.

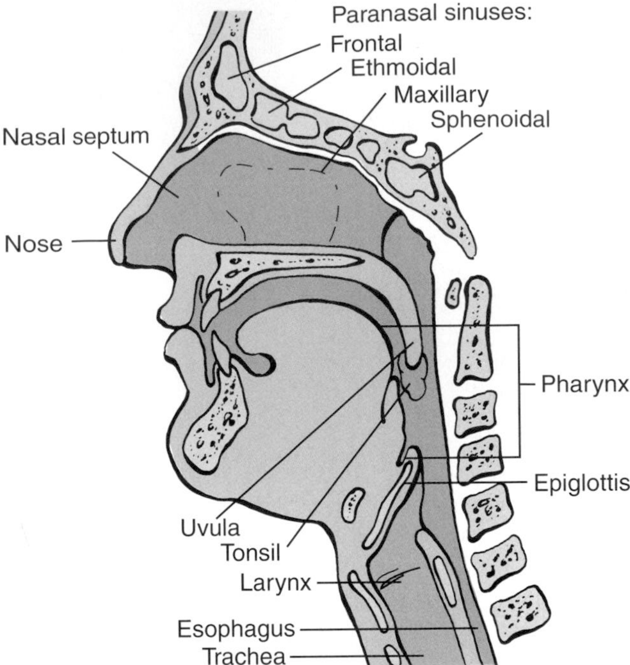

FIGURE 21.1 Major structures of the upper airway.

Paranasal Sinuses

The **paranasal sinuses** are extensions of the nasal cavity located in the surrounding facial bones (see Fig. 21.1). They reduce the weight of the skull and give resonance to the voice. There are four pairs of sinuses. The two **frontal sinuses** lie in the frontal bone extending above the orbital cavities. The ethmoid bone, located between the eyes, contains a honeycomb of small spaces called **ethmoidal sinuses.** The **sphenoidal sinuses** lie behind the nasal cavity. The **maxillary sinuses** are found on either side of the nose in the maxillary bones. They are the largest sinuses and most accessible to treatment.

The lining of the sinuses is continuous with the mucous-membrane lining of the nasal cavity. Mucus traps particles that cilia sweep toward the pharynx. Immunoglobulin A (IgA) antibodies in the mucus protect the lower respiratory tract from infection.

The olfactory area lies at the roof of the nose. The cribriform plate forms part of the roof of the nose and the floor of the anterior cranial fossa. Trauma or surgery in this area carries the risk of injuring or causing infection in the brain.

Turbinate Bones (Conchae)

Turbinates (or **conchae**) are bones that change the flow of inspired air to moisturize and warm it better. As air is inhaled, turbinates deflect it toward the roof of the nose. They have a large, moist, and warm mucous-membrane surface that traps almost all dust and microorganisms. They also contain sensitive nerves that detect odors or induce sneezing to remove irritating particles, such as dust or soot.

Pharynx

The **pharynx,** or throat, carries air from the nose to the larynx, and food from the mouth to the esophagus. The pharynx has three continuous areas: the **nasopharynx** (near the nose and above the soft palate), the **oropharynx** (near the mouth), and the *laryngeal pharynx* (near the larynx). The nasopharynx contains the adenoids and openings of the eustachian tubes, which connect the pharynx to the middle ear. They are the means by which upper respiratory infections spread to the middle ear. The oropharynx contains the tongue. The muscular nature of the pharynx allows for closure of the epiglottis during swallowing and relaxation of the epiglottis during respiration.

Tonsils and **adenoids,** found in the pharynx, do not contribute to respiration but instead protect against infection. Palatine tonsils consist of two pairs of elliptically shaped bodies of lymphoid tissue, located on both sides of the upper oropharynx. Adenoids, or pharyngeal tonsils, also composed of lymphoid tissue, are in the nasopharynx. Chronic throat infections often lead to removal of the tonsils and adenoids. In adults, adenoids may shrink and become nonfunctional.

Larynx

The **larynx,** or voice box, is a cartilaginous framework between the pharynx and trachea. Its primary function is to produce sound. The larynx also protects the lower airway from foreign objects because it facilitates coughing.

Important structures in the larynx include the **epiglottis,** a cartilaginous valve flap covering the opening to the larynx during swallowing; the **glottis,** an opening between the vocal cords; and the **vocal cords** themselves, folds of tissue in the larynx that vibrate and produce sound as air passes through (Fig. 21.2). The pharynx, palate, tongue, teeth, and lips mold the sounds made by the vocal cords into speech.

Lower Airway

The lower respiratory airway consists of the trachea, bronchi, bronchioles, lungs, and alveoli (Fig. 21.3). Accessory structures include the diaphragm, rib cage, sternum, spine, muscles, and blood vessels.

Trachea

The **trachea** is a hollow tube composed of smooth muscle and supported by C-shaped cartilage. The cartilaginous rings are incomplete on the posterior surface. The trachea transports air from the laryngeal pharynx to the bronchi and lungs.

Bronchi and Bronchioles

The trachea divides at the **carina** (lower end of the trachea) to form left and right **bronchi.** Stimulation of

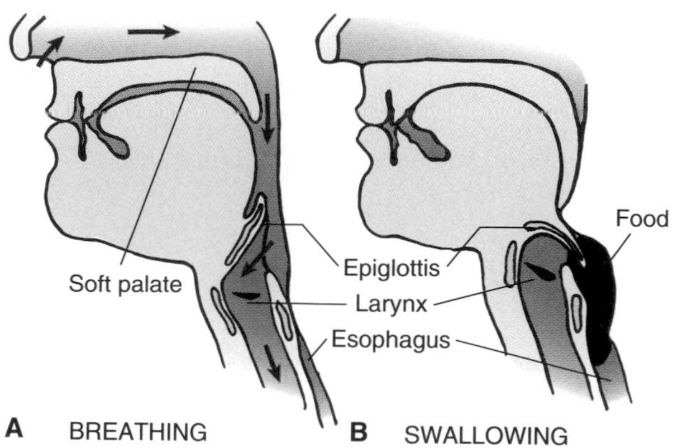

FIGURE 21.2 (**A**) During swallowing, the soft palate elevates to close off air from the nose. Breathing is interrupted momentarily. (**B**) The larynx rises, and the epiglottis shuts off the laryngeal opening until the food has passed down into the esophagus.

the carina causes coughing and *bronchospasm* (bronchial smooth muscle spasm causing narrowing of the lumen). The right mainstem bronchus is shorter, more vertical, and larger than the left. Aspiration of foreign objects is more likely in the right mainstem bronchus and right upper lung. Mucous membrane continues to line this portion of the respiratory tract. Cilia sweep mucus and particles toward the pharynx.

The right and left mainstem bronchi divide into three secondary right bronchi and two secondary left bronchi. Each secondary bronchus supplies air to three right lobes and two left lobes of the lung. The entrance of the bronchi to the lungs is called the **hilus.** The bronchi branch, enter each lobe, and continue to branch to form smaller bronchi and finally terminal **bronchioles** (smaller subdivisions of bronchi).

Lungs and Alveoli

The **lungs** are paired elastic structures enclosed by the thoracic cage. They contain **alveoli,** small, clustered sacs that begin where bronchioles end. Adult lungs contain approximately 300 million alveoli. Each alveolus consists of a single layer of squamous epithelial cells. Capillaries surround these thin-walled alveoli and are the site of oxygen and CO_2 exchange.

The epithelium of the alveoli consists of the following types of cells:

- Type I cells—line most alveolar surfaces
- Type II cells—produce *surfactant,* a phospholipid that alters surface tension of alveoli, preventing collapse during expiration and limiting expansion during inspiration
- Type III cells—destroy foreign material, such as bacteria

The **interstitium** lies between the alveoli and contains pulmonary capillaries and elastic connective tissue. Elastic and collagen fibers allow lungs to have *compliance,*

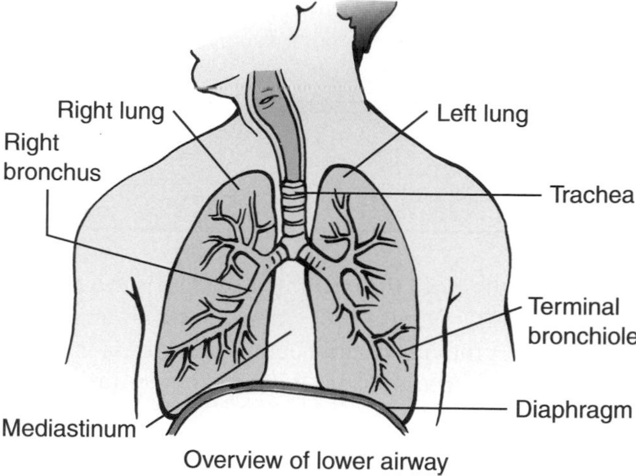

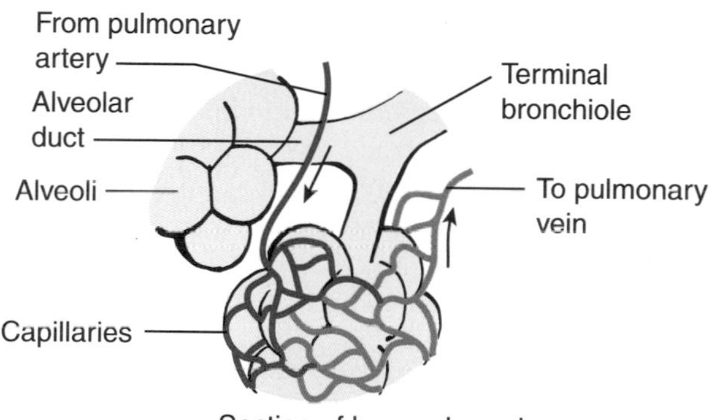

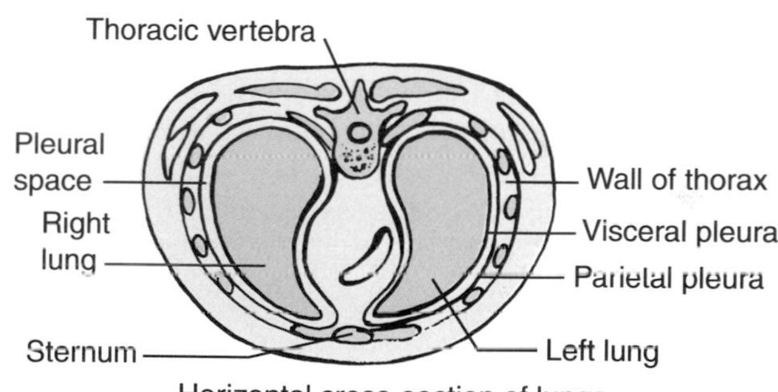

FIGURE 21.3 Lower respiratory tract.

or the ability to expand. Lung expansion creates a negative or subatmospheric pressure, keeping lungs inflated. If air gets into the space between the lungs and thoracic wall, the lungs will collapse.

Accessory Structures

The **diaphragm** separates the thoracic and abdominal cavities. On inspiration, respiratory muscles contract. The diaphragm also contracts and moves downward, enlarging the thoracic space and creating a partial vacuum. On expiration, respiratory muscles relax, and the diaphragm returns to its original position. The **mediastinum** is a wall dividing the thoracic cavity into two halves. This wall has two layers of **pleura,** a saclike serous membrane. The **visceral pleura** covers the lung surface, and the **parietal pleura** covers the chest wall. Serous fluid within the **pleural space** separates and lubricates the visceral and parietal pleurae. Remaining thoracic structures are located between the two pleural layers.

RESPIRATORY PHYSIOLOGY

The main function of the respiratory system is to exchange oxygen and CO_2 between the atmospheric air and blood and between the blood and cells. This process is called **respiration.** Other terms related to respiration are defined in Table 21.1.

Ventilation

Ventilation is the movement of air in and out of the respiratory tract. Air must reach alveoli for gas exchange. This requires a patent airway and intact and functioning respiratory muscles. Pressure gradients between atmospheric air and alveoli enable ventilation. Air flows from an area of higher pressure to an area of lower pressure.

Mechanics of Ventilation

During inspiration, the diaphragm contracts and flattens, expanding the thoracic cage and increasing the thoracic cavity. Pressure in the thorax decreases to a level below atmospheric pressure. As a result, air moves into the lungs. When inspiration is complete, the diaphragm relaxes, and lungs recoil to their original position. The size of the thoracic cavity decreases, increasing pressure to levels greater than atmospheric pressure. Air then flows out of the lungs into the atmosphere (Fig. 21.4).

Neurologic Control of Ventilation

Several mechanisms control ventilation. Respiratory centers in the medulla oblongata and pons control rate and depth. Central chemoreceptors in the medulla respond to changes in CO_2 levels and hydrogen ion concentrations (pH) in the cerebrospinal fluid. They convey a message to the lungs to change the depth and rate of ventilation. Peripheral chemoreceptors in the aortic arch and carotid arteries respond to changes in pH and levels of oxygen and CO_2 in the blood.

Diffusion

Diffusion is exchange of oxygen and CO_2 through the alveolar–capillary membrane. Concentration gradients determine direction of diffusion. During inspiration, oxygen concentration is higher in alveoli than in capillaries. Thus, oxygen diffuses from the alveoli to the capillaries, and is carried to arteries. Oxygen concentration in the arteries is higher than that in cells; thus, oxygen diffuses into cells.

As cellular CO_2 gradients increase, CO_2 diffuses from cells into capillaries and then into the venous circulatory system. As CO_2 travels to the pulmonary circulation, its concentration is higher there than in alveoli, so CO_2 diffuses into alveoli.

Alveolar Respiration

Alveolar respiration determines CO_2 levels in the body. Increased CO_2, present in body fluids primarily as carbonic acid, causes pH to decrease below the normal 7.4. Decreased CO_2 causes pH to increase above 7.4. The pH affects alveolar respiratory rate by direct action of hydrogen ions on the respiratory center in the medulla oblongata.

Kidneys contribute to maintaining normal pH by excreting excess hydrogen ions, keeping serum bicarbonate levels near normal. Lungs and kidneys combine to maintain the ratio of carbonic acid to bicarbonate at 1:20, fixing the pH at approximately 7.4.

In a critically ill client, various homeostatic mechanisms compensate for alterations. Two mechanisms may occur to maintain normal pH:

TABLE 21.1 TERMS RELATED TO RESPIRATION

TERM	DEFINITION
Ventilation	Movement of air in and out of the lungs sufficient to maintain normal arterial oxygen and carbon dioxide tensions
Inspiration	Movement of oxygen into the lungs
Expiration	Removal of carbon dioxide from the lungs
Diffusion	Transfer of a substance from an area of higher concentration or pressure to an area of lower concentration or pressure; exchange of oxygen and carbon dioxide across the alveolar–capillary membrane and at the cellular level
Perfusion	Flow of blood in the pulmonary circulation
Distribution	Delivery of atmospheric air to the separate gas exchange units in the lungs

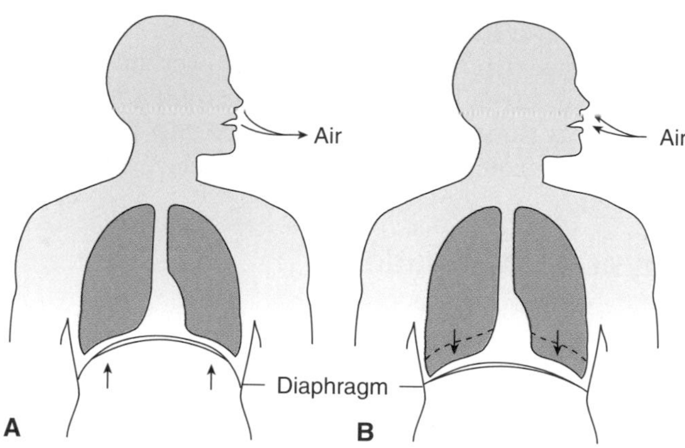

FIGURE 21.4 The mechanics of ventilation. (From Rosdahl, C. B. [2003]. *Textbook of basic nursing* [8th ed.]. Philadelphia: Lippincott Williams & Wilkins.)

- The lungs eliminate carbonic acid by blowing off more CO_2. They also conserve CO_2 by slowing respiratory volume and reabsorbing bicarbonate (HCO_3).
- The kidneys excrete more bicarbonate.

A client's condition remains compensated if the carbonic acid-to-bicarbonate ratio remains 1:20.

Disturbances in pH that involve lungs are considered respiratory. Disturbances in pH involving other mechanisms are termed *metabolic*. At times, respiratory and metabolic disturbances coexist.

Transport of Gases

Oxygen transport occurs in two ways: (1) a small amount is dissolved in water in the plasma, and (2) a greater portion combines with hemoglobin in red blood cells (RBCs; oxyhemoglobin). Dissolved oxygen is the only form that can diffuse across cellular membranes. As this oxygen crosses cellular membranes, oxygen from the hemoglobin rapidly replaces it. Large amounts of oxygen are transported in the blood as oxyhemoglobin.

CO_2 diffuses from the tissue cells to the blood. Bicarbonate ions are then transported to the lungs for excretion. Most CO_2 enters the RBCs, although some combines with hemoglobin to form carbaminohemoglobin. Most CO_2 combines with water in the cells and exits as bicarbonate ions (HCO_3), which the plasma transports to the kidneys. A small portion remains in the plasma and is called *carbonic acid*. The formation of carbonic acid yields hydrogen ions (H^+). The amount of hydrogen ions determines the pH, which also determines the amount of CO_2 for the lungs to excrete. Briefly, acid-base imbalances are compensated in the following ways:

- Respiratory acidosis—kidneys retain more HCO_3 to raise the pH
- Respiratory alkalosis—kidneys excrete more HCO_3 to lower pH
- Metabolic acidosis—lungs "blow off" CO_2 to raise pH
- Metabolic alkalosis—lungs retain CO_2 to lower pH

Pulmonary Perfusion

Perfusion refers to blood supply to the lungs, through which lungs receive nutrients and oxygen. Methods of perfusion are the bronchial and pulmonary circulation.

Bronchial Circulation

Bronchial arteries, which supply blood to the trachea and bronchi, arise in the thoracic aorta and intercostal arteries. Bronchial arteries also supply the lungs' supporting tissues, nerves, and outer layers of the pulmonary arteries and veins. This circulation returns either to the left atrium through the pulmonary veins or to the superior vena cava through the bronchial and azygos veins.

Pulmonary Circulation

The pulmonary artery transports venous blood from the right ventricle to the lungs. It divides into the right and left branches to supply the right and left lungs. Blood circulates through the pulmonary capillary bed, where diffusion of oxygen and CO_2 occurs. Blood then returns to the left atrium through the pulmonary veins.

Pulmonary circulation is referred to as a *low-pressure system* (Smeltzer & Bare, 2004). This means that gravity, alveolar pressure, and pulmonary artery pressure affect pulmonary perfusion. A person in an upright position has less perfusion to the upper lobes. If a person is in a side-lying position, perfusion is greater to the dependent side. Increased alveolar pressure can cause pulmonary capillaries to narrow or collapse, affecting gas exchange. Decreased pulmonary artery pressure results in decreased perfusion to the lungs. Clients with lung and cardiovascular diseases may have decreased pulmonary perfusion.

Problems in Respiratory Physiology

The respiratory system usually has sufficient reserves to maintain normal partial pressures or tension of oxygen and CO_2 in the blood during times of stress. Respiratory insufficiency develops with too much interference with ventilation, diffusion, or perfusion. Abnormalities in these processes can lead to hypoxia, hypoxemia, hypercapnia, and hypocapnia (Table 21.2).

Several factors influence the work of breathing. Pressures needed to overcome the forces interfering with breathing determine the respiratory effort needed. Forces that interfere with breathing include airway resistance and lung compliance.

Airway resistance is related to airway diameter, rate of air flow, and speed of gas flow. As breathing rate increases, so does resistance. A narrowed airway results from increased or thick mucus, bronchospasm, or edema. Conditions that may alter bronchial diameter and affect airway resistance include contraction of bronchial smooth muscle (e.g., asthma); thickening of bronchial mucosa

TABLE 21.2 CONDITIONS RELATED TO ABNORMALITIES IN VENTILATION, PERFUSION, DIFFUSION, AND DISTRIBUTION

CONDITION	DESCRIPTION
Hypoxia	Decreased oxygen in inspired air
Hypoxemia	Decreased oxygen in the blood
Hypercapnia	Increased carbon dioxide in the blood
Hypocapnia	Decreased carbon dioxide in the blood

(e.g., chronic bronchitis); airway obstruction by mucus, a tumor, or a foreign body; and loss of lung elasticity (e.g., emphysema).

Decreased surfactant, fibrosis, edema, and atelectasis (alveolar collapse) affect lung compliance. Greater pressure gradients are needed when lungs are stiff.

ASSESSMENT

Assessment of the respiratory system includes obtaining information about physical and functional issues related to breathing. It also means clarifying how these issues may affect the client's quality of life.

History

Often clients seek medical attention because of respiratory problems related to one or more of the following: dyspnea (labored or difficult breathing), pain on inspiration, increased or more frequent cough, increased sputum production or change in the color/consistency of the mucus, wheezing, or hemoptysis (blood in the sputum). Obtain information about the general health history and family history. Ask clients about the frequency of respiratory illnesses, allergies, smoking history, nature of any cough, sputum production, dyspnea (Box 21-1), and wheezing. Questioning clients about respiratory treatments or medications (prescription and over the counter) is essential. In addition, ask about past pulmonary tests (chest x-ray, tuberculosis test). Include questions about occupation, exercise tolerance, pain, and level of fatigue.

BOX 21-1 ● Questions for the Client With Dyspnea

- What makes you short of breath?
- Do you cough when you are short of breath?
- Do you have other symptoms when you are short of breath?
- Do you get short of breath suddenly or gradually?
- When do you usually have difficulty breathing?
- Can you lie flat in bed?
- Do you get short of breath when you rest? With exercise? Running? Climbing stairs?
- How far can you walk before you get short of breath?

Physical Examination

Physical examination begins with a general examination of overall health and condition. Clients with respiratory problems may show signs of shortness of breath when speaking, or may have a certain posture or position to facilitate breathing. Other observations include skin color; level of consciousness; mental status; respiratory rate, depth, effort, and rhythm; use of accessory muscles; and shape of chest and symmetry of chest movements.

Inspect the nose for signs of injury, inflammation, symmetry, and lesions. Examine the posterior pharynx and tonsils with a tongue blade and light and note evidence of swelling, inflammation, or exudate, and changes in color of the mucous membranes. Also note any difficulty with swallowing or hoarseness.

A physician or nurse practitioner inspects the larynx directly with a laryngoscope or indirectly with a light and laryngeal mirror. Both procedures require local anesthesia to suppress the gag reflex and reduce discomfort.

Inspect and gently palpate the trachea to assess for placement and deviation from the midline. Note any lymph node enlargement. Also examine the chest wall for lesions, symmetry, deformities, skin color, and evidence of muscle weakness or weight loss. Checking contour of the chest walls is important. Normally the anteroposterior diameter of the chest wall is half the transverse diameter; however, some pulmonary conditions (e.g., emphysema) change the chest dimensions (Table 21.3).

An experienced examiner performs percussion of the chest wall to assess normal and abnormal sounds. With the client sitting, the examiner places his or her middle finger on the chest wall and taps that finger with the middle finger of the opposite hand. Table 21.4 describes the types of sounds heard with percussion.

Auscultate breath sounds from side to side, moving from the upper to the lower chest (Fig. 21.5). Listen anteriorly, laterally, and posteriorly. Normal breath sounds include the following:

- Vesicular sounds—Produced by air movement in bronchioles and alveoli, these sounds are heard over the lung fields; they are quiet and low pitched, with long inspiration and short expiration.
- Bronchial sounds—Produced by air movement through the trachea, these sounds are heard over the trachea and are loud with long expiration.
- Bronchovesicular sounds—These normal breath sounds are heard between the trachea and upper lungs; pitch is medium with equal inspiration and expiration.

TABLE 21.3 COMMON ABNORMALITIES OF THE CHEST

CONDITION	DESCRIPTION
Kyphosis	Exaggerated curvature of the thoracic spine; congenital anomaly or associated with injuries and osteoporosis
Scoliosis	Lateral S-shaped curvature of the thoracic and lumbar spine
Barrel chest	Anteroposterior diameter increases to equal the transverse diameter; chest is rounded; ribs are horizontal; sternum is pulled forward; associated with emphysema and aging
Funnel chest	Also known as *pectus excavatum;* the sternum is depressed from the second intercostal space—more pronounced with inspiration; a congenital anomaly
Pigeon chest	Also known as *pectus carinatum;* the sternum abnormally protrudes; the ribs are sloped backward; a congenital anomaly

Adventitious or abnormal breath sounds are categorized as crackles or wheezes. *Crackles* are discrete sounds resulting from delayed opening of deflated airways. They resemble static or sounds made by rubbing hair strands together near one's ear. Sometimes they clear with coughing. They may be present because of inflammation or congestion. Crackles not clearing with coughing may indicate pulmonary edema or fluid in the alveoli.

Wheezes are continuous musical sounds that can be heard during inspiration and expiration. They result from air passing through narrowed or partially obstructed air passages and are heard in clients with increased secretions. Lower pitched wheezes are heard in the trachea and bronchi. Friction rubs are heard as crackling or grating sounds on inspiration or expiration. They occur when the pleural surfaces are inflamed and do not change if the client coughs.

Diagnostic Tests

Arterial Blood Gases

Oxygenation of body tissues depends on the amount of oxygen in arterial blood. Arterial blood gases (ABGs) determine the blood's pH, oxygen-carrying capacity, and levels of oxygen, CO_2, and bicarbonate ion. Blood gas samples are obtained through an arterial puncture at the radial, brachial, or femoral artery, or an indwelling arterial catheter.

ABGs frequently are ordered when a client is acutely ill or has a history of respiratory disorders. If the partial pressure of oxygen in arterial blood (PaO_2) is decreased, body tissues do not receive sufficient oxygen. Table 21.5 presents descriptions and measures of normal ABGs. Clients with respiratory disorders can neither get oxygen into the blood nor get CO_2 out of the blood.

Pulse oximetry is a noninvasive method that uses a light beam to measure the oxygen content of hemoglobin (SaO_2). The monitoring device is attached to the earlobe or fingertip and connects to the oximeter monitor. Wavelengths of light passing through the earlobe or fingertip are registered by the monitor and used to calculate the arterial oxygen saturation, which is displayed on a readout. Normal values are 95% or higher.

Tuberculin Skin Test

The Mantoux test (tuberculin skin test) commonly is done to determine if a client has been infected with *Mycobacterium tuberculosis.* Nurses must remember that this

TABLE 21.4 SOUNDS HEARD WITH CHEST WALL PERCUSSION

SOUND	DESCRIPTION	IMPLICATIONS
Flat	High pitch, little intensity, decreased duration	Heard during percussion of a solid area, such as a mass or pleural effusion
Dull	Medium pitch, medium intensity, medium duration	Heard when no air or fluid is in the lung (e.g., atelectasis, lobar pneumonia)
Tympanic	High pitch, loud intensity, long duration	Normal sounds heard over stomach and bowel; abnormal sounds heard over lungs, such as in a pneumothorax
Resonant	Low pitch, loud intensity, long duration	Normal lung sounds
Hyperresonant	Lower pitch, very loud, longer duration	Abnormal sounds that occur when free air exists in the thoracic cavity (e.g., emphysema, pneumothorax)

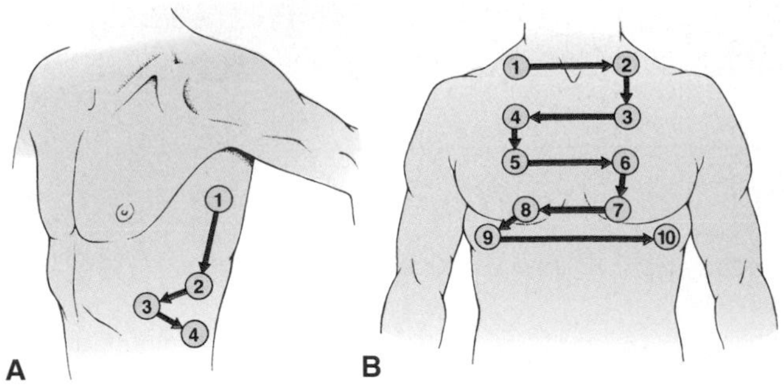

FIGURE 21.5 (**A**) Each side of the chest is auscultated and compared. (**B**) The anterior chest is systematically examined over each lung field.

test does not differentiate between active and dormant disease (Nursing Guidelines 21-1).

Pulmonary Function Studies

Pulmonary function studies measure functional ability of lungs. Measurements are obtained with a spirometer and include:

- Tidal volume—volume of air inhaled and exhaled with a normal breath
- Inspiratory reserve volume—maximum volume of air that normally can be inspired
- Expiratory reserve volume—maximum volume of air that normally can be exhaled by forced expiration
- Residual volume—volume of air left in lungs after maximal expiration
- Vital capacity—maximum amount of air that can be expired after maximal inspiration
- Forced vital capacity—amount of air exhaled forcefully and rapidly after maximal inspiration
- Inspiratory capacity—maximum amount of air that can be inhaled after normal expiration
- Functional residual capacity—amount of air left in the lungs after a normal expiration
- Total lung capacity—total volume of air in the lungs when maximally inflated

Pulmonary function results vary according to age, sex, weight, and height. Maximum lung capacities and volumes are best achieved when the client is sitting or standing. These studies diagnose pulmonary conditions and assess preoperative respiratory status. They also may be used to determine effectiveness of bronchodilators or to screen employees who work in environments hazardous to pulmonary health (Nursing Guidelines 21-2).

Sputum Studies

Sputum specimens are examined for pathogenic microorganisms and cancer cells. Culture and sensitivity tests diagnose infections and determine antibiotics needed. Negative results on examination of sputum smears do not always indicate absence of disease, so collection of sputum for successive days may be done. Sputum is collected by having the client expectorate a specimen, by suctioning the client, or during a bronchoscopy.

Radiography

Chest x-rays show the size, shape, and position of the lungs and other structures of the thorax. Physicians use chest radiography to screen for asymptomatic disease and to diagnose tumors, foreign bodies, and other abnormal conditions. Fluoroscopy helps the physician to view the thoracic cavity with all its contents in motion. It more precisely diagnoses the location of a tumor or lesion. Computed tomography scanning or magnetic resonance imaging may be used to produce axial views of the lungs to detect tumors and other lung disorders during early stages.

Pulmonary Angiography

Pulmonary angiography is a radioisotope study that allows physicians to assess arterial circulation of the lungs, and detect pulmonary emboli. A catheter is introduced into an arm vein and threaded through the right atrium and ventricle into the pulmonary artery. Contrast medium is rapidly injected into the femoral artery, and x-rays are taken to see the distribution of the radiopaque material.

During pulmonary angiography, nurses obtain data about the client's level of anxiety and knowledge of the procedure. They provide additional explanations and inform the client that he or she will experience a feeling of pressure on catheter insertion. When the contrast medium is infused, the client will sense a warm, flushed feeling and an urge to cough.

TABLE 21.5 NORMAL VALUES FOR ARTERIAL BLOOD GASES

BLOOD GAS	NORMAL VALUE
pH, hydrogen ion concentration, acidity or alkalinity of the blood	7.35–7.45
PaO_2, partial pressure of oxygen in arterial blood	80–100 mm Hg
$PaCO_2$, partial pressure of carbon dioxide in arterial blood	35–45 mm Hg
HCO_3, bicarbonate ion concentration in the blood	22–26 mm Hg
SaO_2, arterial oxygen saturation or percentage of the oxygen-carrying capacity of the blood	95%–100%

NURSING GUIDELINES 21-1

Mantoux Test

- Draw up 0.1 mL of intermediate-strength purified protein derivative (PPD) in a tuberculin syringe (½-inch 26- to 27-gauge needle).
- Prepare the injection site on the inner aspect of the forearm, approximately halfway between the elbow and wrist.
- Hold the syringe bevel up, almost parallel to the forearm.
- Inject the PPD to form a pronounced wheal, which indicates proper intradermal injection.
- Record the site, name of PPD, strength, lot number, and date and time of test.
- Read the test site 48 to 72 hours after injection by palpating the site for induration. If induration is present, measure it at its greatest width. Erythema (redness) without induration is not significant. If erythema is present with induration, read the induration only. Interpret the test results as follows:

  Negative reaction—0- to 4-mm induration; no follow-up needed

  Questionable reaction—5- to 9-mm induration; if the client is aware of contact with someone with active tuberculosis, this reaction is seen as significant

  Positive reaction—10 mm or greater induration

Ask if the client has any allergies, particularly to iodine, shellfish, or contrast dye. During the procedure, monitor for signs and symptoms of allergic reactions to the contrast medium, such as itching, hives, or difficulty breathing. Infusion of contrast dye is discontinued immediately if the client has an allergic reaction.

After the procedure, inspect the puncture site for swelling, discoloration, bleeding, or hematoma. Assess distal circulation and sensation to ensure that circulation is unimpaired. If bleeding occurs, apply pressure to the site. Notify the physician about diminished or absent distal pulses, cool skin temperature in the affected limb, poor capillary refill, client complaints of numbness or tingling, and bleeding or hematoma. The client remains on bed rest for 2 to 6 hours after the procedure. The pressure dressing, applied after the catheter is removed, remains in place for this period.

NURSING GUIDELINES 21-2

Pulmonary Function Studies

- Explain the procedure to decrease anxiety and promote cooperation.
- Assure the client that although the spirometry equipment looks complex, the pulmonary function test is simple.
- Explain that the client may be tired after the study.
- Remind the client that the tests should not be performed within 2 hours after a meal.
- Tell the client that bronchodilators may be used during the study.
- Inform the client that he or she will use a nose clip during the study so that air cannot escape through the nose.
- Instruct the client to wear loose-fitting clothing.

Lung Scans

Two types of lung scans may be done for diagnostic purposes: the perfusion scan and the ventilation scan. These procedures may be referred to as a *V-Q scan.* Both require use of radioisotopes and a scanning machine to detect patterns of blood flow and patterns of air movement and distribution in the lungs. V-Q scans are very useful in diagnosing pulmonary emboli. They also detect lung cancer, COPD, and pulmonary edema.

A radioactive contrast medium is administered intravenously for the perfusion scan and by inhalation as a radioactive gas for the ventilation scan. Before the perfusion scan, assess the client for allergies to iodine. During the procedure, the radiologist asks the client to change positions. During inhalation, the client may need to hold his or her breath for short periods as scanning images are obtained. The client needs adequate explanations before the procedure to reduce anxiety. Reassure the client that the amount of radiation from this procedure is less than that used during a chest x-ray.

Bronchoscopy

Bronchoscopy allows for direct visualization of the larynx, trachea, and bronchi using a flexible fiberoptic bronchoscope. The physician introduces the bronchoscope through the nose or mouth or through a tracheostomy or artificial airway. Bronchoscopy is used to diagnose, treat, or evaluate lung disease; obtain a biopsy of a lesion or tumor; obtain a sputum specimen; perform aggressive pulmonary cleansing; or remove a foreign body.

Bronchoscopy is very frightening to clients, who require thorough explanations throughout the procedure. For at least 6 hours before the bronchoscopy, the client abstains from food or drink to decrease risk of aspiration. Risk is increased because the client receives local anesthesia, which suppresses swallow, cough, and gag reflexes.

The client receives medications before the procedure—usually atropine to dry secretions and a sedative or narcotic to depress the vagus nerve. This is important because if the vagus nerve is stimulated during the bronchoscopy, hypotension, bradycardia, or dysrhythmias may occur. Other potential complications include bronchospasm or laryngospasm secondary to edema, hypoxemia, bleeding, perforation, aspiration, cardiac dysrhythmias, and infection. See Nursing Care Plan 21-1 for more information.

Laryngoscopy

Laryngoscopy provides direct visualization of the larynx using a laryngoscope. It is done to diagnose lesions, eval-

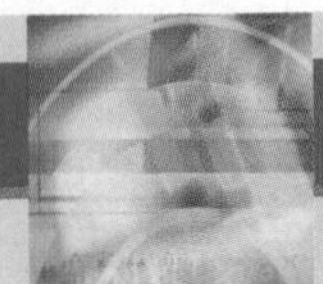

Nursing Care Plan 21-1

THE CLIENT UNDERGOING A BRONCHOSCOPY

Assessment

- Assess level of anxiety and understanding of the procedure.
- Obtain baseline vital signs.
- Assess lung sounds.
- Ask client if he or she wears dentures and when he or she last ate or drank.
- Check record to ensure that consent form is signed and witnessed.

Nursing Diagnosis: **Fear** related to lack of knowledge about what to expect during and after procedure

Expected Outcome: Client will exhibit coping behaviors and follow instructions.

Interventions	*Rationales*
Acknowledge client's fear.	Validating fear communicates acceptance.
Provide simple explanations about the procedure after determining what the client knows and his or her misconceptions.	Acknowledging misconceptions provides a starting point for teaching.
Inform client that he or she will receive medications to alleviate anxiety, reduce secretions, and block the vagus nerve.	Information reduces fear and anxiety.
Explain that a tube will be inserted through the nose and throat and into the lungs and that the medication will assist the client.	Thorough explanations reinforce understanding and reduce fear.
Tell client that after the procedure, food and fluids are withheld until the cough reflex returns.	Preoperative sedation and local anesthesia impair the cough reflex and swallowing for several hours.
Inform client that the throat will be irritated and sore for a few days, and that he or she may cough up blood-tinged mucus.	Knowledge about expected signs and symptoms reduces fear after procedure.

Evaluation of Expected Outcome: Client tolerates procedure without untoward effects, follows instructions, and states that fear is minimal.

Nursing Diagnosis: **Risk for Aspiration** related to diminished gag reflex

Expected Outcomes: (1) Client will maintain a patent airway. (2) Risk of aspiration will decrease.

Interventions	*Rationales*
Assess cough and gag reflexes.	Depressed cough or gag reflex increases risk of aspiration.
Keep client NPO until the gag reflex returns (usually 2 to 8 hours).	NPO status reduces risk of aspiration.
Keep suction equipment available.	If the client aspirates, suctioning helps to maintain a patent airway.
Place client in semi-Fowler's position with the head to one side.	Proper positioning decreases the risk of aspiration.
Encourage client to expectorate secretions frequently into an emesis basin.	Expectoration reduces the risk of aspiration.
After the gag reflex returns, offer sips of water or ice chips initially, then progress the diet to soft foods.	Beginning with sips of water or ice chips ensures that the gag reflex has returned. The client can most easily swallow soft foods.

Evaluation of Expected Outcomes: Airway remains patent. Client does not experience aspiration.

(continued)

Nursing Care Plan 21-1 (Continued)

THE CLIENT UNDERGOING A BRONCHOSCOPY

PC: Pneumothorax: dysrhythmia, bronchospasm

Expected Outcome: The nurse will manage and minimize potential complications.

Interventions	*Rationales*
Monitor vital signs and respiratory status, comparing against baseline assessment data.	Comparison helps the nurse determine if the client is experiencing any respiratory distress.
Observe for symmetric chest movements.	Decreased or asymmetric chest expansion is a sign of pneumothorax.
Report hemoptysis, stridor, or dyspnea immediately.	These findings indicate respiratory distress and probable pneumothorax.

Evaluation of Expected Outcome: Client does not experience postprocedure complications.

uate laryngeal function, and determine any inflammation. Physicians also may dilate laryngeal strictures and biopsy lesions. Refer to the preceding section and Nursing Care Plan 21-1 for more information.

Mediastinoscopy

Mediastinoscopy provides visualization of the mediastinum and is done under local or general anesthesia. The physician makes an incision above the sternum and inserts a mediastinoscope. With this procedure, the physician can visualize lymph nodes and obtain biopsy samples. Possible complications include dysrhythmias, myocardial infarction, pneumothorax, and bleeding.

Thoracentesis

A small amount of fluid lies between the visceral and parietal pleurae. When excess fluid or air accumulates, the physician aspirates it from the pleural space by inserting a needle into the chest wall. This procedure, called **thoracentesis,** is performed with local anesthesia. Thoracentesis also may be used to obtain a sample of pleural fluid or a biopsy specimen from the pleural wall for diagnostic purposes, such as a culture and sensitivity or microscopic examination. Bloody fluid suggests trauma. Purulent fluid is diagnostic for infection. Serous fluid may be associated with cancer, inflammatory conditions, or heart failure. When thoracentesis is done for therapeutic reasons, 1 to 2 L of fluid may be withdrawn to relieve respiratory distress. Medication may be instilled directly into the pleural space to treat infection.

Thoracentesis is done at the bedside or in a treatment or examining room. The client sits at the side of the bed or examining table or is in a side-lying position on the unaffected side. If the client is sitting, a pillow is placed on a bedside table, and the client rests her or his arms and head on the pillow. The physician determines the site for aspiration by x-ray and percussion. The site is cleaned and anesthetized with local anesthesia. When the procedure is done, a small pressure dressing is applied. The client remains on bed rest and usually lies on the unaffected side for at least 1 hour to promote lung expansion on the affected side. A chest x-ray is done after the procedure to rule out a pneumothorax. See Nursing Guidelines 21-3 for specific measures. Complications following a thoracentesis are pneumothorax, subcutaneous emphysema (air in subcutaneous tissue), infection, pulmonary edema, and cardiac distress.

Stop, Think, and Respond ● BOX 21-1

Your client had a thoracentesis 2 hours ago. He begins to complain of feeling short of breath and is very anxious. What should you assess?

NURSING MANAGEMENT

In addition to the nursing management of individual tests, clients require informative and appropriate explanations of any diagnostic procedures they will experience. Remember that for many of these clients, breathing may in some way be compromised. Energy levels may be decreased. For that reason, explanations should be brief yet complete and may need to be repeated. Also help ensure adequate rest periods before and after the procedures. After invasive procedures, carefully assess for signs of respiratory distress, chest pain, blood-streaked sputum, and expectoration of blood. Repeat postprocedure instructions to reduce the client's anxiety and to ensure the best possible recovery.

NURSING GUIDELINES 21-3

Thoracentesis

- Explain the procedure to the client.
- Reassure the client that he or she will receive local anesthesia. Explain that the client will still experience a pressure-like pain when the needle pierces the pleura and when fluid is withdrawn.
- Assist client to an appropriate position (sitting with arms and head on padded table or in side-lying position on unaffected side).
- Instruct client not to move during the procedure, including no coughing or deep breathing.
- Provide comfort.
- Inform client about what is happening.
- Maintain asepsis.
- Monitor vital signs during the procedure—also monitor pulse oximetry if client is connected to it.
- During removal of fluid, monitor for respiratory distress, dyspnea, tachypnea, or hypotension.
- Apply small sterile pressure dressing to the site after the procedure.
- Position client on the unaffected side. Instruct client to stay in this position for at least 1 hour and to remain on bed rest for several hours.
- Check that chest radiography is done after the procedure.
- Record the amount, color, and other characteristics of fluid removed.
- Monitor for signs of increased respiratory rate, asymmetry in respiratory movement, syncope or vertigo, chest tightness, uncontrolled cough or cough that produces blood-tinged or frothy mucus (or both), tachycardia, and hypoxemia.

GENERAL GERONTOLOGIC CONSIDERATIONS

Although numbers of alveoli remain stable with age, alveolar walls become thinner and contain fewer capillaries, resulting in decreased gas exchange. Lungs also lose elasticity and become stiffer. These changes place older adults at increased risk for respiratory disease.

Older clients may have difficulty understanding explanations or directions given by the physician or nurse. Repeating or restating information or directions may be necessary before or during a diagnostic test.

Critical Thinking Exercise

1. *Your client had a thoracentesis today. When he returns to your unit, he begins to complain of pain. What risks are associated with this procedure?*

● NCLEX-STYLE REVIEW QUESTIONS 

1. A 68-year-old client comes to the doctor's office stating that she is having shortness of breath and can hear strange breath sounds when she inhales deeply. Upon auscultation of the lung fields, wheezes are noted. The nurse is most correct in stating that wheezes result from:
   1. Air passing through narrowed passages
   2. Air escaping through a pneumothorax
   3. Air collecting in the pleural cavity
   4. Air between visceral and parietal pleurae
2. The nurse is giving instructions to a client having pulmonary angiography. Which of the following statements is the best evidence that the client understands the nurse's instructions about what will take place during the diagnostic procedure?
   1. "I may have some minor discomfort at the site."
   2. "I may have bleeding or a hematoma following the procedure."
   3. "I will remain on bed rest for 2 to 6 hours following the procedure."
   4. "I will sense a warm, flushed feeling and an urge to cough."

connection

Visit the Connection site at **http://connection.lww.com/go/timbyEssentials** for links to chapter-related resources on the Internet.

References and Suggested Readings

Bullock, B. L., & Henze, R. L. (2000). *Focus on pathophysiology.* Philadelphia: Lippincott Williams & Wilkins.

Carpenito, L. J. (2000). *Nursing diagnosis: Application to clinical practice* (8th ed.). Philadelphia: Lippincott Williams & Wilkins.

Connolly, M. A. (2001). Chest x-ray: Completing the picture. *RN 64*(6), 56–62.

O'Hanlon-Nichols, T. (1998). Basic assessment series: The adult pulmonary system. *American Journal of Nursing, 98*(2), 39–45.

Smeltzer, S. C., & Bare, B. G. (2004). *Brunner & Suddarth's textbook of medical–surgical nursing* (10th ed.). Philadelphia: Lippincott Williams & Wilkins.

chapter 22

Caring for Clients With Upper Respiratory Disorders

Words to Know 

adenoidectomy
adenoiditis
aphonia
coryza
deviated septum
epistaxis
hemoptysis
hypertrophied turbinates
laryngitis
laryngoscopy
laryngospasm
nasal polyps
peritonsillar abscess
pharyngitis
rhinitis
rhinorrhea
sinusitis
stridor
tonsillectomy
tonsillitis
tracheostomy
tracheotomy

Learning Objectives

On completion of this chapter, the reader will:

- Describe nursing care for clients experiencing infectious or inflammatory upper respiratory disorders.
- Discuss assessment data required to provide nursing care to clients with structural disorders of the upper airway.
- Describe airway problems a client may experience following trauma or obstruction to the upper airway.
- Identify risk factors that contribute to development of laryngeal cancer.
- Identify the earliest symptom of laryngeal cancer.
- Discuss treatments for laryngeal cancer.
- Describe measures used to promote alternative methods of communication for clients with a laryngectomy.
- Discuss psychosocial issues that clients may experience following a laryngectomy.
- Relate treatment modalities for clients experiencing short-term or long-term problems with airway management.
- Identify possible reasons for and nursing management of a tracheostomy.
- Explain why a client may require endotracheal intubation.

Disorders of the upper airway range from common colds to cancer. Severity depends on the disorder and the client's physiologic response. Most people experience common colds and sore throats and find them more inconvenient than serious. For others, even the most common disorders of the upper respiratory airway are of great concern because other physical problems compound their effects.

INFECTIOUS AND INFLAMMATORY DISORDERS

The most common upper airway illnesses are infectious and inflammatory disorders. Although dismissing these illnesses as unimportant is easy, the average person experiences three to five upper respiratory infections (URIs) each year. For some individuals, URIs develop into bronchitis or pneumonia, which involves more serious symptoms and may require antibiotics or other treatments (see Chap. 23).

• RHINITIS

Rhinitis is inflammation of the nasal mucous membranes. It also is referred to as the *common cold,* or **coryza.** Rhinitis may be acute, chronic, or allergic, depending on the cause. Rhinovirus is the most common cause. More than 100 strains exist. Colds rapidly spread by inhalation of droplets and direct contact with contaminated articles (e.g., telephone receivers, doorknobs). Allergic rhinitis is a hypersensitive reaction to allergens, such as pollen, dust, animal dander, or food. Rhinitis is usually not serious; however, it may lead to pneumonia and other more serious illnesses for debilitated, immunosuppressed, or older clients.

Symptoms associated with rhinitis include sneezing, nasal congestion, **rhinorrhea** (clear nasal discharge), sore throat, watery eyes, cough, low-grade fever, headache, aching muscles, and malaise. Symptoms may continue for 5 to 14 days. A sustained elevated temperature suggests a bacterial infection or a sinus or ear infection. Symptoms of allergic rhinitis persist as long as the client is exposed to the specific allergen.

For most clients, treatment for rhinitis is minimal (Box 22-1). Unless a specific bacteria infection is identified, antibiotics are not used. Clients may use antipyretics for fever, decongestants for severe nasal congestion, antitussives for prolonged cough, saline gargles for sore throat, or antihistamines for allergic rhinitis. Medications that desensitize or suppress immune responses may also be prescribed for allergic rhinitis.

Teaching clients about URIs helps prevent them and minimizes potential complications. Maintaining a healthy lifestyle of adequate rest and sleep, proper diet, and moderate exercise is the best prevention. Frequent handwashing greatly reduces the spread of infection.

• SINUSITIS

Sinusitis is inflammation of the sinuses. The maxillary sinus is affected most often. Sinusitis can lead to serious complications, such as infection of the middle ear or brain.

Pathophysiology and Etiology

Principle causes are the spread of an infection from the nasal passages to the sinuses and blockage of normal sinus drainage. Interference with sinus drainage predisposes a client to sinusitis because trapped secretions become infected. Allergies frequently cause edema of the nasal mucous membranes, obstructing sinus drainage and leading to sinusitis. Nasal polyps or a deviated septum may also impair sinus drainage. Eating a well-balanced diet, getting plenty of rest, engaging in moderate exercise, avoiding allergens, and seeking medical attention promptly if a cold persists longer than 10 days or nasal discharge is green or dark yellow and foul-smelling help to reduce or prevent sinusitis.

BOX 22-1 • Treating Rhinitis

For all types of rhinitis:
- Rest as much as possible.
- Increase fluid intake to assist in liquefying secretions.
- Use a vaporizer to help liquefy secretions.
- Blow nose with mouth open slightly to equalize pressure.
- Wash hands frequently to avoid spreading infection.
- Use over-the-counter medications as directed; be aware of possible side effects, especially interactions with food and alcohol.

For allergic rhinitis:
- Be tested for allergen sensitivity.
- Avoid specific allergens.
- Use antihistamines and decongestants as ordered.

Assessment Findings

Signs and symptoms depend on which sinus is infected. They include headache, fever, pain over the affected sinus, nasal congestion and discharge, pain and pressure around the eyes, and malaise. A nasal smear or material obtained from irrigation of the sinus for culture and sensitivity testing identifies the infectious microorganism and appropriate antibiotic therapy. Transillumination and x-rays of the sinuses may show a change in the shape of or fluid in the sinus cavity. A thorough history, including an allergy history, usually confirms the diagnosis.

Medical and Surgical Management

Acute sinusitis frequently responds to conservative treatment designed to help overcome the infection. Saline irrigation of the maxillary sinus may be done to remove accumulated exudate and promote drainage. The physician inserts a catheter through the normal opening under the middle concha. Antibiotics are given for severe infections. Vasoconstrictors, such as phenylephrine nose drops, may be used short-term to relieve nasal congestion and aid in sinus drainage.

Surgery is often indicated for chronic sinusitis. Endoscopic sinus surgery opens the inferior meatus to promote drainage. More radical procedures, such as the Caldwell-Luc procedure and external sphenoethmoidectomy, are done to remove diseased tissue and provide an opening into the inferior meatus of the nose for adequate drainage.

Nursing Management

In addition to medical treatment, instruct the client to use mouthwashes and humidification, and increase fluid intake to loosen secretions and increase comfort. Instruct the client to take nasal decongestants and antihistamines as ordered.

If the client has sinus surgery, institute standards for postoperative care. Observe the client for repeated swallowing, a finding that suggests possible hemorrhage. One risk of sinus surgery is damage to the optic nerve. Assess postoperative visual acuity by asking the client to identify the number of fingers displayed. Monitor the client's temperature at least every 4 hours. Assess for pain over the involved sinuses, a finding that indicates postoperative infection or impaired drainage. Administer analgesics and apply ice compresses to involved sinuses to reduce pain and edema.

The client will have nasal packing and a dressing under the nares ("moustache" dressing or "drip pad"). Because nasal packing forces the client to breathe through the mouth, encourage oral hygiene and give ice chips or small sips of fluids frequently. Such measures alleviate dryness caused by mouth breathing. Change the drip pad as needed and report excessive drainage. Postoperative client and family teaching includes telling the client not to blow the nose, lift objects more than 5 to 10 pounds, or do the Valsalva maneuver for 10 to 14 days postoperatively. Urge the client to remain in a warm environment and to avoid smoky or poorly ventilated areas.

Stop, Think, and Respond ● BOX 22-1

A neighbor tells you that she is taking antibiotics for an acute sinus infection. She states that she has severe pain in her sinuses and wonders what she can do other than take analgesics. What advice might you give?

• PHARYNGITIS

Pharyngitis, inflammation of the throat, is associated with rhinitis and other URIs. Viruses and bacteria cause pharyngitis. The most serious bacteria are group A streptococci, which cause a condition commonly referred to as *strep throat.* Strep throat can lead to dangerous cardiac complications (endocarditis and rheumatic fever) and harmful renal complications (glomerulonephritis). Pharyngitis is highly contagious and spreads via inhalation of or direct contamination with droplets.

The incubation period for pharyngitis is 2 to 4 days. The first symptom is a sore throat, sometimes severe, with *dysphagia* (difficulty swallowing), fever, chills, headache, and malaise. Some clients exhibit a white or exudate patch over the tonsillar area and swollen glands. A throat culture reveals the specific bacteria. Rapid identification methods, such as Biostar or Strep A optical immunoassay (OIA), are available to diagnose group A streptococcal infections. These tests are done in clinics and physician offices. Standard 24-hour throat culture and sensitivity tests identify other organisms.

Early antibiotic treatment is the best choice for pharyngitis to treat infection and prevent potential complications. Penicillin or its derivatives are generally the antibiotics of choice. Clients sensitive to penicillin receive erythromycin. The antibiotic regimen is 7 to 14 days.

• TONSILLITIS AND ADENOIDITIS

Tonsillitis is inflammation of the tonsils, and **adenoiditis** is inflammation of the adenoids. These conditions generally occur together—the common diagnosis is tonsillitis. Although both disorders are more common in children, they also may be seen in adults.

Pathophysiology and Etiology

Tonsils and adenoids are lymphatic tissues and common sites of infection. Primary infection may occur in the tonsils and adenoids, or infection can be secondary to other URIs. Chronic tonsillar infection leads to enlargement and partial upper airway obstruction. Chronic adenoidal infection can result in acute or chronic infection in the middle ear (otitis media). If the cause is group A streptococcus, prompt treatment is needed to prevent potential cardiac and renal complications.

Assessment Findings

Sore throat, difficulty or pain on swallowing, fever, and malaise are the most common symptoms. Enlarged adenoids may produce nasal obstruction, noisy breathing, snoring, and a nasal voice quality. Visual examination reveals enlarged and reddened tonsils. White patches may appear on the tonsils if group A streptococci are present. A throat culture and sensitivity test determines the causative microorganism and appropriate antibiotic therapy.

Medical and Surgical Management

Antibiotic therapy, analgesics such as acetaminophen, and saline gargles may be used to treat infection and associated discomfort. Chronic tonsillitis and adenoiditis may require **tonsillectomy,** removal of tonsils, and **adenoidectomy,** removal of adenoids. These are generally done as outpatient surgical procedures. Criteria for performing these procedures are repeated episodes of tonsillitis, hypertrophy of the tonsils, enlarged obstructive adenoids, repeated purulent otitis media, hearing loss related to serous otitis media associated with enlarged tonsils and adenoids, and other conditions (e.g., asthma, rheumatic fever) exacerbated by tonsillitis.

NURSING PROCESS

Tonsillectomy and Adenoidectomy

Assessment

Assess the client's understanding of the procedure and obtain baseline vital signs. Ask if the client wears dentures and when the client last had food or drink. It is essential to take hematocrit, platelet count, and clotting time because of the high risk for postoperative hemorrhage. Ask the client about bleeding tendencies and recent use of aspirin, nonsteroidal anti-inflammatory drugs (NSAIDs), or other medications that prolong bleeding time (see Client and Family Teaching 22-1). Some herbal supplements also prolong bleeding, so ask about use of these supplements.

Diagnosis, Planning, and Intervention

Risk for Aspiration related to impaired swallowing secondary to throat surgery and reduced gag reflex secondary to anesthesia

Expected Outcomes: (1) Client will maintain a patent airway with clear breath sounds. (2) Client will expectorate secretions and vomitus as needed.

- After surgery, position client, until alert, on either side with emesis basin to catch drainage or vomitus. *Retained secretions/vomitus obstruct airway and cause aspiration.*
- Assess gag reflex and ability to swallow. *Depressed gag reflex and inability to swallow increase risk for aspiration.*
- Elevate head of bed 45° when client is fully awake. *Decreases surgical edema and increases lung expansion.*
- Monitor respiratory rate, rhythm, and effort at least every hour. *Increased respiratory rate, decreased breath sounds, or both indicate an increased respiratory effort, possibly related to a partially obstructed airway, aspiration, or both.*
- Auscultate breath sounds for crackles at least every hour. *Aspiration of small amounts may occur without evidence of coughing or respiratory distress.*
- Encourage client to spit secretions/vomitus into the emesis basin. *Removal of secretions/vomitus maintains a clear airway and prevents aspiration.*
- Assess for lethargy, behavior changes, or disorientation. *Decreased level of consciousness indicates poor air exchange.*
- Have oral suction equipment available. *Prompt oral suctioning removes secretions/vomitus from mouth, preventing aspiration.*

Risk for Impaired Tissue Integrity related to injury to the suture line

Expected Outcome: Client will maintain an intact suture line.

- Monitor client for bloody drainage from mouth or frequent swallowing. *These signs indicate increased bleeding from suture site and require immediate attention.*
- Instruct client not to cough, clear throat, blow nose, or use a straw in the first few postoperative days. *These actions increase pressure on suture line and may cause disruption and bleeding.*
- Instruct client to avoid carbonated fluids and fluids high in citrus content. *Such fluids are caustic to surgical site and may traumatize tissue, disrupting suture line.*
- Encourage client to first try ice chips, then small sips of cold fluids, and then popsicles and full liquids as tolerated. *This provides client with an opportunity to slowly try swallowing, without disrupting suture line.*
- Add soft food, such as gelatin and sherbet, as tolerated, after first 24 hours postoperatively. *As diet advances, small amounts of soft foods are less likely to traumatize the suture line.*

Pain related to the surgical incision in the throat

Expected Outcomes: Client will acknowledge relief from pain medications and demonstrate improved ability to swallow.

- Anticipate need for pain relief, medicating client as ordered. *Early treatment of pain assists to decrease its intensity.*
- Apply ice collar as ordered. *Cold reduces swelling and inflammation in soft tissues surrounding surgical incision. The ice pack helps control bleeding, reduce edema and inflammation, and block pain receptors.*
- Encourage client to gently gargle with warm saline three to four times daily. *Gentle gargling cleanses surgical site and helps reduce inflammation and pain, remove thick mucus, and improve swallowing.*

Evaluation of Expected Outcomes

Client maintains a clear airway and expectorates secretions and vomitus. He or she experiences minimal post-

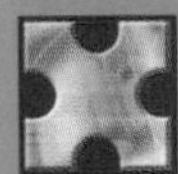

22-1 *Client and Family Teaching* Tonsillectomy and Adenoidectomy

The nurse ensures that the client and family members can manage self-care at home by communicating the following points:

- Report signs of bleeding to physician—this is particularly important in the first 12 to 24 hours, and then 7 to 10 days after surgery as the throat heals.
- Gently gargle with warm saline or alkaline mouthwash to assist in removing thick mucus.
- Maintain a liquid and very soft diet for several days after surgery—avoid spicy foods and rough-textured foods.
- Avoid milk and milk products if client does not tolerate them well.

operative bleeding. Suture line remains intact. Client states relief of pain and ability to swallow.

● PERITONSILLAR ABSCESS

A **peritonsillar abscess** develops in connective tissue between the capsule of the tonsil and constrictor muscle of the pharynx. It may follow a severe streptococcal or staphylococcal tonsillar infection. The client with a peritonsillar abscess experiences difficulty and pain with swallowing, fever, malaise, ear pain, and difficulty talking. On visual examination, the affected side is red and swollen, as is the posterior pharynx. Drainage from the abscess is cultured to identify the microorganism. Sensitivity studies determine appropriate antibiotic therapy.

Immediate treatment of a peritonsillar abscess is recommended to prevent spread of the causative microorganism to the bloodstream or adjacent structures. Penicillin or other antibiotics are given immediately after a culture is obtained and before results of culture and sensitivity tests are known. Surgical incision and drainage of the abscess is done if the abscess partially blocks the oropharynx. The physician sprays or paints local anesthetic on the abscess surface, and evacuates contents. Repeated episodes may require a tonsillectomy.

Nursing management of the client undergoing drainage of an abscess includes placing the client in a semi-Fowler's position to prevent aspiration. An ice collar helps to reduce swelling and pain. The nurse encourages the client to drink fluids. He or she observes the client for signs of respiratory obstruction (e.g., dyspnea, restlessness, cyanosis) or excessive bleeding.

● LARYNGITIS

Laryngitis is inflammation and swelling of the mucous membrane that lines the larynx. Vocal cord edema frequently accompanies laryngeal inflammation. Laryngitis may follow a URI and occurs when infection spreads to the larynx. Other causes include excessive or improper use of the voice, allergies, and smoking.

Hoarseness, inability to speak above a whisper, or **aphonia** (complete loss of voice) are usual symptoms. Clients also have throat irritation and a dry, nonproductive cough. Diagnosis is based on symptoms. If hoarseness persists more than 2 weeks, the larynx is examined (**laryngoscopy**). Persistent hoarseness is a sign of laryngeal cancer and merits prompt investigation. Treatment involves voice rest and treatment or removal of the cause. Antibiotic therapy is used if there is bacterial infection. If smoking is the cause, the nurse encourages smoking cessation and refers the client to a smoking-cessation program.

STRUCTURAL DISORDERS

● EPISTAXIS

Pathophysiology and Etiology

Epistaxis, or nosebleed, is common, resulting from rupture of tiny capillaries in the nasal mucous membrane. It is not usually serious but is frightening. Nosebleeds are usually in the anterior septum, referred to as *Kiesselbach's area.* Causes include trauma, rheumatic fever, infection, hypertension, nasal tumors, and blood dyscrasias. Epistaxis resulting from hypertension or blood dyscrasias is likely to be severe and difficult to control. Those who abuse cocaine may have frequent nosebleeds. Foreign bodies in the nose and deviated septum contribute to epistaxis, along with forceful nose blowing and frequent or aggressive nose picking.

Assessment Findings

Inspection of the nares, using a nasal speculum and light, reveals the area of bleeding. The examiner uses a tongue blade to check the back of the throat and a laryngeal mirror to view the area above and behind the uvula.

Medical and Surgical Management

The severity and location of bleeding determine treatment. One or a combination of the following therapies may be used:

- Direct continuous pressure to nares for 5 to 10 minutes with client's head tilted slightly forward
- Application of ice packs to nose
- Cauterization with silver nitrate, electrocautery, or application of a topical vasoconstrictor such as 1:1000 epinephrine
- Nasal packing with a cotton tampon
- Pressure with a balloon inflated catheter—inserted posteriorly for a minimum of 48 hours

Nursing Management

Monitor vital signs and assess for signs of continued bleeding. Initiate measures to control bleeding, such as applying pressure and ice packs. Other treatments require a physician's order. The client experiencing epistaxis is usually anxious and requires reassurance. If underlying conditions are the cause, refer client for medical follow-up. Also recommend humidification, use of a nasal lubricant to keep mucous membranes moist, and avoidance of vigorous nose blowing and nose picking, or other nose trauma. Teaching about treatment of severe nosebleed includes the following:

- If epistaxis recurs, apply pressure to nares with two fingers. Breathe through mouth and sit with head tipped forward slightly to prevent blood from running down throat.
- Do not swallow blood; spit out any blood oozing from the area. Do not blow the nose.
- If blood is swallowed, diarrhea and black tarry stools may be seen for a few days.
- Do not attempt to remove nasal packing or cut string anchoring the packing.
- Take pain medications as ordered. Do not use aspirin or ibuprofen products until bleeding is controlled.
- Notify physician if bleeding persists or any respiratory problems develop.

● NASAL OBSTRUCTION

Obstruction of the nasal passage interferes with air passage. Three primary conditions lead to nasal obstruction: a deviated septum, nasal polyps, and hypertrophied turbinates.

Pathophysiology and Etiology

A **deviated septum** is an irregularity in the septum that results in nasal obstruction. Deviation may be a deflection from the midline in the form of lumps or sharp projections or a curvature shaped like an "S." Marked deviation can result in complete obstruction of one nostril and interference with sinus drainage. A deviated septum may be congenital, but often results from trauma.

Nasal polyps are grapelike swellings arising from nasal mucous membranes. They result from chronic irritation related to infection or allergic rhinitis. They obstruct nasal breathing and sinus drainage, leading to sinusitis. Most are benign and tend to recur when removed.

Hypertrophied turbinates are enlargements of nasal concha, three bones that project from the lateral wall of the nasal cavity. They hypertrophy, as a result of chronic rhinitis. This interferes with air passage and sinus drainage, and leads to sinusitis.

Assessment Findings

Symptoms include a history of sinusitis, difficulty breathing out of one nostril, frequent nosebleeds, and nasal discharge. Clients report difficulty breathing through one or both sides of the nose. Inspection with a nasal speculum reveals left or right deviation of the nasal septum, number and location of the polyps, or enlarged turbinates.

Medical and Surgical Management

A submucous surgical resection or septoplasty restores normal breathing and permits adequate sinus drainage for the client with a deviated septum. This procedure involves an incision through the mucous membrane and removal of portions of the septum that cause obstruction. After this procedure, both sides of the nasal cavity are packed with gauze, for 24 to 48 hours. A moustache dressing or drip pad is applied to absorb drainage.

Rhinoplasty, reconstruction of the nose, may also be done at the same time. This enhances the client's appearance cosmetically and corrects structural nasal deformities interfering with air passage. The surgeon makes an incision inside the nostril and restructures the nasal bone and cartilage. As with septoplasty, the nasal cavity is packed with gauze, and the nose is taped. Application of a nasal splint maintains shape and structure of the nose and reduces edema. The splint remains in place for at least 1 week.

Treatment for polyps includes a steroidal nasal spray to reduce inflammation or direct injection of steroids into the polyps. If nasal obstruction is severe, the surgeon performs a *polypectomy,* removal of polyps with a nasal snare or laser under local anesthesia. Polyps are examined microscopically to rule out malignant disease.

Hypertrophied turbinates may be treated with application of astringents or aerosolized corticosteroids to shrink them close to the nose. One of the turbinates may be surgically removed (*turbinectomy*).

Nursing Management

Surgery for nasal obstruction is usually done on an outpatient basis. Provide explanations throughout the procedures to alleviate anxiety. It is important to emphasize that nasal packing will be in place postoperatively, necessitating mouth breathing. Application of an ice pack will reduce pain and swelling.

Placing the client in a semi-Fowler's position promotes drainage, reduces edema, and enhances breathing. Inspect nasal packing and dressings frequently for bleeding and ask the client to report excessive swallowing, a sign of bleeding. Monitoring of vital signs is necessary, along with oral hygiene and saline mouth rinses (when permitted) to keep mucous membranes moist. Tell the client that feeling or hearing a sucking noise when swallowing is normal and will resolve when nasal packing is removed.

Teaching measures include preparing the postoperative client for edema and discoloration around the eyes and nose that disappears after a few weeks. Instruct the client in measures to prevent bleeding:

- Do not bend over.
- Do not blow nose.
- If sneezing, keep mouth open.
- Avoid contact with nose or surrounding tissue.
- Keep head elevated with an extra pillow when lying down.
- Avoid heavy lifting.
- Do not use aspirin, ibuprofen, alcohol, or tobacco products.

TRAUMA AND OBSTRUCTION OF THE UPPER AIRWAY

FRACTURES OF THE NOSE

A nasal fracture usually results from direct trauma. It causes swelling and edema of soft tissues, external and internal bleeding, nasal deformity, and nasal obstruction. In severe nasal fractures, cerebrospinal fluid, which is colorless and clear, may drain from the nares. This suggests a fracture in the cribriform plate.

Diagnosis of a nasal fracture may be delayed because of significant swelling and bleeding. As soon as swelling decreases, the examiner inspects the nose internally to rule out a fracture of the nasal septum or septal hematoma. Both conditions require treatment to prevent destruction of septal cartilage. If drainage of clear fluid is observed, a Dextrostix determines the presence of glucose, which is diagnostic for cerebrospinal fluid. X-rays ascertain any other facial fractures.

Medical and Surgical Management

If the fracture is a lateral displacement, the physician applies pressure to the convex portion of the nose to reduce the fracture. Cold compresses control bleeding. If the fracture is more complex, surgery is done after swelling subsides. The surgeon applies a splint postoperatively to maintain alignment.

Nursing Management

Instruct the client to keep head elevated and apply ice four times a day for 20 minutes, to reduce swelling and pain. Give analgesics as ordered to alleviate pain. Postoperatively, assess for airway obstruction, respiratory difficulty (i.e., tachypnea, dyspnea), dysphagia, signs of infection, pupillary responses, level of consciousness, and periorbital edema. Also answer questions and offer reassurance that bruising and swelling will subside and sense of smell will return.

Stop, Think, and Respond ● BOX 22-2

On your way to class, you see a woman suddenly slip on ice and fall on her face. As you approach, she gets to a sitting position. She is wearing a scarf. Blood is pouring from her nose, and your initial impression is that the nose appears deformed. What actions should you take?

LARYNGEAL TRAUMA AND LARYNGEAL OBSTRUCTION

Pathophysiology and Etiology

Laryngeal trauma occurs during motor vehicle accidents when the neck strikes the steering wheel or other blunt trauma occurs in the neck region. Endoscopic and endotracheal intubations are other possible causes. Laryngeal obstruction is a very serious and often life-threatening condition. Causes of upper airway obstruction include edema from an allergic reaction, severe head and neck injury, severe inflammation and edema of the throat, and aspiration of foreign bodies.

Assessment Findings

Laryngeal trauma causes neck swelling, bruising, and tenderness. If tissues surrounding the larynx are greatly swollen, the client exhibits **stridor,** a high-pitched, harsh sound during respiration, indicating airway obstruction. The client also has dysphagia, hoarseness, cyanosis, and possible **hemoptysis** (expectoration of bloody sputum).

Total obstruction prevents passage of air from the upper to the lower respiratory airway; choking clients clutch their throats—the universal distress sign. Unless total obstruction is relieved immediately, death occurs from respiratory arrest. Partial obstruction results in difficulty breathing.

Laryngoscopy reveals the extent of trauma and internal swelling. X-rays and oxygenation studies are performed after a patent airway is established.

Medical and Surgical Management

Maintenance of a patent airway is crucial. If the client has aspirated a foreign body, the Heimlich maneuver is performed to force the object out of the upper respiratory passages. Allergic reactions resulting in severe inflammation and edema may be treated with epinephrine or a corticosteroid and possibly intubation. Severe obstruction requires an emergency *tracheostomy* (surgical opening into the trachea).

Nursing Management

Assess for air movement within the upper respiratory tract. Listen to lung sounds, monitor respiratory patterns, and look for signs of increased nasal swelling and bleeding and symptoms of laryngeal edema. Determine if the airway is obstructed.

Partial or total obstruction of the upper airway requires immediate recognition and intervention. If present when a victim aspirates a foreign body, use the Heimlich maneuver. If this maneuver fails to dislodge the object, a physician may perform an emergency tracheostomy. If edema is the cause of partial upper airway obstruction, oxygen is given until a physician examines the client. Emergency drugs and a tracheostomy tray are available for immediate use. Also take measures to relieve pain and anxiety.

Assess airway patency at least every 2 hours, because maintaining the airway is the highest priority. Auscultate lungs for wheezing or decreased or absent breath sounds every 4 hours. Wheezing indicates increased airway resistance. Decreased or absent breath sounds indicate obstruction. Assess respiratory effort, including respiratory rate, depth, nasal flaring, and use of accessory muscles. Also, check vital signs and monitor for changes at least every 4 hours. Monitor arterial blood gases (ABGs). Increasing $PaCO_2$ and decreasing PaO_2 indicate impending respiratory failure. Place the client in semi-Fowler's position, which promotes maximum lung expansion and improved air exchange. Apply ice to nasal area four times a day for 20 to 30 minutes to reduce inflammation and bleeding. Initiate CPR and prepare for possible airway intubation/tracheostomy if airway is completely obstructed.

LARYNGEAL CANCER

With early detection, cancer of the larynx has great potential for cure. Preventive health measures focus on early consultation for persistent hoarseness and other changes in voice quality.

Pathophysiology and Etiology

Laryngeal cancer is most common in people 50 to 70 years of age. Men are affected more frequently than women. The cause of laryngeal cancer is unknown. Carcinogens, such as tobacco, alcohol, and industrial pollutants, are associated with laryngeal cancer. In addition, chronic laryngitis, habitual overuse of the voice, and heredity may contribute. Most laryngeal malignancies are squamous cell carcinomas, a malignancy arising from epithelial cells lining the larynx. The tumor may be located on the glottis (true vocal cords), above the glottis (supraglottis or false vocal cords), or below the glottis (subglottis).

Assessment Findings

Persistent hoarseness is usually the earliest symptom. At first hoarseness is slight. Later, the client notes a sensation of swelling or a lump in the throat, followed by dysphagia and pain when talking. The client may also complain of burning in the throat when swallowing hot or citrus liquids. If malignant tissue is not removed promptly, symptoms of advancing carcinoma, such as dyspnea, weakness, weight loss, enlarged cervical lymph nodes, pain, and anemia develop.

Visual examination of the larynx (laryngoscopy) and biopsy confirm the diagnosis and identify the type of malignancy. Computed tomography (CT) scanning and chest x-rays are used to detect metastasis and determine tumor size. The physician assesses the mobility of the vocal cords. Limited mobility indicates that tumor growth is affecting surrounding tissue, muscle, and airway.

Medical and Surgical Management

Treatment depends on factors such as size of the lesion, client's age, and metastasis. Medical treatment may include chemotherapy, which has minimal effects, and radiation therapy, either alone or with surgery.

Surgical treatment (Table 22.1) includes laser surgery for early lesions or a partial or total laryngectomy. In more advanced cases, total laryngectomy may be the treatment of choice. If the disease has extended beyond the larynx, a radical neck dissection (removal of the lymph nodes, muscles, and adjacent tissues) is performed. Laser surgery may also be used to relieve obstruction in more advanced cases.

A client with a total laryngectomy has a permanent tracheal *stoma* (opening) because the trachea is no longer connected to the nasopharynx. The larynx is severed from the trachea and removed completely. The only respiratory organs in use are the trachea, bronchi, and lungs. Air enters and leaves through the tracheostomy. The client no longer feels air entering the nose (Fig. 22.1). Because the anterior wall of the esophagus connects with the posterior wall of the larynx, it must be reconstructed. Tube feeding facilitates healing by preventing muscle activity and irritation of the esophagus (see Chap. 46).

TABLE 22.1 DESCRIPTIONS OF LARYNGEAL SURGERY

SURGERY	DESCRIPTION	INDICATION	POSTOPERATIVE EXPECTATIONS
Partial laryngectomy	The affected vocal cord is removed; other structures remain intact	For early-stage laryngeal cancer when only one cord is involved	Voice will be hoarse; intact trachea; no problems with swallowing; high cure rate
Supraglottic laryngectomy	Hyoid bone, glottis, and false cords removed; radical neck dissection done on involved side; remaining structures left intact	For supraglottic tumors	Voice will be hoarse; postoperative tracheostomy until glottic airway functions; nutrition administered through nasogastric tube until surgical sites heal; recurrence is possible
Hemivertical laryngectomy	Thyroid cartilage of trachea is split at midline; one true cord and one false cord are removed along with arytenoid cartilage and half the thyroid cartilage.	When tumor extends beyond the vocal cord but is smaller than 1 cm	Client will have a tracheostomy and nasogastric tube after surgery until healed; voice will be hoarse and diminished; client will have an intact airway and the ability to swallow.
Total laryngectomy	Both vocal cords removed along with the hyoid bone, epiglottis, cricoid cartilage, and two or three rings of the trachea; the tongue, pharyngeal walls, and trachea remain intact; usually a radical neck dissection is done on the affected side.	When the cancer extends beyond the vocal cords	Permanent tracheal stoma; prevents aspiration. No voice but ability to swallow remains. Metastasis to cervical lymph nodes is common.
Radical neck dissection	The neck is opened from the jaw to the clavicle from the midline to the interior border of the trapezius muscle. The following are removed: subcutaneous and soft tissue, sternocleidomastoid muscle, jugular vein, and spinal accessory nerve innervates trapezius muscle—client's shoulder will droop after surgery as the trapezius muscle atrophies). A split-thickness skin graft is applied over the carotid artery.	When cancer has metastasized to cervical lymph nodes	Permanent tracheal stoma. No voice; ability to swallow remains. Client requires physical therapy for neck muscles, along with a prescribed exercise program.

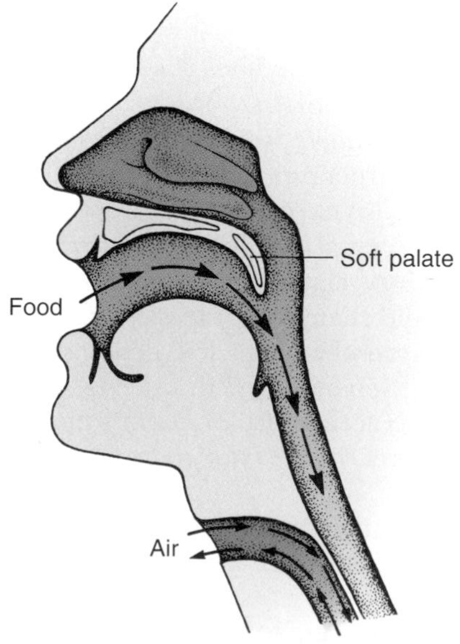

FIGURE 22.1 Air enters and leaves through a permanent tracheal stoma.

Loss of the ability to speak normally is a devastating consequence of laryngeal surgery. Communication with others is a basic need. Clients with a malignancy of the larynx require emotional support before and after surgery and help in understanding and choosing an alternative method of speech. Some methods of alaryngeal speech used after a laryngectomy include the following:

- *Esophageal speech*—requires regurgitation of swallowed air and formation of words with lips
- *Artificial (electric) larynx*—a throat vibrator held against the neck that projects sound into the mouth; words are formed with the mouth
- *Tracheoesophageal puncture (TEP)*—a surgical opening in the posterior wall of the trachea, followed by insertion of a prosthesis (Figure 22.2). Air from the lungs is diverted through the opening in the posterior tracheal wall to the esophagus and out the mouth.

A speech pathologist works with the client to use an artificial speech device, learn esophageal speech, or speak

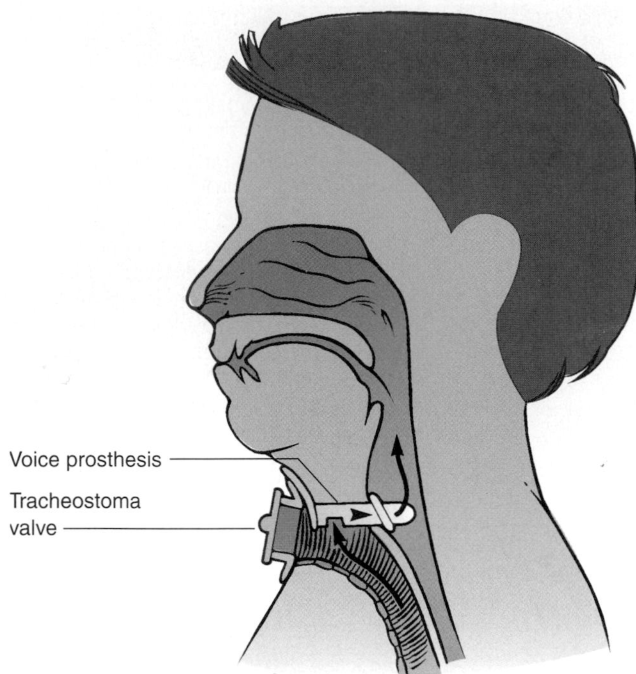

FIGURE 22.2 Schematic representation of TEP. (From Smeltzer, S. C., & Bare, B. G. [2004]. *Brunner & Suddarth's textbook of medical–surgical nursing* [10th ed.]. Philadelphia: Lippincott Williams & Wilkins.)

clearly with a prosthesis. Clients having a partial laryngectomy also may require speech therapy.

NURSING PROCESS

The Client Undergoing Laryngeal Surgery

Assessment

Determine the client's level of understanding of the diagnosis, reason for surgery, and probable outcome. Assess for hoarseness, sore throat, dyspnea, dysphagia, pain, or burning in the throat. Ascertaining the client's level of anxiety is important, as is identifying coping strategies. Also assess the client's ability to communicate in ways other than speaking, such as ability to read and write. Begin preoperative teaching, allowing the client to express fears about surgery, diagnosis, and potential loss of voice postoperatively. Discuss alternative methods of communication and identify which method the client prefers. After surgery, carefully assess for a patent airway and effective airway clearance.

Diagnosis, Planning, and Interventions

Care centers around preventing postoperative complications, managing pain, preventing wound infection, helping the client communicate, and fostering the client's ability to cope with changes in body image. Provide the client and family with the following postoperative instructions:

- Water should not enter the stoma because it will flow from the trachea to the lungs. Thus, avoid swimming, and take care when bathing. Avoid showers until experienced with care of the stoma, and then use a hand-held shower device if possible.
- Wear a scarf or gauze dressing over the stoma to make the opening less obvious.
- Avoid fabrics or dressings that fray to prevent small fibers from being drawn into the stoma.

Ineffective Airway Clearance related to surgical alterations of the airway

Expected Outcome: Client will maintain effective airway clearance as evidenced by clear breath sounds, normal respirations, and effective cough.

- Position client in semi-Fowler's position. *Provides optimal lung expansion and decreases edema in the surgical site.*
- Auscultate breath sounds and respiratory effort at least every 4 hours. *Initial and ongoing assessments provide a baseline for comparison.*
- Assess effectiveness of client's cough. *An effective cough will promote airway clearance.*
- Encourage deep breathing and coughing every 2 hours while client is awake. *Prevents atelectasis and promotes effective gas exchange.*
- Monitor for restlessness, dyspnea, anxiety, and increased heart rate. *These signs indicate ineffective airway clearance.*
- Observe level of consciousness for signs of lethargy or disorientation. *These signs indicate poor gas exchange.*

Impaired Verbal Communication related to removal of larynx and postoperative edema

Expected Outcome: Client will communicate effectively with alternative methods.

- Frequently assess client's need to communicate. *Assessments alleviate client's anxiety.*
- Allow client time to communicate needs. *Promotes acceptance of client and decreases anxiety about ability to communicate.*
- Provide alternative methods of communication: paper and pen, wipe board, or word or picture board. *Having supplies available provides comfort to client.*
- Reinforce instructions regarding use of a voice prosthesis, electrolarynx, or esophageal speech. *Helps client to become more proficient with alternative speech methods.*

Social Isolation related to change in body image, tracheal stoma, and change in or loss of speech

Expected Outcome: Client will demonstrate evidence of adjustment to changes and resume social interactions.

- Demonstrate acceptance of client's changed appearance. *Provides a sense of belonging and promotes positive self-esteem.*
- Encourage client to maintain or reestablish social relationships. *Reduces sense of isolation and increases feelings of acceptance.*
- Provide time for client to express feelings about changes. *Assists client to cope with changes.*

- Refer client to support services such as the International Association of Laryngectomies, and arrange for visits from clients who have had a laryngectomy. *Rehabilitation is lengthy; support from others has a positive effect.*

Evaluation of Expected Outcomes

The client maintains a clear airway, effectively clearing secretions. He or she demonstrates effective alternative communication methods. The client maintains or establishes social interactions and copes with changes.

TREATMENT MODALITIES FOR AIRWAY OBSTRUCTION OR AIRWAY MAINTENANCE

Clients with serious airway conditions require aggressive treatment to maintain an airway or relieve airway obstruction. This section discusses tracheostomy, tracheotomy, endotracheal intubation, and mechanical ventilation.

• TRACHEOSTOMY AND TRACHEOTOMY

A **tracheotomy** is the surgical procedure that makes an opening into the trachea. A **tracheostomy** is a surgical opening into the trachea into which a tracheostomy or laryngectomy tube is inserted. A tracheostomy may be temporary or permanent. A permanent opening in the trachea is required for certain disorders, such as a laryngectomy for laryngeal cancer.

• ENDOTRACHEAL INTUBATION AND MECHANICAL VENTILATION

An endotracheal tube (Fig. 22.3) is inserted through the mouth or nose into the trachea to provide a patent airway for clients who cannot maintain an adequate airway on their own. Examples include those with respiratory difficulty, comatose clients, those undergoing general anesthesia, and clients with extensive edema of upper airway passages.

General Considerations

An endotracheal tube can remain in place for up to 2 weeks. The cuff is inflated to provide a tight seal. The endotracheal tube is attached to a ventilator for control of respirations and ventilation of the lungs. Humidification is necessary because air going to the lungs through an endotracheal tube does not pass through moist mucous membranes of the upper airway.

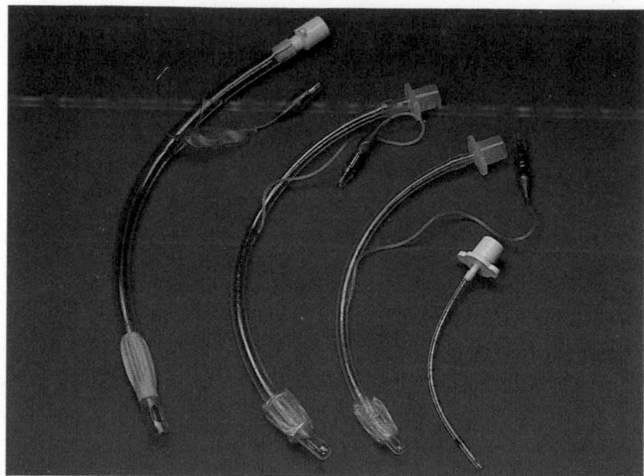

FIGURE 22.3 Endotracheal tubes.

There are several modes of mechanical ventilation, classified according to the manner in which they support ventilation. Two major classifications are negative-pressure and positive-pressure ventilators (Table 22.2). Positive-pressure ventilators are used more commonly. The major difference between the two types is that negative-pressure ventilators exert negative pressure, a pulling or sucking force, on the external chest, while positive-pressure ventilators inflate the lungs by exerting positive pressure, pushing air into the airway. Negative-pressure ventilators are used for clients with chronic respiratory failure related to neuromuscular disease such as poliomyelitis or myasthenia gravis. Positive-pressure ventilators require intubation and are used for clients with acute respiratory failure and primary lung disease, such as cystic fibrosis, or for clients who are comatose, under general anesthesia, or have extensive upper airway edema.

Accidental removal of an endotracheal tube must be prevented because this can result in laryngeal edema or **laryngospasm** (spasm of the laryngeal muscles, resulting in narrowing of the larynx) and subsequent respiratory arrest. The inflated cuff and placement of tape around the tube attached to the client's cheek secures the endotracheal tube. The proximal end of the tube is marked for determining if downward displacement has occurred.

The intubated client has the endotracheal tube removed when vital capacity is adequate and the client can breathe without assistance. Blood gas studies also are used as a guideline for removal. Depending on hospital policy, removal of an endotracheal tube may be done by the nurse, respiratory therapist, or doctor. If

TABLE 22.2 TYPES OF MECHANICAL VENTILATORS

CLASSIFICATION	HOW USED
Negative pressure	Exerts negative pressure on chest; decreases intrathoracic pressure during inspiration, allowing air to flow into lungs; does not require intubation Used for clients experiencing chronic respiratory failure, such as in poliomyelitis, myasthenia gravis, muscular dystrophy, amyotrophic lateral sclerosis
Drinker respirator tank	Also known as the *iron lung;* a negative-pressure chamber; used extensively in the past for clients with poliomyelitis
Body wrap (pneumowrap) and chest cuirass (tortoise shell)	Requires a rigid cage or shell around the thorax to create a negative-pressure chamber
Positive pressure	Exerts positive pressure on airway to inflate lungs; expiration is passive Usually requires endotracheal or tracheal intubation
Pressure-cycled	Inspiration ends when a preset pressure is reached; *cycle* means that ventilator cycles on, delivers flow of air until a certain pressure is reached, and then cycles off Designed for short-term use because volume of air varies as client's airway resistance or compliance changes
Time-cycled	Controls respiration after a preset time; length of inspiration and flow rate of air regulate volume the client receives; usually used on newborns and infants
Volume-cycled	Delivers a preset volume of air with each inspiration; once volume is delivered, ventilator cycles off and client expires air passively Provides consistent adequate breaths despite airway resistance or changes in compliance; most commonly used ventilator for adults
Noninvasive	Ventilation delivered by face masks or other nasal devices; does not require intubation of any kind; used for clients with sleep-related breathing disorders or other chronic respiratory disorders

laryngospasm occurs, air is administered by positive pressure. Reinsertion of the endotracheal tube by the physician or other trained personnel may be necessary if laryngospasm continues. Possible complications with use of endotracheal intubation include ulceration and stricture of the trachea or larynx, atelectasis, and pneumonia.

Nursing Management

Major goals for the intubated client are to improve respirations, maintain a patent airway, and communicate needs to others. Monitor vital signs periodically, depending on the client's condition and the reason for endotracheal tube insertion. Blood gas studies and pulse oximetry provide methods of ongoing evaluation of the client's respiratory status. Review results of these studies and report changes to the physician.

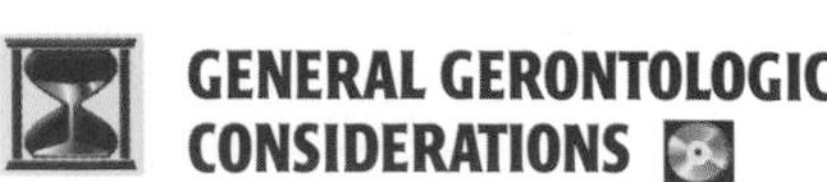

GENERAL GERONTOLOGIC CONSIDERATIONS

If an older adult requires a tracheostomy, be alert to possible confusion after the procedure. If clients are confused or do not understand the purpose of the procedure, they may attempt to pull at the tube or remove it. Restraining measures may be required.

The common cold may be potentially serious for older adults, especially when they have other diseases such as a chronic respiratory disorder or heart disease. Advise older clients to see a physician if cold symptoms are severe or breathing is difficult.

After a laryngectomy, older clients may require extra time and instruction to learn esophageal speech, speak with an electric larynx, or use TEP.

Critical Thinking Exercises

1. *A client with severe pharyngitis is diagnosed with a group A streptococcal infection. The physician prescribes penicillin. What discharge instructions should you give the client?*
2. *Your client is scheduled for a partial laryngectomy. What information must you share to help prepare her for the postoperative period?*

● NCLEX-STYLE REVIEW QUESTIONS 

1. An adult is completing his preoperative tests prior to the scheduled tonsillectomy and adenoidectomy. Which test(s) is most important to review before surgery?
   1. Chest x-ray
   2. Electrocardiogram
   3. Blood count
   4. Blood chemistry

2. The nurse is providing postoperative care for a client who has undergone tonsillectomy. In which position will the nurse place the head of the bed when the client is fully awake?
   1. Flat with the head elevated on a pillow
   2. Slightly raised at a 15° angle
   3. Raised at a 45° angle
   4. Raised at a 90° sitting position

3. A client comes to the doctor's office stating that he has a lump in his throat and is afraid that it is cancer. Which initial question by the nurse addresses the earliest symptom of laryngeal cancer?
   1. "Do you smoke or have you ever smoked?"
   2. "Do you have a burning in your throat?"
   3. "Do you have swollen lymph nodes?"
   4. "Did you notice a persistent cough?"

connection

Visit the Connection site at **http://connection.lww.com/go/timbyEssentials** for links to chapter-related resources on the Internet.

References and Suggested Readings

Carpenito, L. J. (2002). *Nursing diagnosis: Application to clinical practice* (9th ed.). Philadelphia: Lippincott Williams & Wilkins.

Dixon, B., & Tasota, F. J. (2003). Action stat: Inadvertent tracheal decannulation. *Nursing 2003, 33*(1), 96.

Fowler, S. (2000). Know how: Humidification. A guide to humidification. *Nursing Times, 96*(20), 10–11.

Klein, L. (2001). Sinusitis: When to treat and how. *RN, 64*(1), 42–48.

Kunz, M. G. (April 1, 2002). Season for sneezes. *Advance for Nurses,* 25–26.

Putnam, H., & May, K. R. (2001). Relief for patients with severe allergies. *RN, 64*(6), 27–30.

Schreiber, D. (2001). Trach care at home. *RN, 64*(7), 43–46.

Seay, S. J. & Gay, S. L. (2002). Tracheostomy emergencies. *American Journal of Nursing, 102*(3), 59–63.

Sheard, S. (March 18, 2002). Airborne enemies. *Advance for Nurses,* 29–31.

Smeltzer, S. C., & Bare, B. G. (2004). *Brunner & Suddarth's textbook of medical–surgical nursing* (10th ed.). Philadelphia: Lippincott Williams & Wilkins.

chapter 23

Caring for Clients With Disorders of the Lower Respiratory Airway

Words to Know 

acute bronchitis
asbestosis
asthma
atelectasis
bronchiectasis
chronic bronchitis
chronic obstructive pulmonary disease
emphysema
empyema
flail chest
hemoptysis
influenza
lobectomy
lung abscess
pleural effusion
pleurisy
pneumoconiosis
pneumonectomy
pneumonia
pneumothorax
pulmonary contusion
pulmonary edema
pulmonary embolism
segmental resection
septicemia
silicosis
subcutaneous emphysema
thoracentesis
thoracotomy
tracheitis
tracheobronchitis
tuberculosis
wedge resection

Learning Objectives

On completion of this chapter, the reader will:

- Describe infectious and inflammatory disorders of the lower respiratory airway.
- Identify critical assessments needed for a client with an infectious disorder of the lower respiratory airway.
- Define disorders classified as obstructive pulmonary disease.
- Discuss strategies for preventing and managing occupational lung diseases.
- List risk factors associated with the development of pulmonary embolism.
- Discuss conditions that may lead to acute respiratory distress syndrome.
- Differentiate acute and chronic respiratory failure.
- Explain why lung cancer often is diagnosed after the disease is advanced.
- Describe the nursing assessments required for a client who experiences trauma to the chest.
- Explain the purpose of chest tubes after thoracic surgery.
- Describe the preoperative and postoperative nursing management for clients undergoing thoracic care.

Exchange of gases and ventilation occur in the lower respiratory tract, which is subject to various problems compromising its ability to perform primary functions. If untreated, many disorders can lead to respiratory failure or become chronic and affect quality of life.

INFECTIOUS AND INFLAMMATORY DISORDERS

Infectious and inflammatory disorders of the lower airway are medically more serious than those of the upper airway. Inflammation and infection in the alveoli and bronchioles impair gas exchange. Clients may experience difficulty in maintaining a clear airway secondary to retained secretions.

• ACUTE BRONCHITIS

Pathophysiology and Etiology

Inflammation of mucous membranes that line the major bronchi and their branches characterizes **acute bronchitis.** If the inflammatory process involves the trachea, it is referred to as **tracheobronchitis.** Typically, acute bronchitis begins as an upper respiratory infection (URI); the inflammatory process then extends to the tracheobronchial tree. Secretory cells of the mucosa produce increased mucopurulent sputum.

Viral infections most commonly give rise to acute bronchitis. Clients with viral URIs are more vulnerable to secondary bacterial infections, which can lead to acute bronchitis. Sputum cultures identify causative bacterial organisms, the most common of which are *Haemophilus influenzae* and *Mycoplasma pneumoniae*. Chemical irritation from noxious fumes also may induce acute bronchitis. A potential complication is bronchial asthma.

Assessment Findings

Signs and symptoms initially include fever, malaise, and a dry, nonproductive cough later producing mucopurulent sputum, which may be blood streaked if airway mucosa becomes irritated with severe tracheobronchitis and coughing. Clients experience paroxysmal attacks of coughing and may report wheezing. Laryngitis and sinusitis complicate symptoms. Moist inspiratory crackles may be heard on chest auscultation. A sputum sample for culture and sensitivity testing rules out bacterial infection. A chest film may be done to detect additional pathology, such as pneumonia.

Medical Management

Acute bronchitis usually is self-limiting, lasting for several days. Treatment is bed rest, antipyretics, expectorants, antitussives, and increased fluids. Humidifiers assist in keeping mucous membranes moist because dry air aggravates the cough. If secondary bacterial invasion occurs, there is a persistent cough with thick, purulent sputum. Secondary infections usually subside as bronchitis subsides, but may persist for several weeks. The physician orders a broad-spectrum antibiotic when sputum culture results are available.

Nursing Management

Auscultate breath sounds and monitor vital signs every 4 hours, especially if the client has a fever. Encourage the client to cough and deep breathe every 2 hours while awake and to expectorate rather than swallow sputum. Humidification of surrounding air loosens bronchial secretions. Change bedding and the client's clothes if they become damp with perspiration and offer fluids frequently. Teach the client to wash hands frequently, particularly when handling secretions and soiled tissues; cover the mouth when sneezing and coughing; discard soiled tissues in a plastic bag; and avoid sharing eating utensils and personal articles with others to prevent spread of infection.

• PNEUMONIA

Pneumonia is an inflammatory process affecting bronchioles and alveoli. Although usually associated with an acute infection, pneumonia may result from radiation therapy, chemical ingestion or inhalation, or aspiration of foreign bodies or gastric contents.

Pathophysiology and Etiology

Pneumonia is classified according to its etiology and presenting symptoms. Bacterial pneumonias are referred to as *typical pneumonias*. Atypical pneumonias are those caused by mycoplasmas, *Legionella pneumophila* (the causative agent of Legionnaire's disease), viruses, and fungi. *Mycobacterium tuberculosis* also may cause pneumonia. Viruses, usually type A, are the most common etiology. Bacterial pneumonias are less common but more serious. Causative bacterial organisms include *Streptococcus pneumoniae, Pneumocystis carinii, Staphylococcus aureus, Klebsiella pneumoniae, Pseudomonas aeruginosa,* and *H. influenzae*.

Radiation pneumonia results from damage to normal lung mucosa during radiation therapy for breast or lung cancer. Chemical pneumonia results from ingesting kerosene or inhaling volatile hydrocarbons (kerosene or gasoline), which can occur in industrial settings. Aspiration pneumonia may occur when a person inhales a foreign body or gastric contents during vomiting or regurgitation. Hypoventilation of lung tissue over a prolonged period can occur when a client is bedridden and breathing with only part of the lungs. Bronchial secretions subsequently accumulate, which may lead to hypostatic pneumonia.

Bronchopneumonia means that the infection is patchy, diffuse, and scattered. *Lobar pneumonia* means that the inflammation is confined to one or more lobes of the lung (Fig. 23.1).

Another classification of pneumonia refers to where the client acquired it. Community-acquired pneumonia (CAP) means that the client contracted it in a community setting or within 48 hours of admission to a health-

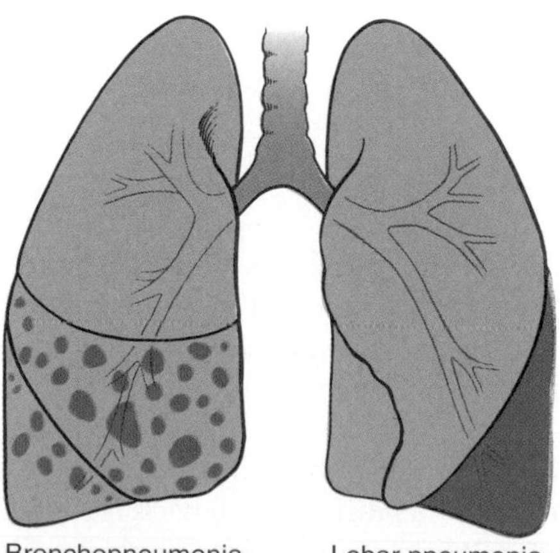

FIGURE 23.1 Distribution of lung involvement in bronchopneumonia and lobar pneumonia.

care facility. Hospital-acquired pneumonia (HAP), or nosocomial pneumonia, occurs in a healthcare setting more than 48 hours after admission. HAP is the most dangerous nosocomial infection (Smeltzer & Bare, 2004).

Organisms that cause pneumonia reach alveoli by inhalation of droplets, aspiration of organisms from the upper airway, or, less commonly, seeding from the bloodstream. When organisms reach alveoli, the inflammatory reaction is intense, producing an exudate that impairs gas exchange. Capillaries surrounding alveoli become engorged and cause alveoli to collapse (atelectasis), further impairing gas exchange and interfering with ventilation. White blood cells (WBCs) move into the area to destroy pathogens, filling interstitial spaces. If untreated, consolidation occurs as inflammation and exudate increase. Hypoxemia results from inability of the lungs to oxygenate blood from the heart. Bronchitis, **tracheitis** (inflammation of the trachea), and spots of *necrosis* (death of tissue) in the lung may follow.

In atypical pneumonias, the exudate infiltrates interstitial spaces rather than alveoli directly. The pneumonia is more scattered, as described for bronchopneumonia, and increasingly interferes with gas exchange. Increased carbon dioxide (CO_2) in the blood stimulates the respiratory center, causing more rapid and shallow breathing.

With any type of pneumonia, the client becomes increasingly ill. If the circulatory system cannot compensate for decreased gas exchange, the client is at risk for heart failure. Death from pneumonia is most common in older adults and those weakened by acute or chronic diseases or disorders or prolonged periods of inactivity. Complications include congestive heart failure (CHF), **empyema** (collection of pus in the pleural cavity), **pleurisy** (inflammation of the pleura), **septicemia** (infective microorganisms in the blood), atelectasis, hypotension, and shock. Septicemia may lead to a secondary focus of infection, such as endocarditis (inflammation of the endocardium), pericarditis (inflammation of the pericardium), and purulent arthritis. Otitis media (infection of the middle ear), bronchitis, or sinusitis also may complicate recovery, especially from atypical pneumonia.

Assessment Findings

Symptoms vary for different types of pneumonia. The onset of bacterial pneumonia is sudden. Clients experience fever, chills, a productive cough, and discomfort in chest wall muscles from coughing, along with general malaise. Sputum may be rust colored. Breathing causes pain, leading to shallow breathing.

Viral pneumonia differs from bacterial pneumonia in that blood cultures are negative, sputum may be more copious, chills are less common, and pulse and respiratory rates are characteristically slow. The course of viral pneumonia usually is less severe than bacterial pneumonia. Mortality rate from viral pneumonia is low but rises when bacterial pneumonia secondarily occurs. Many clients with viral pneumonia are weak and ill for a longer period than those with successfully treated bacterial pneumonia.

Auscultation of the chest reveals wheezing, crackles, and decreased breath sounds. Nail beds, lips, and oral mucosa may be cyanotic. Sputum culture and sensitivity studies help to identify infectious microorganism and effective antibiotics for bacterial pneumonia. A chest film shows areas of infiltrates and consolidation. A complete blood count discloses an elevated WBC count. Blood cultures also may be done to detect any microorganisms in the blood.

Medical Management

Medical management involves prompt initiation of antibiotic therapy for bacterial pneumonia, hydration to thin secretions, supplemental oxygen to alleviate hypoxemia, bed rest, chest physical therapy, bronchodilators, analgesics, antipyretics, and cough expectorants or suppressants, depending on the nature of the client's cough. If a client is hospitalized, treatment is more vigorous, depending on complications. Fluid and electrolyte replacement may be needed secondary to fever, dehydration, and inadequate nutrition. If the client experiences severe respiratory difficulty and thick, copious secretions, he or she may require intubation along with mechanical ventilation.

Nursing Management

Auscultate lung sounds and monitor the client for signs of respiratory difficulty. Check oxygenation status with pulse oximetry and monitor arterial blood gases (ABGs). Assessments of cough and sputum production also are necessary.

Place the client in semi-Fowler's position to facilitate breathing. Increased fluid intake helps to loosen secretions and replace fluids lost through fever and increased respiratory rate. Monitor fluid intake and output, skin turgor, vital signs, and serum electrolytes. Administer antipyretics as indicated and ordered.

Identifying clients at risk for pneumonia provides a means to practice preventive nursing care. Nursing Guidelines 23-1 identifies strategies for clients who are at risk for pneumonia. Nurses encourage at-risk and elderly clients to receive vaccination against pneumococcal and influenza infections. Because the nursing care of clients with infectious lung disorders is similar regardless of the etiology, refer to Nursing Process: Tuberculosis for additional interventions.

NURSING GUIDELINES 23-1

Preventing Pneumonia

- Promote coughing and expectoration of secretions if client experiences increased mucus production.
- Change position frequently if client is immobilized for any reason.
- Encourage deep breathing and coughing exercises at least every 2 hours.
- Administer chest physical therapy as indicated.
- Suction client if he or she cannot expectorate.
- Prevent aspiration in clients at risk.
- Prevent infections.
- Cleanse respiratory equipment on a routine basis.
- Promote frequent oral hygiene.
- Administer sedatives and opioids carefully to avoid respiratory depression.
- Encourage client to stop smoking and reduce alcohol intake.

• PLEURISY

Pleurisy or *pleuritis* refers to acute inflammation of the parietal and visceral pleurae. During the acute phase, the pleurae are inflamed, thick, and swollen, and an exudate forms from fibrin and lymph. Eventually the pleurae become rigid. During inspiration, the inflamed pleurae rub together, causing severe, sharp pain.

Pathophysiology and Etiology

Pleurisy usually occurs secondary to pneumonia or other pulmonary infections. The inflammation spreads from the lungs to the parietal pleura. Pleurisy may develop with tuberculosis (TB), lung cancer, cardiac and renal disease, systemic infections, or pulmonary embolism.

Assessment Findings

Respirations become shallow secondary to excruciating pain. Pleural fluid accumulates as inflammation worsens. Pain decreases as fluid increases because fluid separates the pleura. The client develops a dry cough, fatigues easily, and experiences dyspnea. A *friction rub* (coarse sounds heard during inspiration and early expiration) is heard during auscultation early in the disease process. As fluid accumulates, the pleural friction rub disappears. Decreased ventilation may result in atelectasis, hypoxemia, and hypercapnia.

Chest x-rays show changes in the affected area. Microscopic examination of sputum and a sputum culture may reveal pathogenic microorganisms. If a **thoracentesis** (removal of fluid from the chest) is performed, a pleural fluid specimen is sent to the laboratory for analysis. The physician may perform a pleural biopsy.

Medical Management

The underlying condition dictates treatment. Analgesic and antipyretic drugs provide relief for pain and fever. A nonsteroidal anti-inflammatory drug (NSAID) such as indomethacin (Indocin) provides analgesia and promotes more effective coughing. Severe cases may require a procaine intercostal nerve block.

Nursing Management

When the client has considerable pain with inspiration, instruct the client to take analgesic medications as prescribed. Heat or cold applications provide some topical comfort. Teach the client to splint the chest wall by turning onto the affected side. The client also can splint the chest wall with his or her hands or a pillow when coughing. If the client is very anxious, he or she needs reassurance.

• PLEURAL EFFUSION

Pleural effusion is the collection of fluid between the visceral and parietal pleurae. It may be a complication of pneumonia, lung cancer, TB, pulmonary embolism, and CHF. The amount of accumulated fluid may be so great that the lung partially collapses on the affected side and results in pressure on the heart and other organs of the mediastinum.

Fever, pain, and dyspnea are the most common symptoms. Chest percussion reveals dullness over the involved area. The examiner may note diminished or absent breath sounds over the involved area when auscultating the lungs and may hear a friction rub. Chest x-ray and computed tomography (CT) scan show fluid in the involved area. Thoracentesis may be done to remove pleural fluid for analysis and examination for malignant cells.

The main goal of treatment is to eliminate the cause. Treatment includes antibiotics, analgesics, cardiotonic drugs to control CHF (when present), thoracentesis to remove excess pleural fluid, or surgery for cancer.

If thoracentesis is needed, prepare the client for this procedure (see Nursing Guidelines 21-3). The client usually is frightened and needs support.

● LUNG ABSCESS AND EMPYEMA

A **lung abscess** is a localized area of pus formation in the lung parenchyma. As the abscess increases, the tissue becomes necrotic. Later, the affected area collapses and creates a cavity. The infection can then extend into one or both bronchi and the pleural cavity.

A lung abscess may develop from aspiration, pneumonia, or mechanical obstruction of the bronchi, such as with a tumor. Other causes include necrosis of lung tissue after an infection and necrotic lesions resulting from inhalation of dust particles. Clients with an impaired cough reflex or altered immune function are at risk for lung abscesses.

Empyema is a general term for pus in a body cavity. It generally refers to pus or infected fluid in the pleural cavity (*thoracic empyema*). It may follow chest trauma, such as a stab or gunshot wound, or a pre-existing disease, such as pneumonia or TB. The pus-filled area may become walled off and enclosed by a thick membrane.

Assessment Findings

Signs and symptoms for both conditions include chills, fever, weight loss, anorexia, chest pain, dyspnea, and a productive cough. Sputum may be purulent or blood streaked. Finger clubbing may occur in chronic cases. Chest auscultation reveals dull or absent breath sounds in the affected abscess. Chest x-ray and CT scan usually locate the abscess. Results of blood and sputum cultures may be positive for pathogens. Chest percussion detects an area of dullness. In some instances, thoracentesis may be done, with the aspirated fluid sent to the laboratory for culture and sensitivity tests.

Medical and Surgical Management

For a lung abscess, postural drainage and antibiotics assist in controlling the infection. Occasionally, a lobectomy is performed to remove the abscess and surrounding lung tissue.

A thoracentesis may be done for empyema to aspirate purulent fluid to identify microorganisms, remove pus or fluid, and select appropriate antibiotic therapy. Closed drainage may be used to empty the empyemic cavity. **Thoracotomy** (surgical opening of the thorax) is performed, and one or more large chest tubes are inserted, which are then connected to an underwater-seal drainage bottle. Open drainage, which necessitates the removal of a section of one or more ribs, may be used when pus is thick and the walls of the empyemic cavity are strong enough to keep the lung from collapsing while the chest is opened. One or more tubes may be placed in the opening to promote drainage. The wound is then covered by a large absorbent dressing, which is changed as necessary. The drainage of pus results in a drop in temperature and general symptomatic improvement.

Inadequately treated empyema may become chronic. A thick coating forms over the lung, preventing its expansion. *Decortication* (removal of the coating) and evacuation of the pleural space allow the lung to re-expand.

Nursing Management

Monitor the client for possible adverse effects of antibiotics, administer chest physical therapy as indicated, and encourage the client to deep breathe and cough frequently. A diet high in protein and calories is essential. Provide emotional support, while being honest with the client that lung abscess and empyema take a long time to resolve.

● INFLUENZA

Influenza (flu) is an acute respiratory disease of relatively short duration. Major strains of flu virus are A, B, and C; the strains are related yet different. Each virus can mutate and produce variants within the given strain. Variants are called *subtypes.* Viruses that cause influenza are transmitted through the respiratory tract.

Flu chiefly occurs in epidemics, although sporadic cases may appear. Because viruses change, antibodies produced by those who have had one case of flu are not effective against new subtypes, and a different antibody must be produced annually or during major epidemics. Most clients recover. Fatalities occur from secondary bacterial complications, especially among pregnant women, elderly or debilitated clients, and those with chronic conditions, such as cardiac disease and emphysema.

During a flu epidemic, death from pneumonia and cardiovascular disease rises. Complications include tracheobronchitis, bacterial pneumonia, and cardiovascular disease. Staphylococcal pneumonia is the most serious complication. Table 23.1 lists signs and symptoms of flu. Additional diagnostic studies, such as chest x-ray and sputum analysis, are done to rule out other diseases.

Nursing management focuses on prevention. Annual flu vaccinations are recommended for healthcare workers and people at high risk for complications or exposed daily to many different people. Each year a new vaccine is developed from three different virus strains that are predicted to be present in the coming flu season.

Clients admitted to the hospital with flu need to be isolated from clients who do not have it. Nurses maintain airborne transmission precautions when caring for those clients. If a community is experiencing an epidemic, hospitals and other healthcare facilities usually develop policies regarding visitation and admissions.

TABLE 23.1	SIGNS AND SYMPTOMS OF INFLUENZA
Incubation period	1–3 days
Onset	Sudden Abrupt onset of fever and chills Severe headache Muscle aches
Progression	Anorexia Weakness, apathy, malaise Respiratory symptoms: Sneezing Sore throat, laryngitis Dry cough Nasal discharge–rhinitis Conjunctival irritation
Duration	Fever may persist for 3 days; other symptoms usually continue for 7–10 days. Cough may persist longer.
Period of contagion	2–3 days beginning with onset of symptoms

• PULMONARY TUBERCULOSIS

Pulmonary **tuberculosis** (TB) is a bacterial infectious disease primarily caused by *M. tuberculosis.* It affects the lungs, but may also affect kidneys and other organs. TB is a worldwide health problem, affecting one third of the world's population. It is the leading cause of death from infectious diseases and among people with human immunodeficiency virus (HIV) infection (World Health Organization, 2001). In the United States, there is increased TB, with newer cases found to be resistant to drugs.

Pathophysiology and Etiology

Tubercle bacilli are gram-positive, rod-shaped, acid-fast, and aerobic. They exist in the dark for months as spores in particles of dried sputum, but when exposed to direct sunlight, heat, and ultraviolet light, they are destroyed in a few hours. Spores are difficult to kill with ordinary disinfectants but are destroyed by pasteurization, a process widely used in milk and milk products to prevent spread of TB.

TB is generally transmitted through inhalation of droplets from coughing, sneezing, and spitting from a person with active disease. Brief contact usually does not result in infection. Many factors predispose a client to developing TB, including inadequate healthcare, malnutrition, overcrowding, and poor housing.

TB is characterized by stages of early infection (or primary TB), latency, and potential for recurrence after the primary disease (called *secondary TB*). Bacilli may remain dormant for many years and then reactivate, producing clinical symptoms of TB.

Early Infection

Tubercle bacilli, when inhaled, pass through the bronchial system and implant on the bronchioles or alveoli. Initially, the host has no resistance to this infection. *Phagocytes* (neutrophils and macrophages) engulf the bacilli, which continue to multiply. Bacilli also spread through lymphatic channels to the regional lymph nodes and subsequently to the circulating blood and distant organs. Eventually, the cellular immune response limits further multiplication and dissemination of the bacilli.

IMMUNE ACTIVATION. When immune activation occurs (usually a full response within 2 weeks), a granuloma forms, referred to as the *Ghon tubercle,* from epithelial cells merging with macrophages. Lymphocytes surround the Ghon tubercle, of which the central portion undergoes necrosis. This caseous necrosis has a cheesy appearance and may liquefy and slough into the connecting bronchus, producing a cavity. It also may enter the tracheobronchial system, promoting airborne transmission of infectious particles.

HEALING OF THE PRIMARY LESION. Healing of the primary lesion occurs through resolution, fibrosis, and calcification. Granulation tissue of the primary lesion becomes more fibrous and creates a scar around the tubercle. This is referred to as the *Ghon complex* and is visible on x-ray.

Latent Period

As the lesion heals, the infection enters a latent period that can persist for many years or even an entire lifetime without producing clinical symptoms. If the immune response is inadequate, the affected person eventually will develop clinical disease. Clients at particular risk are those with HIV infection or diabetes and those on chemotherapy or long-term steroids. Only a small percentage of those infected with TB actually develop clinical symptoms.

Secondary Tuberculosis

Secondary TB usually involves reactivation of the initial infection. The person already had an immune response, and thus lesions that form tend to remain in the lungs. The course of this phase usually is as follows:

1. Acute local inflammation and necrosis occur.
2. Infected lung tissue becomes ulcerated.
3. Tubercles cluster together and become surrounded by inflammation.
4. Exudate fills surrounding alveoli.
5. The client develops bronchopneumonia.

6. TB tissue becomes caseous and ulcerates into the bronchus.
7. Cavities form.
8. Ulcerations heal, with scar tissue left around cavities.
9. Pleurae thicken and retract.

The course of TB becomes a cyclical one of inflammation, bronchopneumonia, ulceration, cavitation, and scarring. The TB gradually spreads throughout the lung fields and into the rest of the respiratory structures, as well as to other organs through the lymph system. A client may experience periods of exacerbation, followed by remissions.

Assessment Findings

Signs and Symptoms

The onset of TB is insidious, and early symptoms vary. An infected person may be asymptomatic until the disease is advanced. As symptoms develop, they often are vague and ignored, particularly because they are systemic. Fatigue, anorexia, weight loss, and a slight, nonproductive cough are all symptoms attributable to overwork, excessive smoking, or poor eating habits, but also are early symptoms of TB. Low-grade fever, particularly in late afternoon, and night sweats are common as the disease progresses. The cough typically becomes productive of mucopurulent and blood-streaked sputum. Marked weakness, wasting, **hemoptysis** (expectoration of blood or bloody sputum), and dyspnea are characteristics of later stages. Chest pain may result from spread of the infection to the pleurae.

Diagnostic Findings

Diagnostic tests chiefly consist of tuberculin skin tests (see Chap. 21), chest x-ray, CT scan, magnetic resonance imaging (MRI), and analysis of sputum and other body fluids. A positive tuberculin skin test result is evidence that a TB infection existed at some time, but does not indicate active disease. The chief value of tuberculin skin tests lies in case-finding.

Microscopic examination of sputum and other body fluids identifies the bacilli. The client is instructed to cough deeply so that the specimen does not consist mainly of saliva. Most clients find that it is easier to raise sputum when they first awaken. It may be necessary to collect specimens on several consecutive days.

Gastric lavage, gastric aspiration, or bronchoscopy determines the presence of tubercle bacilli, particularly when a client cannot raise a sputum specimen. Tubercle bacilli may reach the stomach from the lungs when the client raises sputum but swallows rather than expectorates it. Other specimens may be obtained to confirm invasion of tubercle bacilli to other body organs.

Medical and Surgical Management

Although drugs speed recovery and provide a chance to arrest TB in clients with advanced lesions, they do not guarantee a cure. Their usefulness lies in their ability to retard growth and multiplication of tubercle bacilli, giving the body a chance to overcome the disease. Two factors make drug therapy less than ideal: drug toxicity and tendency of the tubercle bacilli to develop drug resistance. Combined therapy with two or more drugs decreases the likelihood of drug resistance, increases the tuberculostatic action of the drugs, and lessens risk for toxic drug reactions (Drug Therapy Table 23.1).

Resistance of bacilli to drugs is an important factor in the lack of response to medical treatment. Clients usually are on drug therapy at home. They need follow-up care for assessment of response to therapy. Culture and sensitivity tests may be done, as well as evaluation of adverse drug effects.

DRUG THERAPY TABLE 23.1 DRUG REGIMEN FOR TUBERCULOSIS

TREATMENT PERIOD	DRUGS PRESCRIBED	LENGTH OF DRUG THERAPY
Initial treatment	isoniazid (INH) rifampin (RIF) pyrazinamide (PZA) (These three medications now in combination tablet.)	INH, RIF, PZA for 4 months INH and RIF for additional 2 months
Suspected drug resistance	isoniazid (INH) rifampin (RIF) pyrazinamide (PZA) ethambutol (EMB) or streptomycin (SM)	If sensitive, continue INH and RIF for 6 more months. If resistant to INH, use other drugs for 6 months. If resistant to RIF, use other drugs for 12–18 months.
Prophylactic treatment	isoniazid (INH) May use pyridoxine (vitamin B_6) to minimize side effects	6–12 months

When the disease is located primarily in one section of the lung, that portion may be removed by **segmental resection** (removal of a lobe segment) or **wedge resection** (removal of a wedge of diseased tissue). If the diseased area is larger, **lobectomy** (removal of a lobe) may be performed. In some cases, the lung is so diseased that **pneumonectomy** (removal of an entire lung) is necessary.

NURSING PROCESS

● Pulmonary Tuberculosis

Assessment

Assess breath sounds, breathing patterns, and overall respiratory status. Ask the client about pain or discomfort experienced with breathing. Inspect the client's sputum for color, viscosity, amount, and signs of blood. Clients with primary TB may have complaints related to fatigue, weakness, anorexia, weight loss, or night sweats. Clients with secondary TB may report chest pain and a cough that produces mucopurulent or blood-tinged mucus or blood, and a low-grade fever.

Diagnosis, Planning, and Interventions

Antitubercular drug regimens extend for long periods and without interruption because healing is slow and interrupted treatment increases drug resistance. The primary focus of nursing management is encouraging the client to adhere to the prescribed medication regimen and teaching.

Instruct the client to take medications exactly as prescribed, observing time interval between doses, not skipping doses or taking more than prescribed amount. Clients need to complete the entire course of drug therapy to control infection. Lapses in taking the prescribed drugs can result in reactivation of the infection. Clients should notify the physician if symptoms worsen or sudden chest pain or dyspnea develops. They should drink plenty of fluids, discontinue smoking immediately, and avoid exposure to secondhand smoke. They need to eat a balanced but light diet.

Ineffective Airway Clearance related to pain with coughing, inability to cough, and abnormal respirations

Expected Outcome: Client will effectively clear secretions.

- Assess cough, noting characteristics of the secretions: color, consistency, amount, and presence of blood. *Coughing is more frequent with increased expectorant; hemoptysis occurs in advanced TB.*
- Encourage client to drink 3 to 4 L/day. *This measure liquefies and thins secretions and facilitates expectoration.*
- Humidify inspired air. *Maintains moisture to assist in liquefying secretions.*
- Encourage deep breathing and coughing every 2 hours while awake. *Promotes lung expansion and mobilization of secretions.*
- Place client in semi-Fowler's position. *Improves breathing and assists client to expectorate mucus.*
- Provide instructions about postural drainage. *Facilitates airway drainage and clearance.*

Activity Intolerance related to general weakness, respiratory difficulties, fever, and severity of illness

Expected Outcome: Client will demonstrate increased activity tolerance.

- Encourage rest periods, particularly before meals, performing activities of daily living (ADLs), and exercise. *Reduces fatigue and spaces activities.*
- Prioritize necessary tasks, eliminating nonessential tasks. *Promotes rest.*
- Assist client with activities as required. *Reduces client's energy expenditure, but allows him or her choices.*
- Keep equipment (e.g., telephone, tissues, wastebasket, bedside commode) close to client. *Reduces energy expenditure.*
- Encourage active range-of-motion (ROM) exercises three times a day. *Maintains muscle strength and joint ROM.*

PC: Side Effects of Medication Therapy—hepatitis, neurologic changes, gastrointestinal (GI) upset

Expected Outcome: Nurse will assist client to minimize side effects of medications.

- Instruct client to take medication 1 hour before or 2 hours after meals. *Food interferes with medication absorption.*
- Instruct clients taking isoniazid (INH) to avoid foods with tyramine and histamine (e.g., tuna, aged cheese, red wine, soy sauce, yeast extracts). *INH, when combined with these foods, may cause light-headedness, flushing, hypotension, headache, and other symptoms.*
- Ask if client is taking any beta blockers or oral anticoagulants. *Rifampin increases metabolism of beta blockers and oral anticoagulants. Dosages may need to be adjusted or medications changed.*
- Inform the client who wears contact lenses that rifampin may color them. *The client may prefer to wear glasses while taking rifampin.*
- Monitor for side effects related to medication regimen. For hepatitis, check liver enzymes. For kidney function, check blood urea nitrogen and serum creatinine levels. For neurologic changes, look for hearing loss and neuritis. Also check for skin rash. *Early identification of side effects promotes prompt treatment of side effects and adjustments in medications.*

Evaluation of Expected Outcomes

The client manages secretions with effective coughing, increased fluid intake, and appropriate postural drainage. He or she reports adequate pain relief and can tolerate increased amounts of time out of bed and perform most ADLs. The client adheres to treatment regimen and schedules tests for liver and kidney function.

Stop, Think, and Respond ● BOX 23-1

A client diagnosed with TB lives in a four-room apartment with his wife. What precautions must the couple follow?

OBSTRUCTIVE PULMONARY DISEASE

Obstructive pulmonary disease describes conditions in which airflow in the lungs is obstructed. Resistance to inspiration is decreased, whereas resistance to expiration is increased, prolonging the expiratory phase of respiration (Bullock & Henze, 2000). **Chronic obstructive pulmonary disease** (COPD) is a broad, nonspecific term describing a group of pulmonary disorders with symptoms of chronic cough and expectoration, dyspnea, and impaired expiratory airflow. Bronchiectasis, atelectasis, chronic bronchitis, and emphysema are categorized as COPDs. Asthma also is an obstructive disorder that is more episodic and usually more acute than the COPDs. Sleep apnea syndrome also can have obstructive causes.

● BRONCHIECTASIS

Bronchiectasis is a COPD characterized by chronic infection and irreversible dilatation of bronchi and bronchioles. Causes include bronchial obstruction by tumor or foreign body, congenital abnormalities, exposure to toxic gases, and chronic pulmonary infections. When airway clearance is impeded, infection can develop in the bronchial walls. Wall tissue structure subsequently changes, resulting in formation of saccular dilatations, which collect purulent material. Airway clearance is further impaired, and purulent material remains, causing more dilatation, structural damage, and more infection (Fig. 23.2).

Assessment Findings

Clients with bronchiectasis experience a chronic cough with expectoration of copious amounts of purulent sputum and possible hemoptysis. Coughing worsens when the client moves. Sputum production varies with the stage of the disease, but it can be several ounces. Clients also experience fatigue, weight loss, anorexia, and dyspnea.

Chest x-ray and bronchoscopy demonstrate the increased size of the bronchioles, possible areas of atelectasis, and changes in pulmonary tissue. Sputum culture and sensitivity tests identify the causative microorganism and effective antibiotics to control the infection. Pulmonary function studies also may be done.

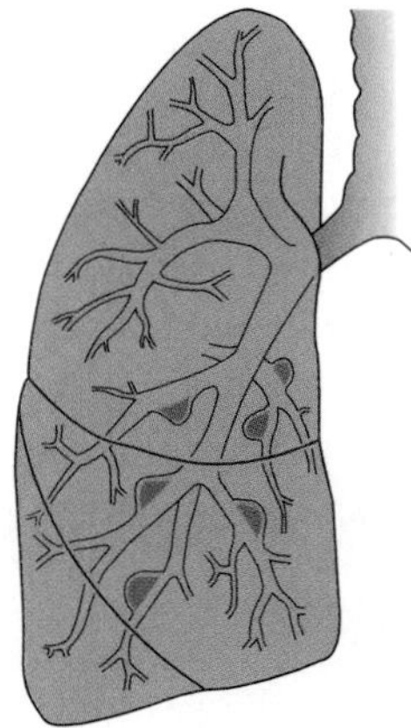

FIGURE 23.2 Bronchiectasis, showing abnormal saccular dilatations of the large bronchi that are filled with inflammatory exudate.

Medical Management

Treatment of bronchiectasis includes drainage of purulent material; antibiotics, bronchodilators, and mucolytics to improve breathing and raise secretions; humidification to loosen secretions; and surgical removal if bronchiectasis is confined to a small area.

Nursing Management

Nursing management focuses on postural drainage techniques, which help the client mobilize and expectorate secretions. Positions for the client to assume depend on the site or lobe to be drained. Figure 23.3 shows positions that drain specific segments of all lobes of the lungs. The client remains in each position for 10 to 15 minutes. Chest percussion and vibration may be performed during this time. When complete, the client coughs and expectorates secretions. This procedure may be repeated. Encourage oral hygiene after treatment.

● ATELECTASIS

Atelectasis is the collapse of alveoli (Fig. 23.4). It may involve a small portion of the lung or an entire lobe. When alveoli collapse, they cannot exchange gas. Atelectasis occurs secondary to aspiration of food or vomitus, a mucus plug, fluid or air in the thoracic cavity, compression on tissue by tumors, an enlarged heart, an aneurysm, or enlarged lymph nodes in the chest. If ill clients are on prolonged bed rest, unable to breathe deeply, cough and raise secretions, or both, they may experience atelectasis.

Assessment Findings

The degree of lung tissue involvement determines symptoms. Small areas of atelectasis may cause few symptoms.

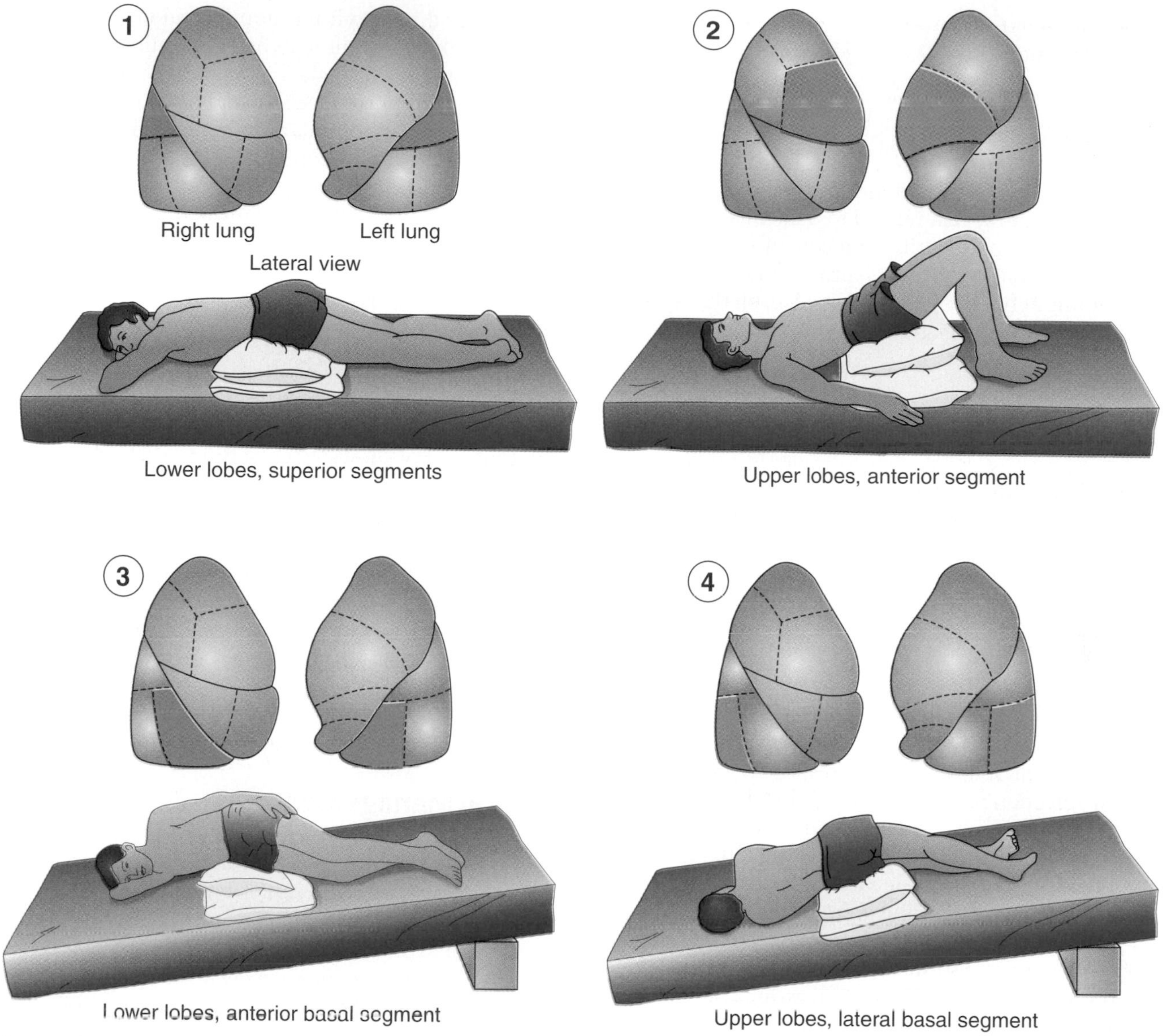

1

Right lung Left lung

Lateral view

Lower lobes, superior segments

2

Upper lobes, anterior segment

3

Lower lobes, anterior basal segment

4

Upper lobes, lateral basal segment

FIGURE 23.3 Lung areas to be drained and the best postural drainage positions for them. (From Smeltzer, S. C., & Bare, B. G. [2004]. *Brunner & Suddarth's textbook of medical–surgical nursing* [10th ed.]. Philadelphia: Lippincott Williams & Wilkins.)

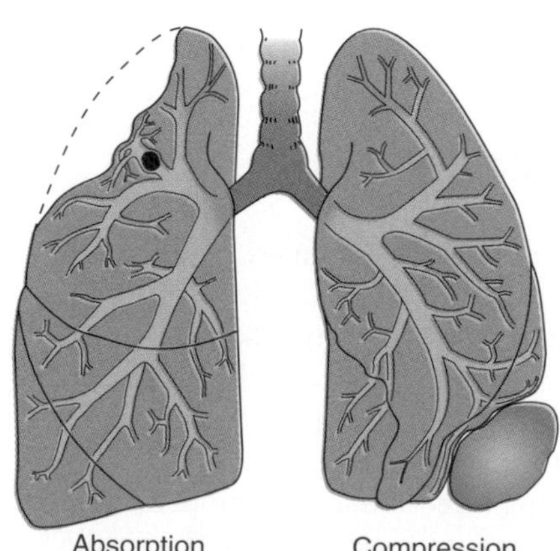

FIGURE 23.4 Atelectasis caused by airway obstruction and absorption of air from the involved lung area on the *left* and by compression of lung tissue on the *right*.

With larger areas, cyanosis, fever, pain, dyspnea, increased pulse and respiratory rates, and increased pulmonary secretions may be seen. Although crackling may be auscultated over affected areas, usually breath sounds are absent. A chest x-ray reveals dense shadows, indicating collapsed lung tissue. Sometimes the x-ray results are inconclusive. ABG and pulse oximetry results may be abnormal.

Medical Management

Treatment includes improving ventilation, suctioning, and deep breathing and coughing to raise secretions. Bronchodilators and humidification assist in loosening and removing secretions. Oxygen is administered for dyspnea. Removing the cause of atelectasis helps to correct the condition.

Nursing Management

Nursing care focuses on preventing atelectasis, especially when the client is at risk related to inadequate aeration. Postoperative deep breathing and coughing can prevent atelectasis. If atelectasis occurs, promote deep breathing and coughing at frequent intervals and teach the client to use an incentive spirometer.

● CHRONIC BRONCHITIS

Chronic bronchitis is a prolonged (or extended) inflammation of bronchi, with a chronic cough and excessive mucus for at least 3 months each year for 2 consecutive years. This serious health problem develops gradually and may go untreated for many years.

Pathophysiology and Etiology

Chronic bronchitis is characterized by hypersecretion of mucus and recurrent or chronic respiratory tract infections. As infection progresses, cilia lining the airway cannot propel secretions upward. Secretions remain in lungs and form plugs in smaller bronchi. These plugs are areas for bacterial growth and chronic infection, increasing mucus secretion and causing areas of focal tissue death. Airway obstruction results from bronchial inflammation.

Development of chronic bronchitis may be insidious or follow a long history of bronchial asthma or acute respiratory tract infections, such as influenza or pneumonia. Air pollution and smoking are significant factors.

Chronic bronchitis develops at any age, but appears most commonly in middle age after years of untreated, low-grade bronchitis. The duration of symptoms, how the disease process began, and history of occupational health hazards, pulmonary disease, and smoking form the basis for diagnosis.

Stop, Think, and Respond ● BOX 23-2

Your client with acute bronchitis smokes two packs of cigarettes per day. What would you advise this client?

Assessment Findings

Signs and Symptoms

The earliest symptom is a chronic cough productive of thick, white mucus. Bronchospasm may occur during severe bouts of coughing. Acute respiratory infections are frequent during winter months and may persist for several weeks. Sputum may become yellow, purulent, copious, and blood streaked after paroxysms of coughing. Expiration is prolonged secondary to obstructed air passages. Cyanosis secondary to hypoxemia may occur, especially after severe coughing. Dyspnea begins with exertion, but later occurs with minimal activity, and then at rest. Right-sided heart failure results from tachycardia in response to hypoxemia, leading to edema in the extremities.

Diagnostic Findings

Results of physical examination, chest x-ray, and pulmonary function tests may be normal. As the disease progresses, these findings become increasingly abnormal. Chest x-ray shows signs of fluid overload and lung consolidation.

As right-sided failure develops, the heart enlarges. Pulmonary function tests demonstrate decreased vital capacity and forced expiratory volume and increased residual volume and total lung capacity. Bronchoscopy, microscopic examination of sputum for malignant cells, and lung scan may be necessary to rule out cancer, bronchiectasis, TB, or other diseases in which cough is a predominant feature.

Medical Management

Goals of treatment are to prevent recurrent irritation of bronchial mucosa by infection or chemical agents, maintain function of the bronchioles, and assist in removal of secretions. Treatment includes smoking cessation, bronchodilators to reduce airway obstruction and bronchospasm, increased fluid intake, maintenance of a well-balanced diet, postural drainage to remove bronchial secretions, steroid therapy if other treatment is ineffective, change in occupation if work involves exposure to dust and chemical irritants, filtration of incoming air to reduce sputum production and cough, and antibiotic therapy.

Nursing Management

Nursing management focuses on educating clients in managing their disease. Help clients identify ways to eliminate environmental irritants. Measures include smoking cessation, occupational counseling, monitoring air quality and pollution levels, and avoiding cold air and wind exposure that can cause bronchospasm.

Preventing infection is also important. Instruct clients to avoid others with respiratory tract infections and to receive pneumonia and flu immunizations. Teach the client to monitor sputum for signs of infection. Also teach proper use of aerosolized bronchodilators and corticosteroids.

Instruct the client in postural drainage techniques and measures to improve overall health, such as eating a well-balanced diet, getting adequate rest, and moderate aerobic activity. For clients with lung disease, dyspnea, not heart rate, should determine aerobic activity. Clients should exercise at the pace and for the length of time they can tolerate without dyspnea. Refer to nursing management of emphysema for nursing diagnoses and additional interventions.

• PULMONARY EMPHYSEMA

Emphysema is a chronic disease characterized by abnormal distention of alveoli. The alveolar walls and capillary beds also show marked destruction. This process of destruction occurs over a long period. By the time of diagnosis, damage to lungs usually is permanent. Emphysema is a common cause of disability and the most common COPD.

Pathophysiology and Etiology

In emphysema, alveoli lose elasticity, trapping air the client normally would expire. On microscopic examination, alveolar walls have broken down, forming one large sac instead of multiple, small air spaces. Capillary beds, previously located within alveolar walls, are destroyed, and fibrous scarring replaces much of the tissue. Formation of fibrous tissue and destruction of alveoli prevent proper exchange of oxygen and CO_2 during respiration.

As the disease progresses, large air sacs (bullae, blebs) may be seen over the lung surface. These sacs can rupture, allowing air to enter the thorax (**pneumothorax**) with each respiration. Emergency thoracentesis must be performed to remove air from the thoracic cavity. A chest tube may be inserted to keep additional air from entering. Recurrent episodes of pneumothorax may require surgery to correct the problem (see section on Thoracic Surgery).

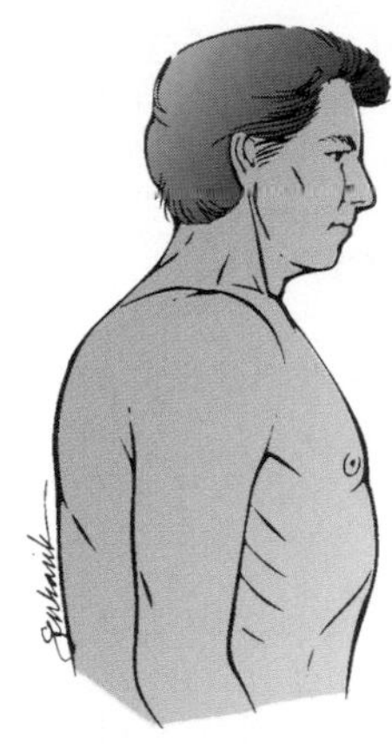

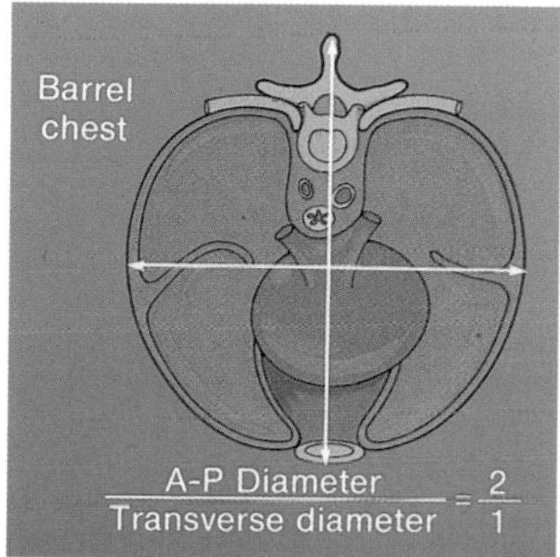

FIGURE 23.5 Characteristics of chest wall in emphysema. (From Smeltzer, S. C., & Bare, B. G. [2004]. *Brunner & Suddarth's textbook of medical–surgical nursing* [10th ed.]. Philadelphia: Lippincott Williams & Wilkins.)

Assessment Findings

Signs and Symptoms

Shortness of breath with minimal activity is called *exertional dyspnea* and often is the first symptom of emphysema. As the disease progresses, breathlessness occurs even at rest. A chronic cough invariably is present and productive of mucopurulent sputum. Inspiration is difficult because of the rigid chest cage. The chest is characteristically barrel shaped (Fig. 23.5).

The client uses accessory muscles of respiration (muscles in the jaw and neck and intercostal muscles) to maintain normal ventilation. Expiration is prolonged, difficult, and often accompanied by wheezing. In advanced emphysema, respiratory function is markedly impaired. Clients with advanced emphysema appear drawn, anxious, and pale, speaking in short, jerky sentences. When sitting up, they lean slightly forward and are markedly short of breath. Neck veins may distend during expiration.

In advanced emphysema, memory loss, drowsiness, confusion, and loss of judgment may result from reduced oxygen that reaches the brain and increased CO_2 in the blood. If the disorder goes untreated, CO_2 content in the blood may reach toxic levels, resulting in lethargy, stupor, and, eventually, coma. This condition is called *carbon dioxide narcosis*. Lung auscultation reveals decreased breath sounds, wheezing, and crackles. Heart sounds are diminished or muffled. Visual inspection shows a barrel-chested person breathing through pursed lips and using accessory muscles of respiration.

Diagnostic Findings

Chest x-ray and fluoroscopy demonstrate hyperinflated lung fields. Pulmonary function studies show a marked decrease in overall function, including increased total lung capacity and residual volume and decreased vital capacity and forced expiratory volume. ABG analysis usually reveals hypoxemia and respiratory acidosis.

Medical Management

Goals of medical management include improving the client's quality of life, slowing disease progression, and treating obstructed airways. Treatment includes the following measures:

- Bronchodilators to dilate airways by decreasing edema and spasms and improving gas exchange
- Aerosol therapy with nebulized aerosols for deep inhalation of bronchodilators and mucolytics in the tracheobronchial tree
- Antibiotics
- Corticosteroids on a limited basis to assist with bronchodilation and removal of secretions
- Physical therapy to increase ventilation—deep breathing, coughing, chest percussion, vibration, and postural drainage

If the prescribed treatment regimen does not help the client, progressive loss of sleep, appetite, weight, and physical strength is likely. As the disease progresses, the client may need to curtail physical activities.

Nursing Management

The respiratory center of the brain is sensitive to CO_2 levels in the blood. If the level increases slightly, respiratory rate and depth increase to eliminate the excess CO_2. If the CO_2 level is chronically elevated, the respiratory center becomes insensitive to CO_2 changes. Under these circumstances, the level of oxygen in the blood becomes a regulatory factor—the hypoxic drive to breathe. As long as the level of oxygen saturation of the blood is low, a client breathes sufficiently to maintain oxygenation. If oxygen is given at or above 32% by mask or other means, the hypoxic drive to breathe is lost and the respiratory rate drops, leading to further retention of CO_2, apnea, and death.

If the client requires oxygen, the safest method of administration is by nasal catheter or cannula, with the oxygen flow rate set at no more than 2 to 3 L/min. If the client's color improves but his or her level of consciousness decreases, discontinue oxygen administration and notify the physician; the client may be approaching a state of respiratory arrest.

Therapeutic breathing exercises effectively use the diaphragm, relieving the compensatory burden on the muscles of the upper thorax. Teach the client to let the abdomen rise when taking a deep breath and to contract abdominal muscles when exhaling. Clients feel the correct way to do this by placing one hand on the chest and the other on the abdomen: during abdominal breathing, the chest should remain quiet and the abdomen should rise and fall with each breath.

Other exercises include blowing out candles at various distances and blowing a small object, such as a pencil, along a tabletop. Encourage the client to exhale more by taking a deep breath and bending the body forward at the waist while exhaling as fully as possible. Pursed-lip breathing (i.e., breathing with lips pursed or puckered on expiration) helps control respiratory rate and depth and slows expiration. This maneuver may decrease dyspnea and reduce anxiety often associated with breathing difficulties. See Client and Family Teaching 23-1 for additional nursing management.

NURSING PROCESS

● Obstructive Pulmonary Disease

Assessment

Assess the client's respiratory effort, rate, and pattern. Determine if the client has diminished breath sounds

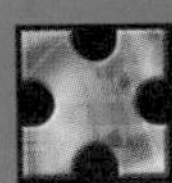

23-1 *Client and Family Teaching* Emphysema

- Education helps clients adjust to their current level of disability and to the potential for increased disability. The primary goal is to prevent or delay progression of emphysema. The nurse explains strategies to slow the disease progression.
- Emphasize that success depends on strict adherence to the treatment regimen. Motivated clients profit more from available treatments and make the best use of their remaining pulmonary function.
- Take medication exactly as prescribed. Observe time intervals between medications. Do not skip doses or take more than what is prescribed.
- Maintain close medical supervision.
- Contact the physician if adverse drug effects occur, drugs fail to relieve symptoms, new symptoms appear, symptoms become more severe, or signs or symptoms of respiratory infection develop.
- Drink extra fluids as indicated, unless restricted.
- Avoid respiratory irritants and people with respiratory infections.
- Eat a well-balanced diet.
- Perform breathing exercises as prescribed.
- Take frequent rests during the day. Space activities to prevent fatigue and shortness of breath.
- Avoid dry-heated areas that can aggravate symptoms.
- Humidify inspired air during the winter months.

and prolonged expiration, and observe for evidence of dyspnea at rest, accentuated accessory neck muscles, and barrel-shaped chest. Ask the client about tolerance for activity and check characteristics of secretions: consistency, quantity, color, or odor. Other assessment data are the client's ability to expectorate secretions, signs and symptoms of infection, and what the client does to relieve pulmonary symptoms.

Diagnosis, Planning, and Interventions

Ineffective Airway Clearance related to bronchoconstriction, increased mucus production, and ineffective cough

Expected Outcome: Client will maintain a patent airway and adequate airway clearance.

- Auscultate breath sounds at least every 8 hours. *Findings may indicate airway obstruction secondary to mucus plug, increasing airway resistance, or fluid in larger airways.*
- Encourage client to cough and clear secretions; suction as needed. *Promotes airway clearance and improves ventilation.*
- Perform postural drainage with percussion and vibration twice a day as indicated. *Assists in mobilizing secretions for expectoration.*
- Observe for dyspnea, restlessness, increased anxiety, or use of accessory muscles. *Such findings indicate possible airway obstruction or ineffective clearance of secretions.*
- Increase fluid intake to 3 L/day if not contraindicated. (Cardiac failure is a contraindication.) Humidify inspired air. *Keeps secretions moist and easier to expectorate.*
- Instruct client in early signs of infection: increased sputum production, change in sputum color and consistency, fever, increased coughing, and increased dyspnea. *Early recognition prevents an infection from progressing to a potentially lethal process.*
- Administer bronchodilators by nebulizer or meter-dose inhaler (MDI) as indicated. *Bronchodilators open airways, facilitating breathing and expectoration of secretions.*
- Teach and encourage use of diaphragmatic and pursed lip breathing. *Improves ventilation and mobilizes secretions.*

Impaired Gas Exchange related to prolonged expiration, loss of lung tissue elasticity, and atelectasis

Expected Outcome: Client will maintain optimal gas exchange.

- Promote more effective breathing patterns through optimal positioning, pursed-lip breathing, and use of abdominal muscles. *High-Fowler's position promotes better lung expansion; turning side-to-side promotes aeration of lung lobes; pursed-lip breathing and other methods open airways and provide for better exhalation.*
- Administer oxygen as prescribed. *Clients with COPD chronically retain CO_2 and depend on hypoxic drive as the stimulus for breathing; accurate oxygen administration is essential for preventing cessation of breathing.*
- Monitor level of consciousness and mental status. *Problems with mentation indicate inadequate oxygenation.*
- Monitor results of ABGs and pulse oximetry. *Changes indicate respiratory deterioration and provide an opportunity for early interventions.*

PC: Atelectasis

Expected Outcome: Nurse will manage and minimize atelectasis.

- Instruct client to do deep breathing and coughing exercises, incentive spirometry, or both. *These techniques promote lung expansion.*
- Encourage client to use abdominal muscles when breathing. *Diaphragmatic breathing promotes lung expansion.*

Evaluation of Expected Outcomes

The client's airway is free of secretions; breath sounds are clear. ABG and pulse oximetry results are within baseline values, and client remains alert and responsive. The client has no signs or symptoms of atelectasis and demonstrates ability to do pulmonary exercises and abdominal breathing as instructed by the nurse.

● ASTHMA

Asthma is a reversible obstructive disease of the lower airway. Airway inflammation and hyperresponsiveness of the airway to internal or external stimuli characterize asthma. Incidence of asthma is increasing, particularly in children and adolescents, and affects almost one fifth of the population at some time. Asthma may be fatal, but for most people it disrupts school and work attendance and affects choices in careers and activities.

Pathophysiology and Etiology

Asthma may develop at any age. There are three types of asthma: *allergic asthma* (extrinsic), which occurs in response to allergens, such as pollen, dust, spores, and animal danders; *idiopathic asthma* (intrinsic) associated with factors such as upper respiratory infections, emotional upsets, and exercise; and *mixed asthma,* which has characteristics of allergic and idiopathic asthma. Mixed asthma is the most common form.

Acute asthma results from increasing airway obstruction caused by bronchospasm and bronchoconstriction, inflammation and edema of the lining of bronchi and bronchioles, and production of thick mucus that can plug the airway (Fig. 23.6). Airways in people with asthma are hyperreactive in response to stimuli. Allergic asthma causes the immunoglobulin E (IgE) inflammatory response (see Chap. 35). These antibodies attach to mast cells within

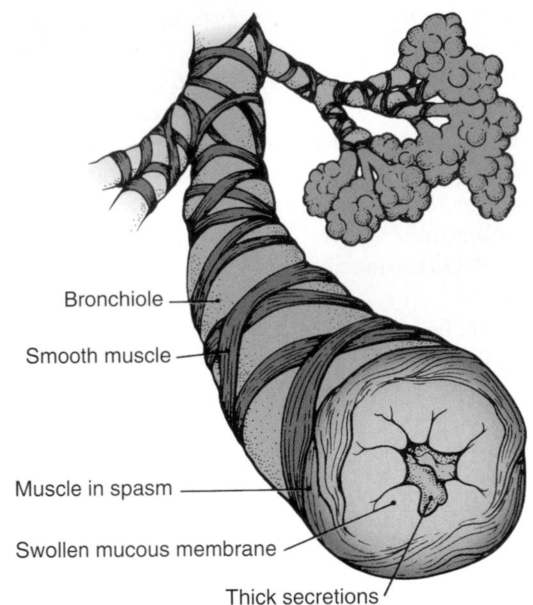

FIGURE 23.6 Bronchial asthma. Muscle spasms, mucosal edema, and thick secretions obstruct the bronchiole on expiration.

the lungs. Re-exposure to the antigen causes it to attach to the antibody, releasing mast cell products such as histamine. Manifestations of asthma become evident as this occurs. Other types of asthma are hyperresponsive to the inflammatory changes.

Because alveoli cannot expel air, they hyperinflate and trap air in the lungs. The client breathes faster, blowing off excess CO_2. The narrowed airway makes it difficult to force air out. Wheezing usually is audible with expiration. Other pathophysiologic changes include interference with gas exchange, poor perfusion, possible atelectasis, and respiratory failure if inadequately treated.

Assessment Findings

Signs and Symptoms

Asthma is typified by paroxysms of shortness of breath, wheezing, and coughing and production of thick, tenacious sputum. Duration of acute episodes varies from less than 1 day to several weeks.

Most clients are aware of wheezing as one of their symptoms. During an acute episode, the work of breathing greatly increases, and the client may suffer from a sense of suffocation. The client frequently assumes a classic sitting position, with the body leaning slightly forward and the arms at shoulder height, which facilitates chest expansion and more effective diaphragmatic excursions. Fear and anxiety often accompany and also intensify the symptoms.

Increased length of expiration phase accompanies the effort to move trapped air. Coughing starts with the onset of the attack but is ineffective in the early stage. When the attack begins to subside the client can expectorate large quantities of thick, stringy mucus. Skin usually is pale. During a severe attack, there may be cyanosis of the client's lips and nail beds. Perspiration often is profuse in an acute attack. An acute attack may intensify and progress to status asthmaticus (persistent state of asthma), which is life-threatening.

Diagnostic Findings

Chest auscultation reveals expiratory and sometimes inspiratory wheezes and diminished breath sounds. Results of pulmonary function studies may be abnormal, with total lung capacity and functional residual volume increased secondary to trapped air. During acute attacks, blood gases show hypoxemia. Partial pressure of carbon dioxide ($PaCO_2$) level may be elevated if the asthma becomes worse, but usually the $PaCO_2$ level is decreased because of the rapid respiratory rate.

Medical Management

Symptomatic treatment is given at the time of the attack. Long-term care involves measures to treat as well as prevent further attacks. If history and diagnostic tests indicate allergy as a causative factor, treatment includes avoidance of the allergen, desensitization, or antihistamine therapy. Oxygen usually is not necessary during an acute attack because most clients are actively hyperventilating.

Pharmacologic management is classified for short-term (rescue) and long-term (maintenance) therapy. Short-term medications treat acute episodes of asthma, whereas maintenance therapy is a daily regimen designed to prevent and control symptoms. Many medications are taken through MDIs. Drug Therapy Table 23.2 lists medications used in maintenance therapy.

Humidification of inspired air is valuable because dehydration of respiratory mucous membranes may lead to asthmatic attacks. Use of steam or cool vapor humidifiers are also effective. Liquefaction of secretions promotes more effective clearing of the airways and a rapid return to normal. Air conditioners may filter offending allergens as well as control temperature and humidity.

Nursing Management

During asthma attacks, clients are extremely anxious. Administer oxygen as indicated and put the client in a sitting position. Rest and adequate fluid intake (both oral and intravenous) are important. Increased fluid intake makes secretions less tenacious. Observe for adverse drug effects, especially when the client is receiving epinephrine or other adrenergic agents, which may cause palpitations, nervousness, trembling, pallor, and insomnia.

DRUG THERAPY TABLE 23.2 MAINTENANCE DRUG THERAPY FOR ASTHMA

DRUG CATEGORY AND EXAMPLES/ MECHANISM OF ACTION	SIDE EFFECTS	NURSING CONSIDERATIONS
Beta Agonists		
albuterol (*Ventolin*) Dilate the smooth muscles of the bronchioles, reduce muscle spasm, and therefore increase the size of the airway	Restlessness, apprehension, anxiety, fear, central nervous system stimulation, nausea, dysrhythmias, sweating, flushing, paradoxical airway resistance with repeated excessive use	Ensure that client understands technique for administering inhalers. Tell client not to exceed recommended dose and to report chest pain, dizziness, irregular heart rate, difficulty breathing, productive cough, or failure to achieve relief.
Anticholinergics		
ipratropium bromide (*Atrovent*) Decrease vagal tone to airways, resulting in bronchodilation	Nervousness, dizziness, headache, nausea, cough, palpitations, exacerbation of glaucoma and urinary retention	Demonstrate proper use of inhaler. Tell client to report eye pain or visual changes, rash, difficulty voiding.
Corticosteroids		
triamcinolone (*Azmacort*) Decrease inflammatory response	Inhalants: oral, laryngeal, and pharyngeal irritation and fungal infections*	Tell client not to use during an acute asthma attack and not to use more often than prescribed. If using an aerosolized bronchodilator, administer the bronchodilator first. Tell client not to discontinue medication abruptly.
Mast Cell Inhibitors		
Inhaled cromolyn (*Intal*) Prevent the release of mast cell products, promoting bronchodilation and decreasing inflammation; ineffective in acute attacks, but very therapeutic if taken regularly	Dizziness, nausea, throat irritation	Tell client not to use during an acute attack, to follow manufacturer's instructions for administration, and not to discontinue abruptly.

*Corticosteroids administered by other routes and in higher dosages are associated with multiple adverse effects.

After the acute asthma attack subsides, assess level of understanding about the disease process, which for many clients may not be clear. Ask if the client has a peak flow meter. If the client does not, obtain one for the client and tell him or her how to use it to monitor the degree of asthma control. Explanations include the following:

- Sit upright in bed or chair or stand and inhale as deeply as possible.
- Form a tight seal around the mouthpiece with lips.
- Exhale forcefully and quickly.
- Note the reading.
- Repeat these steps two more times—write the highest number in the asthma record.
- Explain that best individual peak flows are determined after 2 to 3 weeks of asthma therapy.
- Instruct the client about the zones of peak flow: green—80% to 100% best individual peak flow; yellow—60% to 80%; and red—less than 60%.
- Provide actions for the client to take for each zone.

The client can use the peak flow meter to assess the effectiveness of medication or breathing status. The nurse tells the client to seek care if readings fall below baseline and teaches correct use of inhalers. He or she also helps clients identify triggering events such as dust, smoking, emotional upset, or exposure to irritants such as cleaning fluids or insecticides. The nurse teaches the client relaxation techniques and therapeutic breathing techniques, as discussed previously in the section on nursing management of emphysema.

Stop, Think, and Respond ● BOX 23-3

Your client has asthma caused by extrinsic factors, particularly dust. How can this client reduce asthma attacks?

OCCUPATIONAL LUNG DISEASES

Exposure to organic and inorganic dusts and noxious gases over a long period can cause chronic lung disorders. **Pneumoconiosis** refers to fibrous inflammation or chronic induration of the lungs after prolonged exposure to dust or gases; specifically inhalation of silica (**silicosis**), coal dust (black lung disease, miners' disease), or asbestos (**asbestosis**). Although these conditions are not malignant, they increase the client's risk for development of malignancies. Table 23.2 describes these specific conditions in more detail.

The primary focus is prevention, with frequent examination of those who work in areas of highly concentrated dust or gases. Laws require work areas to be safe in terms of dust control, ventilation, protective masks, hoods, industrial respirators, and other protection. Workers should practice healthy behaviors, such as quitting smoking.

Dyspnea and cough are the most common symptoms of occupational lung diseases. Those exposed to coal dust may expectorate black-streaked sputum. Diagnosis is based on history of exposure to dust or gases. A chest x-ray may reveal fibrotic changes in the lungs. Results of pulmonary function studies usually are abnormal.

Treatment is conservative because the disease is widespread rather than localized. Surgery seldom is of value. Infections are treated with antibiotics. Other treatments include oxygen therapy if severe dyspnea is present, improved nutrition, and adequate rest. Many people with advanced disease are permanently disabled.

Nursing management of clients with occupational lung diseases is similar to emphysema. Many clients require emotional support because these diseases may result in permanent disability at a relatively young age.

PULMONARY EMBOLISM

Pulmonary embolism involves obstruction of one of the pulmonary arteries or its branches. Blockage results from a thrombus that forms in the venous system or right side of the heart.

Pathophysiology and Etiology

An embolus is any foreign substance (blood clot, air, or particle of fat) that travels in venous blood flow to the lungs. The clot occludes one of the pulmonary arteries, causing infarction (necrosis or death) of lung tissue distal to the clot. Scar tissue later replaces the infarcted area.

Clots usually form in the deep veins of the lower extremities or pelvis and are the source for pulmonary emboli. Emboli also arise from the endocardium of the right ventricle when it is the site of an MI or endocarditis. A fat embolus usually occurs after a fracture of a long bone, especially the femur. Other causes include recent surgery, prolonged bed rest, trauma, the postpartum state, and debilitating diseases.

Assessment Findings

When a small area of lung is involved, signs and symptoms usually are less severe and include pain, tachycar-

TABLE 23.2 OCCUPATIONAL LUNG DISEASES

OCCUPATIONAL LUNG DISEASE	PATHOPHYSIOLOGY AND ETIOLOGY	SIGNS AND SYMPTOMS
Coal worker's pneumoconiosis	Referred to as black lung disease, this condition is caused by inhalation of coal dust and other dusts. Initially, lungs clear particles by phagocytosis and transport out of the lungs. When dust inhalation becomes too great, macrophages collect in the bronchioles, leading to clogging of the airways with dusts, macrophages, and fibroblasts. This results in local emphysema and eventually massive blackened lung lesions. Coal macules eventually form, seen as black dots on radiography.	Chronic cough—sputum production Dyspnea Large amounts of sputum containing black fluid (melanoptysis) Respiratory failure
Silicosis	This illness results from inhalation of silica dust and is seen in workers involved with mining, quarrying, stone-cutting, and tunnel building. Silica particles inhaled into the lungs cause nodular lesions that enlarge and form dense masses over time. The results are loss of lung volume and restrictive and obstructive lung disease.	Shortness of breath Hypoxemia Obstruction of airflow Right-sided heart failure Edema
Asbestosis	This illness results from inhalation of asbestos dust. Laws restrict asbestos use, but old materials still contain asbestos. Asbestos fibers enter the alveoli and cause fibrous tissue to form around them. Pleura also have fibrous changes and plaque formation. Results are restrictive lung disease, decreased lung volume, and decreased gas exchange.	Dyspnea Chest pain Hypoxemia Anorexia and weight loss Respiratory failure

dia, and dyspnea. The client also may have fever, cough, and blood-streaked sputum. Larger areas of involvement produce more pronounced signs and symptoms, such as severe dyspnea, severe pain, cyanosis, tachycardia, restlessness, and shock. Sudden death may follow a massive pulmonary infarction when a large embolism occludes a main section of the pulmonary artery.

Serum enzymes typically are very elevated. A chest x-ray may show atelectasis. An ECG rules out a cardiac disorder such as myocardial infarction (MI), which produces similar symptoms. A lung scan, CT scan, or pulmonary angiography may be done to detect involved lung tissue.

BOX 23-1 ● Preventing the Formation of Pulmonary Emboli

Help client practice active and passive leg exercises.
Instruct client to pump muscles (tense and relax) to improve circulation in lower extremities.
Assist client to ambulate as early as possible after a procedure.
Teach client to:

- Wear support hose/elastic hose as directed
- Avoid constrictive clothing
- Avoid sitting for long periods or with legs crossed
- Drink fluids liberally unless contraindicated
- When traveling, move lower legs and feet while sitting, change positions as able, do not cross legs, and ambulate if able

Medical and Surgical Management

Treatment of a pulmonary embolism depends on the size of the area involved and the client's symptoms. IV heparin may be administered to prevent extension of the thrombus and development of additional thrombi in veins from which the embolus arose. IV injection of a thrombolytic drug (one that dissolves a thrombus) such as urokinase, streptokinase, or tissue plasminogen activator also may be used (see Chap. 27). Anticoagulants commonly are given after thrombolytic therapy. Other measures to treat symptoms of pulmonary emboli include complete bed rest, oxygen, and analgesics.

Pulmonary embolectomy, using cardiopulmonary bypass to support circulation while the embolus is removed, may be done if the embolus is lodged in a main pulmonary artery. Insertion of an umbrella filter device (Greenfield filter) in the vena cava prevents recurrent episodes of pulmonary embolus. The umbrella filter is inserted by an applicator catheter inserted into the right internal jugular vein and threaded downward to an area below the renal arteries. Another procedure is placement of Teflon clips on the inferior vena cava. These clips create narrow channels in the vena cava, allowing blood to pass through on its return to the right side of the heart but keeping back large clots.

Nursing Management

The best management of pulmonary emboli is preventing them (Box 23-1). When assessing a client's potential for pulmonary emboli, test for a positive Homan's sign (see Chap. 25). The client lies on his or her back, lifts his or her leg, and dorsiflexes his or her foot. If the client reports calf pain (positive Homan's sign) during this maneuver, he or she may have a deep vein thrombosis.

Pulmonary embolism occurs suddenly, and death can follow within 1 hour. Early recognition of this problem is essential. Start an IV infusion as soon as possible to establish a patent vein before shock becomes profound. Administer vasopressors such as dopamine or dobutamine as ordered to treat hypotension. Provide oxygen for dyspnea and analgesics for pain and apprehension. Close monitoring of vital signs is necessary, as is observing the client at frequent intervals for changes. Institute continuous ECG monitoring because right ventricular failure is a common problem.

Areas for the nurse to monitor include fluid intake and output, electrolyte determinations, and ABGs. Assess the client for cyanosis, cough with or without hemoptysis, diaphoresis, and respiratory difficulty. Monitor blood coagulation studies (i.e., partial thromboplastin time, prothrombin time) when anticoagulant or thrombolytic therapy is instituted.

Assess the client for evidence of bleeding and relief of associated symptoms. Because clients with pulmonary emboli are discharged on oral anticoagulants, they require instruction related to checking for signs of occult bleeding, taking medication exactly as prescribed, reporting missed or extra doses, and keeping all appointments for follow-up blood tests and office visits.

PULMONARY EDEMA

Pulmonary edema is accumulation of fluid in the interstitium and alveoli of the lungs. Pulmonary congestion results when the right side of the heart delivers more blood to the pulmonary circulation than the left side of the heart can handle. The fluid escapes capillary walls and fills airways. A client with pulmonary edema experiences dyspnea, breathlessness, and a feeling of suffocation. He or she also exhibits cool, moist, and cyanotic extremities. Overall skin color is cyanotic and gray. The client has a continual cough productive of blood-tinged, frothy fluid. This condition requires emergency treatment. (See Chap. 30).

RESPIRATORY FAILURE

Respiratory failure describes the inability to exchange sufficient amounts of oxygen and CO_2 for the body's needs. Even when the body is at rest, basic respiratory needs cannot be met. The ABG values that define respiratory failure include a PaO_2 less than 50 mm Hg, a $PaCO_2$ greater than 50 mm Hg, and a pH less than 7.25.

Respiratory failure is classified as acute or chronic. Acute respiratory failure occurs suddenly in a client who previously had normal lung function. In chronic respiratory failure, loss of lung function is progressive, usually irreversible, and associated with chronic lung disease or other disease.

Pathophysiology and Etiology

Table 23.3 describes precipitating factors that can result in respiratory failure. Acute respiratory failure is a life-threatening condition in which alveolar ventilation cannot maintain the body's need for oxygen supply and CO_2 removal. Arterial oxygen falls (hypoxemia) and arterial CO_2 rises (hypercapnia), detected by ABG analysis. Ventilatory failure develops when alveoli cannot adequately expand, when neurologic control of respirations is impaired, or when traumatic injury to the chest wall occurs.

The most common diseases leading to chronic respiratory failure are COPD and neuromuscular disorders. The underlying disease accounts for the pathology seen in respiratory failure. Gas exchange dysfunction occurs over a long period. Symptoms of acute respiratory failure are not apparent in chronic respiratory failure because the client experiences chronic respiratory acidosis over time. Refer to the section on COPD for discussion of diagnostic findings, medical management, and nursing management of chronic respiratory failure.

TABLE 23.3 FACTORS THAT PRECIPITATE RESPIRATORY FAILURE

PRECIPITATING FACTOR	EXAMPLE
Pulmonary infection—especially with COPD	Bacterial, viral, or fungal pneumonia
Trauma	Motor vehicle collision Gunshot/knife wound Burns
Infection	Sepsis Wound infection
Cardiovascular event	Myocardial infarction Aortic aneurysm Pulmonary embolism
Allergic reaction	Transfusion reaction Drug allergy Bee sting or other venom
Pulmonary aspiration	Vomitus Near drowning
Surgical procedure	Abdominal or thoracic surgery
Drug reaction	Overdose of barbiturates or narcotics Reaction to anesthesia
Mechanical factor	Pneumothorax Pleural effusion Abdominal distention
Iatrogenic factor	Endotracheal intubation Failure to clear tracheobronchial secretions
Neuromuscular disorders	Guillain-Barré syndrome Multiple sclerosis Muscular dystrophy

Assessment Findings

Apprehension, restlessness, fatigue, headache, dyspnea, wheezing, cyanosis, and use of accessory muscles of respiration are seen in clients with impending respiratory failure. If untreated, or if treatment fails to relieve respiratory distress, confusion, tachypnea, cyanosis, cardiac dysrhythmias and tachycardia, hypotension, CHF, respiratory acidosis, and respiratory arrest occur.

The client's symptoms, history (e.g., surgery, known neurologic disorder), and ABG results form the basis for a diagnosis of respiratory failure. Additional tests include chest x-ray and serum electrolyte determinations.

Medical Management

Treatment of respiratory failure focuses on maintaining a patent airway (in cases of upper respiratory airway obstruction) with an artificial airway, such as an endotracheal or a tracheostomy tube. Additional treatments include administration of humidified oxygen by nasal cannula, Venturi mask, or rebreather masks. Respiratory failure is managed with mechanical ventilation. When possible, the underlying cause of respiratory failure is treated.

Nursing Management

Because symptoms often occur suddenly, recognition is important. Notify the physician immediately and obtain emergency resuscitative equipment. Assessment and monitoring of respirations and vital signs are necessary at frequent intervals. Pay particular attention to respiratory rate and depth, signs of cyanosis, other signs and symptoms of respiratory distress, and the client's response to treatment. Monitor ABG results and pulse oximetry findings and implement strategies to prevent respiratory complications, such as turning and ROM exercises. Provide explanations to the client and initiate measures to relieve anxiety.

ACUTE RESPIRATORY DISTRESS SYNDROME

Acute respiratory distress syndrome (ARDS) is a clinical condition that follows other clinical conditions. It is not a primary disease. When it occurs, ARDS can lead to respiratory failure and death. Sudden and progressive pulmonary edema, increasing bilateral infiltrates seen on chest radiography, severe hypoxemia, and progressive loss of lung compliance characterize ARDS (Smeltzer & Bare, 2004).

Pathophysiology and Etiology

Factors associated with development of ARDS include aspiration related to near drowning or vomiting; drug ingestion/overdose; hematologic disorders such as disseminated intravascular coagulation or massive transfusions; direct damage to lungs through prolonged smoke inhalation or other corrosive substances; localized lung infection; metabolic disorders such as pancreatitis or uremia; shock; trauma such as chest contusions, multiple fractures, or head injury; any major surgery; embolism; and septicemia (Smeltzer & Bare, 2004). Mortality rate with ARDS is high.

The body responds to injury by reducing blood flow to the lungs, resulting in platelet clumping. Platelets release substances such as histamine, bradykinin, and serotonin, causing localized inflammation of the alveolar membranes. Increased permeability of the alveolar capillary membrane subsequently ensues. Fluid enters the alveoli and causes pulmonary edema. Excess fluid in the alveoli and decreased blood flow through capillaries surrounding them cause many of alveoli to collapse (microatelectasis). Gas exchange decreases, resulting in respiratory and metabolic acidosis. ARDS also causes decreased surfactant production, which contributes to alveolar collapse. Lungs become stiff or noncompliant. Decreased functional residual capacity, severe hypoxia, and hypocapnia result.

Assessment Findings

Severe respiratory distress develops within 8 to 48 hours after onset of illness or injury. In the early stages, few definite symptoms are seen. As the condition progresses, there is increased respiratory rate; shallow, labored respirations; cyanosis; use of accessory muscles; respiratory distress unrelieved with oxygen administration; anxiety; restlessness; and mental confusion, agitation, and drowsiness with cerebral anoxia.

Diagnosis is made according to the following criteria: evidence of acute respiratory failure, bilateral infiltrates on chest x-ray, and hypoxemia as evidenced by PaO_2 less than 50 mm Hg with supplemental oxygen of 50% to 60%. Chest x-rays reveal increased infiltrates bilaterally. There is no evidence of left-sided heart failure (see Chap. 30), such as increased size of the left ventricle.

Medical Management

The initial cause of ARDS must be diagnosed and treated. The client receives humidified oxygen. Insertion of an endotracheal or a tracheostomy tube ensures maintenance of a patent airway. Mechanical ventilation usually is necessary, which provides pressures to the airway that are higher than atmospheric pressures. Mechanical ventilators usually raise airway pressure during inspiration and let it fall to atmospheric or zero pressure during expiration. The client's pulmonary status, determined by ABG findings and pulse oximetry results, dictates the oxygen concentration and ventilator settings.

Hypotension results in systemic hypovolemia. Although the client experiences pulmonary edema, the rest of the circulatory volume is decreased. Pulmonary artery pressure monitors the client's fluid status and assists in determining administration of IV fluids. Colloids such as albumin help pull fluids in from the interstitium to the capillaries. Adequate nutritional support is essential. The first choice is enteral feedings, but total parenteral nutrition may be necessary.

Nursing Management

Nursing management focuses on promotion of oxygenation and ventilation and prevention of complications. Assessing and monitoring a client's respiratory status are essential. Potential complications include deteriorating respiratory status, infection, renal failure, and cardiac complications. The client requires explanations and support. If the client is on a ventilator, verbal communication is impaired. Provide alternative methods for the client to communicate.

LUNG CANCER

Lung cancer is very common, particularly among cigarette smokers and those regularly exposed to secondhand smoke. It remains the number-one cause of cancer-related deaths among men and women in the United States (American Cancer Society, 2001), with more Americans dying each year from lung cancer than from breast, prostate, and colorectal cancers combined. Incidence of lung cancer has markedly increased, related to more accurate methods of diagnosis, growing population of aging people, continued popularity of cigarette smoking, increased air pollution, and increased exposure to industrial pollutants.

Lung cancer is more common in men than in women. The rate of women dying from it continues to increase and indeed is greater than the rate of women dying from breast cancer. Most clients are older than 40 years of age when diagnosed with lung cancer.

Pathophysiology and Etiology

The exact mechanism for the development of lung cancer is unknown, but the link between irritants and lung cancer is well established. Prolonged exposure to carcinogens more than likely will produce cancerous cells. Smokers who quit reduce the risk of lung cancer to that of nonsmokers within 10 to 15 years.

There are four major cell types of lung cancer: large cell or undifferentiated type, small cell or oat cell type, epidermoid or squamous cell type, and adenocarcinoma. Many tumors begin in the bronchus and spread to lung tissue, regional lymph nodes, and other sites, such as the brain and bone. Many tumors have more than one type of cancer cell.

Transformation of an epithelial cell in the airway initiates growth of a lung cancer lesion. As the tumor grows, it partially obstructs the airway or completely obstructs it, resulting in airway collapse distal to the tumor. The tumor may hemorrhage, causing hemoptysis (Bullock & Henze, 2000).

Assessment Findings

The lung cancer cell type, tumor size and location, and presence of metastasis determine signs and symptoms. A cough productive of mucopurulent or blood-streaked sputum is a cardinal sign of lung cancer. The cough may be slight at first and attributed to smoking or other causes. Later, the client may report fatigue, anorexia, and weight loss. Dyspnea and chest pain occur late. Hemoptysis is common.

If pleural effusion occurs from tumor spread to the outside portion of the lungs, the client experiences dyspnea and chest pain. Other indications of tumor spread are symptoms related to pressure on nerves and blood vessels. Symptoms include head and neck edema, pericardial effusion, hoarseness, and vocal cord paralysis.

Early diagnosis of lung cancer is difficult because symptoms often do not appear until disease is well established, making long-term survival rate low. Sputum is examined for malignant cells. Chest films may or may not show a tumor. A CT scan or MRI is done if results from chest x-ray are inconclusive, or to further delineate the tumor area.

Bronchoscopy may be done to obtain bronchial washings and a tissue sample for biopsy. Fine-needle aspiration under fluoroscopy or CT guidance may be done to aspirate cells from a specific area not accessible by bronchoscopy. A lung scan may locate the tumor. A bone scan detects metastasis. Results of a lymph node biopsy may be positive for malignant changes if there is metastasis. Mediastinoscopy provides a direct view of the mediastinal area and possible visualization of tumors that extend into the mediastinal space.

Medical and Surgical Management

The client's prognosis is poor unless the tumor is discovered in its early stages and treatment begins immediately. Because lung cancer produces few early symptoms, its mortality rate is high. Metastasis to the mediastinal and cervical lymph nodes, liver, brain, spinal cord, bone, and opposite lung is common.

Treatment depends on several factors. One major consideration is classification and staging of the tumor. Staging refers to the extent and location of the tumor and absence or presence and extent of metastasis. Other factors that determine treatment are the client's age and physical condition and other diseases or disorders, such as renal disease and CHF.

Surgical removal of the tumor offers the only possibility of cure and usually is successful only in early stages of the disease. The type of lung resection depends on the tumor's size and location.

Radiation therapy may slow the spread of the disease and provide symptomatic relief by reducing tumor size. In turn, pain, cough, dyspnea, and hemoptysis may be relieved. In a small percentage of cases, radiation may be curative, but for most, it is palliative. Complications associated with the use of radiation therapy include esophagitis, fibrosis of lung tissue, and pneumonitis.

Chemotherapy may be used alone or with radiation therapy and surgery. Principal effects of chemotherapy are to slow tumor growth and reduce tumor size and accompanying pressure on adjacent structures. Chemotherapy also is used to treat metastatic lesions. Most chemotherapeutic regimens use a combination of drugs.

New treatments in various stages of development include the following:

- New chemotherapy regimens
- Monoclonal antibodies that target specific cancer proteins
- Photodynamic therapy that is a combination treatment with chemicals and light
- Lung cancer vaccines to stimulate effective immune response (Lungcancer.org, 2001)

Nursing Management

Management of clients with lung cancer is essentially the same as that for any client with a malignant disease. See Chapter 19 for the nursing management of a client with cancer.

Stop, Think, and Respond • BOX 23-4

Your 65-year-old neighbor tells you that he smoked for 25 years but quit 5 years ago. He has experienced a productive cough for 3 weeks. Occasionally, he sees blood in the sputum. What can you advise him?

TRAUMA

All chest injuries are potentially serious. Clients with chest injuries must be observed for dyspnea, cyanosis, chest pain, weak and rapid pulse, and hypotension—signs and symptoms of respiratory distress.

• FRACTURED RIBS

Fractured ribs usually result from a hard fall or a blow to the chest. They are not considered serious, unless accompanied by other injuries.

Pathophysiology and Etiology

Automobile and household accidents are frequent causes of fractured ribs. Rib fractures are painful, but not life-threatening. Other structures may be injured as well; for example, the sharp end of the broken rib may tear the lung or thoracic blood vessels. If injury involves fractured ribs without complications, the client usually returns home after emergency treatment.

Flail chest occurs when two or more adjacent ribs fracture in multiple places (two or more) and the fragments are free-floating (Fig. 23.7). This affects chest wall stability and results in impaired chest wall movement. A paradoxical movement develops: with inspiration the chest expands, but free-floating segments move inward instead of outward. On expiration free-floating segments move outward, interfering with exhalation. Intrathoracic pressures are greatly affected, so movement of air is greatly decreased. Many pathophysiologic phenomena occur as a result: increased dead space, reduced gas exchange, decreased lung compliance, retained airway secretions, atelectasis, and hypoxemia.

Assessment Findings

Symptoms consist primarily of severe pain on inspiration and expiration and obvious trauma. The client experiences shortness of breath. With flail chest, the client has hypotension and inadequate tissue perfusion secondary to decreased cardiac output. Respiratory acidosis occurs because of increased CO_2. Chest x-rays are necessary to confirm the diagnosis.

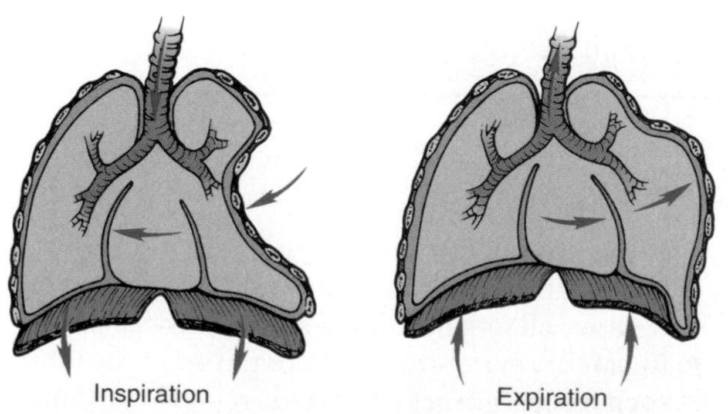

FIGURE 23.7 Flail chest during inspiration and expiration.

Medical Management

Supporting the chest with an elastic bandage or a rib belt assists in immobilizing the rib fractures. These measures lead to decreased lung expansion followed by pulmonary complications such as pneumonia and atelectasis. Therefore, use of these devices usually is limited to multiple rib fractures. Analgesics may be prescribed for pain. Sometimes a regional nerve block is used to relieve pain.

Management of flail chest includes supporting ventilation, clearing lung secretions, and managing pain. Other treatment depends on severity of the flail chest. If a **pulmonary contusion** (crushing bruise of the lung) also exists, fluids are restricted because of the damage to the pulmonary capillary bed. Antibiotics are given to prevent infection. Endotracheal intubation and mechanical ventilation may be necessary if a client's respiratory status is greatly compromised.

Nursing Management

With fractured ribs, apply the immobilization device after the physician examines the client. Instruct the client about application and removal of the rib belt or elastic bandage. Stress the importance of taking deep breaths every 1 to 2 hours, even though breathing is painful. Nurses plan and implement care of clients with more severe injuries based on respiratory needs. Assess and monitor the client for signs of respiratory distress, infection, and increased pain.

• PENETRATING WOUNDS

Gunshot and stab wounds are common types of penetrating wounds to the lungs. They potentially affect cardiopulmonary function and may be life-threatening.

Pathophysiology and Etiology

Penetrating wounds are classified according to velocity of the cause. Stab wounds usually are low velocity because they involve a small area. Knives and switchblades are the most common weapons that cause stab wounds. Gunshot wounds may be low, medium, or high velocity, depending on gun caliber, distance from which the gun was fired, and type of ammunition (Smeltzer & Bare, 2004).

Any type of penetrating wound to the chest is serious because of opening the thorax. On inspiration, the thorax normally is at negative pressure. A penetrating wound creates continuous and direct communication with the outside, which is at positive pressure. Thus, air enters the thoracic cavity, causing a pneumothorax (Fig. 23.8). If not recognized and treated promptly, death may occur. If the wound is large, a sucking noise may be heard as air enters and leaves the chest cavity. Depending on wound size, it takes seconds to hours before the lung collapses as the pressure in the thorax reaches atmospheric pressure. Many chest injuries involve both pneumothorax and hemothorax. **Subcutaneous emphysema** (air in subcutaneous tissues) also may be present. Other trauma may include hemorrhage, lung contusion, damage to surrounding tissues, fractured ribs or other bones, and injury to the heart, blood vessels, or both.

Assessment Findings

Clients exhibit various signs and symptoms, depending on the location and extent of the penetrating wound; dyspnea, pain, and bleeding are common. Clients are at risk for respiratory distress and shock. It is important to thoroughly examine the client to ascertain if there are other injuries, such as more penetrating wounds, particularly in the abdominal area.

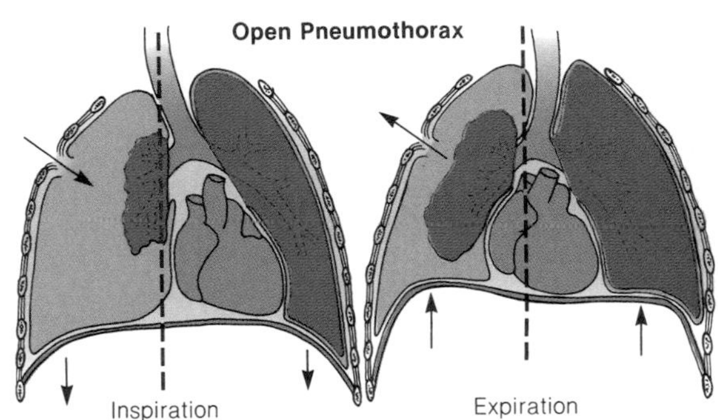

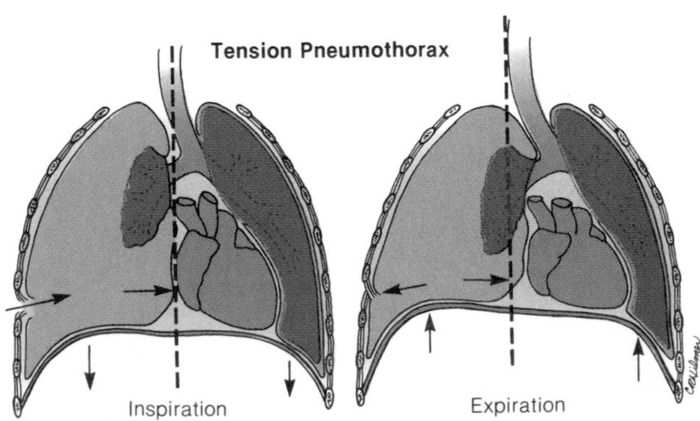

FIGURE 23.8 In open or communicating pneumothorax (*top*), air enters the chest during inspiration and exits during expiration. In tension pneumothorax (*bottom*), air enters but does not leave the chest. As pressure increases, the heart, great vessels, and unaffected lung are compressed, while the mediastinal structures and trachea shift toward the opposite side of the chest.

Diagnosis is based on the injury, physical examination, and auscultation of the lungs. X-rays show the degree of lung collapse and amount of air or blood in the thoracic cavity. The client's cardiopulmonary status is assessed through ABG analysis, pulse oximetry, and ECGs. CT scans or MRI may be done depending on the injuries.

Medical and Surgical Management

Airway management is the first concern. Once an airway is established, other treatment begins. Thoracentesis is done to remove air and blood from the pleural space. A chest tube is inserted and attached to an underwater-seal drainage system. A thoracotomy may be required to repair the injury. Foreign bodies that entered the chest, such as a bullet or a knife, are surgically removed. Their presence in the wound may prevent or slow the entrance of air. Removal before the victim is transported to the hospital may result in continuous sucking of air into the chest, collapse of the lung, compression of the heart and opposite lung, and death. Surgical intervention may be necessary if there is bleeding from the chest tube or indications of injury to other organs or blood vessels.

Emergency treatment of pneumothorax caused by a penetrating wound includes the application of a tight pressure dressing over the injury site to prevent more air from entering the thorax. Immediate evaluation of the client's respiratory status is imperative. Oxygen is given until the physician examines and treats the injury. IV fluids, colloid solutions, or blood are administered to treat or prevent shock. An indwelling catheter is inserted to monitor urine output. A nasogastric tube is placed to prevent aspiration of stomach contents and to decompress the GI tract.

Nursing Management

Care of a client with a penetrating chest wound is similar to that of a client who has thoracic surgery. Refer to the nursing management of a client undergoing thoracic surgery in the next section.

THORACIC SURGERY

A thoracotomy is a surgical opening in the chest wall. It may be done to:

- Remove fluid, blood, or air from the thorax
- Remove tumors of the lung, bronchus, or chest wall
- Remove all or a portion of a lung (Box 23-2)
- Repair or revise structures contained in the thorax, such as open heart surgery or repair of a thoracic aneurysm

BOX 23-2 ● Types of Lung Resections

Lobectomy—single lobe of lung removed
Bilobectomy—two lobes of lung removed
Sleeve resection—cancerous lobe(s) removed and a segment of the main bronchus resected
Pneumonectomy—removal of entire lung
Segmentectomy—segment of lung removed
Wedge resection—removal of small, pie-shaped area of the segment
Chest wall resection with removal of cancerous lung tissue—for cancers that have invaded the chest wall

(Adapted from Smeltzer, S. C., & Bare, B. G. [2004]. *Brunner and Suddarth's textbook of medical-surgical nursing* [10th ed.]. Philadelphia: Lippincott Williams & Wilkins.)

- Repair trauma to the chest or chest wall, such as penetrating chest wounds or crushing chest injuries
- Sample a lesion for biopsy
- Remove foreign objects such as a bullet or metal fragments

A thoracentesis may be done as an emergency procedure to remove blood, fluid, or air from the chest. In some instances, it is necessary to perform a thoracotomy to insert chest tubes (tube thoracotomy) to remove air or fluid from the chest during the preoperative period.

Preoperative Nursing Management

Preparing clients for thoracic surgery includes assessment of vital signs and breath sounds, particularly noting presence or absence of breath sounds. If surgery is an emergency, physical assessment may be limited to a general statement of the client's condition, a list of emergency measures and treatments done, and vital signs.

Postoperative Nursing Management

Opening the thoracic cavity requires special postoperative nursing measures. A significant issue is interference with normal pressures in the thoracic cavity. When the chest is opened, atmospheric air rushes in because of negative pressure that exists in the thoracic cavity on inspiration. Entrance of air under atmospheric pressure causes lungs to collapse and no longer expand or contract. The anesthesiologist ventilates the client during surgery.

After thoracic surgery, draining secretions, air, and blood from the thoracic cavity is necessary to allow lungs to expand. A catheter placed in the pleural space provides a drainage route through a closed or underwater-seal drainage system. Sometimes two chest catheters are placed—one anteriorly and one posteriorly. The anterior catheter (usually the upper one) removes air; the posterior catheter removes fluid.

Chest tubes are securely connected to an underwater-seal system. The tube coming from the client always must be under water. A break in the system, such as from loose or disconnected fittings, allows air to enter the tubing and then the pleural space, further collapsing the lung. When chest tubes are inserted at the end of the surgical procedure, they are connected to an underwater-seal drainage system. All connections are taped carefully to minimize the possibility of air entering the closed system.

It also is essential that the nurse check the underwater-seal drainage system, noting the amount and color of drainage and any bubbling or fluctuation. Assess dressings for drainage and firm adherence to the skin. Inspect the skin around the dressings for signs of subcutaneous emphysema. Assess the client's color, neurologic status, and heart rate and rhythm; monitor respiratory rate, depth, and rhythm; and auscultate the chest for normal and abnormal breath sounds. Also assess levels of pain and anxiety. See Nursing Care Plan 23-1 and Client and Family Teaching 23-2 for additional nursing management.

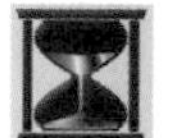

GENERAL GERONTOLOGIC CONSIDERATIONS

Older adults are more prone to pneumonia and may be more acutely ill with this infection because of concomitant health problems, such as heart disease and diabetes.

Before flu season begins, the physician may recommend administration of a vaccine. Older and debilitated clients are more likely to contract the disease and develop complications.

Older adults, who are more subject to falls, may fracture one or more ribs and be more susceptible to pneumonia after a rib fracture.

During the postoperative period, the older client may be confused and attempt to pull out chest tubes. Notify physician if confusion in a client is apparent. An order for soft restraints may be needed.

If confusion occurs, the client requires more frequent observation and assessment of needs.

Older clients may require more detailed explanation of home care management. Adequate time and repeated demonstrations may be necessary.

When possible, teach a family member postoperative exercises to ensure proper return of function to the muscles on the operative side.

For clients older than 50 years of age, nursing home residents, and debilitated clients, vaccination against pneumococcal pneumonia is recommended.

Critical Thinking Exercises

1. *A male client who underwent cholecystectomy (removal of the gallbladder) 2 days ago presses his call button. As you enter his room, he tells you that he is having trouble breathing and has chest pain. What brief questions would you ask the client before you call the physician?*
2. *A client who has bronchiectasis in his left lower lobe attends a pulmonary disease clinic. His physician instructs him to perform postural drainage by lying on the bed, bending at the waist, and lowering his head close to the floor. Two weeks*

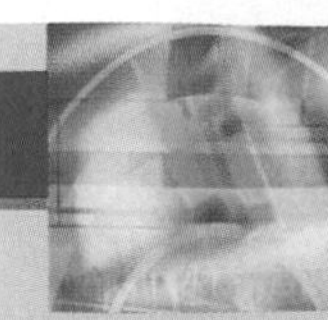

Nursing Care Plan 23-1

THE CLIENT RECOVERING FROM THORACIC SURGERY

Assessment

- Assess respirations: rate, depth, rhythm, and use of accessory muscles.
- Observe skin color, particularly for signs of cyanosis.
- Auscultate breath sounds at least every 4 hours.
- Evaluate mental status.
- Monitor heart rate and rhythm.
- Monitor results of ABGs, pulse oximetry, and other blood tests.
- Assess dressings and incisions for drainage or adherence.
- Check the chest tube drainage system.
- Assess level of pain.

Nursing Diagnosis: **Impaired Gas Exchange** related to decreased lung expansion, impaired lung function, and surgical procedure

Expected Outcome: Client will maintain optimal gas exchange.

Interventions	*Rationales*
Monitor vital signs every 15 minutes for at least 2 hours after return from postanesthesia care unit and then less frequently as condition stabilizes.	Information provides baseline data and early indications of problems.
Reinforce preoperative instructions about deep breathing, coughing, and incentive spirometry. Remind client to do these exercises every 1 to 2 hours.	Exercises expand the alveoli, preventing atelectasis.
Position client with the head of the bed elevated 30° to 40° initially. When the client can tolerate it, position him or her on operative side.	Promotes lung expansion and drainage from operative side.

Evaluation of Expected Outcome: Client demonstrates improved gas exchange, as evidenced by results of ABGs and pulse oximetry and improved efforts with incentive spirometry.

Nursing Diagnosis: **Deficient Fluid Volume** related to surgical procedure, drains, and pain

Expected Outcome: Client will maintain adequate fluid volume.

Interventions	*Rationales*
Monitor and record intake and output hourly.	Provides ongoing information about client's fluid status.
Assess skin turgor and mucous membranes for signs of dehydration.	Provides baseline data about fluid status.
Monitor and document vital signs.	Tachycardia can occur with hypovolemia to maintain adequate cardiac output. Pulse may be weak with hypovolemia. Hypotension occurs with hypovolemia.
Report urine output less than 30 mL/hour for 2 consecutive hours.	Indicates dehydration.
Monitor serum electrolyte and urine osmolality levels, reporting abnormal values.	Elevated hemoglobin, blood urea nitrogen, and urine specific gravity suggest fluid deficit.
Administer parenteral fluids as ordered, and maintain an accurate record of intravenous intake.	Prevents dehydration.
Encourage client to drink at least 30 mL every hour.	Promotes adequate fluid intake.

(continued)

Nursing Care Plan 23-1 (Continued)

THE CLIENT RECOVERING FROM THORACIC SURGERY

Evaluation of Expected Outcome: Client is adequately hydrated as evidenced by urine output greater than 30 mL/hour, stable blood pressure and pulse, and normal skin turgor.

PC: **Blood Loss; Hemorrhage**

Expected Outcome: Nurse will manage and minimize blood loss.

Interventions	*Rationales*
Monitor and record vital signs.	Provides baseline data and information about changes in a client's status.
Assess chest tube drainage and dressings for signs of bleeding.	Bloody drainage from chest tubes may occur initially but should decrease. Increased blood in chest tubes, on dressings, or both indicates a bleeding problem that requires immediate intervention.
Anticipate or prepare client for return to surgery if bleeding is secondary to surgical procedure.	These measures are necessary to resolve the problem.
Increase parenteral fluids as ordered.	Maintains an adequate circulating volume until bleeding stops.
Administer blood products as ordered.	Replace lost blood and volume.

Evaluation of Expected Outcome: Nurse ensures the management of bleeding and its complications.

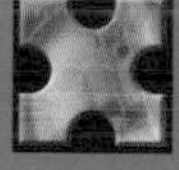

23-2 Client and Family Teaching Care After Thoracic Surgery

The nurse develops a teaching plan that includes instructions given by the physician as well as the following guidelines:

- Perform arm exercises to prevent stiffness and pain.
- Eat a well-balanced diet, or follow the recommended diet.
- Take rest periods throughout the day until fatigue decreases.
- Practice breathing exercises, and take frequent deep breaths.
- Contact the physician if breathing is difficult; drainage, excessive redness, or pain develops around the incision; fever develops; or pain occurs elsewhere in the body.
- Avoid infection or irritants.
- Increase activities slowly and avoid fatigue.
- Take drugs as prescribed, and do not omit, increase, or decrease doses.

later, the client tells you that he cannot tolerate this postural drainage position. Can you think of another way to perform postural drainage for the left lower lobe that may cause less discomfort?

• NCLEX-STYLE REVIEW QUESTIONS 

1. A woman brings her elderly mother to the emergency department. Vital signs are T–102°F, P–88, R–32, and BP–160/86. Upon physical examination, the elderly woman is having difficulty breathing. Which of the following would be **most** appropriate for the nurse to do next?
   1. Instruct the client to take slow deep breaths.
   2. Suction the client's pharynx of secretions.
   3. Apply a pulse oximeter to the client's finger.
   4. Help the client perform postural drainage.
2. A client comes to an urgent care clinic with pleurisy. The nurse is most correct in anticipating that the most common complaint from the client will be:
   1. Thick green sputum
   2. Pain with each breath
   3. Hot flashes with chills
   4. Petechiae on the chest

3. The nurse is caring for a client with tuberculosis. A sputum sample is ordered for the next 3 consecutive days. The nurse is correct to schedule the sputum sample to be obtained:
1. Upon arising in the morning
2. Midmorning following breakfast
3. In the evening
4. At bedtime

connection

Visit the Connection site at **http://connection.lww.com/go/timbyEssentials** for links to chapter-related resources on the Internet.

References and Suggested Readings

American Cancer Society. (2001). *Cancer facts and figures.* Atlanta, GA: Author.

Bullock, B., & Henze, R. L. (2000). *Focus on pathophysiology.* Philadelphia: Lippincott Williams & Wilkins.

Burke, M. S. (November 5, 2001). How to become a champion of smoking cessation. *Advance for Nurses,* 23–25.

Carroll, P. (2001). How to intervene before asthma turns deadly. *RN, 64*(5), 52–58.

Carroll, P. (2002) A guide to mobile chest drains. *RN, 65*(5), 56–60.

Clark, M. V. (February 4, 2002). Respiratory care: Aerosol therapy. *Advance for Nurses,* 34.

Dest, V. M. (2000). Oncology today: Lung cancer. *RN, 63*(5), 32–38.

DiTrapano, C. (August 13, 2001). Antibiotic therapy: Nurses need to remain current about old drugs, new drugs and resistant organisms. *Advance for Nurses,* 15–19.

Dunn, N. A. (2001). Keeping COPD patients out of the ED. *RN, 64*(2), 33–37.

Garvey, C. (December 3, 2001). Asthma management. *Advance for Nurses,* 34, 39.

Goodfellow, L. T., & Jones, M. (2002). Bronchial hygiene therapy. *American Journal of Nursing, 102*(1), 37–43.

Lazzara, D. (2002). Eliminate the air of mystery from chest tubes. *Nursing 2002, 32*(6), 36–43.

Lungcancer.org. (2001). It's time to focus on lung cancer. [On-line.] Available: http://www.lungcancer.org.

Miracle, V. (2002) Action stat: Asthma attack. *Nursing 2002, 32*(11), 104.

Smeltzer, S. C., & Bare, B. G. (2004). *Brunner & Suddarth's textbook of medical-surgical nursing* (10th ed.). Philadelphia: Lippincott Williams & Wilkins.

Trezza, A. (October 22, 2001). TB or not TB? Identifying tuberculosis in health care settings. *Advance for Nurses, 10*(3), 23–25.

Weibelhaus, P., Hansen, S., & Hill, H. (2001). Helping patients survive inhalation injuries. *RN, 64*(10), 28–31.

Woods, A. (2002). Pneumonia. *Nursing 2002, 32*(11), 56–57.

World Health Organization. (2001). Tuberculosis. [On-line.] Available: http://www.who.int.

chapter 24

Introduction to the Cardiovascular System

Words to Know 

angiocardiography
aortography
arteriography
automaticity
cardiac output
central venous pressure
conductivity
contractility
depolarization
dysrhythmias
echocardiography
electrocardiography
electron beam computed tomography
electrophysiology study
excitability
hemodynamic monitoring
isoenzyme
phonocardiography
polarization
refractory period
repolarization
rhythmicity
Starling's law
stroke volume
telemetry
transesophageal echocardiography

Learning Objectives

On completion of this chapter, the reader will:

- Describe normal anatomy and physiology of the cardiovascular system.
- Identify and describe focus assessment criteria when caring for a client with cardiovascular problems.
- List common diagnostic tests used to evaluate the client with suspected heart disease.
- Discuss nursing management of a client undergoing cardiovascular diagnostic tests.

The function of the cardiovascular system is to supply body cells and tissues with oxygen-rich blood and eliminate carbon dioxide (CO_2) and cellular wastes. Damage to and disease in the cardiovascular system greatly jeopardize a person's health. Heart disease is the leading cause of death for adults in the United States. Many advanced treatments are available to treat heart disease. Nevertheless, the primary focus remains preserving the natural heart by preventing heart disease.

ANATOMY AND PHYSIOLOGY

The cardiovascular system consists of the heart, major blood vessels that empty into or exit directly from the heart, and a vast network of smaller peripheral blood vessels. The heart's ability to pump blood is the result of five qualities unique to cardiac tissue:

- **Automaticity**—the ability to initiate electrical stimulus independently
- **Excitability**—the ability to respond to electrical stimulation
- **Conductivity**—the ability to transmit the electrical stimulus from cell to cell in the heart
- **Contractility**—the ability to stretch as a single unit and recoil
- **Rhythmicity**—the ability to repeat the cycle with regularity

Heart Chambers

The heart is a four-chambered muscular pump about the size of a fist (Fig. 24.1). The upper chambers, the right and left *atria* (singular, *atrium*), are receiving chambers for blood. The lower chambers, the right and left *ventricles,* are the heart's pumping chambers. A thick *septum,* or wall, separates the right side of the heart from the left side. The right atrium receives deoxygenated blood from the venous system, and the right ventricle pumps that blood to the lungs to be oxygenated. The left atrium

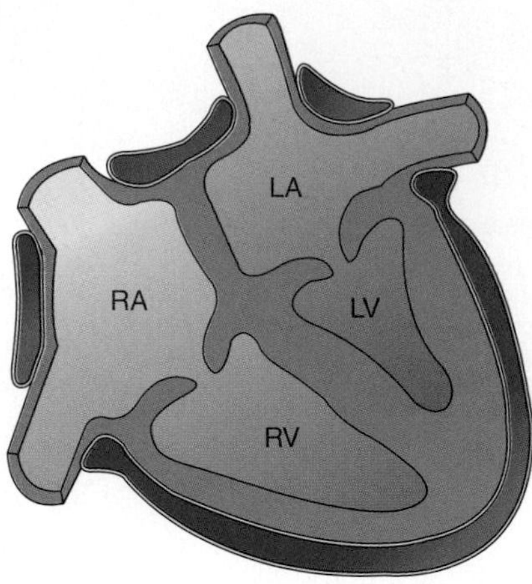

FIGURE 24.1 Layers of the heart, showing the visceral pericardium, the pericardial cavity, and the parietal pericardium. *LA,* left atrium; *LV,* left ventricle; *RA,* right atrium; *RV,* right ventricle.

receives oxygenated blood from the lungs, and the left ventricle pumps that blood to all the cells and tissues of the body. The heart is a double pump—the right side conducts pulmonary circulation, and the left side is responsible for systemic circulation.

The heart lies below and slightly to the left of the midline of the sternum in the mediastinum, a portion of the thoracic cavity that also contains the trachea and blood vessels. The upper portion of the heart is the base, and the tip is the apex. The right ventricle is directly under the sternum, a location that is significant in cardiopulmonary resuscitation. The lower border of the right ventricle rests on the diaphragm and forms a blunt point that angles to the left side of the body.

Cardiac Tissue Layers

Three distinct layers of tissue make up the heart wall. The outer layer is the *epicardium,* composed of fibrous and loose connective tissue. The middle layer, the *myocardium,* consists of muscle tissue. It is the force behind the heart's pumping action (see previous discussion). The inner layer, the *endocardium,* is composed of a thin, smooth layer of endothelial cells. Folds of endocardium form the heart valves. The endocardium is in direct contact with blood that passes through the heart.

The *pericardium* is a saclike structure surrounding and supporting the heart. Two membranous layers form the pericardium. The outer, tougher layer is called the *parietal pericardium.* The inner serous layer is called the *visceral pericardium* (also called the *epicardium*), which adheres to the heart itself. Density of the parietal pericardium safeguards the heart from invasion by infectious microorganisms. Serous fluid fills the pericardial space between the two layers, lubricating the heart and reducing friction with each heartbeat.

Heart Valves

Valves of the heart are membranous structures that ensure that blood passes through the heart in a one-way, forward direction. In a normal heart, valves do not allow blood to backflow, or regurgitate, into the chamber from which it came.

Two *atrioventricular valves* separate the atria from the ventricles. They prevent blood from returning to the atria when the ventricles contract. These valves are cusped, or leaflike. The valve between the right atrium and right ventricle is the tricuspid valve, which has three cusps. The valve between the left atrium and left ventricle is the bicuspid (two-cusped) valve, or *mitral valve.*

Attached to the mitral and tricuspid valves are cordlike structures known as *chordae tendineae,* which attach to the *papillary muscles,* two major muscular projections from the ventricles. When the ventricles contract, the papillary muscles also contract, applying tension to the atrioventricular valves. Contraction of the papillary muscles and firm support of the chordae tendineae prevent eversion of the valves and regurgitation of blood back into the atria.

The other two valves, called *semilunar valves* because they resemble portions of the moon, prevent blood from flowing back into the ventricles after the heart contracts. The valves are named for the blood vessel into which the blood is deposited. The valve between the right ventricle and pulmonary artery is called the *pulmonary,* or *pulmonic, valve.* The valve between the left ventricle and aorta is called the *aortic valve.* Contraction of the ventricles forces blood into the pulmonary artery and aorta. Relaxation follows, and the fall in pressure in the ventricles causes the pulmonic and aortic valves to close, preventing backflow into the ventricles.

Stop, Think, and Respond ● BOX 24-1

Where are the following cardiac valves located?— A, mitral valve; B, tricuspid valve; C, pulmonic valve. 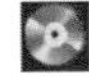

Arteries and Veins

Arteries carry oxygenated blood from the heart, and veins return deoxygenated blood to the heart. The smallest arteries are called *arterioles,* and the smallest veins are called *venules.* Arteries and arterioles are elastic and dilate or constrict to accommodate changes in blood flow. Veins have thinner walls than arteries because venous pressure is lower than arterial pressure. Veins have larger diameters than corresponding arteries.

Arterioles branch into *capillaries*, which are microscopic vessels that form a connecting network between arterioles and venules. Capillaries are one cell layer thick and in direct contact with cells of all tissues. This complex circulatory network delivers oxygen and metabolic substances to cells. The thin walls, tremendous surface area, and tiny size of the capillaries allow for rapid exchange of gases and metabolic substances between blood and cells. After this exchange, venules and veins transport blood back to the heart.

Heart contraction moves blood from the heart into arteries and arterioles; skeletal muscle contraction compresses veins and propels blood back to the heart. Closure of successive sets of valves in veins keeps blood from pooling under the influence of gravity.

Cardiopulmonary Circulation

The largest veins, the *inferior* and *superior venae cavae*, bring venous (deoxygenated) blood from all areas of the body into the right atrium. The right atrium fills with blood, and the tricuspid valve opens. Blood then travels into the right ventricle and is pumped into the *pulmonary artery* (the only artery in an adult that carries deoxygenated blood). The pulmonary artery branches to deliver venous blood to the right and left lungs. Lungs exchange oxygen in inspired air for CO_2 in the venous blood. CO_2 is transferred into alveoli and exhaled. Pulmonary veins then bring oxygenated blood into the left atrium. Oxygenated blood leaves the left atrium through the bicuspid, or mitral, valve. The left ventricle then pumps blood through the aorta to all body cells and tissues.

Stop, Think, and Respond ● BOX 24-2

Give the next location of blood when it is in the following structures: A, right ventricle; B, inferior vena cava; C, left ventricle; D, pulmonary veins. 

Blood Supply to the Heart

The *left and right coronary arteries* supply oxygenated blood to cardiac muscle. Openings to coronary arteries lie just inside the aorta. The myocardium is the first tissue to be supplied with oxygenated blood with each heartbeat (Fig. 24.2).

The left coronary artery and its branches, the *left anterior descending artery* and *left circumflex artery*, are critical for maintaining the pumping function of the heart. They keep the left atrium and most of the left ventricle perfused with oxygen, enabling the left side of the heart to forcefully pump oxygen-rich blood to the body. The right coronary artery and its branches maintain heart rhythm, because they nourish the nerve tissue of the conduction system.

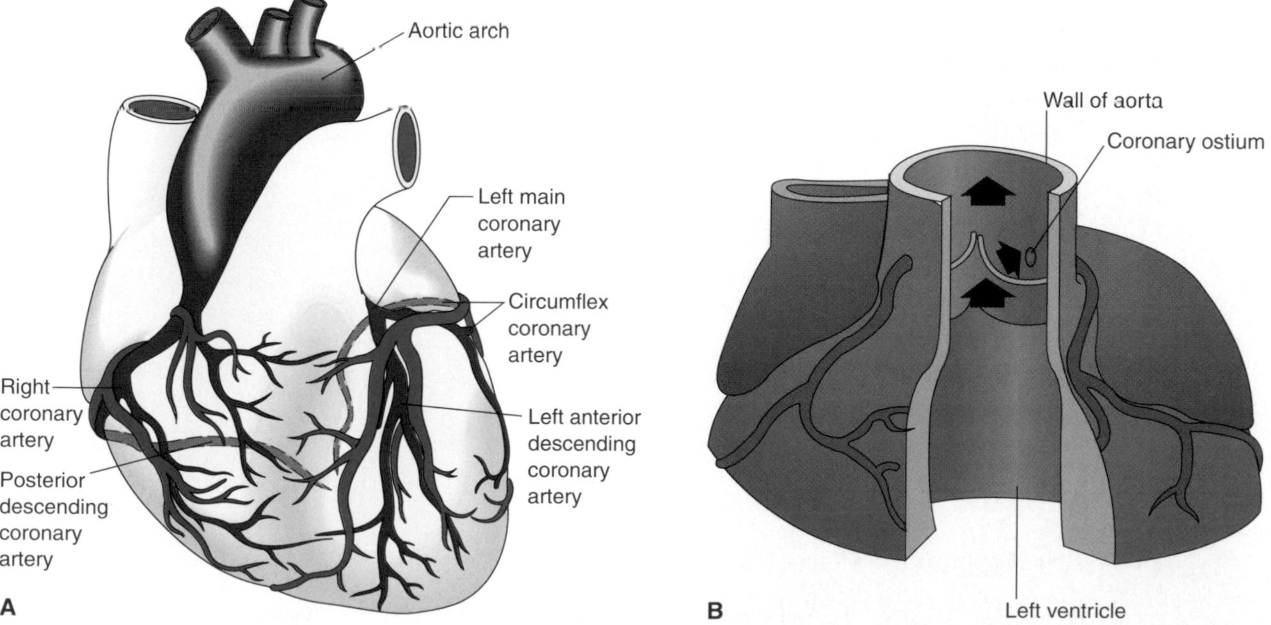

FIGURE 24.2 (**A**) Coronary arteries (*red vessels*) arise from the aorta and encircle the heart; coronary veins (*blue vessels*). (**B**) The orifices of the coronary arteries lie just beyond the aortic valve.

After having distributed oxygenated blood to myocardial cells, the coronary veins carry away CO_2 produced by cellular metabolism. Coronary veins empty into the coronary sinus in the right atrium. Blood then mixes with blood from the inferior and superior venae cavae and is recirculated to the lungs.

Cardiac Cycle

The term *cardiac cycle* refers to contraction (systole) and relaxation (diastole) of both atria and both ventricles (Fig. 24.3). The atria contract simultaneously; then, as they relax, the ventricles contract and relax. Contraction of the left ventricle can be felt as a wavelike impulse (the pulse) in peripheral arteries. The pause between pulsations is ventricular diastole. Contraction of the atria and then the ventricles can be heard with a stethoscope as "lub-dub" sounds. Sounds are created when the atrioventricular and semilunar valves alternately snap shut.

Both sides of the heart work in unison to accomplish different goals. Blood enters both atria and as pressure builds from the increasing volume of blood in the atria, the atrioventricular valves open, depositing blood into the ventricles. During atrial systole, contraction of the upper chambers squeezes remaining blood into the ventricles. When pressure builds in ventricles, the atrioventricular valves snap shut.

During ventricular systole, blood is pumped through semilunar valves into major vessels exiting the heart. The greater the stretch of the myocardium as the ventricles fill with blood, the stronger the ventricular contraction. This phenomenon is called **Starling's law.** It can be compared to the effect created by stretching a rubber band: the more the rubber band is stretched, the greater the snap when it is released.

Conduction System

The conduction system sustains electrical activity of the heart. It consists of the sinoatrial (SA) node, atrioventricular (AV) node, bundle of His, bundle branches, and Purkinje fibers.

The *SA node* is an area of nerve tissue located in the posterior wall of the right atrium. It is called the *pacemaker of the heart,* because it initiates electrical impulses that cause the atria and ventricles to contract. Normally, it produces between 60 and 100 impulses per minute; the average is approximately 72 impulses per minute. The SA node initiates impulses faster in response to sympathetic nervous system stimulation and slows impulses in response to parasympathetic stimulation. Other areas in the conduction pathway may initiate an electrical impulse if the SA node malfunctions, but they do so at rates slower than that of the SA node.

In the normal sequence of events, the cardiac impulse starts in the SA node (Fig. 24.4). It spreads throughout the atria over internodal and interatrial pathways. Waves of stimulation through the heart resemble rings that a pebble makes when dropped into a pond. Once cells in the atria are excited, they contract in unison. When the impulse reaches the *AV node,* it is delayed a few hundredths of a second. The impulse then stimulates the ventricles. While ventricles fill with blood, the impulse travels from the AV node to the *bundle of His,* to the *right and left bundle branches,* and eventually to the *Purkinje fibers.* Then, both ventricles contract.

During diastole, while myocardial cells are at rest and before an impulse is generated, the cells are in a polarized state (**polarization**). Positive ions predominate outside myocardial cell membranes; negative ions predominate inside. When an electrical impulse is initiated, it spreads from cell membrane to cell membrane, causing a transfer

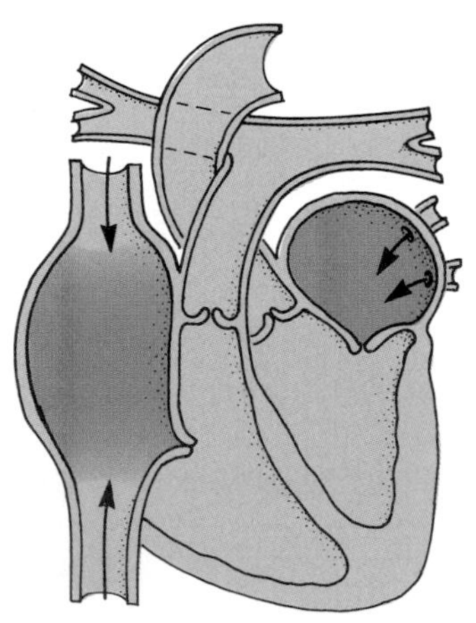
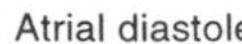

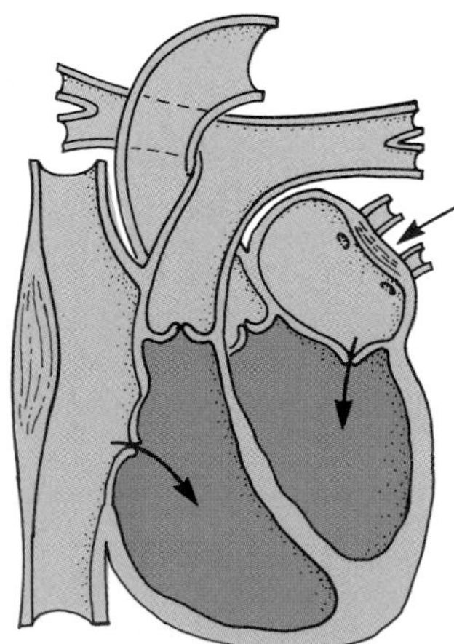

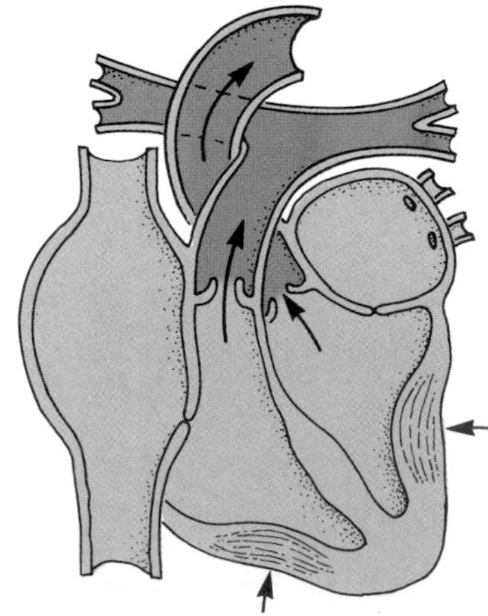

FIGURE 24.3 Pumping cycle of the heart. During atrial diastole, blood from the venae cavae and pulmonary veins fills the atria. During atrial systole, blood is delivered to the ventricles. When the ventricles contract, blood is pumped into the aorta and pulmonary arteries.

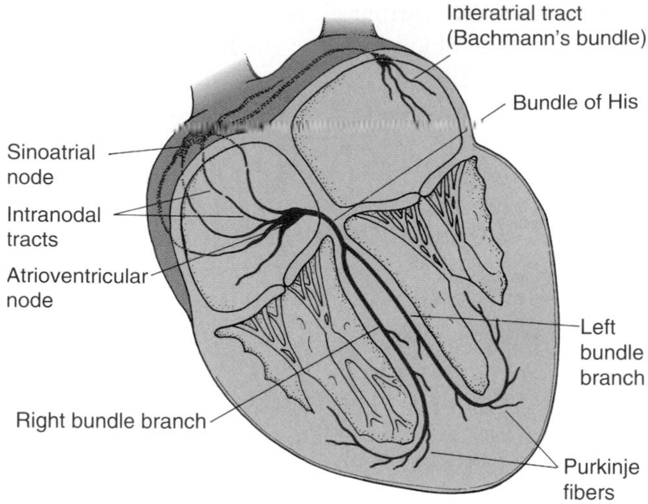

FIGURE 24.4 Electrical conduction system of the heart.

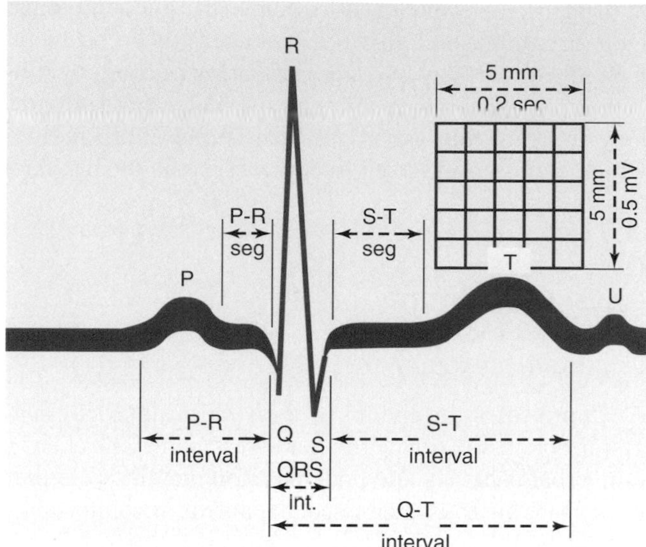

FIGURE 24.5 ECG graph and commonly measured complex components. Each small box represents 0.04 seconds on the horizontal axis and 1 mm or 0.1 millivolt on the vertical axis. The PR interval is measured from the beginning of the P wave to the beginning of the QRS complex; the QRS complex is measured from the beginning of the Q wave to the end of the S wave; the QT interval is measured from the beginning of the Q wave to the end of the T wave. (From Smeltzer, S. C. & Bare, B. G. [2004]. *Brunner & Suddarth's textbook of medical–surgical nursing* [10th ed.]. Philadelphia: Lippincott Williams & Wilkins.)

of ions. Positive ions move inside the myocardial cell membranes, and negative ions move outside. This process, which corresponds with cardiac muscle contraction, is called **depolarization.** It occurs first in the atria and then in the ventricles. Once depolarization occurs, ions realign themselves in their original position and wait for another electrical impulse. This process is called **repolarization.** Another normal cardiac impulse cannot be carried out until ions are again in polarized alignment. The time during which cells are resistant to electrical stimulation is called the **refractory period.**

Electrolyte balance is important for proper functioning of all cells in the body. Normal ranges of potassium and calcium ions are particularly essential for maintaining heart function. Excess potassium ions decrease heart rate and strength of contraction. Abnormally low potassium levels disturb cardiac rhythm. Excess calcium ions increase and prolong heart contraction. Low serum calcium levels reduce heart function.

Depolarization and repolarization produce electrical changes. Because body tissues conduct current easily, this electrical activity is detected by electrodes placed on the external surface of the body and recorded by a machine known as the *electrocardiograph (ECG)* (Fig. 24.5).

Cardiac Output

Cardiac output is the amount of blood pumped out of the left ventricle each minute. In a healthy adult, cardiac output ranges from 4 to 8 L/min (the average is approximately 5 L/min). Volume varies according to body size. The heart adjusts cardiac output to the body's changing needs. During active exercise, athletes may have a cardiac output that is five to seven times the normal amount. Cardiac output increases in two ways: by increasing heart rate and increasing stroke volume. **Stroke volume** is the amount of blood pumped per contraction of the heart. Stroke volume averages about 65 to 70 mL. The following formula is used to calculate cardiac output:

$$\text{Cardiac output} = \text{heart rate} \times \text{stroke volume}$$

Stop, Think, and Respond ● BOX 24-3

If a person's heart rate is 72 beats per minute (bpm), what is the cardiac output?

ASSESSMENT

History

Initial assessment includes the client's (or family member's) description of symptoms the client experienced before and during admission. A past medical history of angina, myocardial infarction (MI), or any cardiac surgeries is important to note at this time. Family medical history is important because many cardiac disorders have a familial or genetic predisposition. If close blood relatives are no longer living, it is important to ask about cause of death, age at death, and relationship to the client.

Ask the client to identify prescription and nonprescription drugs that he or she is taking. Adverse effects or drug interactions can contribute to cardiac symptoms. Note drug and food allergies because future diagnostic procedures may involve administration of drugs or substances, such as radiopaque dyes. An allergy to seafood may indicate that the client also is allergic to iodine, which commonly is used in contrast media during various x-rays.

Physical Examination

General Appearance

An appraisal of the client's general appearance may suggest problems requiring further assessment. The client's nonverbal behavior and body position may indicate that he or she is anxious, depressed, in pain, or uncomfortable.

Pain

Poor circulation, a common problem in clients with cardiovascular disorders, causes ischemia (reduced blood supply) to body organs. A classic sign of ischemia is pain, resulting from a lack of oxygen in the tissue. Chest pain is a sign of ischemia to the heart muscle. Leg pain, especially with activity, can indicate inadequate oxygenation to leg muscles.

When pain is present, evaluate it carefully. Obtaining as much information as possible is essential. Rapid treatment of pain is extremely important.

Vital Signs

TEMPERATURE. Fever is characteristic in some types of heart disease. It can accompany the inflammatory response when myocardial cells are damaged after an acute MI (heart attack) or infections such as rheumatic fever and bacterial endocarditis.

PULSE. When taking a client's pulse, note rate, rhythm, and quality. Pulse rhythm is the pattern of pulsations and pauses between them. A normal pulse is felt regularly with a similar length of pause. Pulse quality refers to its palpated volume. Pulse volume is described as feeling full, weak, or thready, meaning barely palpable. Also determine pulse deficit by counting heart rate through auscultation at the apex while a second nurse simultaneously palpates and counts the radial pulse for a full minute. The difference, if any, is the pulse deficit.

RESPIRATORY RATE. Count respiratory rate for 60 seconds. Observe character of the respirations, noting whether the client's breathing is easy or labored (dyspneic), deep or shallow, noisy or quiet. Use of accessory muscles (neck or abdominal muscles) during respiration indicates that the client is having difficulty breathing.

BLOOD PRESSURE. Cardiac disorders often are associated with changes in blood pressure (BP). If the client is not acutely ill, take BP with the client in standing, sitting, and lying positions (orthostatic vital signs). These baseline determinations help to monitor effects of cardiovascular diseases and drugs that can alter BP during position changes. To ensure an accurate assessment, select the cuff width most appropriate for the diameter of the client's arm.

Take the BP in both arms on admission and at least once daily thereafter, reporting a marked difference in pressure between left and right arms. When charting, identify the arm used to measure BP and the client's position at the time it was measured. Question the client about dizziness or light-headedness when changing positions, such as rising from a sitting or lying position. These symptoms may indicate postural (or orthostatic) hypotension.

Cardiac Rhythm

Electrical activity that produces heart rhythm can be observed continuously with bedside cardiac monitoring. Electrodes are attached to the chest and connected to a machine that displays cardiac rhythm on an oscilloscope. Components of an ECG are discussed later in the chapter. A paper strip of the cardiac rhythm can be printed and attached to the client's record. Most cardiac monitors sound an alarm and automatically print out tracings of abnormal rhythms, called **dysrhythmias** (or arrhythmias).

A cardiac monitor does not reveal the heart's mechanical activity. The healthcare provider must palpate a peripheral pulse or auscultate apical heart rate to obtain this information. Comparing heart rate and rhythm with information displayed on the monitor is important because the ECG pattern may appear normal in some clients even when mechanical function is abnormal.

Cardiac **telemetry** sends ECG information over radio waves to a monitor distant from the client. Telemetry communicates information to a hospital emergency room from an ambulance, or to a central station when a client requires continuous monitoring. When telemetry is used, electrodes are attached to a battery pack, secured inside a pocket on the client's hospital gown or clothing.

Heart Sounds

NORMAL HEART SOUNDS. Auscultation of the heart requires familiarization with normal and abnormal heart sounds. The first heart sound ("lub"), referred to as S_1, is the closing of the mitral and tricuspid valves. S_1 is heard loudest over the apex of the heart and occurs nearly simultaneously with the palpated pulse. The second heart sound ("dub"), referred to as S_2, is the closing of the aortic and pulmonic valves. S_2 is heard loudest with the stethoscope at the second intercostal space to the right of the sternum.

ABNORMAL HEART SOUNDS. All other heart sounds are abnormal and take considerable practice to recognize. A sound that follows S_1 and S_2 is called an S_3 heart sound or a ventricular gallop. When the three sounds are heard together, some say the cadence sounds like "Ken-tuck-y" or "lub-dub-dee." An S_3, although normal in children, often is an indication of heart failure in an adult. An extra sound just before S_1 is an S_4 heart sound, or atrial gallop. Some say this sound resembles the word "Ten-nes-see" or "lub-lub-dub." An S_4 sound often is associated with hypertensive heart disease.

Auscultation may also reveal other abnormal sounds, such as murmurs and clicks caused by turbulent blood flow through diseased heart valves. A friction rub may cause a rough, grating, or scratchy sound indicative of pericarditis (inflammation of the pericardium).

Peripheral Pulses

Palpate radial arteries and major arteries of the leg bilaterally during physical assessment. Record presence or absence of these pulses and their strength.

Skin

Many clients with cardiac disorders exhibit changes in skin color (e.g., cyanosis, pallor). A good light is necessary when assessing skin color. Cyanosis can be detected by carefully noting color changes in oral mucous membranes as well as on lips, earlobes, skin, and nail beds. In light-skinned clients, extreme pallor is easy to detect because skin appears almost bloodless. In dark-skinned clients, a grayish cast to the skin usually indicates pallor.

During assessment of skin, note if skin is warm or cold, or dry or clammy. If the client has a problem with peripheral circulation, inspect arms and legs for variations in skin color and temperature and compare bilateral findings with other areas of the body. Sparse hair growth on the legs and thick toenails can indicate poor circulation. Also note any varicosities (enlargement of veins).

Peripheral Edema

Edema occurs when blood is not pumped efficiently or plasma protein levels are inadequate to maintain osmotic pressure. When right-sided heart failure occurs, blood accumulates in great vessels and backs up in peripheral veins. Because it has nowhere else to go, extra fluid enters the tissues. Particular areas for examination are the dependent parts of the body, such as feet and ankles. Other areas prone to edema are fingers, hands, and over the sacrum. To assess for edema, the examiner gently presses his or her fingers into the skin and then quickly releases. If marks of the fingers remain, the effect is termed *pitting edema.* Edema is evaluated on a scale of +1 to +4, depending on the depth of the pit and the amount of time it takes the pit to disappear. The higher the number, the more pronounced in the edema.

Weight

Weight gain can indicate edema. A rapid gain in weight often means that edema is increasing. A 2-pound weight gain in a short period indicates that the client has an additional liter of fluid in the body. Weight loss often reflects loss of excess fluid from tissues and is used to evaluate effectiveness of drug therapy, especially diuretics. If weight is recorded daily, the client is weighed at the same time, with the same amount of clothing, using the same scale, each day. Weight is recorded as accurately as possible.

Jugular Veins

If the right side of the heart fails to pump efficiently, blood becomes congested in the neck veins (Fig. 24.6). With the client sitting at a 45° angle, the client turns his or her head to the left or right so the nurse can inspect the external jugular vein. Distention of this vein usually indicates increased fluid volume and pressure in the right side of the heart (see Chap. 30).

Lung Sounds

If the left side of the heart fails to pump efficiently, blood backs up into pulmonary veins and lung tissue. The nurse auscultates lungs for abnormal and normal breath sounds. With left-sided congestive heart failure, auscultation reveals a crackling sound and possibly wheezes and

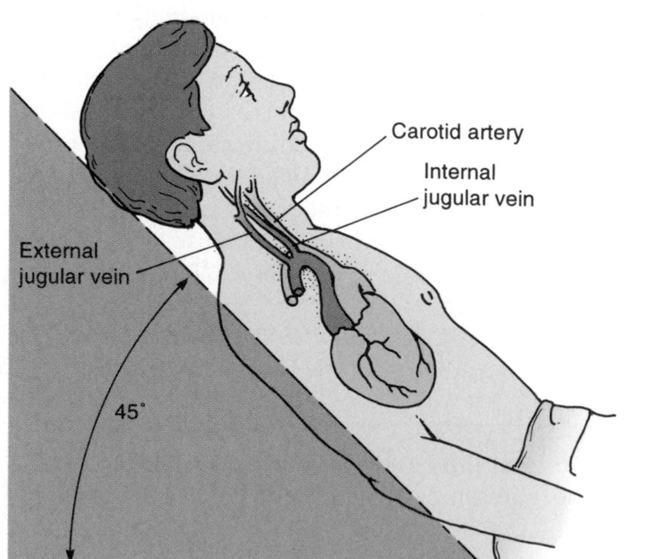

FIGURE 24.6 Jugular vein distention is assessed with the client at a 45° angle.

gurgles. Wet lung sounds are accompanied by dyspnea and an effort to sit up to breathe. If uncorrected, left-sided heart failure is followed by right-sided heart failure because the circulatory system is a continuous loop.

Sputum

Clients with cardiac disease may have a productive or nonproductive cough. Note the type and frequency of the cough and the amount and appearance of sputum. These findings are important in diagnosing heart failure or other pulmonary complications.

Mental Status

Some clients with cardiac disorders may be alert and oriented—others confused and disoriented. Confusion or disorientation can result from a decrease in oxygen supply to the brain (cerebral ischemia) as a result of poor circulation. Chest pain and impaired breathing creates anxiety. Report extremes of emotion or disturbances in thought processes because such effects interfere with the client's safety, diagnostic testing, and prescribed therapy.

Diagnostic Tests

Laboratory Tests

Various laboratory tests are used to diagnose heart disease and monitor the client's progress and response to therapy. Laboratory tests may be performed daily or every few days.

BLOOD CHEMISTRY. Blood chemistries, such as fasting blood glucose and serum electrolyte, cholesterol, and triglyceride levels, may be used as part of the diagnostic analysis. Hyperglycemia (elevated blood glucose) and hypertriglyceridemia (elevated triglyceride level) indicate undiagnosed or unsuccessful control of diabetes mellitus. Diabetes mellitus (see Chap. 52) is associated with accelerated pathologic changes leading to coronary artery disease. Elevated serum sodium is associated with fluid retention and hypertension; abnormal sodium, potassium, calcium, and magnesium levels may cause dysrhythmias. A total serum cholesterol level above 200 mg/dL, a low-density lipoprotein level above 130 mg/dL, or a high-density lipoprotein level below 25 mg/dL suggests potential for developing atherosclerotic heart disease.

SERUM ENZYMES AND ISOENZYMES. Enzymes are complex proteins produced by living cells that function as catalysts, substances that produce chemical changes without being changed themselves. An **isoenzyme** is one of several forms of the same enzyme that may exist in cells and is capable of being identified separately from others.

When tissues and cells break down, are damaged, or die, great quantities of certain enzymes are released into the bloodstream. The following enzymes are important in cardiac disease:

- Troponin, an enzyme in myocardial contractile tissue
- Creatine kinase (CK), formerly creatine phosphokinase, and its isoenzymes
- Lactate dehydrogenase (LDH) and its isoenzymes
- Aspartate aminotransferase (AST), formerly serum glutamic oxaloacetic transaminase

Troponin is present only in myocardial tissue and is specific for determining heart damage in the early stages of an MI (see Chap. 27). Other enzymes can be elevated in response to cardiac or other organ damage. Therefore, the isoenzymes CK-MB, LDH_1, and LDH_2 are evaluated for their cardiac specificity.

Electron Beam Computed Tomography

Electron beam computed tomography (EBCT) is a radiologic test that produces x-rays of the coronary arteries using an electron beam. This noninvasive test scans the heart quickly and produces clear images. It can detect and quantify calcified plaque in the coronary arteries before clients are symptomatic. There is a high degree of correlation between the amount of calcium plaque identified by EBCT and future risk of MI. If test results demonstrate heart disease, treatment interventions are instituted earlier than with conventional diagnostic regimens. The test is repeated at 1-year or longer intervals.

Radiography and Radionuclide Studies

Chest x-ray and fluoroscopy are used to determine the size and position of the heart and condition of the lungs. These studies also are used to guide insertion and confirm placement of cardiac catheters and pacemaker wires. CT scanning and magnetic resonance imaging determine heart size and detect lung involvement.

Radionuclides are radioactive chemical elements that are injected into the bloodstream, sometimes referred to as *nuclear cardiology*. The radionuclide technetium 99m detects areas of myocardial damage. The radionuclide thallium 201 diagnoses ischemic heart disease during a stress test.

Echocardiography

Echocardiography uses ultrasound waves to determine left ventricular functioning and to detect cardiac tumors, congenital defects, and changes in the tissue layers of the heart. High-frequency sound waves pass through the chest wall (transthoracic) and are displayed on an oscilloscope. The image is recorded and kept as a permanent record.

A second ultrasound technique is **transesophageal echocardiography** (TEE). It involves passing a tube with a small transducer internally from the mouth to the esophagus, which lies behind the heart. Images of the posterior heart and its internal structures are obtained. TEE is an alternative to standard transthoracic echocardiography and provides superior views not possible using conventional technique. It also is an adjunct for assessing intraoperative complications in the heart during cardiothoracic surgery. Clients whose chests are rotund or who are obese are candidates for TEE. Because the throat is anesthetized locally, the nurse cautions the client to avoid eating or drinking until sensation and the gag reflex return, which may take 1 hour or longer after removal of the tube containing the transducer.

Phonocardiography

Phonocardiography is the graphic representation of normal and abnormal heart sounds. It is used in diagnosing valvular and other cardiac disorders. Microphones placed on the chest pick up heart sounds, which then are amplified and converted to electrical impulses. These impulses are relayed to a recorder, which produces a graph of the heart sounds.

Electrocardiography

Electrocardiography is the graphic recording of electrical currents generated by heart muscle. It helps to identify cardiac dysrhythmias and detect myocardial damage. Color-coded electrodes matched to corresponding lead wires connect the client to the recording machine. Electrodes are coated with conductive gel and applied to the skin surface of the wrists, ankles, and chest (Fig. 24.7).

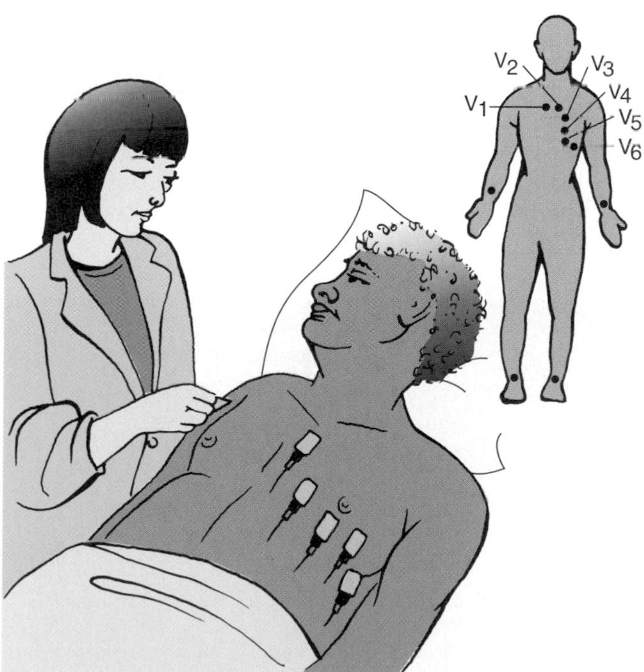

FIGURE 24.7 The nurse attaches electrodes to the client's chest and limbs before an ECG.

Computerized ECG machines immediately interpret the tracings, or rhythm strips. A physician later interprets the rhythm strips. He or she uses the 12-lead ECG to aid in diagnosing heart disease. The nurse can continuously monitor a client's cardiac activity by observing one or more leads.

The ECG pattern consists of waves, intervals, segments, and complexes. The P wave represents initiation of the electrical impulse that causes depolarization of the atria. The PR interval is the time it takes for the impulse to travel from its point of initiation, through the atrial conduction pathways, to the AV node. The QRS complex, the collective term for the Q, R, and S waves, is the measurement of time that it takes for the impulse to spread throughout the ventricles from the AV node to the Purkinje fibers, causing its subsequent depolarization. The ST segment represents early repolarization of the ventricular muscle, which ends after the T wave. The ST segment is a particularly sensitive indicator of ischemia and myocardial damage. Ischemia causes the ST segment to sag below the baseline (isoelectric line). An elevated ST segment indicates muscle injury. The QT interval represents ventricular depolarization and repolarization.

AMBULATORY ELECTROCARDIOGRAPHY. Ambulatory ECG, or Holter monitoring, is the recording of an ambulatory client's cardiac rate and rhythm over 24 to 48 hours as the client performs daily activities. The Holter monitor, worn on a belt or carried on a shoulder strap, consists of a tape recorder connected to ECG leads attached to the client's chest. During the test period, the client keeps a diary of activities and associated symptoms. At the end of the recording period, the monitor is returned to the hospital or physician and the tape is analyzed. The client's written notes are compared with recorded information. Ambulatory ECG helps to detect dysrhythmias and myocardial ischemia that occur sporadically during activity or rest.

EXERCISE-INDUCED STRESS TESTING. Stress testing is done to evaluate how the heart functions during exercise. Electrical activity of the heart is assessed with an ECG monitor while the client walks on a treadmill, pedals a stationary bicycle, or climbs stairs.

A resting ECG is taken as a baseline before the test is started. During the test, the speed of the treadmill, the force required to pedal the bicycle, or the pace of stair climbing is gradually increased. The goal is to increase the heart's workload until a predetermined target heart rate is reached. The client's heart rate and rhythm are monitored continuously, and ECG waveforms are recorded periodically. The client's BP and respiratory rate also are assessed. The client is instructed to report chest pain, dizziness, leg cramps, or weakness. The stress test is stopped if the client develops chest pain, severe dyspnea, elevated BP, confusion, or dysrhythmias. The physician interprets ECG tracings obtained during the test. A radionuclide such as thallium may be injected intravenously (IV) during the test, followed by a heart scan.

DRUG-INDUCED STRESS TESTING. Drugs may be used to stress the heart for clients with sedentary lifestyles or those with a physical disability, such as severe arthritis, that interferes with exercise testing. Drugs such as adenosine (Adenocard), dipyridamole (Persantine), or dobutamine (Dobutrex) may be administered singularly or in combination by the IV route. The drugs dilate the coronary arteries, similar to the vasodilation that occurs when a person exercises to increase the heart muscle's blood supply. When thallium, a radionuclide, is injected a few minutes later, a scan of the heart can detect compromised blood flow, which indicates coronary artery disease.

Cardiac Catheterization

Cardiac catheterization provides a means for measuring fluid pressures in heart chambers and collecting blood samples to analyze oxygen and CO_2 content. A long, flexible catheter is inserted from a peripheral blood vessel in the groin, arm, or neck into one of the great vessels and then into the heart. Cardiac catheterization may be done on the left side of the heart by way of an artery or on the right side by way of a vein.

The usual length of stay is at least 5 to 9 hours or overnight. The client needs to consult the physician about which prescribed medications to take or omit the day of the cardiac catheterization. Food and fluids usually are withheld. If the test is late in the day, light food may be permitted. Allergies must be identified; those of primary concern before a cardiac catheterization are iodine, shellfish, radiographic dye, and latex. IV fluids are administered before the test to maintain hydration and to administer any necessary medications. A sedative is administered before the test, but anesthesia is not necessary.

While the client lies on the examination table, the site where the catheter is inserted, usually the groin or arm, is scrubbed and covered with a sterile cloth. Electrode patches with wires are attached to the chest to monitor heart rhythm. The physician injects local anesthesia at the insertion site and threads a catheter while watching its progress toward the heart on an imaging screen that also is visible to the client. Dye is instilled when the catheter reaches its destination. The client feels a brief warm sensation as the dye is administered. He or she must report chest discomfort, nausea, or difficulty breathing. Several images are taken for future evaluation. The catheter is removed and the site is covered with a pressure dressing to control bleeding; sometimes sutures also are used.

After the test, discuss the following with the client and family:

- Keep extremity straight and avoid movement for several hours.
- Monitor BP and pulse frequently to detect changes.
- Check dressing over insertion site frequently for signs of bleeding.
- Check pulses, color in all extremities, and temperature.
- Report any warm, wet feeling that may indicate oozing blood, numbness, tingling, or sharp pain in the extremity.
- Drink a large volume of fluid to relieve thirst and promote the excretion of the dye.
- Follow discharge instructions (Box 24-1) for home care.

Electrophysiology Studies

Clients who experience dysrhythmias may be candidates for electrophysiology studies. An **electrophysiology study** is a procedure that enables the physician to examine electrical activity of the heart, produce actual dysrhythmias by stimulating structures in the conduction pathway, determine the best method for preventing further dysrhythmic episodes, and, in some cases, eradicate the precise location in the heart that is producing the dysrhythmia.

Preparation, management, and recovery for the client undergoing an electrophysiology study are similar to those for a client undergoing a heart catheterization. Usually, the client is monitored for a full day and discharged the following day if no bleeding or vascular complications occur.

Arteriography

CORONARY ARTERIOGRAPHY. A left-sided cardiac catheterization is used to determine the degree of blockage of the coronary arteries by performing arteriography while the catheter is in place. An **arteriography** is a diagnostic procedure that involves instilling dye, referred to as *contrast medium,* into an artery. In this case, it is instilled into the catheter and deposited into each coronary artery. Occlusive heart disease is indicated if one or more coronary

BOX 24-1 ● Discharge Instructions for Clients Having Cardiac Catheterization

- Rest for the next 3 days, and avoid heavy lifting, strenuous activity, or sports during this time.
- Do not drive or climb stairs for the next 24 hours.
- Do not take a tub bath until the puncture site is healed.
- Change the bandage in 24 hours; continue changing the bandage until a crust or scab forms over the puncture site.
- You may experience some soreness at the puncture site; however, if it becomes worse, notify your physician.
- If pain or swelling of the puncture site occurs, notify your physician.
- If the puncture site begins to bleed, hold pressure over the site and call 911 or another emergency services number.

arteries appear narrow or do not fill. Clients with coronary artery disease who are considered candidates for invasive treatment procedures must undergo cardiac catheterization and coronary arteriography.

After removal of the catheter, inspect the insertion site for bleeding, tenderness, hematoma formation, and inflammation. The client remains on bed rest for the rest of the day. He or she must avoid flexion, or bending, of the arm or leg used for catheter insertion. Vascular assessments distal to the insertion site continue at frequent intervals. Absent distal peripheral pulses, cool toes, and pale or cyanotic arms and legs indicate arterial occlusion, usually from a blood clot. These signs as well as a rapid or irregular pulse rate indicate a medical emergency that the nurse must report immediately to the physician.

ANGIOCARDIOGRAPHY. In **angiocardiography,** a radiopaque dye is injected into a vein, and its course through the heart is recorded by a series of radiographic pictures taken in rapid succession. The pictures reveal the size and shape of the heart chambers and great vessels and the sequence and time of their filling with dye. Angiocardiography is used to diagnose congenital abnormalities of the heart and great vessels. It usually is performed when simpler diagnostic measures fail to provide the necessary information. The client fasts for at least 3 hours before the test. A sedative and an antihistaminic medication usually are administered before the client is taken to the x-ray department.

AORTOGRAPHY. **Aortography** detects aortic abnormalities such as aneurysms (abnormal dilatation of a blood vessel wall) and arterial occlusions. When aortography is performed, contrast medium is injected and radiographic films are taken of the abdominal aorta and major arteries in the legs. Distribution of the contrast medium also may be observed as it circulates to other vessels, such as the renal arteries.

PERIPHERAL ARTERIOGRAPHY. Peripheral arteriography diagnoses occlusive arterial disease in smaller arteries. Contrast medium is injected into an artery, and x-ray films are taken. After the procedure, the chance for bleeding is greater than after a venipuncture. A pressure dressing is applied and client activity is restricted for about 12 hours. Observe the client for bleeding and cardiac dysrhythmias and assess adequacy of peripheral circulation by frequently checking peripheral pulses.

Hemodynamic Monitoring

Hemodynamic monitoring is used to assess volume and pressure of blood in the heart and vascular system by means of a surgically inserted catheter. Such monitoring assesses cardiac function and circulatory status, detects fluid imbalances, adjusts fluid infusion rates, and evaluates the client's response to therapeutic measures, such as drug therapy. Methods for hemodynamic monitoring include direct BP monitoring, **central venous pressure** (CVP) monitoring, and pulmonary artery pressure monitoring.

NURSING PROCESS

● Diagnostic Procedures of the Cardiovascular System

Assessment

For both outpatients and inpatients, perform a thorough initial assessment of clients undergoing diagnostic testing to establish accurate baseline data for use before, during, and after the procedure. Weigh the client and measure vital signs. Measure BP in both arms and compare findings. Assess apical and radial pulses, noting rate, quality, and rhythm. Check peripheral pulses in the lower extremities.

Ask the client to describe any symptoms. If the client is experiencing chest pain, a history of its location, frequency, and duration is necessary, as is a description of the pain, if it radiates to a particular area, what precipitates its onset, and what brings relief. Another important area of questioning is whether the client is experiencing pressure, fluttering, or palpitations in the chest. Ask if the client has episodes of dyspnea, dizziness, or fainting. Assess the lower extremities for edema and toes for color and temperature.

Auscultate heart and lung sounds and obtain family history of heart disease or other chronic diseases related to cardiovascular disorders such as diabetes mellitus. Another important area is identification of current prescribed medications, herbal preparations, and over-the-counter drugs used for self-treatment. Also determine the client's anxiety and knowledge level about the procedure.

Diagnosis, Planning, and Interventions

Deficient Knowledge related to the test's purpose, performance, and after-care

Expected Outcome: Client and family will demonstrate sufficient knowledge from which to provide informed consent and perform self-care afterward.

- Assess client's and family's knowledge of the diagnostic procedure. *Clarifying misconceptions or misinformation and building on what is already known are important interventions.*
- Provide both verbal and written information concerning the test's purpose, procedure, and after-care. *Written information enables the client to further process the verbal information and serves as a basis for recalling verbal instructions.*
- Use language that the client can easily understand. *Medical terminology that is not part of the client's vocabulary may heighten anxiety and intimidate the client to the extent that he or she may not ask further questions.*

- Ask client, family, or both to paraphrase information. *The ability to paraphrase provides evidence as to whether they understood information the nurse provided.*

Pain and **Activity Intolerance** related to ischemia

Expected Outcomes: (1) Pain will be relieved or controlled within a tolerable level during the diagnostic procedure. (2) Activity will be limited to that which avoids dyspnea or tachycardia.

- Assess pain level frequently before, during, and after the diagnostic procedure. *Pain is a subjective symptom that the nurse can reliably assess only by asking the client to rate and describe it.*
- Allow for rest periods. *Rest reduces heart rate and demand for increased oxygenated blood.*
- Stop the procedure, assess vital signs, give a short-acting prescribed vasodilator such as nitroglycerin, and administer oxygen if chest pain occurs. *Monitoring and treating chest pain with prescribed interventions that improve blood flow to the heart are within the interdependent nursing domain.*
- Notify the physician if rest, oxygen, or prescribed medications do not provide relief. *Sustained chest pain may require medical assessment and additional interventions.*

Risk for Injury related to untoward reactions during or after diagnostic tests

Expected Outcome: The client's condition will remain stable during and after diagnostic tests.

- Assess for dyspnea, hypotension or hypertension, cardiac dysrhythmias, mental changes, pain or discomfort, and cyanosis. *Post-test findings that differ significantly from pretest results are highly suggestive of a cause-and-effect relationship between the test's physiologic requirements and the client's response.*
- Implement nursing measures to stabilize the client, such as ensuring a patent IV access and administering oxygen and prescribed medications. *The nurse's role includes independent, interdependent, and dependent nursing actions.*
- Collaborate with the physician to restore client to a stable condition. *The physician's role is to manage complications medically; the nurse assists the physician.*

Evaluation of Expected Outcomes

The test is performed uneventfully or the client is stabilized when complications are managed successfully. The client and family have an accurate understanding of the diagnostic testing process and discharge instructions.

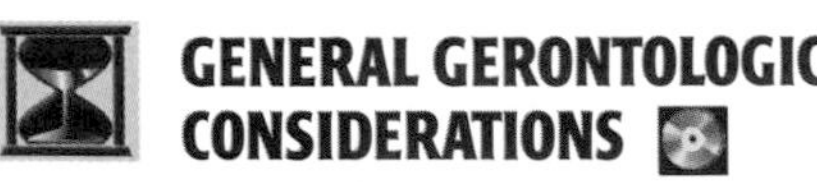

GENERAL GERONTOLOGIC CONSIDERATIONS

Older clients are more likely to experience confusion and disorientation because of advanced arteriosclerotic and atherosclerotic age-related changes that cause decreased perfusion to the brain. Repeated explanations and reassurances throughout all phases of the nursing process are indicated.

The aging heart is less able to meet demands placed on it during times of stress and requires more time to return to baseline levels after stress. This inability to handle stress results from decreased cardiac output and contractile strength and delayed conduction in the heart.

The older adult who has renal impairment or is chronically dehydrated is at increased risk for complications during and after diagnostic studies requiring the use of a dye because the iodinated contrast is nephrotoxic.

The incidence of cardiac dysrhythmias increases with age because of anatomic changes that accompany aging. Dysrhythmias also are more serious and difficult to treat in the older adult because organs that already are impaired by aging can be further compromised by the lack of adequate blood supply caused by the dysrhythmia.

Critical Thinking Exercises

1. *An outpatient client is scheduled to have a cardiac catheterization. The client's spouse asks you what the catheter is for and what will happen once it is placed. How will you respond?*
2. *You are assisting a client who is undergoing an exercise-induced stress test. What assessments would indicate that the client is responding adversely to the exercise?*

● NCLEX-STYLE REVIEW QUESTIONS 

1. A 70-year-old man comes to the emergency department complaining of chest pain. Which question is most important for the nurse to ask initially?
    1. "When did your pain begin?"
    2. "Have you had this type of pain before?"
    3. "Do you have any food or drug allergies?"
    4. "Do you have pain in any other place?"
2. A hospitalized client takes an antihypertensive medication and complains of being light-headed when getting out of bed. Which nursing intervention is most appropriate at this time?
    1. Notify the client's primary care physician.
    2. Take the client's blood pressure while she is lying, sitting, and standing.
    3. Ask the client if this has happened before.
    4. Hold the client's medication until she feels better.
3. Which client is it most important for the nurse to assess for complications following a cardiac catheterization?
    1. A 75-year-old man with an elevated blood urea nitrogen (BUN) level
    2. A 50-year-old woman who experiences occasional numbness and tingling in her hands
    3. A 25-year-old who complains of chest pain
    4. A 38-year-old with a family history of a bleeding disorder

connection

Visit the Connection site at **http://connection.lww.com/go/timbyEssentials** for links to chapter-related resources on the Internet.

References and Suggested Readings

American Heart Association. (2001). Calcium scan predicts heart attack risk in physically fit people. [On-line.] Available: http://www.americanheart.org.

Bickley, L. S. (2003). *Bates' guide to physical examination and history taking* (8th ed.). Philadelphia: Lippincott Williams & Wilkins.

Bullock, B. L., & Henze, R. L. (2000). *Focus on pathophysiology.* Philadelphia: Lippincott Williams & Wilkins.

Darty, S. N., Thomas, M. S., Neagle, C. M., et al. (2002). Cardiovascular magnetic resonance imaging. *American Journal of Nursing, 102*(12), 34–38.

Gehring, P. E. (2002). Perfecting your skills: Vascular assessment. *RN,* 4, 16–24.

He, Z., Hedrick, T. D., Pratt, C. M., et al. (2000). Severity of coronary artery calcification by electron beam computed tomography predicts silent myocardial ischemia. [On-line.] Available: http://circ.ahajournals.org/cgi/content/abstract/101/3/244.

Ide, B., & Drew, B. (2001). EKG clinical questions: How a rhythm strip aids in clinical diagnosis. *Progress in Cardiovascular Nursing, 16*(2), 88.

Khorovets, A. (2000). What is an electrocardiogram (ECG)? *Internet Journal of Advanced Nursing Practice, 4*(2), 6.

Nazzaro, C. (2002). Cardiac MRI comes of age. *Advance for Nurses, 4*(23), 29–30.

Ott, K., Johnson, K., & Ahrens, T. (2001). New technologies in the assessment of hemodynamic parameters. *Journal of Cardiovascular Nursing, 15*(2), 41–55.

Tasota, F. J., & Tate, J. (2000). Eye on diagnostics: Understanding transesophageal echocardiography. *Nursing, 30*(8), 26.

Way, S., Redeker, N. S., Moreyra, A. E., et al. (2001). Comparison of comfort and local complications after cardiac catheterization. *Clinical Nursing Research, 10*(1), 29–39.

chapter 25

Caring for Clients With Infectious and Inflammatory Disorders of the Heart and Blood Vessels

Words to Know 

cardiac tamponade
cardiomyopathy
decortication
deep vein thrombosis
effusion
emboli
Homans' sign
impedance plethysmography
infective endocarditis
intermittent claudication
murmur
myocardial disarray
myocarditis
myofibrils
pericardiectomy
pericardiocentesis
pericardiostomy
pericarditis
petechiae
postphlebitic syndrome
precordial pain
pulmonary embolus
pulsus paradoxus
rheumatic carditis
splinter hemorrhages
syncope
thrombectomy
thrombophlebitis
vegetations
vena caval filter
vena caval plication procedure
venography
Virchow's triad

Learning Objectives

On completion of this chapter, the reader will:

- Identify inflammatory conditions of the heart.
- Describe organisms that cause infectious conditions of the heart.
- Explain treatments for inflammatory and infectious heart disorders.
- Discuss nursing management of clients with infectious or inflammatory heart disorders.
- Compare the types of cardiomyopathy.
- List interventions that reduce the risk of thrombophlebitis.
- Discuss nursing management of clients with inflammatory disorders of peripheral blood vessels.

The body uses many defense mechanisms to combat the effects of trauma, disease, and microorganisms. The inflammatory response, skin and mucous membranes, and immune system work together to protect the body's cardiovascular system. Despite these protective mechanisms, infectious and inflammatory disorders may compromise the heart and blood vessels.

INFECTIOUS AND INFLAMMATORY DISORDERS OF THE HEART

• INFECTIVE ENDOCARDITIS

Infective endocarditis (formerly called *bacterial endocarditis*) is inflammation of the inner layer of heart tissue as a result of an infectious microorganism. Endocarditis is initially considered an autoimmune response—not an infection—because no microorganism can be isolated from blood or other cultured specimens. Valvular changes associated with rheumatic carditis increase a client's susceptibility to endocardial colonization by pathogens. **Rheumatic carditis** refers to inflammatory cardiac manifestations of rheumatic fever in either the acute or later stage. Cardiac structures usually affected include (1) heart valves, particularly the mitral valve; (2) endocardium; (3) myocardium; and (4) pericardium. Other susceptible clients include those with nonrheumatic valve disease or artificial heart valves, repaired congenital heart defects, a prolapsed mitral valve, or hypertrophic cardiomyopathy (discussed later); IV drug users; and immunosuppressed clients with central venous catheters.

Pathophysiology and Etiology

Microorganisms that cause infective endocarditis include bacteria and fungi (Box 25-1). *Streptococcus viridans* and *Staphylococcus aureus* are the most common causes. They are found abundantly on skin and mucous membranes of the mouth, nose, throat, and other cavities.

Most pathogens find their way into the bloodstream through trauma caused by invasive procedures involving mucous membranes or other tissues that harbor microorganisms. Although anyone can contract endocarditis, clients with a history of rheumatic carditis are especially susceptible. Prolonged IV therapy, insertion of cardiac pacemakers, cardiac catheterization, tracheal intubation, cardiac surgery, genitourinary instrumentation (Foley catheters and cystoscopy), and IV drug abuse create portals of entry for causative microorganisms. Once microorganisms migrate to the endocardial surface, they attach themselves to **vegetations** composed of fibrin and platelets surrounding heart valves, chordae tendineae, and papillary muscles (Fig. 25.1). Microorganisms bury themselves in the vegetative mass, making them difficult to destroy with natural defenses or antibiotic therapy. The cycle continues with layer upon layer of imbedded microorganisms and fibrin/platelet deposits.

The endocardium on the left side of the heart is affected more often than on the right. The mitral valve is the most common location of vegetations and microbial deposits. If valve leaflets erode and slough, blood leaks between the heart chambers, diminishing the heart's efficiency as a pump. Heart failure often is a consequence. Vegetations can break off to form **emboli,** mobile masses of fibrin and clusters of platelets that circulate in the bloodstream. Emboli may occlude small blood vessels and interfere with an organ's blood supply.

BOX 25-1 ● Microorganisms That Cause Endocarditis

Streptococci	Account for 55% of cases of endocarditis
Group A beta-hemolytic	Attack normal or damaged heart valves and may cause rapid destruction
S. bovis	Related to GI malignancy
S. viridans	Tend to affect previously damaged heart valves
Staphylococci	Cause 30% of cases of endocarditis
S. aureus	Virulent strain with high mortality rate
S. epidermidis	Associated with dental procedures and valve replacements
S. faecalis	Cause both acute and subacute infections Associated with urologic instrumentation in men, bacteremia, respiratory tract infections, pneumonia, sinusitis, otitis media, and epiglotitis
Enterococci	Normal inhabitants of the GI tract, anterior urethra, and occasionally the mouth
E. faecalis and *E. faecium*	Relatively resistant to single antibiotics; require combination of antibiotic therapy for a minimum of 4 weeks
HACEK Group	Slow-growing gram-negative bacilli
***H**aemophilus parainfluenzae* and *Haemophilus aphrophilus*	Require culture for 2 weeks or longer when initial culture is negative Cause subacute presentations Associated with very large vegetations
***A**ctinobacillus actinomycetemcomitans*	
***C**ardiobacterium hominis*	
***E**ikenella corrodens*	
***K**ingella kingae*	
Fungi	Increased incidence in IV drug users
Candida	Risk increased with improper use of antibiotics and steroids
Gram-negative bacteria	May travel from GI or genitourinary tracts
Escherichia coli	Increased risk in older adults
Klebsiella	
Pseudomonas	

GI, gastrointestinal.

Assessment Findings

Infective endocarditis can have an acute onset (less than 1 week). The client has fever, chills, muscle aches in the lower back and thighs, and joint pain. Subacute infections progress slowly over weeks to months with vague signs such as headache, malaise, fatigue, and sleep disturbances. As the condition advances, purplish, painful nodules may appear on the pads of the fingers and toes. Black longitudinal lines (**splinter hemorrhages**) can be seen in the nails. The spleen may be enlarged and tender. A heart murmur may be present from malfunctioning valves. **Petechiae,** tiny, reddish hemorrhagic spots on the skin and mucous membranes, indicate embolization. Pronounced weakness, anorexia, and weight loss are common. Symptoms change suddenly if embolization or

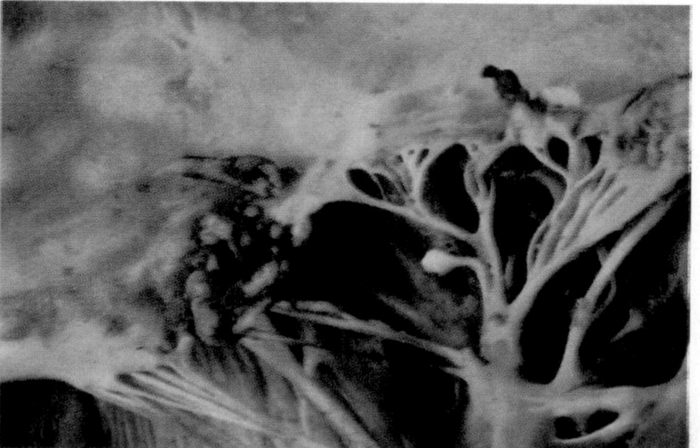

FIGURE 25.1 Bacterial endocarditis. The mitral valve shows destructive vegetations. (Rubin E., & Farber J. L. [1999]. *Pathology* [3rd ed., p. 572]. Philadelphia: Lippincott Williams & Wilkins.)

heart failure occurs. Emboli to the brain cause cerebrovascular accidents (see Chap. 40); emboli to the kidneys cause flank pain and renal failure (see Chap. 58); pulmonary emboli result in sudden chest pain and dyspnea (see Chap. 23). Clients with heart failure present with dyspnea, hypotension, and peripheral or pulmonary edema.

Anemia and slight leukocytosis are common findings. A series of three blood cultures collected over 1 to 24 hours usually identifies the microorganism circulating in the blood. Vegetations may be cultured. Echocardiography reveals vegetations, altered valvular function, and impaired pumping quality of the ventricles. ECG may reveal abnormalities in heart rhythm if vegetations involve a valve close to conduction tissue.

Medical and Surgical Management

High doses of an appropriate IV antibiotic are prescribed initially (Drug Therapy Table 25.1). Antibiotic therapy lasts 2 to 6 weeks. It is resumed if the infection recurs. Bed rest is ordered initially. When the client begins to

DRUG THERAPY TABLE 25.1 AGENTS USED TO TREAT ENDOCARDITIS

DRUG	MECHANISM OF ACTION	SIDE EFFECTS	NURSING CONSIDERATIONS
penicillin G (Pfizerpen, Pentids, Wycillin, Bicillin)	Inhibits cell wall synthesis of organisms sensitive to penicillin G, killing the organisms	Allergic reaction: rash, fever, wheezing; possibly anaphylaxis and death Nausea, vomiting, diarrhea, abdominal pain, glossitis, stomatitis, gastritis, furry tongue	Be sure to check client's allergy history before administering. In acute care settings, retrieve the antibiotic from the refrigerator 15 minutes before administration. Evaluate the IV site for phlebitis before and after administration. Administer IM penicillin deep into the muscle mass.
nafcillin (Unipen)	Inhibits cell wall synthesis of organisms sensitive to nafcillin, killing the organisms	Lethargy, hallucinations, seizures, glossitis, stomatitis, gastritis, furry tongue, anemia, nephritis	Use cautiously in clients with renal disorders. If giving IM, alternate sites. Repeated use of the same site can result in atrophy. Be sure to administer oral forms 1 hour before or 2 hours after meals. Do not administer with soft drinks or fruit juices.
gentamicin (Garamycin, Gentacidin)	Inhibits protein synthesis in gram-negative, susceptible strains Appears to disrupt function of bacterial cell membranes, killing the bacteria	Tinnitus, dizziness, vertigo, nausea, vomiting, palpitations, purpura, rash, fever, apnea, irreversible ototoxicity, nephrotoxicity	Give by IM route if possible. Ensure that the client receives adequate hydration throughout therapy. Monitor results of renal function tests, complete blood counts, and serum drug levels.
ceftriaxone (Rocephin)	Inhibits cell wall synthesis of bacteria sensitive to ceftriaxone, killing the organisms	Nausea, vomiting, diarrhea, anorexia, abdominal pain, flatulence, rash, fever, pain, superinfections	Advise clients to avoid alcohol and substances that contain alcohol to prevent a disulfiram-like reaction. Protect the drug from exposure to light. For clients with renal or hepatic impairment, monitor blood levels of the drug to prevent toxicity.
vancomycin (Vancocin)	Inhibits cell wall synthesis of bacteria sensitive to vancomycin, killing the organisms	Ototoxicity, nausea, nephrotoxicity, urticaria (hives)	When clients are receiving long-term therapy, continually monitor results of renal function tests. Advise the client not to discontinue the drug without notifying the physician.
rifampin (Rifadin)	Inhibits RNA polymerase activity in sensitive bacterial cells	Headache, drowsiness, fatigue, dizziness, heartburn, epigastric distress, eosinophilia, thrombocytopenia, rash, "flulike syndrome"	Administer this drug to a client with an empty stomach 1 hour before or 2 hours after meals. Advise client that this drug will color body fluids orange-red. Tell the client to report fever, chills, muscle and bone pain, fatigue, anorexia, yellow skin or eye, or unusual bruising, bleeding, rash, or itching.

improve, bathroom privileges and increased activity are allowed. If a heart valve is severely damaged and drug therapy does not adequately support the heart in failure, valve replacement may be necessary (see Chaps. 26 and 31).

Nursing Management

Many clients cannot appreciate the danger of the disease without seeing external signs of damage. Remind the client to limit activity. Continually assess for changes in weight and pulse rate and rhythm and note and report new symptoms. Administer prescribed antibiotics around the clock to sustain therapeutic blood levels of the medication at all times. Inform clients that periodic antibiotic therapy is a lifelong necessity because they are vulnerable to the disease for the rest of their lives.

Stop, Think, and Respond ● BOX 25-1

If a client asks why he or she needs to take an antibiotic before having dental work done, what information is appropriate to provide?

• MYOCARDITIS

Pathophysiology and Etiology

Myocarditis is inflammation of the myocardium (the muscle layer of the heart). A viral, bacterial, fungal, or parasitic infection causes most cases; a viral origin is most common in the United States. Typical viral agents are coxsackie virus A and B, influenza A and B, measles, adeno virus, mumps, rubella, rubeola, Epstein-Barr virus, and cytomegalovirus (Lewandowski, 1999). The myocardium also can become inflamed from toxins of microorganisms, chronic alcohol and cocaine abuse, radiation therapy, or autoimmune disorders.

Whatever the cause, an inflammatory response causes cardiac muscle tissue to swell, which interferes with the myocardium's ability to stretch and recoil. Cardiac output is reduced and blood circulation is impaired, predisposing the client to CHF (see Chap. 30). The myocardium becomes ischemic from a reduced supply of oxygenated blood, predisposing the client to tachycardia and dysrhythmias. Cardiomyopathy, atypical changes in the myocardial wall, may develop as a complication of myocarditis and other disorders.

Assessment Findings

Clients may complain of general chest discomfort relieved by sitting up, low-grade fever, tachycardia, dysrhythmias, dyspnea, malaise, fatigue, and anorexia. Skin may be pale or cyanotic. If the heart's pumping activity is impaired, neck vein distention, ascites, and peripheral edema may be noted, indicating right-sided heart failure. Crackles may be heard in the lungs if the left side fails. An S_3 galloping rhythm or a pericardial friction rub may be heard.

Serum electrolyte levels and thyroid function studies help rule out other causes for the symptoms. The WBC count is slightly elevated. C-reactive protein, a nonspecific antigen–antibody test, is elevated in inflammatory conditions. Cardiac isoenzyme levels are elevated, and results of ECG may be abnormal. Chest x-rays show overall heart enlargement and fluid infiltration in the lungs. Echocardiography demonstrates structural and functional abnormalities in the ventricles, such as impaired motion of the ventricular wall and reduced ejection of blood from the heart. Radionuclide studies reveal areas where the myocardial wall is enlarged, thickened, or scarred. A myocardial biopsy may be done to obtain a definitive diagnosis.

Medical and Surgical Management

Management aims at treating the underlying cause and preventing complications. Antibiotics are prescribed if the infecting microorganism is bacterial. Bed rest, a sodium-restricted diet, and cardiotonic drugs (digitalis and related drugs) are prescribed to prevent or treat heart failure. In severe cases of cardiomyopathy, a heart transplant is necessary.

Nursing Management

Monitor the client's cardiopulmonary status to assess for possible complications such as CHF or dysrhythmias. Assessments include vital signs, daily weights, intake and output, heart and lung sounds, pulse oximetry measurements, and dependent edema. The client is on bed rest to reduce cardiac workload and promote healing. If the client is febrile, administer a prescribed antipyretic; minimize layers of bed linen, promoting air circulation and evaporation of perspiration; and offer oral fluids. Administer supplemental oxygen to relieve tachycardia that develops from hypoxemia. Elevating the client's head promotes maximal breathing potential. Use a bedside cardiac monitor or telemetry unit to assess heart rhythm, which determines if and when antidysrhythmic medications are necessary, or the client's response to their use.

• CARDIOMYOPATHY

Cardiomyopathy is a chronic condition characterized by structural changes in heart muscle. Three major types of cardiomyopathies are (1) dilated cardiomyopathy, (2) hypertrophic cardiomyopathy, and (3) restrictive cardiomyopathy (Table 25.1).

TABLE 25.1 TYPES OF CARDIOMYOPATHY

TYPE	CAUSES	DESCRIPTION	TREATMENT
Dilated	Viral myocarditis Autoimmune response Chemicals (e.g., chronic alcohol ingestion)	The cavity of the heart is stretched (dilated).	Drug therapy to minimize symptoms and prevent complications Abstinence from alcohol Salt restriction Weight loss Possible heart transplantation
Hypertrophic	Hereditary Unknown	The muscle of the left ventricle and septum thickens, causing heart enlargement.	Drug therapy to reduce heart rate and force of contraction Antidysrhythmic drugs Artificial pacemaker Alcohol ablation: injection of alcohol into an artery supplying the extra tissue to destroy excess heart muscle (currently experimental) Ventriculomyotomy, a surgical procedure to reduce muscle tissue
Restrictive	Deposits of amyloid Scleroderma, a connective tissue disorder Granulomatous tumors Hemochromatosis, iron stores in tissue Scar tissue that forms after a myocardial infarction	Heart muscle stiffens, which interferes with its ability to stretch and fill with blood.	No specific treatment; drugs such as diuretics and antihypertensives used to control symptoms

Pathophysiology and Etiology

In some cases, there is no explanation for cardiomyopathy. In others, cardiomyopathy accompanies or follows another medical problem, such as myocarditis, connective tissue disorders like systemic lupus erythematosus, muscular dystrophy, chronic alcoholism, or cancer chemotherapy. Regardless of the cause, heart muscle loses its ability to pump blood efficiently. When a client's medical history includes disorders that are bacterial or viral in origin, a family history of early cardiac deaths, or any of several other conditions that correlate with heart involvement, the possibility of cardiomyopathy is considered. For some affected clients, their condition remains stable for a long period before disabling symptoms develop; others are unaware of their condition until there is a potentially fatal cardiac event like a sudden dysrhythmia or heart failure.

Assessment Findings

Manifestations of cardiomyopathy vary slightly according to the type that develops:

- *Dilated cardiomyopathy,* the most common type, is accompanied by dyspnea on exertion and when lying down. Clients feel fatigued and their legs swell. They may experience palpitations and chest pain.
- *Hypertrophic cardiomyopathy* is associated with **syncope** (sudden loss of consciousness) or near-syncopal episodes, which clients describe as "graying out." They also may feel fatigued, become short of breath, and develop chest pain. Many are asymptomatic and the disorder is not discovered until the client dies or becomes acutely ill after strenuous exercise.
- *Restrictive cardiomyopathy,* which is the least common type in the United States but more common in tropical locales of Africa, India, South and Central America, and Asia, has symptoms of exertional dyspnea, dependent edema in the legs, ascites (fluid in the abdomen), and hepatomegaly (enlarged liver).

A heart **murmur,** which is an atypical heart sound, may be the first abnormal sign detected. Forceful heart contractions may be palpated over the left chest wall.

Cardiomyopathy sometimes is detected among asymptomatic clients during other diagnostic tests. Chest x-ray may show heart enlargement. An exercise, chemical, or ambulatory ECG provides evidence of abnormal cardiac rhythm. Definitive diagnosis is determined by performing an echocardiogram and cardiac catheterization. During cardiac catheterization, elevated pressures are detected in the heart ventricles. In some cases, an endomyocardial biopsy is performed, which may reveal **myocardial disarray** (Fig. 25.2), an alteration in the usual alignment of

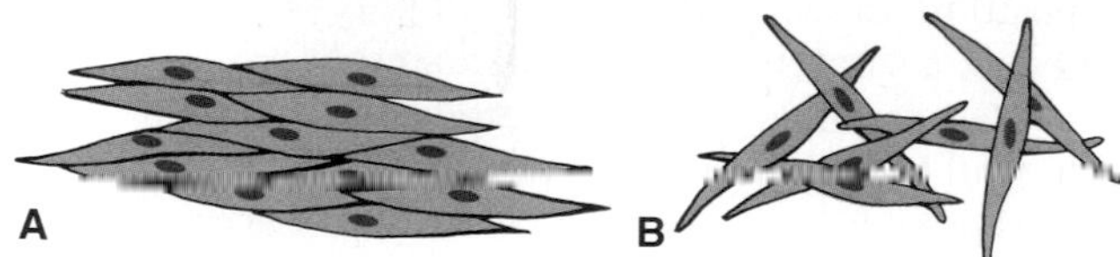

FIGURE 25.2 (**A**) Normal muscle structure. (**B**) Myocardial disarray.

myofibrils, the contractile component of muscle tissue. The result is a lack of coordination during systole (ventricular contraction) and impaired diastole, the period of ventricular relaxation (Porth, 2002). Radionuclide studies show the heart muscle's inability to contract efficiently when stressed during exercise.

Medical and Surgical Management

Treatment depends on the type of cardiomyopathy. See Table 25.1 for more information.

Nursing Management

Obtain a comprehensive medical and family history and ask clients to describe any symptoms. Outpatients may be attached to an ambulatory cardiac monitor; nurses teach such clients to keep a journal of their symptoms. Perform a physical examination that includes taking vital signs, auscultating heart and lung sounds, and checking for peripheral edema and abdominal enlargement. Note an irregular pulse, tachycardia, or reduced levels of oxygen saturation (SpO_2) on pulse oximetry, which may occur during postural changes or exercise. Clients are usually monitored.

Oxygen is administered either continuously or when dyspnea or dysrhythmias develop. Administer prescribed medications and collect data to evaluate their effectiveness. Ensure that the client's activity level is reduced and sequence any activity that is slightly exertional between periods of rest.

Support clients emotionally as they cope with a chronic, perhaps life-threatening illness. Help clients identify realistic limitations, yet avoid becoming invalids as a consequence of fear. Depending on the type of cardiomyopathy, encourage family members to undergo diagnostic testing to determine if they also have the same disorder. A teaching plan includes the following components:

- Achieve a healthy weight by following dietary instructions, limiting sodium to reduce fluid retention, and avoiding beverages containing caffeine, which contributes to tachycardia.
- Stop using tobacco products because nicotine is a vasoconstrictor and cardiac stimulant.
- Stay within exercise tolerance limits or stop activity immediately if dyspnea or chest pain develops.
- Restrict driving or operating equipment if syncope is a common symptom.
- Keep appointments for medical follow-up to evaluate the status of the disease and symptom control.
- Receive the pneumonia vaccine and yearly influenza vaccinations to avoid pulmonary complications that may compromise cardiopulmonary function.
- For female clients, seek co-consultation with a cardiologist and an obstetrician if pregnancy is desired.

• PERICARDITIS

Pericarditis, inflammation of the pericardium, can be a primary condition (develops independently of any other condition) or a secondary condition (develops because of another condition). Inflammation can occur with or without **effusion,** the accumulation of fluid between two layers of tissue.

Pathophysiology and Etiology

Pericarditis usually is secondary to endocarditis, myocarditis, chest trauma, or myocardial infarction (MI; heart attack) or develops after cardiac surgery. Other causes include tuberculosis, malignant tumors, uremia, and connective tissue disorders. When pericardial cells become inflamed, their membranes become more permeable and intracellular fluid leaks into the interstitial spaces. The exudate or effusion can be serous, resembling clear serum, fibrinous, like thick, congealed liquid; purulent, containing pus; or sanguineous, containing blood.

Pericardial fluid accumulation results in **cardiac tamponade,** acute compression of the heart. Pericardial fluid occupies space the heart needs to accommodate for filling with blood (Fig. 25.3). Impaired filling is reflected by a condition called *pulsus paradoxus* or *paradoxical pulse.* **Pulsus paradoxus** is a difference of 10 mm Hg or more between the first Korotkoff sound heralding systolic blood pressure (BP) heard during expiration and the first that is heard during inspiration. The normal difference between the two is 4 to 5 mm Hg. The technique for detecting pulsus paradoxus is described in Nursing Guidelines 25-1. Pulsus paradoxus develops because reduction in the volume capacity of the left ventricle during inspiration is greater, combined with an impaired ability of the left ventricle to expand because of the rigid pericardium. The smaller capacity reduces stroke volume from the left ventricle. As cardiac tamponade progresses, stroke volume is diminished, cardiac output is compromised, and death may result.

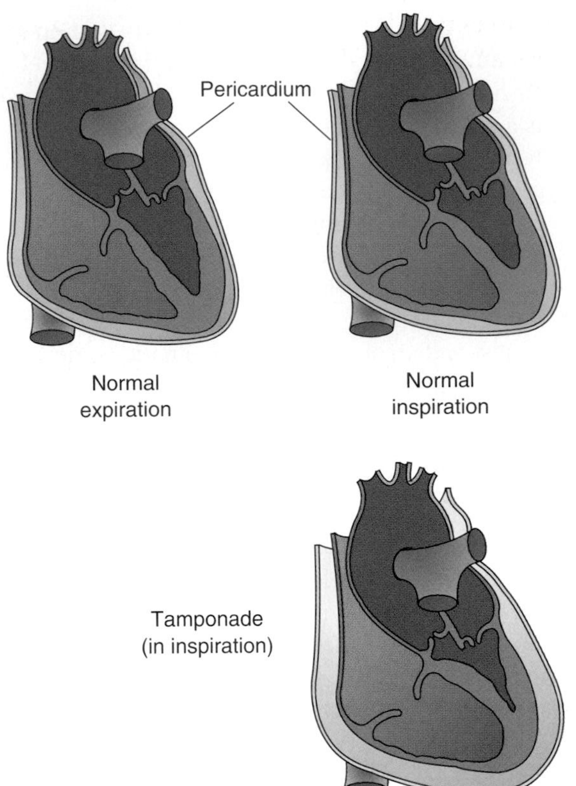

FIGURE 25.3 Effects of respiration and cardiac tamponade on ventricular filling and cardiac output.

Assessment Findings

Typical signs and symptoms that accompany an inflammatory response, such as fever and malaise, are present. The client is dyspneic or complains of heaviness in the chest. One chief characteristic is **precordial pain** (pain in the anterior chest overlying the heart). It may be slight or severe and mistaken for esophagitis, indigestion, pleurisy, or MI. Moving and breathing deeply worsen the pain; sitting upright and leaning forward relieve it, whereas pain of acute MI remains unchanged regardless of position, movement, or breathing. A pericardial friction rub, a scratchy, high-pitched sound, is a diagnostic sign. Heart sounds are difficult to hear because accumulating fluid muffles them. Respiratory symptoms occur as the enlarged heart crowds the airway passages and lung tissue and respirations become rapid and labored. Hypotension is severe, and pulse quality is weak.

The ST segment of the ECG is elevated, but cardiac isoenzyme levels are normal. The heart may appear enlarged on chest x-ray. Echocardiography demonstrates a wide gap between the pericardium and epicardium, indicating that the space is filled with fluid. Hemodynamic monitoring values are abnormal. Pericardial fluid may be cultured, but it is a nonbacterial cause, test results often are nondiagnostic. The WBC count and ESR often are elevated.

NURSING GUIDELINES 25-1

Assessment of Pulsus Paradoxus

- Advise client to breathe normally throughout the assessment.
- Inflate BP cuff 20 mm Hg above systolic pressure.
- Deflate the cuff slowly, noting that sounds are audible during expiration but not inspiration.
- Note when the first BP sound (Korotkoff's) is heard.
- Continue to deflate the cuff until BP sounds are heard during both inspiration and expiration.
- Measure the difference in mm Hg between the first BP sound heard during expiration and the first BP sound heard during both inspiration and expiration.

Medical and Surgical Management

MI (see Chap. 27) must be ruled out. Treatment of pericarditis depends on the underlying cause. Rest, analgesics, antipyretics, nonsteroidal anti-inflammatory drugs, and sometimes corticosteroids are prescribed. **Pericardiocentesis,** needle aspiration of fluid from between the visceral and parietal pericardium, may be necessary when cardiac output is severely reduced. A small drainage catheter can be left in place. Needle aspiration is hazardous because the needle can puncture the myocardium, a branch of a coronary artery, or the pleura.

When pericardiocentesis and catheter drainage are inadequate, a **pericardiostomy,** a surgical opening or window, is made in the pericardium to allow fluid to drain. Constrictive pericarditis is treated surgically by removing the pericardium (**pericardiectomy** or **decortication**) to allow more adequate filling and contraction of the heart chambers.

NURSING PROCESS

● The Client With Pericarditis

Assessment

Ask the client about the incidence and nature of the pain and what worsens or relieves it. Assess for a pericardial friction rub by asking the client to briefly hold his or her breath while you auscultate heart sounds; a pericardial friction rub does not disappear when the client holds the breath. Note additional signs and symptoms that further suggest cardiac tamponade and decreased cardiac output (Fig. 25.4).

Diagnosis, Planning, and Interventions

Pain related to pericardial inflammation and decreased myocardial perfusion

Expected Outcome: Client will be free of pain or pain will be tolerable 30 minutes after a nursing intervention.

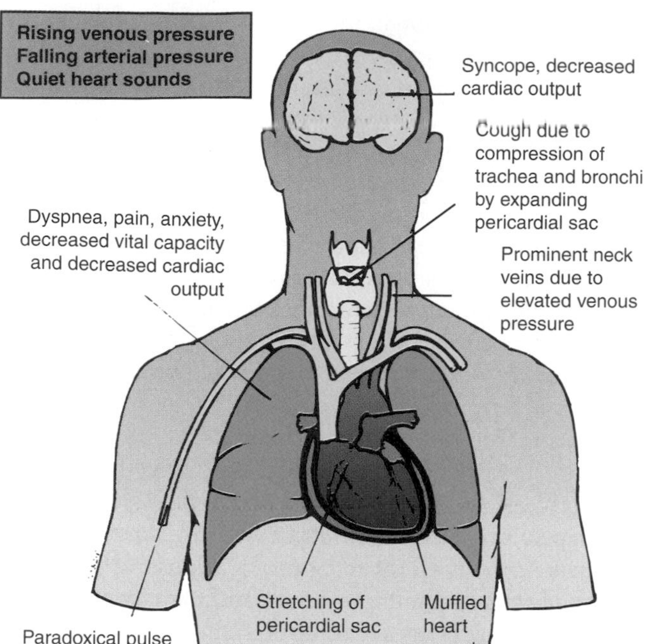

FIGURE 25.4 Signs and symptoms of cardiac tamponade. (From Smeltzer, S. C. & Bare, B. G. [2004]. *Brunner & Suddarth's textbook of medical–surgical nursing* [10th ed.]. Philadelphia: Lippincott Williams & Wilkins.)

- Assess pain status as often as vital signs. *Pain is considered the fifth vital sign. When pain exists, the nurse must implement interventions targeted for its relief.*
- Assist client to a position of comfort such as sitting upright and leaning forward. *Sitting up and leaning forward positions the stretched pericardium away from the pleura, which relieves discomfort.*
- Administer anti-inflammatory drugs and analgesics as prescribed. *Reduced inflammation and pain transmission promote comfort.*
- Reassure client that pericardial pain does not indicate an MI. *Clarifying the reality and significance of pain may reduce the workload of the heart and acuity of discomfort.*

Decreased Cardiac Output related to inability of the heart muscle to stretch completely, fill with appropriate amount of blood, and eject a sufficient volume during ventricular systole

Expected Outcome: Client will (1) maintain normal arterial BP, (2) remain alert, (3) be free of chest pain, and (4) eliminate at least 35 mL of urine per hour.

- Monitor vital signs every 4 hours and as needed. *Hypotension and tachycardia are signs of decreased cardiac output.*
- Measure urine output every hour unless output is greater than 35 mL/hour. *Kidneys cannot form urine when renal artery blood supply is reduced secondary to decreased cardiac output. An output of at least 35 mL/hour is necessary to eliminate nitrogen wastes and other toxic substances.*
- Monitor for cardiac dysrhythmias. *Hypoxemia is a leading cause of dysrhythmias. Inadequate cardiac output creates potential for myocardial ischemia and disturbances in electrical conduction.*
- Assess orientation. *Confusion and disorientation are signs of compromised cerebral arterial blood flow secondary to decreased cardiac output.*
- Instruct client to report chest pain. *It is a consequence of inadequate blood supply to the myocardium.*
- Maintain bed rest. *Activity increases demand for myocardial oxygenation, which depends on cardiac output.*
- Administer supplemental oxygen as prescribed. *Giving more than the 20% oxygen that is present in room air helps reduce hypoxemia that results from inadequate cardiac output.*
- Provide six small meals a day; avoid gas-forming foods. *Abdominal distention crowds the thoracic cavity and compresses space the heart needs to fill with blood and the lungs need to fill with air.*
- Restrict caffeine and sodium. *Caffeine increases heart rate and sodium increases circulating blood volume, both of which increase myocardial work and need for cardiac output.*
- Collaborate with physician regarding a stool softener. *Bearing down during bowel movements interferes with cardiac filling and output. Stool softeners promote ease of eliminating stool.*
- Administer prescribed medications such as sedatives, anxiolytics, vasodilators, diuretics, antidysrhythmics. *Reducing anxiety, keeping the client calm and quiet, reducing BP and volume, and facilitating normal heart conduction help avoid exceeding the heart's ability to eject an adequate cardiac output.*

Evaluation of Expected Outcomes

The client states pain is relieved. Vital signs are stable, and cardiac rhythm is normal. The client is alert and oriented. Urine output exceeds 35 mL/hour. See Client and Family Teaching 25-1.

> **Stop, Think, and Respond ● BOX 25-2**
>
> *While caring for a client with pericarditis, you measure the client's BP and hear the first Korotkoff sound during expiration at 110 mm Hg. The sounds continue throughout auscultation, and you note that when the manometer is at 98 mm Hg, you hear sounds during both inspiration and expiration. Is this client manifesting pulsus paradoxus?*

INFLAMMATORY DISORDERS OF THE PERIPHERAL BLOOD VESSELS

● THROMBOPHLEBITIS

Thrombophlebitis is an inflammation of a vein accompanied by clot or thrombus formation. Although clots can form in any blood vessel, veins deep in the lower

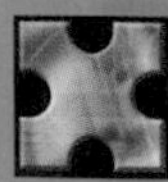

25-1 *Client and Family Teaching* Infectious and Inflammatory Heart Disorders

The nurse performs the following teaching components:

- Explains procedures required during therapy and the importance of each treatment modality
- Informs clients of need for continued follow-up care because they are always at risk for endocarditis
- Advises those with a history of rheumatic fever, congenital valve disorders, or prosthetic valve replacements to see physician if fever, malaise, or other symptoms of infection occur
- Instructs clients with damaged heart valves about need for antibiotics before and after an event that can cause bacteremia, such as dental surgery
- Ensures that clients who are prescribed antibiotics understand that they must take the full dose for the full time because noncompliance with the drug regimen hinders complete destruction of the pathogen
- Explains how to take medications, potential adverse effects, and signs to report
- Provides written instructions or pamphlets explaining prescribed drugs in language the layperson can understand
- Finds discreet ways to quiz client, such as asking, "How often must you take this drug?" to evaluate if the client has understood the instructions
- Documents information provided and evidence of the client's understanding

extremities are most commonly affected. In such cases, the condition is referred to as **deep vein thrombosis** (DVT). Thrombi that form in or above the popliteal vein of the leg are at high risk for migration toward the pulmonary circulation; these cases are referred to as a **pulmonary embolus** (PE).

Pathophysiology and Etiology

When the inner lining of a vein is irritated or injured, platelets clump together, forming a clot. The clot interferes with blood flow, causing congestion of venous blood distal to the blood clot. Sometimes collateral vessels recirculate the blood blocked by the clot. Accumulated waste products in the blocked vessel irritate the vein wall, initiating an inflammatory response. Increased permeability of cells and convergence of leukocytes and lymphocytes cause the area to swell, redden, and feel warm and tender.

Development of a PE may complicate thrombophlebitis if the clot in the extremity becomes mobile and moves in the venous circulation to the lungs (see Chap. 23). Despite appropriate and successful treatment of thrombophlebitis, some clients experience a vascular complication referred to as **postphlebitic syndrome** for up to 5 years after the initial episode (Church, 2000). For example, valvular impairment in the affected vein may follow the original thrombotic event. Incompetent valves are less efficient at returning venous blood to the heart. When venous pressure increases because of pooled blood, some fluid leaks from capillaries into subcutaneous tissue, causing leg ulcers.

Venous stasis (slowed circulation), altered blood coagulation, and trauma to the vein, referred to as **Virchow's triad,** predispose clients to thrombosis and thrombophlebitis. Factors contributing to clot formation include inactivity, reduced cardiac output, compression of veins in the pelvis or legs, and injury. Some IV drugs and chemicals also irritate the vein. Thrombi are prone to form in arm, subclavian, or jugular veins cannulated for extended IV use. Older adults with heart and blood vessel disease are susceptible to thrombophlebitis because of impaired mobility, reduced activity, and compromised circulation. Risk for clot formation is increased among women who take oral contraceptives, although the exact trigger is not known. Women who take oral contraceptives and smoke are at even higher risk.

Assessment Findings

Clients with thrombophlebitis frequently complain of discomfort in the affected extremity. Calf pain that increases on dorsiflexion of the foot is referred to as a positive **Homans' sign.** Heat, redness, and swelling develop along the length of the affected vein. Capillary refill takes less than 2 seconds because of venous congestion. The client often has a fever, malaise, fatigue, and anorexia.

Most cases of thrombophlebitis are diagnosed according to clinical findings alone. **Venography,** using radiopaque dye instilled into the venous system, indicates a filling defect in the area of the clot. Doppler ultrasound may detect an area of venous obstruction. Results of Doppler ultrasound sometimes are difficult to interpret because there are so many collateral vessels, and deep veins are especially difficult to assess. **Impedance plethysmography** (IPG) is the preferred test for diagnosing clots in deep veins. During IPG, a sensor records blood volume in the arm or leg before and after inflating a BP cuff to stop venous blood flow. If a clot is present, blood volumes are nearly the same because the clot impairs venous return.

Medical and Surgical Management

Complete rest of the arm or leg is essential to prevent the thrombus from breaking free and floating in the circulation (embolus). Anticoagulant therapy with heparin, oral anticoagulants, or drugs that prevent platelet aggregation (clustering) are prescribed to decrease the incidence of future clot formation (Drug Therapy Table 25.2). Low–molecular-weight heparins such as enoxaparin (Lovenox) enable clients with thrombophlebitis with small thrombi to be treated at home. People with repeated episodes may be placed on oral anticoagulant therapy for 3 to 6 months.

Continuous warm, wet packs are ordered to improve circulation, ease pain, and decrease inflammation. Surgical intervention may be necessary when a clot occludes a large vein or the danger of a PE arises. **Thrombectomy,** surgical removal of a clot, is performed if the clot interferes with venous drainage from a large vein such as the femoral vein. With danger of PE, surgery on the inferior vena cava may be necessary to reduce the possibility of a clot traveling from the legs to the lungs. Several surgical procedures may be performed on the vena cava: ligation, insertion of an umbrella-like **vena caval filter** (Fig. 25.5) to trap emboli before they reach the heart and lungs, or plication. A **vena caval plication procedure** changes the lumen of the vena cava from a single channel to several small channels through the use of a suture or Teflon clip.

NURSING PROCESS

The Client With Thrombophlebitis

Assessment

Determine if the client has a history of blood clots or other risk factors that predispose to thrombus formation, such as cardiovascular disorders or recent surgery, especially

DRUG THERAPY TABLE 25.2 ANTICOAGULANTS

DRUG	MECHANISM OF ACTION	SIDE EFFECTS	NURSING CONSIDERATIONS
heparin sodium (Hepalean)	Inhibits thrombus and clot formation by blocking the conversion of prothrombin to thrombin and fibrinogen to fibrin	Hemorrhage, bruising, thrombocytopenia, alopecia, chills, fever Chance of hemorrhage increases with oral anticoagulants	Monitor PTT test range between 1½ to 2½ times normal. Apply pressure to all IM injection sites. Monitor for epistaxis and other forms of bleeding. Have protamine sulfate readily available in case of overdose.
low–molecular-weight heparin enoxaparin (Lovenox), dalteparin (Fragmin), andeparin (Normiflo)	Inhibits thrombus and clot formation by blocking factors Xa and IIa	Bruising, hemorrhage, fever, pain, local irritation	Note that laboratory monitoring is not done. Provide devices like a soft toothbrush and electric razor to protect against bleeding. Ensure the availability of protamine sulfate in case of overdose. Ensure that the client avoids foods with vitamin K. Monitor PT ratio or INR regularly to adjust dosage.
warfarin (Coumadin)	Interferes with the hepatic synthesis of vitamin K–dependent clotting factors	Nausea, alopecia, urticaria, dermatitis, prolonged bleeding	Evaluate client regularly for signs of blood loss—petechiae, dark stools and urine, bruises, bleeding gums. Keep vitamin K on hand in case of overdose. Monitor WBC count before and during therapy to assess for neutropenia.
ticlopidine (Ticlid)	Inhibits binding of fibrinogen and interactions of platelets	Diarrhea, nausea, vomiting, abdominal pain, neutropenia, phlebitis	Administer with food.
aspirin	Inhibits platelet aggregation	Nausea, epigastric pain, occult blood loss, anaphylaxis, tinnitus, dizziness, increased risk of bleeding, especially with other anticoagulants	Give with food. Advise client not to crush or chew enteric-coated or sustained-release tablets.
glycoprotein IIb/IIIa inhibitors tirofiban (Aggrastat)	Binds to the platelet receptor glycoprotein, preventing fibrinogen from binding	Dizziness, weakness, bleeding, hypotension	Use in conjunction with heparin. Assess complete blood count, PT, aPTT, and active clotting time before and periodically during therapy.

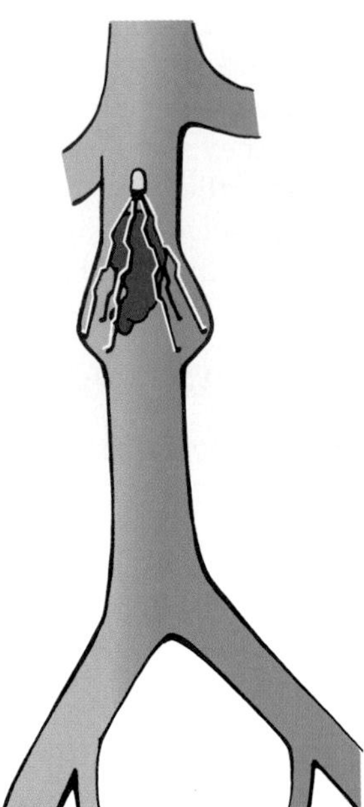

FIGURE 25.5 A permanently implanted vena caval filter allows blood to circulate to the lungs but traps blood clots before they enter the pulmonary circulation.

repair of a hip fracture or hip joint replacement; self-imposed inactivity as a result of obesity or sedentary lifestyle; immobility from a medical condition, pain, or treatment regimen; current use of an oral contraceptive; use of tobacco products; dehydration that may decrease fluid volume of blood; or recent trauma to an extremity. Assess for Homans' sign by asking the client whether he or she experiences pain or tenderness in the calf of the affected extremity when dorsiflexing the foot, or if movement causes or aggravates pain. Inspect the color, temperature, and capillary refill of extremities and measures leg (or arm) circumference at various areas and compare findings with the unaffected extremity. Regularly check for a low-grade fever. Ask the client about chest pain and dyspnea, which are hallmarks of PE, a complication of thrombophlebitis. If drug therapy is prescribed, monitor the laboratory test results associated with anticoagulant therapy.

Diagnosis, Planning, and Interventions

An important role is to prevent venous stasis and thrombophlebitis by promoting activity and exercise for at-risk clients. Ankle-pumping exercises are imperative for clients on bed rest. For inactive clients, the nurse applies knee- or thigh-high elastic stockings or uses a pneumatic venous compression device that alternately inflates and deflates to support vein walls and promote venous circulation (Fig. 25.6). He or she assists the client to change positions frequently and avoid restricting venous blood flow from prolonged sitting or gatching the bed at the knees (Client and Family Teaching 25-2). Additional nursing management includes the following measures.

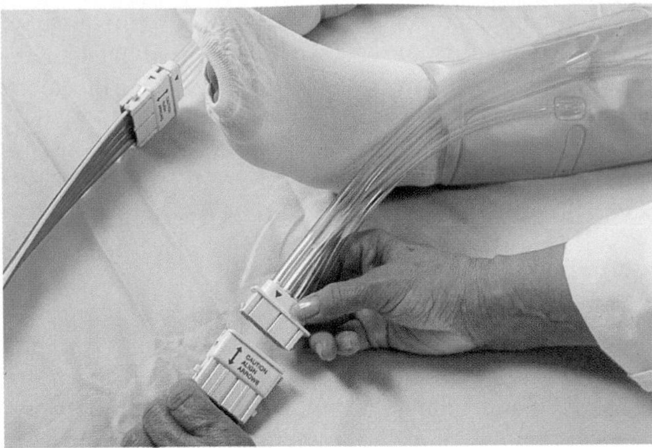

FIGURE 25.6 Pneumatic compression device.

Pain related to venous inflammation
Expected Outcome: Discomfort will be relieved or reduced to a tolerable level.

- Administer prescribed non-narcotic analgesics and anti-inflammatory agents. *Non-narcotic agents inhibit prostaglandin, a chemical that sensitizes nerve receptors that transmit pain. Relief of inflammation interferes with release of cellular chemicals that contribute to pain and localized swelling.*
- Support and handle the extremity gently. *Movement and muscle contraction increase pain.*

Ineffective Tissue Perfusion related to localized swelling secondary to the inflammatory response and impaired venous circulation
Expected Outcomes: Client's venous circulation will be adequate as evidenced by (1) reduced localized edema, (2) capillary refill less than 3 seconds in the toes of the affected extremity, (3) skin color in affected extremity similar to that of the unaffected extremity.

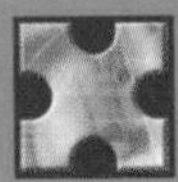

25-2 *Client and Family Teaching* Thrombophlebitis

The nurse teaches clients with thrombophlebitis and their families the following:

- Methods to prevent recurrences: avoiding prolonged sitting and crossing the legs at the knee, performing active movement, elevating the legs periodically, wearing support hose, and drinking fluids liberally
- The importance of taking long-term anticoagulant therapy exactly as prescribed and keeping appointments for the ordered laboratory tests to determine the effectiveness of therapy
- Signs that indicate impaired clotting: nosebleeds, bleeding gums, rectal bleeding, easy bruising, and prolonged oozing from minor cuts

- Elevate affected extremity 20° or more in a straight plane on pillows (do not bend the knees). *Relieves swelling and promotes venous circulation; bending the knees interferes with venous circulation and may increase the size of the existing clot or contribute to formation of additional thrombi.*
- Apply warm, moist compresses to the area of discomfort or apply an aquathermia pad over protected skin at a setting of approximately 105°F (40.5°C). Remove compresses and reapply after 20 minutes or sooner if cooling occurs. Remove aquathermia pad every 2 hours for 20 minutes to assess skin. *Warmth dilates blood vessels, improves circulation, and relieves swelling, all of which relieve discomfort. Moist heat is more comforting than dry heat. Skin assessments are standard care to avoid injury.*
- Promote a liberal intake (2000 to 2500 mL/24 hours) of oral fluid unless contraindicated. *Dilutes blood cells in plasma and reduces risk for platelet aggregation.*

PC: Bleeding

Expected Outcome: The nurse will manage and minimize blood loss.

- Monitor laboratory test findings that reflect coagulation status such as partial thromboplastin time (PTT), prothrombin time (PT), and international normalized ratio (INR); report values that exceed therapeutic levels. *With the exception of low–molecular-weight heparin, doses of anticoagulant drug therapy are adjusted according to laboratory test results.*
- Keep antidotes for overdose of anticoagulants (protamine sulfate for unfractionated heparin and vitamin K for warfarin) available. *Antidotes reverse effects of anticoagulant therapy.*
- Inspect skin for signs of bruising. *Tendency to bruise suggests the client could easily bleed internally.*
- Provide client with a soft-bristled toothbrush for oral hygiene; advise using an electric razor for shaving. *Reduces potential for skin and soft tissue trauma leading to bleeding.*
- Test stools, emesis, urine, and nasogastric drainage for blood. *Detects blood not obvious to the naked eye.*
- Protect client from falls or other trauma. *Any injury may precipitate excessive or prolonged bleeding if client is receiving anticoagulant therapy.*
- Perform neurologic assessments every 1 to 2 hours if the client experiences a head injury (see Chap. 41). *Changes in level of consciousness, size and response of pupils to light, and verbal responses suggest intracranial bleeding.*
- Apply direct pressure to the site of external bleeding. *Pressure compresses vascular walls and decreases blood flow, providing time for an initial clot to form.*
- Place an ice pack at site of prolonged oozing of blood. *Causes vasoconstriction and decreases volume of blood loss.*
- Prepare for IV fluid, blood, or blood product administration. *Parenteral fluids replace lost fluid volume; blood and blood products replace cells and fluid.*

Evaluation of Expected Outcomes

Expected outcomes include reduced or eliminated pain. Venous circulation improves and adequate blood flow to the heart is maintained; both extremities are comparable in size, temperature, and color. Homans' sign is negative. Bleeding is prevented or controlled.

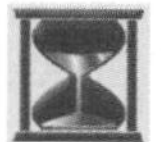

GENERAL GERONTOLOGIC CONSIDERATIONS

Older adults are at increased risk for infectious or inflammatory disorders of the cardiovascular system. A decreased inflammatory and immune response may prolong recovery.

Discourage older adults from using electric heating devices because of decreased temperature perception resulting from impaired circulation. Burns are more likely to occur. Thermal underwear and blankets are alternatives to electric blankets and heating pads.

Encourage older clients who are inactive to move every hour during the day to promote circulation. Such movement is especially important during long automobile or airplane trips.

Rheumatic heart disease may occur in the older adult who had rheumatic fever at an earlier age, or an acute episode may develop later in life.

Joint inflammation is more disabling in the older adult who may have some joint deformity or damage from chronic disorders such as osteoarthritis.

Many older adults have peripheral vascular insufficiency that is manifested in weak or absent pedal pulses; cold, clammy feet; thickened toenails; and shiny skin on the lower extremities.

Risk of hemorrhage during heparin therapy is greater in clients 60 years of age or older.

Critical Thinking Exercises

1. *A client complains of **intermittent claudication**, pain when the legs are elevated, and cold, numb feet. The nurse notes several dry ulcerations of the feet. Does the client suffer from venous or arterial insufficiency? What additional assessment data must the nurse collect? What lifestyle habits might predispose the client to this disorder?*
2. *What health teaching is important for a client with a history of thrombophlebitis?*

• NCLEX-STYLE REVIEW QUESTIONS 

1. A client comes to the emergency department complaining of dyspnea and heaviness in the chest. Pericarditis is suspected, and further investigation reveals severe precordial pain. When auscultating the client's chest, the nurse should anticipating hearing:
   1. A friction rub
   2. Well-defined S_1 S_2 heart sounds
   3. Expiratory wheezing
   4. A bounding apical pulse
2. A client diagnosed with thrombophlebitis receives instruction regarding her condition. Which statement made by the client indicates a need for further teaching?

1. "When I go back to work, I need to change my position often."
2. "I will need to take anticoagulants for a while."
3. "I will notify the nurse if I have any trouble breathing."
4. "When I feel cramping in my calf, I should rub it until the pain goes away."

3. A client is diagnosed with endocarditis. When obtaining the client's medical history, which question asked by the nurse is most important initially?

1. "Have you recently been treated for strep throat?"
2. "Have you recently had flu-like symptoms?"
3. "Do you have any skin rashes?"
4. "Have you had any recent cuts or bruises?"

connection

Visit the Connection site at **http://connection.lww.com/go/timbyEssentials** for links to chapter-related resources on the Internet.

References and Suggested Readings

Alderman, L. M. (2000). At risk: Adolescents and adults with congenital heart disease. *Dimensions in Critical Care Nursing, 19*(1), 2–14.

Allen, J. K. (2000). Genetics and cardiovascular disease. *Nursing Clinics of North America, 35,* 653–662.

Benton, L. (2000). A question of practice: DVT prevention . . . deep vein thrombosis. *American Journal of Nursing, 100*(2), 84.

Breen, P. (2000). DVT: What every nurse should know . . . deep vein thrombosis. *RN, 63*(4), 58–63.

Brenner, Z. R. (2000). Preventing postoperative complications: What's old, what's new, what's tried-and-true. *Nursing Management, 31*(12), 17–23.

Bryant, J. L., & Turkoski, B. B. (1999a). Critical care extra. New drugs. Cilostazol (Pletal): New treatment for intermittent claudication. *American Journal of Nursing, 99*(6), 24NN.

Bryant, J. L., & Turkoski, B. B. (1999b). Relieving intermittent claudication: A nursing approach. *Journal of Vascular Nursing, 17*(4), 81–85.

Carroll, P. (2000). Treating deep venous thrombosis at home with molecular weight heparin. *Home Healthcare Nurse,* (January Suppl.), 3–15.

Church, V. (2000). Staying on guard for DVT and PE. *Nursing 2000, 30*(2), 34–42.

Epley, D. (2000). Pulmonary emboli risk reduction. *Journal of Vascular Nursing, 18*(2), 61–70.

Fort, C. W. (2002). Get pumped to prevent DVT. *Nursing 2002, 32*(9), 50–52.

Gargiulo, J. (2000). Critical care extra. Hypertrophic cardiomyopathy: Preventing tragic endings. *American Journal of Nursing, 100*(8), 24JJ, 24LL.

Gehring, P. E. (April, 2002). Perfecting your skills: Vascular assessment. *RNs TNT,* 16–24.

Goldrick, B. A. (2003). Emerging infections: Endocarditis associated with body piercing. *American Journal of Nursing, 103*(1), 26–27.

Gorski, L. A. (2000). A clinical pathway for deep vein thrombosis. *Home Healthcare Nurse, 18,* 451–462.

Guglielmo, B. J. (1999). Use of antimicrobial agents in patients with cardiovascular disease. *Journal of Cardiovascular Nursing, 13*(2), 23–30.

Harris, G. D., & Steimle, J. (2000). Compiling the identifying features of bacterial endocarditis. [On-line.] Available: http://www.postgradmed.com/issues/2000/01_00/harris.htm.

Lewandowski, D. M. (1999). Clinical snapshot: Myocarditis. *American Journal of Nursing, 99*(8), 44–45.

Molitor, L. (2000). Triage decisions: A 64-year-old woman with a swollen and painful leg . . . deep vein thrombosis. *Journal of Emergency Nursing, 26,* 278–279.

Porth, C. M. (2002). *Pathophysiology: Concepts of altered states* (6th ed.). Philadelphia: Lippincott Williams & Wilkins.

Wackel, J. (2000). Altered coagulation: A diagnosis for the problem of deep vein thrombosis. *Nursing Diagnosis, 11*(2), 69–79.

Wallis, M., & Autar, R. (2001). Deep vein thrombosis: Clinical nursing management. *Nursing Standard, 15*(18), 47–54.

chapter 26

Caring for Clients With Valvular Disorders of the Heart

Words to Know 

annuloplasty
aortic regurgitation
aortic stenosis
balloon valvuloplasty
commissures
mitral regurgitation
mitral stenosis
mitral valve prolapse
point of maximum impulse
pulmonary hypertension
sequela
valvular incompetence
valvular regurgitation
water-hammer pulse

Learning Objectives

On completion of this chapter, the reader will:

- Explain five disorders that commonly affect heart valves.
- Discuss assessment findings common among clients with valvular disorders.
- Describe diagnostic tests used to confirm valvular disorders.
- Identify consequences of valvular disorders.
- Name categories of drugs used to treat valvular disorders.
- Give examples of treatments other than drug therapy to correct valvular disorders.
- Discuss nursing management of clients with valvular disorders.

Each heart structure helps to maintain normal cardiac function. The four cardiac valves—aortic, mitral, tricuspid, and pulmonic—promote forward circulation of blood to sustain adequate cardiac output (Fig. 26.1). Malformations at birth, inflammatory and infectious disorders (see Chap. 25), age-related degeneration, structural damage after myocardial infarction (MI), or injury during an intracardiac procedure can alter structure and function of cardiac valves. The aortic and mitral valves, located on the left side of the heart, where fluid pressures are higher than on the right side, are most commonly affected. Less common are disorders involving pulmonic and tricuspid valves.

DISORDERS OF THE AORTIC VALVE

The aortic valve has three cusps, or leaflets, and is described as a *semilunar* valve because each cusp appears like a half-moon. The left ventricle pumps blood from the heart through the aortic valve. When a nondiseased aortic valve opens during contraction of the left ventricle, it facilitates unrestricted passage of oxygenated blood into the arterial vascular system. Coronary arteries supplying the myocardium are the first blood vessels perfused. After ejection of left ventricular blood, the aortic valve closes tightly to prevent backflow of blood. Two valvular conditions interfere with unidirectional blood flow from the left side of the heart: aortic stenosis and aortic regurgitation.

• AORTIC STENOSIS

Stenosis means *narrowing.* **Aortic stenosis** describes narrowing of the opening in the aortic valve when valve cusps become stiff and rigid.

Pathophysiology and Etiology

In older adults without predisposing cardiac conditions, narrowing of the aortic valve is an age-related degenerative change from progressive calcium deposits in valve cells. In young adults, aortic stenosis usually is a later consequence of a congenital defect in which the valve has two instead of three cusps. At birth and throughout childhood, this defect does not produce symptoms. Symptoms appear after several decades, when the same calcification process

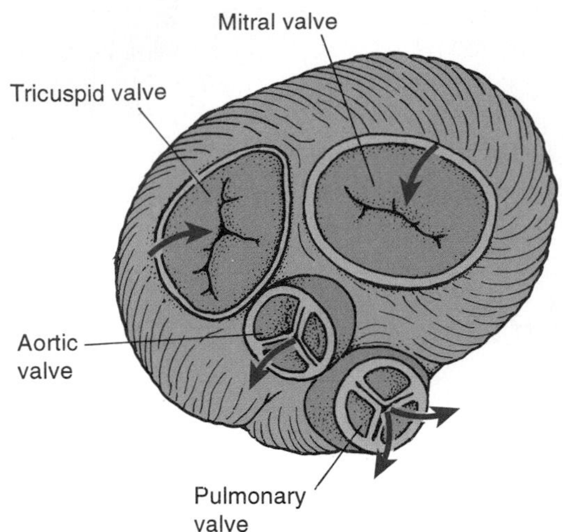

FIGURE 26.1 The tricuspid and mitral valves, located between the atria and ventricles, prevent blood from returning to the atria during ventricular contraction. The aortic and pulmonary valves, referred to as semilunar valves, open as blood is ejected from the ventricles.

that affects older adults causes the valves to harden. In others, aortic stenosis results directly from valvular damage related to rheumatic carditis and infective endocarditis (see Chap. 25).

The stiff, calcified valve cannot open properly and needs more force to push blood through its narrowed opening (Fig. 26.2). The muscular wall of the left ventricle enlarges and thickens (*hypertrophies*) in response. Blood volume passing through the narrowed valve eventually becomes insufficient to nourish the myocardium and other organs. Exercise or any circumstance that increases heart rate can cause myocardial ischemia, affecting the heart's ability to contract effectively. Left-sided heart failure (see Chap. 30) may develop because the heart cannot fully empty during systole and becomes more fatigued as it tries

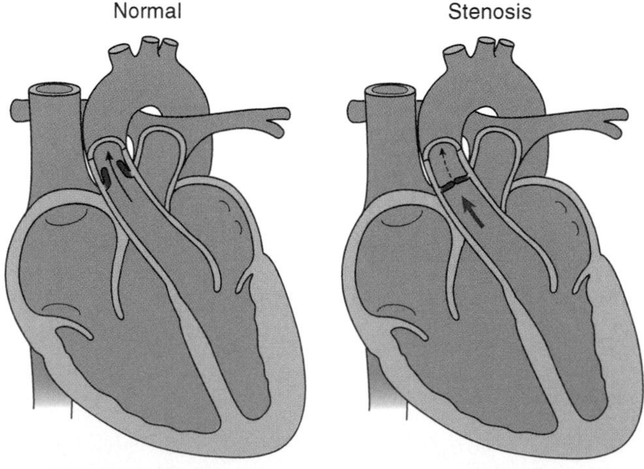

FIGURE 26.2 Aortic stenosis. Blood pools in the left ventricle, and cardiac output is reduced because the blood cannot completely pass through the narrowed valve opening.

to overcome resistance created by the narrowed valve. Should the adult with aortic stenosis develop coronary artery disease (CAD) and MI (see Chap. 27), the infarct may enlarge. Risk of mortality increases because of the valve's compromised ability to perfuse the myocardium with oxygen.

Assessment Findings

A client with aortic stenosis may be asymptomatic for several decades. When symptoms develop, they include dizziness, fainting, and angina because of insufficient cardiac output. At first, clients experience dyspnea and fatigue during activity. With ventricular enlargement, heart pulsations are displaced laterally or distally on the chest wall from the usual **point of maximum impulse** (PMI) at the fifth intercostal space medial to the left midclavicular line. The carotid pulse feels weak because of a low stroke volume.

The S_2 heart sound is split with a definite separation between the sounds of the aortic valve and pulmonic valve closing. Usually these sounds occur in unison or are so closely timed that they seem as one. While listening at the second intercostal space to the right and left of the sternum, the S_1 and split S_2 sounds like "lub-t-dub." The split persists throughout inspiration and expiration and does not disappear when the client sits up during auscultation. This finding distinguishes the split S_2 from a normal, physiologic splitting. Sometimes auscultation identifies other abnormal sounds (e.g., systolic murmur, click).

Ventricular enlargement is evident on a chest x-ray. An echocardiogram validates ventricular thickening and diminished transvalvular size. The height of the R wave on the electrocardiogram (ECG) may be increased, reflecting the large mass and force of contracting muscle. During left-sided cardiac catheterization, the pressure of blood in the left ventricle is higher than usual.

Medical and Surgical Management

Medical treatment may begin while the client is asymptomatic and focuses on maintaining adequate cardiac output by supporting the heart's pumping activity. Digitalis, an antihypertensive, antidysrhythmic drug particularly for atrial fibrillation with rapid ventricular response (see Chap. 28), and a diuretic may be prescribed. Sodium is restricted. Antibiotics are prescribed to prevent recurrences of infective endocarditis, which compound valvular damage. Nitrates or beta-adrenergic blockers are beneficial for relieving chest pain.

To increase survival, additional treatment eventually becomes critical. **Balloon valvuloplasty** is an invasive, nonsurgical procedure to enlarge a narrowed valve opening. A catheter with a deflated balloon is threaded through a peripheral blood vessel into the heart until the tip is located in the stenotic valve. When in position, the balloon is inflated to stretch the opening. Balloon valvuloplasty is considered temporary for clients whose conditions are too unstable for immediate surgery, yet whose symptoms cannot be adequately controlled more conservatively. The stretched valve opening will narrow within 6 to 12 months. Surgical aortic valve replacement eventually becomes necessary. Ideally, aortic valve replacement is performed before the client reaches the late stages of heart failure (see Chap. 30). A coronary arteriogram is performed to identify CAD; if present, valve replacement and surgical measures to improve vascular supply to the myocardium may be performed at the same time.

Nursing Management

Monitor subjective and objective symptoms and explain the purposes and techniques of diagnostic tests. Administer prescribed medications and monitor for therapeutic or adverse responses. Institute measures to ensure adequate cardiac output and tissue oxygenation. Assist the client to comply with dietary modifications to reduce fluid volumes and work placed on the heart (Nursing Care Plan 26-1).

● AORTIC REGURGITATION

Aortic regurgitation occurs when the aortic valve does not close tightly, a condition called **valvular incompetence.**

Pathophysiology and Etiology

Valvular incompetence can result from damage to valve cusps or papillary muscles. It may result from various disorders such as rheumatic carditis, endocarditis, syphilis, age-related stretching of the proximal aorta, and systemic inflammatory conditions.

When blood is pumped through the incompetent aortic valve, some leaks backward (**valvular regurgitation**) into the left ventricle. This backflow reduces cardiac output and causes fluid overload in the left ventricle, which becomes chronically stretched, hindering its ability to pump effectively (see Chap. 30). High fluid pressure in the left ventricle causes the mitral valve to shut early, interfering with left atrial emptying. Blood in the left atrium backs up into the pulmonary circulation. Left ventricular enlargement increases the heart's need for oxygen. When coronary arteries cannot supply the heart muscle with enough oxygen because of decreased cardiac output, the myocardium becomes ischemic and the client experiences angina. Dizziness, confusion, and left ventricular failure may develop.

Assessment Findings

The client remains asymptomatic as long as the left ventricle can sustain adequate circulation. Tachycardia is a first sign. When valve damage affects the left ventricle, the client becomes aware of forceful heart contractions (palpitations). At first, palpitations occur only when lying flat or on the left side. In later stages, the client experiences dyspnea and chest pain.

During physical examination, skin may be flushed and moist, especially in the upper body. The radial pulse may be very strong, with quick, sharp beats followed by a sudden collapse of force, a characteristic called a **water-hammer pulse** or *Corrigan's pulse.* Often, pulse pressure is wide because systolic blood pressure (BP) tends to be extremely high, whereas diastolic BP usually remains low or normal. The enlarged heart displaces the PMI. The chest may heave or rock from forceful contractions of the enlarged left ventricle. A heart murmur, caused by turbulence of blood falling back through the dilated aortic valve, also may be heard.

Cardiac catheterization reveals high left ventricular pressure and backward movement of blood. A chest x-ray reveals heart enlargement, and the aortic valve appears dilated. The ECG presents with tall R waves; depressed ST segments indicate myocardial ischemia (see Chap. 24). A radionuclide scan comparing blood flow through the heart at rest and during exercise reveals severity of the disease. Standard or transesophageal echocardiography provides images of atypical valvular and myocardial function. A computed tomography or magnetic resonance imaging scan may be performed if echocardiographic images are inconclusive.

Medical and Surgical Management

Because aortic regurgitation is mild and only slowly progressive in most people, clients are sustained with cardiac glycosides or beta blockers and diuretics. When taken appropriately, prophylactic antibiotics prevent recurrences of infective endocarditis. Clients are advised to modify their lifestyles to avoid excessive demands on the heart, such as those that may result from strenuous exercise and emotional stress. When a client becomes symptomatic, replacement of the diseased aortic valve is considered (see Chap. 31). The less heart damage that occurs before surgery, the better the outcome. If the aorta is diseased, the procedure is more involved because repair involves a vascular graft.

Nursing Management

Prepare the client for diagnostic procedures and monitor responses. Report changes in heart rate and rhythm, dyspnea, chest pain, and loss of consciousness to the physician immediately. Administer prescribed medications and evaluate the client's response. Ensuring that physical activity is balanced according to the client's tolerance is important. Before discharge, explain the need for antibiotic therapy before medical and dental procedures and teach how to assess BP regularly as well as methods to control hypertension. See Nursing Care Plan 26-1 for more information.

Stop, Think, and Respond ● BOX 26-1

A client with an aortic valvular disorder experiences chest pain while performing bathing and hygiene. What nursing actions are appropriate? 

DISORDERS OF THE MITRAL VALVE

The mitral valve, which lies between the left atrium and left ventricle, is a bicuspid valve. The two cusps are

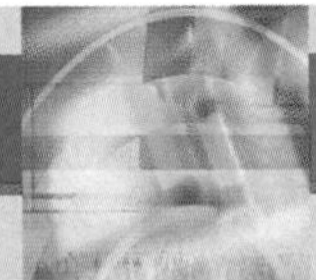

Nursing Care Plan 26-1

THE CLIENT WITH A VALVULAR DISORDER

Assessment

Determine the following:

- Vital signs, noting tachycardia, rapid respirations, dyspnea, hypotension, or hypertension
- Episodes of dizziness or fainting with or without confusion
- Chest pain and its characteristics
- Normal or abnormal lung and heart sounds
- Fluid intake and output
- Current weight and fluctuations during treatment
- Level of activity tolerance
- Social aspects (e.g., occupational activities) as they relate to physical energy requirements
- Knowledge of medical condition and current and future treatment protocols

Nursing Diagnosis: **Risk for Decreased Cardiac Output** related to diminished cardiac muscle contractility, tachycardia, and hypertension

Expected Outcome: Cardiac output will be adequate as evidenced by no chest pain, hypotension, or dizziness.

Interventions	*Rationales*
Monitor cardiac rhythm and rate.	Heart rate tachydysrhythmias compromise cardiac output.
Measure urine output every 8 hours or more often if less than 500 mL/day.	Renal output reflects heart's ability to perfuse renal arteries.
Maintain client on bed rest.	Lowers heart rate, which increases diastolic filling volume.
Reduce anxiety by responding to requests for attention or assistance.	Reduces tachycardia and hypertension.
Provide substitutes for dietary sources of caffeine and sodium.	Caffeine increases heart rate and promotes vasoconstriction; sodium contributes to fluid retention.
Promote ease in eliminating stool through such measures as increasing fiber and administering a prescribed stool softener.	Bearing down to eliminate stool interferes with cardiac filling; reduced cardiac filling decreases cardiac output.
Reduce any fever by changing to lighter or fewer bed linens, assisting with tepid sponge baths, or administering prescribed antipyretics.	Increased heart rate accompanies fever and adds to the heart's workload, which may compromise cardiac output.

Evaluation of Expected Outcome: Client is pain free; heart rate, BP, and urine output are within normal ranges.

(continued)

Nursing Care Plan 26-1 (Continued)

THE CLIENT WITH A VALVULAR DISORDER

Nursing Diagnosis: **Activity Intolerance** related to decreased cardiac output

Expected Outcome: Client will tolerate activity without dyspnea or heart rate above 100 beats/min.

Interventions	*Rationales*
Provide complete or partial assistance with activities of daily living.	Activity taxes endurance and results in increased heart rate and blood pressure.
Allow adequate time for client to perform self-care.	Activity that is done without urgency is less physically demanding.
Intersperse periods of activity with rest.	Rest helps heart recover from demands that increase its rate or force of contraction.

Evaluation of Expected Outcome: Client manages self-care and moderate activity without becoming breathless, hypotensive, or tachycardic.

Nursing Diagnosis: **Pain** related to myocardial ischemia

Expected Outcome: Pain will be reduced to client's self-described tolerance level within 30 minutes of a nursing intervention.

Interventions	*Rationales*
Provide rest immediately.	Slows the heart rate and decreases myocardium's need for oxygen.
Administer oxygen temporarily.	Promotes myocardial cellular oxygenation.
Give prescribed short-acting nitrate or analgesic.	Nitrates cause vasodilatation and increase blood flow from the coronary arteries to the myocardium; analgesics block transmission or perception of pain.
Assist clients with mitral valve prolapse to lie flat and elevate the legs 90° for 3 to 5 minutes.	Elevating the legs facilitates volume changes in the heart.

Evaluation of Expected Outcome: Client is free of pain.

PC: **Congestive Heart Failure**

Expected Outcome: The nurse will monitor for, manage, and minimize heart failure.

Interventions	*Rationales*
Auscultate lung and heart sounds at least once per shift or more often if abnormal sounds are evident.	Crackles, rhonchi (gurgles), and an S_3 heart sound are signs of cardiopulmonary complications such as left-sided congestive heart failure.
Weigh client daily at the same time, with similar clothing, on the same scale.	A weight gain of 2 lb or more in 24 hours suggests fluid retention equal to 1 L.
Support compliance with prescribed sodium and fluid restrictions.	Such restrictions decrease the work and sustain the ability of the heart to contract efficiently.

Evaluation of Expected Outcome: The nurse documents appropriate assessment findings, reports critical information to the physician, and implements prescribed interventions.

attached on the ventricular surface to strands of fibrous tissue called *chordae tendineae,* which are projections from papillary muscles. The papillary muscles contract in unison with the ventricle, pull on the chordae tendineae, and prevent cusps from ballooning into the left atrium. Functions of the mitral valve are to open widely to allow oxygenated blood to fill the left ventricle and close tightly to prevent blood from re-entering the left atrium after the left ventricle is filled. As long as the mitral valve remains structurally sound, blood exits the left ventricle through the aortic valve, where the aorta receives a 50- to 70-mL bolus of oxygenated blood, referred to as the *stroke volume.* The valve may become rigid (stenotic), incompetent (inadequate closure), or prolapsed (floppy). Mitral valve prolapse is the most common valvular disorder.

• MITRAL STENOSIS

Pathophysiology and Etiology

Mitral stenosis means that the valve does not open properly to facilitate filling of the left ventricle (Fig. 26.3). It is primarily a **sequela** (a condition that follows a disease) of rheumatic carditis (see Chap. 25). Mitral stenosis worsens with each recurrence of endocarditis. Inflammation causes the cusps to stick together and form a thick, rigid, calcified scar at the **commissures,** the area where the cusps contact each other, and the chordae tendineae fuse and shorten. The mitral valve cannot open completely, leading to incomplete emptying of the left atrium. Pooled blood from incomplete emptying contributes to clot formation, which puts the client at risk for arterial emboli. The left atrium enlarges because it has to contract more forcibly to empty. Pressure from overfilling is conveyed backward through blood vessels to the lungs, creating **pulmonary hypertension** and potential pulmonary edema (see Chap. 30). Pulmonary hypertension increases the work of the right ventricle as it pumps against high pressure in the pulmonary vascular system.

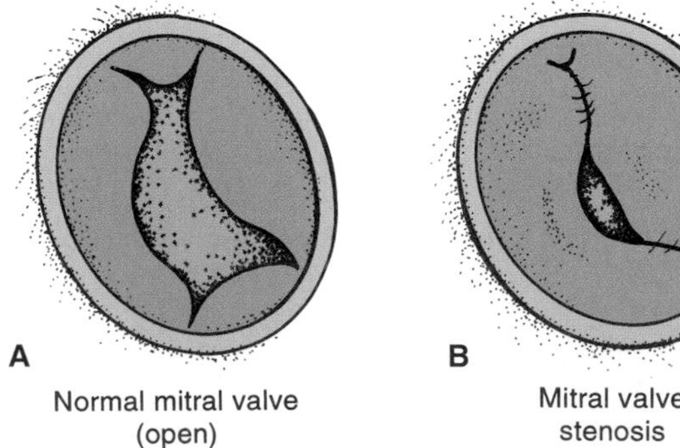

FIGURE 26.3 (**A**) The normal mitral valve opens widely to allow blood to pass from the left atrium to the left ventricle. (**B**) Following what is generally an infectious process, the mitral valve leaflets become fused with scar tissue, causing a partially obstructed pathway for the passage of blood.

Because blood flows in a circuit, disease on the left side of the heart eventually affects the right side. The right ventricle may enlarge in response to its increased workload. When contraction of the right ventricle can no longer overcome pulmonary resistance, right-sided heart failure develops. Excess blood accumulates in the venous circulation, the liver becomes congested, and edema occurs in the legs.

Assessment Findings

It may take 20 to 40 years for a client who has had rheumatic fever to develop mitral stenosis. At that time, clients report fatigue and dyspnea after slight exertion. Symptoms become disabling approximately 10 years after onset; they are accentuated when unusual demands are placed on the heart (e.g., fever, emotional stress, pregnancy). Later, clients experience heart palpitations caused by *tachydysrhythmias* (rapid dysrhythmias). With onset of pulmonary hypertension, clients may become more dyspneic at night and must sleep in a sitting position. They may develop a cough productive of pink, frothy sputum. Crackles heard in the bases of the lungs are a sign of pulmonary congestion.

Changes in heart sounds may be the earliest indication of mitral valve stenosis. S_1 may be extremely loud if cusps are fused, or muffled or absent if cusps have calcified and are immobile. A murmur, described as sounding like a rumbling underground train, can be heard at the heart's apex, especially when the client assumes a left lateral position. The systolic BP is low from reduced cardiac output. If backward pressure through the pulmonary circulation is sufficient to affect the right ventricle, the client's face is flushed; neck vein distention is evident; the liver is enlarged; and there is peripheral edema.

A chest x-ray reveals an enlarged left atrium and mitral valve calcification. In advanced stages, evidence of pulmonary edema is found. A standard or esophageal echocardiogram demonstrates decreased movement of the mitral valve cusps and changes in the size of the atrial chamber. On ECG, the P wave is notched, showing that the left atrium takes longer to depolarize than the right atrium because of its increased size.

Medical and Surgical Management

Antibiotic therapy is prescribed to prevent future episodes of infective endocarditis. Preventing or relieving symptoms of heart failure is essential. A daily aspirin, dipyridamole (Persantine), or other oral anticoagulant may be ordered to avoid clot formation. Dysrhythmias, such as *atrial fibrillation* (quivering of the atrial muscle with insufficient force to pump blood), are treated with drugs or cardioversion. Cardioversion stops the heart momentarily to allow the sinoatrial node to re-establish itself as the pacemaker.

Not all clients with mitral stenosis are suitable candidates for surgery. Those whose condition is so slight that it does not cause symptoms or so severe or of such long duration that profound changes in the heart and lungs have occurred usually are excluded. The earlier surgery is performed, the greater is the likelihood that it will relieve symptoms.

Percutaneous balloon valvuloplasty, also called *valvotomy,* is a nonsurgical alternative to *commissurotomy,* a surgical technique to separate the fused leaflets (see Chap. 31). When percutaneous balloon valvuloplasty is performed, a catheter with an uninflated balloon is passed through the femoral vein and threaded into the right atrium. The septum is then punctured between the right and left atria. When the catheter is in the mitral valve, it is inflated. Clients often are discharged on the same day as the procedure. The atrial puncture allows some blood to shunt from the left atrium to the right, but the opening usually closes within 6 months. Complications, although rare, include mitral regurgitation (discussed next), residual atrial-septal defect, perforation of the left ventricle, embolization, and MI. Management of the client after percutaneous balloon valvuloplasty includes the following:

- Echocardiogram within 72 hours to detect mitral regurgitation, left ventricular dysfunction, or pronounced atrial-septal defect
- Oral anticoagulation therapy within 1 to 2 days for clients who have a history of atrial fibrillation or instituted for others if atrial fibrillation develops in the future
- Prophylactic antibiotic protocols to prevent infective endocarditis
- Yearly medical follow-up that includes echocardiography, chest radiography, and ECG

Nursing Management

Monitor the client's physical condition, prepare him or her for diagnostic testing, and provide post-treatment care. Discharge teaching includes information regarding drug therapy, activity modification, signs and symptoms of complications, and when to contact the physician. See Nursing Care Plan 26-1 for additional discussion.

• MITRAL REGURGITATION (INSUFFICIENCY)

Mitral regurgitation, sometimes referred to as *mitral insufficiency,* occurs when the mitral valve does not close completely (Fig. 26.4). Some clients present with severe acute symptoms; others, whose heart muscle increases in size to compensate, remain asymptomatic or develop symptoms gradually over many years.

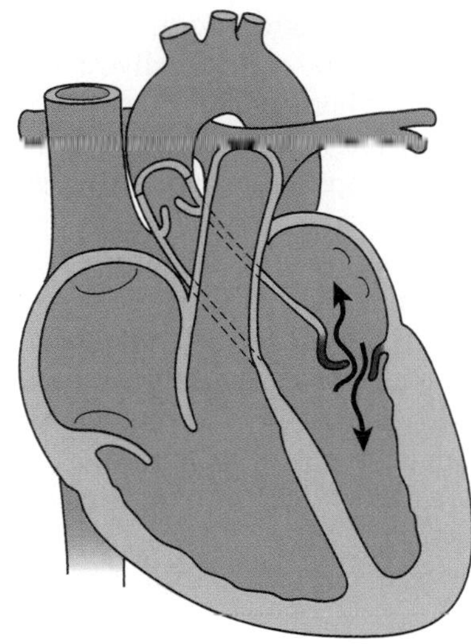

FIGURE 26.4 Mitral insufficiency. The incompetent atrioventricular valve allows blood to return to the left atrium.

Pathophysiology and Etiology

Mitral regurgitation is associated with rheumatic carditis and mitral valve prolapse (discussed next). It also is linked with damage to papillary muscles, impaired myocardial function after MI, connective tissue disorders, stretching of the valve opening from an enlarged left ventricle, and malfunction of a replaced valve. It also can develop after balloon valvuloplasty. Use of anorectic drugs identified in discussion of aortic regurgitation also are associated with mitral valve regurgitation.

When the mitral valve becomes incompetent (i.e., does not close completely), blood flows backward into the left atrium during ventricular systole and leaks into the left ventricle during atrial diastole. The heart usually can compensate for a small amount of blood that is regurgitated backward and forward by increasing the size of the left ventricle and left atria. The larger size facilitates ejection of blood from the heart, in which case pulmonary congestion does not occur. If regurgitation occurs rapidly, the heart is less able to compensate. Forward output from the left ventricle is diminished, and the client develops signs of shock. Accumulation of blood in the left atrium results in pulmonary congestion.

Assessment Findings

The client typically experiences chronic fatigue and dyspnea on exertion. He or she may notice heart palpitations caused by forceful contraction of the left ventricle as it attempts to empty excess blood from its chamber. The S_1 heart sound is diminished because of incomplete closure of the mitral valve. An S_3 heart sound, if heard, is an early sign of impending heart failure. Hypertension may develop when reduced cardiac output triggers the renin-angiotensin-aldosterone cycle. Tachycardia is a compensatory mechanism when stroke volume decreases. A loud, blowing murmur often is heard throughout ventricular systole at the heart's apex. If pulmonary congestion occurs, the client develops shortness of breath and moist lung sounds typical of left ventricular failure (see Chap. 30).

Standard transthoracic or transesophageal echocardiography is the best technique to identify structural changes in the mitral valve. Chest x-ray shows enlarged chambers on the left side of the heart. Radionuclide angiography provides information on the volume of regurgitated blood. ECG reflects cardiac enlargement, papillary muscle or chordae tendineae dysfunction, and various associated dysrhythmias (e.g., atrial fibrillation).

Medical and Surgical Management

Asymptomatic clients are monitored through physical examination and annual echocardiograms. Exercise is not limited until mild symptoms develop. An angiotensin-converting enzyme inhibitor like quinapril (Accupril) reduces afterload, preserving the left ventricle's ability to eject blood effectively. Digitalis, calcium channel blockers, beta blockers, or other antidysrhythmic drugs control tachycardia. Some clients are given drugs to prevent intracardiac thrombi, a common complication of blood stasis that accompanies atrial fibrillation. Prophylactic antibiotics are prescribed to prevent recurrences of infective endocarditis. An intra-aortic balloon pump, which provides counterpulsation to the contraction of the left ventricle, can be used in an emergency to stabilize a client in left ventricular failure (see Chap. 30).

Surgery to correct mitral regurgitation includes **annuloplasty,** repair of the valve leaflets and their fibrous ring. Implantation of a biologic or prosthetic valve to restore unidirectional blood flow may accompany annuloplasty (see Chap. 31).

Nursing Management

Closely monitor BP, heart rate and rhythm, heart sounds, and lung sounds. Weigh the client to determine changes in fluid balance. If sodium is restricted, work with the client and dietitian to find palatable seasonings and foods. Administer medications to treat symptoms and report signs of left- or right-sided heart failure immediately. Emphasize the need for prophylactic antibiotics and periodic health assessments. Refer to Nursing Care Plan 26-1 for more specific interventions.

• MITRAL VALVE PROLAPSE

In **mitral valve prolapse,** valve cusps enlarge, become floppy, and bulge backward into the left atrium (Fig. 26.5). Mitral regurgitation may occur, but not in all cases. Besides being the most common valvular disorder, mitral valve prolapse is the leading cause of mitral regurgitation. It is more common in young women than men, and is considered to be a more benign disease for people affected.

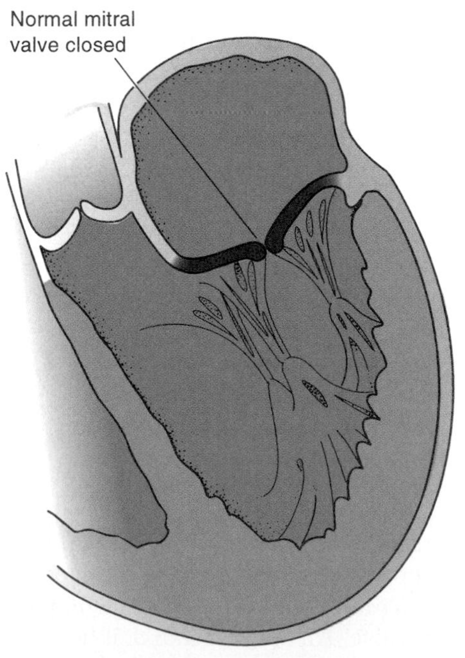

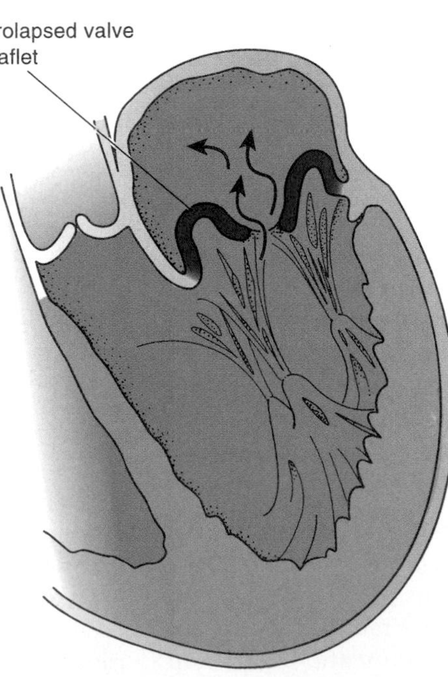

FIGURE 26.5 In mitral valve prolapse, the floppy valve leaflets allow blood to regurgitate, or move in retrograde fashion, from the left ventricle to the left atrium.

Pathophysiology and Etiology

The cause of mitral valve prolapse is not completely understood, and it often is classified as idiopathic (having no known cause). Some clients develop mitral valve prolapse in association with CAD, although it is questionable that an etiologic relationship actually exists. There is strong evidence that mitral valve prolapse accompanies valvular changes of rheumatic carditis, and structural changes predispose the valve to further damage if infective endocarditis develops.

Assessment Findings

Many clients with mitral valve prolapse are asymptomatic. When symptoms are present, they include chest pain, palpitations, and fatigue. Chest pain differs from that of angina: its onset does not correlate with physical exertion, its duration is prolonged, and it is not easily relieved. Some clients also experience symptoms that resemble anxiety or panic, such as a rapid and irregular heart rate, shortness of breath, light-headedness, difficulty concentrating, and fear that symptoms indicate impending death. Auscultation of heart sounds reveals a characteristic "click" during ventricular systole caused by tightening of the chordae tendineae. A systolic murmur is associated with mitral regurgitation. The presumptive diagnosis of mitral valve prolapse is strong if the murmur disappears or diminishes when the client squats during auscultation. Additional symptoms of mitral regurgitation also may be manifested.

Echocardiography shows abnormal movement of one or more mitral valve leaflets during systole. The ECG (resting, exercise, chemical, or ambulatory) is essentially normal, eliminating MI as a cause for the chest pain. ECG, however, may detect other causes.

Medical and Surgical Management

Many clients with mitral valve prolapse require no treatment except periodic antibiotic therapy before invasive procedures. Drugs such as digitalis, beta blockers, and calcium channel blockers control tachydysrhythmias; all but digitalis also control hypertension. Medications to reduce platelet aggregation (e.g., a single daily aspirin, ticlopidine [Ticlid]) are prescribed to prevent thrombus formation. If symptoms become severe, valve replacement is indicated.

Nursing Management

One measure to relieve chest pain is to have the client lie flat with the legs elevated and supported against a wall or couch at a 90° angle for 3 to 5 minutes to facilitate volume changes in the heart. Other recommendations include increasing activity when tachycardia occurs to eliminate initiation of extra, ineffective beats, and make up for reduced cardiac output. To relax or decrease shortness of breath, instruct the client to breathe deeply and slowly and then exhale through pursed lips. Advise the client to avoid caffeinated beverages and over-the-counter medications that contain stimulating chemicals to avoid contributing to an already rapid heart rate. If hypertension is not a problem, encourage the client to drink adequate fluid and continue moderate use of salt to maintain intravascular fluid volume. Discourage the use of alcohol because of its dehydrating effects and because withdrawal after chronic use can cause cardiac stimulation. Warn clients who are prescribed minor tranquilizers not to stop the medication abruptly or they may experience stimulating withdrawal symptoms. Additional nursing management depends on other assessment data. See Nursing Care Plan 26-1.

Stop, Think, and Respond ● BOX 26-2

Explain why clients with valvular disorders may need exercise modifications. 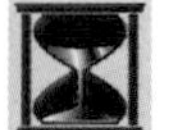

GENERAL GERONTOLOGIC CONSIDERATIONS

Older adults may require lower doses of cardiac glycosides than younger clients because of age-related metabolic changes. The more medications older adults take, the more likely they are to have dangerous interactions. Monitor the heart rate and BP of older adults taking beta blockers closely; adverse effects of bradycardia and hypotension can cause confusion and falls.

Fluid and electrolyte imbalances resulting from diuretic therapy can cause fatigue and weakness, which older adults may confuse as a worsening of symptoms related to valvular disease.

Calcification of heart structures, especially valvular tissue and the proximal aorta, increases with aging, putting older adults at increased risk for dangerous dysrhythmias and heart failure with subsequent alterations in cardiac output.

Syncope and falls resulting from decreased cardiac output occur more often in older adults.

Critical Thinking Exercises

1. *Compare and contrast stenosis and regurgitation of the aortic and mitral valves.*
2. *You are assisting a newly admitted client with a diagnosis of mitral stenosis into his hospital room. The individual in the next bed is diagnosed with tracheobronchitis, has a humidifier at the bedside, and receives frequent aerosol breathing treatments. What is the potential problem? What measures are appropriate to correct it?*

● NCLEX-STYLE REVIEW QUESTIONS 

1. The nurse assesses the client diagnosed with aortic regurgitation. The nurse should notify the primary care physician when:
    1. The heart rate is above 120 beats per minute.
    2. The skin becomes pale and dry.
    3. The S_2 sounds become split.
    4. The point of maximum impulse is at the fifth intercostal space.
2. When auscultating the chest of a client diagnosed with mitral valve prolapse, what is the nurse most likely to hear?
    1. A clicking sound during systole
    2. Heart rate less that 60 beats per minute
    3. Moist breath sounds on inspiration
    4. Respiratory rate less than 12 per minute
3. Mitral valve regurgitation secondary to mitral valve prolapse is the admitting diagnosis for a client. The nurse should frequently assess for which complication?
    1. Thrombus formation
    2. Infection
    3. Decreased urine output
    4. Ascites

connection

Visit the Connection site at **http://connection.lww.com/go/timbyEssentials** for links to chapter-related resources on the Internet.

References and Suggested Readings

Baptiste, M. M. (2001). Aortic valve replacement. *RN, 64*(1), 58–64.

Linden, B. (2000). Systems and diseases: The heart, part seven. Valvular heart disease. *Nursing Times, 96*(4), 49–52.

Linden, B. (2000). Systems and diseases: The heart, part eight. Valvular heart disease. *Nursing Times, 96*(8), 49–52.

chapter 27

Caring for Clients With Disorders of Coronary and Peripheral Blood Vessels

Words to Know 

aneurysm
angina pectoris
apolipoproteins
arteriosclerosis
atherectomy
atheroma
atherosclerosis
bruit
cardiac rehabilitation
cholesterol
collateral circulation
coronary artery bypass graft
coronary artery disease
coronary occlusion
coronary stent
coronary thrombosis
embolus
high-density lipoprotein
homocysteine
hyperlipidemia
infarct
ischemia
laser angioplasty
low-density lipoprotein
percutaneous transluminal coronary angioplasty
peripheral vascular disease
phlebothrombosis
phytoestrogens
plaque
thrombolytic agents
thrombosis
thrombus
topical hyperbaric oxygen
transmyocardial revascularization
varicose veins
vein ligation
vein stripping
venous insufficiency
venous reflux
venous stasis ulcer

Learning Objectives

On completion of this chapter, the reader will:

- Distinguish between arteriosclerosis and atherosclerosis.
- Identify risk factors associated with coronary artery disease.
- Discuss symptoms, diagnosis, treatment, and nursing management of myocardial infarction.
- Explain symptoms, diagnosis, and treatment of Raynaud's disease, thrombosis, phlebothrombosis, and embolism.
- Describe nursing management of clients with an occlusive disorder of peripheral blood vessels.
- Discuss symptoms, diagnosis, and treatment of varicose veins.
- Describe nursing management of clients undergoing surgery for varicose veins.
- Discuss symptoms, diagnosis, treatment, and nursing management of clients with an aortic aneurysm.

Uninterrupted blood flow is essential to cells and tissues. Cardiovascular disease is the leading cause of death in the United States. Occlusive disorders of the coronary arteries and resulting complications are largely responsible. Occlusive disorders of peripheral blood vessels also affect many. The most common causes of occlusive vascular diseases are atherosclerosis, arteriosclerosis, clot formation, and vascular spasm. Venous insufficiency and valvular incompetence also contribute to peripheral vascular disorders.

ARTERIOSCLEROSIS AND ATHEROSCLEROSIS

Arteriosclerosis refers to loss of elasticity or hardening of the arteries. **Atherosclerosis** is a condition in which the lumen of the artery fills with fatty deposits (chiefly composed of cholesterol) called **plaque.** Arteriosclerosis and atherosclerosis affect many blood vessels that supply body organs and tissues (i.e., heart, brain, kidneys, extremities). Consequently, these two conditions contribute to several disorders (myocardial infarction [MI], cerebrovascular accidents, renal failure).

To some degree, arteriosclerosis and atherosclerosis normally accompany the aging process. The rate at which arterial changes occur varies. Many factors affect rate of onset and overall severity of these conditions. As cells in arterial tissue layers degenerate with aging, calcium is deposited in the cytoplasm. Calcium causes arteries to lose elasticity. As the left ventricle contracts, sending oxygenated blood from the heart, the rigid arterial vessels fail to stretch. The potential result is a reduced volume of oxygenated blood delivered to organs.

Hyperlipidemia, or high levels of blood fat, triggers atherosclerotic changes. Factors such as sex, heredity, diet, and activity individually or collectively contribute to hyperlipidemia. For example, some clients inherit genetic codes that replicate cells with reduced numbers of receptors for binding with cholesterol; therefore, they are more likely to develop high lipid levels. Clients who consume a high-fat diet may saturate all available cholesterol receptors, which also results in hyperlipidemia. Above-normal cholesterol levels have been linked to a byproduct of methionine, an amino acid present in meat, called **homocysteine.** High levels of homocysteine also are implicated in thickening, narrowing, and scarring of arterial walls.

A current hypothesis is that atherosclerosis is linked with prior infections with *Chlamydia pneumoniae,* a bacterium that commonly causes respiratory infections (Fong, 2000; Ross, 1999). *C. pneumoniae* may accelerate the atherosclerotic process or destabilizes one that already exists, leading to an area of local inflammation. *C. pneumoniae* has been cultured from the **atheroma** (fatty mass) in the arterial wall. Results of blood tests such as C-reactive protein levels and white blood cell (WBC) counts, which reflect inflammation and infection, are elevated among clients hospitalized for coronary events. It is safe to assume that multiple factors contribute to arterial disease. A client with elevated lipid levels who also has other risk factors (cigarette smoking, stressful lifestyle, diabetes mellitus, hypertension, or a previous infection with *C. pneumoniae* or other microorganisms) is predisposed to the accelerated accumulation of fatty plaque within the arteries.

The body responds to microscopic injury in arterial walls by activating the inflammatory response. Monocytes migrate to the injury and deposit themselves under endothelial cells of the tunica intima. Monocytes then attract and accumulate lipid (fatty) material. The enlarging lesion elevates the endothelium of the artery wall and narrows the lumen (Fig. 27.1). Atherosclerotic vessels cannot produce endothelial-derived relaxing factors, impairing the ability of the artery to dilate. As subendothelial atheroma enlarges, the intimal layer may split and expose the lesion. Platelets become trapped in the roughened wall, initiating the clotting cascade. When this occurs in a coronary artery, the resulting mass is called a *coronary thrombosis.*

OCCLUSIVE DISORDERS OF CORONARY BLOOD VESSELS

Coronary occlusion, the closing of a coronary artery, reduces or totally interrupts blood supply to the distal muscle area. Coronary artery disease precedes coronary occlusion, which can lead to MI. Symptoms usually do not occur until at least 60% of the arterial lumen is occluded.

• CORONARY ARTERY DISEASE

Coronary artery disease (CAD) refers to arteriosclerotic and atherosclerotic changes in coronary arteries supplying the myocardium. It may not be diagnosed until clients are in late middle age or older, but vascular changes most likely begin much earlier. CAD occurs 10 to 15 years earlier in men than in women (Halm & Penque, 1999).

Pathophysiology and Etiology

CAD results from many factors rather than a single cause. Several inherited and behavioral risk factors contribute to the development of CAD (Box 27-1). Although men are affected earlier than women, incidence rises in postmenopausal women and becomes similar to that in men.

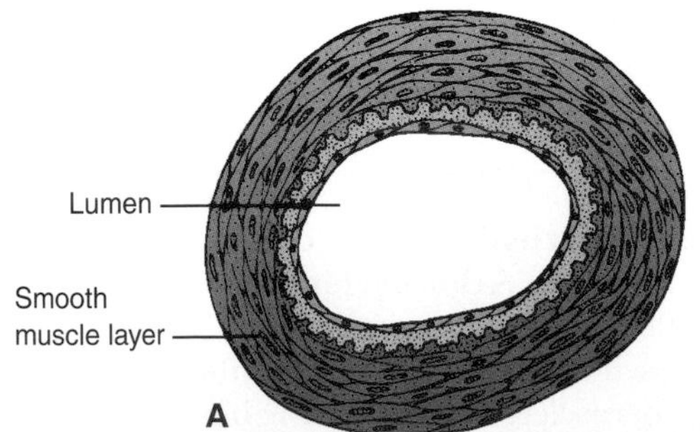

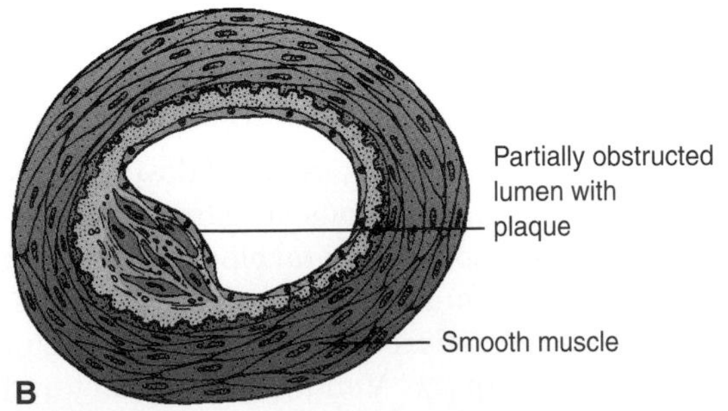

FIGURE 27.1 (**A**) Cross-section of a normal artery in which the lumen is fully patent, or open. (**B**) Cross-section of an atherosclerotic artery. (From Smeltzer, S. C. & Bare, B. G. [2004]. *Brunner & Suddarth's textbook of medical–surgical nursing* [10th ed.]. Philadelphia: Lippincott Williams & Wilkins.)

BOX 27-1 ● Risk Factors for Coronary Artery Disease

Inherited	Behavioral
Middle age or older	Smoking
Male sex	Sedentary lifestyle
Diabetes mellitus	Obesity
Increased lipid levels	Competitive, aggressive personality
Genetic predisposition	High-fat diet
Hypertension	

At rest, ample blood flow may be maintained despite considerable CAD. The condition may go unrecognized, particularly among those with a sedentary lifestyle. During situations that increase myocardial oxygen demand (i.e., exercise, emotional stress), the compromised coronary arteries cannot adequately oxygenate the myocardium. When myocardial tissue becomes *ischemic* (deprived of oxygen), clinical manifestations of CAD, such as **angina pectoris** (chest pain of cardiac origin) occur. Death of heart muscle does not accompany angina.

Assessment Findings

Signs and Symptoms

In mild CAD, clients are asymptomatic or complain of fatigue. The classic symptom is chest pain (angina) or discomfort during activity or stress. Such pain or discomfort typically is manifested as sudden pain or pressure centered over the heart (precordial) or under the sternum (substernal). Pain may radiate to the shoulders and arms, especially on the left side, or to the jaw, neck, or teeth. Some clients describe discomfort other than pain, such as indigestion or a burning, squeezing, or crushing tightness in the upper chest or throat.

Some clients present with signs suggesting hyperlipidemia. They may be obese and hypertensive. An obese person with an apple-shaped body (carries most weight in the abdomen) is at higher risk for CAD than one with a pear-shaped body (carries most weight below the hips). The pulse may be high at rest and become irregular with exercise. An opaque white ring about the periphery of the cornea, called *arcus senilis* (Fig. 27.2), results from a deposit of fat granules but may be apparent only in older adults. *Xanthelasma,* a raised yellow plaque on the skin of the upper and lower eyelids (Fig. 27.3), suggests lipid accumulation. Some research suggests a relationship between a diagonal crease in the earlobe and the risk for CAD.

Diagnostic Findings

The level of total serum **cholesterol,** a fatty (lipid) substance, is elevated; sometimes the level of triglycerides, which are chains of fatty acids, is increased as well. Proteins transport lipids (cholesterol) in the blood. **Low-density lipoprotein** (LDL) has a higher ratio of cholesterol than protein; **high-density lipoprotein** (HDL) is the opposite—it has more protein than cholesterol. In clients with CAD, the level of LDL, sometimes referred to as "bad cholesterol" because it sticks to arteries, exceeds recommended amounts. The level of HDL, or "good cholesterol" because it carries cholesterol to the liver for removal, is lower than desirable. Cardiac risk is estimated by dividing total serum cholesterol level by the HDL level; a result greater than 5 suggests a potential for CAD.

Apolipoproteins are proteins on the surface of cholesterol molecules that bind to enzymes that direct cholesterol to sites for metabolism. They often are low or absent among clients genetically prone to hyperlipidemia and are considered better direct indicators of CAD in women than are other standard blood fat profile measurements (HeartCenterOnline, 2001).

Exercise electrocardiogram (ECG) or stress testing may reveal ST segment depression, dysrhythmias, or exercise-induced hypertension. Narrowing of one or more coronary arteries is documented during coronary

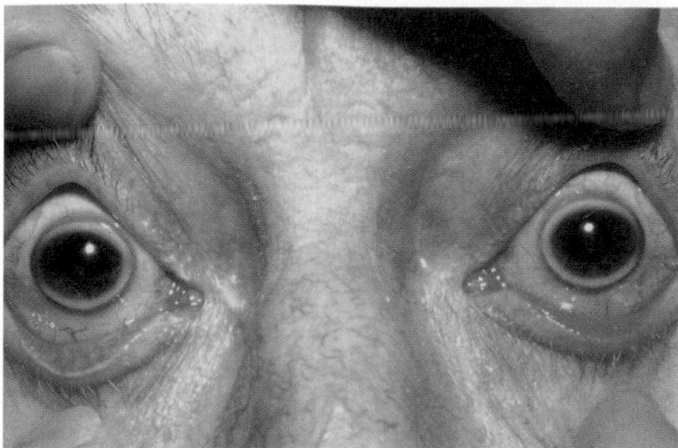

FIGURE 27.2 Arcus senilis, an opaque ring in the periphery of the cornea, is a sign of systemic fat deposits. (Courtesy of Patrick J. Saine, CRA.)

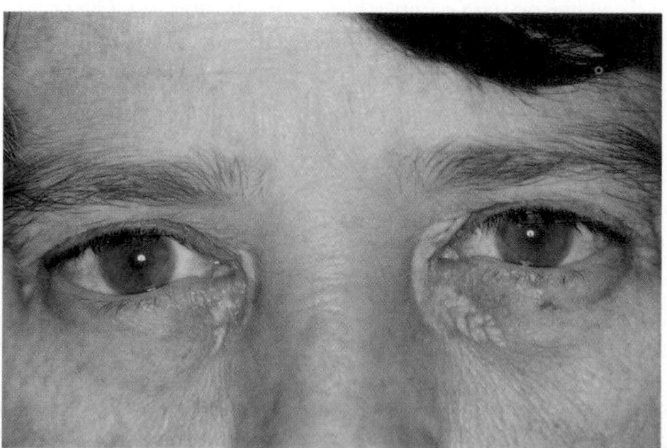

FIGURE 27.3 Xanthelasma, yellowish plaques about the eyelids, is a sign of lipid accumulation. (Courtesy of Patrick J. Saine, CRA.)

arteriography. Electron-beam computed tomography detects calcified plaque in one or more coronary arteries in asymptomatic clients.

Medical and Surgical Management

The first line of defense is lifestyle changes such as smoking cessation, weight loss, stress management, and exercise. When these are inadequate, drug therapy and other noninvasive, nonsurgical, or surgical interventions are indicated.

Drug therapy includes medications that produce arterial vasodilation, such as nitrates (e.g., nitroglycerin, isosorbide dinitrate). Beta-adrenergic blocking agents, which decrease consumption of myocardial oxygen by reducing heart rate, also are used. Calcium channel blocking agents may be used as well, although research shows they are less beneficial than beta-adrenergic blocking agents. Ongoing research is testing the use of antibiotic therapy. Drugs such as angiotensin-converting enzyme inhibitors and diuretics, as well as stress management, are used to control hypertension. Nicotinic acid (niacin) in pharmacologic doses (i.e., not the dosage in multivitamins) helps increase HDL and lower LDL. Daily intake of food sources or supplements of folate or folic acid, vitamin B_6 (pyridoxine), and vitamin B_{12} (cyanocobalamin) reduce homocysteine levels.

Blood glucose is kept regulated, and weight loss is encouraged. Prevention of further plaque formation is attempted by lowering elevated cholesterol and triglyceride levels through diet, exercise, and, in extreme cases, lipid-lowering drugs such as HMG CoA reductase inhibitors, known as *statins,* and bile acid sequestrants. Some physicians advise taking one aspirin tablet (325 mg or less) daily to prevent thrombi from developing. Because soy products are classified as **phytoestrogens,** plant sources of estrogen, some clients are increasing consumption of soy as a cardioprotective strategy.

Stop, Think, and Respond ● BOX 27-1

A person with a family history of CAD asks what he or she can do to reduce the risk of developing a similar problem. What information might you provide?

Invasive Perfusion Techniques

Invasive nonsurgical procedures can reopen narrowed coronary arteries and include percutaneous transluminal coronary angioplasty, coronary stent, and atherectomy. Surgical procedures include coronary artery bypass graft and transmyocardial revascularization.

PERCUTANEOUS TRANSLUMINAL CORONARY ANGIOPLASTY. For clients who fit specific criteria, **percutaneous transluminal coronary angioplasty** (PTCA), referred to as *balloon angioplasty,* is performed. In PTCA, which uses sedation and local anesthesia, a balloon-tipped catheter is inserted through the skin and threaded from a peripheral artery into the diseased coronary artery (Fig. 27.4). As passage of the catheter is monitored under fluoroscopy, the catheter is positioned in the area of stenosis and the balloon is inflated with carbon dioxide (CO_2) from several seconds to several minutes. Inflation of the balloon compresses the atherosclerotic plaque against the arterial wall, increasing the diameter of the artery. Arterial rupture, MI, and abrupt reclosure are complications of PTCA. Repeating PTCA often is necessary because the artery tends to reocclude in 40% to 50% of clients who undergo the procedure. Clients who have not had an accompanying MI but have had PTCA or any procedure that uses a percutaneous catheter are provided with the following discharge instructions for self-care:

- Avoid lifting more than 10 pounds for at least 3 days if the groin was used for catheter insertion. Avoid lifting more than 1 pound for at least 3 days if a site in the upper extremity was used.
- Refrain from riding a bicycle, driving a vehicle, or mowing the lawn for at least 3 days.
- Refrain from sexual activity for 1 week.
- Shower rather than bathe until the catheterization site heals.
- Clean site with soap and water; remove any dressing.
- Take a mild analgesic like acetaminophen (Tylenol) to relieve discomfort; numbness at the site is temporary and not unusual.
- Expect to see a bruise, which may last 1 to 3 weeks, at catheter insertion site.
- Report any signs of infection or impaired circulation: fever, swelling, redness, drainage, acute pain in the extremity, cold or pale skin.
- Notify cardiologist immediately if there is pain or tightness in the chest, which could indicate obstructed blood flow through the coronary artery.

CORONARY STENT. A **coronary stent** is a small metal coil with meshlike openings placed in the coronary artery during PTCA (Fig. 27.5). The stent prevents the coronary artery from collapsing shortly after the procedure and keeps the lumen open for a longer period than traditional PTCA alone. The stent remains permanently in the enlarged artery, and endothelial tissue is incorporated into the mesh within 4 to 6 weeks. Restenosis usually is a problem even with placement of a stent, resulting from an overgrowth of cells accompanying inflammation caused by local trauma to the tissue. A newly developed stent known as *CYPHER* is coated with an anti-inflammatory/antibiotic substance called sirolimus (Rapamune). It is still in clinical trials.

ATHERECTOMY. Clients whose atherosclerotic plaque is no longer soft and pliable may benefit from an **atherec-**

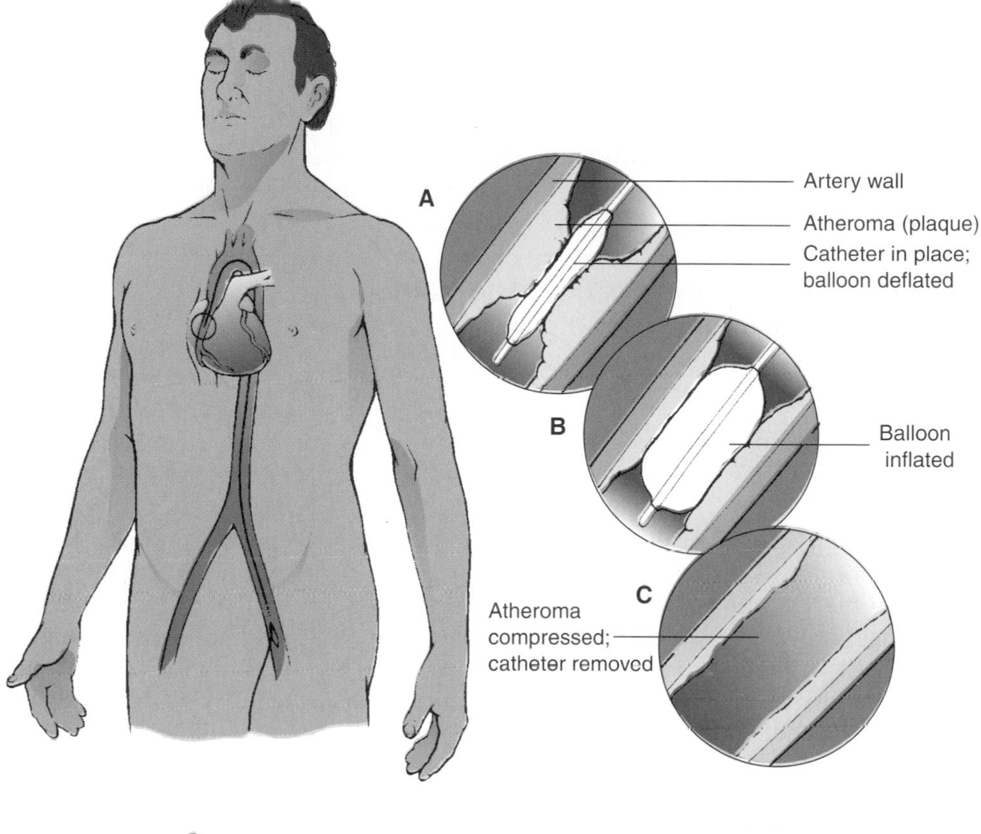

FIGURE 27.4 Percutaneous transluminal coronary angioplasty. (**A**) A balloon-tipped catheter is passed into the affected coronary artery and placed within the area of the atheroma (plaque). (**B**) The balloon is then rapidly inflated and deflated with controlled pressure. (**C**) After the atheroma is compressed, the catheter is removed, and blood flow improves. (From Smeltzer, S. C., & Bare, B. G. [2004]. *Brunner & Suddarth's textbook of medical–surgical nursing* [10th ed.]. Philadelphia: Lippincott Williams & Wilkins.)

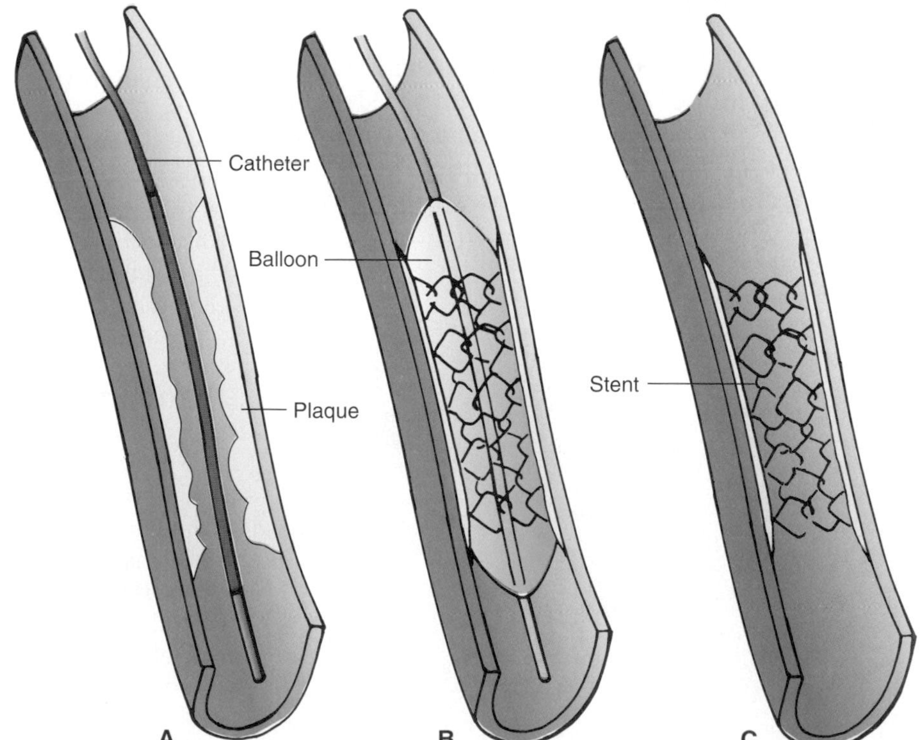

FIGURE 27.5 Insertion of a cardiac stent. (**A**) The stent is collapsed and placed over a balloon-tipped catheter. The catheter is threaded through a blood vessel in the groin and into the artery. (**B**) The balloon is inflated, and the stent expands. (**C**) The stent locks and forms a scaffold to keep the artery open. The balloon is deflated, and the catheter is withdrawn.

tomy, removal of fatty plaque. The plaque is removed by either inserting a cardiac catheter with a cutting tool at the tip (Fig. 27.6) or performing **laser angioplasty,** which uses short pulses of light that vaporize plaque without creating heat that is intense enough to damage the arterial wall. Atherectomy usually is followed by PTCA and placement of a stent.

CORONARY ARTERY BYPASS GRAFT SURGERY. **Coronary artery bypass graft** (CABG) surgery is a technique for revascularizing the myocardium. See Chapter 31.

TRANSMYOCARDIAL REVASCULARIZATION. A **transmyocardial revascularization** (TMR) laser procedure, which improves oxygenation of myocardial tissue, may improve quality of life for clients with chest pain that does not respond to medication and who are not candidates for CABG surgery. TMR may be performed for the following reasons:

- Occluded coronary arteries are too narrow or distal to permit catheter insertion.
- There are so many occlusions that risks from a lengthy surgical procedure are unreasonable.
- The client has end-stage (seriously advanced) CAD, which increases potential for life-threatening complications or death.

Nursing Management

Assess characteristics of chest pain and administer prescribed drugs that dilate coronary arteries or reduce the work of the heart. Encourage rest and administer oxygen to improve available oxygen supply to the heart muscle. If drugs, rest, and oxygen do not relieve pain, notify the physician.

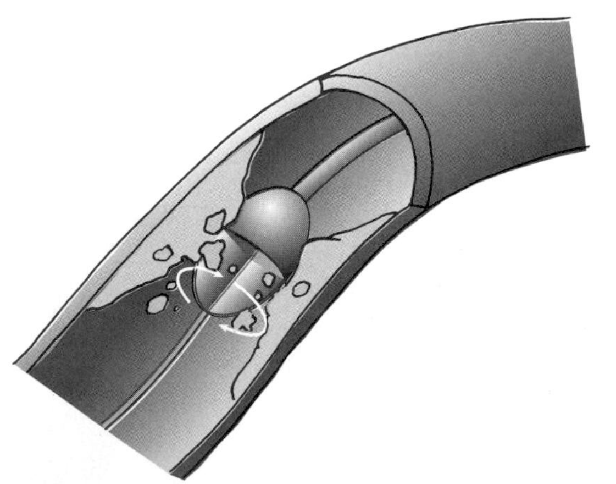

FIGURE 27.6 An atherectomy catheter removes plaque with either a circular blade or an abrasive material. A balloon catheter opens the coronary artery by compressing soft plaque.

Help clients learn how to reduce modifiable CAD risk factors, which improve not only cardiac health but overall well-being. Explain that a low-fat diet and regular aerobic exercise (e.g., walking, swimming) significantly reduce risks. Arrange a consultation with a dietitian and provide written material about a heart healthy diet. Refer clients to smoking cessation programs and discuss medications that can help.

Teach about the administration and side effects of antianginal drugs (Client and Family Teaching 27-1). Emphasize that severe, unrelieved chest pain indicates a need to be examined by a physician without delay. Advise the client to report changes in the usual pattern of angina, like increased frequency or severity or occurrence with rest or during sleep.

Inform clients about diagnostic tests or treatment procedures. Withhold anticoagulant therapy before the procedure to decrease chance of hemorrhage. Monitor all vascular sites for bleeding after a procedure and assess distal pulses. Observe mental status because cerebral emboli can occur. Monitor urine output and administer analgesics for discomfort. Report any of the following immediately: severe chest pain, abnormal heart rate or rhythm, mental confusion or loss of consciousness, hypotension, urine output less than 30 to 50 mL/hour, or a cold, pulseless extremity.

• MYOCARDIAL INFARCTION

An **infarct** is an area of tissue that dies from inadequate oxygenation (*necrosis*). An MI or heart attack occurs when there is prolonged total occlusion of coronary arterial blood flow. The larger the necrotic area is, the more serious the damage. Each coronary artery supplies oxygenated blood to a different area of the myocardium. The location of the infarction depends on the area where the blood supply to the myocardium is interrupted by the respective occluded coronary artery (Fig. 27.7).

Pathophysiology and Etiology

The most common cause of MI is a **coronary thrombosis,** a blood clot within a coronary artery. Thrombosis usually is secondary to arteriosclerotic and atherosclerotic changes. Arterial spasms also may cause an MI. Once part of the myocardium is damaged and destroyed, cells there lose their special functions of automaticity, excitability, conductivity, contractility, and rhythmicity. Dysrhythmias and heart failure are common consequences (see Chaps. 28 and 30).

Injury to the myocardium triggers the inflammatory response. Proinflammatory chemicals disrupt the permeability of cell membranes. Damaged cells release serum

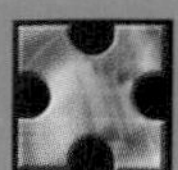

27-1 *Client and Family Teaching* Use of Short-Acting Nitroglycerin

The nurse discusses the following points with clients who are prescribed short-acting nitroglycerin and their families.

For sublingual nitroglycerin:

- Sit down and rest before self-administering nitroglycerin. Decreased activity may relieve chest pain; sitting will prevent injury should the nitroglycerin lower BP and cause fainting.
- Place one nitroglycerin tablet under the tongue if 2 to 3 minutes of rest fails to relieve pain.
- Expect to feel dizzy or flushed or to develop a headache.
- Let the tablet dissolve slowly; there should be slight tingling or burning under the tongue.
- Take a second nitroglycerin tablet in 5 minutes if chest pain is still present.
- Take a third nitroglycerin tablet in 5 more minutes if chest pain is still present.
- Call 911 if chest pain continues; do not drive to an emergency department. Discuss the chest pain with the physician if self-management relieved it or its usual characteristics changed.
- Keep a few nitroglycerin tablets in a dark, dry container with you at all times; consult with the pharmacist about a sealed metal container that you can wear around the neck.
- Do not place other medications in the container with the nitroglycerin.
- Replace nitroglycerin tablets every 6 months or after any container has been opened six times.

For nitroglycerin spray:

- Assume a sitting position.
- Hold the canister upright.
- Spray the nitroglycerin onto the tongue without inhaling.
- Close the mouth immediately afterward.
- Expect to feel dizzy or flushed or to develop a headache.
- Repeat spraying every 5 minutes for a second and third time if chest pain is unrelieved.
- Call 911 if chest pain continues.
- Discuss the chest pain with the physician if self-management relieved it or its usual characteristics changed.
- Expect a new canister of nitroglycerin to deliver approximately 200 doses.
- Check the amount of nitroglycerin in the canister by floating it in a bowl of water; the higher the canister floats, the less medication it contains. Obtain a reserve canister when the present canister shows signs of becoming empty.

cardiac markers (intracellular enzymes) and electrolytes into extracellular fluid. Loss of intracellular potassium and accumulation of lactic acid from anaerobic cellular metabolism affect depolarization and repolarization of myocardial cells. Dangerous dysrhythmias can develop during this time because affected areas are electrically unstable.

The infarction process can take up to 6 hours. Thrombolytic drugs (clot busters) are given during this 6-hour window of opportunity to re-establish blood flow and save as much myocardial tissue as possible.

Leukocytosis and slightly elevated body temperature follow in 3 to 7 days. New capillaries begin to grow to establish **collateral circulation** to the infarcted area. It takes 2 or 3 weeks before such flow is significant. A "cardiac patch" of collagen fibers begins to form within the first 2 weeks of the infarct, but it takes as long as 3 months for the scar to grow firm. Scar tissue is less effective than the myocardium it is replacing, because it does not stretch and contract like the original tissue. Lack of resiliency impairs the heart's ability to pump effectively. Consequently, cardiomyopathy (see Chap. 25) and heart failure (see Chap. 30) are lifelong, potential complications.

Complications

Any number of *dysrhythmias* (see Chap. 28) may occur during the acute phase. More than 50% of deaths from MI occur within 72 hours for this reason. Some abnormal rhythms can be fatal within a few minutes. Early detection and treatment of them reduce the fatality rate.

Cardiogenic shock, which has a high mortality rate, occurs when 40% of the left ventricle loses the ability to pump effectively (see Chap. 20). Onset may be sudden, or may develop over hours or days. The sooner shock is detected and treatment is instituted, the better are the chances of survival. This complication has been successfully treated with medications, ventricular assist devices, and an intra-aortic balloon pump (see Chap. 30).

Ventricular rupture occurs when a soft necrotic area ruptures. Dyspnea, rapid right-sided heart failure, and shock result. *Hemopericardium* (blood in the pericardium) and cardiac tamponade follow. Prognosis is poor, although survival is possible.

A *ventricular aneurysm* is a bulging of the portion of the heart affected by the MI. This area of poorly contrac-

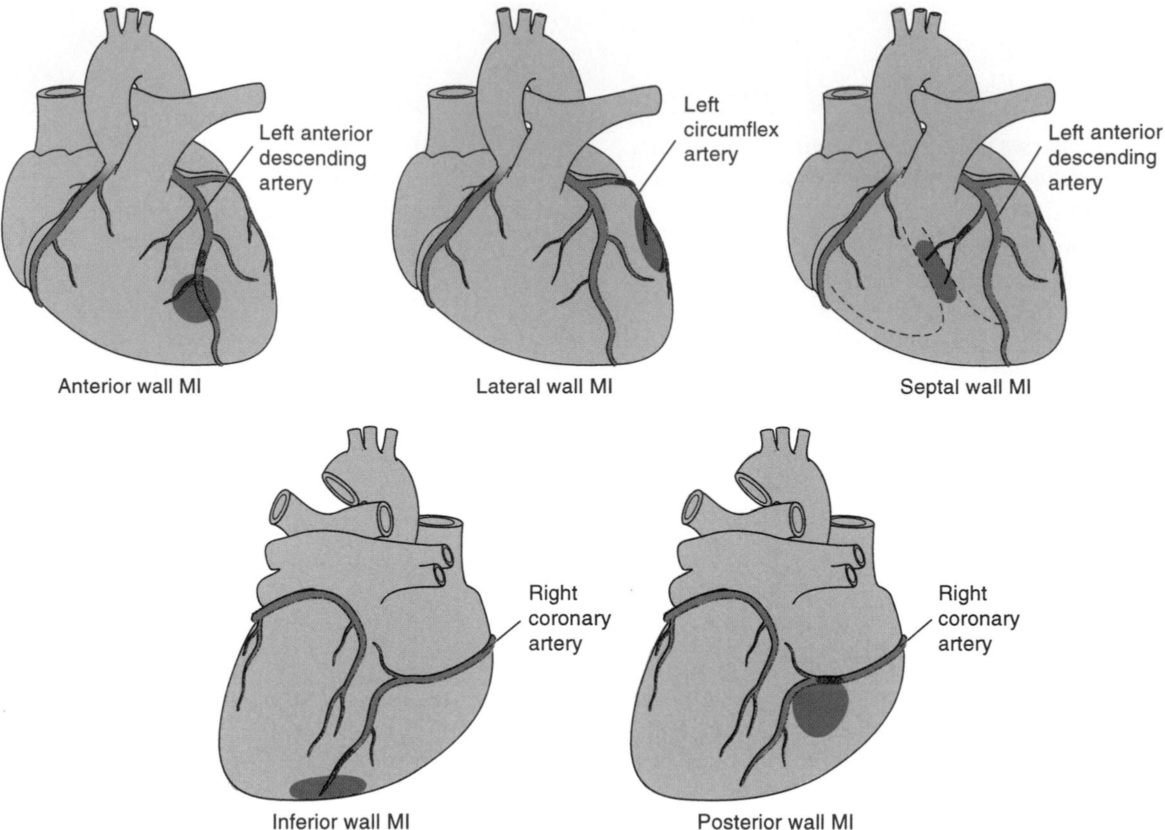

FIGURE 27.7 Zones of myocardial infarction based on the artery that becomes occluded.

tile tissue predisposes the heart to failure. Blood trapped in the projection tends to form thrombi, which may be released into arterial circulation. The aneurysm may burst, resulting in hemorrhage and death.

Clots can form in the cavity of the ventricular aneurysm, or tissue debris can break free. If clots enter the systemic arterial circulation, they may occlude a peripheral artery. Symptoms depend on the location of the affected artery. Arteriotomy (opening of an artery) and embolectomy (removal of an embolus) may be necessary. A client who has recently had an MI is a poor surgical risk.

Venous thrombosis arises mostly in the veins of the lower extremities and pelvis. Use of antiembolism stockings and regular performance of foot and leg exercises help to prevent thrombus formation. Antiplatelet medications and anticoagulants also are given.

Most *pulmonary emboli* arise from venous thrombi in the lower extremities and pelvis (see Chap. 23). They also may arise from the right ventricle after an MI. The onset of a pulmonary embolism usually is sudden, with chest pain, dyspnea, and cyanosis being the first symptoms. Sputum may be tinged with blood. Treatment depends on the size of the infarcted pulmonary area, the age and condition of the client, and the seriousness (or extent) of the MI.

Pericarditis may be mild or severe. The mild form may not require treatment (see Chap. 25). If pericardial effusion develops, the client is observed closely for signs of cardiac tamponade; pericardiocentesis is done to remove excess fluid.

If papillary muscles are involved in an MI and mitral valve leaflets are compromised, *mitral regurgitation* may occur. In this condition, blood not only flows forward into the aorta but backward into the left atrium through an incompetent mitral valve (see Chap. 26).

Assessment Findings

Symptoms vary but typically include sudden, severe chest pain, which usually is substernal and may radiate to the shoulder, arm, teeth, jaw, or throat. Most clients are aware of its seriousness and are apprehensive. Pain is more severe and lasts longer than anginal pain. Some clients describe it as squeezing or crushing. Unlike anginal pain, rest and sublingual nitrates do not relieve MI pain. If untreated, it may last for several hours or 1 or 2 days. Finally, it becomes sore or achy before disappearing entirely. A few clients experience little or no pain and may never know that they had an MI until an ECG detects it weeks, months, or years later. Clients appear pale and diaphoretic. They may experience nausea and vomiting or be hypotensive and faint. Pulse is rapid and weak and may be irregular. Signs of left-sided heart failure (dyspnea, cyanosis, cough) may appear if left ventricular pumping is sufficiently impaired.

Laboratory tests include a series of serum cardiac markers, substances that damaged myocardial cells release during an infarct (Table 27.1). They include myoglobin and cardiospecific troponin subunits known as troponin T and troponin I. The subunit troponin C is the same for cardiac and skeletal muscle and therefore is not measured. Fractions or isoforms of cardiac enzymes such as creatine kinase and lactate dehydrogenase are measured initially and every 8 hours for 24 hours to determine elevated levels. The WBC count, C-reactive protein, and erythrocyte sedimentation rate increase on about the third day because of the inflammatory response that injured myocardial cells triggered. Blood glucose level may be elevated in clients with diabetes (and those without) because of the body's response to a major stressor. After an MI, characteristic changes appear on the ECG within 2 to 12 hours. They may, however, take as long as 3 days to develop. These changes include ST segment elevation, T-wave inversion, and a Q wave (Fig. 27.8).

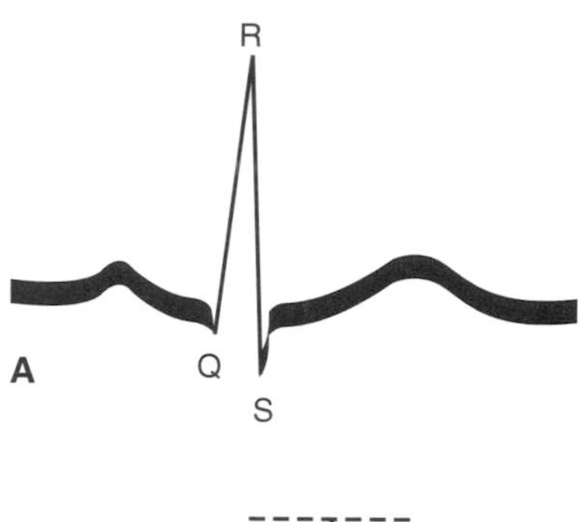

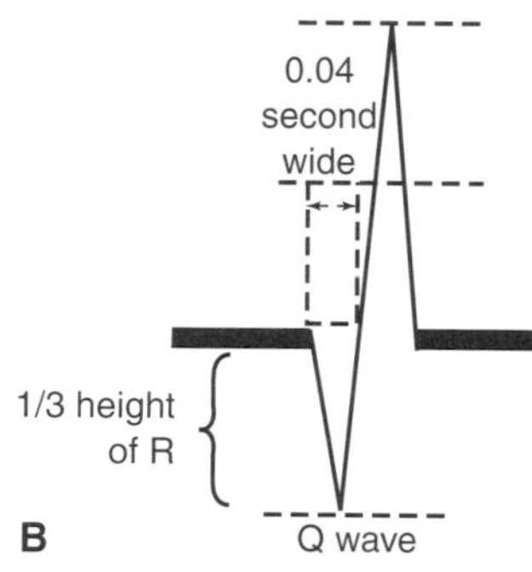

FIGURE 27.8 (**A**) Normal QRS complex. (**B**) A pathologic Q wave indicates a transmural myocardial infarction.

Medical Management

Thrombolytic Therapy

If the client is seen within 6 hours of the onset of the occlusion, re-establishing coronary artery blood flow can reduce the zone of necrosis. Treatment may include administration of **thrombolytic agents,** drugs that dissolve blood clots, unless the client is disqualified on the following bases:

- BP greater than 180/110 mm Hg
- History of a hemorrhagic stroke
- History of cerebral thrombotic stroke within 1 year
- Head trauma within past 2 to 4 weeks
- Known bleeding disorder; does not include menses
- Active internal bleeding in the past 2 weeks; active peptic ulcer
- Noncompressible vascular punctures
- Traumatic or prolonged (>10 minutes) cardiopulmonary resuscitation in past 2 to 4 weeks
- Surgery or trauma within the past 2 to 4 weeks
- Pregnancy
- Terminal illness
- Jaundice, hepatitis, kidney failure
- Use of anticoagulants in therapeutic doses

Drugs such as streptokinase, urokinase, and recombinant tissue plasminogen activator dissolve the thrombus occluding the coronary artery, thus restoring circulation of oxygenated blood to the myocardium. Depending on how stable the client's condition is, PTCA or CABG may follow thrombolytic therapy after risk for bleeding is reduced. Clients who are not candidates for thrombolytic therapy should undergo PTCA within 1 to 2 hours of admission or within 12 hours from the onset of symptoms (American College of Cardiology [ACC] and American Heart Association [AHA], 1999).

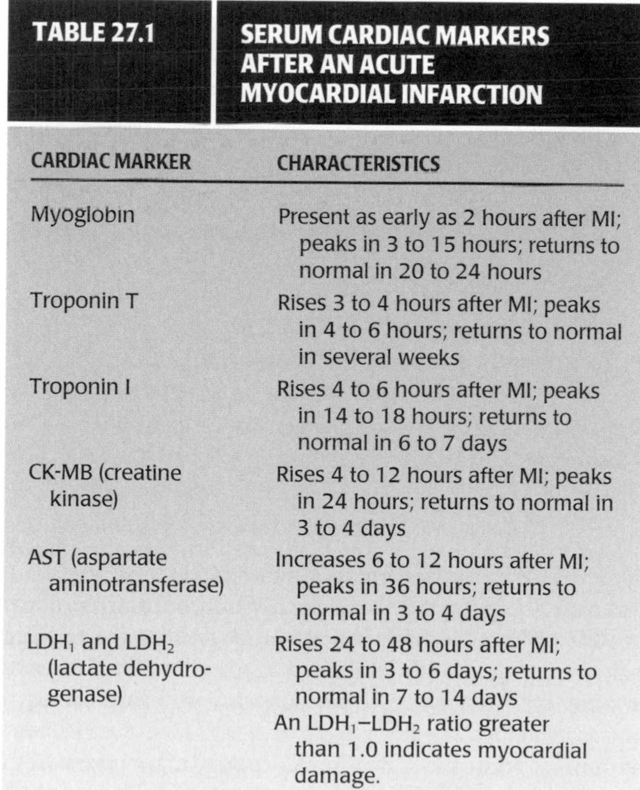

TABLE 27.1 SERUM CARDIAC MARKERS AFTER AN ACUTE MYOCARDIAL INFARCTION

CARDIAC MARKER	CHARACTERISTICS
Myoglobin	Present as early as 2 hours after MI; peaks in 3 to 15 hours; returns to normal in 20 to 24 hours
Troponin T	Rises 3 to 4 hours after MI; peaks in 4 to 6 hours; returns to normal in several weeks
Troponin I	Rises 4 to 6 hours after MI; peaks in 14 to 18 hours; returns to normal in 6 to 7 days
CK-MB (creatine kinase)	Rises 4 to 12 hours after MI; peaks in 24 hours; returns to normal in 3 to 4 days
AST (aspartate aminotransferase)	Increases 6 to 12 hours after MI; peaks in 36 hours; returns to normal in 3 to 4 days
LDH_1 and LDH_2 (lactate dehydrogenase)	Rises 24 to 48 hours after MI; peaks in 3 to 6 days; returns to normal in 7 to 14 days An LDH_1–LDH_2 ratio greater than 1.0 indicates myocardial damage.

Symptomatic Treatment

An intravenous (IV) infusion is initiated to provide fluid while eating is restricted. The IV route also is used to administer parenteral medications. Drug therapy includes analgesics for pain, nitrates or other vasodilating drugs to improve blood flow, diuretics to reduce circulating blood volume, sedatives to promote rest and reduce anxiety, anticoagulants to prevent additional thrombus formation, and drugs to treat dysrhythmias (Drug Therapy Table 27.1). Oxygen is ordered to treat or prevent hypoxemia. Complete bed rest is prescribed initially but not recommended for uncomplicated MIs after the first 12 hours. Activity is adjusted according to the extent of the MI, complications, and response to therapy. When chest pain is controlled, a clear liquid diet is allowed and progressed to a heart-healthy diet thereafter. Clients who regularly consumed caffeine before an MI are allowed up to 400 mg/day, which equals two to four cups of coffee, without danger of increasing BP (ACC/AHA, 1999). A stool softener is prescribed to prevent increased BP from straining with the passage of stool. Permanent smoking cessation is imperative. The intra-aortic balloon pump may be used for clients who develop severe left ventricular failure (see Chap. 30).

Surgical Management

CABG surgery (see Chap. 31) is done to revascularize the myocardium surgically. In clients who are experiencing cardiogenic shock, a ventricular assist device may be implanted, or cardiomyoplasty, a new procedure for grafting skeletal muscle to replace a dysfunctional area of myocardium, may be used (see Chap. 30).

Cardiac Rehabilitation

After a significant cardiac event like an MI or heart surgery, clients are encouraged to participate in a medically supervised **cardiac rehabilitation** program, which combines exercise and educational activities to speed recovery and reduce or prevent recurring episodes. Cardiac rehabilitation usually begins before discharge but continues on an outpatient basis. The plan is designed according to the client's unique needs. Some clients may achieve goals of therapy by meeting two to three times a week for 1 hour or more over a few weeks. Other clients may require therapy for 3 to 4 months. Activities and educational topics include the following:

- Gradual exercise that increases according to the client's tolerance
- Establishment of physical limitations such as the maximum amount the client can lift
- Recognition and management of depression
- Medication regimen: importance of drug therapy, dose, time taken, adverse drug effects
- Smoking cessation
- When and how to resume sexual activity (Box 27-2)
- Diet modifications, how to read food labels, what food labels indicate
- How to monitor pulse rate and BP
- Symptoms to report to a physician as soon as possible
- How to avoid or minimize stressors
- Importance of continued medical supervision

NURSING PROCESS

The Client With Acute Myocardial Infarction

Assessment

Ask the client to describe the pain. Check vital signs every 30 minutes until stable and then every 4 hours and as needed (PRN). Assess for any nausea, vomiting, diaphoresis, and anxiety. Check oxygen saturation level with pulse oximeter. Determine the cardiac rhythm via cardiac monitor or ECG. Auscultate heart and lung sounds, and check for the presence and quality of peripheral pulses. Review the results of serum cardiac markers. Conduct a thorough history to establish baseline data about disorders such as diabetes mellitus, hypertension, recent streptococcal infection or allergic reaction to streptokinase and findings that may disqualify client from thrombolytic therapy. Include a drug history for prescribed, over-the-counter, and herbal products.

Diagnoses, Planning, and Interventions

Acute Pain related to diminished myocardial oxygenation
Expected Outcome: Pain will be within client's identified comfort level within 30 minutes.

- Administer prescribed sublingual or spray nitroglycerin every 5 minutes, up to three doses, if pain is unrelieved. *Nitroglycerin dilates blood vessels, improving blood flow through coronary arteries, and lowers BP, which decreases cardiac afterload.*
- Administer prescribed IV morphine sulfate. *Reduces pain perception and anxiety. Reduced anxiety decreases heart rate and BP, alleviating heart's demand for oxygenation.*
- Administer oxygen at 2 L/minute by nasal cannula or as prescribed. *Supplemental oxygen raises hemoglobin saturation and oxygen in plasma. Adequate myocardial oxygen diminishes angina.*

Anxiety or **Fear** related to perception of impending doom, concern over actual/potential lifestyle changes, worry concerning family situation
Expected Outcome: Client will report decreased anxiety and fear.

- Allow client to express fears and anxiety. *Relieves or reduces emotional distress.*

DRUG THERAPY TABLE 27.1 AGENTS USED TO TREAT MYOCARDIAL INFARCTION

DRUG CATEGORY AND EXAMPLES	MECHANISM OF ACTION	SIDE EFFECTS	NURSING CONSIDERATIONS
Vasodilators			
nitroglycerin	Relieve chest pain by dilating coronary arteries Reestablish blood flow around thrombi	Headache, dizziness, orthostatic hypotension, tachycardia, flushing, nausea	Assess for hypotension. Monitor for pain relief, headache, and flushed skin.
Beta-Adrenergic Blockers			
propranolol (Inderal)	Prevent or inhibit sympathetic stimulation, decreasing myocardial oxygen demand Are used to prevent anginal attacks	Hypotension, bradycardia, bronchospasm, CHF, depression, erectile dysfunction, hypoglycemia	Administer with meals. Advise client not to discontinue medication abruptly. Monitor for fluid retention, rash, and difficulty breathing. Monitor blood glucose level in clients with diabetes.
Thrombolytics			
alteplase (Activase); recombinant tissue plasminogen activator (r-TPA)	Reestablish blood flow to ischemic areas by dissolving thrombi Are contraindicated in clients with history of cerebrovascular accident or bleeding tendencies	Cardiac dysrhythmias, hypotension, bleeding at venous or arterial access sites, nausea, vomiting	Use caution when administering with heparin because of increased risk for hemorrhage. Monitor PT and PTT. Apply pressure to control superficial bleeding.
Anticoagulants			
heparin sodium (Hepalean)	Inhibit thrombus and clot formation by blocking conversion of prothrombin to thrombin and fibrinogen to fibrin	Hemorrhage, bruising, thrombocytopenia, alopecia, chills, fever	Monitor closely for bleeding or hemorrhage when combined with oral anticoagulants. Give subcutaneously or IV. Apply pressure to all intramuscular injection sites. Monitor for epistaxis and other bleeding. Ensure protamine sulfate is on the unit in case of overdose.
Calcium Channel Blockers			
diltiazem (Cardizem)	Relieve angina by dilating arteries, which improves blood supply to myocardium and reduces myocardial oxygen demand by decreasing myocardial contractility and heart rate Reduce dysrhythmias	Hypotension, dizziness, CHF, pulmonary edema, nausea	Check BP and heart rate before each dose. Withhold drug in the presence of hypotension. Observe for signs and symptoms of CHF and fluid overload.
Diuretics			
furosemide (Lasix)	Decrease work of heart by promoting excretion of sodium and water, thus reducing circulating blood volume	Dizziness, dehydration, nausea, diarrhea, nocturia, polyuria, orthostatic hypotension, hypokalemia	Weigh client daily. Measure intake and output. Monitor serum potassium level, and replace potassium with bananas, orange juice, or prescribed supplement.

CHF, congestive heart failure; PT, prothrombin time; PTT, partial thromboplastin time.

BOX 27-2 ● Sexual Guidelines After Myocardial Infarction

- Check with physician before resuming sexual activity.
- Avoid sex with anyone other than your usual partner.
- Avoid positions that require supporting your own weight.
- Get adequate rest before sexual intercourse.
- Have sex in the same environment as before the MI.
- Postpone sex for 2 to 3 hours after eating a heavy meal or consuming alcohol.
- Use a short-acting nitrate, if the physician approves, before intercourse.
- Begin with moderate sexual foreplay.
- Use medium water temperatures when bathing or showering before or after sexual activity.

- Explain all procedures before performing them. *Eliminates element of surprise or misinterpretation of nursing activities.*
- Carry out procedures in a calm, relaxed manner. *A client who senses confidence in the nurse may experience less apprehension.*
- Promote uninterrupted blocks of time for rest, sleep, or visits with family members. *Physical rest and support from others promote ability to cope.*
- Check client frequently, and answer call lights promptly. *Relieves fear.*
- Acknowledge grief over perceived or actual changes in lifestyle. *Dealing with reality facilitates grieving.*
- Administer prescribed sedatives and anxiolytic drugs as indicated. *They block sympathetic nervous system responses, which reduces anxiety and fear.*

PC: Hemorrhage related to thrombolytic therapy

Expected Outcome: The nurse will monitor client to detect, manage, and minimize bleeding.

- Observe closely for bleeding during thrombolytic therapy and until sufficient half-lives reduce pharmacodynamic effects. *Client is at risk for bleeding when thrombolytic drugs change plasminogen to plasmin.*
- Check for blood in stool or urine, bruising, epistaxis, abdominal pain, or altered neurologic status. *Thrombolytic drugs dissolve blood clots and interfere with their formation.*
- Avoid intramuscular, IV, and arterial punctures during therapy and until risk for excessive bleeding subsides. *Controlling bleeding may be difficult while an active level of thrombolytic drug remains in bloodstream.*
- Keep client on bed rest; pad side rails if agency policy mandates. *Trauma can cause excessive blood loss.*
- Have aminocaproic acid (Amicar) available as an antidote for bleeding. *Aminocaproic acid is an antiplasmin agent that inhibits plasminogen activator.*

PC: Dysrhythmias related to reperfusion of myocardium with thrombolytic therapy and instability of the conduction system

Expected Outcome: The nurse will monitor client to detect, manage, and minimize dysrhythmias.

- Place client on a cardiac monitor and closely observe for dangerous dysrhythmias. *A cardiac monitor continuously displays heart rate and rhythm; it sounds an alarm to call attention to a dysrhythmic event.*
- Be prepared to perform CPR if a life-threatening dysrhythmia or asystole occurs. *CPR provides basic life support.*
- Assist with endotracheal intubation, defibrillation, and administration of antidysrhythmic drugs. *Advanced cardiac life support may resuscitate a client.*

Evaluation of Expected Outcomes

Pain is eliminated or reduced to a tolerable level. Anxiety is reduced as evidenced by normal heart rate and BP, no nervous activity, and self-reported tolerance of stressors. Client shows no evidence of bleeding. Dysrhythmias are controlled.

OCCLUSIVE DISORDERS OF PERIPHERAL BLOOD VESSELS

Peripheral vascular disease is a term for disorders affecting blood vessels distant from large central blood vessels supplying the myocardium or that circulate blood directly in and out of the heart. Common peripheral vascular disorders which occlude blood flow by various mechanisms include Raynaud's disease, thrombosis, phlebothrombosis, and embolism.

RAYNAUD'S DISEASE

Raynaud's disease is characterized by periodic constriction of arteries that supply extremities. The disorder is most common in young women.

Pathophysiology and Etiology

Raynaud's disease is characterized by brief spasms of the arteries and arterioles in the fingers (most common site), toes, nose, ears, or chin. Spasms last approximately 15 minutes and cause temporary **ischemia** (impaired oxygenation) to tissues. Vessels then dilate widely, apparently to compensate for restriction. Patchy areas of necrosis occur with prolonged ischemia.

The underlying cause of Raynaud's disease is not entirely clear. In some clients, it seems *idiopathic* (no explainable reason); in others, it is secondary to connective tissue diseases, such as scleroderma, systemic lupus erythematosus, or rheumatoid arthritis (see Chap. 61).

The anatomy of the arteries and arterioles is normal. One theory explaining vasospasms is impaired release of *prostaglandins* (chemicals stored in cellular membranes).

Some prostaglandins cause vasoconstriction; others cause vasodilation. The type that accompanies an inflammatory response causes vasodilation.

Assessment Findings

Attacks are intermittent and of varying frequency but especially common after exposure to cold. When the condition occurs in the hands, they become cold, blanched, and wet with perspiration. Numbness and tingling also may occur. The client may note awkwardness and fumbling, especially when attempting fine movements. After initial pallor, the hands, especially the fingers, become deeply cyanotic and begin to ache. Hallmark symptoms of arterial insufficiency include ischemia, pain, and paresthesia. Placing the affected part in warm water or going to a warm area can relieve an attack. Eventually the vasospasm is relieved, and blood rushes to the affected part. Skin in the deprived areas becomes flushed, swollen, and warm, and the person has a sensation of throbbing pain.

In early stages of the disease, hands usually appear normal between attacks. The disease does not necessarily progress to cause severe disability. Symptoms often are mild and may even improve spontaneously. When the disease is severe and of long standing, cyanosis of the fingers persists between attacks and skin changes gradually develop. Painful ulcers and superficial gangrene may appear at the fingertips. Fingers are especially vulnerable to infection. Healing of even minor lesions often is slow and uncertain.

No specific laboratory studies can confirm Raynaud's disease. Diagnosis is made by a history of symptoms and examination of the involved part. Laboratory blood tests are ordered to confirm or rule out an accompanying connective tissue disorder (see Chap 61).

Medical and Surgical Management

Treatment involves avoiding factors that precipitate attacks. Smoking is contraindicated because it causes vasoconstriction. Drug therapy with peripheral vasodilators, such as isoxsuprine (Vasodilan), may be attempted, but results usually are less favorable than desired. Other drugs, such as nifedipine (Procardia), are being used investigationally. An IV infusion of prostaglandin E may provide temporary relief. Gangrenous areas are amputated.

Nursing Management

Once an episode of pain occurs, there are several ways the attack can be aborted. If warming hands in water is impossible, encourage the client to imagine warming them in some way such as holding them near a roaring fire. The mind can alter physiology of blood flow. Another technique is to teach clients to imitate an exercise snow skiers use called the McIntyre maneuver: while standing, clients swing their arms behind and then in front of their bodies at a rate of about 180 times per minute. The swinging motion distributes blood to the distal areas of the fingers.

Instruct clients to avoid situations that contribute to ischemic episodes. Explain that injuries may heal slowly. If clients smoke, they must stop because nicotine causes vasoconstriction and increases frequency of episodes. Advise clients to wear wool socks and mittens during cold weather. Clients should avoid over-the-counter decongestants, cold remedies, and drugs for symptomatic relief of hay fever because of their vasoconstrictive qualities. Advise clients to wear work gloves during household chores like gardening and washing dishes to prevent accidental injury. Inform clients how to perform nail care to avoid injury, like soaking the hands or feet before trimming nails, trimming nails straight across, and seeing a podiatrist for the treatment of corns or calluses. Applying cream to prevent excessive skin dryness may be helpful.

● THROMBOSIS, PHLEBOTHROMBOSIS, AND EMBOLISM

A **thrombus** is a stationary clot. **Thrombosis** is a state in which a clot forms in a blood vessel. **Phlebothrombosis** is the development of a clot within a vein without inflammation. Phlebothrombosis and thrombophlebitis have similar symptoms and treatment (see Chap. 25). An **embolus** is a moving mass (clot) of particles, either solid or gas, in the bloodstream.

Pathophysiology and Etiology

Thrombosis in the venous system usually occurs in lower extremities and is associated with disorders or circumstances that cause venous stasis (inactivity, immobility, or trauma to a blood vessel). Orthopedic surgical procedures increase incidence of deep vein thrombosis (DVT) of the lower extremities. Atherosclerosis, endocarditis, pooling of blood in a ventricular aneurysm, and dysrhythmias like atrial fibrillation can precipitate arterial thrombosis and subsequent embolization. When a thrombus forms or an embolus reaches a blood vessel too small to permit its passage, blood flow is partly or totally occluded.

Assessment Findings

When an arterial clot is present, symptoms arise from ischemia to tissues that depend on the obstructed vessel for their oxygenated blood supply. With total occlusion, the extremity suddenly becomes white, cold, and extremely painful. Arterial pulsations are absent below the obstructed area. Numbness, tingling, or cramping also may be present, and surrounding blood vessels spasm. Loss of sensation and ability to move the part follows. Symptoms of shock frequently result if a large vessel is obstructed. When a small vessel is occluded, symptoms of ischemia, such as pallor and coldness, occur but are less severe. Unless blood flow is restored, gangrene develops.

Clients with phlebothrombosis may have few, if any, symptoms because inflammation is absent. Signs and symptoms of DVT usually include mild fever and pain, swelling, and tenderness of the affected extremity. A positive *Homans' sign,* pain on dorsiflexion of the foot, may be present. A thrombus may become a mobile embolus and lodge in a distal blood vessel, like the pulmonary capillaries, causing symptoms related to the organ to which circulation is impaired. (See discussions of pulmonary embolism in Chap. 23 and cerebral embolism in Chap. 40.)

Arteriography or venography (also called *phlebography*) uses a contrast dye to identify the point of obstruction. Doppler ultrasonography is used to detect abnormalities in peripheral blood flow. Plethysmography measures volume changes in the venous or arterial system.

Medical and Surgical Treatment

Treatment depends on whether an artery or a vein is occluded and the degree of occlusion (partial or complete).

Arterial Occlusive Disease

If an artery is completely occluded, treatment cannot be delayed. The physician may order an immediate IV injection of heparin to prevent development of further clots or extension of those already present. Administration of vasodilating drugs may improve circulation. A sympathetic nerve block (injection of a local anesthetic into the sympathetic ganglia) may relieve vasospasm. Narcotics may relieve pain and ease the client's apprehension. A thrombolytic agent may be given if the client experiences a pulmonary embolism or the embolus is occluding a large arterial vessel. If circulation to the extremity cannot be restored, a thrombectomy, embolectomy, *endarterectomy* (removal of the lining of an artery), or CABG is necessary. Nursing management of thrombectomy, embolectomy, endarterectomy, and bypass grafting is discussed in Chapter 31.

Venous Occlusive Disease

Venous thrombosis is treated with bed rest, elevation of the extremity, local heat, analgesics for pain, and intermittent subcutaneous injections or continuous IV heparin therapy, followed by oral anticoagulants once heparin has achieved a therapeutic effect. DVT may necessitate surgical removal of the clot (*thrombectomy*).

Nursing Management

Obtain a history of symptoms and identify characteristics of the pain. Assess for Homans' sign by having the client dorsiflex each foot. Examine extremities and compare skin color, temperature, capillary refill time, and tissue integrity; also measure each calf. Palpate peripheral pulses or use a Doppler ultrasound device if pulses cannot be palpated. Mark the location of each peripheral artery with a soft-tipped pen to facilitate its relocation. Immediately report any change in quality of a peripheral pulse or its sudden absence. Outlining any color change (line of demarcation) above or below the occluded area with a soft-tipped pen is useful to establish a baseline for future comparison.

Monitor the client's response to anticoagulation therapy. If heparin is administered, assess IV infusions hourly. Monitor partial thromboplastin time (PTT), prothrombin time (PT), and international normalized ratio (INR) when concurrent oral anticoagulation is prescribed. These values help determine therapeutic response and daily dosage. Be alert for signs of bleeding and keep protamine sulfate on hand for reversing heparin and vitamin K on hand for reversing oral anticoagulants. Additional nursing management is directed at increasing arterial or venous blood flow, relieving pain, and preventing complications.

To prevent recurrence of thrombosis, phlebothrombosis, or embolism, inform clients to avoid prolonged inactivity (especially sitting), elevate the legs periodically, and walk or do isometric leg exercises frequently if sitting is unavoidable. Recommend wearing antiembolism stockings to prevent venous stasis (especially if the client has venous leg ulcers). Instruct clients to apply stockings before assuming a dependent position or after elevating the extremities for several minutes. The client needs to remove and reapply antiembolism stockings twice a day or as recommended by the physician. Inform those who must take continued anticoagulants to observe for signs of unusual bleeding and keep appointments for laboratory tests.

• VENOUS INSUFFICIENCY

Venous insufficiency is a peripheral vascular disorder in which flow of venous blood is impaired through deep or superficial veins (or both). The condition usually affects lower extremities, most often the medial aspect of the leg or around the ankle.

Pathophysiology and Etiology

Venous insufficiency may be a consequence of varicose veins (discussed later) or valvular damage from a previous venous thrombosis. When forward movement of venous blood is affected, venous congestion develops from accumulating blood volume. Increased hydrostatic fluid pressure causes fluid to leave the veins and enter interstitial spaces. Localized edema is evident; skin becomes shiny and hard. The fluid-filled space acts as a barrier between cells in surrounding tissue and their capillary blood supply. Consequently, cells are subjected to accumulating amounts of CO_2. As unoxygenated cells die, they release inflammatory chemicals that cause *dermatitis,* inflammation of the dermis layer of skin. Skin becomes red and "hot." Hemoglobin from blood cells also escapes into extravascular space, causing tissue to appear dark brown, deep purple, or black. Serous fluid oozes from the skin when there is no outlet for vascular or lymphatic circulation. Eventually skin becomes impaired. A lesion referred to as a **venous stasis ulcer** forms. Without adequate circulation, healing is retarded. Some ulcers may be present for years. The skin is fragile and easily retraumatized in the healing process. Secondary infections often occur in the ulceration.

Assessment Findings

The foot or feet appear swollen. Testing for pitting is difficult because congested fluid cannot be displaced. Superficial veins are dilated and obvious during inspection. Skin color is not uniform; there usually is a red or darkly pigmented area. If a lesion is present, its margin usually is irregular. Serous fluid may have collected in a pocket beneath the skin, or there are beads of fluid on its surface that return after being wiped away. If an infection is present drainage may change from clear to opaque. Most clients report moderate pain. Pedal and tibial pulses may be difficult to palpate because of venous fluid congestion.

Doppler ultrasound demonstrates a reversed direction of blood flow, indicating valvular incompetence in superficial or deep veins. *Photoplethysmography,* a diagnostic test for venous pathology, measures light that is not absorbed by hemoglobin and consequently is reflected back to the machine. When clients with venous insufficiency undergo photoplethysmography during exercise and rest, light reflection is greater during rest, showing that the client has decreased oxygen-bound hemoglobin and increased volume of **venous reflux** (downward flow of venous blood). Air plethysmography measures venous pressure by filling a cuff with air after it is applied to the calf while the client is supine with legs elevated. When the client stands, pressure is measured again and venous pressure increases, indicating an increased volume of venous reflux.

Medical and Surgical Management

A major goal of therapy is to promote venous circulation. This is accomplished by applying elastic compression stockings such as *Jobst* stockings that maintain venous pressure at 40 mm Hg. The client wears the stockings at all times except when lying down. Because older adults have difficulty applying elastic compression stockings, the physician may apply a nonelastic gauze dressing soaked in zinc paste and glycerine known as an *Unna boot.* Pneumatic compression pump therapy, similar to EECP, also may be implemented. The compression pump promotes venous blood flow more efficiently than compression stockings but is more expensive and time-consuming. It also interferes with performance of daily activities during its use. Mild analgesics are recommended for pain. Vascular surgery can be performed in which the valves in larger veins are repaired or incompetent valves are bypassed using a length of vein with healthy valves from elsewhere in the body.

A stasis ulcer is managed by keeping the skin and ulcer clean with soap and water or a diluted solution of a disinfectant like Hibiclens. Necrotic tissue is debrided. Any infection is treated by applying Silvadene, an antibacterial cream, or an antibiotic ointment. The wound is covered with an occlusive transparent dressing like Tegaderm that traps moisture, which speeds healing. Chronic, nonhealing skin lesions also are treated with **topical hyperbaric oxygen** (THBO) therapy. This approach delivers oxygen above atmospheric pressure directly to the wound rather than to the full body as with other disorders like carbon monoxide poisoning. Oxygen accelerates the healing process. THBO is applied by covering the area with an inflatable boot that confines the oxygen at low hyperbaric pressure at the wound site. The boot remains in place for approximately 90 minutes a day for 4 consecutive days. The treatment is repeated after 3 days of nontreatment in a cycle over 8 to 10 weeks.

Nursing Management

Assess the appearance of the extremities and quality of circulation. If an ulcer is present, measure it and describe its appearance. Ask the client to rate his or her pain and administer an analgesic if warranted. Measure the diameter of the calf and ankle and length of the leg from heel to knee to obtain accurately fitting compression stockings. Help apply stockings each morning before the client lowers the legs to the floor. Implement wound care according to physician orders.

Teach the client to do the following:

- Purchase more than one pair of compression stockings so one pair is worn while the other is laundered.
- Dry elastic stockings by laying them flat rather than hanging them, which stretches elastic.

- Lose weight if necessary.
- Elevate legs periodically for at least 15 to 20 minutes.
- Walk or do isometric calf muscle pumps hourly to promote venous circulation.
- Raise foot of the bed to promote venous drainage during sleep.
- Avoid morning showers or sitting in front of a fire because heat dilates blood vessels and contributes to venous congestion.
- Wear shoes with laces rather than slippers or sandals to reduce pooling of blood in the feet.

DISORDERS OF BLOOD VESSEL WALLS

● VARICOSE VEINS

Varicose veins or varicosities are dilated, tortuous veins. Both sexes suffer equally from this disorder. Saphenous leg veins commonly are affected because they lack support from surrounding muscles. Varicose veins also may occur in other body parts, such as the rectum (hemorrhoids) and esophagus (esophageal varices).

Pathophysiology and Etiology

Varicose veins have a familial tendency. Valves of the veins become incompetent in early adulthood, resulting in varicosities. In others, anything constricting or interfering with venous return contributes to the formation of varicose veins. Prolonged standing compromises venous return as blood pools distally with gravity. Obesity and pressure on blood vessels from an enlarging fetus, liver, or abdominal tumor contribute to venous congestion. Thrombophlebitis may lead to varicose veins because the inflammatory process may damage vein valves.

Normally, the action of leg muscles during movement and exercise aids venous return (Fig. 27.9). When valves in veins are incompetent, blood accumulates rather than being propelled efficiently to the heart. The congestion stretches veins. Over time, they cannot recoil and remain chronically distended. Venous hypertension then forces some fluid to move into the interstitial spaces of surrounding tissue. Venous congestion and local edema may diminish arterial blood flow, impairing cellular nutrition. Even minor skin or soft tissue injuries easily become infected and ulcerated. Healing of such lesions is slow and uncertain.

Assessment Findings

Often the condition first manifests itself when other factors impair venous return. The legs feel heavy and tired, particularly after prolonged standing. The client may say that activity or elevation of the legs relieves the discomfort. Leg veins look distended and torturous and can be seen under the skin as dark blue or purple, snakelike elevations. Feet, ankles, and legs may appear swollen. The

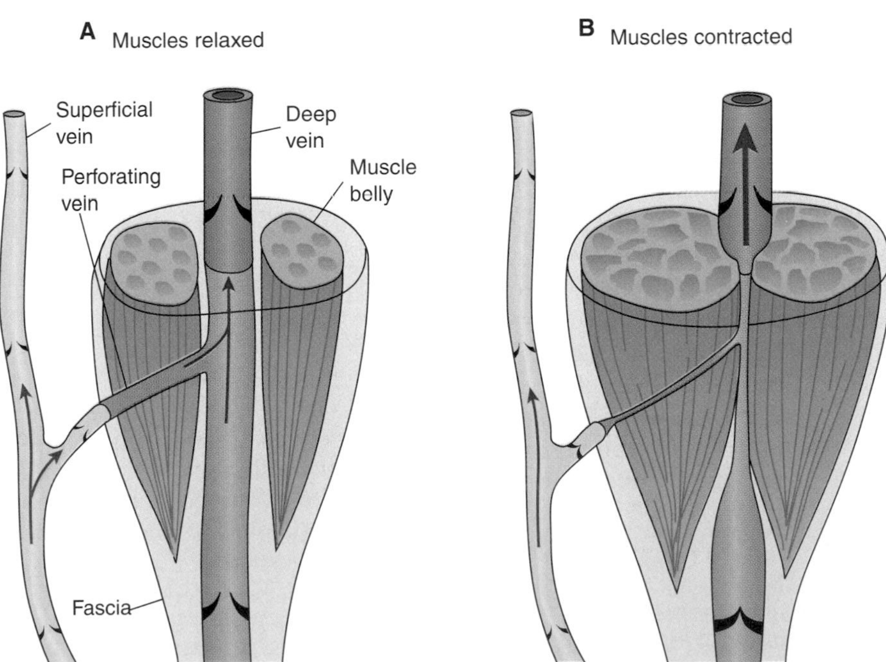

FIGURE 27.9 The skeletal muscle pumps and promotes blood flow in the deep and superficial calf vessels. Most perforating veins lie below the knee. When the calf muscle is relaxed (**A**), blood moves from the superficial to the deep veins. Muscle contraction (**B**) propels blood in the deep veins toward the heart; closure of the venous valves prevents backflow. (Margolis, D. J. [1992]. Management of venous ulcerations. *Hospital Practice, 27*[5], 37. © 1992, The McGraw-Hill Companies.)

skin may be slightly darker in the areas of impaired circulation. There may be signs of skin ulcerations in various stages of healing. Capillary refill may be abnormal.

The Brodie-Trendelenburg test is performed for diagnostic purposes. The client lies flat and elevates the affected leg to empty the veins. A tourniquet is then applied to the upper thigh, and the client is asked to stand. If blood flows from the upper part of the leg into the superficial veins when the tourniquet is released, the valves of the superficial veins are considered incompetent. Ultrasonography and venography also are used to detect impaired blood flow.

Medical Management

Treatment of mild varicose veins includes exercising (walking, swimming), losing weight (if needed), wearing elastic support stockings, and avoiding prolonged periods of sitting or standing. The defective vein may be sclerosed or occluded by injecting a chemical that sets up an inflammation in the vein wall. Eventually adhesions form, and blood flow must find an alternate route through collateral veins.

Surgical Management

Surgical treatment for severe or multiple varicose veins consists of vein ligation with or without vein stripping. A **vein ligation** is a procedure in which the affected veins are ligated (tied off) above and below the area of incompetent valves, but the dysfunctional vein remains. For better results, a **vein stripping** is performed; in this procedure the ligated veins are severed and removed. The entire great saphenous vein, which extends from groin to ankle, or the small saphenous vein may be removed.

Nursing Management

Assess skin, distal circulation, and peripheral edema. Ask the client to rate the level of discomfort and ability to do active and isometric leg exercises.

When the client returns from surgery with a gauze dressing covered by elastic roller bandages on the operative leg, monitor for swelling and its effect on circulation. Remove and rewrap the roller bandage to facilitate blood flow. Inspect the dressing for signs of active bleeding. In the immediate postoperative period, elevate the foot of the bed to aid venous circulation to the heart and remind the client to alternately contract and relax lower leg muscles. If active exercise is inadequate, consult with the physician about using pneumatic venous compression stockings, which cover the leg from foot to thigh and periodically inflate and release air, simulating isometric muscle contraction. Help the client ambulate as soon as possible to promote venous circulation, reduce edema, and prevent venous thrombosis. When bleeding is no longer a problem, apply elastic antiembolism stockings in place of the elastic roller bandage. Provide adequate fluid to decrease potential thrombosis.

When teaching the client and family, identify factors that impair venous circulation: wearing elastic girdles or tight belts, using round garters or rolling and twisting nylon stockings, standing or sitting for prolonged periods, and sitting with the knees crossed. Describe appropriate foot and nail care to facilitate tissue integrity. Explain that any open areas on the feet or lower legs require examination and treatment by the physician. Recommend active or isometric exercises and elevation of the extremities frequently during the day. Demonstrate how to apply and remove elastic support stockings. Refer the client to the dietitian if weight loss is indicated.

• ANEURYSMS

An **aneurysm** is stretching and bulging of an arterial wall. Aneurysms of the aorta (aortic arch, thoracic, abdominal) are the most common, but aneurysms can be found in other arteries, such as those in the leg and brain.

Pathophysiology and Etiology

Arteriosclerosis, hypertension, trauma, or a congenital weakness can affect elasticity of the *tunica media* (middle layer of the artery wall), causing part of the vessel to bulge. Once formed, some aneurysms lay down layers of clots, blocking the vessel until blood flow stops. Most aneurysms enlarge until they rupture. Loss of a large volume of arterial blood leads to shock and death if not controlled. Some aneurysms tear and leak blood into surrounding cavities, like the thorax or abdomen. Blood in a dissecting aneurysm is unavailable to arteries that branch off the aorta. When blood flow decreases or stops, tissue necrosis occurs.

Assessment Findings

Many aneurysms go unnoticed until found during physical examination or the client has a massive hemorrhage. Some cause pain, discomfort, and symptoms related to pressure on nearby structures. For example, a thoracic aortic aneurysm can cause bronchial obstruction, *dysphagia* (difficulty swallowing), and dyspnea. An abdominal aortic aneurysm can produce nausea and vomiting from pressure exerted on intestines, or it may cause back pain from pressure on vertebrae or spinal nerves. Most clients are hypertensive. A pulsating mass may be felt or even seen around the umbilicus or to the left of midline over the abdomen. A **bruit** (purring or blowing sound) can be auscultated over the mass. Circulation to tissue may be impaired.

Symptoms of a dissecting aneurysm vary and depend on whether a branching artery has been occluded or a tear has occurred in the aortic wall. Many clients become suddenly and acutely ill. Difference in the BPs of the left and right arms may be marked, or the BPs of the left and right legs may be unequal. Severe pain and signs of shock usually are present, but symptoms can be less severe in some instances. Because symptoms vary, diagnosis may be difficult.

X-rays can demonstrate aneurysms when the arterial wall contains calcium deposits. Aortography identifies the size and exact location of the aneurysm.

Medical and Surgical Management

Medical treatment includes administering antihypertensive drugs to keep BP within normal range. Aneurysms are treated surgically whenever possible; no other cure exists. They are repaired by bypass or replacement grafting. A dissecting or ruptured aneurysm is a surgical emergency.

Nursing Management

Help control hypertension by keeping activity and stress to a minimum. The client should avoid straining during bowel movements, coughing, and holding breath while changing positions. Monitor BP, pulse, hourly urine output, skin color, level of consciousness, and characteristics of pain for signs of hemorrhage or dissection. Prepare the client for diagnostic testing and operative interventions. Afterward, monitor for shock and adequate tissue perfusion. See Chapter 31 for nursing management of a client undergoing cardiovascular surgery.

GENERAL GERONTOLOGIC CONSIDERATIONS

Incidence of arteriosclerosis and other vascular disorders rises with age.

Older clients who take medication can ask their pharmacists to dispense the drug in a container without a childproof cap. This cap usually is difficult to remove when the client has arthritis or limited vision.

General physiologic changes of aging predispose clients to vascular occlusive disorders, especially as a result of atherosclerotic plaque formation. In addition, the heart's pumping ability decreases with age, increasing the risk of heart failure after an MI.

CAD is the most common cause of death in older adults. Less than 50% of older adults report chest pain with acute MI, whereas approximately 80% of younger adults report chest pain. Older adults are more likely to have nonspecific symptoms such as dyspnea, confusion, and syncope.

Use of calcium channel blockers, such as nifedipine and verapamil, to treat angina causes a peripheral vasodilating effect. Therefore, they are given cautiously to older adults who are at increased risk for hypotension.

Older adults are more sensitive to the hypotensive effects of nitrates, probably because of impaired venous valves, diminished baroreceptor reflex, and decreased vascular volume.

Critical Thinking Exercises

1. *A client presents in the emergency department complaining of substernal chest pain. He has a history of angina. What assessment criteria will help you differentiate between an anginal attack and an MI? What diagnostic tests will confirm an MI?*
2. *A client with Raynaud's disease relates that she has difficulty reducing attacks during the winter. What client teaching is indicated? How can the client reduce the ischemic episodes?*
3. *A client who has had a ligation of varicose veins returns to her room after surgery. What assessments are a priority? How can you teach the client to reduce the incidence of further varicose vein formation?*

● NCLEX-STYLE REVIEW QUESTIONS 

1. A visitor in a hospital complains of severe chest pain and tells the nurse that he has a history of angina pectoris. Which of the following is the most appropriate action the nurse can take next?
   1. Ask the client to lie down.
   2. Help the client relax.
   3. Encourage the client to rest.
   4. Help the client perform exercises.
2. The nurse advises a client recovering from a myocardial infarction to decrease fat and salt in her diet. Which food choice would the nurse include in the client's diet?
   1. Oatmeal and apple juice
   2. Bacon and scrambled eggs
   3. Pepperoni pizza and beer
   4. Cheeseburger and french fries
3. A client with venous stasis in the lower extremities complains to the nurse that the elastic compression stockings are "too tight." Which response by the nurse is most appropriate?
   1. "The stockings used are designed to improve the circulation in your legs."
   2. "I will call the doctor and see about discontinuing them."
   3. "Do you feel numbness and tingling in your toes?"
   4. "I can see if Central Supply can send up a larger pair of stockings."

connection

Visit the Connection site at **http://connection.lww.com/go/timbyEssentials** for links to chapter-related resources on the Internet.

References and Suggested Readings

American College of Cardiology and American Heart Association. (1999). 1999 Update: ACC/AHA guidelines for the management of patients with acute myocardial infarction. [On-line.] Available: http://www.acc.org/clinical/guidelines/nov96/1999/index.htm.

Anderson, L. A. (2001). Abdominal aortic aneurysm. *Journal of Cardiovascular Nursing, 15*(4), 1–14.

Ayers, D. M. (2002). Preparing a patient for cardiac catheterization. *Nursing 2002, 32*(9), 82.

Beattie, S. (2002). New biomarkers may predict CAD. *RN, 65*(9), 47–54.

Church, V. (2000). Staying on guard for DVT & PE . . . deep vein thrombosis . . . pulmonary embolism. *Nursing 2000, 30*(2), 34–44.

Di Trapano, C., & Mege, J. (February 3, 2003). Alleviating angina. *Advance for Nurses,* 24–25, 38.

Fong, I. W. (2000). Emerging relations between infectious diseases and coronary artery disease and atherosclerosis. *Canadian Medical Association Journal, 163,* 49–56.

Gehring, P. E. (2002). Perfecting your skills: Vascular assessment. *RN's TNT, 4,* 16–24.

Hadaway, L. C. (2002). What you can do to decrease catheter-related infections. *Nursing 2002, 32*(9), 46–48.

Halm, M. A., & Penque, S. (1999). Heart disease in women. *American Journal of Nursing, 99*(4), 26–32.

HeartCenterOnline. (2001). Women and cholesterol. [On-line.] Available: http://www.heartcenteronline.com.

Kunimoto, B., Cooling, M., Gulliver, W., et al. (2001). Best practices for the prevention and treatment of venous leg ulcers. *Ostomy/Wound Management, 47*(2), 34–44.

Littrell, K. (September 24, 2001). Cardiac markers in acute coronary syndromes. *Advance for Nurses,* 17–19.

McCaffrey, E. (November 25, 2002). Battling cholesterol. *Advance for Nurses,* 12–13, 37.

Patterson, S. (1999). Percutaneous myocardial revascularization: New treatment option for patients with angina. *Critical Care Nurse, 19*(5), 27–33, 35–36.

Platek, Y. M. (1999). PTMR . . . percutaneous transluminal myocardial revascularization. *American Journal of Nursing, 99*(7), 64–66.

Pope, W. (2002). Angioplasty and stenting. *RN, 65*(6), 55–59.

Reilly, P. J. (May 27, 2002). Cholesterol-lowering agents. *Advance for Nurses,* 18–20.

Ross, R. (1999). Mechanisms of disease: atherosclerosis: An inflammatory disease. *New England Journal of Medicine, 340,* 115–126.

Rudolph, D. (2001). Standards of care for venous leg ulcers; compression therapy and moist wound healing. *Journal of Vascular Nursing, 19*(1), 20–27.

Ryan, D. (2000). Is it an MI? A lab primer. *RN, 63*(1), 26–31.

Sullivan, C. (2000). Easing severe angina with laser surgery. *Nursing 2000, 30*(4), Crit Care 32cc1–32cc2, 32cc4.

The cholesterol connection: Homocysteine: the cholesterol for the 21st century. *National Women's Health Report, 22*(4), 7.

Tuite, L. (September 30, 2002). Women and heart disease. *Advance for Nurses,* 21–23.

U.S. Prevention Services Task Force. (2002). Aspirin for primary prevention of cardiovascular events: Recommendations and rationale. *American Journal of Nursing, 102*(3), 67–70.

U.S. Prevention Services Task Force. (2002). Screening for lipid disorders in adults: Recommendations and rationale. *American Journal of Nursing, 102*(3), 91–95.

Wackel, J. (2000). Altered coagulation. A diagnosis for the problem of deep vein thrombosis. *Nursing Diagnosis, 11*(2), 17–23.

Woods, A. (2002). High cholesterol (hyperlipidemia). *Nursing 2002, 32*(6), 56–57.

chapter **28**

Caring for Clients With Cardiac Dysrhythmias

Words to Know 

asystole
atrial fibrillation
atrial flutter
automatic implanted cardiac defibrillator
bigeminy
bradydysrhythmia
chemical cardioversion
couplets
defibrillation
demand (or synchronous) mode pacemaker
dysrhythmia
ectopic site
elective electrical cardioversion
fixed-rate (or asynchronous) mode pacemaker
heart block
implanted pacemaker
Maze procedure
multifocal PVCs
pacemaker
premature atrial contraction
premature ventricular contraction
radiofrequency catheter ablation
R on T phenomenon
sinus bradycardia
sinus tachycardia
supraventricular tachycardia
tachydysrhythmias
transcutaneous pacemaker
transthoracic pacemaker
transvenous pacemaker
ventricular fibrillation
ventricular tachycardia

Learning Objectives

On completion of this chapter, the reader will:

- Describe common dysrhythmias.
- Identify medications to control or eliminate dysrhythmias.
- Explain the purpose and advantages of elective cardioversion.
- Discuss when defibrillation is used to treat dysrhythmias.
- Describe the purpose for implanting an automatic internal cardiac defibrillator.
- Name various types and purposes of artificial pacemakers.
- Describe nursing management of the client with a dysrhythmia treated by drug therapy, elective cardioversion, defibrillation, or pacemaker insertion.

Cardiac rhythm refers to the pattern (or pace) of the heartbeat. The conduction system of the heart and inherent rhythmicity of cardiac muscle produce a rhythm pattern, which greatly influences the heart's ability to pump blood effectively. Cardiac conduction and electrocardiogram (ECG) waveforms are discussed in Chapter 24. The usual cardiac rhythm is called *normal sinus rhythm* (Box 28-1; Fig. 28.1).

A **dysrhythmia** (also called an *arrhythmia*) is a conduction disorder resulting in an abnormally slow or rapid heart rate or one that does not proceed through the conduction system as it should. Some dysrhythmias do not require treatment; others require immediate intervention because they are potentially fatal. The most common cause of dysrhythmias is ischemic heart disease (see Chap. 27). Drug therapy, electrolyte disturbances, metabolic acidosis, hypothermia, and degenerative age-related changes are other conditions that cause dysrhythmias.

BOX 28-1 • Characteristics of Normal Sinus Rhythm

- Heart rate is between 60 and 100 beats/minute.
- The SA node initiates the impulse (upright P wave before each QRS complex).
- Impulse travels to the AV node in 0.12 to 0.2 second (the PR interval).
- The ventricles depolarize in 0.12 second or less (the QRS complex).
- Each impulse occurs regularly (evenly spaced).

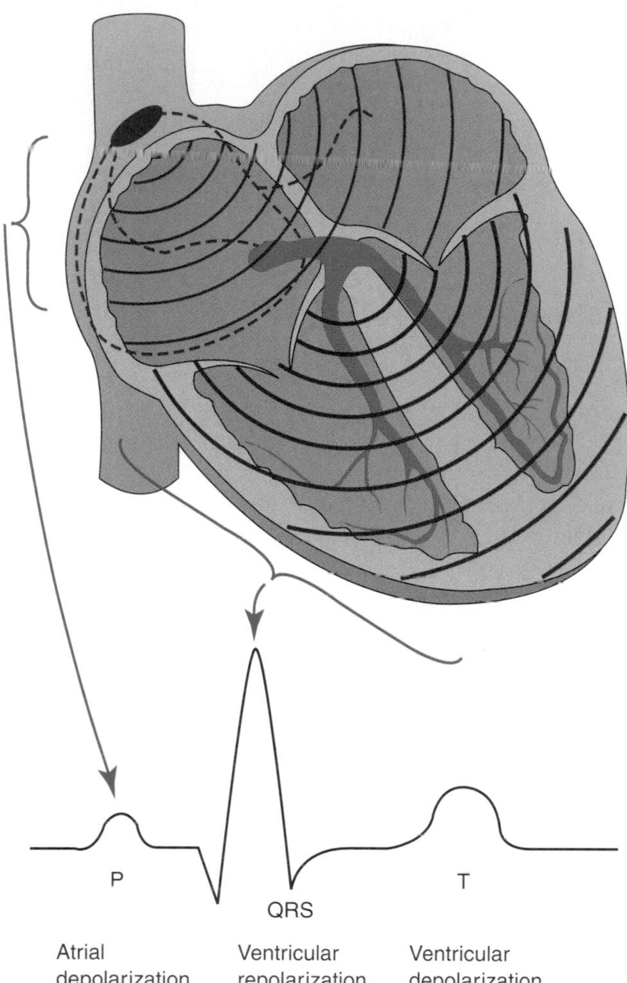

FIGURE 28.1 Normal conduction and ECG waveforms.

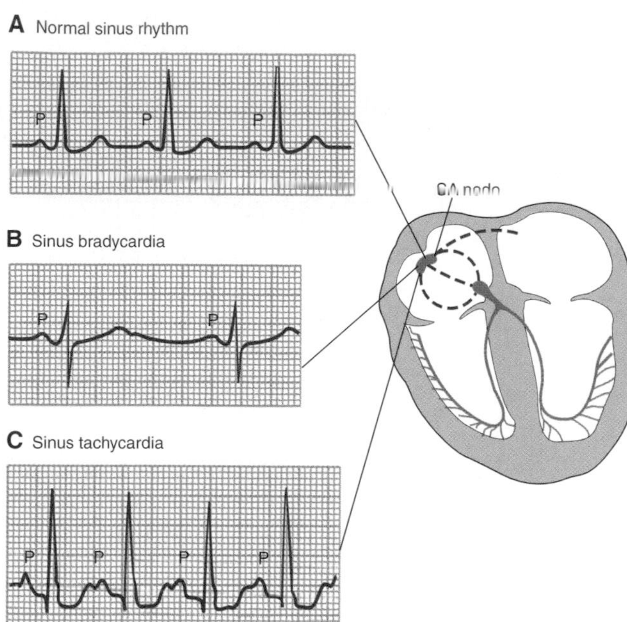

FIGURE 28.2 (**A**) In sinus rhythm, the SA node initiates impulses (P waves) 60 to 100 times/min. (**B**) In sinus bradycardia, the SA node initiates impulses at 40 to 60 times/min. (**C**) In sinus tachycardia, the SA node initiates impulses at 100 to 150 times/min.

CARDIAC DYSRHYTHMIAS

Dysrhythmias Originating in the Sinoatrial Node

Sinus Bradycardia

Sinus bradycardia is a dysrhythmia that proceeds normally through the conduction pathway but at a slower than usual rate (≤60 beats/minute; Fig. 28.2). Healthy athletes and others who are physically fit often have heart rates below 60 beats/minute; however, this finding reflects a well-toned heart conditioned through regular exercise. Such a heart rate is pathologic in clients with heart disorders, increased intracranial pressure, hypothyroidism, or digitalis toxicity. The danger in sinus bradycardia is that the slow rate may be insufficient to maintain cardiac output. Atropine sulfate is given intravenously (IV) to increase a dangerously slow heart rate.

Sinus Tachycardia

Sinus tachycardia is a dysrhythmia that proceeds normally through the conduction pathway but at a faster than usual rate (100 to 150 beats/minute; see Fig. 28.2). It occurs in clients with healthy hearts as a physiologic response to strenuous exercise, anxiety and fear, pain, fever, hyperthyroidism, hemorrhage, shock, or hypoxemia.

Premature Atrial Contractions

Occasionally, neural tissue in the atrial conduction system initiates an early electrical impulse called a **premature atrial contraction** (PAC), which is identified by an irregularity in the underlying rhythm (Fig. 28.3). The P wave of the waveform may look similar to other conducted impulses or may differ slightly because it is initiated somewhere in the atria other than the sinoatrial (SA) node. PACs can occur for various reasons: consumption of caffeine, use of nicotine or other sympathetic nervous system stimulants, or in response to heart disease or metabolic disorders like hyperthyroidism. When PACs are isolated or infrequent, there is no cause for alarm. Eliminating

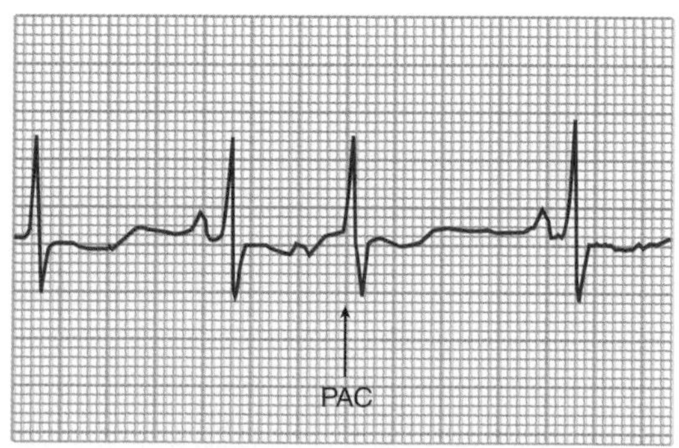

FIGURE 28.3 Normal sinus rhythm with 1 PAC.

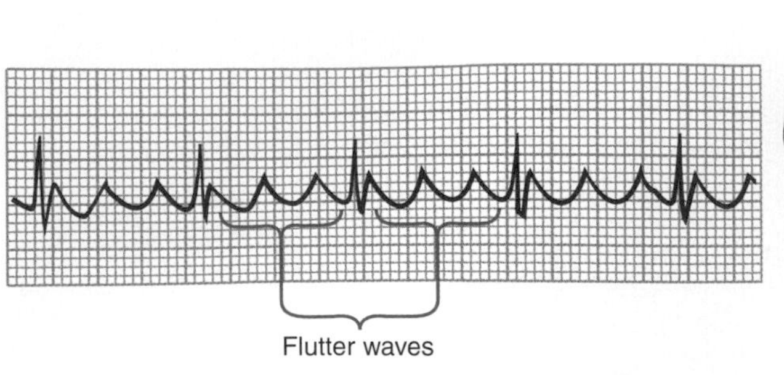

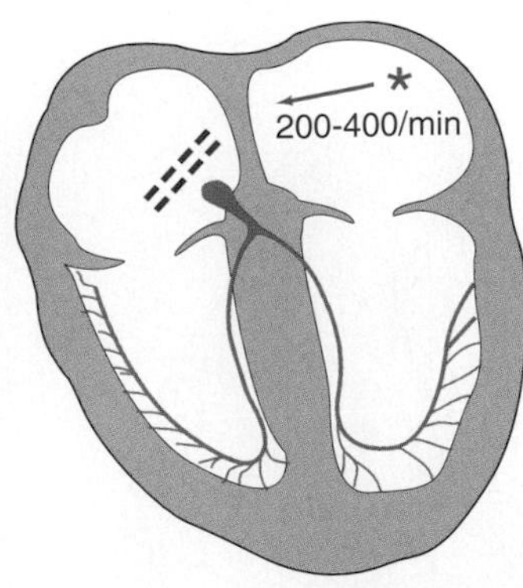

FIGURE 28.4 Atrial flutter produces sawtooth flutter waves. Most of the atrial impulses are not conducted to the ventricles.

the cause usually controls PACs. Occasionally, the **ectopic site,** one that initiates an electrical impulse independently of the SA node, can lead to more serious dysrhythmias like supraventricular tachycardia.

Supraventricular Tachycardia

Supraventricular tachycardia (SVT) is a dysrhythmia in which the heart rate is dangerously high (≥150 beats/minute). Diastole is shortened and the heart does not have sufficient time to fill. Cardiac output drops dangerously low and heart failure can occur, especially in clients with pre-existing heart disease or damage. Clients with coronary artery disease (CAD) and SVT can develop chest pain because coronary blood flow cannot meet the increased need of the myocardium imposed by the fast rate. Besides tachycardia and angina, hypotension, syncope, and reduced renal output are signs and symptoms of low cardiac output and impending heart failure. Digitalis, adrenergic blockers, and calcium channel blockers are used to slow heart rate.

Atrial Flutter

Atrial flutter (Fig. 28.4) is a disorder in which a single atrial impulse outside the SA node causes the atria to contract at an exceedingly rapid rate (200 to 400 contractions/minute). The atrioventricular (AV) node conducts only some impulses to the ventricle, resulting in a ventricular rate that is slower than the atrial rate. The atrial waves in atrial flutter have a characteristic sawtooth pattern.

Atrial Fibrillation

In **atrial fibrillation,** several areas in the right atrium initiate impulses resulting in disorganized, rapid activity. The atria quiver rather than contract (Fig. 28.5). The ventricles respond to the atrial stimulus randomly, causing irregular ventricular heart rates, which may be too infrequent to maintain adequate cardiac output. Ibutilide (Corvert) is an antidysrhythmic drug used to convert new-onset atrial fibrillation into sinus rhythm; flecainide (Tambocor) and propafenone (Rythmol) also treat and prevent atrial fibrillation. Use of drugs to eliminate a dysrhythmia is referred to as **chemical cardioversion.** Atrial fibrillation also is treated with elective cardioversion (discussed later) or digitalis if the ventricular rate is not too slow. Clients who are not candidates for cardioversion and fail to respond to conventional measures may be candidates for a surgical intervention referred to as the **Maze procedure.** During the Maze procedure, the surgeon creates a new conduction pathway that eliminates rapid firing of ectopic pacemaker sites in the atria. Some individuals with atrial fibrillation continue to experience chronic atrial fibrillation or episodic events.

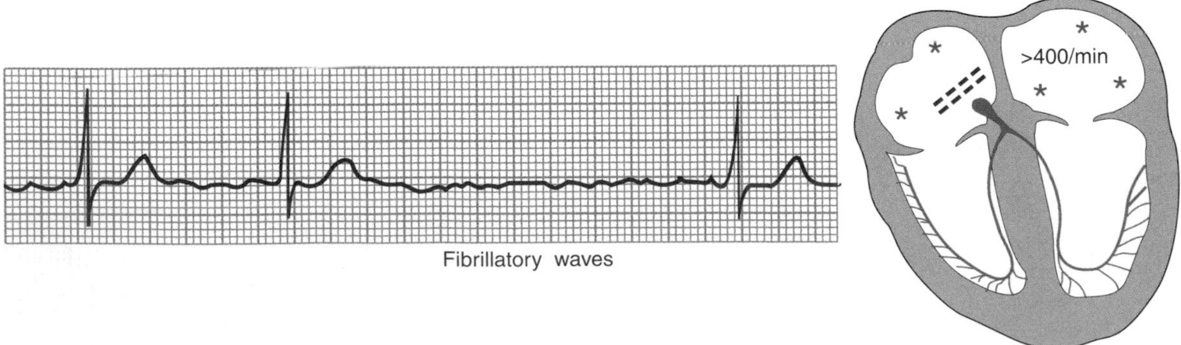

FIGURE 28.5 There are no identifiable P waves in atrial fibrillation. The atrial impulses look like a fine, undulating line.

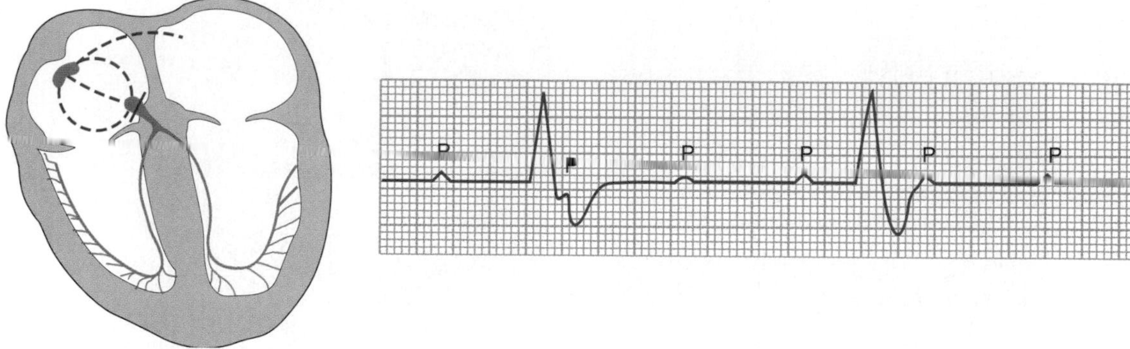

FIGURE 28.6 In heart block, SA-initiated impulses are delayed at the AV node or fail to progress altogether. In this example of complete heart block, the ventricles are beating independently of the atria.

Dysrhythmia Originating in the Atrioventricular Node: Heart Block

Heart block refers to disorders in the conduction pathway that interfere with transmission of impulses from the SA node through the AV node to the ventricles. Heart block may be first degree, second degree, or third degree (also called *complete*). In first- and second-degree heart block, the impulse is delayed. In complete heart block (Fig. 28.6), the atrial impulse never gets through, and ventricles develop their own rhythm independent of atrial rhythm. Ventricular rate usually is slow (30 to 40 beats/minute). Pacemaker insertion (discussed later) is the treatment for complete heart block.

Dysrhythmias Originating in the Ventricles

Premature Ventricular Contractions

Premature ventricular contraction (PVC) is a ventricular contraction that occurs early and independently in the cardiac cycle before the SA node initiates an electrical impulse. No P wave precedes the wide, bizarre-looking QRS complex (Fig. 28.7). If the heart rate is very slow, the ventricles can repolarize after a PVC in sufficient time to receive the atrial stimulus precisely when it is due. PVCs often cause a flip-flop sensation in the chest, sometimes described as "fluttering." Associated signs and symptoms include pallor, nervousness, sweating, and faintness. Many people experience occasional PVCs, which usually are harmless. They may be related to anxiety, stress, fatigue, alcohol withdrawal, or tobacco use. Although PVCs normally are not associated with a specific heart disorder, thorough examination is important to ensure no heart disease exists.

In the presence of acute heart injury, such as after surgery or with acute myocardial infarction (MI), PVCs in certain patterns suggest myocardial irritability and are precursors of lethal dysrhythmias (Fig. 28.8):

- Six or more PVCs per minute
- Runs of **bigeminy** (every other beat is a PVC)
- Two PVCs in a row (**couplets**)
- Runs of PVCs (three or more in a row)
- **Multifocal PVCs** (originating from more than one location)
- A PVC whose R wave falls on the T wave of the preceding complex (**R on T phenomenon**)

When dangerous PVCs occur, the client is given an IV bolus of lidocaine, followed by an IV infusion of the drug.

Ventricular Tachycardia

Ventricular tachycardia is caused by a single, irritable focus in the ventricle that initiates the heartbeat (see

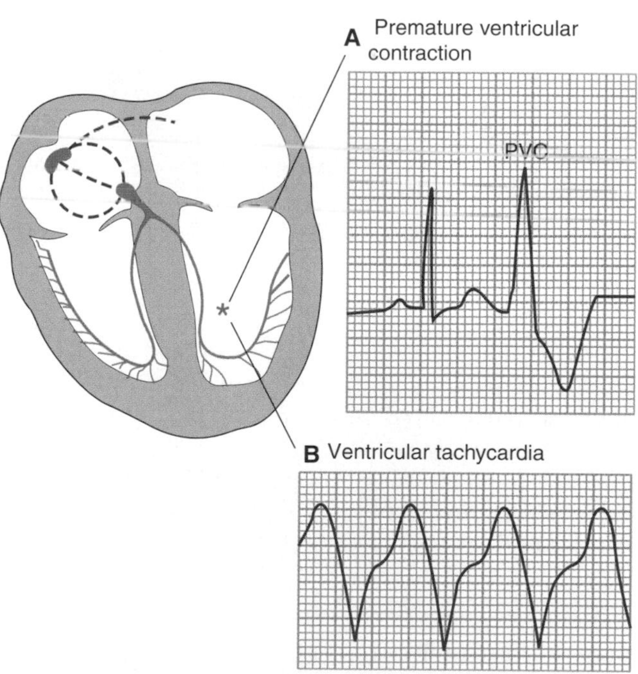

FIGURE 28.7 (**A**) An area outside the normal conduction pathway in the ventricles initiates a PVC. (**B**) Continuous generation of impulses results in ventricular tachycardia.

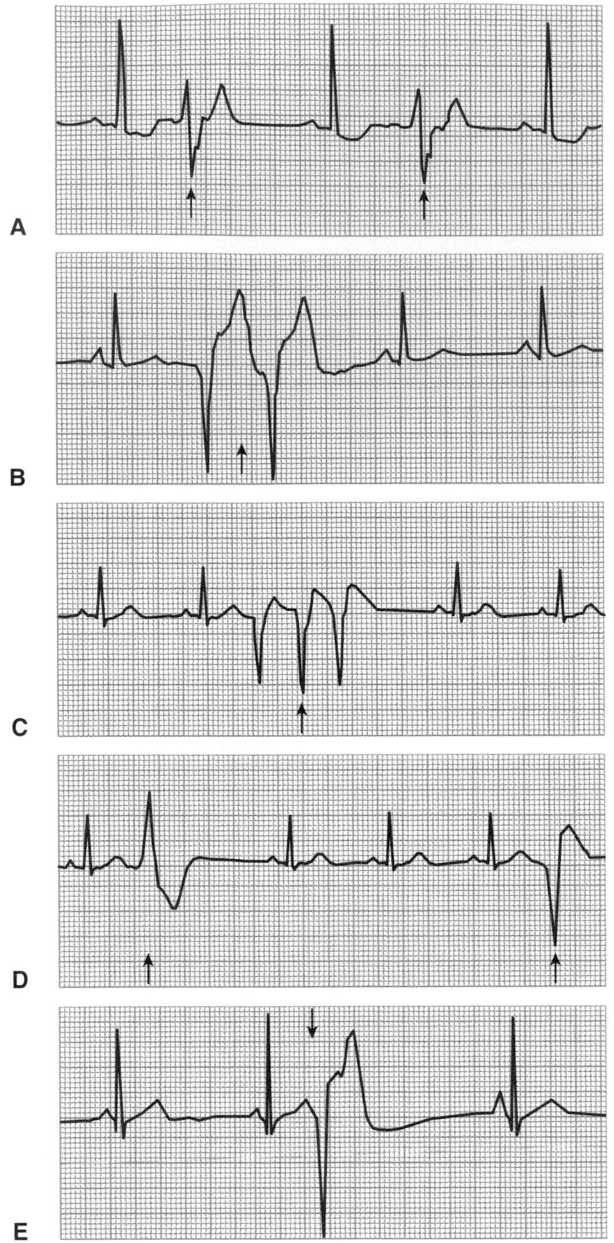

FIGURE 28.8 Dangerous forms of PVCs: (**A**) bigeminy, (**B**) couplets, (**C**) run, (**D**) multifocal, and (**E**) R on T phenomenon.

Fig. 28.7). The ventricles beat very fast (150 to 250 beats/minute), and cardiac output is decreased. Depending on how long the dysrhythmia is present, the client may lose consciousness and become pulseless. Ventricular tachycardia sometimes ends abruptly without intervention but often requires defibrillation. It may progress to ventricular fibrillation.

Ventricular Fibrillation

Ventricular fibrillation (Fig. 28.9) is the rhythm of a dying heart. PVCs or ventricular tachycardia can precipitate it. Ventricles do not contract effectively and there is no cardiac output. Ventricular fibrillation is an indication for cardiopulmonary resuscitation (CPR) and immediate defibrillation.

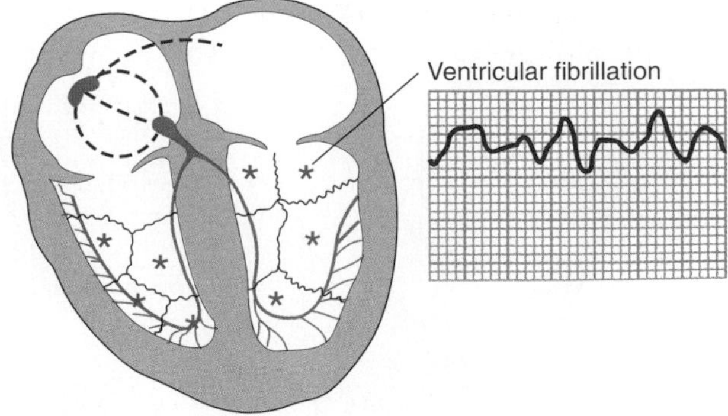

FIGURE 28.9 The ventricles quiver during ventricular fibrillation, as shown by a wavy line.

Pathophysiology and Etiology of Cardiac Dysrhythmias

Many clinical states predispose clients to dysrhythmias. One of the most common causes of serious dysrhythmias is myocardial ischemia, lack of oxygenated blood to heart muscle, which can occur secondary to CAD, congestive heart failure, inadequate ventilation, and shock. The conduction system also is susceptible to disturbances from anxiety, pain, endocrine disorders, electrolyte imbalances, valvular heart disease, placement of invasive catheters in the heart, and drug effects. Because of altered rate and rhythm, all dysrhythmias affect the heart's pumping action and cardiac output to some degree.

Assessment Findings

A client whose dysrhythmia causes decreased cardiac output is likely to feel weak and tired, experience anginal pain, or faint. Some clients with **tachydysrhythmias** (abnormally fast rhythms) describe palpitations or flutterings in their chest. Blood pressure (BP) usually is low. Pulse is irregular or difficult to palpate; the rate is unusually fast or slow. Apical and radial pulse rates may differ. Skin may be pale and cool. The client may be disoriented and confused if the brain is not adequately oxygenated, or there may be loss of consciousness and even clinical death. A monitor rhythm strip or 12-lead ECG can identify dysrhythmias. Electrophysiology studies can locate their origin.

Medical and Surgical Management

Some dysrhythmias are not life-threatening and may not require treatment. Many are treated with drug therapy and electrical modalities such as elective electrical cardioversion, defibrillation, or temporary or permanent pacing.

Drug Therapy

Oral and IV antidysrhythmic drugs are used to treat clients with dysrhythmias, but not all clients require medication. Usually, long-term antidysrhythmic drug therapy is based on the degree of hemodynamic compromise and potential for the client to develop a life-threatening dysrhythmia. During resuscitation efforts, one or more various drugs used in cardiac emergencies is administered (Drug Therapy Table 28.1).

Elective Electrical Cardioversion

Elective electrical cardioversion is a nonemergency procedure done by a physician to stop rapid atrial, but

Drug Therapy Table 28.1 ANTIDYSRHYTHMICS

DRUG CATEGORY AND EXAMPLES	MECHANISM OF ACTION	SIDE EFFECTS	NURSING CONSIDERATIONS
Class I Antidysrhythmics			
lidocaine hydrochloride (Xylocaine)	Suppress ventricular dysrhythmias by decreasing ventricular excitability	Dizziness, fatigue, drowsiness, nausea, vomiting, vision changes, seizures, hypotension	Monitor cardiac rhythm and vital signs. Keep life support equipment available.
procainamide hydrochloride (Pronestyl)	Slow electrical conduction, suppressing ventricular dysrhythmias	Hypotension, rash	Monitor cardiac rhythm and BP frequently.
Class III Antidysrhythmic			
bretylium tosylate (Bretylol)	Inhibit the release of norepinephrine Used for ventricular dysrhythmias resistant to other antidysrhythmic agents	Nausea, vomiting, hypotension, pain at IV site	Monitor cardiac rhythm and BP continuously. Keep client recumbent.
Class IV Antidysrhythmics			
verapamil hydrochloride (Calan)	Suppress tachydysrhythmias by inhibiting the movement of calcium across cell membranes	Dizziness, headache, bradycardia, hypotension, heart block	Monitor BP, heart rate, rhythm, and output. Keep client flat for 1 hr after administration. Have equipment for cardioversion and pacing available.
adenosine (Adenocard)	Slow rapid conduction through the AV node, restoring sinus rhythm	Headache, dizziness, nausea, other dysrhythmias, facial flushing, dyspnea, chest pain	Monitor BP and cardiac rhythm continuously, and have emergency equipment nearby. Monitor client frequently, especially those with underlying asthma or chronic obstructive pulmonary disease.
Vasopressors			
epinephrine hydrochloride (Adrenalin)	Increase heart rate, force of contraction, and BP Used in asystole	Hypertension, dysrhythmias, pallor, oliguria	Administer every 5 min during cardiac resuscitation. Monitor vital signs and cardiac rhythm.
Cholinergic Antagonists			
atropine sulfate	Block the effects of vagus nerve stimulation Increase heart rate Used for bradydysrhythmias	Palpitations, tachycardia, urinary retention	Monitor for therapeutic and adverse effects. Document heart rate before and after administration.
Other			
calcium chloride	Increase cardiac contraction in cases of cardiac standstill Improve weak or ineffective myocardial contractions when epinephrine fails	Slowed heart rate, tingling, hypotension with rapid IV administration	Give intravenously. Avoid extravasation. Monitor cardiac response.

not necessarily life-threatening, dysrhythmias. It is similar to defibrillation (Table 28.1). One difference is that the machine delivering electrical stimulation waits to discharge until it senses the appearance of an R wave. By doing so, the machine prevents disrupting the heart during the critical period of ventricular repolarization.

The client is sedated for the procedure. Electrodes lubricated with a special gel or moist saline pads are applied to the chest wall. When the discharge button on the paddles is depressed and the heart is in ventricular depolarization, electrical energy is released. The electric current completely depolarizes the entire myocardium. As the heart repolarizes, the normal pacemaker regains control and restores continued normal conduction through the heart.

Defibrillation

The only treatment for a life-threatening ventricular dysrhythmia is immediate **defibrillation,** which has the same effect as cardioversion except defibrillation is used when there is no functional ventricular contraction. Without defibrillation, the client will die. The defibrillator discharges its electrical energy when the discharge button is depressed. It is used during pulseless ventricular tachycardia, ventricular fibrillation, and **asystole** (cardiac arrest) when no identifiable R wave is present. The American Heart Association recommends public access defibrillation—that is, automatic electrical defibrillators (AEDs) be located in public places such as worksites and locations where large numbers of people gather. AEDs are carried on some airplanes and police cars. If defibrillation is performed within the first 5 minutes of ventricular fibrillation or cardiac arrest, potential for survival is 50%; after 10 minutes without defibrillation, the chance for resuscitation is unlikely (American Heart Association, 2000).

AUTOMATIC IMPLANTED CARDIAC DEFIBRILLATOR. The **automatic implanted cardiac defibrillator** (AICD) is an internal electrical device used for selected clients with recurrent life-threatening tachydysrhythmias. Candidates for an AICD include those who (1) have survived at least one episode of cardiac arrest from a ventricular dysrhythmia, (2) experience recurrent episodes of ventricular tachycardia, or (3) are at risk for sudden cardiac death because of structural heart disease like cardiomyopathy (see Chap. 25) with poor ventricular function.

An AICD consists of a generator with a battery and one (sometimes two) electrical lead that resembles a wire (Fig. 28.10). The generator is placed in a pocket under the skin near the clavicle, and the lead wire is inserted transvenously through the subclavian or cephalic vein to the apex or septum of the right ventricle. The lead senses the cardiac rhythm, which it transmits to the generator. The generator, programmed for various responses depending on the sensed rhythm, delivers an electrical shock through the lead to restore a life-sustaining cardiac rhythm, records the data, and then resets itself. A conscious client perceives the defibrillating shock as a thump or "kick" to the chest. AICDs also can pace the heart to obliterate a tachydysrhythmia and perform low-energy cardioversion. It has been shown that AICDs reduce death rates among at-risk clients far better than drug therapy alone.

The AICD is checked and reprogrammed every 3 to 4 months. Stored information can be retrieved. AICDs deliver approximately 200 to 250 discharges and last approximately 3 to 6 years before the battery requires replacement. Although AICDs are highly safe, some forms of electrical interference may adversely affect their function. Clients are instructed to avoid devices with a magnetic field. Examples include magnetic resonance imaging devices, extracorporeal shock-wave lithotripsy machines (see Chap. 58), electrocautery and diathermy

TABLE 28.1 COMPARISON OF CARDIOVERSION AND DEFIBRILLATION

CARDIOVERSION	DEFIBRILLATION
Scheduled procedure 1 to several days in advance	Emergency procedure performed during resuscitation
Used to eliminate atrial dysrhythmias (e.g., atrial flutter, atrial fibrillation, supraventricular tachycardia)	Used to eliminate ventricular dysrhythmias (e.g., ventricular fibrillation, asystole)
Client sedated before procedure	Client not sedated but unresponsive
Uses less electrical energy (50–100 joules) than defibrillation, but higher levels can be administered if initial outcome is unsuccessful	Uses more electrical energy (200–360 joules) than cardioversion
Delivers electrical energy when the machine senses the R wave of the ECG	Delivers electrical energy whenever the buttons on the paddles are pressed

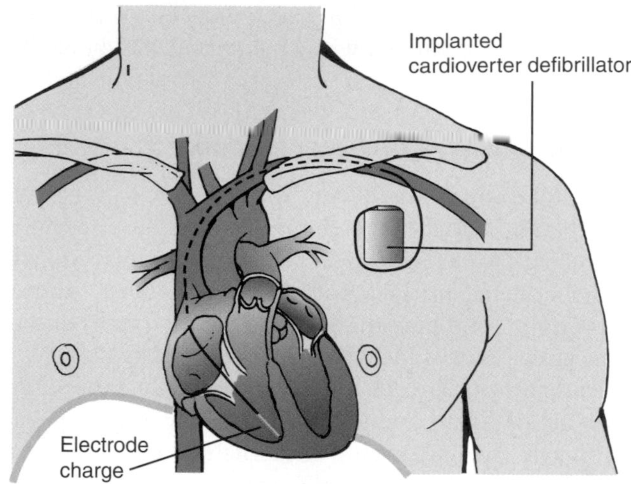

FIGURE 28.10 The automatic implanted cardiac defibrillator (AICD).

devices, peripheral nerve stimulators, large industrial electrical motors, and arc welding equipment. Analog cellular telephones are safe, but electrical signals from digital cellular telephones can mimic an abnormal heart rhythm, activating the AICD. Most power tools and microwave ovens have shields or are grounded, making them safe. A hand search is preferable to a scan with a metal detector at airports. Placing a donut magnet over the generator deactivates the device and should be done only if equipment is available to use an external defibrillator.

Clients with AICDs are advised to carry information about the device on their person, including names of physicians involved in their care. Driving usually is restricted for at least 6 months. Clients are told to report episodes in which they sense AICD activity. If the AICD discharges repeatedly or the client is symptomatic, immediate assessment by a cardiologist or electrophysiologist is warranted. The AICD may need to be reprogrammed, additional therapy with antidysrhythmic drugs may be initiated, or current medications may be adjusted.

Stop, Think, and Respond ● BOX 28-1

Explain why ventricular dysrhythmias are more serious than most atrial dysrhythmias.

Pacemakers

A **pacemaker** provides an electrical stimulus to the heart muscle to treat an ineffective **bradydysrhythmia** (slow abnormal rhythm). There are two major types of pacemakers: temporary or permanent. Temporary pacing is done under urgent or emergency circumstances. They include transcutaneous, transthoracic, and transvenous. An internal pacemaker is totally implanted and designed for permanent use.

Pacemakers function in either a demand (synchronous) or fixed-rate (asynchronous) mode. **Demand (synchronous) mode pacemakers** self-activate when the client's pulse falls below a certain level. If the pacemaker is set at 72 beats/minute, it will not activate until the client's natural heart rate falls below 72 beats/minute. **Fixed-rate (asynchronous) mode pacemakers,** used less frequently, produce an electrical stimulus at a preset rate (usually 72 to 80 beats/minute) despite the client's natural rhythm.

TEMPORARY PACEMAKERS. An external **transcutaneous pacemaker** is an emergency measure for maintaining adequate heart rate. It uses disposable, self-adhering leads attached to the chest wall (transcutaneous; Fig. 28.11). Heart rate is paced from an external generator. Use of a transcutaneous pacemaker is temporary until either a transvenous or permanent pacemaker can be placed, or the client is stabilized with medication.

A **transvenous pacemaker** is a temporary pulse-generating device that sometimes is necessary to manage transient bradydysrhythmias such as those that occur during acute MIs or after coronary artery bypass graft surgery, or to override tachydysrhythmias. The electrical lead is introduced through the subclavian, external or internal jugular, or cephalic vein and threaded first into the right atrium, then into the right ventricle. Fluoroscopy and a cardiac monitor are used to determine correct placement of the tip of the pacemaker lead.

Leads of a **transthoracic pacemaker,** which extend from the chest incision, are inserted during open heart surgery for emergency use. If a client requires cardiac pacing, leads are connected to a temporary pacing unit.

PERMANENT PACEMAKERS. An **implanted pacemaker** is an electrical device used to manage a chronic bradydysrhythmia. Inserting a permanent pacemaker is usually for

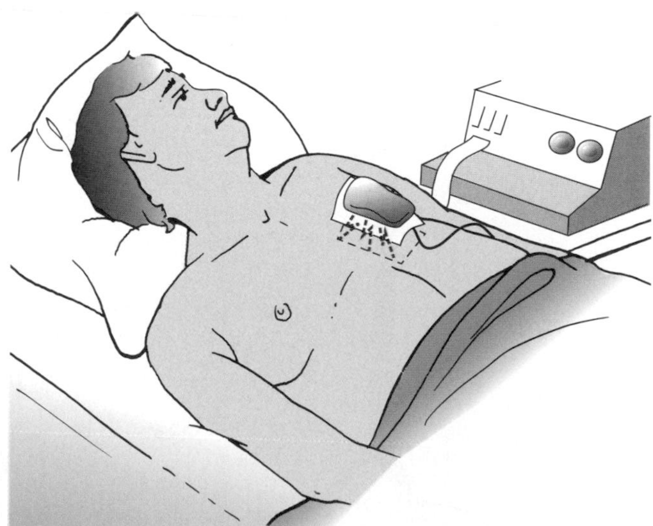

FIGURE 28.11 Transcutaneous pacemaker with electrode pads connected to the anterior and posterior chest walls.

complete or second-degree heart block accompanied by a slow ventricular rate. Permanent pacing may be used to treat certain tachydysrhythmias that do not respond to treatment or whose treatment results in bradycardia.

The lead of an implanted pacemaker is inserted transvenously, and the pacing threshold, voltage, and rate are set. One type of pacemaker has leads in both the right atrium and right ventricle (dual chamber); the lead of a single-chamber pacemaker is in either the right atrium or right ventricle. The implantable pacemaker generator, about the size of a half-dollar coin and three times as thick, is positioned under the skin below the right or left clavicle. The small incision is closed with sutures. PVCs are more frequent during the early postimplantation period, and drug therapy is used to suppress this dysrhythmia.

Mercury, lithium, or nuclear-powered (plutonium) batteries provide power for the pacemaker. The mercury battery has the shortest life (5 to 7 years); the nuclear-powered has the longest (8 to 10 years). Externally charged batteries also are used. Pacemaker batteries do not fail suddenly. The physician regularly monitors the status of their power. When the battery is nearing its end, the entire generator is replaced and leads are connected to the new generator. After the pacemaker is inserted, the client is reassessed in 3 months and every 6 months thereafter. If the client redevelops original symptoms or suddenly shows dyspnea, vertigo, syncope, unexplained fatigue, edema in upper or lower extremities, muscle twitching, or extended hiccuping in the interim, the pacemaker is checked over the telephone. Routine telephone checks are scheduled every 2 to 4 months for the first 3 years and every month after. If a problem develops, the pacemaker is reprogrammed with an external wand just like the AICD.

Radiofrequency Catheter Ablation

Radiofrequency catheter ablation is a procedure in which a heated catheter tip destroys dysrhythmia-producing tissue. A catheter is threaded transvenously into the heart, initially for electrophysiology studies (see Chap. 24). Once the location of the dysrhythmia-generating tissue is identified, electrical energy is sent to the catheter tip (Fig. 28.12). Heat destroys errant tissue, allowing impulse conduction to travel over appropriate pathways. Accompanying risks include bleeding from insertion site, perforation of catheterized vein, and vascular complications like thrombus formation. When the catheter is in the heart itself, it may pierce the myocardium, leading to pericardial tamponade. The heated tip may obliterate normal conductive tissue, requiring a permanent pacemaker to ensure heart contraction.

Nursing Management

Clients with symptomatic dysrhythmias require careful monitoring and documentation of symptoms. Clients with serious dysrhythmias are potentially unstable, making frequent rhythm analyses important. Administering and monitoring effects of antidysrhythmic drugs are key nursing responsibilities. Drugs given to restore or con-

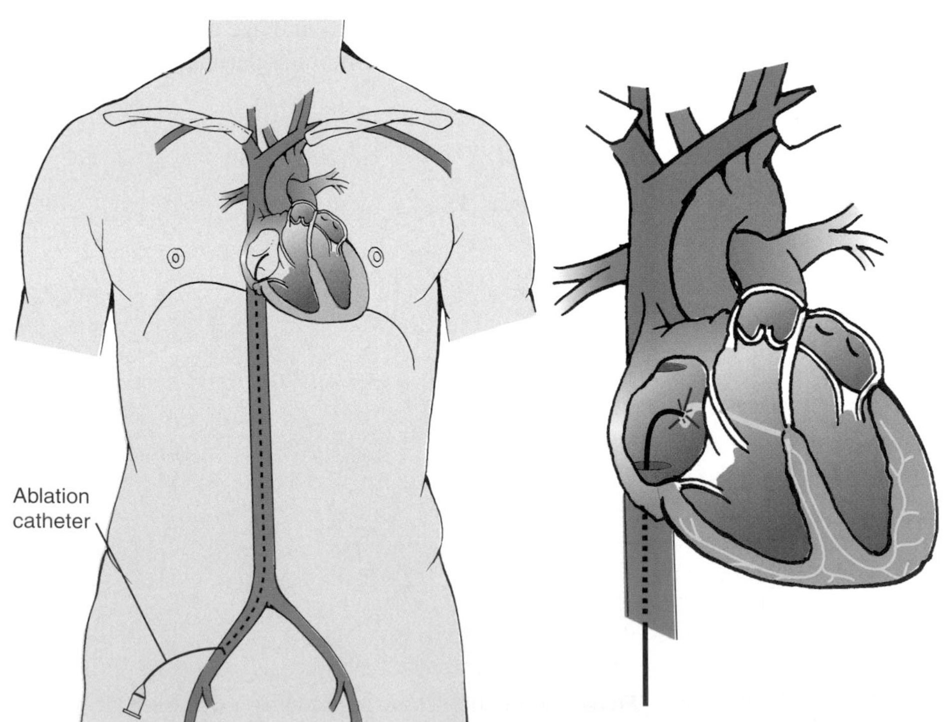

Figure 28.12 A catheter is guided to the heart, and radiofrequency ablation destroys the defective conducting tissue.

trol cardiac rhythm are powerful, and their therapeutic levels often are close to toxic levels. Many of these drugs cause unwanted side effects and are contraindicated in certain conditions. Assist with medical procedures that help restore normal sinus rhythm and manage postprocedural care. Provide health teaching to promote the client's ability to maintain safe self-management after discharge.

Elective Electrical Cardioversion

Prepare the client for electrical cardioversion similarly to preparing a client for a surgical procedure. There must be a signed consent form. Food and oral fluids are restricted. Ensure a patent IV line and check with the physician to determine if scheduled drugs should be withheld and if drugs to decrease anxiety are to be administered. The physician may order a sedative 30 to 60 minutes before the procedure. Digitalis and diuretics are withheld for 24 to 72 hours before cardioversion because these drugs in myocardial cells may decrease the ability to restore normal conduction and increase chances of a fatal dysrhythmia developing after cardioversion.

Place the cardioverter in the client's room. Check that emergency equipment such as an oral airway, oxygen, suction, and emergency drugs are on hand. Just before the procedure, assist the client with bladder or bowel elimination. Administer an IV tranquilizer, usually diazepam (Valium) or midazolam (Versed), as prescribed and insert an oral airway once the client is sedated. The desired response to elective cardioversion is a normal sinus rhythm, normal or adequate BP, and strong peripheral pulses in all extremities. After cardioversion, monitor vital signs every 15 minutes for the first 1 or 2 hours and then as ordered. Observe the cardiac monitor to evaluate heart rate and rhythm continuously and compare ECG changes with those before the procedure.

Defibrillation

Defibrillation is instituted as soon as possible after a dangerous dysrhythmia is detected. Until such time, administer CPR to maintain oxygenation and circulation of blood. Defibrillation is performed by a nurse or some other health team member who is trained in the use of the defibrillator (Nursing Guidelines 28-1).

After successful defibrillation, frequently monitor level of consciousness, ECG pattern, BP, and pulse and respiratory rates. Review laboratory results, such as arterial blood gas analyses and serum electrolyte levels. Check paddle application sites for redness and impaired skin integrity. The defibrillator is kept on standby because repeat defibrillation may be necessary. Even when cardiac activity is restored, potential remains that oxygen deprivation affected one or more organs. Monitor urine output to detect kidney failure and assess for motor weakness or paralysis, memory impairment, and level of consciousness to detect for possible effects from cerebral anoxia.

NURSING GUIDELINES 28-1

Steps in Defibrillation

When performing defibrillation, the nurse:

- Determines that there is no breathing or pulse
- Checks the ECG rhythm
- Facilitates CPR until the client is prepared for defibrillation
- Applies gel or saline pads to skin of the upper right chest near the sternum and apical area
- Charges paddles to 200 joules of energy while stating "Charging"
- Selects the nonsynchronized mode on the defibrillator (the synchronized mode is used for cardioversion)
- Places the paddles on the chest over the gel or pads with firm pressure
- Shouts "All clear" to ensure that no one is in contact with the client or bed
- Presses discharge buttons on each paddle with thumbs while stating "Shocking now"
- Evaluates postdefibrillation cardiac rhythm
- Repeats defibrillation using 200 joules one more time and 360 joules for subsequent defibrillation attempts if there is no improvement in the cardiac rhythm
- Continues CPR as IV medications are administered and between defibrillation attempts

Pacemakers

When a client has a temporary or permanent pacemaker, ensure that temporary pacemakers are attached appropriately to the external pacemaker unit, position the unit so that there is no tension on pacemaker leads, and observe rhythm strips for pacemaker's characteristic electrical artifact or "spike," identified by a thin, vertical stroke.

Instructions for a permanent implantation include the following:

- Avoid strenuous movement especially of the arm on the side where the pacemaker is inserted.
- Keep the arm on the side of the pacemaker lower than the head except for brief moments when dressing or performing hygiene.
- Delay for at least 8 weeks such activities as swimming, bowling, playing tennis, vacuum cleaning, carrying heavy objects, chopping wood, mowing or raking, and shoveling snow.
- Avoid sources of electrical interference similar to those problematic for people with AICDs.

Client and Family Teaching 28-1 highlights maintenance and care instructions for clients with permanent pacemakers.

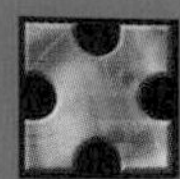

28-1 *Client and Family Teaching* Permanent Pacemakers

The nurse instructs clients with permanent pacemakers and their families as follows:

- Maintain follow-up care.
- Report if the suture line becomes inflamed or sore.
- Avoid injury to area where pacemaker is inserted.
- Follow physician's advice regarding lifting, sports, and exercise.
- Palpate pulse and count rate for a full minute daily or when feeling ill.
- Obtain and wear a Medic Alert bracelet or tag identifying that a pacemaker is implanted.
- Be cautious of situations that can cause pacemaker malfunction: gravitational force during airplane departures or landings, bumpy car rides, high-tension wires, short-wave radio transmissions, telephone transformers, and nuclear magnetic resonance imaging. Move to another location and check pulse rate if dizziness or palpitations occur.
- Request hand scanning during airport security checks; some pacemakers trigger alarms.
- Maintain at least 6 inches between a cellular phone and pacemaker generator or 12 inches if cellular phone transmits over 3 watts.
- Check with physician concerning transtelephonic pacemaker checks or when a pacemaker battery change will be necessary in the future.

NURSING PROCESS

● The Client With a Dysrhythmia

Assessment

Review the client's medical history, including allergy and drug history. In addition to performing a general cardiovascular assessment (see Chap. 24), note trends in heart rate, cardiac rhythm, BP, level of consciousness, urinary output, and physiologic changes in response to activity. If hemodynamic monitoring devices like an arterial line, central venous pressure manometer, or pulmonary artery catheter are used, analyze results of pressure readings and measurements of cardiac output. Record any symptoms the client reports, such as dizziness, fainting, or chest pain. Determine the client's knowledge level about drug therapy or other treatment measures such as elective cardioversion or use of an AICD or a pacemaker.

Diagnosis, Planning, and Interventions

Decreased Cardiac Output related to ineffective heart contraction secondary to dysrhythmia or ineffective response to treatment measures

Expected Outcome: Client will maintain adequate cardiac output as evidenced by stable vital signs; no chest pain, dizziness, or syncope; and urine output of at least 1500 mL per 24 hours.

- Maintain physical and emotional rest. *Reduces tachycardia and may relieve consequences of a tachydysrhythmia.*
- Provide supplemental oxygen for dyspnea, chest pain, or syncope. *Supplemental oxygen by inhalation diffuses at the alveolar-capillary level and increases oxygen concentration in blood, making more oxygen available for cellular metabolism.*

PC: Life-Threatening Dysrhythmia

Expected Outcome: The nurse will monitor to detect dysrhythmias and manage and minimize any that occur.

- Monitor cardiac rhythm continuously. *Cardiac monitors display real-time heart rate and rhythm and alert nurse to potentially life-threatening dysrhythmias.*
- Ensure a patent IV access. *Emergency medications are usually given by the IV route.*
- Administer antidysrhythmic drugs as prescribed. *Restore normal sinus rhythm by interfering with ectopic pacemaker sites.*
- Prepare client for elective cardioversion or use of a temporary pacemaker (see earlier discussion). *An alert client will be less anxious when given an explanation of the purpose and techniques for measures to restore normal cardiac rhythm.*
- Summon the team who will provide advanced cardiac life support measures such as defibrillation, and administer CPR. *CPR provides supportive breathing and circulates blood by heart compression to facilitate resuscitation. Advanced cardiac life support provides endotracheal intubation, positive pressure ventilation, and electrical defibrillation to enhance the potential for resuscitation (see earlier discussion for specifics on defibrillation).*

Risk for Ineffective Management of Therapeutic Regimen related to unfamiliarity with treatment measures

Expected Outcome: Client will describe ways to manage self-care before discharge.

- Explain action, side effects, dosage, route, administration, and importance of medications used to control the dysrhythmia. *Promotes safety and adherence.*
- Teach client the technique for assessing the radial pulse. *Helps the client evaluate his or her response to treatment measures.*
- Identify guidelines for withholding specific drugs and reporting symptoms to physician. *Enhances early intervention when complications develop.*
- Provide information about precautions for an AICD or pacemaker. *Electrical interference and magnetization can impair the function of these devices.*
- Stress importance of continued medical follow-up. *Ensures that the client's condition remains stable or facilitates early modifications to treatment.*

Evaluation of Expected Outcomes

Expected outcomes are restoration and maintenance of adequate cardiac output. Any life-threatening dysrhythmias are effectively treated. The client and family accurately relate the treatment plan and postdischarge care.

GENERAL GERONTOLOGIC CONSIDERATIONS

Age increases risk for dysrhythmias because of several degenerative changes. Cells in the SA node of older adults continue to decrease and accumulate fat and calcium.

In older adults, stress, exercise, or illness may cause dysrhythmias and other cardiac disorders, such as congestive heart failure and myocardial ischemia.

Sinus bradycardia and heart block are common dysrhythmias in older clients.

Critical Thinking Exercises

1. *A client for whom an antidysrhythmic drug has been prescribed returns for a follow-up examination. How would you determine if the client has followed the drug therapy regimen?*
2. *What information is essential to document when helping to resuscitate a client who has experienced a cardiac arrest?*

● NCLEX-STYLE REVIEW QUESTIONS

1. A client in the intensive care unit (ICU) is noted to have ventricular fibrillation. Which nursing action is most appropriate initially?
   1. Performing immediate defibrillation using an AED
   2. Preparing the client for pacemaker insertion
   3. Assessing the client for electrolyte imbalance
   4. Taking temperature, pulse, and blood pressure
2. After taking a sublingual nitroglycerin tablet, a client newly diagnosed with angina pectoris complains of a headache and feeling lightheaded. The nurse teaches the client that:
   1. Nitroglycerin causes vasodilation of the blood vessels resulting in hypotension.
   2. Nitroglycerin causes the client's blood pressure to rise.
   3. The client's carotid arteries are occluded resulting in stroke-like symptoms.
   4. The client's nitroglycerin dose is too high.
3. A client receives digoxin (Lanoxin) for heart failure. The nurse monitors for signs and symptoms related to digoxin toxicity, which include:
   1. Ringing in the ears, dizziness, and facial flushing
   2. Weakness, fatigue, and orthostatic hypotension
   3. Frequent seizures, headache, and oliguria
   4. Nausea, vomiting, and visual disturbances

connection

Visit the Connection site at **http://connection.lww.com/go/timbyEssentials** for links to chapter-related resources on the Internet.

References and Suggested Readings

American Heart Association. (2000). Early defibrillation. [On-line.] Available: http://216.185.112.5/presenter.jhtml?identifier=7252.

Bausbach-Aballo, S., Henry-Kamen, D., & Padre, I. (November 5, 2001). And the beat goes on . . . *Advance for Nurses,* 25–27.

Chart Smart. (2002). Keeping tabs on arrhythmias. *Nursing 2002, 32*(10), 82.

Dhala, A., Sra, J., Blanck, Z., et al. (1999). Ventricular arrhythmias, electrophysiologic studies, and devices. *Critical Care Nursing Clinics of North America, 11,* 375–382.

Docherty, B., & Roe, J. (2001). Cardiac arrhythmias: Recognition and care. *Professional Nurse, 16,* 1492–1496.

Dwyer, D. (2000). Pacing your patients. *Nursing 2000, 30*(3), 82.

Hatchett, R., Arundale, K., & Francis-Reeme, L. (1999). Systems and diseases. The heart, part four: Basic cardiac arrhythmias. *Nursing Times, 95*(43), 44–47.

Konick-McMahan, J. (December 3, 2001). Antiarrhythmic medications: News from the front lines. Advance for Nurses, 16–17.

Kraus, E., Shamp, J., & Bensing, K. (October 22, 2001). Cardiac rehabilitation: After the crisis. Advance for Nurses, 15–17.

Morris, E. R. (March 4, 2002). Keeping pace. Advance for Nurses, 23–24.

Palatnick, A., & Kates, R. (2002). Could that medication cause bradycardia? *Nursing 2002, 32*(8), 32hn1–32hn4.

Shaffer, R. S. (2002). ICD therapy: The patient's perspective. *American Journal of Nursing, 102*(2), 46–49.

Sims, J. M., & Miracle, V. A. (2001). Fast facts about supraventricular tachycardia. *Nursing 2001, 31*(6), 44–45.

Teplitz, L. (2000). Zapping tachyarrhythmias with radiofrequency catheter ablation. *Nursing 2000, 30*(2), Crit Care: 32cc1–32cc2, 32cc4, 32cc6.

Thomas, S. A., Friedmann, E., & Kelley, F. J. (2001). Living with an implantable cardioverter–defibrillator: A review of the current literature related to psychosocial factors. *AACN Clinical Issues: Advanced Practice in Acute and Critical Care, 12*(1), 156–163.

Woods, A. (2001). Calling all pacemakers. *Nursing 2001, 31*(7), 46–47.

Wooten, J. M. (2002). Drug-induced arrhythmias. *RN, 65*(1), 37–44.

Wooten, J. M., Earnest, J., & Reyes, J. (2000). Review of common adverse effects of selected antiarrhythmic drugs. *Critical Care Nursing Quarterly, 22*(4), 23–38.

chapter 29

Caring for Clients With Hypertension

Words to Know 

accelerated hypertension
diastolic blood pressure
essential hypertension
hypertension
hypertensive cardiovascular disease
hypertensive heart disease
hypertensive vascular disease
malignant hypertension
natriuretic factor
papilledema
secondary hypertension
systolic blood pressure

Learning Objectives

On completion of this chapter, the reader will:

- Identify physiologic components that create blood pressure.
- List factors that influence and structures that physiologically control arterial pressure.
- Explain systolic and diastolic arterial pressure.
- Describe hypertension and its risk factors.
- Differentiate essential and secondary hypertension.
- List consequences of chronic hypertension.
- Discuss assessment findings and treatment of hypertension.
- Discuss nursing management of clients with hypertension.
- Differentiate accelerated and malignant hypertension.
- Identify potential complications of uncontrolled malignant hypertension.
- Discuss the medical and nursing management of the client with malignant hypertension.

Blood pressure (BP) is the force produced by the volume of blood in arterial walls. It is represented by the formula:

$$BP = CO \text{ (cardiac output)} \times PR \text{ (peripheral resistance)}$$

Measured BP reflects ability of arteries to stretch and fill with blood, efficiency of the heart as a pump, and volume of circulating blood. Blood pressure is affected by age, body size, diet, activity, emotions, pain, position, gender, time of day, and disease states. Studies of healthy persons show that BP can fluctuate within a wide range and remain normal. Thus, obtaining several measurements for comparison is important.

ARTERIAL BLOOD PRESSURE

The autonomic nervous system, kidneys, and various endocrine glands regulate arterial pressure. When measured, pressure during systole and diastole is expressed as a fraction. The top number is systolic BP; the bottom number is diastolic BP. Normal BP for adults ranges from 100/60 to 139/89 mm Hg. BP tends to increase with age, most likely from arteriosclerotic and atherosclerotic changes in blood vessels or other effects of chronic diseases. Screening BP is an important method for identifying people at risk for heart failure, renal failure, and stroke. Those at highest risk are older adults, African Americans, and clients with diabetes mellitus.

Systolic Blood Pressure

Systolic blood pressure is determined by force and volume of blood that the left ventricle ejects during systole and ability of the arterial system to distend at the time of ventricular contraction. Arterial walls are normally elastic and yield to the force and volume of ventricular contraction. In older clients, systolic BP may be elevated because of loss of arterial elasticity (arteriosclerosis). Narrowing of arterioles, either from arteriosclerosis or some other mechanism causing vasoconstriction, increases peripheral resistance, which in turn increases systolic BP. This resistance can be compared to the narrowing of a tube, such as a drinking straw. The narrower the lumen is, the greater the pressure needed to move air or liquid through it.

Diastolic Blood Pressure

Diastolic blood pressure reflects arterial pressure during ventricular relaxation. It depends on resistance of arterioles and diastolic filling times. If arterioles are resistant (constricted), blood is under greater pressure.

HYPERTENSIVE DISEASE

The term **hypertension** refers to a sustained elevation of systolic arterial BP of 140 mm Hg or higher, a sustained diastolic arterial BP of 90 mm Hg or higher, or both. The Joint National Committee on Detection, Evaluation, and Treatment of High Blood Pressure (1997) identified three stages of hypertension (Table 29.1). When elevated BP causes a cardiac abnormality, the term **hypertensive heart disease** is used. When vascular damage is present without heart involvement, the term **hypertensive vascular disease** is used. When both heart disease and vascular damage accompany hypertension, the appropriate term is **hypertensive cardiovascular disease.**

ESSENTIAL AND SECONDARY HYPERTENSION

Hypertension is divided into two main categories: essential (primary) and secondary. **Essential hypertension,** about 95% of cases, is sustained elevated BP with no known cause. **Secondary hypertension** is elevated BP that results from or is secondary to some other disorder.

Pathophysiology and Etiology

The exact cause of essential hypertension is unknown. BP often increases with age; hypertension may run in families. Essential hypertension affects African Americans at a higher rate than it does other ethnic groups. Obesity, inactivity, smoking, excessive alcohol intake, and ineffective stress management are risk factors.

Research into specific factors that contribute to development of essential hypertension continues. It is well documented that hypernatremia (elevated serum sodium level) increases blood volume, which raises BP. A low serum potassium level may cause sodium retention as kidneys try to maintain a balanced number of cations (positively charged electrolytes) in body fluid. Scientists are also investigating the role of calcium in hypertension because serum calcium levels are low in some hypertensive clients.

Essential hypertension also may develop from alterations in other body chemicals. Defects in BP regulation may result from an impairment in the renin-angiotensin-aldosterone mechanism. Renin is a chemical that kidneys release to raise BP and increase vascular fluid volume. For those with a heightened stress response, hypertension may be correlated with a higher than usual release of catecholamines, such as epinephrine and norepinephrine, which elevate BP. Last, some researchers theorize that a deficiency of **natriuretic factor,** a hormone produced by the heart, causes arteries and arterioles to remain in a state of sustained vasoconstriction.

Secondary hypertension may accompany any primary condition that affects fluid volume or renal function or

TABLE 29.1 RECOMMENDATIONS FOR BLOOD PRESSURE FOLLOW-UP*

CATEGORY	SYSTOLIC (mm Hg)	DIASTOLIC (mm Hg)	RECOMMENDED FOLLOW-UP
Optimal†	<120 and	<80	Recheck in 2 years.
Normal	<130 and	<85	Recheck in 2 years.
High normal	130–139 or	85–89	Recheck in 1 year.
Hypertension			
Stage 1 (mild)	140–159 or	90–99	Confirm within 2 months.
Stage 2 (moderate)	160–179 or	100–109	Evaluate within 1 month.
Stage 3 (severe)	≥180 or	≥110	Evaluate immediately or within 1 week, depending on clinical situation.

*Classification of BP for adults 18 years of age or older, with recommended follow-up.
†Optimal blood pressure with respect to cardiovascular risk is <120/80 mm Hg; however, unusually low readings should be evaluated for clinical significance.
(From Joint National Committee on Detection, Evaluation, and Treatment of High Blood Pressure. [1997]. The Sixth Report of the Joint National Committee on Detection, Evaluation, and Treatment of High Blood Pressure. *Archives of Internal Medicine, 157,* 2413–2446.)

causes arterial vasoconstriction. Predisposing conditions include kidney disease, pheochromocytoma (a tumor of the adrenal medulla), hyperaldosteronism, atherosclerosis, use of cocaine or other cardiac stimulants (e.g., weight control drugs, caffeine), and use of oral contraceptives.

Regardless of whether a person has essential or secondary hypertension, accompanying organ damage and complications are the same. Hypertension causes the heart to work harder to pump against increased resistance. The size of the heart muscle increases. When the heart no longer can pump adequately to meet the body's metabolic needs, heart failure occurs (see Chap. 30). The extra work and greater mass increase the heart's need for oxygen. If the myocardium does not receive sufficient oxygenated blood, myocardial ischemia occurs and the client experiences angina.

In addition to its direct effects on the heart, high BP damages the arterial vascular system. It accelerates atherosclerosis. Increased resistance of arterioles to the flow of blood causes serious complications in other body organs, including the eyes, brain, heart, and kidneys. Hemorrhage of tiny arteries in the retina may cause marked visual disturbances or blindness. A cerebrovascular accident may result from hemorrhage or occlusion of a blood vessel in the brain. Myocardial infarction (MI) may result from occlusion of a branch of a coronary artery. Impaired circulation to the kidneys may result in renal failure.

Assessment Findings

Clients with hypertension may be asymptomatic. Onset of hypertension, considered "the silent killer," often is gradual. It can exist for years but be discovered only during a routine physical examination or when the client experiences a major complication. As BP becomes elevated, clients may identify symptoms such as a throbbing or pounding headache, dizziness, fatigue, insomnia, nervousness, nosebleeds, and blurred vision. Angina or dyspnea may be the first clue to hypertensive heart disease.

The most obvious finding during a physical assessment is a sustained elevation of one or both BP measurements. The pulse may feel bounding from the force of ventricular contraction. Clients may be overweight. They may have a flushed face from engorgement of superficial blood vessels. Peripheral edema may be present. An ophthalmic examination may reveal vascular changes in the eyes, retinal hemorrhages, or edema of the optic nerve, known as **papilledema.**

Diagnostic tests are performed to determine the extent of organ damage. Electrocardiography, echocardiography, and chest x-ray may reveal an enlarged left ventricle. Blood tests may show elevated blood urea nitrogen and serum creatinine levels, indicating impaired renal function, findings that excretory urography (intravenous [IV] pyelography) may further validate. Fluorescein angiography, an ophthalmologic test using IV dye, often reveals leaking retinal blood vessels.

If the cause of hypertension is a renal vascular problem, renal arteriography demonstrates narrowing of the renal artery. If the cause is related to dysfunction of the adrenal gland, a 24-hour collected urine specimen detects elevated catecholamines. Blood studies reveal elevated cholesterol and triglyceride levels, indicating that atherosclerosis is an underlying factor.

Medical Management

The primary objective of therapy for either type of hypertension is to lower BP and prevent major complications. Recommended follow-up is based on BP measurements (see Table 29.1). Initial management depends on the stage of hypertension; however, nonpharmacologic interventions usually are used first. For mild elevations, weight reduction, decreased sodium intake (Box 29-1), moderate exercise, and reduced contributing factors (e.g., smoking, alcohol use) may return the BP to normal levels. A diet low in saturated fats is recommended if cholesterol and triglyceride levels are high.

Depending on the client's response to nonpharmacologic therapy, one of several drugs may be prescribed (Drug Therapy Table 29.1). If BP remains elevated, the dosage may be increased or a second, third, or fourth antihypertensive agent may be added. Secondary hypertension often resolves by treating its cause.

BOX 29-1 ● Recommendations for Limiting Sodium

- Consume no more than 2.4 g (2400 mg) of sodium per day in the form of salt (sodium chloride) or other compounds such as monosodium glutamate (MSG) or sodium bicarbonate. One teaspoon of table salt contains 2300 mg of sodium.
- Read food labels to determine the sodium content per serving.
- Prepare fresh rather than canned products, or buy those that are labeled as "unsalted, no salt, sodium-free, low sodium, or reduced sodium."
- Prepare food from "scratch" without adding salt, as opposed to purchasing premade entrées, which usually are highly salted.
- Drain and rinse canned foods.
- Avoid or limit consumption of frankfurters, ham, bacon, and processed meat products, which often contain sodium nitrate as a preservative.
- Substitute healthy snacks like fresh or dried fruit for those that are salted.
- Experiment with seasonings like lemon, garlic, and onion powder as alternatives to salt.
- Eliminate or restrict items that contain significant sodium like pickles, green olives, sauerkraut, mustard, catsup, barbecue sauce, pizza sauce, canned soup, and packaged mixes.

(Adapted from U.S. Department of Agriculture and U.S. Department of Health and Human Services. [1995]. Dietary guidelines for Americans. [On-line.] Available: http://www.nalusda.gov/fnic/dga95/cover.html.)

DRUG THERAPY TABLE 29.1 ANTIHYPERTENSIVE AGENTS

DRUG CATEGORY AND EXAMPLES	MECHANISM OF ACTION	SIDE EFFECTS	NURSING CONSIDERATIONS
Alpha-Adrenergic Blockers			
prazosin (Minipress)	Relax vascular smooth muscle by blocking $alpha_1$ receptor sites for epinephrine and norepinephrine	Hypotension, dizziness, drowsiness, nausea, palpitations	Administer first dose just before bedtime to reduce potential for syncope. Monitor client for postural hypotension. Caution client to change positions slowly.
Beta-Adrenergic Blockers			
propranolol (Inderal)	Blocks $beta_1$ and $beta_2$ adrenergic receptors Decrease renin levels	Hypotension, bradycardia, bronchospasm, CHF, depression, erectile dysfunction, hypoglycemia	Administer with meals. Advise client not to discontinue medication abruptly. Monitor for fluid retention, rash, and difficulty breathing. Monitor blood glucose level in clients with diabetes. These drugs are contraindicated in clients with chronic respiratory disorders.
Alpha-Beta Blockers			
labetalol (Normodyne)	Block $alpha_1$-, $beta_1$-, and $beta_2$-adrenergic receptors	Dizziness, GI symptoms, dyspnea, cough, erectile dysfunction, decreased libido	Administer with meals. Caution client to avoid discontinuing drug therapy abruptly and to inform anesthesiologist of use before surgery to avoid drug–drug interaction.
Diuretics			
furosemide (Lasix)	Promote sodium and water excretion, thus reducing circulating blood volume	Dizziness, dehydration, blurred vision, anorexia, diarrhea, nocturia, polyuria, thrombocytopenia, orthostatic hypotension, hypokalemia	Weigh client daily. Measure intake and output. Monitor serum potassium level. Advise client to replace lost potassium with bananas, orange juice, or prescribed supplement.
ACE Inhibitors			
captopril (Capoten)	Block ACE from converting angiotensin I to angiotensin II (a potent vasoconstrictor) Promote fluid and sodium loss and decrease peripheral vascular resistance	Tachycardia, hypotension, GI irritation, pancytopenia, proteinuria, rash, cough, dry mouth, hyperkalemia	Excretion is reduced in clients with renal failure. First-dose hypotension is common in older adults. Administer 1 hour before or 2 hours after meals. Monitor serum potassium blood urea nitrogen and creatinine.
Angiotensin II Receptor Antagonists			
losartan (Cozaar)	Block effects of angiotensin II Relax vascular smooth muscle Increase salt and water excretion Reduce plasma volume	Orthostatic hypotension; GI disturbances; hyperkalemia; respiratory congestion; swelling of face, lips, eyelids, tongue in hypersensitive persons	Assess BP for postural changes. Monitor serum potassium levels. Observe for allergic reactions when drug therapy begins.
Calcium Channel Blockers			
nifedipine (Procardia XL)	Decrease BP by dilating coronary and peripheral arteries	Hypotension, dizziness, CHF, edema, atrioventricular block, nausea	Check BP and heart rate before each dose. Withhold drug in cases of hypotension. Observe for signs and symptoms of CHF and fluid overload.

ACE, angiotensin-converting enzyme; *BP,* blood pressure; *CHF,* congestive heart failure; *GI,* gastrointestinal.

NURSING PROCESS

• The Client With Hypertension

Assessment

Initially take BP in both arms with client in a standing, sitting, and then supine position, using an appropriately sized cuff (Table 29.2). Thereafter, use the same arm and place client in the same position each time you take a reading. Ask questions to determine if client is following the treatment regimen. Perform additional cardiac assessments (see Chap. 24) depending on the client's medical history and current symptoms. Teach about nonpharmacologic and pharmacologic methods for restoring and maintaining BP below hypertensive levels, as well as techniques for self-management (Client and Family Teaching 29-1). Collaborate with a dietitian to provide information on dietary modifications such as Dietary Approaches to Stop Hypertension (DASH diet).

Diagnosis, Planning, and Interventions

Risk for Decreased Cardiac Output related to excessive or prolonged systemic vascular resistance

Expected Outcome: Client will maintain an adequate cardiac output as evidenced by reduced BP to normal or near-normal levels, heart rate between 60 and 100 beats/minute, effortless breathing, clear lung sounds, alert mental status, and urine output that approximates or slightly exceeds intake.

- Promote physical rest. *Decreases BP and reduces resistance the heart must overcome to eject blood.*
- Relieve emotional stress. *Reduced stress decreases production of neurotransmitters that constrict peripheral arterioles.*
- Instruct client to avoid bearing down against a closed glottis (Valsalva maneuver). *Straining or bearing down against a closed glottis momentarily increases BP.*
- Encourage compliance with salt/sodium restrictions. *Decreases blood volume and improves potential for greater cardiac output.*
- Recommend smoking cessation. *Nicotine raises heart rate, constricts arterioles, and reduces heart's ability to eject blood.*
- Enforce prescribed fluid restrictions. *Ultimately decreases circulating blood volume and systemic vascular resistance.*
- Help client reduce or eliminate caffeine. *Caffeine increases heart rate and causes vasoconstriction.*
- Administer prescribed antihypertensives. *They use various mechanisms to control BP, including increasing urine elimination, blocking production of angiotensin, and dilating blood vessels.*

Risk for Injury related to syncope and dizziness secondary to antihypertensive drugs

Expected Outcome: The client will be injury free.

- Monitor postural changes in BP by assessing client while he or she is lying, sitting, and standing. *BP usually falls when assuming an upright position. Assessment validates whether drop in BP is significant.*
- Encourage client to rise slowly from a sitting or lying position. *Gradual changes in position provide time for the heart to increase its rate of contraction to resupply oxygen to the brain.*
- Help client to sit or lie down if he or she is dizzy. *Support of a chair or bed reduces potential for falling.*

Evaluation of Expected Outcomes

Expected outcomes are that adequate cardiac output is maintained or improved when systolic and diastolic BP are reduced. The client does not experience syncope or fall from postural changes in BP.

Stop, Think, and Respond • BOX 29-1

A neighbor asks you to take her BP. The measurement is 160/90 mm Hg. What questions will you ask? What recommendations will you make for follow-up?

TABLE 29.2 RECOMMENDED BLADDER DIMENSIONS FOR BLOOD PRESSURE CUFFS

ARM CIRCUMFERENCE AT MIDPOINT* (cm)	CUFF NAME	BLADDER WIDTH (cm)	BLADDER LENGTH (cm)
27–34	Adult	13	30
35–44	Wide adult	16	38
45–52	Thigh	20	42

*Midpoint of arm is defined as half the distance from the acromion to the olecranon processes. (American Heart Association. [1993]. Human blood pressure determined by sphygmomanometry. [On-line]. Available: http://www.216.185.112.5/presenter.jhtml?identifier=3000894.)

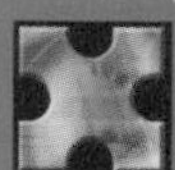

29-1 *Client and Family Teaching* Hypertension

The nurse instructs as follows:

- Adhere to treatment regimen even if you have few, if any, symptoms and feel well. Hypertension is a chronic condition requiring lifelong management and treatment.
- Learn to regularly monitor BP using a home sphygmomanometer or arrange for monitoring by a community agency that provides this service at no or low cost.
- Keep a log of BP measurements for follow-up visits.
- Comply with treatment regimen involving diet, exercise, and drug therapy.
- Consult cookbooks published or endorsed by the American Heart Association, American Diabetes Association, or other reliable sources for "heart smart" recipes.
- Follow directions for medications; never increase, decrease, or omit a prescribed drug unless first conferring with the primary care provider.
- Report adverse effects from medications to the prescribing provider. Get medical approval before taking nonprescription drugs. Inform all physicians and dentists of medications that you are taking.
- Avoid tobacco and beverages containing caffeine or alcohol, unless permitted by the provider.

● ACCELERATED AND MALIGNANT HYPERTENSION

Accelerated and malignant hypertension are more serious forms of elevated BP. **Accelerated hypertension** describes markedly elevated BP, accompanied by hemorrhages and exudates in the eyes. If untreated, accelerated hypertension may progress to **malignant hypertension,** dangerously elevated BP accompanied by papilledema.

Pathophysiology and Etiology

Accelerated and malignant hypertension occur in clients with undiagnosed hypertension or in those who fail to maintain follow-up or comply with medical therapy. They usually have an abrupt onset; if untreated, severe symptoms and complications follow rapidly. Malignant hypertension is fatal unless BP is quickly reduced. Even with intensive treatment, the kidneys, brain, and heart may be permanently damaged.

Consequences are life-threatening when BP in the vascular system becomes extremely elevated. Some arterial blood vessels already may have ruptured or will soon. Retinal hemorrhages can lead to blindness. A stroke occurs if vessels in the brain rupture and bleed. If an aneurysm has developed in the aorta from chronic hypertension, it may burst and cause hemorrhage and shock. Cardiac effects include left ventricular failure with pulmonary edema or MI. Renal failure also may be forthcoming if pressure is not reduced.

Assessment Findings

Some clients may present with confusion, headache, visual disturbances, seizures, and, possibly, coma. Sudden, marked rise in BP may cause chest pain, dyspnea, and moist lung sounds. Renal failure is evidenced by less than 30 mL/hour of urine. Onset of sudden, severe back pain accompanied by hypotension (abnormally low BP) indicates that an aortic aneurysm is dissecting or has ruptured (see Chap. 27).

Systolic BP is 160 mm Hg or higher, diastolic BP is 115 mm Hg or higher, or both. The optic disk (nerve) appears to bulge forward into the posterior chamber from swelling of the brain. The retinal blood vessels are obscured where they radiate from the bulging disk, making identification of their continuous pathway difficult. The retinas may show flame-shaped hemorrhages or fluffy white exudates.

Diagnostic studies that may reveal abnormalities include computed tomographic scan, positron emission tomography scan, and magnetic resonance imaging. Reducing BP is a priority, and neurologic tests may be postponed until emergency treatment is instituted.

Medical Management

In true hypertensive emergencies, the goal is to lower BP within 1 to 2 hours by using potent IV drugs, such as diazoxide (Hyperstat IV), nitroprusside (Nitropress), nitroglycerin, or labetalol (Normodyne). If the client's condition is not extremely critical, alternative antihypertensive drugs, such as nifedipine (Procardia), verapamil (Isoptin), captopril (Capoten), and prazosin (Minipress), are prescribed for oral administration. Oxygen is ordered to reduce hypoxia-induced tachycardia.

Nursing Management

Implement medical orders promptly to lower BP as quickly and safely as possible. Apply an automatic BP recording machine to the arm to measure BP every few minutes, or assess BP directly if using an arterial catheter. Report a systolic BP of 160 mm Hg or higher or a diastolic BP of 115 mm Hg or higher immediately. While awaiting medical orders, restrict client activity and monitor the client closely for neurologic, cardiac, and renal complications. Keep emergency equipment and drugs ready in case complications develop. See Nursing Process: The Client With Hypertension for additional nursing management.

GENERAL GERONTOLOGIC CONSIDERATIONS

Hypertension caused by arteriosclerosis or atherosclerosis is not uncommon in older adults. It may go undiagnosed unless the client sees a physician regularly. Encourage older adults to have their BP checked at least every 6 months. Older adult centers and pharmacies frequently offer free BP monitoring.

Because postural hypotension is common in older adults, correct BP measurement is particularly important. Measurements are obtained while the older person is supine or sitting, and immediately after he or she stands.

Older adults are at increased risk for development of hypokalemia from diuretic drugs. Lower doses of hydrochlorothiazide or chlorthalidone can control hypertension and minimize the risk of hypokalemia.

Critical Thinking Exercises

1. *On admission, a client's BP is 210/112 mm Hg in a supine position. What additional data would be pertinent to collect before reporting the finding to the nurse in charge and physician?*
2. *To which community resources in your locale would you refer a client with hypertension for support or care after discharge?*

• NCLEX-STYLE REVIEW QUESTIONS 

1. At a community center, the nurse instructs middle-aged men and women about the signs and symptoms of hypertension. Of the following people who are present at the discussion, whose blood pressure is most important for the nurse to assess?
    1. A 75-year-old African-American man
    2. A 50-year-old executive who lifts weights
    3. A 35-year-old woman who weighs 120 pounds
    4. A 60-year-old man who is being treated for a dysrhythmia
2. A client diagnosed with hypertension comes to the clinic for a routine visit and reports to the nurse that he stopped taking his medication because it made him tired and restless. Which of the following is the best response from the nurse?
    1. "Continue taking your medication, because it was a physician's order and must be followed without question."
    2. "Continue taking your medication, because hypertension can increase the size of the heart and result in congestive heart failure."
    3. "Continue taking your medication, because hypertensive medications decrease sodium in the blood."
    4. "Continue taking your medication, because hypertension can lead to retinal detachment and blindness."
3. A client diagnosed with hypertension begins drug therapy using an antihypertensive agent. The nurse instructs the client's spouse to remove any objects in the home that can lead to falls. The nurse knows that teaching has been successful when the client restates which of the following?
    1. "Antihypertensive drugs can lead to hypotension, resulting in falls."
    2. "Blurred vision is a common side effect of antihypertensive therapy."
    3. "Fatigue and weakness are manifestations of antihypertensive medications."
    4. "A sudden drop in blood pressure can lead to confusion and subsequent falls."

connection

Visit the Connection site at **http://connection.lww.com/go/timbyEssentials** for links to chapter-related resources on the Internet.

References and Suggested Readings

Avvampato, C. S. (2001). Effect of one leg crossed over the other at the knee on blood pressure in hypertensive patients. *Nephrology Nursing Journal, 28,* 325–328.

Baldwin, C. M., Bevan, C., & Beshalske, A. (2000). At-risk minority populations in a church-based clinic: Communicating basic needs. *Journal of Multicultural Nursing and Health, 6*(2), 26–28.

Barker, E. (2001). What's your patient's stroke risk? *Nursing 2001, 31*(4), Hospital Nursing: 32hn1, 32hn4–32hn5.

Bruni, K. R. (2001). Renovascular hypertension. *Journal of Cardiovascular Nursing, 15*(4), 78–90.

Clark, M. J., Curran, C., & Noji, A. (2000). The effects of community health nurse monitoring on hypertension identification and control. *Public Health Nursing, 17,* 452–459.

Collins, N. (2002). Take the guesswork out of sodium restrictions. *Nursing 2002, 32*(8), 32hn7–32hn8.

Feather, C. (2001). Blood pressure measurement. *Nursing Times, 97*(4), 33–34.

Fleury, J., & Keller, C. (2000). Cardiovascular risk assessment in elderly individuals. *Journal of Gerontological Nursing, 26*(5), 30–37.

Frazier, L. (2000). Factors influencing blood pressure: Development of a risk model. *Journal of Cardiovascular Nursing, 15*(1), 62–79.

Graham-Garcia, J., Raines, T. L., Andrews, J. O., et al. (2001). Race, ethnicity, and geography: disparities in heart disease in women of color. *Journal of Transcultural Nursing, 12*(1), 56–67.

Halm, M. A., & Penque, S. (2000). Heart failure in women. *Progress in Cardiovascular Nursing, 15*(4), 121–133.

Karch, A. M., & Karch, F. E. (2000). Practice errors: When a blood pressure isn't routine. *American Journal of Nursing, 100*(3), 23.

Kozuh, J. L. (2000). NSAIDs and antihypertensives: An unhappy union. *American Journal of Nursing, 100*(6), 40–43.

Lahdenper, T. S., & Kyngs, H. A. (2000). Compliance and its evaluation in patients with hypertension. *Journal of Clinical Nursing, 9,* 826–833.

Mansfield, J., & Daley, K. (2000). Hypertensive emergencies. *American Journal of Nursing, 100*(9, Suppl.), 20–26.

Marcolongo, E. (2003). Isolated systolic hypertension—not your usual silent killer. *Nursing 2003, 33*(1), 32hn1–32hn3.

Mulrow, C. D., Chiquette, E., Angel, L., et al. (2001). Dieting to reduce body weight for controlling hypertension in adults. *Nursing Times, 97*(20), 42.

Munson, B. L. (2002). . . . About beta-blockers and hypertension. *Nursing 2002, 32*(10), 84.

Palatnik, A. (2002). Could that medication cause bradycardia? *Nursing 2002, 32*(8), 32hn1–32hn4.

Robinson, A. W., & Sloan, H. L. (2000). Healthy people 2000: Heart health and older women. *Journal of Gerontological Nursing, 26*(5), 38–45.

Woods, A. D. (2001). Improving the odds against hypertension. *Nursing 2001, 31*(8), 36–42.

chapter 30

Caring for Clients With Heart Failure

Words to Know 

acute heart failure
afterload
aldosterone
cardiac resynchronization therapy
cardiomyoplasty
chronic heart failure
congestive heart failure
cor pulmonale
digitalization
exertional dyspnea
heart failure
hemoptysis
intra-aortic balloon pump
left-sided heart failure
myocardial oxygen demand
orthopnea
paroxysmal nocturnal dyspnea
pitting edema
preload
pulmonary edema
pulmonary hypertension
pulmonary vascular bed
right-sided heart failure
ventricular assist device

Learning Objectives

On completion of this chapter, the reader will:

- Discuss the pathophysiology and etiology of heart failure.
- Distinguish between acute and chronic heart failure.
- Identify differences between left-sided and right-sided heart failure.
- Describe symptoms, diagnosis, and treatment of left-sided and right-sided heart failure.
- Discuss nursing management of clients with heart failure.
- Explain the pathophysiology, etiology, symptoms, diagnosis, and treatment of pulmonary edema.
- Discuss nursing management of clients with pulmonary edema.

The heart is a double pump: the right side pumps deoxygenated blood to the lungs for oxygenation, and the left side pumps oxygen-rich blood into the systemic circulation (see Chap. 24). This process provides a continuous supply of oxygen and nutrients for cellular metabolism and a mechanism to eliminate carbon dioxide (CO_2) and metabolic wastes. Disturbances in one part of the heart, if they are severe or last long enough, eventually affect the entire circulation.

HEART FAILURE

Heart failure is the inability of the heart to pump sufficient blood to meet the body's metabolic needs. **Congestive heart failure** (CHF) describes the accumulation of blood and fluid in organs and tissues from impaired circulation.

Types

Heart failure is classified as acute or chronic, and as right-sided or left-sided. Many cardiologists classify heart failure based on the amount of activity restriction it imposes (Table 30.1).

Acute and Chronic Heart Failure

Acute heart failure, a sudden change in the heart's ability to contract, can cause life-threatening symptoms and pulmonary edema (discussed later). **Chronic heart failure** occurs when another chronic disorder gradually compromises the heart's ability to pump effectively.

Left-Sided and Right-Sided Heart Failure

The heart is a double pump and either the left or right ventricle (or both) can become impaired. **Left-sided heart failure** results from various conditions that impair the left ventricle's ability to eject blood into the aorta. **Right-sided heart failure** occurs when the right ventricle fails to eject its total diastolic filling volume into the pulmonary artery, causing congestion of blood in the venous vascular system. The major cause of right-sided heart failure is left-sided heart failure.

TABLE 30.1 NEW YORK HEART ASSOCIATION FUNCTIONAL CLASSIFICATION OF HEART FAILURE

CLASS	LIMITATIONS
I	No symptoms and no limitation in ordinary physical activity
II	Mild symptoms and slight limitation during ordinary activity; comfortable at rest
III	Marked limitation in activity from symptoms, even during less-than-ordinary activity; comfortable only at rest
IV	Severe limitations; symptoms even while at rest

Pathophysiology and Etiology

The primary reason for failure of either the left or right ventricle is inability of the heart muscle to contract because of direct damage to the muscular wall. Myocardial infarction (MI) usually affects the pumping ability of the left or right ventricle and contributes to acute heart failure, which may immediately follow an MI or develop some time after the initial episode. A second reason for failure occurs when the pumping chambers enlarge and weaken, as in cardiomyopathy. It is impossible for the ventricles to eject all the blood they receive.

When the left ventricle fails, heart muscle cannot contract forcefully enough to expel blood into the systemic circulation (cardiac output). Blood becomes congested in the left ventricle, left atrium, and finally the pulmonary vasculature. Fluid accumulates and creates congestion in the **pulmonary vascular bed** (the capillary network surrounding the alveoli). Increased pressure causes fluid to move from the pulmonary capillaries into the alveoli. Gas exchange is impaired, cells become hypoxic (a state of insufficient oxygen), and CO_2 accumulates in the blood.

Hypertension, tachydysrhythmias, valvular disease, cardiomyopathy, and renal failure contribute to chronic heart failure. These conditions reduce cardiac output by:

1. Increasing afterload or systemic vascular resistance. **Afterload** is the force the ventricle must overcome to empty its diastolic volume.
2. Reducing ventricular ejection volume because diastole, when the ventricle fills with blood (**preload**), is shortened
3. Causing a loss of elasticity in the muscle

When right ventricular failure develops, the right ventricle cannot forcefully contract and push blood into the pulmonary artery. Congestion of blood and backflow accumulate in the right ventricle, the right atrium, the superior and inferior vena cava, and finally the venous vasculature. MIs that affect the right ventricle can cause right ventricular failure. Clients with chronic respiratory disorders tend to develop right-sided failure as a consequence of **cor pulmonale,** a condition in which the heart (*cor*) is affected by lung damage (*pulmonale*). Pulmonary disease impairs oxygen and CO_2 exchange in the alveoli, leading to increased CO_2 in the blood. Pulmonary arterial vasoconstriction then occurs. Prolonged pulmonary arterial vasoconstriction results in **pulmonary hypertension** (elevated pressure in the pulmonary arterial system), forcing the right ventricle to pump against a high-pressure gradient. The right ventricle enlarges and weakens under increased workload, leading to failure. When the right ventricle fails to empty completely, blood is trapped in the venous vascular system. Eventually, fluid is forced to move in retrograde fashion into interstitial spaces and cells of other organs and tissues.

The body can compensate for changes in heart function (Fig. 30.1). When cardiac output falls, compensatory mechanisms increase stroke volume and maintain blood pressure (BP) and temporarily improve cardiac output. Ultimately they fail when contractility is further compromised.

As cardiac output falls, the client becomes hypotensive, stimulating the sympathetic nervous system to release catecholamines (e.g., epinephrine, norepinephrine) to raise heart rate and BP. Increased force and contraction of the heart maintain the client's BP but increase **myocardial oxygen demand** (the amount of oxygen the heart needs to perform its work). Epinephrine also causes blood vessels to constrict in an effort to raise BP. As the sympathetic nervous system is stimulated, more blood is shunted to the brain and heart, decreasing blood supply to kidneys. The kidneys secrete renin in response to decreased blood flow, initiating the renin-angiotensin-aldosterone mechanism. Renin activates angiotensin, which causes vasoconstriction and increases BP. Angiotensin also stimulates the adrenal gland to secrete **aldosterone,** a hormone causing retention of sodium and water, which raises BP by increasing the amount of blood returning to the heart.

Ultimately, compensatory mechanisms further compromise the client's status by increasing the blood volume the heart must pump and the resistance it must overcome from arterial constriction. If cardiac output continues to fall, the body's cells are deprived of oxygen and switch from aerobic metabolism to less efficient

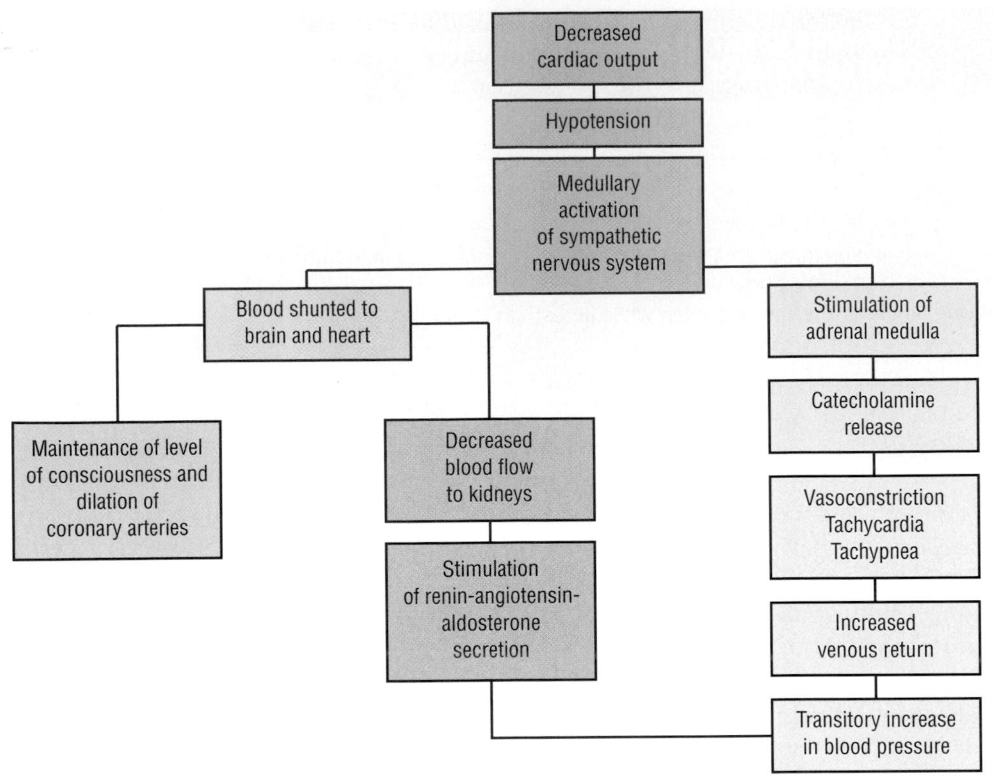

FIGURE 30.1 Compensatory mechanisms of the sympathetic nervous system. Decreased cardiac output triggers a series of compensatory mechanisms in the body in an effort to maintain level of consciousness and blood pressure.

anaerobic metabolism. This results in an accumulation of lactic acid, which lowers blood pH and eventually causes metabolic acidosis.

Assessment Findings

Signs and Symptoms

Severity of symptoms depends on the body's ability to adjust to decreased cardiac output. Initial signs and symptoms reflect the ventricle of the heart experiencing dysfunction. When a client has chronic heart failure, he or she develops signs and symptoms of both right-sided and left-sided heart failure. Table 30.2 highlights clinical differences between left and right ventricular heart failure.

In left-sided heart failure, hypoxemia occurs as a result of reduced cardiac output of arterial blood and respiratory symptoms. Clients notice unusual fatigue with activity. **Exertional dyspnea** (effort at breathing when active) may be the first symptom. Inability to breathe unless sitting upright (**orthopnea**) or being awakened by breathlessness (**paroxysmal nocturnal dyspnea**) may prompt clients to use several pillows in bed or sleep in a chair or recliner. Pulse may be rapid or irregular and BP elevated from sympathetic nervous system stimulation. A cough, **hemoptysis** (blood-streaked sputum), and moist crackles on auscultation are typical respiratory findings. Urine output is decreased. If acute left-sided heart failure with pulmonary edema develops, the client suddenly becomes hypoxic, restless, and confused.

Clients with right-sided heart failure may have a history of gradual unexplained weight gain from fluid retention. Dependent **pitting edema** (Fig. 30.2) in feet and ankles can be observed. The edema seems to disappear overnight but actually is redistributed by gravity to other tissues. Fluid may distend the abdomen (ascites), and the liver may be enlarged (hepatomegaly). Jugular veins often are distended from increased central venous pressure. Enlarged abdominal organs can restrict ventilation, creating dyspnea. Clients observe that rings, shoes, or clothing

TABLE 30.2 SIGNS AND SYMPTOMS OF LEFT AND RIGHT VENTRICULAR FAILURE

LEFT VENTRICULAR FAILURE	RIGHT VENTRICULAR FAILURE
Fatigue	Weakness
Paroxysmal nocturnal dyspnea	Ascites
Orthopnea	Weight gain
Hypoxia	Nausea, vomiting
Crackles	Dysrhythmias
Cyanosis	Elevated central venous pressure
S_3 heart sound	Jugular vein distention
Cough with pink, frothy sputum	
Elevated pulmonary capillary wedge pressure	

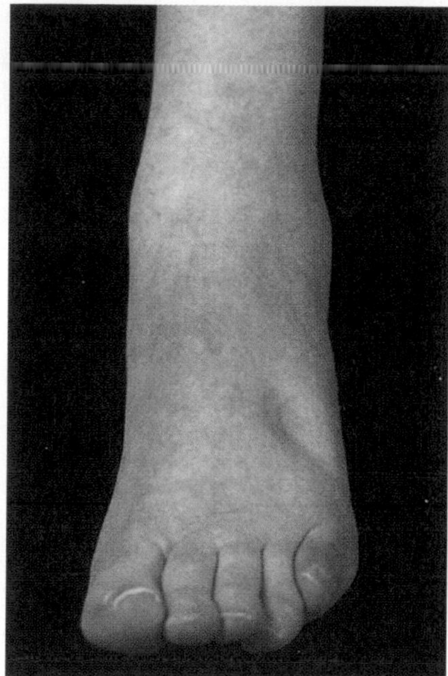

FIGURE 30.2 Example of pitting edema.

have become tight. Accumulation of blood in abdominal organs may cause anorexia, nausea, and flatulence.

> **Stop, Think, and Respond ● BOX 30-1**
>
> *Which type of heart failure is evidenced by the following assessment findings? Client A has swollen ankles. His clothes fit poorly, and he has purchased larger pants and shirts. When he is weighed, he remarks that he has gained 10 pounds in the last month, but his diet has not changed. He says he feels "full," can't eat as much as usual, and "works hard" to breathe. Client B becomes breathless while changing into a gown before the assessment. She reports sleeping better when sitting up in a recliner. Her cough is "wet." She is tachycardic and says she has noticed less frequent urination.*

Diagnostic Findings

In left-sided heart failure, chest x-ray shows cardiac enlargement and fluid accumulation in the lungs. An echocardiogram reveals an increased left ventricle and ineffective pumping of the heart. At first, arterial blood gas (ABG) analysis may reveal respiratory alkalosis as a result of rapid, shallow breathing. Later, there is a shift to metabolic acidosis as gas exchange becomes more impaired. Serum sodium levels may be elevated. Elevated blood urea nitrogen indicates impaired renal perfusion. Sicker clients will have a pulmonary artery catheter inserted which shows decreased cardiac output and elevated pulmonary artery pressure.

For right-sided failure, a chest x-ray, electrocardiogram (ECG), and echocardiogram reveal right ventricular enlargement. A lung scan and pulmonary arteriography confirm cor pulmonale. Liver enzymes are elevated if the liver is impaired.

Medical Management

Goals of medical management of heart failure are to reduce workload of the heart and improve cardiac output, primarily through dietary modifications, drug therapy, and lifestyle changes. A low-sodium diet is prescribed, and fluids may be restricted. Activity is limited according to the condition's severity. Sedatives or tranquilizers reduce dyspnea and relieve anxiety. In acute or worsening heart failure, a device for resynchronizing the heart's contraction or an intra-aortic balloon pump may be used to support left ventricular function.

Drug Therapy

Drug therapy with one or more medications aims at improving cardiac output (Drug Therapy Table 30.1). Digoxin is the primary drug used to slow and strengthen the heart. Giving large doses of digoxin at the beginning of therapy to build up therapeutic blood levels is termed **digitalization.** In acute heart failure or pulmonary edema (discussed later), physicians may prescribe a potent inotropic agent, one that increases the force of contraction and improves stroke volume. Diuretic therapy reduces the heart's workload. Loop diuretics like furosemide (Lasix) or thiazide diuretics like chlorothiazide (Diuril) increase sodium and therefore water excretion, but also increase potassium excretion. Digitalis toxicity is more likely in clients with hypokalemia (low serum potassium). Vasodilators also reduce afterload. Clients with a history of heart failure may receive a drug like an angiotensin-converting enzyme (ACE) inhibitor (captopril [Capoten]) or another category of drug causing vasodilatation.

> **Stop, Think, and Respond ● BOX 30-2**
>
> *A client with a possible bowel obstruction has a history of chronic heart failure. He has been taking digoxin (Lanoxin) at home. What nursing actions are appropriate?*

Other Medical Options

Cardiac resynchronization therapy (CRT) restores synchrony in the contractions of the right and left ventricles. CRT is used primarily for clients whose heart failure is caused by dilated cardiomyopathy. It is achieved with a biventricular pacemaker, which is inserted transvenously similarly to a traditional pacemaker, with electrical leads in the right atrium and right ventricle and the battery placed beneath the skin of the chest. It has an

DRUG THERAPY TABLE 30.1 HEART FAILURE AGENTS

DRUG CATEGORY AND EXAMPLES	MECHANISM OF ACTION	SIDE EFFECTS	NURSING CONSIDERATIONS
Cardiac Glycosides *digoxin (Lanoxin)*	Increase cardiac output by slowing heart rate (negative chronotropic action) and increasing force of contraction (positive chronotropic action)	Fatigue, generalized muscle weakness, anorexia, nausea, vomiting, yellow-green halos around visual images, dysrhythmias	Monitor pulse rate before each dose. Withhold if pulse is <60 or >120 beats/min. Provide dietary sources of potassium.
Diuretics *furosemide (Lasix)*	Promote sodium and water excretion, thus reducing circulating blood volume and decreasing heart's workload	Dizziness, dehydration, blurred vision, anorexia, diarrhea, nocturia, polyuria, thrombocytopenia, orthostatic hypotension, hypokalemia	Weigh client daily. Measure intake and output. Monitor serum potassium levels. Replace lost potassium with bananas, orange juice, or prescribed supplement.
Vasodilators *nitroglycerin*	Improve stroke volume by reducing afterload; reduce preload by dilating veins and arteries	Headache, dizziness, orthostatic hypotension, tachycardia, flushing, nausea, hypersensitivity	Assess for hypotension. Monitor for headache and flushed skin.
ACE Inhibitors *captopril (Capoten)*	Block ACE from converting angiotensin I to angiotensin II (a potent vasoconstrictor); promote fluid and sodium loss and decrease peripheral vascular resistance	Tachycardia, hypotension, GI irritation, pancytopenia, proteinuria, rash, cough, dry mouth, hyperkalemia, increased BUN and creatinine	Excretion is reduced in clients with renal failure. First-dose hypotension is common in older adults. Administer 1 hr before or 2 hr after meals.
Nonglycoside Inotropic Agents *dobutamine (Dobutrex)*	Relieve cardiogenic shock by strengthening force of myocardial contraction and increasing cardiac output	Headache, hypertension, tachycardia, angina, nausea	Monitor for increased heart rate, elevated BP, and dysrhythmias.

ACE, angiotensin-converting enzyme; *BP*, blood pressure; *BUN*, blood urea nitrogen; *GI*, gastrointestinal.

additional internal third lead that is placed outside the left ventricle. The dual ventricular leads stimulate the right and left ventricles to contract at the same time. When ventricles contract simultaneously, the force of contraction improves and more blood is ejected with each heartbeat.

If cardiogenic shock accompanies acute left ventricular heart failure, an **intra-aortic balloon pump** (IABP) may be used. This acts as a temporary, secondary pump to supplement ineffectual contraction of the left ventricle. It is inserted as a catheter into the left femoral artery and threaded up to the descending aortic arch (Fig. 30.3). The IABP is connected to a machine that inflates the balloon portion during ventricular diastole and deflates during systole, a process known as *counterpulsation.* Inflation of the IABP increases coronary artery, renal artery, and myocardial perfusion. Deflation actually keeps the aorta distended so that cardiac output is improved; the work of the left ventricle is decreased, and peripheral organs are more adequately perfused with oxygenated blood. The IABP is intended only for a few days' use.

Surgical Management

When medical treatment alone is unsuccessful, clients may require surgical treatment options such as the insertion of a VAD, cardiomyoplasty, or an implantable artificial heart. Human heart transplantation is discussed in Chapter 31.

Ventricular Assist Device

Some clients awaiting heart transplants are treated with a **ventricular assist device,** an auxiliary heart pump enhancing the heart's ability to eject blood. If the VAD supports left ventricular function, it is referred to as a *left ventricular assist device* or LVAD, designed to be used for weeks to months. Some clients have relied on LVADs for more than 1 year. The natural heart remains in place and continues to function at whatever capacity is possible. Most LVADs use an outflow and inflow cannula to carry blood from the left ventricle into the aorta (Fig. 30.4). They are battery operated through an external power

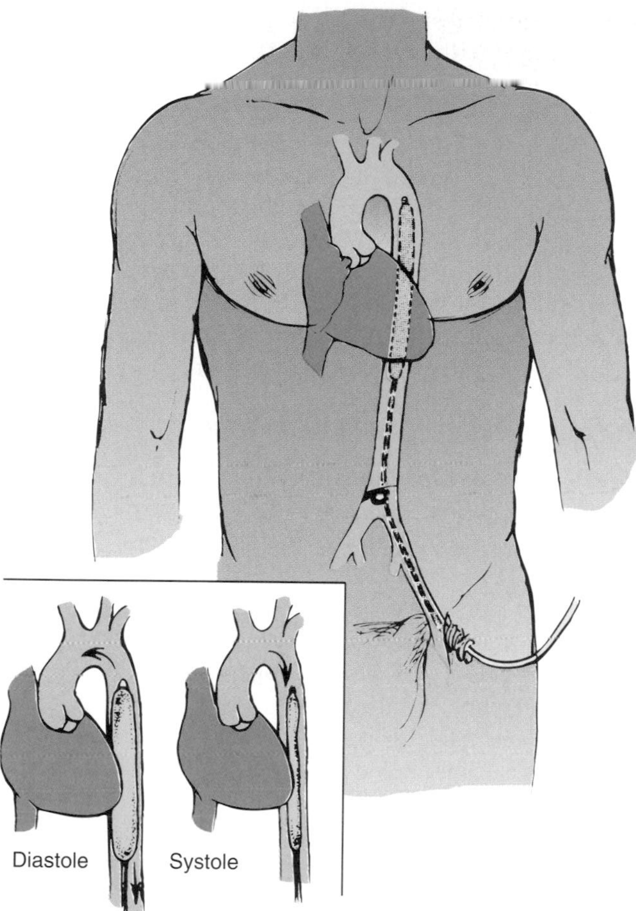

FIGURE 30.3 The intra-aortic balloon pump (IABP).

source worn about the waist, allowing most clients to be at home. By assisting the weak, ineffective left ventricle, LVADs maintain cardiac output at normal volumes. One double-assist device can be used for left-sided, right-sided, or biventricular heart failure. A large external driver powers this device, necessitating continuous hospitalization for its use.

Cardiomyoplasty

Cardiomyoplasty is a surgical procedure in which the client's own chest muscle (latissimus dorsi) is grafted to the aorta and wrapped around the heart. An electrical stimulator placed in a subcutaneous pouch triggers skeletal muscle contraction. The contraction acts as a counterpulsation mechanism similar to the IABP. It augments ineffective myocardial muscle contraction.

Artificial Heart

Adults younger than 55 years are candidates for heart transplantation when medical treatment is unsuccessful (see Chap. 31). An artificial heart may be used while the client awaits a donor organ, although long-term use has not been successful. It is hoped that future use of artificial hearts will provide a viable alternative to human heart transplantation (Fig. 30.5).

Nursing Management

Most clients manage chronic heart failure at home. Many medications, lifestyle changes, and diet restrictions help

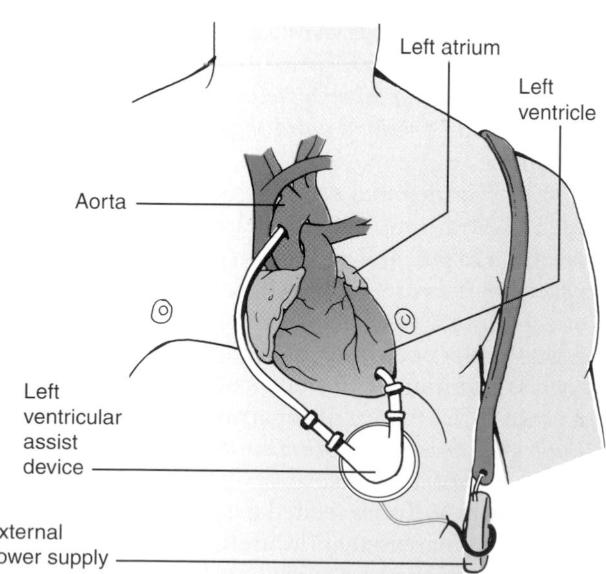

FIGURE 30.4 The LVAD pump weighs 1.5 lb. It is implanted below the diaphragm; its battery pack is carried outside the body. Tubes connect the pump to the left ventricle and aorta.

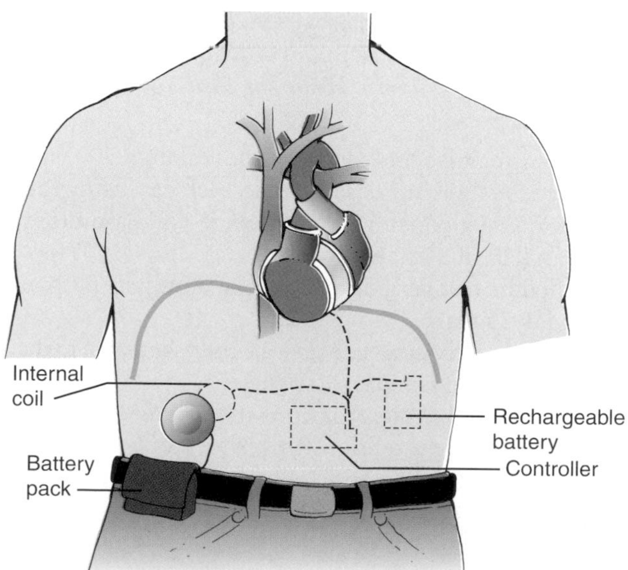

FIGURE 30.5 The newest artificial heart fits inside the chest with no external wires or tubes. An external battery pack transmits power to the internal coil and keeps the backup battery charged.

control heart failure. During acute illness, usual methods may not control symptoms, and clients will need hospitalization. Nurses in various settings administer prescribed medications and monitor for therapeutic and adverse effects. They implement interventions promoting the heart's ability to eject as much blood as possible, monitor for signs of excess fluid volume and evidence of electrolyte imbalance, promote oxygenation, balance activity according to the client's tolerance, and support family members who may be the usual primary caregivers (Client and Family Teaching 30-1).

NURSING PROCESS

● The Client With Congestive Heart Failure

Assessment

Obtain client's history of symptoms and medications and perform an initial physical assessment to establish baseline data. Observe for dyspnea, auscultate apical heart rate and count radial heart rate, measure BP, observe for distended neck veins, and note any signs of peripheral edema, lethargy, or confusion. Obtain an admission weight and thereafter weigh the client daily on the same scale, at the same time of day, with the client wearing similar clothing.

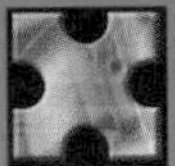

30-1 *Client and Family Teaching* Heart Failure

The nurse instructs about the disease process, meaning of the term failure, *signs and symptoms of impending CHF (weight gain, ankle swelling, fatigue, dyspnea), and importance of taking all medications regularly. He or she also covers the following points:*

- Measure pulse and blood pressure daily.
- Check weight at the same time each day using the same scale; consult a physician if you gain more than 2 lb in 24 hours.
- Schedule rest periods to reduce or eliminate fatigue and dyspnea.
- Increase activities such as walking when able to do so without dyspnea or fatigue.
- Identify and avoid occasions that produce stress.
- Elevate the legs while sitting.
- Follow the diet prescribed by the physician.
- Avoid extreme heat, cold, or humidity.
- Report a heart rate less than 60 or more than 120 beats/minute before taking digitalis.
- Contact the physician if symptoms return or swelling in the legs, ankles, or feet suddenly increases.
- Maintain follow-up care.

Note laboratory test results of serum electrolytes because drug therapy with certain diuretics depletes potassium blood levels. Initiate intake and output measurements and evaluate fluid volumes at least every 8 hours. Measure abdominal girth to determine if the client is developing ascites or responding to therapeutic measures. Note respiratory difficulties during activity and rest. Question the client about nocturnal dyspnea (asking how many pillows normally used for sleep) and listen for crackles on auscultation of lungs. While auscultating the chest, listen for additional heart sounds. Monitor oxygenation status with pulse oximetry or review results of ABG studies.

Diagnosis, Planning, and Interventions

Decreased Cardiac Output related to ineffective ventricular contraction, tachycardia, reduced stroke volume, hypertension, and increased vascular volume

Expected Outcome: Client will have increased cardiac output as evidenced by heart rate between 60 to 100 beats/minute, urinary output between 1500 to 3000 mL/day, systolic BP below 140 mm Hg, diastolic BP below 90 mm Hg, and no mental confusion.

- Assess apical heart rate before administering a cardiac glycoside (digitalis) or other drug that slows heart rate. *Cardiac output is related to heart rate and stroke volume. Withhold a cardiac glycoside until the physician is consulted when heart rate is less than 60 or more than 120 beats/minute.*
- Administer prescribed medications such as cardiac glycosides (digitalis), diuretics, and antihypertensives. *Cardiac glycosides slow heart rate and increase force of contraction. Diuretics decrease afterload by reducing circulating fluid volume. Antihypertensives promote vasodilatation, thus reducing afterload. One or a combination of these drugs reduces the workload of the left ventricle.*
- Promote rest. *Reduces heart contraction (ventricular work). Increasing diastole helps increase the volume in the ventricles (preload) and the ejected volume (stroke volume).*
- Avoid activities that engage the Valsalva maneuver, such as straining with bowel elimination or using the arms to pull and reposition oneself. *The Valsalva maneuver increases intrathoracic pressure, reduces right atrial filling, triggers tachycardia, and increases BP.*
- Assist with procedures that improve cardiac output, such as insertion of a biventricular pacemaker, cardiomyoplasty, LVAD, IABP, or artificial mechanical heart. *Improving the heart's force of contraction or stroke volume improves cardiac output.*

Excess Fluid Volume related to reduced renal function secondary to increased antidiuretic hormone and aldosterone production and reduced cardiac output

Expected Outcome: Fluid volume will be reduced as evidenced by reduced weight and peripheral edema, normal BP measurements, increased urine output, and no adventitious lung sounds.

- Administer prescribed diuretic. *Promotes excretion of sodium and water.*
- Provide sodium-restricted diet as prescribed. *Sodium attracts water; reduced sodium decreases water retention.*
- Apportion oral fluids according to prescribed limitations. *Reduces circulating volume.*

PC: Hypokalemia related to excretion of potassium secondary to diuretic therapy

Expected Outcome: The nurse will monitor for evidence of hypokalemia and prevent or manage low serum potassium levels.

- Monitor for clinical signs of hypokalemia: fatigue, muscle weakness, and abnormal sensations like tingling or numbness. *Potassium is necessary for normal nerve and muscle activity; neuromuscular changes, anorexia, nausea, and vomiting are signs of a low potassium level.*
- Observe the ECG, cardiac monitor, or cardiac rhythm strip for a U wave or cardiac dysrhythmia. *A U wave is associated with hypokalemia. The heart is a muscle that may develop a dysrhythmia if the potassium level is not within normal range.*
- Provide foods and beverages that are good sources of potassium, like bananas and orange juice, within the client's dietary and fluid restrictions. *Dietary intake of foods and beverages that are rich in potassium affect serum potassium levels.*
- Administer a prescribed potassium supplement. *They ensure potassium replacement.*

Evaluation of Expected Outcomes

Expected outcomes are that BP and heart rate return to baseline, with no evidence of excess fluid. Fluid intake approximates output. Serum potassium level remains within or is restored to normal range.

PULMONARY EDEMA

Pulmonary edema is fluid accumulation in the lungs, which interferes with gas exchange in the alveoli. It represents an acute emergency and is a frequent complication of left-sided heart failure. Cardiac dysrhythmias and cardiac or respiratory arrest are associated complications. Noncardiogenic pulmonary edema, also referred to as *acute respiratory distress syndrome,* develops when a pulmonary embolism, infection, or blast injury alters the pulmonary capillary membrane (see Chap. 23). The following discussion focuses on cardiogenic pulmonary edema.

Pathophysiology and Etiology

In cardiogenic pulmonary edema, the left ventricle is incapable of maintaining sufficient output of blood with each contraction. The right ventricle continues to pump blood toward the lungs and the left ventricle has difficulty emptying. Fluid accumulates in the left atrium and pulmonary veins. Pulmonary capillaries and alveoli become engorged with blood. Lungs rapidly fill with fluid, and acute respiratory distress develops. As CO_2 accumulates, respiratory rate and depth increase. Without treatment, hyperventilation becomes insufficient to prevent respiratory acidosis. Metabolic acidosis follows.

Assessment Findings

Clients with acute pulmonary edema exhibit sudden dyspnea, wheezing, orthopnea, restlessness, cough (often productive of pink, frothy sputum), cyanosis, tachycardia, and severe apprehension. Respirations sound moist or gurgling. Cardiac output is reduced. While the body responds with arterial vasoconstriction, it may temporarily sustain adequate BP; however, the client eventually becomes hypotensive and peripheral pulses disappear. Chest x-rays show pulmonary infiltration with fluid. ABGs indicate severe hypoxemia (low PaO_2), hypercapnia (high $PaCO_2$), and a pH below 7.35.

Medical Management

Every effort is made to relieve lung congestion quickly because pulmonary edema can be fatal. Inotropic medications, which improve myocardial contractility, are administered to relieve symptoms. Supplemental oxygen or mechanical ventilation supports breathing. If the cause of heart failure and pulmonary edema can be corrected surgically (e.g., a mitral valve disorder), the client is supported medically while being prepared for surgery.

Drug Therapy

Inotropic agents, such as dopamine (Intropin), dobutamine (Dobutrex), and amrinone (Inocor), or digitalis are administered IV to improve ventricular contraction. To reduce myocardial oxygen consumption, drugs that reduce venous return to the heart (diuretics) and promote vasodilatation (nitrates, ACE inhibitors, calcium channel blockers) are prescribed. IV morphine sulfate is given because it relieves respiratory symptoms by depressing higher cerebral centers, thus relieving anxiety and slowing respiratory rate. It also promotes muscle relaxation and reduces the work of breathing.

Oxygenation

To facilitate gas exchange, oxygen is administered. A mask rather than nasal cannula is needed to deliver maximum percentages of oxygen. If respiratory failure occurs, the client is intubated and oxygen is administered under continuous positive airway pressure or with mechanical ventilation with positive end-expiratory pressure.

Invasive Measures

If the client does not respond to drug therapy and oxygenation, additional interventions such as the insertion of an IABP, biventricular pacemaker, or LVAD are used to sustain life. Cardiomyoplasty, use of an artificial heart, and subsequent heart transplantation are further treatments.

Nursing Management

Effective resolution of pulmonary edema requires both medical and nursing management. Nursing diagnoses, interventions, and expected outcomes for clients with pulmonary edema are similar to those for clients experiencing CHF. Clients with pulmonary edema need close assessment in an intensive care unit.

Establish an IV line for medication administration, such as IV diuretics and inotropic agents. Monitor the therapeutic and adverse effects of medication therapy. Bedside ECG monitoring is standard, as are continuous pulse oximetry and automatic BP and pulse measurements approximately every 15 to 30 minutes. Critically ill clients may have a pulmonary artery catheter inserted. A urinary catheter is inserted to evaluate response to diuretics. Assess for proper placement/adherence of electrodes and ascertain that electronic monitoring equipment is functioning properly. The client receives oxygen to maintain normal blood gases. If the client requires mechanical ventilation, suction the airway as needed, provide frequent mouth care, and establish an alternative method for verbal communication.

GENERAL GERONTOLOGIC CONSIDERATIONS

Dyspnea on exertion is the earliest symptom of heart failure in many older clients. They also may experience a change in mental status, particularly confusion.

The heart is not exempt from aging. Cardiac reserve is lessened, and the heart becomes less able to withstand the effects of injury or disease.

Vascular changes can lead to heart failure by interfering with the blood supply to the heart muscle and causing the heart to pump blood through vessels that have become narrowed and inflexible.

A thorough drug history from a new client or the family is essential because many older adults take digitalis preparations for cardiac disorders. Age-related changes in the gastrointestinal, renal, and hepatic systems necessitate careful monitoring for therapeutic effects and adverse reactions. Older adults are at increased risk for toxicity because of the decreased ability of the kidneys to excrete the drug.

If limited finances prevent a client from preparing or purchasing special foods and needed medications, contact a social service worker or other community agent for assistance.

Critical Thinking Exercises

1. *Discuss how the care of a client with right-sided heart failure differs from the care of a client with left-sided heart failure.*
2. *A client diagnosed with heart failure presents with the following assessment data: temperature 99.1°F, pulse 100 beats/minute, respirations 42 breaths/minute, BP 110/50 mm Hg; crackles in both lung bases; nausea; pulse oximeter reading of 89%; enlarged, soft abdomen. Which assessment findings need immediate attention? Why?*

• NCLEX-STYLE REVIEW QUESTIONS 

1. A client comes to the clinic complaining of shortness of breath, pink-tinged sputum, and a cough. The nurse suspects congestive heart failure. Which assessment finding further confirms the diagnosis?
   1. Moist crackles in the lung fields
   2. Bradycardia less than 60 bpm
   3. Blood pressure 90/60 mm Hg
   4. Increased urine output
2. A client diagnosed with congestive heart failure is admitted to the hospital for treatment. Which nursing intervention requires priority?
   1. Administer three liters O_2 per nasal cannula.
   2. Give a loading dose of digoxin (Lanoxin).
   3. Draw blood for baseline electrolytes.
   4. Assess for distended neck veins
3. Prior to giving a client his morning dosage of digoxin (Lanoxin), the nurse assesses the apical pulse and finds the pulse to be less than 55 beats/minute. Which nursing action is the priority?
   1. Call the physician and report the finding.
   2. Hold the drug and assess for toxic effects.
   3. Take the client's blood pressure.
   4. Recheck the pulse in 30 minutes.

connection

Visit the Connection site at **http://connection.lww.com/go/timbyEssentials** for links to chapter-related resources on the Internet.

References and Suggested Readings

Baker, S., & Graziano, J. (2003). A new device for heart failure. *RN, 66*(3), 32–35.

Barold, S. S. (2001). What is resynchronization therapy? *The American Journal of Medicine, 111,* 224–232.

Bausbeck-Aballo, S., Eyerman, T., Henry-Kamen, D. & Padre, I. (November 5, 2001). And the beat goes on . . . *Advance for Nurses,* 25–27.

Beattie, S. (2000). Heart failure with preserved LV function: Pathophysiology, clinical presentation, treatment, and nursing implications. *Journal of Cardiovascular Nursing, 14*(4), 24–37.

Bond, A. E., Nelson, K., Germany, C. L., & Smart, A. N. (2003). The left ventricular assist device. *American Journal of Nursing, 103*(1), 32–40.

Bosen, D. M. (2002). What you need to know about the new heart failure guidelines. *Nursing 2002, 32*(6), 32cc8–32cc9.

Bradley, C. (2000). Drug therapy review. Spironolactone in heart failure: A revived role for an old drug. *Intensive and Critical Care Nursing, 16,* 403–404.

Chojnowski, D. (February 3, 2003). Chronic heart failure. *Advance for Nurses,* 17–19.

Christensen, D. M. (July 22, 2002). Ventricular assist devices. *Advance for Nurses,* 17–19.

Christensen, D. M. (2000). The ventricular assist device: an overview. *Nursing Clinics of North America, 35,* 945–959.

Davis, S. L. (2002). How the heart failure picture has changed. *Nursing 2002, 32*(11), 36–44.

DeWald, T., Gaulden, L., Beyler, M., et al. (2000). Current trends in the management of heart failure. *Nursing Clinics of North America, 35,* 855–875.

Dwyer, D. (2002). Monitoring temporary pacemaker connections. *Nursing 2002, 32*(9), 76.

Gever, M. P. (2002). Carvedilol: Test your drug IQ. *Nursing 2002, 32*(6), 32cc10–32cc11.

Henrick, A. (2001). Cost-effective outpatient management of persons with heart failure. *Progress in Cardiovascular Nursing, 16*(2), 50–56.

Incredibly Easy. (2002). What to do when a temporary pacemaker fails. *Nursing 2002, 32*(12), 72.

Lazzara, D. (2001). Respiratory distress: Loosening the grip. *Nursing 2001, 31*(6), 58–64.

MacKlin, M. (2001). Managing heart failure: A case study approach. *Critical Care Nurse, 21*(2), 36–38, 40–46, 48, 50–51.

Martens, K. H. (2000). Home care nursing for persons with congestive heart failure: Description and relationship to hospital readmission. *Home Healthcare Nurse, 18,* 404–409.

Martin, T. (2002). How heart failure complicates care. *Nursing 2002, 32*(7), 32hn1–32hn5.

McConnell, E. A. (2002). Using an automated external defibrillator. *Nursing 2002, 32*(10), 18.

Mendzef, S. D. (2000). Neurohormonal factors in heart failure. *Nursing Clinics of North America, 35,* 841–853.

Morris, E. R. (March 4, 2002). Keeping pace. *Advance for Nurses,* 23–24.

Pope, B. B. (2002). Heart failure. *Nursing 2002, 32*(8), 50–51.

Pugh, L. C., Havens D. S., Xie, S., et al. (2001). Case management for elderly persons with heart failure: The quality of life and cost outcomes. *MEDSURG Nursing, 10*(2), 71–78.

Shaffer, S. (2002). ICD therapy: The patient's perspective. *American Journal of Nursing, 102*(2), 46–49.

Shatzer, M., & Saul, L. (2003). Using a BNP test to identify heart failure. *Nursing 2003, 33*(1), 68.

Tedesco, C., Reigle, J., & Bergin, J. (2000). Sudden cardiac death in heart failure. *Journal of Cardiovascular Nursing, 14*(4), 38–56.

chapter 31

Caring for Clients Undergoing Cardiovascular Surgery

Words to Know 

annuloplasty
cardioplegia
cardiopulmonary bypass
commissurotomy
coronary artery bypass graft
embolectomy
endarterectomy
extracorporeal circulation
myocardial revascularization
thrombectomy
valvuloplasty

Learning Objectives

On completion of this chapter, the reader will:

- Identify the purpose of cardiopulmonary bypass.
- Describe disadvantages of cardiopulmonary bypass.
- Explain indications for cardiac surgery.
- Describe how coronary artery blood flow is surgically restored.
- Name four surgical procedures for revascularizing the myocardium.
- Identify three techniques to correct valvular disorders.
- Describe methods for controlling bleeding from heart trauma.
- List problems associated with heart transplantation.
- Discuss the preoperative preparation of a client undergoing cardiovascular surgery.
- Discuss the nursing management of clients undergoing cardiac surgery.
- List types of surgery performed on central or peripheral blood vessels.
- Discuss the nursing management of clients undergoing vascular surgery.

Cardiac surgery is a relatively new process. In the 1960s, the technique for mechanically circulating and oxygenating blood outside the body, called **extracorporeal circulation** or **cardiopulmonary bypass** (Fig. 31.1), was developed. Removing blood from the venae cavae, circulating it through an oxygenator, and returning it to the aorta or femoral artery provides a nearly bloodless area while the beating heart is stopped.

Although most forms of cardiac surgery use cardiopulmonary bypass, some new surgical techniques have eliminated its use. Surgery on the beating heart without cardiopulmonary bypass reduces the potential for negative "pump" consequences (Box 31-1).

CARDIAC SURGICAL PROCEDURES

Cardiac surgery is used to correct and treat various cardiac disorders. It is done to revascularize the myocardium, repair or replace cardiac valves, repair ventricular aneurysm, remove heart tumors, manage heart trauma, and replace the heart with one from a human donor.

Myocardial Revascularization

Myocardial revascularization refers to surgical techniques that improve delivery of oxygenated blood to the myocardium for clients with coronary artery disease (CAD). It is accomplished with one or more **coronary artery bypass grafts** (CABG) that improve myocardial oxygenation by bypassing or detouring around the occluded portion of one or more coronary arteries with a relocated blood vessel. The saphenous vein in the leg is most often used for grafting. The surgeon makes a long incision on the medial aspect of the leg or removes the vein endoscopically through one to three small (1-inch) leg incisions. An endoscopically removed vein results in less muscle and tissue damage, decreased pain, and reduced scarring. Alternative graft vessels include the

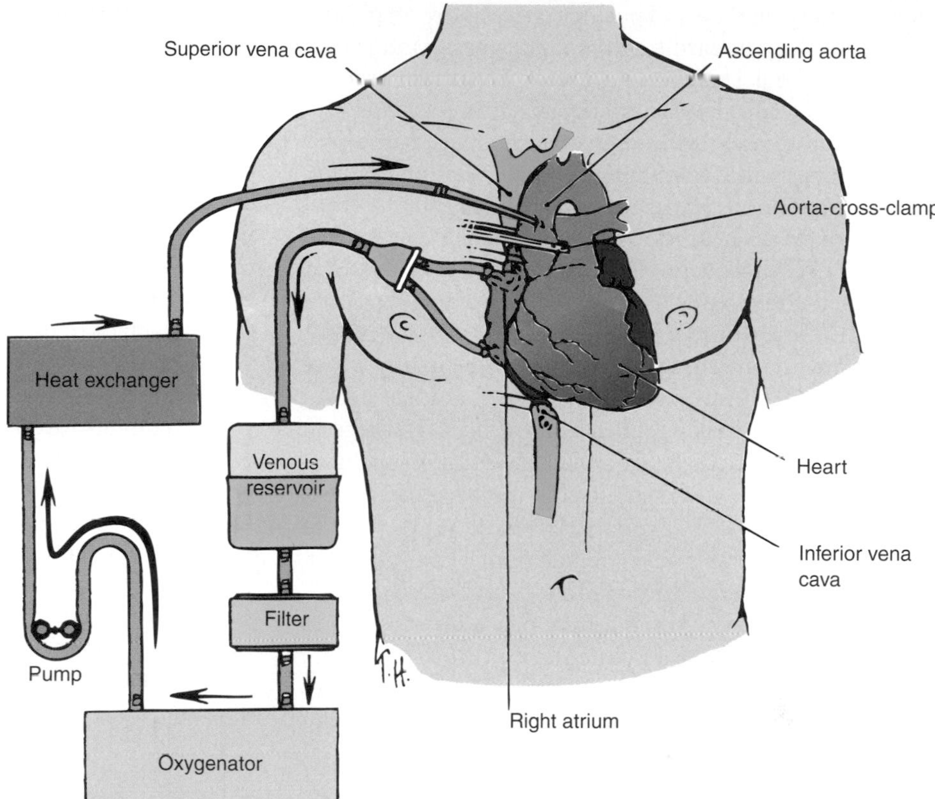

FIGURE 31.1 The cardiopulmonary bypass system. Cannulae are placed into the superior and inferior vena cava to divert blood from the body and into the bypass system. The pump creates a vacuum and pulls blood into the venous reservoir. The filter clears the blood of air bubbles, clots, and particulates. The blood then passes through the oxygenator, to the pump, and to the heat exchanger, which regulates the blood's temperature. The blood is then returned to the body. (From Smeltzer, S. C. & Bare, B. G. [2004]. *Brunner & Suddarth's textbook of medical–surgical nursing* [10th ed.]. Philadelphia: Lippincott Williams & Wilkins.)

basilic and cephalic veins in the arm, internal mammary and internal thoracic arteries in the chest, radial artery in the arm, and, in some cases, the gastroepiploic artery from the stomach. The advantage of using chest arteries is that doing so avoids making a second operative incision elsewhere on the body. The disadvantage is that the portion of the chest arteries available for graft use is shorter than other graft vessels.

CABG is used for clients with CAD who are not candidates for less invasive procedures. CABG is performed when (1) the client has multiple coronary artery occlusions, (2) the atheromas are calcified and noncompressible, or (3) the anatomic location of the occlusion(s) interferes with safe insertion of a coronary artery catheter.

BOX 31-1 ● Disadvantages of Cardiopulmonary Bypass

- Long operative period (6 hours)
- Necessity for anticoagulation
- Hypotension
- Need for postoperative blood replacement
- Overall decline in mental function, perhaps because of an inflammatory response triggered by blood circulating through plastic tubing or gaseous bubbles in the circulated blood
- Risk for stroke, dysrhythmias, and renal failure

The most conventional technique for performing CABG involves a mid-chest incision, use of a cardiopulmonary bypass machine, and **cardioplegia** (stopping the heart) during surgery. One or several occluded areas can be bypassed during the surgical procedure, which is referred to as a *double, triple,* or *quadruple* bypass depending on the number of vessels that are grafted.

Off-pump coronary artery bypass (OPCAB) is similar to conventional CABG except that the heart remains beating at a slow rate, eliminating use of the cardiopulmonary bypass machine. The OPCAB chest incision is somewhat less than in a conventional CABG procedure. OPCAB reduces risks associated with using the coronary bypass machine and decreases postoperative recovery time spent in the hospital. OPCAB procedures have only been done in recent years. It is too early to know if long-term success is as good or better than with conventional CABG.

Minimally invasive direct coronary artery bypass (MIDCAB) is also a "beating heart" procedure. It is *minimally invasive* because the incision, made between the ribs, is only about 3 to 5 inches long. The surgeon uses an endoscope to view the heart while grafting the vessels. Some surgeons are learning to use a robotic instrument inside the chest cavity rather than their hands. This type of procedure is limited to grafting only one or two vessels on the anterior surface of the heart in clients who are not obese or whose coronary arteries are not heavily calcified. Despite these limitations, the MIDCAB procedure shortens surgical time and postoperative recovery period, eliminates risks of cardiopulmonary bypass, and is cosmetically more acceptable because of the smaller scar.

Port access coronary artery bypass (PACAB) is a coronary artery bypass technique that uses the cardiopulmonary bypass machine, but eliminates the long sternal incision common in conventional CABG. The surgeon gains access to the heart through several small incisions on the left lateral chest near the axilla, which facilitate insertion of metal tubes approximately the diameter of a pencil (Fig. 31.2). It is through these tubes, or ports, that surgical instruments are inserted. A fourth and slightly larger incision in the chest permits insertion of a video camera attached to an endoscope called a *thorascope.* The surgeon uses the image from the video camera and transesophageal echocardiography to visualize the operative area after the heart is stopped. A robotic hand, activated by the surgeon's voice command, manipulates the surgical instruments that are inserted through the ports (Fogoros, 2001).

PACAB shortens the operative procedure from 3 to 6 hours to 2 hours and reduces mortality rates from complications. Clients stay in the hospital only 2 to 3 days after the procedure, compared with 7 to 10 days after conventional CABG. Full recovery is much faster as well.

Valvular Repairs

Heart valves need surgical repair or replacement if they become narrowed (stenosed) or stretched (incompetent) (see Chap. 26). One method of repair is **commissurotomy** (opening adhesions in the valve cusps), done without direct visualization of the valve. This procedure is performed through a thoracotomy (chest incision). The surgeon places a purse-string suture in the wall of the heart, makes an incision, and inserts his or her finger or a metal dilator into the narrowed valve, stretching its opening. The surgeon then pulls the purse-string suture tight to prevent blood from escaping. Cardiopulmonary bypass is not required but is kept available for immediate use if complications develop or direct visualization is required to repair the valve. **Valvuloplasty** (valve repair) and **annuloplasty** (repair of the fibrous ring that encircles the valve) tighten an incompetent valve (Fig. 31.3). The diseased valve also can be excised and replaced with a mechanical valve or a bioprosthetic valve (Fig. 31.4).

Surgeons also are using minimally invasive approaches when replacing heart valves. Some of these approaches are performed through a mini-sternotomy, or parasternal incision, or a port access approach. Although cardiopulmonary bypass is required, proponents of minimally invasive approaches to valve replacement cite the advantages of reduced surgical trauma, mechanical ventilation, blood loss, and postoperative pain; faster mobility; decreased length of hospital stay and perioperative costs; and improved cosmetic appearance.

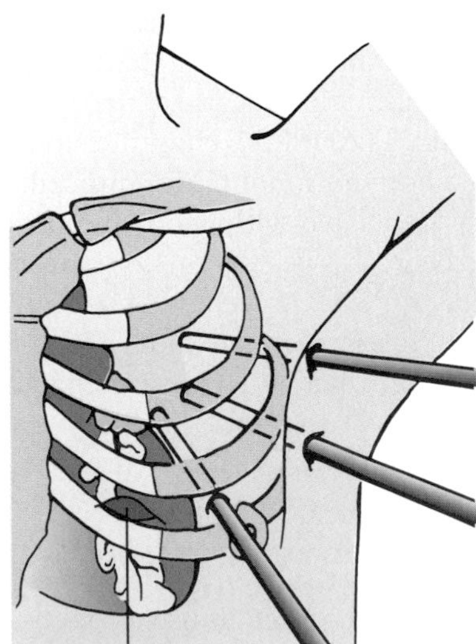

FIGURE 31.2 In a PACAB technique, the surgeon makes three small incisions in the chest near the axilla. He or she inserts surgical instruments through the ports and an endoscope through a larger incision. The surgeon then views the surgical field.

Repair of Ventricular Aneurysm

An aneurysm of the ventricular wall develops when an infarcted area of myocardium balloons outward. Thrombi commonly form in the crater of the bulging tissue. A ventricular aneurysm is the most lethal complication among clients who survive the acute stage of a myocardial infarction (MI). Because motion of the myocardium may rupture the aneurysm, an emergency procedure may be performed to suture the weakened area. If waiting is possible, stretched tissue is excised 4 to 8 weeks after the MI when scar tissue has formed. If surgery is performed too early, it is difficult to differentiate healthy from necrotic tissue, and sutures placed in necrotic tissue usually are not retained.

Removal of Heart Tumors

Primary tumors of the heart, both benign and malignant, are rare. The clinical course and operative procedure depend on the type of tumor and its location in the heart. Benign tumors typically extend from a pedicle or stem, making their removal uncomplicated. Malignant tumors are more difficult to remove, and the prognosis is extremely poor.

Repair of Heart Trauma

A nonpenetrating injury of the chest, such as being crushed against a steering wheel, may cause bruising and

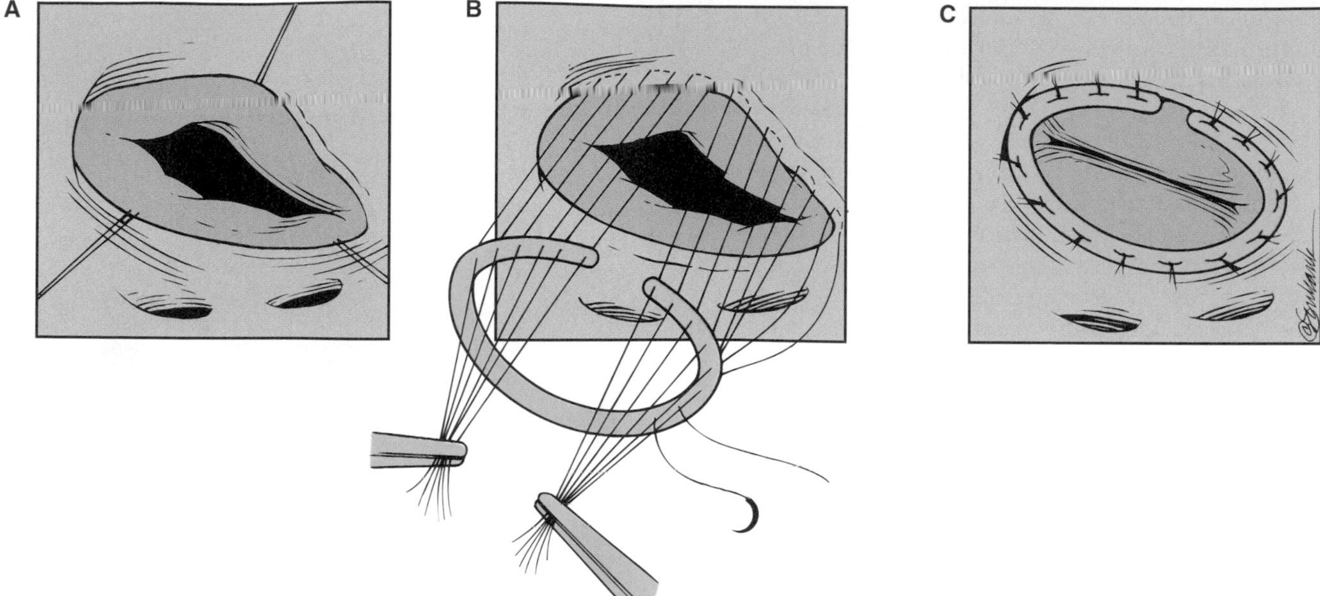

FIGURE 31.3 Annuloplasty ring insertion. (**A**) Mitral valve regurgitation; leaflets do not close. (**B**) Insertion of an annuloplasty ring. (**C**) Completed valvuloplasty; leaflets close.

bleeding of the heart. Because the pericardium encloses the heart, blood accumulates in the pericardial space, resulting in cardiac tamponade. Somctimes traumatic cardiac tamponade is treated conservatively with bed rest. Inactivity and increased pressure from blood in the pericardium may stop the bleeding. The client may need to have blood aspirated from the pericardial sac, in which case pericardiocentesis is performed (see Chap. 25). One aspiration is sufficient in most cases, but if bleeding continues, open thoracotomy is indicated to control blood loss.

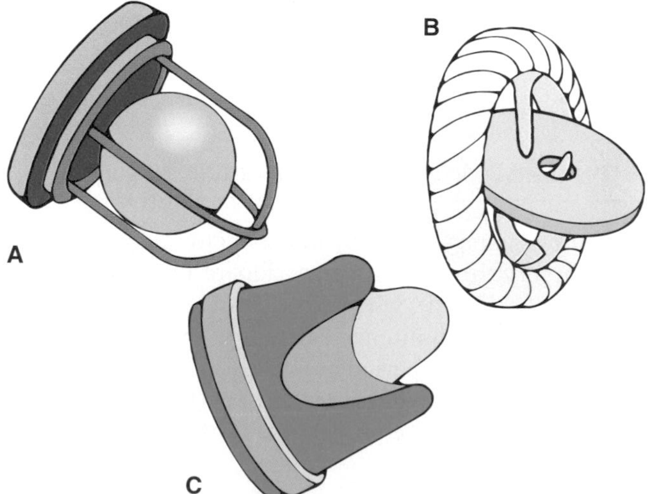

FIGURE 31.4 Common mechanical and biologic valve replacements. (**A**) Caged ball valve (Starr-Edwards, mechanical). (**B**) Tilting-disk valve (Medtronic-Hall, mechanical). (**C**) Porcine heterograft valve (Carpenter-Edwards, biologic).

A penetrating injury, such as a stab wound, also causes blood to leak into the pericardium. A pericardial tear often seals with a clot, whereas a myocardial tear continues to bleed. Large tears necessitate surgery. If the wound is severe enough to cause immediate shock from hemorrhage, the prognosis is poor.

Heart Transplantation

In adults, heart transplantation is indicated for cardiomyopathy (see Chap. 25) and end-stage coronary artery disease (see Chap 27). In newborns and infants, heart transplantation is indicated for a severe congenital cardiac defect. It is performed when other treatment modalities fail.

The National Organ Transplant Act, which Congress passed in 1984, outlaws sale of human organs. The United Network for Organ Sharing (UNOS) is the organization that maintains a computerized database with which to match organs with recipients. Once a client is certified as a candidate for transplantation, his or her name and tissue type are placed on a computerized recipient list. Tissue typing is necessary to match recipient with donor. Problems associated with heart transplantation include scarcity of donor organs, tissue rejection, postoperative infection, postoperative psychosis, and cost. When a donor heart becomes available, it must be removed from the donor and transplanted within 6 hours of being harvested.

The most common method of heart transplantation is an orthotopic heart transplant. The recipient's failing heart is removed and the donor heart is sutured onto the native great vessels of the heart. Recipients are given immunosuppressive drugs such as cyclosporine (Sandimmune), azathioprine (Imuran), and prednisone (Meticorten) to prevent organ rejection. The client is closely observed for signs of organ rejection (e.g., elevated white blood cell count, electrocardiographic [ECG] changes, fever), and is placed in protective isolation because an infection can be life-threatening. Throughout the client's lifetime, a heart biopsy in which cardiac tissue is obtained by an instrument attached to a venous catheter inserted into the heart is performed to detect rejection. Heart biopsies are performed every week for the first 3 to 6 weeks after surgery, then every 3 months for 1 year, and every year thereafter (National Heart, Lung, and Blood Institute, 1997). When signs of rejection occur, the dose or number of immunosuppressives is increased.

The transplanted heart beats faster than the client's natural heart, averaging about 100 to 110 beats/minute, because nerves that affect heart rate have been severed. The new heart also takes longer to increase the heart rate in response to exercise. CAD is a common problem among heart transplant recipients. They do not experience angina because the transplanted heart's nerve supply is no longer intact.

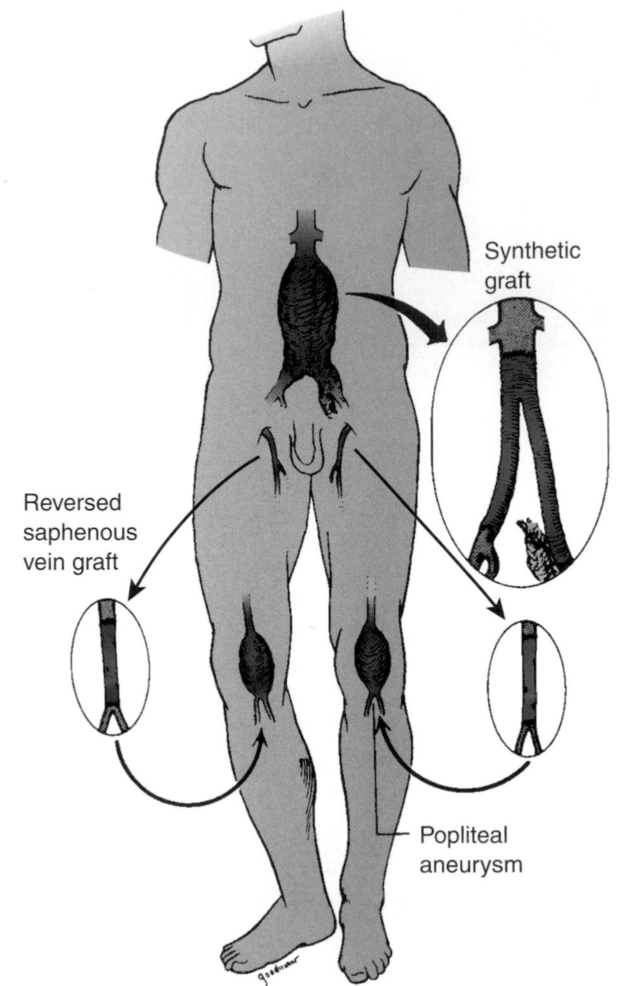

FIGURE 31.5 Surgical repair of an abdominal aneurysm and bilateral popliteal aneurysms. (From Smeltzer, S. C. & Bare, B. G. [2004]. *Brunner & Suddarth's textbook of medical–surgical nursing* [10th ed.]. Philadelphia: Lippincott Williams & Wilkins.)

CENTRAL OR PERIPHERAL VASCULAR SURGICAL PROCEDURES

Vascular Grafts

Vascular grafts are used to bypass or replace diseased sections of major systemic blood vessels such as the aorta or femoral arteries. The replacement graft may be made of synthetic fiber, such as Dacron or Teflon, or may be human tissue harvested from cadavers. A clamp is placed above and below the affected area, and the diseased blood vessel is removed. The replacement graft is then sewn in place, and clamps are removed (Fig. 31.5). Depending on the area involved, cardiopulmonary bypass may be necessary.

Embolectomy and Thrombectomy

When thrombi or emboli occlude a major vessel, a **thrombectomy** (removal of a thrombus) or **embolectomy** (removal of an embolus) is performed. The vessel is opened above the clot, the clot is removed, and the vessel is sutured closed. This type of surgery may be an emergency because complete occlusion results in loss of blood supply to an area.

Endarterectomy

Endarterectomy is the resection and removal of the lining of an artery (see Chap. 40). This type of surgery is performed to remove obstructive atherosclerotic plaques from the carotid, femoral, or popliteal arteries (Fig. 31.6).

NURSING PROCESS

● The Client Undergoing Cardiac or Vascular Surgery

The nurse manages the care of the client undergoing cardiac surgery throughout the perioperative and rehabilitation phases. Clients who undergo cardiovascular surgery are cared for in an intensive care unit during the immediate postoperative period because of their unstable condition and need for nurses with expertise in managing complex monitoring equipment (Fig. 31.7).

Assessment

Obtain the client's medical and surgical history and perform a physical examination (see Chap. 24). Obtain a drug history to determine if the client has any drug aller-

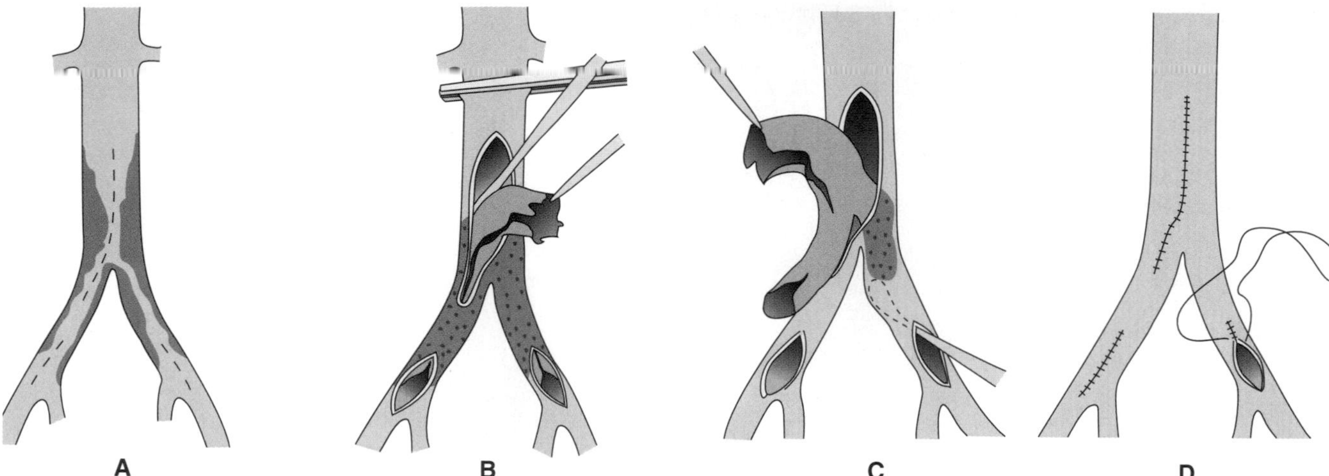

FIGURE 31.6 In an aortoiliac endarterectomy, the vascular surgeon (**A**) identifies the diseased area, (**B**) clamps off blood supply to the vessel, (**C**) removes the plaque, and (**D**) sutures the vessel shut, after which blood flow is restored. (Adapted with permission from Rutherford, R. B. [1995]. *Vascular surgery* [4th ed., Vols. I and II]. Philadelphia: W. B. Saunders.)

gies. Weigh the client, record vital signs regularly, and measure intake and output. Prepare the client for extensive diagnostic assessment tests such as chest x-ray, ECG, exercise ECG (stress test), pulmonary function studies, echocardiography, laboratory blood tests, and coronary arteriography, and carefully check results.

Take time to assess the client's understanding of the scheduled procedure. After open heart surgery, the anesthetist and other members of the operating team send many clients directly from the operating room to the intensive care unit. Obtain a comprehensive surgical report from the anesthetist or anesthesiologist and check all invasive monitoring devices. Thoroughly and systematically assess for signs and symptoms of potential complications, such as hemorrhage and shock, thrombus or embolus formation, cerebral anoxia, cardiac dysrhythmias, fluid overload, electrolyte imbalance, respiratory failure, and cardiac tamponade.

Palpate peripheral pulses or use a Doppler ultrasound device if the pulses are not palpable. Check for inadequate tissue perfusion, such as a weak or absent pulse, cold or cyanotic extremity, or skin mottling. Assess blood pressure (BP) and pulse rate in both arms after thoracic surgery. Inspect intravenous (IV) sites and monitor rates of infusing solutions. Calculate urine output and other fluid intake hourly. Perform a neurologic assessment every 30 minutes, including evaluation of level of consciousness, size of pupils and their reaction to light, movement in both arms and legs, verbal response, and status of orientation.

Diagnosis, Planning, and Interventions

Risk for Impaired Gas Exchange related to retained secretions, hypoventilation secondary to pain, displacement of chest tubes

Expected Outcome: Client maintains adequate gas exchange as evidenced by arterial blood gases (ABGs) within normal limits and no dyspnea or tachycardia.

- Assess lung sounds, heart rate, level of consciousness, pulse oximetry, and ABG results as often as necessary. *Abnormal findings are indicators of developing hypoxemia.*
- Notify physician if oxygen saturation falls below 90%. *This finding indicates that the client requires supplemental oxygenation.*
- Administer oxygen as prescribed. *Prevents hypoxemia or relieves oxygen deficits.*
- Elevate head of bed as much as possible. *Facilitates maximum chest/lung expansion, promotes comfort, and decreases the work of breathing.*
- Hyperoxygenate with 100% oxygen before suctioning; do not suction for more than 10 to 15 seconds. *Suctioning removes oxygen and can cause hypoxemia, myocardial ischemia, and dysrhythmias. Hyperoxygenation saturates the blood and hemoglobin to compensate for temporary removal during suctioning.*
- Promote rest and administer prescribed sedatives. *Rest reduces oxygen consumption; sedatives promote rest and are sympathetic antagonists.*
- Inspect chest tubes frequently to ensure they are not kinked or compressed. *Obstructed chest tubes interfere with removal of air from the pleura, which interferes with lung expansion.*

Risk for Decreased Cardiac Output related to impaired ventricular contraction

Expected Outcome: Client will maintain adequate cardiac output as evidenced by stable vital signs, alertness, adequate urine output, and no dysrhythmias, chest pain, dyspnea, confusion, or dizziness. Cardiac output readings are within normal limits.

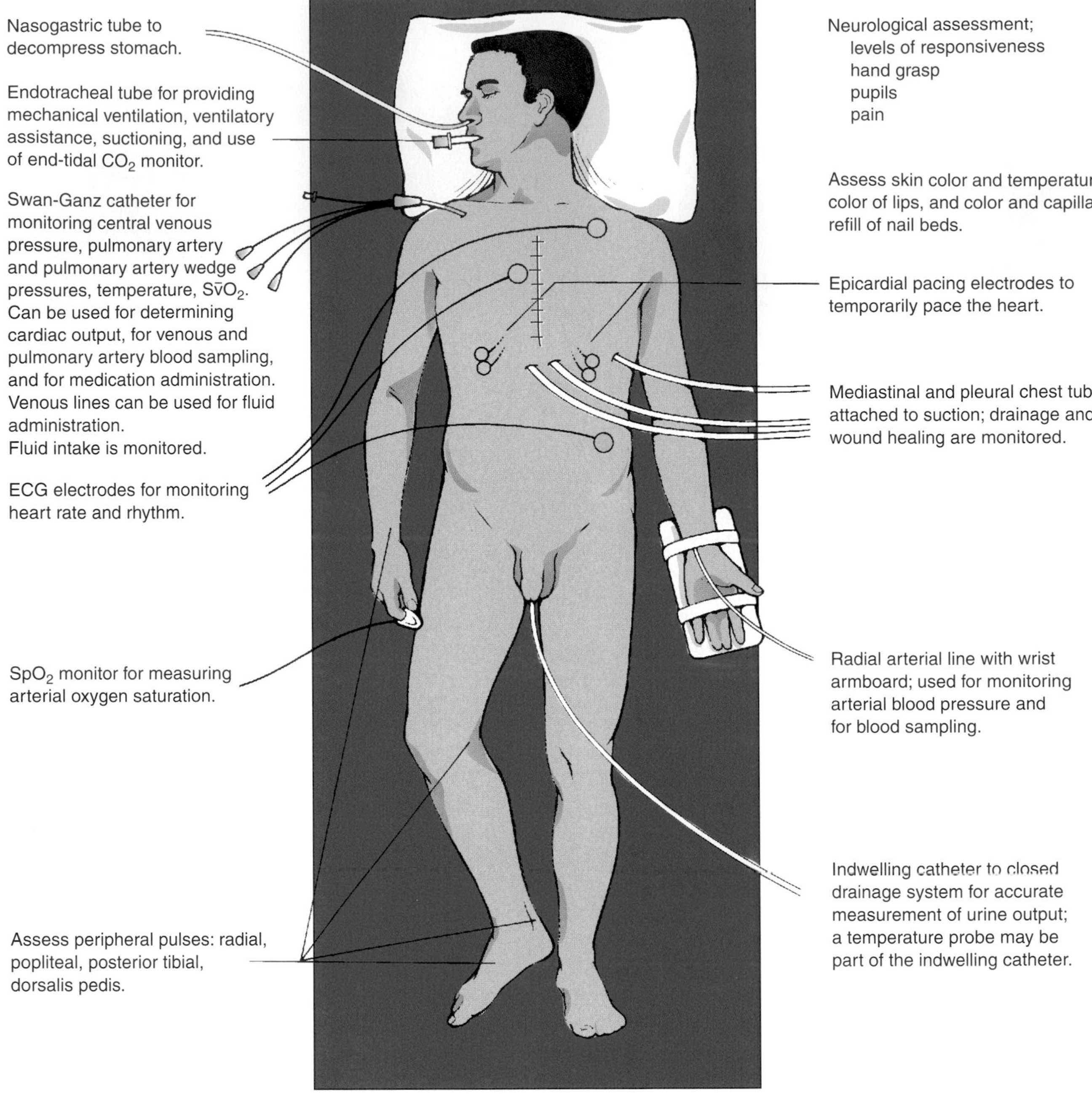

FIGURE 31.7 Postoperative care of the client undergoing cardiac surgery. (From Smeltzer, S. C. & Bare, B. G. [2004]. *Brunner & Suddarth's textbook of medical–surgical nursing* [10th ed.]. Philadelphia: Lippincott Williams & Wilkins.)

- Assess hemodynamics with direct BP monitoring by arterial line, pulmonary artery catheter and cardiac output measurements, vital signs, heart and lung sounds, intake and output, pulse rhythm and quality, mental status, and signs of peripheral edema as often as necessary. *Focused assessments that reflect the heart's ability to circulate intravascular fluid are an indication of an adequate or inadequate cardiac output.*
- Administer IV fluids and blood replacement at rate prescribed. *Parenteral fluids increase intravascular volume to facilitate adequate cardiac output.*
- Administer prescribed inotropic medications. *They increase the force of heart contraction.*
- Administer prescribed vasodilators or diuretics. *They decrease afterload and promote optimum cardiac output.*
- Administer prescribed antidysrhythmics. *They promote normal conduction, depolarization, and repolarization of myocardial tissue to ensure normal cardiac output.*
- Be prepared to use a transcutaneous or transvenous pacemaker. *A temporary pacemaker ensures a heart rate that is compatible with life.*

PC: Hemorrhage

Expected Outcome: The nurse will monitor for, manage, and minimize hemorrhage.

- Assess incisional drainage; sites used for cardiopulmonary bypass cannulation; volume and color of chest tube drainage; BP and pulse rate; urinary output; mental status; partial thromboplastin time, prothrombin time, and international normalized ratio (INR); presence of occult blood in stool; bruising; bleeding gums; and hemodynamic measurements as often as necessary. *Abnormal findings of such focused assessments are indicators of bleeding.*
- Report to the physician a cluster of symptoms that suggest significant blood loss. *The nurse works collaboratively to manage complications.*
- Be prepared to administer parenteral fluids, blood replacement, fresh frozen plasma, or antidotes for anticoagulants. *Fluids, blood, and blood products increase blood volume. Fresh frozen plasma replaces clotting factors. Antagonists of anticoagulants restore endogenous clotting mechanisms.*
- Apply direct pressure to bleeding sites. *Promotes stasis of blood.*

Risk for Ineffective Tissue Perfusion: Peripheral related to compromised collateral circulation in extremity used to harvest donor vein, cannulation of peripheral artery and vein for cardiopulmonary bypass, venous stasis secondary to inactivity

Expected Outcome: Client's donor extremities will be adequately perfused with oxygenated blood; venous blood circulation will be adequate.

- Assess peripheral pulses, dependent edema, capillary refill, skin color and temperature, urinary output, mental status, and Homans' sign as often as necessary. *Focused assessment of these data reflects status of peripheral blood flow.*
- Position extremity above level of heart. *Gravity promotes venous return to heart. Reducing edema facilitates potential space for arterial circulation.*
- Encourage leg exercises every hour while awake. *Contraction of skeletal leg muscles propels venous blood toward the heart.*
- Apply elastic stockings or use a mechanical compression device. *Elastic stockings support valves in leg veins to prevent venous stasis. Mechanical compression devices apply pressure to tissues of the legs to propel venous blood.*
- Assist client to ambulate several times a day. *Walking contracts leg muscles that promote venous blood return.*
- Ensure client avoids prolonged sitting or crossing legs at the knee. *Gravity and pressure contribute to venous stasis.*
- Encourage oral fluids within prescribed limits. *Adequate fluid volume decreases potential for hemoconcentration and thrombus formation.*

Evaluation of Expected Outcomes

The client ventilates adequately to maintain adequate gas diffusion; cardiac output is sufficient to maintain vital signs and renal output within normal ranges. No significant bleeding develops. Extremities are warm and nonedematous, reflecting adequate arterial and venous circulation.

Stop, Think, and Respond ● BOX 31-1

Mr. Jones has been in the intensive care unit for the past 4 days after CABG surgery. Normally alert and oriented, he is very confused, restless, and agitated. What could be possible reasons for this new-onset confusion? What other data will you need to collect? What can you do to help Mr. Jones right now?

GENERAL GERONTOLOGIC CONSIDERATIONS

Narcotics must be given with caution in older adults because the respiratory system of the older adult is more sensitive to the depressant effect of narcotic analgesics. Anticholinergic drugs such as atropine and scopolamine are used cautiously (if at all) in older adults because they are at greater risk for adverse reactions.

The older adult is prone to postoperative confusion. This confusion may manifest as disorientation, paranoia, aggression, or visual hallucinations.

Many older adults are poor surgical risks and have other concurrent medical problems, such as diabetes, heart failure, cardiac dysrhythmias, hypertension, and poor renal function. These clients require close observation during the postoperative period.

Critical Thinking Exercises

1. *What information would you offer to a person with CAD who says the physician has advised myocardial revascularization but the thought of a long mid-chest incision and leg incision are very frightening?*
2. *While caring for a client who is recovering from CABG surgery, you gather the following data: the client has leg pain, which he rates as 8 on a scale of 1 to 10; his respiratory rate is 30 breaths/minute at rest; there is dried blood on the thoracic dressing; the client's throat is sore after being weaned from mechanical ventilation; and he is concerned because he has not had a bowel movement in 3 days. Which assessment finding should be the major concern at this time?*
3. *What teaching would you do on seeing a client with a conventional CABG using a saphenous vein graft sitting in a chair with his or her legs crossed at the knee?*

● NCLEX-STYLE REVIEW QUESTIONS

1. A client returns to the intensive care unit after a coronary artery bypass graft (CABG) where the saphenous vein was removed. During the immediate postoperative period, which nursing intervention is most important?
   1. Inspect the IV site and infusion rate.
   2. Assess the client for peripheral edema.
   3. Palpate the peripheral pulses.
   4. Administer an anticoagulant.

2. A client is recovering from cardiovascular surgery and has decreased cardiac output. The nurse reviews the client's care plan where an expected outcome is to maintain adequate cardiac output. Which sign or symptom best demonstrates the expected outcome?
   1. The client's urine output is 25 mL/kg/hour.
   2. The client has fixed, dilated pupils.
   3. The client has frequent palpitations.
   4. The client's vital signs are within normal limits.

connection

Visit the Connection site at **http://connection.lww.com/go/timbyEssentials** for links to chapter-related resources on the Internet.

References and Suggested Readings

Allen, S. (2000). Off-pump bypass technique gets high praise from patients. *Nursing Spectrum* (Greater Chicago/NE Illinois & NW Indiana Edition), *13*(23), 14–15.

Augustine, S. M. (2000). Heart transplantation: Long-term management related to immunosuppression, complications, and psychosocial adjustments. *Critical Nursing Clinics of North America, 12,* 69–77.

Baptiste, M. M. (2001). Aortic valve replacement. *RN, 64*(1), 58–64.

Becker, C., & Petlin, A. (1999). Heart transplantation. *American Journal of Nursing, 99*(5, Suppl.), 8–14, 50–52.

Bogan, L. M., Rosson, M. W., & Petersen, F. F. (2000). Organ procurement and the donor family. *Critical Care Nursing Clinics of North America, 12,* 23–33.

Cope, S., & Hawley, R. (2001). Needs of the older patient in the intensive care unit following heart surgery. *Progress in Cardiovascular Nursing, 16*(2), 44–48.

Drug Watch. (1999). Post-transplant immunosuppression. *American Journal of Nursing, 99*(2), 14.

Fogoros, R. (2001). Robotic heart surgery—a status report. [On-line.] Available: http://heartdisease.about.com/library/weekly/aa060401a.htm.

Hadaway, L. C. (2002). What you can do to decrease catheter-related infections. *Nursing 2002, 32*(9), 46–48.

Henke, K., & Eigsti, J. (2003). After cardiopulmonary bypass: Watching for complications. *Nursing 2003, 33*(3), 32cc1–32cc4.

Holmquist, M., Chabalewski, F., Blount, T., et al. (1999). A critical pathway: Guiding care for organ donors. *Critical Care Nurse, 19*(2), 84–88, 90–100.

Kaba, E., Thompson, D. R., & Burnard, P. (2000). Coping after heart transplantation: A descriptive study of heart transplant recipients' methods of coping. *Journal of Advanced Nursing, 32,* 930–936.

Krause, E., Shamp, J., & Bensing, K. (October 22, 2001). Cardiac rehabilitation: After the crisis. *Advance for Nurses,* 15–17.

Lewis, D. D., & Valerius, W. (1999). Organs from non-heart-beating donors: An answer to the organ shortage. *Critical Care Nurse, 19*(2), 70–74.

Ley, S. J. (2001). Keeping pace. Cardiac surgery 2001: What's hot, what's not. *Progress in Cardiovascular Nursing, 16*(3), 132–133.

Mann, D. (2001). Moving toward better bypass surgery: Surgeons report better results when they operate on beating hearts. [On-line.] Available: http://www.my.webmd.com/content/Article/30/1728_72285.htm.

Mason, V. F., & Miller, K. H. (2001). Optimizing outcomes: Nurses caring for patients after cardiac surgery can promote early transfers. *American Journal of Nursing, 101*(5, Suppl.), 13–15, 48–50.

Morse, C. J. (2001). Advance practice nursing in heart transplantation. *Progress in Cardiovascular Nursing, 16*(1), 21–24, 38.

National Heart, Lung, and Blood Institute. (1997). Facts about heart and heart-lung transplants. [On-line.] Available: http://www.nhlbi.nih.gov/health/public/heart/other/hrt_lung.htm.

Popernack, M. L. (2000). Are we overlooking a hidden source of organs? *Nursing 2000, 30*(1), 44–47.

Rembacz, J. M., & Abel, C. J. (2000). Pericardial tamponade. *American Journal of Nursing, 100*(9, Suppl.), 10–14.

chapter 32

Introduction to the Hematopoietic and Lymphatic Systems

Words to Know 

agranulocytes
basophils
eosinophils
erythrocytes
erythropoietin
granulocytes
hematopoiesis
hemoglobin
leukocytes
leukocytosis
leukopenia
lymph
lymphatics
lymph nodes
lymphocytes
neutrophils
phagocytosis
plasma
platelets
pluripotential stem cells

Learning Objectives

On completion of this chapter, the reader will:

- Describe the process of hematopoiesis.
- Name the types and function of blood cells produced by bone marrow.
- List components of plasma.
- Describe the function of plasma proteins.
- Discuss the importance of transfusing compatible blood types.
- Explain the function of the lymphatic system and its role in hematopoiesis.
- Discuss pertinent assessments of the hematopoietic and lymphatic systems when obtaining a health history and conducting a physical examination.
- Describe laboratory and diagnostic tests for disorders of the hematopoietic and lymphatic systems.
- Discuss the nursing management of clients with hematopoietic or lymphatic disorders.

Hematopoiesis is the manufacture and development of blood cells. The hematopoietic system consists of bone marrow, where most blood cells are produced, and the lymphatic system, which includes the thymus gland and spleen.

Bone marrow is the substance in the interior of the long bones and spongy bones of the skeleton. The types of bone marrow are (1) red marrow and (2) yellow marrow. Red marrow is primarily found in the ribs, sternum, skull, clavicle, vertebrae, proximal ends of the long bones, and iliac crest. It manufactures blood cells and hemoglobin. Yellow marrow consists primarily of fat cells and connective tissue. It does not participate in blood cell production, but can form blood cells under conditions involving intense stimulation, such as after significant blood loss (hemorrhage). Lymphoid tissue, which includes the thymus gland and spleen, also plays a role in hematopoiesis.

HEMATOPOIETIC SYSTEM

• ANATOMY AND PHYSIOLOGY

Blood consists of cells suspended in a fluid called plasma (Fig. 32.1). All blood cells are produced from undifferentiated precursors called **pluripotential stem cells** in the bone marrow. Myeloid stem cells are converted to (1) **erythrocytes,** which are red blood cells (RBCs); (2) several types of **leukocytes,** or white blood cells (WBCs); and (3) **platelets,** also known as *thrombocytes* because they help control bleeding by forming a loose blood clot.

Lymphoid stem cells are converted to **lymphocytes,** WBCs with immune functions. Each component of blood has specialized functions (Table 32.1).

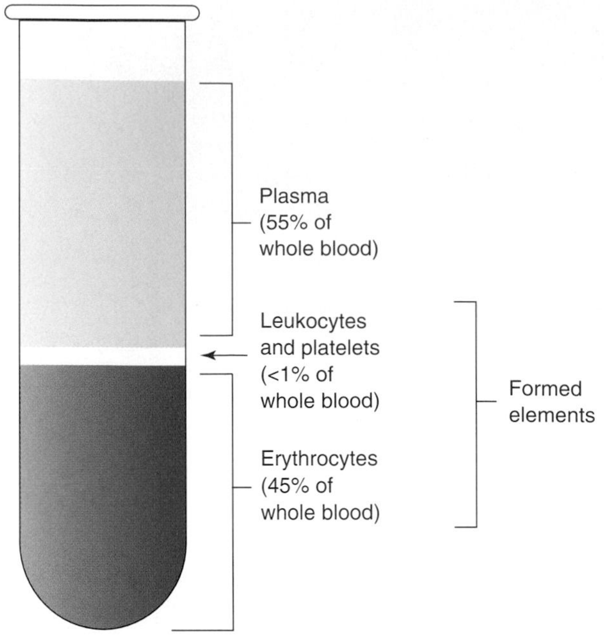

FIGURE 32.1 Components of blood.

TABLE 32.1 COMPONENTS OF BLOOD

COMPONENT	FUNCTION
Blood Cells	
Erythrocytes (red blood cells)	Transport oxygen
Leukocytes (white blood cells)	Protect against infection
Platelets (thrombocytes)	Participate in clotting blood
Plasma	
Water	Circulates blood cells and noncellular components Contributes to blood pressure Relocates to other fluid compartments as needed
Plasma proteins	
Albumin	Affects intravascular osmotic pressure
Fibrinogen	Participates in clotting blood
Globulin	Carries other protein substances, for example, those that are involved in inflammatory and immune responses
Clotting factors	Convert a loose blood clot to a stabilized blood clot
Nutrients	
Glucose	Provides a source of immediate energy
Amino acids	Provide components for cell growth and repair
Lipids	Provide a reserve for cellular energy in the absence of glucose
Vitamins	Participate in essential physiologic functions
Electrolytes	Facilitate a variety of biochemical actions
Hormones	Perform multiple endocrine functions
Wastes (carbon dioxide, drug metabolites)	Prevent toxicity when biotransformed and excreted

Erythrocytes

Erythrocytes are flexible, anuclear (lacking a nucleus), biconcave disks covered by a thin membrane through which oxygen and carbon dioxide (CO_2) pass freely. The flexibility of erythrocytes allows them to change shape as they travel through capillaries. Their major function is to transport oxygen to and remove CO_2 from tissues.

Production of erythrocytes is called *erythropoiesis.* The rate of erythrocyte production is regulated by **erythropoietin,** a hormone released by the kidneys. Erythrocytes arise from myeloid stem cells, which requires iron and B vitamins such as B_{12}, B_6, and folic acid to mature properly. Immature erythrocytes, known as *erythroblasts,* go through several intermediary stages of maturation before being released into the blood. In their immature state, erythroblasts contain a nucleus; mature erythrocytes have no nucleus.

The normal number of erythrocytes varies with age, sex, and altitude but is between 3.6 and 5.4 million/µL. Infants have more erythrocytes than adults; women have fewer erythrocytes than men. People who live at high altitudes or engage in strenuous activity have an increased number of erythrocytes.

The red color of blood is caused by **hemoglobin,** an iron-containing pigment attached to erythrocytes. The heme portion of the molecule freely binds with oxygen, forming a substance called *oxyhemoglobin.* Hemoglobin carries oxygen to the cells. In adults, normal hemoglobin is 12 to 17.4 g/dL. As erythrocytes pass through the lungs, hemoglobin picks up oxygen and releases CO_2. Oxygenated blood is bright red and carried by arteries, arterioles, and capillaries to all body tissues. After hemoglobin releases oxygen for use by the tissues, it is called *reduced* (or *deoxygenated*) *hemoglobin.* The blood becomes dark red and returns by way of veins to the heart and lungs, where CO_2 is released and blood is reoxygenated.

Erythrocytes circulate in the blood for about 120 days, after which the spleen removes them; the liver removes severely damaged erythrocytes. When erythrocytes are destroyed, the iron component of hemoglobin is returned to the red marrow and reused. Residual pigment is stored in the liver as bilirubin and excreted in bile.

Leukocytes

Leukocytes perform various protective functions such as engulfing invading microorganisms and cellular debris,

TABLE 32.2 DIFFERENTIAL WHITE BLOOD CELL COUNT

	PERCENT OF TOTAL WBCs	NUMERIC RANGE (mL)
Neutrophils	60–70	3000–7000
Basophils	1–4	50–400
Eosinophils	0.5–1	25–100
Lymphocytes	20–40	1000–4000
Monocytes	2–6	100–600

and manufacturing antibodies (see Chap. 35). They circulate in blood but also migrate from the blood into body tissues to search for and destroy potentially harmful substances.

Normal leukocyte count is between 5000 and 10,000/mm^3. An increased number of leukocytes is called **leukocytosis;** a decreased number is called **leukopenia.** Table 32.2 shows the differential leukocyte count. The life span of leukocytes is only 1 to 2 days; consequently, demand for the production of WBCs is continuous, and even greater with an infection. Leukocytes are divided into two categories: **granulocytes,** which contain cytoplasmic granules, and **agranulocytes,** which do not contain granules (Fig. 32.2).

Granulocytes, or *polymorphonuclear leukocytes,* are divided into three subgroups: neutrophils, basophils, and eosinophils. **Neutrophils,** a major component of the inflammatory response and defense against bacterial infection, are also called *microphages.* They protect the body by **phagocytosis,** the ingestion and digestion of bacteria and foreign substances (Fig. 32.3). Immature neutrophils, called *band cells,* circulate in peripheral blood.

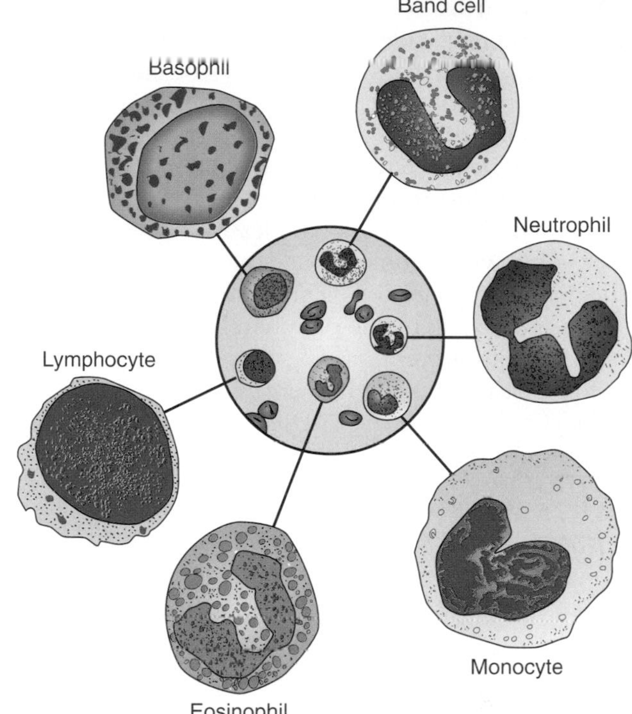

FIGURE 32.2 White blood cells.

Basophils are also capable of phagocytosis and are active in allergic contact dermatitis (immediate hypersensitivity) and some delayed hypersensitivity reactions. **Eosinophils** phagocytize foreign material. Their numbers increase in allergies, some dermatologic disorders, and parasitic infections.

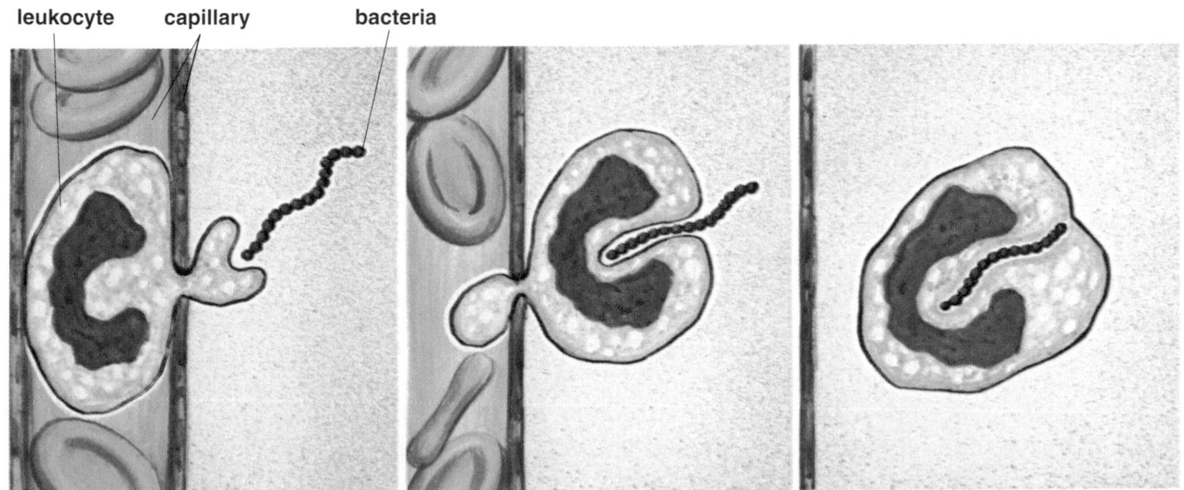

FIGURE 32.3 Phagocytosis. The cell membrane of the neutrophil surrounds and pinches off the bacteria or dead tissue. Enzymes within the cell destroy the foreign material. (From Smeltzer, S. C. & Bare, B. G. [2004]. *Brunner & Suddarth's textbook of medical-surgical nursing* [10th ed.]. Philadelphia: Lippincott Williams & Wilkins.)

Agranulocytes are divided into two groups: *lymphocytes* and *monocytes.* Lymphocytes are divided into *B lymphocytes* (or B cells), which provide humoral immunity by producing antibodies (immunoglobulins), and *T lymphocytes* (or T cells), which provide cellular immunity (or cell-mediated response). B lymphocytes produce antibodies against foreign antigens, and T lymphocytes interact with foreign cells and release a substance called *lymphokine,* which enhances actions of phagocytic cells. Some lymphoid stem cells mature in the bone marrow, whereas others migrate to peripheral lymphoid tissue to complete their maturation.

Monocytes, also known as *macrophages* because they phagocytize large-sized debris, fight severe infections and are part of the immune response.

Platelets

Platelets (*thrombocytes*), disklike, non-nucleated cell fragments with a life span of approximately 7.5 days, are manufactured in the red bone marrow. Approximately two thirds of the total 150,000 to 350,000/mm^3 platelets circulate in the blood and contribute to hemostasis. The remaining one third are in the spleen, where they remain unless needed in cases of significant bleeding. When a blood vessel is injured, platelets migrate to the injury site. They release a substance known as glycoprotein IIb/IIIa, causing the platelets to adhere (platelet aggregation) and form a plug, or clot, that occludes the injured vessel.

Plasma

Plasma is the liquid, or serum, portion of blood, consisting of 90% water and 10% proteins. Besides blood cells, plasma contains and transports proteins (albumin, globulins, and fibrinogen), clotting factors like prothrombin, pigments, vitamins, glucose, lipids, electrolytes, minerals, enzymes, and hormones.

Plasma Proteins

Albumin, formed in the liver, is the most abundant protein in plasma. Under normal conditions, albumin cannot pass through a capillary wall. Consequently, albumin helps maintain the osmotic pressure that retains fluid in the vascular compartment.

Globulins are divided into three groups: alpha, beta, and gamma. The gamma globulins are also called *immunoglobulins.* Globulins function primarily as immunologic agents, preventing or modifying some types of infectious diseases. They also help maintain osmotic pressure in the vascular compartment.

Fibrinogen, the largest plasma protein, plays a key role in forming blood clots. It can be transformed from a liquid to fibrin, a solid that controls bleeding.

Blood Groups

There are four blood groups or types, A, B, AB, and O, determined by heredity. Blood is typed by identifying the protein, or *antigen,* on the red cell membranes. Group A has A antigen, group B has B antigen, group AB has A and B antigen, and group O has no antigen. *Antibodies,* immunoglobulins in plasma that inactivate any substance that is nonself, react with incompatible RBC antigens. People with type O blood are universal donors because they do not have antigens on the red cell membrane. People with type AB blood are universal recipients because they are compatible with blood types A, B, and O.

The Rh factor is a specific protein on the RBC membrane. If the protein is present, the person is Rh positive. If the protein is absent, the person is Rh negative. When blood is transfused, donor blood must be type and Rh compatible with the recipient's blood. The donor's blood is typed and labeled at the time of donation. The recipient's blood is typed and crossmatched (matched for compatibility with donor blood). Donor and recipient blood are considered compatible if there is no clumping or *hemolysis* (destruction of erythrocytes) when both samples are mixed in the laboratory. In an emergency, type O blood is given to recipients with type A, B, AB, or O. People with Rh-positive blood can receive Rh-positive or Rh-negative blood because Rh negative indicates the Rh factor is missing; those with Rh-negative blood, however, must never receive Rh-positive blood.

Stop, Think, and Respond ● BOX 32-1

When you go to the hospital's blood bank to obtain a unit of blood for a client with blood type A, Rh-positive blood, you receive a unit of blood that is blood type A, Rh negative. Is this unit of blood compatible? Explain your answer.

LYMPHATIC SYSTEM

● ANATOMY AND PHYSIOLOGY

The lymphatic system includes the thymus gland, spleen, and a network of lymphatic vessels, lymph nodes, and lymph. This system of **lymphatics** circulates interstitial fluid and carries it to the veins (Fig. 32.4). Along the pathway, the lymphatic system filters and destroys pathogens and removes other potentially harmful substances.

Thymus Gland

The thymus gland is lymphatic tissue in the upper chest that contains undifferentiated stem cells released from

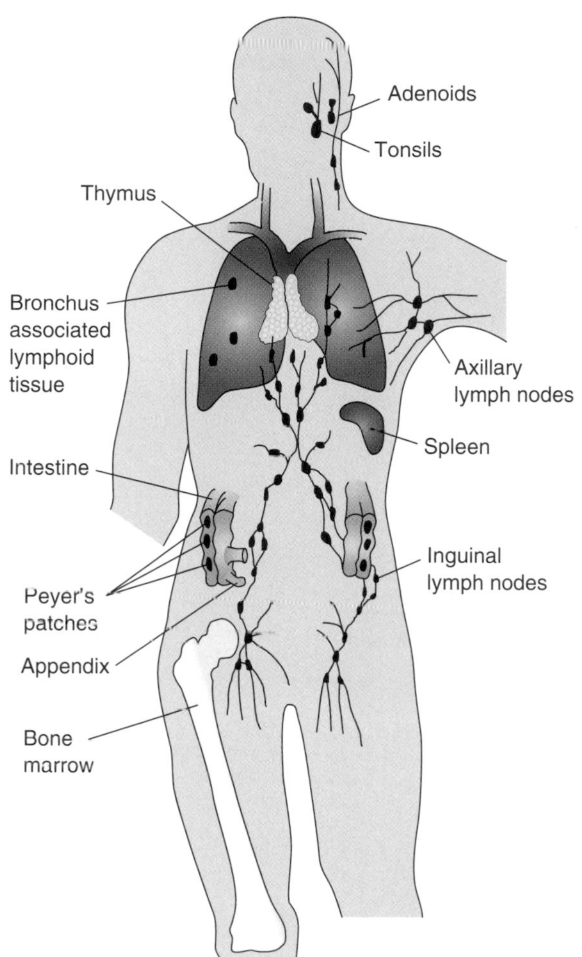

FIGURE 32.4 Central and peripheral lymphoid organs and tissues.

bone marrow. Once the undifferentiated cells migrate to the thymus gland, they develop into *T lymphocytes* because they are thymus derived (Fig. 32.5).

Spleen

The spleen is the largest lymphatic structure. It lies in the abdomen beneath the diaphragm and behind the stomach. The spleen is a reservoir of blood and contains phagocytes that engulf damaged erythrocytes and foreign substances.

Lymph Nodes

Lymph nodes, glandular tissue along the lymphatic network, are clustered in the axilla, groin, neck, and large vessels of the thorax and abdomen. Lymphatic ducts, through which lymph flows, connect the nodes. The nodes contain both T and B lymphocytes in the smaller nodules of each lymph node.

Lymph

Lymph is fluid with a similar composition to plasma. It flows through lymphatics by contraction of skeletal muscles. Lymph enters each node by way of the afferent lymph duct, passes through the node, and leaves by the efferent lymph duct. As lymph passes through the node, macrophages attack and engulf foreign substances like bacteria and viruses, abnormal body cells, and other debris.

ASSESSMENT

The nurse collects data by taking a health history, examining the client, and monitoring results of laboratory tests.

History

The health history includes the client's description of signs and symptoms. If abnormalities are present, determine when the signs or symptoms began, their severity, and frequency. In relation to the hematopoietic and lymphatic systems, it is especially important to establish if the client experiences prolonged bleeding from an injury; has unexplained blood loss as in rectal bleeding, nosebleeds, bleeding gums, or vomiting blood; feels fatigued with normal activities; becomes dizzy or faints; bruises easily; is easily chilled; has frequent infections; feels discomfort in the axilla, groin, or neck; has difficulty swallowing with localized throat tenderness; or has had surgery with lymph node removal or splenectomy, is undergoing treatment for cancer, or has renal failure—all of which may affect blood cell volume or lymphatic circulation.

Take a drug history of prescribed and nonprescribed medications. Some antibiotics and cancer drugs contribute to hematopoietic dysfunction. Aspirin and anticoagulants can contribute to bleeding and interfere with clot formation. Because industrial materials, environmental toxins, and household products also can affect blood-forming organs, the nurse explores any exposure to these agents. Ask about foreign travel to countries where infectious agents may cause anemia (malaria) or occlude lymph vessels (roundworms). Obtain a dietary history because compromised nutrition interferes with production of blood cells and hemoglobin.

Physical Examination

Physical examination includes inspection of the skin with particular attention to color (e.g., normal, extreme redness, pallor), temperature, and ecchymosis or other lesions. A rapid pulse rate can indicate reduced erythrocytes or inadequate hemoglobin levels.

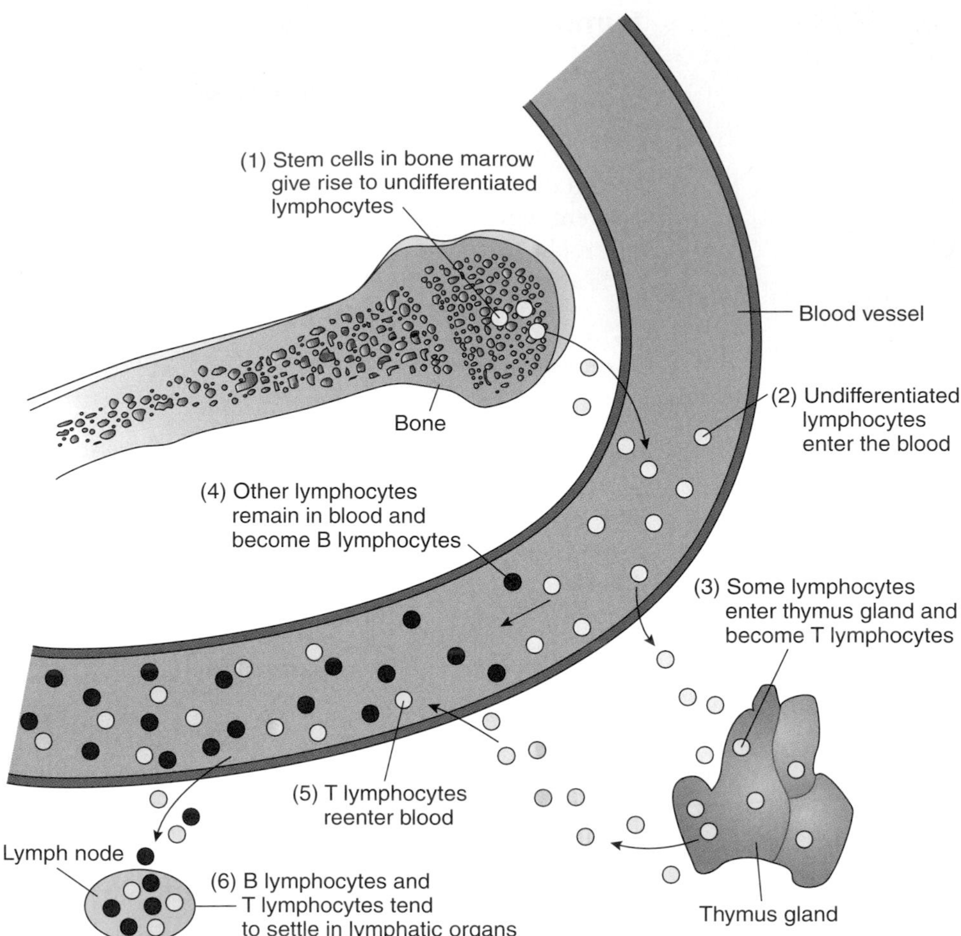

FIGURE 32.5 Transformation of T and B lymphocytes.

Palpate lymph nodes in the neck for tenderness or swelling and note size, location, and characteristics of symptomatic lymph nodes. Examine skin adjacent to the node for redness, streaking, and swelling. Inspect the tonsils for size and appearance. Examine extremities to determine if they are of similar size—obstruction of lymphatic circulation can cause unilateral enlargement.

Diagnostic Tests

Laboratory tests include a complete blood count and tests that reflect the client's blood clotting status such as prothrombin time, fibrinogen level, activated partial thromboplastin time, D-dimer test for fibrin, fibrin degradation products, and factor assays.

A bone marrow aspiration is performed to determine the status of blood cell formation. The marrow is examined for the types and percentage of immature and maturing blood cells. The nurse assists the physician, supports the client during a bone marrow aspiration, and monitors his or her status afterward (Nursing Guidelines 32-1).

The Schilling test is performed to diagnose pernicious anemia, macrocytic anemia, and malabsorption syndromes. Radioactive vitamin B_{12} is given orally, followed in 1 hour by an injection of nonradioactive B_{12}. All urine is collected for 24 to 48 hours after the client receives the nonradioactive B_{12}. Little or no vitamin B_{12} in the urine indicates absence of the intrinsic factor or defective absorption of vitamin B_{12} from the intestinal tract.

Lymphatic disorders are diagnosed using procedures such as lymph node biopsy, ultrasound of the spleen or selected lymph nodes, and lymphangiography (radiographic examination using contrast media). Additional diagnostic tests include radiography, computed tomography, bone scan, and magnetic resonance imaging. Although they are not specific for hematologic or lymphatic disorders, they are used to rule out other disorders or note changes in organs that have a direct or indirect relationship to a hematologic or lymphatic disorder.

NURSING MANAGEMENT

Collect appropriate data to assist the physician in diagnosing hematologic or lymphatic disorders and the client's response to treatment. Before any diagnostic testing, determine the client's knowledge of the procedure and offer a description of the test routine, what tasks are necessary to participate in the test, and what discomfort is likely.

NURSING GUIDELINES 32-1

Assisting With a Bone Marrow Aspiration

- Inform the client of the plan and approximate time for the bone marrow aspiration. Allow time to answer questions.
- Witness the client's signature on a consent form.
- Check the client's medical record for history of allergies, especially to local anesthetics or latex.
- Obtain a sterile bone marrow aspiration tray and add the type and strength of local anesthetic according to the physician's orders.
- Determine the site from which the physician intends to obtain the sample of bone marrow.
- Position the client on his or her back or side to facilitate access to the aspiration site.
- Suggest distraction techniques to avoid focusing on the pressure or discomfort associated with puncturing the bone.
- Label the specimen and ensure its delivery to the laboratory.
- Follow Standard Precautions when there is a potential for contact with blood from the client, equipment, and bedside environment.
- Limit the client's activity for approximately 30 minutes after the procedure.
- Monitor the puncture site frequently for continued bleeding; change or reinforce the dressing as needed.
- Report prolonged bleeding, unusual pain at the site, and signs of an infection.

Wear gloves when collecting specimens. After collection, check the specimen for the correct label and immediately take it to the laboratory. When the test involves a puncture, assess the area for excessive bleeding and apply pressure or a pressure dressing to the site as needed. Monitor vital signs to assess the client's recovery, notify the physician regarding adverse responses, and analyze and report test results promptly.

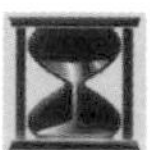

GENERAL GERONTOLOGIC CONSIDERATIONS

The components of blood change only slightly with age. RBCs become slightly less flexible and fewer in number.

With age, lymphocytes decrease in number, causing a decreased resistance to infection.

The Schilling test may pose a problem in older adults if proper collection of the 24-hour specimen is not possible as a result of cognitive problems or urinary incontinence.

Critical Thinking Exercises

1. *Describe the process of blood cell formation.*
2. *Describe the nurse's responsibilities when assisting with bone marrow aspiration.*
3. *Three clients have the following blood count values:*
   Client A = 80,000 platelets
   Client B = 2,400,000 RBCs
   Client C = 24,500 WBCs
   After notifying the physician, what precautions are appropriate to institute?

• NCLEX-STYLE REVIEW QUESTIONS 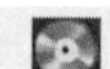

1. A physician tells a client that her body is not making enough blood cells. After the physician leaves, the client appears very upset and states, "I do not even know how my body is supposed to make blood cells." The simplest, yet correct, instruction for the nurse to give the client at this time is that:
   1. Complex mechanisms within the body make blood cells.
   2. The bone marrow produces blood cells.
   3. Blood cells originate from a healthy immune system.
   4. The lymphatic system produces blood cells.
2. After completion of a bone marrow aspiration, it is essential that the nurse monitor:
   1. Fluctuations in the blood pressure
   2. Bleeding from the puncture site
   3. Changes in the client's pulse
   4. The client's level of consciousness

connection

Visit the Connection site at **http://connection.lww.com/go/timbyEssentials** for links to chapter-related resources on the Internet.

References and Suggested Readings

Call-Schmidt, T. (2001). Interpreting lab results: A primer. *MEDSURG Nursing, 10,* 179–184.

Cohen, B. J., & Wood, D. L. (1999). *Memmler's the human body in health and disease* (9th ed.). Philadelphia: Lippincott Williams & Wilkins.

Fischbach, F. T. (1999). *A manual of laboratory and diagnostic tests* (6th ed.). Philadelphia: Lippincott Williams & Wilkins.

Malloy, B. J. (2000). Hematopoiesis, stem cells, and transplantation: What have we learned for the new millennium? *Journal of Intravenous Nursing, 23,* 298–303.

Martini, F. H. (2001). *Fundamentals of anatomy and physiology* (5th ed.). Englewood Cliffs, NJ: Prentice Hall.

McConnell, E. A. (2000). Clinical do's and don'ts: Infusing packed RBCs. *Nursing 2000, 30*(2), 17.

Porth, C. M. (2002). *Pathophysiology: Concepts of altered health states* (6th ed.). Philadelphia: Lippincott Williams & Wilkins.

Wolf, S. (1999). Evolutions/revolutions: Another source of stem cells. *RN, 62*(9), 30–34.

chapter 33

Caring for Clients With Disorders of the Hematopoietic System

Words to Know 

agranulocytosis
anemia
aplasia
blood dyscrasias
coagulopathies
erythrocytosis
heme
leukocytosis
leukopenia
pancytopenia
thrombocytopenia

Learning Objectives

On completion of this chapter, the reader will:

- List types of anemia, including examples of inherited types.
- Identify nutritional deficiencies that can lead to anemia.
- Discuss clinical problems that clients with any type of anemia experience.
- Explain *erythrocytosis,* with characteristics of the disease, and possible complications.
- Explain how forms of leukemia are classified.
- List clinical problems or nursing diagnoses common among clients with leukemia.
- Explain the term *pancytopenia* and give one example of a disorder that represents this condition.
- Discuss the meaning of coagulopathy.
- Discuss nursing responsibilities when managing the care of clients with thrombocytopenia.

This chapter discusses common **blood dyscrasias,** abnormalities in the numbers and types of blood cells, and **coagulopathies,** bleeding disorders that involve platelets or clotting factors. These disorders develop from various pathologic processes, some of which are life-threatening. Despite their differences, many blood disorders have similar symptoms and require similar diagnostic tests.

ANEMIA

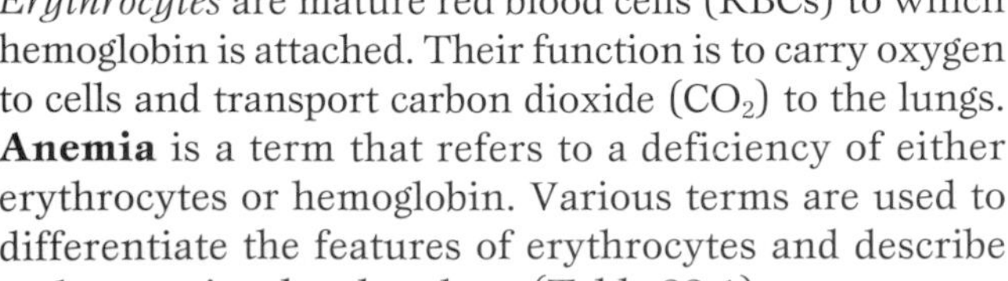

Erythrocytes are mature red blood cells (RBCs) to which hemoglobin is attached. Their function is to carry oxygen to cells and transport carbon dioxide (CO_2) to the lungs. **Anemia** is a term that refers to a deficiency of either erythrocytes or hemoglobin. Various terms are used to differentiate the features of erythrocytes and describe pathogenesis related to them (Table 33.1).

Most anemias result from (1) blood loss, (2) inadequate or abnormal erythrocyte production, or (3) destruction of normally formed RBCs. The most common types include hypovolemic anemia, iron deficiency anemia, pernicious anemia, folic acid deficiency anemia, sickle cell anemia, and hemolytic anemias. Although each form of anemia has unique manifestations, all share a common core of symptoms (Fig. 33.1).

• HYPOVOLEMIC ANEMIA

Hypovolemia is caused by loss of blood volume, resulting in fewer blood cells. Because erythrocytes are the most abundant type of blood cell, a consequence of blood loss is *hypovolemic anemia.*

Pathophysiology and Etiology

Hypovolemic anemia results from a sudden loss of a large volume of blood (e.g., trauma from a knife wound) or a

TABLE 33.1 TERMS USED TO DESCRIBE ERYTHROCYTES AND ERYTHROCYTE PATHOLOGY

DESCRIPTOR	MEANING
Normocytic	Normal cell size
Microcytic	Small cell size
Macrocytic	Large cell size
Megaloblastic	Large immature cell
Normochromic	Normal hemoglobin concentration
Hypochromic	Low hemoglobin concentration
Hyperchromic	High hemoglobin concentration
Aplastic	Decreased cell production
Hemolytic	Premature destruction
Pernicious	Potentially injurious

chronic loss of small amounts of blood (e.g., gastric bleeding from a peptic ulcer). When blood is lost, bone marrow responds by increasing its number of erythrocytes. Cells are smaller (microcytic) and contain less **heme** (hypochromic), the pigmented, iron-containing portion of hemoglobin. If formation of new RBCs cannot compensate for the loss, cellular function is compromised from inadequate oxygen supply and accumulated CO_2.

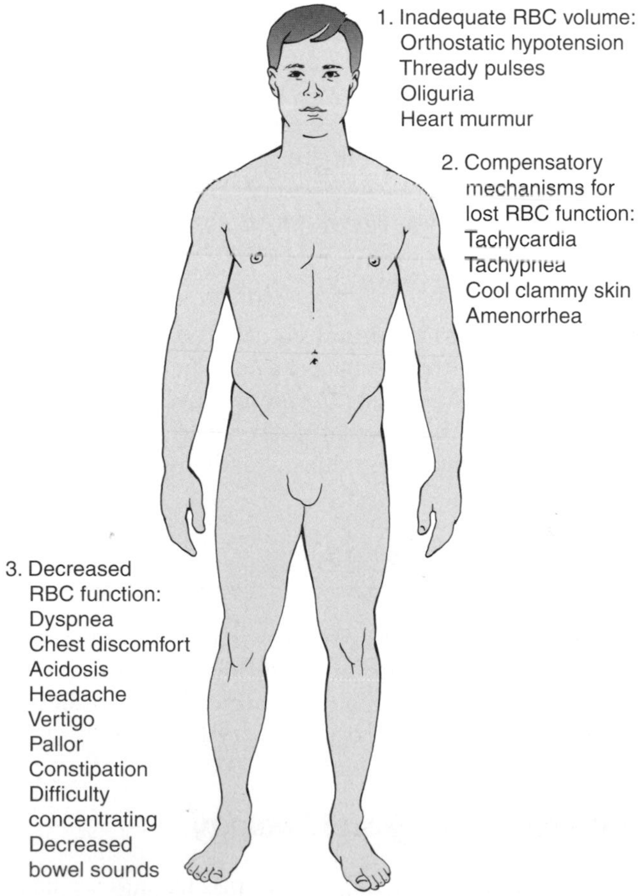

FIGURE 33.1 Clinical manifestations of anemia.

Assessment Findings

Acute hypovolemic anemia from severe blood loss is evidenced by signs and symptoms of hypovolemic shock: extreme pallor, tachycardia, hypotension, reduced urine output, and altered consciousness (see Chap. 20). Symptoms of chronic hypovolemic anemia include pallor, fatigue, chills, postural hypotension, and rapid heart and respiratory rates.

Laboratory confirmation of acute or chronic hypovolemic anemia is detected through a complete blood count (CBC), which demonstrates decreased erythrocytes, increased *reticulocytes* (erythrocytes in the process of maturation), and low hemoglobin and hematocrit levels (Table 33.2). Mean cell volume is lower than normal as a result of the smaller size of the erythrocytes. The mean cell hemoglobin concentration is below normal, reflecting the reduced hemoglobin level.

Medical Management

Treatment of sudden, severe bleeding involves replacement of blood by transfusions. If blood loss is chronic (e.g., from bleeding uterine tumors, peptic ulcer disease, hemorrhoids), the underlying condition is treated. Depending on how much blood is lost, treatment includes blood transfusion or administration of oral, intravenous (IV), or intramuscular (IM) iron to help the body compensate for the lost hemoglobin. Oxygen therapy sometimes is necessary if the anemia is severe.

NURSING PROCESS

● The Client With Hypovolemic Anemia

Assessment

Question the client to determine possible reasons for the presenting symptoms, obtain vital signs, review laboratory test results, prepare the client for diagnostic tests such as endoscopic examinations, and perform a physical examination to detect sources of bleeding.

Diagnosis, Planning, and Interventions

PC: Hypovolemia

Expected Outcome: The nurse will monitor to detect hypovolemia and manage and minimize blood loss.

- Monitor the results of CBC, especially RBC count and hematocrit and hemoglobin levels. *Lower than normal RBCs and hemoglobin level reflect blood cell loss. The*

TABLE 33.2 NORMAL CBC VALUES

COMPONENT	ADULT MALES	ADULT FEMALES
Red blood cells (erythrocytes)	4.6–6.2 million/mm³	4.2–5.4 million/mm³
Hematocrit	40%–54%	38%–47%
Hemoglobin	13.5–18 g/dL	12–16 g/dL
Mean cell volume (MCV)	80–94 µg/m³	81–99 µg/m³
Mean cell hemoglobin (MCH)	27–31 picograms/cell	27–31 picograms/cell
Mean cell hemoglobin concentration (MCHC)	32–36 g/dL	32–36 g/dL
Reticulocytes	0.5%–2.0% of RBCs	Slightly higher in females
White blood cells (leukocytes)	5000–13,000/mm³	5000–10,000/mm³
Neutrophils	3000–7500/mm³	3000–7500/mm³
Eosinophils	50–400/mm³	50–400/mm³
Basophils	25–100/mm³	25–100/mm³
Monocytes	100–500/mm³	100–500/mm³
Lymphocytes	1500–4500/mm³	1500–4500/mm³
T lymphocytes	60%–80% of lymphocytes	60%–80% of lymphocytes
B lymphocytes	10%–20% of lymphocytes	10%–20% of lymphocytes
Platelets	150,000–450,000/mm³	150,000–450,000/mm³

hematocrit level indicates the percentage of RBCs in the volume of whole blood.

- Report systolic blood pressure (BP) below 90 mm Hg and heart rate above 100 beats/minute (bpm). *Hypotension and tachycardia are signs of hypovolemia.*
- Report urine output less than 30 to 50 mL/hour. *Low urine volume reflects decreased circulating blood volume and inadequate renal perfusion. The kidneys must excrete 30 to 50 mL/hour or 500 mL/24 hours to eliminate wastes sufficiently.*
- Use Standard Precautions to examine and test stool and body fluids for evidence of blood. *Blood may be occult (hidden) rather than obvious. Nurses commonly perform tests to detect blood in stool and body fluids.*
- In cases of hemorrhage, apply direct pressure to the bleeding site. Alternatively, apply pressure to a proximal artery. *Compression of blood vessels decreases blood loss.*
- Place the client in a modified Trendelenburg position if hypovolemic shock develops. *Facilitates blood flow to the brain.*
- Supplement parenteral fluids with oral fluids, if possible. *Oral fluids contribute to intravascular fluid replacement.*

PC: Hypoxemia

Expected Outcome: The nurse will monitor to detect hypoxemia and manage and minimize inadequate oxygenation.

- Monitor oxygen saturation with a pulse oximeter. *It measures the percentage of oxygen bound to hemoglobin.*
- Report a sustained oxygen saturation value below 90%. *Normal oxygen saturation is 95% to 100%; clients become compromised when oxygen saturation falls below 90%.*
- Give oxygen per nasal cannula or simple mask to maintain oxygen saturation at or above 90%. *Supplemental oxygen delivers more than the 21% oxygen of room air.*

Activity Intolerance related to reduced cellular capacity to carry oxygen

Expected Outcomes: The client will (1) tolerate essential activity as evidenced by a heart rate below 100 bpm and (2) have a respiratory rate less than 28 breaths/minute.

- Limit the client's nonessential activities. *Reduces demand for oxygen.*
- Distribute essential tasks over a long period. *Promotes endurance.*
- Provide periods of rest. *Prevents acute hypoxemia.*
- Administer supplemental oxygen during periods of rapid breathing or tachycardia. *Short-term, periodic oxygen administration relieves brief episodes of hypoxemia.*

Evaluation of Expected Outcomes

Blood volume loss is minimized, RBC count and hematocrit level are within normal ranges. The client has 90% or greater saturation of hemoglobin. The client's BP and heart rate are within normal target ranges before, during, and after performing activities of daily living (ADLs).

● HEMOLYTIC ANEMIA

The term *hemolytic anemia* refers to the consequence of a widely diverse group of conditions, some acquired, some hereditary, and some idiopathic, in which there is chronic premature destruction of erythrocytes.

Pathophysiology and Etiology

Examples of conditions that can produce hemolytic anemia are the use of cardiopulmonary bypass during surgery;

arsenic or lead poisoning; invasion of erythrocytes by the malaria parasite, infectious agents; or toxins and exposure to hazardous chemicals. Other causes include the production of antibodies that destroy erythrocytes. Antibodies can be produced against antigens from another person, such as is seen in blood transfusion reactions, as well as against the body's own erythrocytes. As the number of destroyed blood cells increases, the potential for hyperbilirubinemia (excess bilirubin) and jaundice also increases.

Assessment Findings

Symptoms are similar to those associated with hypovolemic anemia. In more severe forms of hemolytic anemia, the client is jaundiced and the spleen is enlarged. In some cases, hemolysis is so extensive that it causes shock.

Microscopic examination reveals erythrocyte fragments. When an erythrocyte survival study is performed using radioactive chromium, the life span of erythrocytes is 10 days or less. Reaction on a direct Coombs' test (direct antiglobulin test) is positive when the hemolytic anemia results from a transfusion reaction, use of certain drugs, or production of antibodies against the erythrocytes.

Medical and Surgical Management

Treatment includes removing the cause (when possible) and administering corticosteroids. In some cases the steroid dose can be reduced and then discontinued after several weeks. Blood transfusions often are necessary. Splenectomy is performed if the client fails to respond to medical treatment.

Nursing Management

Obtain a comprehensive health history to help determine the cause of the hemolysis. Until the cause is determined, provide supportive care to help the client meet basic needs. When the diagnosis is confirmed, implement the medical regimen for treatment and prepare the client for discharge by teaching measures for self-care. Arrange the plan for follow-up evaluations and share the information with the client.

• PERNICIOUS ANEMIA

Pernicious anemia develops when a client lacks intrinsic factor, which normally is present in stomach secretions. Intrinsic factor is necessary for absorption of vitamin B_{12}. Vitamin B_{12}, the extrinsic factor in blood, is required for the maturation of erythrocytes.

Pathophysiology and Etiology

The production of intrinsic factor decreases with aging and gastric mucosal atrophy. It also decreases secondary to surgical removal of the stomach or small bowel resection, in which the ileum (site for vitamin B_{12} absorption) is removed. Without adequate vitamin B_{12}, erythrocytes remain in an immature form. If the condition is not recognized and treated promptly, degenerative changes in the nervous system develop. Sometimes permanent damage occurs before treatment begins.

Assessment Findings

In addition to the usual symptoms of anemia, some clients with pernicious anemia develop stomatitis (inflammation of the mouth) and glossitis (inflammation of the tongue), digestive disturbances, and diarrhea. Anemia may be so severe that dyspnea occurs with minimal exertion. Jaundice, irritability, confusion, and depression are present when the disease is severe. Mental changes usually disappear with treatment. Numbness and tingling in the arms and legs and ataxia are common signs of neurologic involvement. Some affected clients lose vibratory and position senses.

Diagnosis is established by the client's history, symptoms, and blood and bone marrow studies. The Schilling test is used to confirm the diagnosis. Microscopic examination of a blood smear reveals many large, immature erythrocytes.

Medical Management

Vitamin B_{12} is given IM in a dose adequate to control the disease. Therapy must continue for life. No toxic effects have been noted from the use of vitamin B_{12}. Oral vitamin B_{12} seldom is effective, except for short intervals. Iron therapy seldom is needed because mature erythrocytes are manufactured and the hemoglobin level is normal when the condition is corrected. Clients with permanent neurologic deficits benefit from physical therapy.

Nursing Management

If glossitis and stomatitis are present, a soft, bland diet relieves the discomfort associated with eating. Most clients better tolerate small, frequent meals than three large meals. Meticulous oral care after eating is essential to remove particles of food that may irritate the mucosal lining and increase soreness.

If a permanent neurologic deficit has occurred, encourage the client to move about as much as possible to prevent complications associated with immobility, such as contractures and pressure ulcer formation. Assistance with ambulation is necessary because some clients have difficulty walking and are prone to falling. If behavioral changes occur, close supervision is necessary. Emphasize the importance of lifelong administration of vitamin B_{12}. Teach a family member of the client how to administer vitamin B_{12} injections or refer the client to a home health nursing service.

FOLIC ACID DEFICIENCY ANEMIA

Folic acid deficiency causes anemia that is characterized by immature erythrocytes.

Pathophysiology and Etiology

A folic acid deficiency commonly is related to an insufficient dietary intake of folic acid (vitamin B_9). Older adults and clients with alcoholism, intestinal disorders that affect food absorption, malignant disorders, and chronic illnesses often have a folic acid deficiency because of poor nutrition. Certain drugs, such as anticonvulsants and methotrexate, are folic acid antagonists and interfere with folic acid absorption. Because pregnant women and clients with chronic hemolytic anemias have increased folic acid requirements, they can experience a folic acid deficiency even when they follow a normal diet. Prolonged IV therapy and total parenteral nutrition also can result in a folic acid deficiency.

Assessment Findings

Severe fatigue, a sore and beefy-red tongue, dyspnea, nausea, anorexia, headaches, weakness, and lightheadedness occur. Blood test results reveal low hemoglobin and hematocrit levels. The serum folate level is decreased. A Schilling test differentiates pernicious anemia and anemia caused by a folic acid deficiency.

Medical Management

Oral or parenteral folic acid supplements are provided. Parenteral administration is required for clients with an intestinal malabsorption disorder. A well-balanced diet that includes foods high in folic acid content such as beef liver, peanut butter, red beans, oatmeal, asparagus, and broccoli is recommended.

Nursing Management

Encourage the client to eat foods high in folic acid. Encourage the eating of soft, bland foods and the performance of good oral hygiene. If fatigue is a prominent symptom, plan adequate rest periods between activities.

ERYTHROCYTOSIS: POLYCYTHEMIA VERA

There are some conditions in which one of the primary characteristics is **erythrocytosis,** an increase in circulating erythrocytes. One of these conditions is *polycythemia vera,* which is characterized by a greater than normal number of erythrocytes, leukocytes, and platelets. For people who live at high altitudes, erythrocytosis is a normal phenomenon and usually requires no treatment.

Pathophysiology and Etiology

Polycythemia vera is associated with a rapid proliferation of blood cells produced by the bone marrow. The cause of this accelerated production is unknown. Polycythemia vera usually has an insidious onset and a prolonged course. Despite the abundance of erythrocytes, their life span is shorter. The dead erythrocytes release intracellular potassium, which can cause hyperkalemia, and uric acid, which causes goutlike joint symptoms. The oxygen-combining capacity of the erythrocytes is impaired, which compromises cellular oxygenation. The increased number of erythrocytes makes the blood more viscous than normal and increases the likelihood for the development of thrombi in small blood vessels. Compli cations include hypertension, congestive heart failure, stroke, areas of infarction, and hemorrhage.

Assessment Findings

The face and lips are reddish-purple. Fatigue, weakness, headache, pruritus, exertional dyspnea, and dizziness are common. Excessive bleeding after minor injuries, perhaps because of engorgement of the capillaries and veins, occurs. Hemorrhoids develop. Splenomegaly (enlargement of the spleen) is common. The joints become swollen and painful because of elevated uric acid levels.

The blood cell count, especially erythrocytes, is elevated, with a similar rise in hemoglobin and hematocrit levels. The platelet and WBC counts are increased. Levels of serum potassium and uric acid are above normal.

Medical Management

Treatment involves measures to reduce the volume of circulating blood, lessen its viscosity, and curb the excessive production of erythrocytes. A phlebotomy (opening a vein to withdraw blood) is done several times a week; 500 mL of blood is removed each time. Anticoagulants are given to reduce potential for forming clots. Radiophosphorus and radiation therapy can be used to decrease production of erythrocytes in the bone marrow. Antineoplastic drugs such as mechlorethamine (Mustargen) are given to curb excessive bone marrow activity.

Nursing Management

Observe the client for complications and provide information about drug therapy and techniques to promote circulation and reduce potential thrombi formation. The plan of care includes the following measures:

- Advise drinking 3 quarts (L) of fluid per day. *Promotes venous return and ensures sufficient urine production.*
- Teach client to avoid crossing the legs at the knee and wearing tight clothing. *Reduces risk for thrombus formation.*
- Encourage the client to be physically active, change positions frequently, and elevate the lower extremities as much as possible. *Promotes the circulation of venous blood.*
- Teach the client how to perform isometric exercises such as contracting and relaxing the quadriceps and gluteal muscles during periods of inactivity. *Compresses the walls of veins and increases the circulation of venous blood as it returns to the heart.*
- Help the client don thromboembolic stockings or support hose during waking hours. *Promotes venous circulation and prevents the formation of thrombi.*
- Tell the client to rest immediately if chest pain develops. *Chest pain indicates myocardial ischemia. Rest reduces the work of the heart and restores sufficient oxygenated blood flow to overcome the temporary deficiency.*

LEUKOCYTOSIS

Leukocytosis is an increased number of leukocytes above normal limits. In wound healing, increased leukocytes serve as a protective mechanism. In some disease conditions such as leukemia the proliferation of leukocytes is detrimental.

• LEUKEMIA

Leukemia refers to any malignant blood disorder in which proliferation of leukocytes, usually in an immature form, is unregulated. There often is an accompanying decrease in production of erythrocytes and platelets. There are four general types of leukemia, classified according to the bone marrow stem cell line that is dysfunctional (Table 33.3). Acute and chronic lymphocytic leukemias result from bone marrow dysfunction that affects lymphoid stem cells; the primary marrow dysfunction in acute and chronic myelocytic leukemia is in myeloid stem cells (Fig. 33.2).

Pathophysiology and Etiology

The cause of leukemia is unknown, although exposures to toxic chemicals and radiation, viruses, and certain drugs are known to precipitate the disorder. In some cases there is a genetic correlation. Although the increase in leukocytes is rampant, there are many more immature than mature cells. Because of their immaturity, the leukocytes are ineffective at fighting infections. Rapid proliferation of leukocytes results in decreased production of erythrocytes and platelets. The client eventually develops severe anemia, and the reduction in platelets leads to bleeding. Excessive leukocytes infiltrate the spleen, liver, lymph nodes, and brain if unchecked.

TABLE 33.3 TYPES OF LEUKEMIA

TYPE	CELLULAR CHARACTERISTICS	AGE OF ONSET (YR)
Acute lymphocytic (ALL)	Increased immature lymphocytes Normal or decreased granulocytes Decreased erythrocytes Decreased platelets	Younger than 5; uncommon after 15
Chronic lymphocytic (CLL)	Same as above, but erythrocyte and platelet counts may be normal or low	Older than 40; most common type in adults
Acute myelogenous (AML)	Decrease in all myeloid formed cells: monocytes, granulocytes, erythrocytes, and platelets	Occurs in all age ranges
Chronic myelogenous (CML)	Same as above, but greater number of normal cells than in acute form	Older than 20, but incidence increases with age; genetic link in 90% to 95% of cases

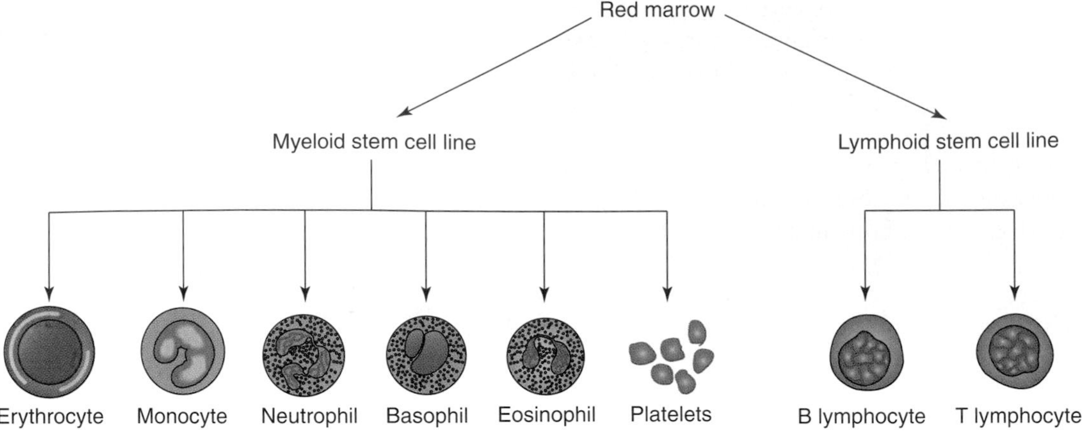

FIGURE 33.2 Maturation of myeloid and lymphoid stem cells.

Assessment Findings

Infections, fatigue from anemia, and easy bruising are hallmarks of leukemia. At the onset of leukemia, particularly in acute lymphocytic leukemia (ALL), a fever is present, the spleen and lymph nodes enlarge, and internal or external bleeding develops. Common sites of bleeding include the nose, mouth, and gastrointestinal tract. The leukocyte count is low, normal, or high, but the number of normal leukocytes is decreased. Consequently, the number of erythrocytes and platelets decreases as well.

Medical Management

Drug therapy is the primary weapon for arresting leukemia. Years of research have led to the development of successful drug protocols using one or combinations of antineoplastic drugs. The type of drug or combination of drugs depends on the form of leukemia.

Erythrocyte and platelet transfusions are necessary to treat the anemia and decreased platelets. Antibiotics are given when secondary infections develop.

Bone marrow transplantation and stem cell transplantation have increased survival for some clients. Their source is either *autologous* (from oneself) or *allogenic* (from another; see Chap. 19). Stem cells are harvested by removing them from peripheral blood, obtaining bone marrow, or collecting cord blood from a newborn. Malignant stem cells are removed from an autologous specimen before transplantation. Toxic drugs or radiation are administered before transplantation, making the client extremely susceptible to infection. The client remains hospitalized for several weeks to observe if normal blood cells are eventually produced, to detect signs of *graft-versus-host disease,* in which the foreign donor cells destroy the recipient's tissues and organs, and to protect the client who is immunosuppressed from acquiring a life-threatening infection (see Chap. 19).

NURSING PROCESS

● The Client With Leukemia

Assessment

First, obtain a history of symptoms. Look for a cluster of symptoms that includes weakness and fatigue, frequent infections, nosebleeds or other prolonged bleeding events, and joint pain. Also look for symptoms associated with leukocyte infiltration of the central nervous system, such as headache and confusion.

Examine the client's body, looking for evidence of bruising. Palpate the abdomen to detect enlargement and tenderness over the liver and spleen. Review laboratory test results, noting the numbers and types of blood cells. Calculate the absolute neutrophil count to determine the client's potential for infection. Also assess the outcome of bone marrow aspiration.

Diagnosis, Planning, and Interventions

Risk for Infection related to compromised immunity

Expected Outcome: Client will be free of infection as evidenced by normal temperature and no signs of an infectious disorder.

- Implement neutropenic precautions (Box 33-1). *Reduces exposure to pathogens that are dangerous when immunity is suppressed.*
- Ensure that any staff person, family member, or visitor who is ill temporarily discontinues direct contact with the client. *Reduces the potential for transmitting microorganisms to the client.*
- Monitor temperature at lease once per shift and continually assess for signs of infection, such as swelling and tenderness, which can appear in any area or organ of the body. *Progressive hyperthermia occurs in some types of infections, and fever (unrelated to drugs or blood products) occurs in most clients with leukemia. Early intervention is essential to prevent sepsis/septicemia in*

BOX 33-1 ● Neutropenic Precautions

To help prevent infection in clients with neutropenia:

- Place the client in a private room.
- Always wash hands before touching the client; encourage client to remind all staff and visitors to wash hands.
- Tell client to wash his or her hands before and after eating and after using the bathroom.
- Encourage the client to shower daily.
- Place a mask over client's mouth and nose if leaving the room; minimize time client spends in crowded areas.
- Ensure that no raw fruits or vegetables are served.
- Minimize invasive procedures (schedule all blood work to be drawn at one time of the day; discontinue invasive lines as soon as possible).
- Tell client not to handle flowers.

immunosuppressed persons. (Note: Septicemia may occur without fever.)

PC: Hemorrhage

Expected Outcome: The nurse will monitor for hemorrhage; if bleeding is detected, the nurse will manage and minimize it.

- Monitor the platelet count. *Suppression of bone marrow and platelet production places the client at risk for spontaneous and uncontrolled bleeding.*
- Inspect the skin for signs of bruising and petechiae; report melena, hematuria, or epistaxis (nosebleeds). *Fragile tissues and altered clotting mechanisms can result in hemorrhage after even minor trauma.*
- Handle client gently when assisting with care and encourage use of electric razors. *Trauma and microabrasions from razors can contribute to anemia from bleeding.*
- Apply prolonged pressure to needle sites or other sources of external bleeding. *Reduced platelet production results in a delayed clotting process.*
- Implement physician orders for transfusions of blood and platelets. *Transfusion restores and normalizes the cell count and oxygen-carrying capacity of RBCs to correct anemia and prevent and treat hemorrhage.*

Evaluation of Expected Outcomes

Expected outcomes include that the client does not acquire an infection and experiences no or minimal blood loss. He or she tolerates activity between periods of rest. The client adapts to changes in body image and copes with anxiety and fears. See Client and Family Teaching 33-1.

MULTIPLE MYELOMA

Multiple myeloma is a malignancy involving plasma cells, which are B-lymphocyte cells in bone marrow. The prognosis is poor, with an estimated survival of 1 to 5 years after diagnosis.

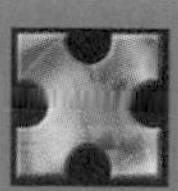

33-1 *Client and Family Teaching* Leukemia

If the client is to take medication at home, the nurse explains the dosage schedule because compliance is essential to treat the disease successfully. If untoward effects occur, the healthcare team will make every effort to control the symptoms while continuing chemotherapy. The nurse includes the following points in a teaching plan:

- Frequent examinations of the blood and sometimes the bone marrow are necessary to monitor the results of therapy. (The nurse emphasizes the importance of these examinations to promote wellness rather than focusing on possible complications from drug therapy.)
- Take precautions to avoid physical injury.
- Avoid exposure to people who have infections (e.g., colds).
- Seek medical care promptly if excessive bleeding or bruising or symptoms of illness or infection occur.
- Obtain sufficient rest and eat an adequate diet to prevent secondary infections.
- When feeling well, continue usual activities unless the physician instructs otherwise.
- If sores in the mouth occur, contact the physician as soon as possible. Do not self-treat this problem.
- Contact the physician immediately about any of the following: severe nausea with prolonged vomiting, severe diarrhea, fever, chills, excessive bleeding or bruising, cough, chest pain, cloudy urine, rash, blood in the stool or urine, severe headache, extreme fatigue, increased respiratory rate or difficulty breathing, and rapid pulse rate.
- Follow the physician's recommendations to monitor temperature and weight.
- Keep all clinic or office appointments.

Pathophysiology and Etiology

The exact triggering mechanism for the disorder is unknown. Multiple myeloma is associated with aging, recurrent infections, drug allergies, and exposure to occupational toxins and radiation (Porth, 2002). Onset is rare before age 40 years. The abnormal plasma cells proliferate in the bone marrow, where they release osteoclast-activating factor. This in turn causes osteoclasts to break down bone cells, resulting in increased blood calcium and pathologic fractures. The plasma cells also form single or multiple *osteolytic* (bone-destroying) tumors that produce a "punched-out" or "honeycombed" appearance in bones such as the spine, ribs, skull, pelvis, femurs, clavicles, and scapulae. Weakened vertebrae lead to compression of the spine accompanied by significant pain.

Malignant plasma cells release two types of abnormal proteins. In the process of being excreted by the kidneys, Bence Jones proteins impair renal tubules, causing renal failure. The other protein, called *M-type globulin,* compromises production of functional immunoglobulins (also known as *antibodies*), thus interfering with an optimal immune response (see Chap. 35). Excess production of plasma cells reduces formation of erythrocytes and platelets, causing anemia and increasing risk for bleeding. In addition to infection, which may cause death, those with multiple myeloma experience thrombotic complications such as clot formation in the deep veins of the legs, pulmonary embolism, and stroke caused by increased viscosity of the blood.

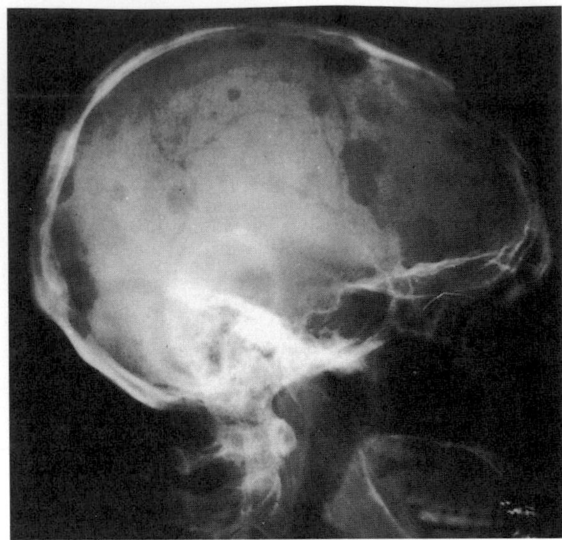

FIGURE 33.3 Multiple myeloma. A radiograph of the skull shows numerous "punched out" radiolucent areas (From Rubin, E., & Farber, J. L. [1999]. *Pathology* [3rd ed.]. Philadelphia: Lippincott Williams & Wilkins.)

Assessment Findings

The first symptom usually is vague pain in the pelvis, spine, or ribs. As the disease progresses, the pain becomes more severe and localized. Pain intensifies with activity and is relieved by rest. When tumors replace bone marrow, pathologic fractures develop. The client may have an unusually high incidence of infection, especially pneumonia, caused by decreased production of appropriate antibodies. The client may experience symptoms typically associated with anemia: weakness, fatigue, and chills. Bruising and nosebleeds are evidence of decreased platelets. Renal calculi (stones) may develop from hypercalcemia and renal failure.

Skeletal radiographic studies reveal characteristic bone lesions (Fig. 33.3). Blood cell counts are abnormally low. Serum calcium levels are elevated from bone destruction. Urine samples are positive for Bence Jones protein. Bone marrow aspiration demonstrates increased atypical plasma cells. The uric acid level is elevated from cellular destruction.

Medical Management

Steroids and anticancer drugs, like melphalan (Alkeran) and cyclophosphamide (Cytoxan), and radiation are used to decrease the tumor mass and lessen bone pain. Remission occurs in approximately 60% of clients (Copstead & Banasik, 1999). Analgesics control pain; stronger narcotic analgesics are reserved for terminal stages of the disease. Allopurinol (Zyloprim) is used to prevent uric acid crystallization and subsequent renal calculus formation. See Chapter 58 for a discussion of the management of renal failure.

Anemia is treated with blood transfusions, and infections are managed with antibiotics. Back braces are necessary when the spine is involved, and body casts are used when involvement is extensive and causes pathologic fractures.

Autologous bone marrow and peripheral stem cell transplants are considered standard care for clients with multiple myeloma. Since October 2000, Medicare pays for transplants for those newly diagnosed, younger than 78 years, and who have not responded to prior therapy (International Myeloma Foundation, 2000). Those who receive a bone marrow or stem cell transplant early in the disease have approximately 39 months of disease-free survival.

Nursing Management

Assess the client frequently for pain, signs of infection, excessive fatigue, bleeding, thrombus formation, and changes in the quantity or quality of urine production. Administer prescribed analgesics for effective pain management. Assist the client with ambulation because immobility can worsen loss of calcium from the bone. Provide up to 4000 mL of fluid to prevent renal damage from hypercalcemia and precipitation of protein in the renal tubules. Document and report signs suggestive of calculus formation in the kidney, ureters, or bladder (see Chaps. 58 and 59).

Safety is paramount because any injury, no matter how slight, can result in a fracture. When pain is severe, delay position changes and bathing until an administered analgesic has reached its peak concentration level and the client is experiencing maximum pain relief. Take measures to reduce the potential for infection.

AGRANULOCYTOSIS

Agranulocytosis refers specifically to a decreased production of granulocytes, including neutrophils, basophils, and eosinophils. This is opposed to **leukopenia,** which is a general reduction in all WBCs. Decreased granulocytes place the client at risk for infection.

Pathophysiology and Etiology

The most common cause of agranulocytosis is toxicity from drugs such as sulfonamides, chloramphenicol (Chloromycetin), antineoplastics, and some psychotropic medications.

Assessment Findings

Fatigue, fever, chills, headache, and opportunistic infections in the mouth, throat, nose, rectum, or vagina can develop.

Medical Management

Treatment includes removal of the cause, such as discontinuing the drug that is producing agranulocytosis. Prognosis is related to the condition's cause and severity. When the cause is determined and promptly removed, the client usually recovers. Some clients improve after receiving filgrastim (Neupogen), a drug that supplies human granulocyte colony-stimulating factor.

Nursing Management

Determine the names of all drugs (prescription and nonprescription) the client has used in the past 6 to 12 months. Protective isolation is necessary if the leukocyte count is extremely low. Visitors or staff with any type of an infection are restricted from close client contact until the infection has cleared.

PANCYTOPENIA

Pancytopenia refers to conditions such as aplastic anemia in which numbers of all marrow-produced blood cells are reduced.

• APLASTIC ANEMIA

Aplastic anemia is more than just a deficiency of erythrocytes. Its name is derived from the word **aplasia,** which means "failure to develop." There are usually insufficient numbers of erythrocytes, leukocytes, and platelets, collectively described as *pancytopenia.*

Pathophysiology and Etiology

Aplastic anemia is a consequence of inadequate stem cell production in the bone marrow. In some cases, the cause of the disorder is never determined, but it may be autoimmune (self-destroying) in nature (see Chap. 36). In many cases, bone marrow becomes dysfunctional from exposure to toxic chemicals, radiation, and drug therapy with anticancer drugs and some antibiotics. Clients with aplastic anemia are very ill, and the death rate is high if the bone marrow is severely damaged.

Assessment Findings

Clients with aplastic anemia experience all the typical characteristics of anemia (weakness and fatigue). They also have frequent opportunistic infections and coagulation abnormalities manifested by unusual bleeding, small skin hemorrhages called *petechiae,* and *ecchymoses* (bruises). The spleen becomes enlarged with an accumulation of the client's blood cells destroyed by lymphocytes that failed to recognize them as normal cells, or with an accumulation of dead transfused blood cells. The blood cell count shows insufficient numbers of blood cells. A bone marrow aspiration confirms suppressed production of stem cells.

Medical Management

In some instances, withdrawal of the causative agent allows bone marrow to regenerate and assume normal function. Transfusions of whole blood, packed cells, and platelets are given to boost circulating blood cells. Antibiotics are administered to prevent or treat infection. High doses of corticosteroids that suppress the immune system are given in cases of an autoimmune connection. Bone marrow transplantation is considered if a matching donor can be found; otherwise, stem cell transplantation is an alternative.

Nursing Management

Assess for signs of severe anemia, infection, and bleeding tendencies. Make every effort to prevent infection. If the leukocyte count is extremely low, implement special isolation procedures, such as restricting visitors and using a laminar airflow room.

Include soft foods in the diet and modify oral hygiene techniques to prevent bleeding from the gums. Apply pressure to any punctures from injections or IV sites. Monitor the client closely during blood transfusions because risk for reaction increases with repeated introduction of foreign cells from multiple blood donors.

COAGULOPATHIES

The term *coagulopathy* refers to conditions in which a clotting factor or other component is necessary to control bleeding is missing or inadequate. One example is hemophilia, which is covered in Unit 2: Pediatric Nursing. Another example is **thrombocytopenia,** a lower than normal number of platelets or thrombocytes.

Pathophysiology and Etiology

Thrombocytopenia occurs when there is decreased platelet production by the bone marrow or increased platelet destruction by the spleen. It accompanies leukemia and other malignant blood diseases and is caused by severe infections and certain drugs. *Idiopathic thrombocytopenic purpura* is thrombocytopenia without a known cause.

Assessment Findings

Thrombocytopenia is evidenced by *purpura,* small hemorrhages in the skin, mucous membranes, or subcutaneous tissues. Bleeding from other parts of the body, such as the nose, oral mucous membrane, and the gastrointestinal tract, also occurs. Severe and even fatal internal hemorrhage is possible.

Diagnosis is based on symptoms, a low platelet count, and abnormal bleeding and clotting times. Bone marrow aspiration may be performed. A health history sometimes reveals agents associated with drug-induced thrombocytopenia.

Medical and Surgical Management

When possible, the cause is eliminated. Corticosteroids provide symptomatic relief until the platelet count returns to normal. Transfusions of platelets or whole blood are given in a hemorrhagic emergency. If spontaneous recovery does not occur, splenectomy is necessary to stop destruction of platelets in the spleen. Removal of the spleen results in a rise in the platelet count and relief of symptoms.

Clients with idiopathic thrombocytopenia often recover spontaneously. If the cause can be removed or treated, prognosis is good. Thrombocytopenia in conjunction with illnesses such as leukemia has a poor prognosis.

Nursing Management

Refer to nursing interventions for managing and minimizing bleeding and hemorrhage discussed with leukemia. If instituting corticosteroid therapy, observe the client for adverse drug effects. Gradually taper the dose and frequency of steroid medication before discontinuing it to avoid adrenal insufficiency or crisis (see Chap. 51).

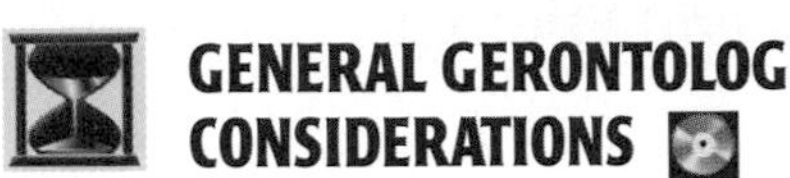

GENERAL GERONTOLOGIC CONSIDERATIONS

Iron deficiency anemia is unusual in older adults. Normally, the body does not eliminate excessive iron, causing total body iron stores to increase with age. If an older adult is anemic, blood loss from the gastrointestinal or genitourinary tract is suspected.

Although rare, iron deficiency anemia can develop in older adults for many reasons: living on a fixed income, being unable to shop for food, and lacking energy or motivation to prepare complete meals. These clients require a thorough evaluation of their dietary habits and education in the methods of preventing iron deficiency anemia.

Although treatments have the most success in young clients, acute leukemia is primarily a disease of older adults. ALL occurs at a rate four times higher in older adults than in children.

Pernicious anemia (vitamin B_{12} deficiency) accounts for approximately 9% of all anemias in older adults. Because neurologic damage and dementia may occur before any hematologic changes are found, early detection is critical. Be sure to assess the older adult with neurologic decline or dementia for pernicious anemia.

Older adults are particularly susceptible to drug-induced hemolytic anemia because they often take more drugs than young people. Discontinuing the offending drug usually corrects the anemia.

Because older adults could forget to take medicine or could take more than prescribed, instruction or supervision in drug taking is important.

Critical Thinking Exercises

1. *List hematopoietic disorders associated with anemia and an etiology of each.*
2. *Discuss the problems that clients with anemia, leukemia, or thrombocytopenia share. What interventions can nurses use regardless of the particular disorder?*

NCLEX-STYLE REVIEW QUESTIONS

1. A 28-year-old client arrives at the emergency department after a motorcycle accident. Vital signs are T–97.7°F, P–122, R–28, and BP–96/54. The client has suffered profuse blood loss. From the clinical picture, the nurse would be correct in placing this client in which position?
    1. Semi-Fowler's
    2. Modified Trendelenburg
    3. Reverse Trendelenburg
    4. Lithotomy
2. A client has been diagnosed with pernicious anemia. She exclaims, "Oh my, my grandmother died of the disease years ago." The nurse is most accurate in explaining that:

1. "We have come a long way in furthering life expectancy."
2. "We now give vitamin B_{12} to control the disease."
3. "Regular blood transfusions keep the disease in remission."
4. "Bone marrow transfusion is the only cure for the disease."

3. A client is being admitted to a medical–surgical floor with diagnosis of acute lymphocytic leukemia. Which nursing intervention is most important in the acute phase of the disease?
1. Implement neutropenic precautions.
2. Monitor blood chemistry results.
3. Institute standard precautions.
4. Use a low air flow mattress.

connection

Visit the Connection site at **http://connection.lww.com/go/timbyEssentials** for links to chapter-related resources on the Internet.

References and Suggested Readings

Baldino, M. J. (March 18, 2002). I've got plenty of iron. *Advance for Nurses,* 32–33.

Benvenato, D. (April 29, 2002). Platelet transfusion therapy. *Advance for Nurses,* 37–39.

Bullock, B. A., & Henze, R. L. (2000). *Focus on pathophysiology.* Philadelphia: Lippincott Williams & Wilkins.

Call-Schmidt, T. (2001). Interpreting lab results: A primer. *MEDSURG Nursing, 10*(4), 179–184.

Cook, L. S. (2000). A simple case of anemia: Pathophysiology of a common symptom. *Journal of Intravenous Nursing, 23,* 271–281.

Copstead, L. C., & Banasik, J. L. (1999). *Pathophysiology: Biological and behavioral perspectives.* Philadelphia: W. B. Saunders.

Derivan, M., & Ferrante, C. (2001). Clinical focus: Aplastic anemia. *Clinical Journal of Oncology Nursing, 5,* 227–229.

Fukuyama, S. N., & Itano, I. (1999). Thrombocytopenia secondary to myelosuppression. *American Journal of Nursing,* April Suppl., 5–8, 34–36.

Goldman, D. (2000). Test your knowledge: Chronic lymphocytic leukemia and its impact on the immune system. *Clinical Journal of Oncology Nursing, 4,* 233–234, 236.

Holcomb, S. S. (2001). Anemia: Pointing the way to a deeper problem. *Nursing 2001, 31*(7), 36–43.

Horrell, C. J., & Rothman, J. (2001). The etiology of thrombocytopenia. *Dimensions of Critical Care Nursing, 20*(4), 10–16.

International Myeloma Foundation. (2000). Medicare breakthrough for patients seeking a transplant for myeloma. *Blood and Marrow Transplant Newsletter, 11*(3), 1–3.

Loney, M., & Chernecky, C. (2000). Anemia. *Oncology Nursing Forum, 27,* 951–966.

Mackey, H. T., & Klemm, P. (2000). Leukemia: Aggressive therapies predispose patients to a host of side effects. *American Journal of Nursing,* April Suppl., 27–31, 52–54.

Maloy, B. J. (2000). Hematopoiesis, stem cells, and transplantation: What have we learned for the new millennium? *Journal of Intravenous Nursing, 23,* 298–303.

McDaniel, P. (2000). Focus on (clotting) factors. *Journal of Intravenous Nursing, 23,* 282–289.

Medoff, E. (2000). Oncology today: New horizons. Leukemia. *RN, 63*(9), 42–46, 49–50.

Porth, C. M. (2002). *Pathophysiology: Concepts of altered health states* (6th ed.). Philadelphia: Lippincott Williams & Wilkins.

Smeltzer, S. C., & Bare, B. G. (2004). *Brunner & Suddarth's textbook of medical–surgical nursing* (10th ed.). Philadelphia: Lippincott Williams & Wilkins.

Tasota, F. J., & Tate, J. (2001). Eye on diagnostics: Interpreting the highs and lows of platelet counts. *Nursing 2001, 31*(2), 25.

Wright, S. M., & Finical, J. (2000). Beyond leeches: Therapeutic phlebotomy today. *American Journal of Nursing, 100*(7), 55–56, 58–59, 61+.

chapter 34

Caring for Clients With Disorders of the Lymphatic System

Words to Know 

Epstein-Barr virus
Hodgkin's disease
infectious mononucleosis
lymph
lymphadenitis
lymphangitis
lymphatics
lymphedema
lymph nodes
lymphoma
non-Hodgkin's lymphomas
Reed-Sternberg cells

Learning Objectives

On completion of this chapter, the reader will:

- Explain the cause and characteristics of lymphedema.
- Discuss the role of the nurse when managing the care of clients with lymphedema.
- Describe nursing interventions that promote resolution of lymphangitis and lymphadenitis.
- Explain the nature and transmission of infectious mononucleosis.
- List suggestions the nurse can offer to those who acquire infectious mononucleosis.
- Define the term *lymphoma* and name two types.
- Name the type of malignant cell diagnostic of Hodgkin's disease.
- List three forms of treatment used to cure or promote remission of lymphomas.
- Name at least four problems that nurses address when caring for clients with Hodgkin's disease and non-Hodgkin's lymphoma.

The lymphatic system is a network of vessels, known as **lymphatics,** which transport **lymph,** the watery fluid derived from plasma that exits capillary walls and enters interstitial spaces. The lymphatic vessels carry lymph to and through **lymph nodes,** clusters of bean-sized structures located primarily in the neck, axilla, chest, abdomen, pelvis, and groin. Lymph nodes contain lymphocytes and macrophages, specialized immune defensive cells that trap, destroy, and remove infectious microorganisms, cellular debris, and cancer cells. The tonsils, thymus gland, and spleen are accessory lymphatic structures.

Most lymphatic fluid circulates with the help of skeletal muscle contraction and is returned to venous circulation through one of two ducts. The *thoracic duct,* located in the posterior abdominal cavity, collects lymph from all body areas except that which circulates above the right diaphragm and deposits fluid into the left subclavian vein. The *right lymphatic duct* returns lymph from the right side of the head, neck, chest, and right arm and empties it into the right subclavian vein (Fig. 34.1).

Occlusive, inflammatory, infectious, or malignant disorders of the lymphatic system result in fluid distribution problems, tender and painful lymph node enlargement, compromised immune functions, or a combination of these. This chapter discusses such disorders.

OCCLUSIVE, INFLAMMATORY, AND INFECTIOUS DISORDERS

• LYMPHEDEMA

Pathophysiology and Etiology

Lymphedema is a condition resulting from obstructed lymph circulation. Primary lymphedema usually is con-

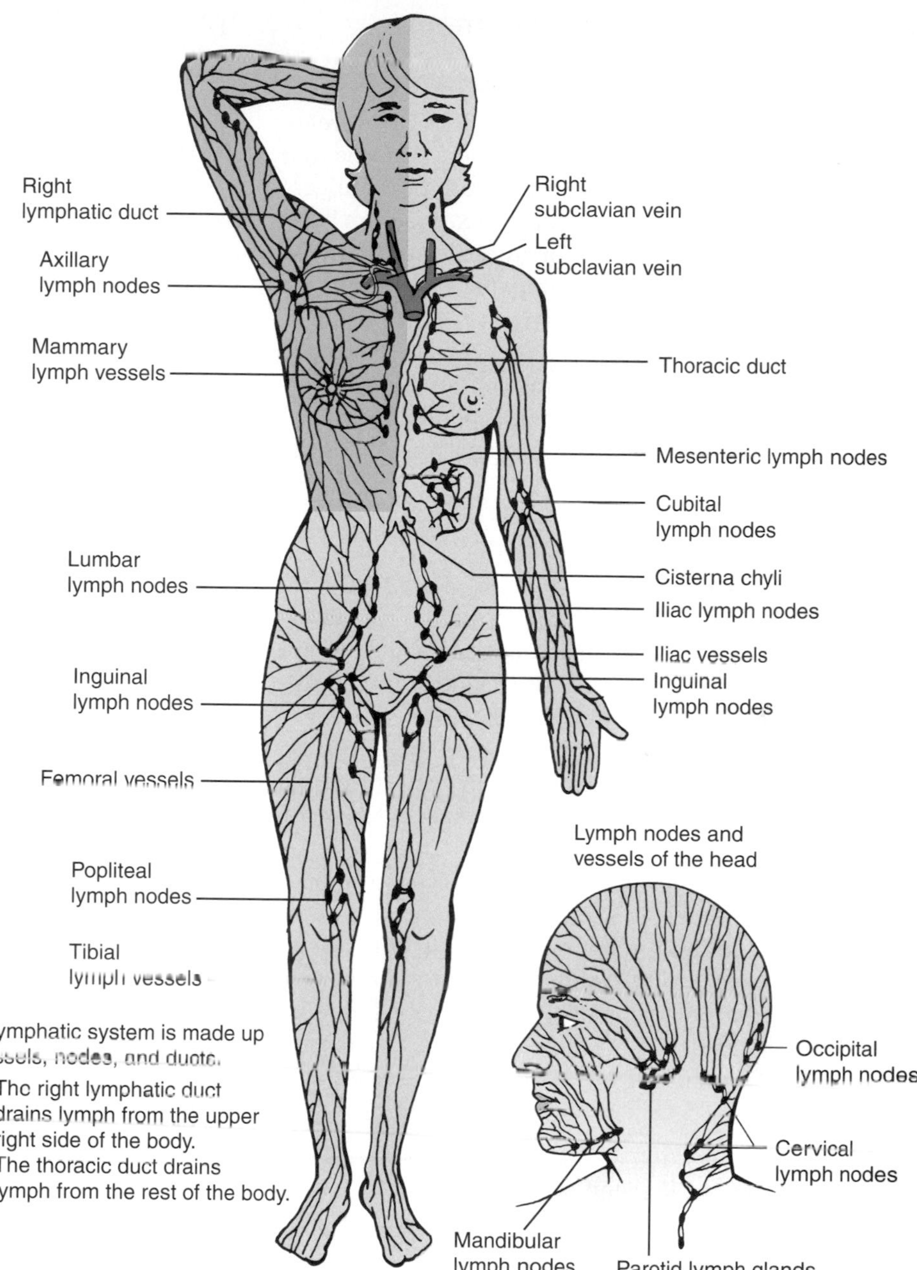

FIGURE 34.1 Lymphatic system.

genitally acquired. Symptoms usually do not appear until adolescence or early adulthood. It affects women more often than men. Secondary lymphedema develops (1) as a complication of other disorders such as repeated bouts of phlebitis and streptococcal infection, burns, or elephantiasis (an obstructive lymphatic disorder caused by a parasite); or (2) as a consequence of treatment such as mastectomy (see Chap. 54) or radiation for cancer. The causative disorder leads to occlusion of affected lymphatic vessels, which impairs lymph circulation and causes lymph to accumulate in the lymphatic system. Resulting edema, when massive, results in chronic deformity in locations such as the arms, legs, and genitalia, with subsequent poor nutrition to tissues.

Assessment Findings

Skin in the affected area swells, especially in a dependent position. Pitting is evident, but the tissue remains soft in the early stages. Skin eventually becomes firm, tight, and shiny. Elevation does not diminish the swelling. Skin also appears thickened, rough, and discolored. Because tissue nutrition is impaired from the stagnation of lymph fluid, ulcers and infection can develop in the edematous area. The area can appear red and feel warm and painful. *Lymphangiography* (a special examination in which an intravenous [IV] dye and radiography are used to detect lymph node involvement in certain diseases or conditions) reveals the degree and extent of blockage in the lymph system.

Medical and Surgical Management

Treatment usually is symptomatic. The affected part is elevated to promote lymphatic drainage. The client wears an elastic stocking or sleeve when the leg or arm is in a dependent position. Massage starting at the toes or fingers and moving toward the body and active exercises are helpful. A mechanical pulsating compression device is applied to the arm or leg at prescribed intervals. The alternating filling and emptying "milk" the lymph toward the duct, leading to venous drainage.

Sometimes surgery relieves obstruction of lymphatics. Congenital lymphedema responds poorly to surgical intervention. In some cases, lymphedema persists despite treatment.

Nursing Management

Inspect and measure the affected area to assess the extent of enlargement and condition of the skin. Encourage the client to move and exercise the affected arm or leg to enhance flow of lymph from the affected area. Instruct the client to elevate affected extremities when sitting and teach how to apply and use elastic garments and mechanical devices.

Extensive emotional support is necessary when the edema is severe. The client's self-esteem often is decreased, which can lead to social withdrawal. Support the client's self-image by suggesting certain styles of clothing that conceal abnormal enlargement of an arm or leg. For information on client teaching, see the discussion that follows nursing management for clients after a mastectomy in Chapter 54.

Stop, Think, and Respond ● BOX 34-1

Why is a client at increased risk for lymphedema after a mastectomy?

● LYMPHANGITIS AND LYMPHADENITIS

Lymphangitis is inflammation of lymphatic vessels. When such inflammation affects the lymph nodes near the lymphatics, the condition is called **lymphadenitis.**

Pathophysiology and Etiology

An infectious agent, commonly streptococcal microorganisms, usually causes both lymphangitis and lymphadenitis. The lymph nodes and lymph vessels show typical signs of inflammation: redness, swelling, discomfort, and compromised function.

Assessment Findings

Red streaks follow the course of the lymph channels and extend up the arm or leg. Fever also may be present. When lymphadenitis is present, lymph nodes along the lymphatic channels are enlarged and tender on palpation. Diagnosis is made by visual inspection and palpation.

Medical Management

A broad-spectrum antibiotic commonly is ordered.

Nursing Management

Inspect the area two to three times daily and note the client's response to antibiotic therapy. Give assistance if the discomfort interferes with activities of daily living. Elevation reduces swelling. Warmth promotes comfort and enhances circulation. Notify the physician if the affected area appears to enlarge, additional lymph nodes become involved, or temperature remains elevated. In cases with persistent swelling, teach the client how to apply an elastic sleeve or stocking.

● INFECTIOUS MONONUCLEOSIS

Infectious mononucleosis is a viral disease affecting lymphoid tissues such as tonsils and spleen. It can involve other organs such as the brain, meninges, and liver as well.

Pathophysiology and Etiology

The **Epstein-Barr virus** causes infectious mononucleosis. This contagious disorder spreads by direct contact with saliva and pharyngeal secretions from an infected person. It is transmitted at the time of kissing; through oral spray during coughing, talking, or sneezing; or through sharing food, cigarettes, or other items containing oral secretions. The incubation period can be as long as 30 to 50 days. The virus most commonly affects young adults, especially those in close living quarters, such as the armed services and college dormitories.

At the time of infection, macrophages engulf the virus, resulting in a display of the antigen on the cell surface. Active production of T lymphocytes follows. T lymphocytes trigger production of B-cell lymphocytes and antibodies. They also infiltrate tissue, particularly the spleen, causing it to enlarge. Force to the abdomen can cause the spleen to rupture when it is enlarged.

Symptoms resolve in approximately 1 to 2 weeks unless complications develop. One episode of infectious mononucleosis produces subsequent immunity, but the virus remains in the body for the person's lifetime. The Epstein-Barr virus is believed to trigger Hodgkin's lymphoma (discussed later in the chapter) in approximately 40% of people with this disease.

Assessment Findings

Fatigue, fever, sore throat, headache, and cervical lymph node enlargement typically occur. Tonsils ooze white or greenish gray exudate. Pharyngeal swelling can compromise swallowing and breathing. Some clients develop a faint red rash on their hands or abdomen. The liver and spleen become enlarged. Symptoms persist for several weeks.

The leukocyte and differential cell counts demonstrate lymphocytosis. A positive slide agglutination test (Monospot, Mono-Test, Monosticon) is presumptive evidence that the Epstein-Barr virus is causing the symptoms. A rise in the Epstein-Barr virus antibody titer and a heterophil agglutination test result of 1:224 or greater is conclusive for infectious mononucleosis.

Medical Management

The infection usually is self-limiting. Bed rest, analgesic and antipyretic therapy, and increased fluid intake are recommended. Corticosteroid therapy is prescribed if complications such as hepatic involvement occur. If a bacterial infection such as sinusitis or streptococcal pharyngitis accompanies mononucleosis, an antibiotic is prescribed.

Nursing Management

Inspect the client's throat for the extent of inflammation or edema. Gently palpate lymph nodes to detect swelling and encourage fluids. Advise the client to rest as much as possible. If the client expresses concern over prolonged time off from work or school, listen and help the client cope with anxiety. Advise the client to withhold donating blood for at least 6 months after recovering from the illness.

LYMPHOMAS

The term **lymphoma** applies to a group of cancers that affect the lymphatic system. Lymphoma is classified by the microscopic appearance of the malignant cells and how quickly the malignancy spreads. Two of the most common forms of lymphoma are Hodgkin's disease and **non-Hodgkin's lymphoma** (Table 34.1). Acquired immunodeficiency syndrome–related lymphoma occurs in those who have been infected with the human immunodeficiency virus.

HODGKIN'S DISEASE

Hodgkin's disease is a malignancy that produces enlargement of lymphoid tissue, the spleen, and the liver, with invasion of other tissues such as the bone marrow and lungs. It may appear in several forms: acute, localized, latent with relapsing pyrexia (elevated temperature), splenomegaly (enlarged spleen), and as lymphogranulomatosis (multiple granular tumors or growths composed of lymphoid cells).

Pathophysiology and Etiology

Although the exact cause of Hodgkin's disease is unknown, it appears that a virus, particularly the Epstein-Barr virus (the etiologic agent of infectious mononucleosis), causes mutations in some, but not all, lymphocytes, creating a malignant cell type known as **Reed-Sternberg cells.** Reed-Sternberg cells are nearly immortal, continue to reproduce prolifically, and are somehow shielded from being destroyed by killer T cells. The virus also appears

TABLE 34.1 COMPARISON OF LYMPHOMAS

HODGKIN'S	NON-HODGKIN'S
Four subtypes	Thirty subtypes
Two peaks of onset: ages 15 to 40 and older than age 55 years	Peaks after age 50 years
Reed-Sternberg cells	No Reed-Sternberg cells
Forty percent of affected clients test positive for Epstein-Barr virus	More common in industrial countries; common among clients with immunosuppression
B-cell origin	B- and T-cell origin
Usually starts in lymph nodes above the clavicle, commonly in the neck and chest; 15% are below the diaphragm; spreads downward from initial site	Common in abdomen, tonsils; can develop in areas other than lymph nodes (e.g., brain, nasal passages)
More orderly growth from one node to adjacent nodes	Less predictable growth; spreads to extranodal sites
More curable	Less curable

to inactivate the immune system's ability to suppress tumor growth. The malignant cells release chemicals known as *cytokines* (see Chap. 35), causing inflammatory symptoms such as pain and fever. Some clients develop generalized itching and a skin rash because of the release of histamine from an atypical allergic/immune response.

The disease is more common in men than in women and most frequently occurs during late adolescence and young adulthood. Some clients survive 10 or more years; others die in 4 to 5 years. A cure is possible when the disease is localized to one section of the body. Clients who receive treatment usually have remissions that last for months or even years. Death results from respiratory obstruction, cachexia (state of ill health, malnutrition, and wasting), or secondary infections.

TABLE 34.2 STAGES OF HODGKIN'S DISEASE

STAGE	INVOLVEMENT
I	Single lymph node region
II	Two or more lymph node regions on one side of the diaphragm
III	Lymph node regions on both sides of the diaphragm but extension is limited to the spleen
IV	Bilateral lymph nodes affected and extension includes spleen plus one or more of the following: bones, bone marrow, lungs, liver, skin, gastrointestinal structures, or other sites

Assessment Findings

Early symptoms of Hodgkin's disease include painless enlargement of one or more lymph nodes. Cervical lymph nodes are the first to be affected. As nodes enlarge, they press on adjacent structures, such as the esophagus or bronchi. As retroperitoneal nodes enlarge, there is a sense of fullness in the stomach and epigastric pain. Marked weight loss, anorexia, fatigue, and weakness occur. Low-grade fever, pruritus, and night sweats are common. Sometimes marked anemia and thrombocytopenia develop, causing a tendency to bleed. Resistance to infection is poor, and staphylococcal skin infections and respiratory tract infections often complicate the illness.

A complete blood count demonstrates low red blood cell count, elevated leukocytes, and decreased lymphocytes. Reed-Sternberg cells, characterized as giant multinucleated B lymphocytes, are microscopically identifiable in lymph node biopsies. Results of blood chemistry tests such as erythrocyte sedimentation rate are elevated, suggesting a current inflammatory process. Liver enzymes such as alkaline phosphatase are elevated. Lymphangiography, chest radiography, computed tomography, magnetic resonance imaging, or a laparotomy to obtain abdominal nodes for biopsy demonstrate size of lymph nodes and spread of the disease in the thorax, abdomen, or pelvis. A bone marrow aspiration and biopsy indicate abnormalities of other blood cells. After diagnosis, the disease is staged from stage I to IV, based on the number of positive lymph nodes and the involvement of other organs (Table 34.2). Staging helps determine treatment.

Stages I, II, III, and IV adult Hodgkin's disease are subclassified into A and B categories: B for those with defined general symptoms and A for those without B symptoms. The B designation is given to clients with any of the following symptoms*:

- Unexplained loss of more than 10% of body weight in the 6 months before diagnosis
- Unexplained fever with temperatures above 38°C
- Drenching night sweats

(*Note: The most significant B symptoms are fever and weight loss. Night sweats alone do not confer an adverse prognosis.) Careful staging and treatment planning by a multidisciplinary team of cancer specialists is required to determine optimal treatment of patients with this disease.

Medical Management

Treatment of Hodgkin's disease includes localized radiation to affected lymph nodes and chemotherapy with combinations of antineoplastic drugs (Table 34.3). Antibiotics are given to fight secondary infections. Transfusions are prescribed to control anemia. If resistance to treatment develops, autologous bone marrow or peripheral stem cells are harvested, followed by high doses of chemotherapy that destroy the bone marrow (see Chaps. 19 and 33). A transplant is performed after separating normal stem cells from malignant cells in the harvested specimen.

TABLE 34.3 CHEMOTHERAPY REGIMENS FOR HODGKIN'S DISEASE

REGIMEN	DRUGS
ABVD	doxorubicin (Adriamycin), bleomycin (Blenoxane), vinblastine (Velban), dacarbazine (DTIC)
MOPP	mechlorethamine (Mustargen), vincristine (Oncovin), prednisone (Meticorten), procarbazine (Matulane)
MOPP/ABVD	Alternation of drugs from both regimens
For partial remission or relapse within 1 year	
CBV	cyclophosphamide (Cytoxan), carmustine (BiCNU), etoposide (VePesid)
BEAM	carmustine (BiCNU), etoposide (VePesid), cytosine arabinoside-e (Cytosar-U), melphalan (Alkeran)

NURSING PROCESS

The Client With Hodgkin's Disease

Assessment

Look for a history of infectious mononucleosis or symptoms resembling this disorder. Assess for location, size, and characteristics of enlarged lymph nodes, such as whether they are fixed or mobile. Ask how long the client has noticed the enlarged lymph nodes and check for presence and extent of tenderness in the area of lymph node enlargement. Ask about fever, chills, or night sweats. Check the client's current weight and deviation from usual weight, enlargement of the liver and spleen, and level of energy and appetite. Inspect the appearance of the skin, ask about any itching, and discuss any additional symptoms caused by lymph node enlargement (e.g., coughing, breathlessness, nausea, vomiting).

Diagnosis, Planning, and Interventions

Client and Family Teaching 34-1 describes instructions for nurses to communicate to clients with Hodgkin's disease. Other nursing care includes, but is not limited to, the following:

Risk for Ineffective Airway Clearance and **Risk for Impaired Gas Exchange** related to compression of trachea secondary to enlarged cervical lymph nodes

Expected Outcome: Breathing will remain adequate to maintain blood oxygen saturation of 90% or greater.

- Assess respiratory status each shift and prn. Note quality, rate, pattern, depth, flaring of nostrils, dyspnea on exertion, evidence of splinting, use of accessory muscles, and position for breathing. *Any deviation from quiet, effortless breathing indicates compromised ventilation.*
- Keep the neck in midline and place the client in high Fowler's position if respiratory distress develops. *Avoiding unnecessary pressure on the trachea and positioning for increased lung expansion improve air exchange.*
- Administer oxygen per physician's orders if blood saturation is consistently less than 90%. *Reduces deficits in the blood oxygen level.*
- Place an endotracheal tube, laryngoscope, and bag–valve mask at the bedside for intubation. *Ensures that medical intervention and emergency assistance are not delayed.*

Risk for Infection related to immunosuppression secondary to impaired lymphocytes and drug or radiation therapy

Expected Outcome: Client will remain free of infection as evidenced by no fever and symptoms of secondary infection.

- Restrict visitors or personnel with infections from contact with the client. *Reduces transmission of pathogens to the client.*
- Practice conscientious handwashing and follow other principles of medical and surgical asepsis. *Reduces risk of transmitting pathogens from one location to another.*
- Institute infectious disease precautions if normal white blood cells are suppressed to dangerous limits. *Protective isolation techniques provide an environmental barrier against pathogens while a client is highly susceptible to disease.*

Activity Intolerance and **Self-Care Deficit** related to anemia and generalized weakness from disease

Expected Outcome: Client will tolerate essential activities as evidenced by heart and respiratory rates within normal limits.

- Divide care into manageable amounts. *Reduces energy expenditures.*
- Provide rest periods between activities. *Allows time for body to recover before the next demand for energy.*
- Perform priority activities first. *Client completes most important or necessary activities while energy levels are highest.*
- Assist client with whatever activities of daily living are independently unmanageable. *Reduces the client's energy expenditure.*

Evaluation of Expected Outcomes

Breathing is noiseless and effortless. The client shows no signs or symptoms of infection. He or she can perform essential activities.

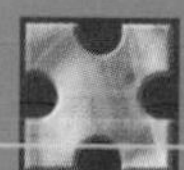

34-1 *Client and Family Teaching* Hodgkin's Disease

The nurse instructs the client as follows:

- Keep appointments for medical follow-up.
- Take prescribed medications as directed. Report side effects to the physician.
- Avoid crowds or people who have infectious diseases.
- Wash hands frequently.
- Avoid oral contact with germ-laden objects.
- Contact physician if breathing becomes labored.
- Eat small amounts frequently or include a liquid nutritional supplement between meals and at bedtime.
- Reduce work schedule or rest frequently to avoid exhaustion.
- Consult with employer about sick-leave considerations or a representative from the Social Security Administration about unemployment benefits and disability payments.
- Obtain a disability sticker to facilitate easy access to public buildings to lessen fatigue.

NON-HODGKIN'S LYMPHOMAS

Non-Hodgkin's lymphomas are a group of 30 subclassifications of malignant diseases that originate in lymph glands and other lymphoid tissue. Examples include lymphosarcoma, Burkitt's lymphoma, and reticulum cell sarcoma. The incidence of non-Hodgkin's lymphomas is six to seven times that of Hodgkin's disease, and the number of cases continues to rise.

Pathophysiology and Etiology

There is no single definitive cause for non-Hodgkin's lymphomas, although a genetic link is strongly implicated in some types. An environmental "trigger," such as a viral agent, chemical herbicides, pesticides, or hair dye, could induce the disease. Administration of immunosuppressive drugs to prevent transplant rejection also is correlated with cases of non-Hodgkin's lymphoma.

In non-Hodgkin's lymphoma, chromosomal changes occur in affected lymphocytes, and lymphoid tissue enlarges to accommodate proliferative production of malignant cells. Non-Hodgkin's lymphoma is classified as either (1) *indolent,* meaning the client is relatively asymptomatic at diagnosis and the disorder is relatively responsive to radiation and chemotherapy; or (2) *aggressive* because the condition has a shorter onset with acute symptoms. Nevertheless, 30% to 60% of aggressive forms of non-Hodgkin's lymphoma are curable with intensive treatment.

Assessment Findings

Symptoms of non-Hodgkin's lymphoma depend on site of lymph node involvement. Lymph node enlargement, which usually is diffuse rather than localized, occurs in cervical, axillary, and inguinal regions. Diagnosis and differentiation of the subtypes of non-Hodgkin's lymphoma from Hodgkin's disease depend on microscopic examination of lymphoid tissue biopsies. Additional tests are performed to determine the stage of the lymphoma.

Medical Management

Non-Hodgkin's lymphoma is treated with radiation, chemotherapy, or both. The physician may adopt a "watch and wait" approach for clients with indolent forms of non-Hodgkin's lymphoma, choosing to treat the client once the disease accelerates. Immunotherapy with monoclonal antibodies (MABs) and bone marrow transplants is being used to cure lymphomas or extend the lives of clients with these diseases. See Chapter 19 for more information on cancer treatment.

Research continues on the use of biologic therapy (immunotherapy) with MABs to eliminate malignant cells and induce remission. With MABs, human cancer cells are injected into laboratory animals such as mice. The mice make lymphocytes that produce antibodies against cancer cells. The mouse lymphocytes are harvested and fused with a laboratory-grown cell, creating clones that, when administered to a client with cancer, continue to produce tumor-fighting antibodies. The MABs are used alone or are bound to a chemotherapeutic or radioactive agent. The advantage of combining MABs with drugs or radiation is that they target and destroy cancer cells while sparing normal cells. One MAB drug, rituximab (Rituxan), is now approved for treating non-Hodgkin's lymphoma. Others are in clinical trials.

Nursing Management

Nursing care is similar for all clients with lymphoma, whether they have non-Hodgkin's lymphoma or Hodgkin's disease. Because chemotherapy and radiation kill many cells, encourage clients to drink extra fluids (=2500 mL/day) to facilitate excretion of the cells destroyed by therapy.

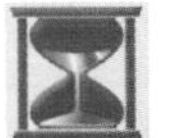

GENERAL GERONTOLOGIC CONSIDERATIONS

Risk of malignancies (e.g., lymphoma) is increased in older adults primarily because of the immunologic changes of aging and prolonged exposure to carcinogens.

Older adults do not tolerate doxorubicin and methotrexate well because these drugs have toxic effects on the kidney.

Older adults respond less well to chemotherapy than younger persons because older clients cannot tolerate maximum doses.

The benefits of chemotherapy must be weighed against the adverse reactions that occur in older adults. Treatment modalities, however, are not based on age alone.

Critical Thinking Exercises

1. *List the differences between lymphedema and lymphoma.*
2. *What teaching is indicated for a person diagnosed with lymphedema?*

NCLEX-STYLE REVIEW QUESTIONS 

1. A college student reports to the school infirmary and is diagnosed with infectious mononucleosis. She asks the health nurse how she acquired the condition. The best response by the nurse is that the virus is transmitted by:
    1. Contact with microorganisms in the blood
    2. Direct contact with the infected person
    3. Consuming contaminated food or water
    4. The bite of an insect such as a mosquito
2. A 45-year-old man with Hodgkin's disease is admitted to the hospital. In discussing the client's care with the nurse's aide, the nurse is most correct in instructing that the chief manifestation of the disease process is:

1. Severe itching
2. Tonic–clonic seizure activity
3. Frequent loose stools
4. Enlarged cervical lymph nodes

3. The nurse is teaching a 65-year-old woman with lymphedema how to correctly wear her elastic leg stockings. The nurse is correct in instructing that the stockings are to promote:
   1. Circulation in the lower extremities
   2. Support of the lower legs during ambulation
   3. Lymphatic drainage of the lower extremities
   4. Tissue healing of the lower extremities

connection

Visit the Connection site at **http://connection.lww.com/go/timbyEssentials** for links to chapter-related resources on the Internet.

References and Suggested Readings

Barnes, L. (2000). Non-Hodgkin's lymphoma. *Rehabilitation Oncology, 18*(2), 14–16.

Capriotti, T. (2001). Monoclonal antibodies: drugs that combine pharmacology and biotechnology. *MEDSURG Nursing, 10*(2), 89–95.

Davis, B. S. (2001). Lymphedema after breast cancer treatment. *American Journal of Nursing, 101*(4), Continuing Care Extra, 24AAAA–DDDD.

Kotsits, C., & Callaghan, M. (2000). Rituximab: A new monoclonal antibody therapy for non-Hodgkin's lymphoma. *Oncology Nursing Forum, 17*(1), 51–59.

Lin, R. Z. (April 29, 2002). Hodgkin's disease. *Advance for Nurses,* 33–34.

Paskett, E. D., & Stark, N. (2000). Lymphedema: Knowledge, treatment, and impact among breast cancer survivors. *Breast Journal, 6,* 373–378.

Radina, M. E., & Armer, J. M. (2001). Post-breast cancer lymphedema and the family: A qualitative investigation of families coping with chronic illness. *Journal of Family Nursing, 7,* 281–299.

Samdani, S., Lachmann, E., & Nagler, W. (2001). Unilateral extremity swelling in female patients with cancer. *Journal of Women's Health and Gender-Based Medicine, 10,* 319–326.

Smith, L. (July 8, 2002). Lymphedema. *Advance for Nurses, 31,* 35.

Stremick, K. & Gallagher, E. (2000). Malignant lymphomas: Hodgkin's disease and non-Hodgkin's lymphoma. *American Journal of Nursing,* (April Suppl.), 18–22, 52–54.

Whitman, M. (2000). Controlling lymphedema-related swelling. *Clinical Journal of Oncology Nursing, 4,* 101–102.

chapter 35

Introduction to the Immune System

Words to Know 

anergy
antibodies
antigens
artificially acquired active immunity
cell-mediated response
colony-stimulating factors
complement system
cytokines
cytotoxic T cells
effector T cells
helper T cells
humoral response
immune response
immunoglobulins
interferons
interleukins
lymphokines
macrophages
memory cells
microphages
monocytes
natural killer cells
naturally acquired active immunity
neutrophils
passive immunity
phagocytes
phagocytosis
plasma cells
regulator T cells
stem cells
suppressor T cells
tumor necrosis factor

Learning Objectives

On completion of this chapter, the reader will:

- Explain the meaning of an immune response.
- List components of the immune system.
- Discuss the role of T-cell and B-cell lymphocytes.
- Differentiate between an antigen and an antibody.
- Name examples of lymphoid tissue.
- List some cells and chemicals that enhance the function of the immune system.
- Describe types of immunity and how each develops.
- Discuss techniques for detecting immune disorders.
- Describe the role of the nurse when caring for a client with an immune disorder.

Although all humans have the same types of cells, each person's cells are unique and different from those of all others. Body cells are coded with distinct histocompatibility (tissue cell) markers, which act as a "fingerprint" for the immune system to differentiate "self" from "nonself." When it detects a nonself substance, the immune system protects, defends, and destroys what it perceives as atypical or abnormal. The immune system primarily targets infectious, foreign, or cancerous cells. The **immune response,** a target-specific system of defense, is carried out primarily by lymphocytes, specialized cells located in blood and lymphoid tissue. Hyperactivity of the immune system, as in allergic or autoimmune disorders (see Chap. 36), or a decrease in its function, as in acquired immunodeficiency syndrome (AIDS; see Chap. 37), can be life-threatening.

STRUCTURES OF THE IMMUNE SYSTEM

The immune system is a collection of specialized white blood cells and lymphoid tissues that cooperate to protect a person from external invaders and the body's own altered cells. Function of these structures is assisted and supported by activities of natural killer (NK) cells, antibodies, and nonantibody proteins like cytokines and the complement system (Fig. 35.1).

White Blood Cells

White blood cells (leukocytes) are produced in bone marrow. Initially all blood cells are nonspecific **stem cells** that

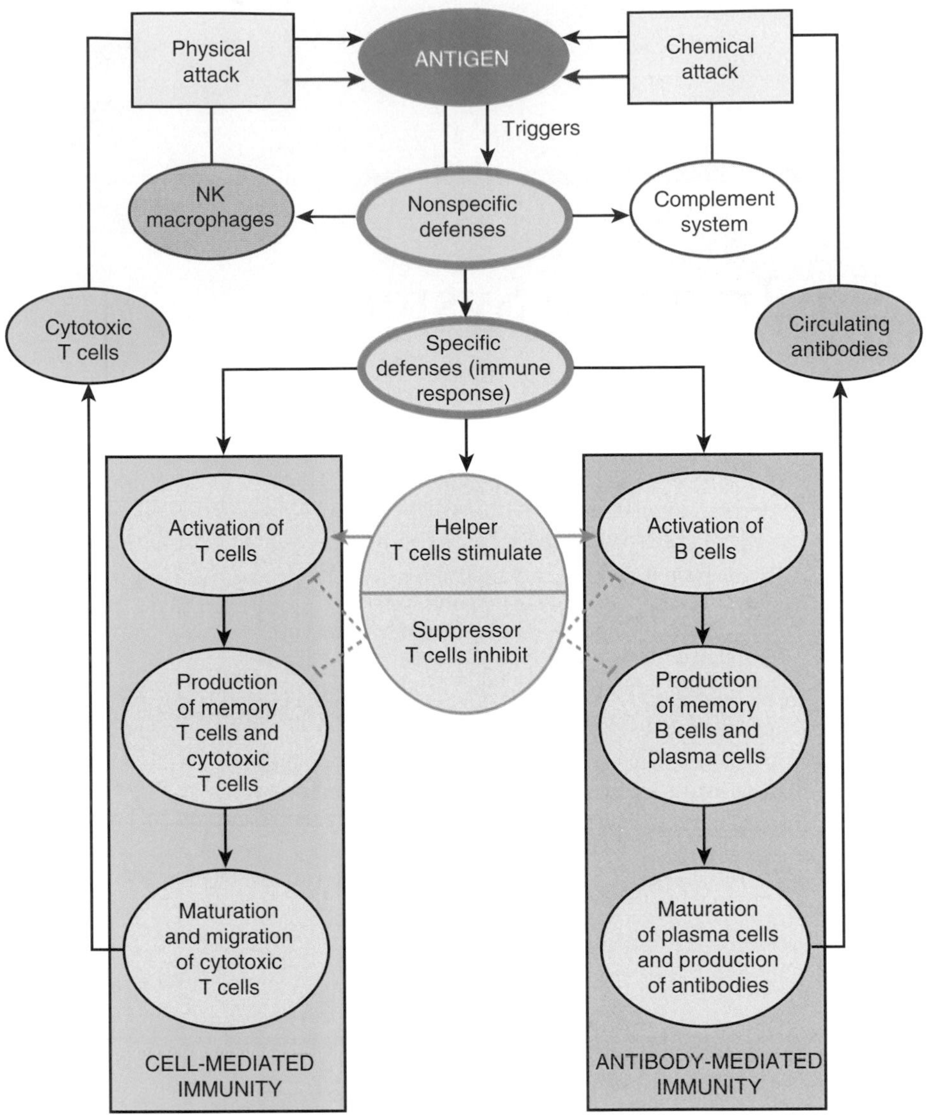

FIGURE 35.1 Schematic representation of the immune response.

later differentiate into various types of cells including lymphocytes, neutrophils, and monocytes. Figure 35.2 shows the development of various types of blood cells.

Lymphocytes

Lymphocytes, which are either T-cell or B-cell lymphocytes, comprise 20% to 30% of all leukocytes. T-cell and B-cell lymphocytes are primary participants in the immune response. They distinguish harmful substances and ignore those natural and unique to the individual. Table 35.1 identifies various types of lymphocytes and the role they play in the immune response.

T-cell lymphocytes are manufactured in bone marrow and travel to the thymus gland, to become either regulator T cells or effector T cells. **Regulator T cells** include helper and suppressor cells; **effector T cells** are killer (cytotoxic) cells. **Helper T cells** are very important in fighting infection. They recognize **antigens,** protein markers on cells, and form additional T-cell clones to stimulate B-cell lymphocytes to produce antibodies against foreign antigens. **Antibodies** are chemical substances that destroy foreign agents such as microorganisms. Helper T cells also are called T4 cells or CD4 cells.

Cytotoxic T cells bind to invading cells, destroy the targeted invader by altering their cellular membrane and intracellular environment, and release chemicals called lymphokines. **Lymphokines,** a type of cytokine (discussed later in this chapter), attract neutrophils and monocytes to remove debris. They also promote maturation of more T cells when they detect antigens and direct B-cell lymphocytes to multiply and mature.

Suppressor T cells limit or turn off the immune response in the absence of continued antigenic stimulation. Because surface molecules of suppressor and killer T cells differ from those of helper T cells, they may be referred to as T8 or CD8 cells.

The immune response that T-cell lymphocytes perform is called a **cell-mediated response.** It occurs when

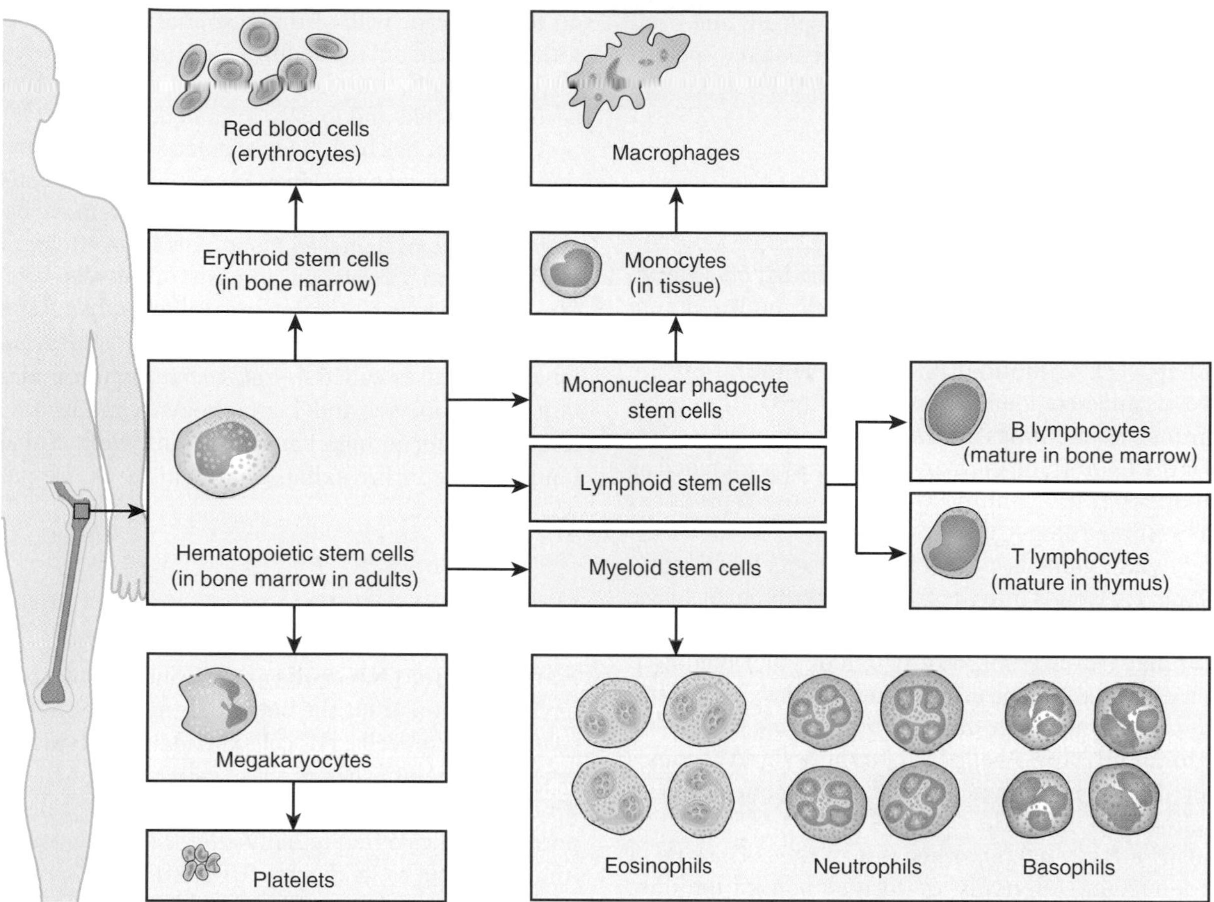

FIGURE 35.2 Origin of blood cells.

T cells survey proteins in the body, actively analyze the surface features, and respond to those that differ from the host by directly attacking the invading antigen. An example of a cell mediated response is one that occurs when an organ is transplanted.

TABLE 35.1	TYPE AND FUNCTIONS OF LYMPHOCYTES
TYPE	**FUNCTION**
T Cells	
Regulator T cells	
Helper T cells	Recognize antigens; stimulate B cells to produce antibodies
Suppressor T cells	Turn off the immune response
Effector cells	
Cytotoxic cells	Bind to and destroy invader cells; stimulate the release of lymphokines
B Cells	
Plasma cells	Produce antibodies
Memory cells	Convert to plasma cells that will produce antibodies when re-exposed to an antigen

B cell lymphocytes mature in bone marrow and migrate to the spleen and other lymphoid tissues such as the lymph nodes. When stimulated by T cells, B cells become either plasma or memory cells. **Plasma cells** produce antibodies. Formation of antibodies is called a **humoral response.**

Memory cells convert to plasma cells on re-exposure to a specific antigen. When activated, B cells accumulate in lymphoid tissues, which explains the phenomena of swollen and tender lymph nodes that accompany infectious disorders and an enlarged spleen in various immune disorders.

Stop, Think, and Respond ● BOX 35-1

Explain the difference between a cell-mediated response and a humoral response.

Neutrophils and Monocytes

Neutrophils and **monocytes** are **phagocytes,** which are cells that perform **phagocytosis,** the process of engulfing and digesting bacteria and foreign material. Phagocytes are stationary (fixed) or mobile. Neutrophils, also called **microphages** because they are small, are present in blood and migrate to tissue as necessary. Monocytes, also called **macrophages** because they are large, are present in tissues such as the lungs, liver, lymph nodes, spleen, and peritoneum. They also migrate after a cell-mediated response. The mononuclear phagocyte system was formerly known as the *reticuloendothelial system.*

Lymphoid Tissues

Lymphoid tissues (Fig. 35.3), such as the thymus gland, tonsils and adenoids, spleen, and lymph nodes, play a role in the immune response and prevention of infection (see Chap. 32). Lymphoid tissue also is found on the surface of mucous membranes of the intestine, alveolar membranes in the lungs, and in the lining of the sinusoids of the liver. Bone marrow sometimes is included as a component of the immune system because it produces undifferentiated stem cells.

The thymus gland is located in the neck below the thyroid gland. It extends into the thorax behind the top of the sternum and produces lymphocytes during fetal development. It may be the embryonic origin of other lymphoid structures such as the spleen and lymph nodes. After birth, the thymus gland programs T lymphocytes to become regulator or effector T cells. The thymus gland becomes smaller during adolescence but retains some activity throughout the life cycle.

Tonsils are located on either side of the soft palate of the oropharynx. Adenoids are located behind the nose on the posterior wall of the nasopharynx. These tissues filter bacteria from tissue fluid. Because they are exposed to pathogens in the oral and nasal passages, they can become infected and locally inflamed.

The spleen has both hematopoietic and immune functions. It acts as an emergency reservoir of blood and filters blood as well. Macrophages in the spleen remove bacteria and old, dead, or damaged blood cells from circulation.

The lymphatic system consists of vessels similar to capillaries that drain tissue fluid, called *lymph.* At various areas in the body, lymphatics converge and drain into larger structures called *lymph nodes.* Lymph nodes contain B lymphocytes and T lymphocytes and remove bacteria and other foreign particles from lymph. Superficial lymph nodes in the axilla, groin, and neck are palpable when enlarged.

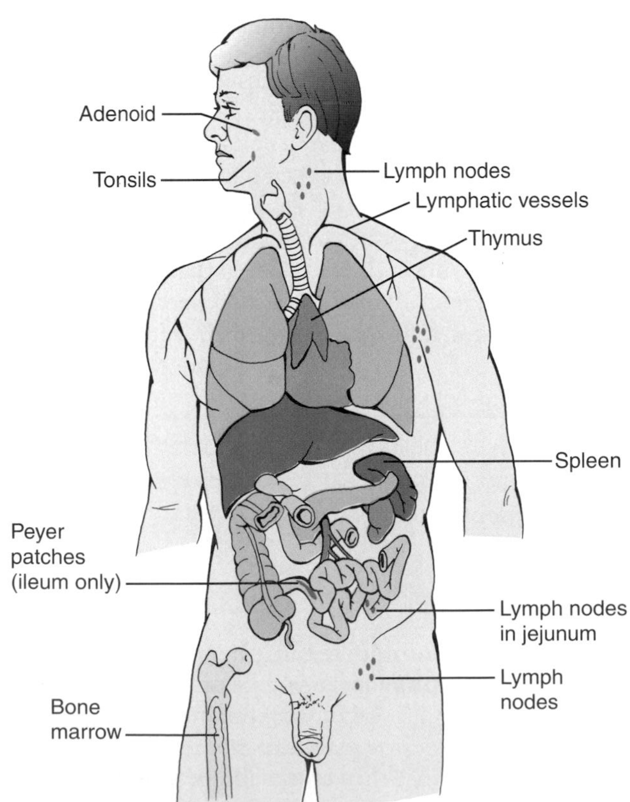

FIGURE 35.3 Lymphoid tissues.

Natural Killer Cells

Natural killer (NK) cells are lymphocyte-like cells that circulate throughout the body looking for virus-infected cells and cancer cells. NK cells can identify atypical markers on the membranes of these cells without the help of T or B cell lymphocytes. Once identified, NK cells release potent chemicals that lethally alter the target cell's membrane, leading to its demise. Unfortunately, cancer cells can escape NK cell surveillance, which explains how cancer is able to become established and spread beyond its primary site.

Antibodies

Antibodies, proteins produced by B lymphocyte plasma cells, are more correctly referred to as **immunoglobulins** (Ig). There are five classes of immunoglobulins: IgA, IgD, IgE, IgG, and IgM. Each immunoglobulin has a separate role in ensuring the maintenance of a healthy state (Table 35.2).

Immunoglobulins bind with antigens and promote destruction of invading cells. They may hinder antigens physically by (1) neutralizing their toxins; (2) linking antigens together in a process called *agglutination;* and (3) causing antigens to precipitate, or become soluble. Antibodies also facilitate destruction of antigens with other mechanisms such as those performed by nonantibody proteins like the complement system and cytokines.

Nonantibody Proteins

Nonantibody proteins provide additional methods for disabling antigens and further protecting the body. There are two groups of nonantibody proteins.

TABLE 35.2 TYPES OF IMMUNOGLOBULINS

TYPE	PERCENTAGE OF TOTAL	LOCATION	FUNCTION
IgG	75%	Intravascular and intercellular fluid	Neutralizes bacterial toxins; accelerates phagocytosis
IgA	15%	Body secretions such as saliva, sweat, tears, mucus, bile, colostrum	Interferes with entry of pathogens through exposed structures or pathways
IgM	10%	Intravascular serum	Agglutinates (clusters) antigens and lyses (dissolves) cell walls
IgD	0.2%	Surface of lymphocytes	Binds to antigens; promotes secretion of other immunoglobulins
IgE	0.004%	Surface of basophils and mast (connective tissue) cells	Promotes release of vasoactive chemicals such as histamine and bradykinin in allergic, hypersensitivity, and inflammatory reactions

Complement System

The **complement system** is made up of many different proteins activated in a chain reaction when an antibody binds with an antigen. Collectively, proteins cooperate with antibodies to attract phagocytes, coat antigens to make them more recognizable for phagocytosis, and stimulate inflammation through release of histamine from mast cells and basophils.

Cytokines

Cytokines are chemical messengers released by lymphocytes, monocytes, and macrophages. There are many subgroups of cytokines, including interleukins, interferons, tumor necrosis factor, and colony-stimulating factors.

Interleukins carry messages between leukocytes and tissues that form blood cells. Some interleukins enhance the immune response, whereas others suppress it. Interleukin activity can include the following: promotion of inflammation and fever; formation of scar tissue by fibroblasts; growth and activation of NK cells and additional T cells; production of mast cells; growth of B cells, formation of plasma cells, and production of antibodies; formation of new blood vessels known as *angiogenesis;* and stimulation of the anterior pituitary gland to secrete corticotropin.

Interferons are chemicals that primarily protect cells from viral invasion. They enable cells to resist viral infection and slow viral replication. They are used as adjunctive therapy in the treatment of AIDS. Interferons also are used to treat some forms of cancer like leukemia because they stimulate NK cell activity.

Tumor necrosis factor (TNF) initially showed promise in shrinking tumors. Although TNF reduced tumors in laboratory animals, it caused toxic effects among humans. Research is ongoing to determine if the antitumor effect can be achieved and toxic side effects limited by injecting TNF directly into the tumor.

Research shows that TNF helps in cellular repair when administered in small doses. Excess amounts destroy healthy tissue. Consequently, TNF is being used to regulate various autoimmune (see Chap. 36) and inflammatory disorders.

Colony-stimulating factors (CSFs) regulate production, maturation, and function of blood cells (Nevidjon & Sowers, 2000). Growth factors enable stem cells in bone marrow to differentiate into specific types of cells such as leukocytes, erythrocytes, and platelets. Pharmacologic preparations of cytokines, such as epoetin alfa (Epogen), filgrastim (Neupogen), and sargramostim (Leukine), are used to promote natural production of blood cells in people whose own hematopoietic functions are compromised. Clients with cancer who are receiving antineoplastic drugs may avoid interrupting treatment by reducing their risk for infection. Persons who undergo bone marrow transplantation may recover sooner, and individuals with chronic renal failure can avoid repeated blood transfusions to compensate for their anemia.

TYPES OF IMMUNITY

Three types of immunity are naturally acquired active immunity, artificially acquired active immunity, and passive immunity (Fig. 35.4). Both forms of active immunity

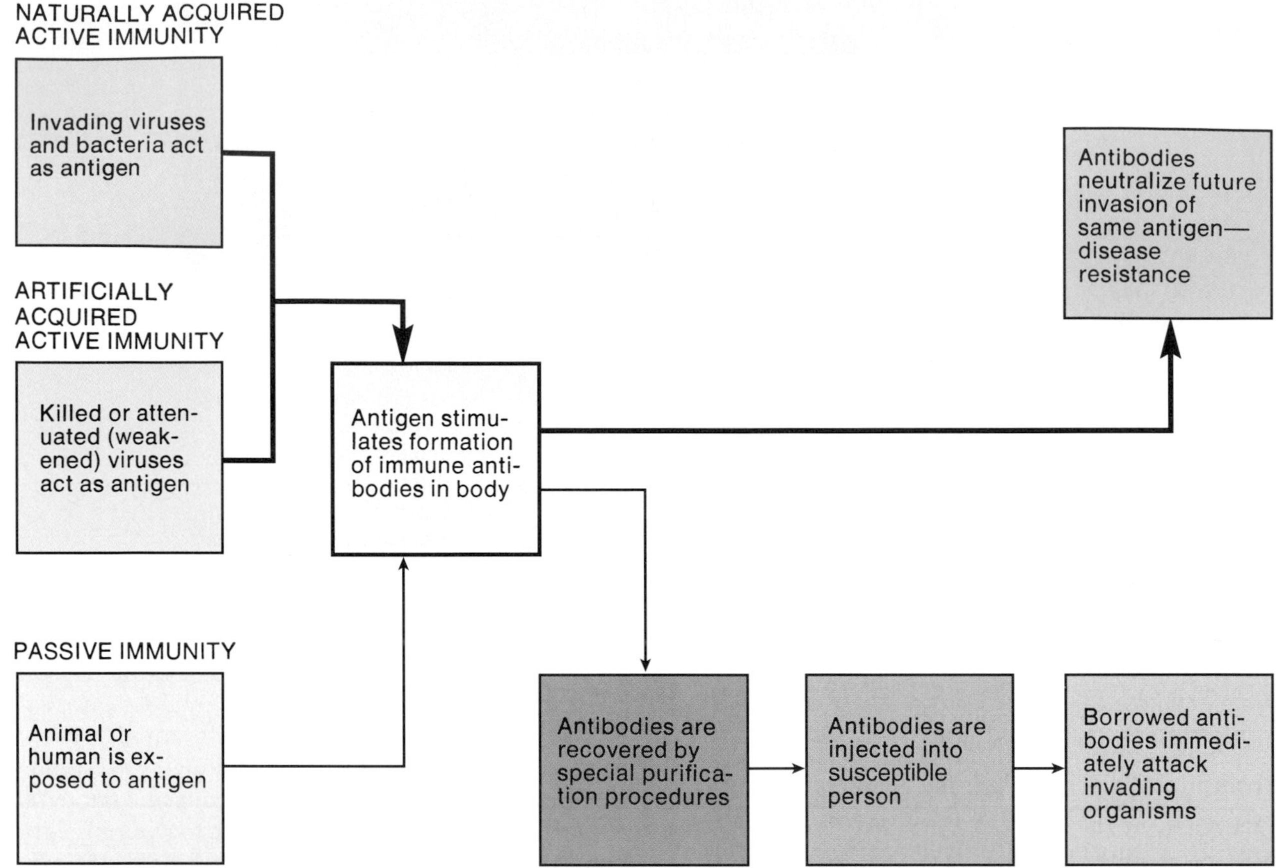

FIGURE 35.4 Active and passive immunity.

require the individual's own production of plasma and memory cells. Passive immunity occurs when ready-made antibodies are provided.

Naturally acquired active immunity occurs as a direct result of infection by a specific microorganism. An example is immunity to measles that develops after initial infection. Not all invading microorganisms produce a response that gives lifelong immunity.

Artificially acquired active immunity results from the administration of a killed or weakened microorganism or toxoid (attenuated toxin). Memory cells manufactured by the B lymphocytes "remember" the killed or weakened antigen and recognize it if a future invasion occurs. Immunizations not administered or completed during childhood are recommended for adults. Some immunizations, such as those for tetanus and influenza, require re-administration to maintain adequate immunity.

Passive immunity develops when ready-made antibodies are given to a susceptible individual. The antibodies provide immediate but short-lived protection from the invading antigen. No memory cells are produced, and the level of the injected antibodies diminishes over a period of several weeks to a few months.

Ready-made antibodies are obtained from the serum of another organism, either animal or human. Immune serum globulin, also called *gamma globulin* or *immunoglobulin,* is recovered from pooled human plasma. Because the pool comprises plasma from more than one donor, the serum is likely to contain a variety of specific antibodies. Human immune serum is used for passive immunization against measles (rubella), pertussis (whooping cough), hepatitis B, chickenpox (varicella), and tetanus.

Newborns receive passive immunity to some diseases for which their mothers have manufactured antibodies. The circulating maternal antibodies cross the placental barrier. As with other forms of passive immunity, infants are protected for only a few months after birth.

> **Stop, Think, and Respond ● BOX 35-2**
>
> *Identify the type of immunity that develops from (1) receiving a vaccine for hepatitis B, (2) having chickenpox, and (3) receiving an injection of gamma globulin.*

ASSESSMENT

History

Obtain a history of immunizations, recent and past infectious diseases, and recent exposure to infectious diseases. Review the client's drug history because certain drugs (e.g., corticosteroids) suppress inflammatory and immune responses. Investigate the client's allergy history and question the client about practices that put him or her at risk for AIDS (see Chap. 37).

Physical Examination

During the initial appraisal of the client's health, note if the client appears healthy, acutely or mildly ill, malnourished, extremely tired, or listless. Record vital signs and weight. Then examine the skin for rashes or lesions; assess the abdomen for an enlarged liver or spleen; inspect the pharynx for large, red tonsils and purulent drainage; and palpate the lymph nodes in the neck, axilla, and groin for enlargement and tenderness.

Diagnostic Tests

Laboratory tests to identify immune system disorders usually include a complete blood count with differential. Protein electrophoresis screens for diseases associated with a deficiency or excess of immunoglobulins. T-cell and B-cell assays (or counts) and the enzyme-linked immunosorbent assay (see Chap. 37) may be performed. Additional tests are performed if autoimmune or genetic immune disorders are suspected (see Chap. 36).

Skin tests may be administered. Disease-specific antigens, such as purified protein derivative of the tuberculin toxin, are injected intradermally on the inner aspect of the forearm. The injection area swells if the client has developed antibodies against the antigen in the past (see Chap. 23). The client is not necessarily actively infectious if test results are positive (see Chap. 23). Skin tests using various common disease antigens like mumps are administered if **anergy** (the inability to mount an immune response) is suspected. It is common among clients with AIDS or those who are immunosuppressed for other reasons.

NURSING MANAGEMENT

Clear identification of any substances to which the client is allergic is essential. Consult drug references to verify that prescribed medications do not contain substances to which the client is hypersensitive. Explain diagnostic skin testing procedures to the client and inform the client when to return for interpretation of the results. Ensure that written consent is obtained before testing for human immunodeficiency virus (HIV) and keeps results of HIV testing confidential. Standard Precautions are required whenever there is the potential for contact with blood or body fluids. Follow agency guidelines for controlling infectious diseases or protecting the client who is immunosuppressed. Client teaching includes information about immunizations and instructions regarding drug therapy prescribed for disorders involving the immune system.

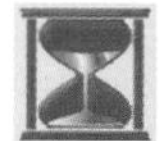

GENERAL GERONTOLOGIC CONSIDERATIONS

The older client is more likely to have problems related to the immune system because the activity of the immune system declines with the natural aging process.

Older adults with chronic diseases such as respiratory disorders or cardiac disease should have an annual influenza vaccine and a one-time pneumococcal vaccine.

Although vaccination against viral disorders is recommended for older adults, vaccines are less effective in an older adult than in a younger adult, probably because of the decreased immune response that occurs with age.

Critical Thinking Exercises

1. *How would you respond to a friend who tells you that her sister has an immune disorder and asks what this means?*
2. *Discuss the benefit of obtaining immunizations for common childhood diseases.*

● NCLEX-STYLE REVIEW QUESTIONS

1. A 26-year-old client had a splenectomy following a violent motor vehicle accident. The parents ask the nurse if there are any special considerations following the surgical removal of the spleen. The nurse is most correct to begin instruction stating that the spleen's main function is:
   1. To produce red blood cells
   2. To maintain acid-base balance
   3. To synthesize vitamin K
   4. To filter the blood
2. A client is suspected of having an immune system disorder. What laboratory study would the nurse expect to be ordered during the initial blood studies?
   1. Blood chemistry
   2. Complete blood count
   3. Complete blood count with differential
   4. Liver enzyme studies

connection

Visit the Connection site at **http://connection.lww.com/go/timbyEssentials** for links to chapter-related resources on the Internet.

References and Suggested Readings

Alcoser, P. W., & Burchett, S. (1999). Bone marrow transplantation: Immune system suppression and reconstitution. *American Journal of Nursing, 99*(6), 26–32.

Bliss, D. Z., & Lehmann, S. (1999). Tube feeding: immune-boosting formulas. *RN, 62*(8), 26–28, 32.

Bullock, B., & Henze, R. L. (2000). Focus on pathophysiology. Philadelphia: Lippincott Williams & Wilkins.

Cohen, B. J. (1999). *Memmler's the human body in health and disease* (9th ed.). Philadelphia: Lippincott Williams & Wilkins.

Copstead, L. C., & Banasik, J. L. (1999). *Pathophysiology: Biological and behavioral perspectives* (2nd ed.). Philadelphia: W. B. Saunders.

Decker, G. M. (2000). Integrated care. Pharmacologic and biologic therapies in cancer care: Part II. *Clinical Journal of Oncology Nursing, 4,* 283–284, 287.

Dudek, S. G. (2001). *Nutrition handbook for nursing practice* (4th ed.). Philadelphia: Lippincott Williams & Wilkins.

Fischbach, F. T. (2004). *A manual of laboratory diagnostic tests* (7th ed.). Philadelphia: Lippincott Williams & Wilkins.

Kaye, J. (2000). Stress, depression, and psychoneuroimmunology. *Journal of Neuroscience Nursing, 32*(2), 93–100.

Moldawer, N., & Carr, E. (2000). The promise of recombinant interleukin-2. *American Journal of Nursing, 100*(5), 35–40.

Nevidjon, B. M., & Sowers, K. (2000). *A nurse's guide to cancer care.* Philadelphia: Lippincott Williams & Wilkins.

Smeltzer, S. C., & Bare, B. G. (2004). *Brunner & Suddarth's textbook of medical-surgical nursing* (10th ed.). Philadelphia: Lippincott Williams & Wilkins.

chapter 36

Caring for Clients With Immune-Mediated Disorders

Words to Know 

allergen
allergic disorder
alloimmunity
anaphylaxis
angioneurotic edema
autoantibodies
autoimmune disorder
chronic fatigue syndrome
desensitization
exacerbation
fibromyalgia
histocompatible cells
mast cells
neurally mediated hypotension
remission
sensitization
tilt-table test
urticaria

Learning Objectives

On completion of this chapter, the reader will:

- Describe an allergic disorder.
- Discuss allergic signs and symptoms.
- Explain categories of allergens, giving an example of each.
- Describe allergic reactions.
- Describe diagnostic skin testing.
- Name methods for treating allergies.
- Discuss the nursing management of a client with an allergic disorder.
- Explain the meaning of autoimmune disorder, naming examples of related diseases.
- Discuss at least one theory that explains the development of an autoimmune disorder.
- Name categories of drugs used in the treatment of autoimmune disorders.
- Discuss the nursing management of a client with an autoimmune disorder.
- Give explanations for how chronic fatigue syndrome develops.
- List common symptoms experienced by people with chronic fatigue syndrome.
- Discuss the nursing management of a client with chronic fatigue syndrome.

The immune system may respond aggressively and destructively to substances not necessarily harmful. Examples of such a response include allergic and autoimmune disorders. This chapter discusses allergic and autoimmune disorders and appropriate nursing care for clients who have them. It also explores chronic fatigue syndrome, a consequence of an immune-mediated disorder, and the nursing management of this condition.

ALLERGIC DISORDERS

An **allergic disorder** is a hyperimmune response to weak antigens or **allergens** that usually are harmless (Table 36.1). Allergens have a protein component and gain entry to the host from the environment. Allergies occur at any age. Allergic responses can vary in the same person during his or her life. For example, a person may suddenly develop an allergic reaction to a substance like latex, even though he or she has had multiple prior contacts with latex and no past problems. See Box 36-1 for products that contain latex. On the other hand, an allergic response to one agent may gradually disappear or be replaced by sensitivity to another substance. The reason for these changes is unclear.

Types of Allergies

Allergic disorders occur in different ways depending on how the allergen gains entry to the body and the intensity of the response. Organs and structures primarily involved in allergic reactions include the skin, respiratory

TABLE 36.1 COMMON ALLERGENS

TYPE OF ALLERGEN	EXAMPLES	COMMON REACTION
Ingestants	Food, drugs (especially penicillin)	Gastroenteropathy, dermatitis, asthma, anaphylaxis, urticaria, angioedema, serum sickness
Inhalants	House dust and mites, insect excrement, animal products (dander, saliva, urine), pollens, spores	Allergic asthma, rhinitis, hypersensitivity pneumonitis
Contactants	Plant oils, topical medications, occupational chemicals, cosmetics, metals in jewelry and clothing fasteners, hair dyes, latex	Contact dermatitis, urticaria or anaphylaxis (rare)
Injectants	Drugs, bee venom	Anaphylaxis, angioedema, acute urticaria

passageways, gastrointestinal tract, blood, and vascular system (Table 36.2). Some types of allergic manifestations cause temporary, localized discomfort, whereas others are life-threatening.

Stop, Think, and Respond ● BOX 36-1

List substances to which you or others you know are allergic.

Pathophysiology and Etiology

Approximately 10% to 15% of the population develops allergies. The tendency can be inherited, although members of the same family may not all be sensitive to the same allergens. Allergy-prone individuals may react to more than one type of antigen. For example, a person may be sensitive to ragweed pollen and eggs.

The first exposure to an allergen does not produce symptoms, but causes **sensitization,** the process by which cellular and chemical events follow during a second or subsequent exposure to an allergen. Once sensitization occurs, the hypersensitivity reaction can be immediate or delayed depending on the time it takes for the immune system to mount a response.

An *immediate hypersensitivity response* occurs rapidly. **Anaphylaxis,** a rapid and profound allergic response characterized by shock, laryngeal edema, wheezing, stridor, tachycardia, and generalized itching, occurs seconds to minutes after exposure to the sensitizing allergen. Immediate hypersensitivity responses result from activation of B-cell lymphocytes and subsequent production of immunoglobulin E (IgE) antibodies. IgE antibodies attach to basophils or **mast cells,** which are constituents of connective tissue that contain granules of heparin, serotonin, bradykinin, and histamine (the most potent chemical of this group). With subsequent exposures to the allergen, mast cells and basophils release their vasoactive granules, causing various allergic and inflammatory manifestations. Localized reactions include watery eyes, increased nasal and bronchial secretions, sneezing, vomiting, and diarrhea. Additional symptoms include hives (called **urticaria**), itching, and localized redness (e.g., in the conjunctiva of the eyes). A massive release of histamine causes vasodilation; increased capillary permeability; **angioneurotic edema** (acute swelling of the face, neck, lips, larynx, hands, feet, genitals, and internal organs); hypotension; and bronchoconstriction (Fig. 36.1).

A *delayed hypersensitivity response* may develop over several hours or reach maximum severity days after exposure. Examples include a blood transfusion reaction that occurs days to weeks after blood administration, or rejection of transplanted tissues. T-cell lymphocytes mediate delayed hypersensitivity reactions.

Several mechanisms can suppress the allergic response. One method involves release of *eosinophil chemotactic factor* (ECF), a chemical mediator from mast cells. ECF

BOX 36-1 ● Products That Contain Latex

Household	Medical
Carpet backing	Gloves
Feeding nipples	Face masks
Pacifiers	Mattresses
Elastic in clothing	Patient-controlled analgesia syringes
Sports equipment	Ambu bags
Balloons	Stethoscope
Erasers	Blood pressure cuff tubing
Toys	Dental devices
Shoe soles	Urinary catheters
Condoms/diaphragms	Tourniquets
Computer mouse pads	Electrode pads
Buttons on electronic equipment	Bulb syringes
Food handled with powdered latex gloves	Syringe stoppers and medication vial stoppers
Handles on racquets, tools, and similar items	Adhesive tape
	Bandages
	Injection ports
	Wound drains

TABLE 36.2 TYPES OF ALLERGIES

ALLERGY TYPE	SIGNS AND SYMPTOMS	MEDICAL MANAGEMENT
Allergic rhinitis	Sneezing, itching, nasal congestion, watery nasal discharge, itching and redness of the eyes	Antihistamines, nasal decongestants, corticosteroid nasal spray, immunotherapy, allergen avoidance, eye drops
Contact dermatitis	Itching, burning, redness, rash on contact with substance	Allergen avoidance, wearing gloves, topical or oral antihistamines and corticosteroids
Dermatitis medicamentosa	Sudden generalized bright red rash, itching, fever, malaise, headache, arthralgias	Discontinuation of drug, antihistamines and topical corticosteroids
Food allergy	Nausea, vomiting, diarrhea, abdominal cramping, malaise, itching, wheezing, rash, cough	Identification and avoidance of allergenic food
Urticaria	Itching, swelling, redness, wheals of superficial skin layers	Topical or oral antihistamines and corticosteroids
Angioedema	Itching, swelling, redness of deeper tissues and mucous membranes	Intubation, subcutaneous epinephrine, aminophylline

attracts eosinophils, which suppress inflammation by degrading histamine and other vasoactive chemicals. Epinephrine, a neurotransmitter, interferes with release of vasoactive chemicals from mast cells. Corticosteroids, anti-inflammatory hormones produced by the adrenal cortex, block synthesis of leukotrienes, also known as *slow reactive substance of anaphylaxis,* and prostaglandins, both of which contribute to vascular permeability and smooth muscle contraction.

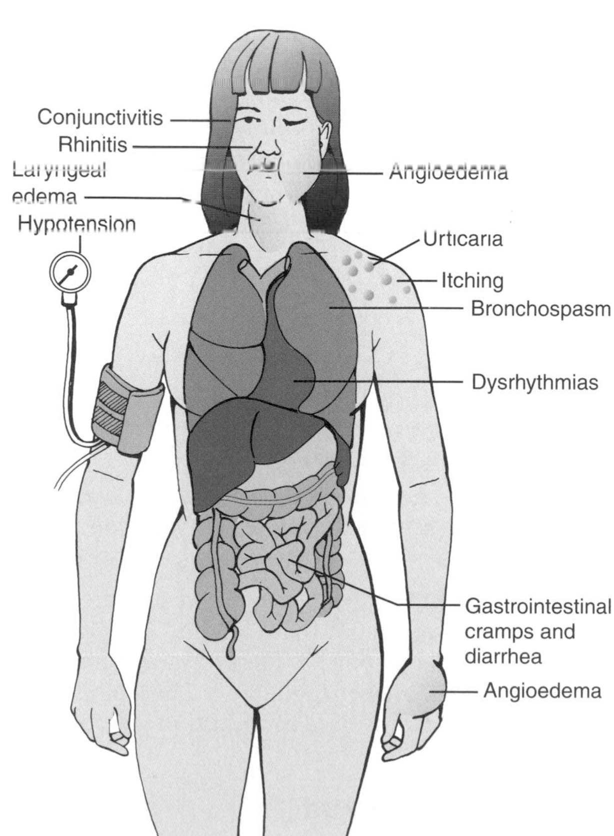

FIGURE 36.1 Manifestations of allergic reactions.

Assessment Findings

Signs and Symptoms

Clients often identify a cause-and-effect relationship between particular substances and their allergic symptoms. Clinical symptoms often correlate with the manner in which the allergen enters the body. For example, inhaled allergens usually cause respiratory symptoms and often trigger asthma (see Chap. 23). Contactants cause skin reactions such as hives, rash, and localized itching. Cramping, vomiting, and diarrhea are associated with ingested food allergens. Injectants, such as bee venom, and some other allergens can produce systemic and potentially fatal effects, including shock and airway obstruction caused by laryngeal swelling.

Diagnostic Findings

Diagnosis of an allergy may be clear or require multiple tests and extensive history-taking. Diagnosis is difficult when a client is allergic to more than one substance or when symptoms vary with fatigue, emotional stress, or the seasons.

Various abnormalities in blood test results suggest an allergic disorder. For example, the eosinophil count may be elevated. The radioallergosorbent blood test (RAST) measures IgE. On a scale of 0 to 5, a score of 2 or greater is significant for an allergic disorder. The RAST does not identify the cause of the allergy, but does validate that the person is potentially hypersensitive to antigenic substances.

Specific allergens can be identified by skin testing with extracts of various substances (antigens), such as pollens, animal danders, food, dust, and stinging insects. Methods of skin testing are the scratch or prick test, the patch test, and the intradermal injection test.

The *scratch* or *prick test* involves scratching the skin and applying a small amount of liquid test antigen to the scratch. The tester applies one allergen per scratch over the client's forearm, upper arm, or back. The back is more sensitive than the arms. It also provides a larger area for testing because each substance being tested should be distributed at least 3 cm and preferably up to 5 cm (slightly more than 1 to 2 inches) from one another. Results from a scratch test are identifiable in as little as 20 minutes. If a raised wheal or localized erythema appears, the tester measures its length and width in millimeters. The larger the reaction, the greater is the likelihood that the tested allergen causes symptoms in the tested individual.

The *patch test* is used to identify the offending substance in allergic contact dermatitis. The tester applies a concentrated form of the substance to the skin and covers the area with an occlusive dressing. After 48 hours, the tester removes the dressing and examines the area for erythema, edema, and vesicles.

In the *intradermal injection test,* which usually is performed only when results of a scratch test are negative for allergies, the tester injects a dilute solution of an antigen intradermally. A positive reaction is based on the size of a raised wheal and localized erythema (redness) that forms where the antigen was injected (Fig. 36.2).

To identify food allergens, the client fasts for 1 to 2 days, consuming only distilled water. He or she is then monitored for symptoms as new foods are added to the diet. Nursing Guidelines 36-1 explains the process of identifying food allergens in more detail.

Complications

Clients with inhalant allergies such as seasonal or allergic rhinitis (also known as *hay fever*) may develop nasal

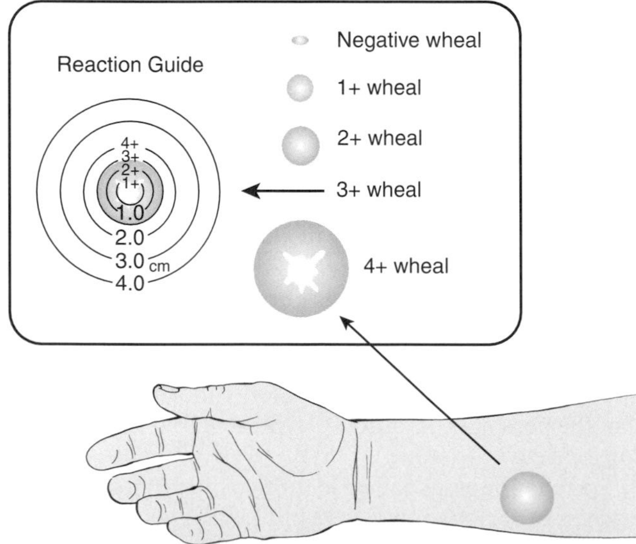

FIGURE 36.2 The wheal that forms after an intradermal skin test is measured to interpret the allergic response. The following scale is used: Negative = soft wheal and minimal redness; 1+ = 5–8 mm wheal and redness; 2+ = 7–20 mm wheal and redness; 3+ = 9–15 mm asymmetric wheal and redness; 4+ = >12 mm asymmetric wheal and diffuse redness.

NURSING GUIDELINES 36-1

Identifying Food Allergens

- Have the client fast for 1 to 2 days, drinking only distilled water.
- Introduce hypoallergenic foods (e.g., rice, tapioca) one at a time.
- Introduce allergenic foods (e.g., wheat, peanuts) one at a time in small quantities.
- Observe client for allergic symptoms after introducing each new food.

polyps from chronic inflammation. They also are prone to sinus infections related to chronic nasal congestion. Secondary pulmonary infections such as bronchitis also occur. Asthma develops in some clients. The most severe complication is anaphylactic shock and angioneurotic edema, which can be lethal without immediate medical interventions.

Medical Management

Treatment used to relieve allergic symptoms depends on the type of allergy. Besides avoiding the allergen if possible, many clients experience symptomatic relief with drug therapy (Drug Therapy Table 36.1).

Another option is **desensitization,** a form of immunotherapy. The individual receives weekly or twice-weekly injections of dilute but increasingly higher concentrations of an allergen without interruption. Repeated exposure to the weak antigen promotes production of IgG, an antibody that blocks IgE so it cannot stimulate mast cells. When the maximum dose is achieved after 2 to 4 months of treatment, maintenance injections are administered at longer intervals, usually every 2 to 4 weeks. It may take several years before a person treated with desensitization experiences significant relief. After a desensitization injection, the client is observed for 30 minutes to assess for allergic symptoms. Epinephrine (Adrenalin) is administered if a severe reaction occurs.

Stop, Think, and Respond ● BOX 36-2

List signs and symptoms that suggest a person who is undergoing desensitization needs epinephrine.

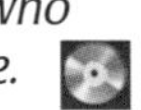

Clients with severe allergies to bee venom are advised to carry an emergency kit that contains a premeasured dose of injectable epinephrine. The syringe autoinjects the epinephrine when pressed to the skin. The lateral thigh is the site most commonly used for injection (Fig. 36.3).

Nursing Management

Throughout the client's care, observe for signs of an allergic reaction, especially when administering medica-

DRUG THERAPY TABLE 36.1 ALLERGIC DISORDERS

DRUG CATEGORY AND EXAMPLES	MECHANISM OF ACTION	SIDE EFFECTS	NURSING CONSIDERATIONS
Antihistamines *diphenhydramine (Benadryl), hydroxyzine (Atarax), fexofenadine (Allegra), astemizole (Hismanal), loratidine (Claritin), cetirizine (Zyrtec)*	Block histamine (H_1) receptors	Sedation, dryness of mucous membranes; rare: heart dysrhythmias	Caution client not to drive or operate machinery until sedative effects of medication are known.
Nasal Decongestant Agents *flunisolide (Nasalide), oxymetazoline hydrochloride (Afrin)*	Vasoconstrict nasal membranes	Headache, transient nasal burning, nasal congestion, sneezing, epistaxis, rebound nasal congestion	Advise client to pump spray three to four times before first use and one to two times before each daily use to prime. Caution clients using Afrin to avoid using for longer than 3 to 5 days in a row or rebound nasal congestion may occur.
Nasal Steroid Spray and Inhalant *beclomethasone dipropionate (Beconase), fluticasone propionate (Flonase), fluticasone propionate (Flovent)*	Anti-inflammatory	Headache, fungal infection, nasal irritation, cough, flulike illness	Examine nares. Avoid contact with the eyes. Several weeks of therapy may be necessary for full benefit. Report sore throat or signs of oral fungal infection.
Oral Corticosteroids *dexamethasone (Decadron), hydrocortisone (Cortef), methylprednisolone (Medrol)*	Regulate immune response; control inflammatory response	Euphoria, insomnia, gastrointestinal irritation, increased appetite, weight gain, hyperglycemia	Taper doses when discontinuing; abrupt discontinuation may lead to acute adrenal insufficiency. Give doses in the morning with food. Monitor blood sugar levels. Assess for peripheral edema.
Oral Decongestant Agents *pseudoephedrine hydrochloride (Sudafed), albuterol (Proventil), metaproterenol (Alupent), ipratropium (Atrovent), terbutaline (Brethine)*	Vasoconstrict nasal membranes (sympathomimetics)	Anxiety, nervousness, palpitations, headache, dizziness, tremors, sleeplessness, hypertension	Use cautiously in clients with severe hypertension, diabetes, glaucoma, hyperthyroidism, prostatic hyperplasia, coronary artery disease, those taking monoamine oxidase inhibitors, and women who are breast-feeding. Avoid taking within 2 hours of bedtime. Brethine interferes with labor and delivery.
Bronchodilating Inhaled Agents *epinephrine (Primatene Mist)*	Stimulate adrenergic receptors or block cholinergic receptors	Nervousness, tremor, euphoria, palpitations, hypertension, dysrhythmias, headache	Monitor blood pressure and heart rate. Use caution in those with hypertension, heart disease, diabetes, cirrhosis, or those using digitalis glycosides. Teach proper technique for using inhaler.
Oral or Parenteral Sympathomimetic Agents *epinephrine (Adrenalin chloride), theophylline (Theo-Dur, Elixophyllin), theophylline (Aminophylline)*	Act on alpha or beta receptors	Nausea, anxiety, restlessness, headache, trembling, tachycardia, hypertension, increased urination, increased gastric secretions	Use cautiously in clients with gastritis or peptic ulcer disease, congestive heart failure, hyperthyroidism, or seizure disorders. Monitor vital signs regularly. Give oral drugs with food to decrease gastric irritation.
Leukotriene Antagonists *montelukast (Singulair), zileuton (Zyflo)*	Block receptors for leukotrienes (slow-reacting substance of anaphylaxis)	Headache, nausea, abdominal upset, flulike symptoms such as fatigue, hepatotoxicity	Avoid if breast-feeding. Monitor for infections. Administer on an empty stomach.

1. Carefully uncap the Epipen device, holding it so that the injecting end is upright.

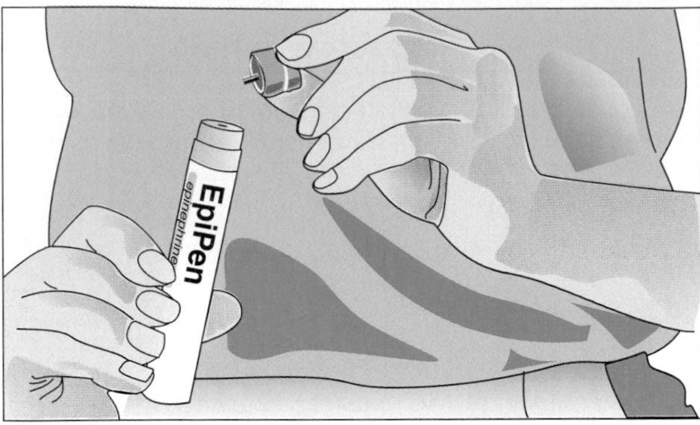

2. Position the device at the middle portion of the thigh.

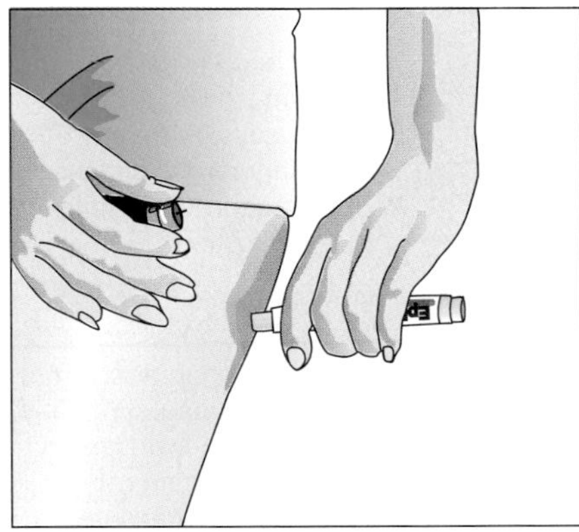

3. Push the device into the thigh as far as possible. The Epipen device will autoinject a premeasured dose of epinephrine into the subcutaneous tissue.

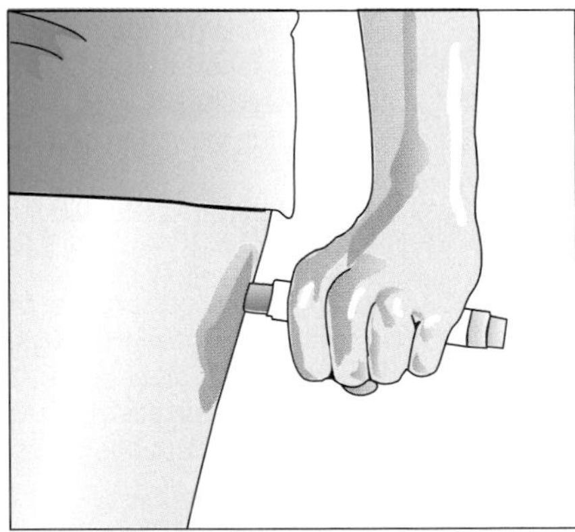

FIGURE 36.3 To avoid an anaphylactic reaction, a premeasured dose of epinephrine is autoinjected into subcutaneous tissue.

tions, applying substances like adhesive patches to the skin, or caring for a client receiving contrast media for diagnostic testing. If you suspect a mild allergic reaction, remove or withhold the offending substance and notify the physician. If a client has an anaphylactic reaction, immediately stop the client's exposure to the allergen and provide life support while summoning the code team or calling the 911 operator.

Instruct clients undergoing diagnostic skin testing to avoid taking prescribed or over-the-counter antihistamine or cold preparations for at least 48 to 72 hours before testing. Doing so reduces potential for false-negative test results. Clients must temporarily discontinue some medications for even longer. Assist the provider who performs diagnostic testing and help to document findings. Once the test is completed, monitor the client's response until it is safe for the person to return home.

For clients who elect to undergo desensitization, administer the serial doses and monitor the client for 30 minutes after administration. Teach clients who are being desensitized and those who choose drug therapy for relief of their allergy symptoms how to self-administer prescribed medications, especially those delivered by metered dose or dry powder inhalers. Make clients aware of possible side effects and when medical follow-up is necessary.

Techniques for avoiding or reducing exposure in the client's home and work environment are nursing areas for health teaching. Some examples include the following:

- Insist that the environment be "smoke free" when a person manifests inhalant allergies or respiratory symptoms
- Keep pets outdoors or at least in one confined area of the home
- Bathe pets weekly or at frequent intervals
- Cover the mattress and box springs with an impervious material to reduce dust mites
- Eliminate area rugs
- Contract with an exterminator if cockroaches or other vermin are present
- Clean humidifiers and heating and cooling ducts to remove mold spores

For other health teaching information, see Client and Family Teaching 36-1.

Stop, Think, and Respond ● BOX 36-3

Discuss ways to avoid inhaled and ingested allergens. 

AUTOIMMUNE DISORDERS

Autoimmune disorders involve killer T cells and autoantibodies that attack or destroy natural cells—those cells that are "self." **Autoantibodies,** antibodies against self-antigens, are immunoglobulins. They target **histocompatible cells,** whose antigens match the individual's own genetic code. Autoimmune disorders are characterized by unrelenting, progressive tissue damage without any verifiable etiology.

The term **alloimmunity** is used to describe an immune response that is waged against transplanted organs and

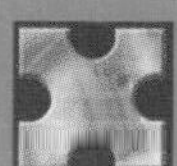

36-1 *Client and Family Teaching* Allergies

The nurse teaches clients who have allergic disorders and their family members the following guidelines:

- Never begin smoking or quit if you are currently smoking if your allergy causes respiratory symptoms.
- Treatment for chronic allergic disorders, such as allergic rhinitis and food allergies, may extend over several years.
- Follow the medical regimen as instructed by the physician.
- Do not overuse nose drops or sprays for nasal congestion. Use only prescribed or recommended drugs and only in the dosage suggested by the physician.
- Keep a record of symptoms or lack of symptoms. Bring the record to the physician's office or clinic. The record will help the physician determine therapy.
- Keep a record of symptoms or absence of symptoms each time you add a new food to the diet. Add new foods to the diet slowly and one at a time.
- Avoid environmental substances that cause allergic reactions.
- Seek immediate medical attention if symptoms worsen or new symptoms occur.
- Carry identification, such as a MedicAlert card or bracelet, to inform medical personnel of allergies, especially if you have a history of anaphylactic reactions.
- Do not miss an immunotherapy appointment; missed appointments may necessitate restarting the series of injections.
- Check prefilled syringes that contain epinephrine for an expiration date. You must refill the prescription and discard the old prescription on or immediately before this date. Keep the directions for use with the product.

tissues that carry nonself antigens. See Chapters 25 and 52 for more information.

Pathophysiology and Etiology

Although several theories have been proposed to explain the cause of autoimmune disorders, none appears to explain autoimmunity completely. This suggests that more than one mechanism is responsible.

In many autoimmune disorders, there tends to be a triggering event, such as an infection or trauma. One hypothesis is that the triggering event upsets the immune system's tolerance or recognition of self-antigens. A cause-and-effect relationship exists between some viral and bacterial infections (e.g., measles) and the development of a blood disorder called *thrombocytopenic purpura* (see Chap. 33). Another cause-and-effect relationship is found between streptococcal infections and disorders like rheumatic heart disease (see Chap. 25). Despite such relationships, no scientific evidence supports the hypothesis. It may be that the antigenic surface of the microorganism so closely resembles the person's histocompatible cell markers that antibodies cannot differentiate between host and invader.

Certain individuals may be genetically predisposed to autoimmune disorders. Theorists propose that histocompatible markers are genetically inherited and act as receptors for disease-causing microorganisms, making certain cells more vulnerable than others. Another possibility is that some people inherit a trait for suppressor T-cell dysfunction. Suppressor T cells mediate immune responses. Without adequate suppressor T-cell function, killer T cells can destroy healthy cells, tissues, and organs without restraint. Consequently, genetic factors may also explain why autoimmune disorders have a tendency to occur among blood relatives.

Another interesting phenomenon supports the sequestered antigen theory. Evidence shows that when a person experiences trauma followed by inflammation to the iris, ciliary body, and choroid layer of one eye, the vision in the untraumatized eye is also affected. This is referred to as *sympathetic uveitis.* During fetal development, cells and tissues of the eye are not exposed to the lymphatic drainage system. The lymphocytes never learned to recognize ocular cells as having self-antigens. When trauma occurs and these cells are no longer sequestered, or hidden, from the lymphocytes, the immune system attacks what it perceives to be foreign.

Regardless of theoretical premises, the outcome is clear. The immune system fails to recognize histocompatible cells. Consequently, T and B cells mount a cell-mediated or humoral response (see Chap. 35). The attack may be localized to one organ or type of tissue or it may be systemic (Box 36-2). Cells, tissues, and organs under attack are damaged or destroyed.

Assessment Findings

Autoimmune disorders produce various signs and symptoms depending on the tissues and organs affected. Symptoms are characteristic of an acute inflammatory response. They develop as antibodies attack normal tissue mistakenly identified as nonself. In some cases, inflammatory symptoms are episodic. Periods of acute flare-ups (known as **exacerbations**) alternate with periods of **remission** (asymptomatic periods). Duration of these periods is completely unpredictable. During acute exacerbations, clients often experience a low-grade fever, malaise, or fatigue, and may lose weight.

BOX 36-2 • Examples of Autoimmune Disorders

ORGAN SPECIFIC

Blood
- Hemolytic anemia
- Thrombocytopenia purpura

Central nervous system
- Multiple sclerosis
- Guillain-Barré syndrome

Heart
- Endocarditis

Muscles
- Myasthenia gravis

Endocrine
- Hashimoto's thyroiditis
- Type 1 diabetes mellitus

Eye
- Uveitis

Joint
- Ankylosing spondylitis

Gastrointestinal
- Ulcerative colitis

Renal
- Glomerulonephritis

SYSTEMIC
- Systemic lupus erythematosus
- Scleroderma
- Rheumatoid arthritis
- Sjögren's syndrome

Diagnostic testing depends on the autoimmune disorder. Elevated circulating antibodies are the hallmark findings for autoimmune disorders. Some examples include elevated erythrocyte sedimentation rate, antistreptolysin-O titer, antinuclear antibody titer, and rheumatoid factor.

Medical Management

Autoimmune disorders are rarely cured. The goal of therapy is to induce a remission or slow the immune system's destruction. Drug therapy using anti-inflammatory and immunosuppressive agents is the mainstay for alleviating symptoms (Drug Therapy Table 36.2). Some antineoplastic (cancer) drugs also are used for their immunosuppressant effects. Controlling or limiting side effects of the drugs, one of which is increased susceptibility to infection, is a major concern. Even with remission, most people must continue taking prescribed medications to avoid another acute exacerbation.

NURSING PROCESS

• The Client With an Autoimmune Disorder

Assessment

During the initial interview with the client, obtain a family history and be alert to information about family members who have had chronic diseases with an inflammatory component that involves cardiac, urinary, neurologic, or connective tissues. During acute exacerbations, the client is quite ill. Vital signs may reveal elevated temperature, a finding supporting an infectious or inflammatory process. Examine the client for signs of localized inflammation and compromised body functions such as changes in the skin, joints, gait, heart, and renal function. Ask about the client's level of energy because fatigue is common. Review laboratory test findings for evidence that correlates with an inflammatory process or immunologic changes typical of one of many autoimmune disorders. Teaching points for those with autoimmune disorders are discussed in Client and Family Teaching 36-2.

Diagnosis, Planning, and Interventions

Activity Intolerance related to joint pain secondary to inflammation, malaise, and fatigue

Expected Outcome: The client will perform activities of daily living (ADLs) without extreme fatigue or discomfort.

- Encourage rest during periods of severe exacerbation and regular exercise during periods of remission. *Activity levels within a client's level of endurance promote well-being. Endurance is related to the frequency, duration, and intensity of activity (Carpenito, 2004).*
- Provide nonpharmacologic and pharmacologic pain management as ordered by the physician. *Nonpainful stimuli (e.g., massage, activity, heat, cold, imagery, pleasant sounds) can reduce or relieve pain. Analgesic anti-inflammatory medications block neurotransmitters that carry pain stimuli to the brain; narcotic analgesics dull the brain, making it less perceptive to pain transmission; corticosteroids suppress the immune response.*

Disturbed Personal Identity related to coping with chronic illness and physical changes associated with autoimmune disorders

Expected Outcome: The client will maintain a positive self-concept.

- Interact with and frequently show genuine interest in the client. *A person's concept of "self" is determined to a great extent by the response of others. The client may interpret lack of interest and avoidance as rejection and being unworthy of attention.*
- Refer client to community organizations and support groups. *Sharing problems and experiences with others similarly affected dispels the idea that a person's symptoms and feelings are unique. A person can more easily resolve and tolerate problems when he or she shares the burden with others.*

Evaluation of Expected Outcomes

The client participates in self-care and ADLs without overwhelming fatigue. The client perceives himself or herself realistically with more positive attributes than negative.

CHRONIC FATIGUE SYNDROME

Chronic fatigue syndrome (CFS), also called *chronic fatigue* and *immune dysfunction syndrome,* is a complex of symptoms characterized by profound fatigue with no identifiable cause. Fatigue worsens with physical activ-

DRUG THERAPY TABLE 36.2 IMMUNOSUPPRESSIVE DRUGS

DRUG CATEGORY AND EXAMPLES	MECHANISM OF ACTION	SIDE EFFECTS	NURSING CONSIDERATIONS
Corticosteroids			
prednisone (Meticorten) *methylprednisolone (Medrol)*	Initiates many immunosuppressive and anti-inflammatory cellular responses	Euphoria, insomnia, gastrointestinal irritation, increased appetite, weight gain	Dose must be tapered. Abrupt withdrawal may cause acute adrenal insufficiency.
Cytotoxic Drugs			
azathioprine (Imuran)	Suppresses cell-mediated hypersensitivity and alters antibody production	Oral ulceration, nausea, vomiting, pancreatitis, leukopenia, bone marrow suppression, hepatotoxicity, immunosuppression, thrombocytopenia, rash, hair thinning	Follow facility policy on administration of cytotoxic drugs. Instruct clients not to take aspirin. Warn client to report signs of infection and to use effective birth control during treatment and for 4 months after.
cyclophosphamide (Cytoxan)	Interferes with replication of lymphocytes	Cardiotoxicity, anorexia, nausea, vomiting, oral ulceration, hemorrhagic cystitis, leukopenia, thrombocytopenia, anemia, pulmonary fibrosis, reversible alopecia	Advise clients to void every 1 to 2 hours while awake and to drink at least 3 L of fluid per day to reduce risk of cystitis. Do not give drug at bedtime.
methotrexate (Folex-PFS, Mexate-AQ, Rheumatrex)	Inhibits cellular replication	Stomatitis, diarrhea, nausea, vomiting, tubular necrosis, anemia, leukopenia, thrombocytopenia, hepatotoxicity, pulmonary fibrosis, urticaria, photosensitivity, alopecia	Follow facility policy on administration of cytotoxic drugs. Advise client to use birth control while on medication and to report signs of infection immediately.
Immunosuppressives			
cyclosporine (Sandimmune)	Inhibits lymphocytes; exact mechanism of action unknown	Tremor, gum hyperplasia, nausea, vomiting, diarrhea, nephrotoxicity, leukopenia, thrombocytopenia, hepatotoxicity	Warn client to report signs of infection, take drug at same time every day, take with meals if it causes nausea, avoid pregnancy, and not to stop medication without physician approval. Risk for anaphylaxis is high with injection form. Advise clients to report signs of infection immediately.
tacrolimus (Prograf)	Inhibits T-cell activation; exact mechanism of action unknown	Hypersensitivity, headache, tremor, insomnia, hypertension, diarrhea, nausea, abnormal renal function, anemia, leukocytosis, thrombocytopenia, hyperkalemia, hyperglycemia, hypomagnesemia, pleural effusion, pain, fever, asthenia	Monitor for anaphylaxis for 30 minutes after starting an infusion and frequently thereafter. Have epinephrine (1:1000) and oxygen available at the bedside. Check blood cell counts for suppression. Inform client of an increased risk for cancer. Store diluted solution in glass or polyethylene (not polyvinyl chloride) containers and discard if unused after 24 hours.

ity and does not improve with rest. *Chronic* refers to the fact that the duration of fatigue is unrelenting for 6 or more months. Some believe that CFS is associated with **fibromyalgia,** pain in fibrous tissues of the body such as muscles, ligaments, and tendons, because both conditions share many symptoms.

The Centers for Disease Control and Prevention estimates that over 500,000 people in the United States have symptoms that correspond with CFS (National Center for Infectious Diseases, 2003), with white women 20 to 50 years of age most likely to seek treatment. CFS also occurs in men and among other races. Some clients experience improvement, but not a cure, after 1 year of treatment; most suffer with their symptoms for years and may feel worse. When the duration of symptoms is lengthy, the prognosis is less optimistic.

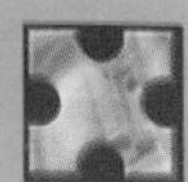

36-2 Client and Family Teaching Autoimmune Disorders

The nurse teaches clients who have autoimmune disorders and their family members the following guidelines:

- Notify a healthcare practitioner of any sign of infection such as cough, fever, severe diarrhea, mouth lesions, or sore throat.
- Notify a healthcare practitioner of any new side effects to prescribed medications.
- Do not stop taking any medications abruptly.
- Avoid crowds or people with infections if you are taking an immunosuppressant drug.
- Limit stress and use stress reduction techniques such as progressive relaxation or breathing exercises.
- Maintain close follow-up with a physician.

Pathophysiology and Etiology

One cause of CFS may be related to immune system dysfunction, in which the immune system remains activated long after an infection. However, there is not a clear connection between CFS and viral infections. Another theory centers around low cortisol levels found in CFS clients. Cortisol suppresses inflammation and immune activity. The hypothalamus secretes corticotropin-releasing factor, which tells the pituitary to release adrenocorticotropic hormone (ACTH). When ACTH stimulates the adrenal glands, they make corticosterone (cortisol). Impaired regulation interferes with immune suppression and allows the hyperfunctioning immune processes to continue unabated. This may explain why those with CFS experience **neurally mediated hypotension** (NMH), a condition in which individuals experience hypotension with fatigue after standing for more than 10 minutes. It may be due to pooling of blood in the lower limbs, resulting in decreased cerebral oxygenation.

Assessment Findings

Signs and Symptoms

Many clients with CFS report having had a recent illness with flulike symptoms or an upper respiratory infection. Most clients do not describe their initial symptoms as being extraordinarily severe. In fact, the opposite is true. Thereafter severe, ongoing fatigue lasts for at least 6 months without any explanation. Even though fatigue is constant, it worsens after physical activity. It is so debilitating that it usually interferes with a person's ability to work in or outside the home.

In addition to fatigue, the client exhibits at least four or more of the following:

- Low-grade fever
- Sore throat
- Tender cervical or axillary lymph nodes
- Muscle weakness
- Myalgia (muscle pain)
- Headaches
- Migrating joint pain without any accompanying swelling or redness
- Unrefreshing sleep
- Neurologic symptoms like photophobia, defects in the visual field, irritability, forgetfulness, confusion, difficulty concentrating, and depression

Stop, Think, and Respond ● BOX 36-4

Discuss possible consequences among people who suffer unrelenting fatigue and pain.

Diagnostic Findings

Findings of the medical history and physical examination are unremarkable. Although the client may have other physical or psychological conditions, they are unrelated to the client's presenting symptoms. Results from a battery of blood tests specific for diagnosing diseases associated with fatigue such as alkaline phosphatase; blood urea nitrogen; serum calcium, glucose, and thyroid-stimulating hormone levels; and tests for antinuclear antibodies all fail to reveal an explanation for the client's symptoms. The exhaustive medical workup excludes all diagnoses except CFS.

A **tilt-table test,** one in which the client lays horizontally on a table whose incline is elevated to approximately 70° for 45 minutes, may be done. During the test, the blood pressure and pulse are monitored. The test tends to provoke hypotension in 96% of those eventually diagnosed with CFS (National Center for Infectious Diseases, 2003).

Medical Management

Treatment focuses on relieving the client's symptoms because nothing, as yet, holds promise for a cure. One drug, polyl:polyC12U (Ampligen), is producing modest improvement among individuals with CFS. This drug is a synthetic nucleic acid that stimulates production of interferons, which have antiviral functions and modify the immune response. Manufacturers of nicotinamide adenine dinucleotide (NADH), a nutritional supplement known as Enada, claim it stimulates the production of adenosine triphosphate, which provides cellular energy. Approximately one third of participants with CFS using Enada in clinical trials report more endurance and less fatigue.

Without any definitive drug treatment, the client is advised to balance activity with rest. An employed client may need to resign from his or her job or negotiate for a less physically demanding position. The physician may prescribe a modest exercise program under the supervision of a physical therapist to avoid muscle atrophy that contributes to weakness. The client is to avoid overexertion at all costs.

Mild pain and fever are treated with aspirin, acetaminophen (Tylenol), or nonsteroidal anti-inflammatory agents like ibuprofen (Motrin, Advil) or naproxen sodium (Naprosyn, Aleve). Even low doses of tricyclic antidepressants like amitriptyline (Elavil), doxepin (Sinequan), or nortriptyline (Pamelor) can relieve pain and improve sleep.

Clients who experience hypotension are advised to increase salt and water intake as long as doing so is not contraindicated by cardiac or renal disease. Some clients also experience greater blood pressure stability when fludrocortisone (Florinef), a corticosteroid, is prescribed. An antihypotensive agent like midodrine (ProAmatine) may be prescribed to increase vascular tone and elevate blood pressure.

Nursing Management

Educate the client about his or her disease process and the limitations that it requires (see Client and Family Teaching 36-3 and Nursing Care Plan 36-1).

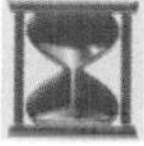

GENERAL GERONTOLOGIC CONSIDERATIONS

T-cell lymphocytes decrease with age, which may be the result of gradual degeneration of the thymus gland.

With age, the body's autoimmune response increases, which subsequently raises the risk for the older adult to develop autoimmune disorders, such as food or environmental allergies or rheumatoid arthritis.

Antihistamines are used cautiously in older men with prostatic hypertrophy because these clients may experience difficulty voiding while taking an antihistamine.

Adverse reactions to antihistamines, such as dizziness, sedation, and confusion, are more common in older adults. Careful monitoring of the older adult by the nurse or, if an outpatient, by a family member may be necessary.

When an older adult reports chronic fatigue, evaluate the client for depression.

Critical Thinking Exercises

1. *A client complains about being delayed from going home for 30 minutes after receiving a desensitizing injection to control his allergies. How would you respond?*
2. *Explain why allergies, autoimmune diseases, and CFS are classified as immune-mediated disorders.*

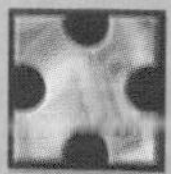

36-3 Client and Family Teaching Chronic Fatigue Syndrome

The nurse teaches clients who have CFS and their family members the following guidelines:

- When using over-the-counter analgesics, follow the recommended dosages and frequency for administration. Excess use can lead to increased potential for bleeding, liver, and kidney damage.
- Herbal products also have potential side effects; therefore, consult with the physician and keep him or her informed of any alternative therapeutic approaches you are using.
- Many companies make herbal and health-related supplements, but there is no standard among them for safe, effective dosages. Read and compare labels and ask the physician for his or her opinion on a product's efficacy.
- No scientific evidence demonstrates that vitamins or minerals alter the course of CFS; however, they are not harmful taken in recommended dosages.
- When searching for a support group, be wary of organizations that
  - Promise a cure for CFS
  - Use meetings as an opportunity to criticize specific physicians or treatment programs
  - Advise abandoning standard treatment regimens
  - Recommend an untested, unresearched, unscientific approach for managing CFS
  - Press participants to discuss information of a personal nature
  - Charge unreasonable fees for membership
  - Do not tolerate differences of opinion among group participants
  - Sell health-related items for a profit
- A strong network of family and supportive friends is an important factor in coping with the chronicity of CFS.

• NCLEX-STYLE REVIEW QUESTIONS 

1. A young client who is symptomatic after having been stung by a bee is brought to the emergency department. The initial priority nursing assessment is:
   1. Respiratory status
   2. Level of consciousness
   3. Heart rate
   4. Urinary output
2. The nurse is directing care and providing teaching for a child with an autoimmune disorder. Which statement by the child's mother demonstrates a correct understanding of the expected outcome for this child?
   1. "My child will be cured of the autoimmune disorder."

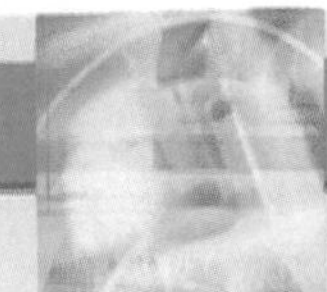

Nursing Care Plan 36-1

THE CLIENT WITH CHRONIC FATIGUE SYNDROME

Assessment

- Ask client to rate his or her energy level using a scale of 0 to 10, with 10 being the highest level. Have the client keep an energy diary to track periods during the day when energy levels are highest and lowest to determine any predictable pattern.
- Assess blood pressure and pulse in resting and sitting positions to detect postural changes.
- Have client report his or her estimation of the quality of sleep.
- Determine client's pain level and location of discomfort.

Nursing Diagnosis: **Fatigue** related to chronic immune response secondary to CFS

Expected Outcome: Client's fatigue will be reduced sufficiently so that he or she can manage ADLs.

Interventions	*Rationales*
Have client identify ADLs of high priority.	Keeps physical and mental stress manageable.
Determine ADLs that the client can delegate.	Ensures completion of ADLs without the client expending personal energy.
Help client perform one or more priority ADLs during a period of peak energy.	Minimizes fatigue and avoids overexertion, which contributes to a relapse.
Schedule 5- to 10-minute rest periods every hour or more.	Relaxation can be more restorative than long naps.
Assist client to perform gentle stretching exercises in a chair followed by low-grade active exercises recommended by the physician or physical therapist for 2 to 5 minutes daily.	Promotes blood circulation to muscles and eases the response to exercise.
Increase exercise periods by ½ to 1 minute every 2 to 3 weeks according to client's response.	Increases endurance.

Evaluation of Expected Outcome: Client performs hygiene and essential ADLs between periods of rest.

Nursing Diagnosis: **Chronic Pain** related to unknown etiology

Expected Outcome: Client's pain will be reduced to a tolerable level.

Interventions	*Rationales*
Apply a covered hot or cold pack to joints or muscles for 20 minutes; reapply after allowing the skin some recovery time.	Heat improves circulation and relieves muscle spasm and pain. Cold prevents swelling, numbs sensation, and relieves pain.
Encourage client to float in a pool or tub of tepid water (85°F) for 15 minutes as desired.	Cool temperatures reduce metabolic processes, including the immune response. Submersion in water results in buoyancy, a feeling of weightlessness, and relaxation. Movement and exercise are easier to perform in water.
Massage painful areas gently.	Releases endorphins and enkephalins that inhibit neurotransmission of pain.
Administer prescribed analgesics, corticosteroids, and antidepressants.	Relieves pain through several physiologic mechanisms.

Evaluation of Expected Outcome: Client's pain is reduced to a level of 5, which is within the client's tolerable range.

(continued)

Nursing Care Plan 36-1 (Continued)

THE CLIENT WITH CHRONIC FATIGUE SYNDROME

Nursing Diagnosis: **Risk for Injury** related to neurally mediated hypotension

Expected Outcome: The client will remain injury free.

Interventions	*Rationales*
Advise client to salt food liberally and to consume at least eight full glasses of fluid per day.	Sodium attracts water. An adequate amount of fluid maintains circulating blood volume, reducing the potential for hypotension.
Apply elastic stockings or thigh-high support hose before client lowers legs below the level of the heart.	Elastic fibers compress vein walls and prevent pooling of blood in the extremities.
Have client dangle and flex his or her lower limbs before getting out of bed.	Muscle contraction promotes circulation of blood from distal body areas to the heart and brain. Adequate blood flow to the brain reduces hypotensive episodes.
Instruct client to use a shower chair and avoid hot water when performing hygiene.	Reduces potential for injury from a fall. Hot water causes vasodilation and a drop in blood pressure.
Administer prescribed antihypotensive or corticosteroid medications.	Raising vascular tone and promoting sodium and water retention reduce the potential for low blood pressure.

Evaluation of Expected Outcome: Client's blood pressure is within normal limits and no fainting or injuries have occurred.

2. "My child will need no more pharmacologic therapy."
3. "My child will be asymptomatic by avoiding immunologic triggers."
4. "My child will be in remission or have occasional exacerbations."

3. During an initial physical assessment, an older adult client reports chronic fatigue. When all the assessment findings are normal, it is most appropriate for the nurse to further evaluate the client for:
   1. Depression
   2. Anxiety
   3. Fear
   4. Confusion

connection

Visit the Connection site at **http://connection.lww.com/go/timbyEssentials** for links to chapter-related resources on the Internet.

References and Suggested Readings

Bowyer, R. V. S. (1999). Latex allergy: How to identify it and the people at risk. *Journal of Clinical Nursing, 8*(2), 144–149.

Carpenito, L. J. (2004). *Nursing diagnosis: Application to clinical practice* (10th ed.). Philadelphia: Lippincott Williams & Wilkins.

Carroll, P. (1999). Latex allergy: What you need to know. *RN, 62*(9), 40–42, 45–46.

Castillo, B. (2000). Overcoming fatigue . . . "Chronic fatigue syndrome: Do you know what it means?" *American Journal of Nursing, 100*(1), 14.

Gehring, L. L., & Ring, P. (1999). Latex allergy: Creating a safe environment. *MEDSURG Nursing, 8*(6), 358–362.

Graves, P. B. (April 1, 2002). Itching for more information? *Advance for Nurses,* 27–29.

National Center for Infectious Diseases. (2003). Chronic fatigue syndrome, demographics. [On-line.] Available: http://www.cdc.gov/ncidod/diseases/cfs/demographics.htm.

Shute, N. (2000). Allergy epidemic. *U.S. News & World Report, 128*(18), 46–50, 52–53.

chapter 37

Caring for Clients With AIDS

Words to Know 

acquired immunodeficiency syndrome
acute retroviral syndrome
AIDS dementia complex
AIDS drug assistance program
autologous blood
candidiasis
capsid
directed donor blood
distal sensory polyneuropathy
drug cross-resistance
drug resistance
enzyme-linked immunosorbent assay
highly active anti-retroviral therapy
human immuno-deficiency virus
integrase
Kaposi's sarcoma
mortality
opportunistic infection
p24 antigen test
Pneumocystis pneumonia
polymerase chain reaction
protease
protease inhibitor
reverse transcriptase
reverse transcriptase inhibitor
reverse transcription
safer sex practices
Western blot

Learning Objectives

On completion of this chapter, the reader will:

- Explain the term *acquired immunodeficiency syndrome (AIDS).*
- Identify the virus that causes AIDS.
- Discuss the characteristics of a retrovirus.
- Explain how human immunodeficiency virus (HIV) is transmitted.
- Describe methods for preventing transmission of HIV.
- List criteria for diagnosing AIDS.
- Discuss the pathophysiologic process of AIDS.
- Define manifestations characteristic of acute retroviral syndrome.
- Explain laboratory tests used to test for HIV antibodies and confirm a diagnosis of AIDS.
- Discuss the purpose of laboratory tests used to measure viral load.
- Identify categories of drugs used to treat individuals infected with HIV, giving an example of a specific drug in each category.
- Give the criterion for successful drug therapy.
- Discuss the nursing management of a client with AIDS.
- Give examples of information to provide clients infected with HIV.
- Describe techniques for preventing HIV infection among healthcare workers who care for infected clients.

Acquired immunodeficiency syndrome (AIDS) is an infectious and eventually fatal disorder that profoundly weakens the immune system. AIDS is acquired from a pathogen known as the **human immunodeficiency virus** (HIV). People can remain well, sometimes up to 10 years or longer, despite being infected with HIV before the initial infection develops into AIDS (Fig. 37.1). In the asymptomatic interim, the infected person can infect others.

HIV/AIDS is a disease infecting large numbers of people throughout the world. Based on statistics compiled at the end of 2002 by the Joint United Nations Programme on HIV/AIDS, CUNAIDS and the World Health Organization (WHO) estimate that 42 million people are living with HIV or AIDS worldwide (AIDS Epidemic Update, 2003). Of that number, greater than 90% live in underdeveloped countries.

In the early history of the disease in developed countries, HIV occurred more often among homosexual men and intravenous (IV) drug users, but that is no longer the case. Increasing numbers of heterosexual women are being infected, which leads to transmission of HIV to newborns. To date, nurses are the largest group of healthcare workers to have occupationally acquired HIV infection (CDC, 1999).

Globally, 2.8 million deaths were due to AIDS in 1999 (AIDS Education and Research Trust, 2000). This figure represents the highest **mortality** or death rate from AIDS since AIDS statistics have been compiled. AIDS continues to be a major public health problem in the United States. Currently, it is the leading cause of death among African-American men aged 25 to 44 years and the fifth leading cause of death among people of all races and both sexes

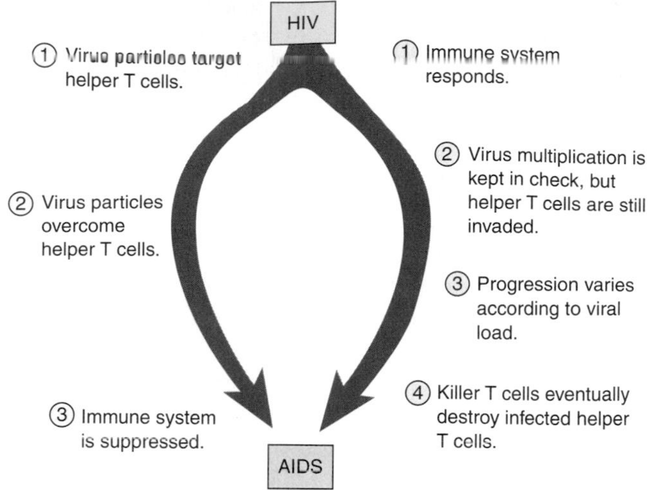

FIGURE 37.1 Cycle of HIV infection and development of AIDS.

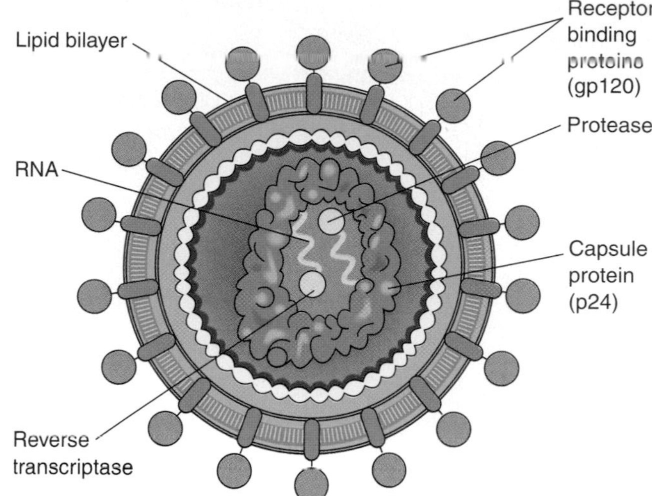

FIGURE 37.2 Structure of a retrovirus.

in this same age range (National Center for Health Statistics, 2001).

HUMAN IMMUNODEFICIENCY VIRUS

It is speculated that HIV is an altered genetic form of simian (monkey) immunodeficiency virus (SIV). It is believed that the transformation facilitated viral transmission from chimpanzees to humans.

Subtypes

Two HIV subtypes have been identified: HIV-1 and HIV-2. HIV-1 mutates easily and frequently, producing multiple substrains that are identified by letters from A through O. HIV-2 is less transmittable, and the interval between initial infection with HIV-2 and development of AIDS is longer. HIV-1 is more prevalent in the United States, where approximately 650,000 to 900,000 people are infected with it. Fewer than 100 Americans are known to be infected with HIV-2. Western Africa is the primary site of infection for HIV-2.

Structural Characteristics

Viruses require a living host cell for survival and duplication. Like all viruses, HIV is genetically incomplete. A double layer of lipid material surrounds the incomplete HIV, referred to as a **capsid.** Surface-binding proteins, called gp120, project in all directions from the lipid bilayer. Inside the capsid are three important enzymes—reverse transcriptase, integrase, and protease—and strands of RNA (Fig. 37.2).

When HIV encounters a helper T-cell lymphocyte, one of the binding proteins fuses with the T cell's receptor, called a *CD4 receptor.* The fusion provides a means by which the capsid can insert its contents into the helper T cell.

Stop, Think, and Respond ● BOX 37-1

What is the role of helper T cells in the immune response?

Replication

To replicate, which means to produce more copies, HIV becomes a parasite of helper T cells (also known as *T4* or *CD4 cells* because of their CD4 receptor; see Chap. 35). HIV alters the T cell's genetic code to make more viral particles. To do this, the enzyme **reverse transcriptase** copies the RNA into DNA, a process called **reverse transcription.** A second viral enzyme, **integrase,** incorporates the reprogrammed DNA with its new viral code into the host cell's DNA.

The altered DNA tells the cell how to assemble amino acids to form protein substances, like the virus. The transformed DNA provides the blueprint or cookbook for making clones of HIV along with the enzymes the virus needs to continue reinfecting additional cells.

The cell follows the DNA's directions and forms long chains of viral particles enclosed within its membrane. **Protease,** the third viral enzyme, cuts the long chains, freeing replicated viral particles into the cytoplasm of the cell. Some migrate to the cell wall and form buds. When the buds rupture, they release many copies of the virus, which reinfect other helper T cells (Fig. 37.3).

More than 10 billion viral particles are released daily. Mutations occur frequently, complicating drug therapy and making production of a vaccine nearly impossible.

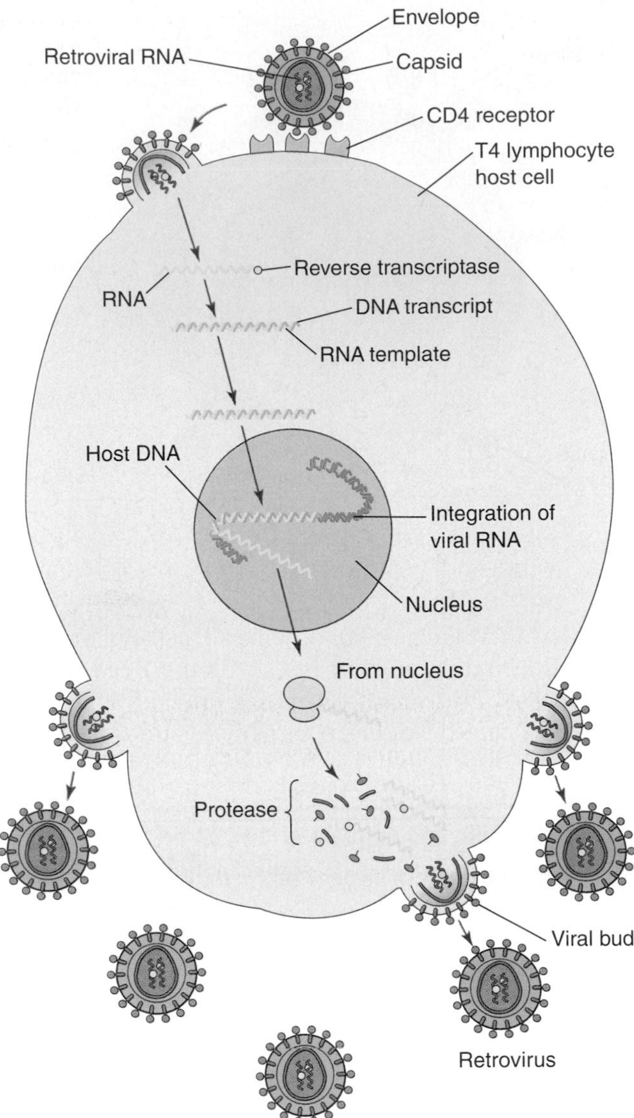

FIGURE 37.3 HIV replication.

Transmission

Human immunodeficiency virus is not transmitted by casual contact. There are only four known body fluids through which HIV is transmitted: blood, semen, vaginal secretions, and breast milk. HIV may be present in saliva, tears, and conjunctival secretions, but transmission of HIV through these fluids has not been implicated. HIV is not found in urine, stool, vomit, or sweat.

> **Stop, Think, and Respond ● BOX 37-2**
>
> *How would you respond to those who avoid drinking from a common cup, such as those used in Christian church services, because they fear acquiring AIDS?*

Certain behaviors increase the risk for acquiring HIV from infectious body fluids (Box 37-1). Unprotected sexual intercourse and multiple sexual partners increase the risk for HIV infection and other sexually transmitted diseases. Using a condom is one of the most effective ways to reduce risk of HIV infection. Condoms are available for both men and women (Fig. 37.4).

Blood and blood products were a major source of transmission before 1984, but now an HIV screening test is performed on donated blood. Screening donated blood for HIV antibodies reduces risk of transfusion-related infection with HIV, but it is not flawless. Antibody screening cannot identify infected blood from donors who have yet to produce significant antibodies. The window of time between infection (entrance of HIV into the body) and production of antibodies varies from 1 to 6 weeks. A recently infected person with HIV could donate blood containing the virus, even though screening test results are negative for HIV. Other potential methods of transmission include receiving infected semen from a sperm bank or infected organs or tissues for transplantation.

ACQUIRED IMMUNODEFICIENCY SYNDROME

Acquired immunodeficiency syndrome is the end stage of HIV infection. Certain events establish conversion of HIV infection to AIDS: (1) markedly decreased T4 cell count from a normal level of 800 to 1200/mm^3; and (2) development of certain cancers and **opportunistic infections,** that usually do not occur in individuals with a healthy immune system. In 1993, the CDC devised a classification system involving two categories that constitute an AIDS diagnosis: (1) Category 1, 2, or 3, and (2) Category A, B, or C (Table 37.1).

> **Stop, Think, and Respond ● BOX 37-3**
>
> *What classification would be assigned to an HIV-positive person with a T4 cell count of 350/mm^3 who develops* Pneumocystis carinii *pneumonia?* 

BOX 37-1 ● High-Risk Factors for HIV Infection

- Unprotected vaginal, anal, or oral sex
- Contact with blood and infectious body fluids during medical, surgical, dental, or nursing procedures
- Sharing intravenous needles or syringes
- Receiving nonautologous transfusions of blood or blood products
- Receiving plasma or clotting factors that have not been heat treated
- Contact with infected blood on body-piercing, tattoo, and dental equipment
- Transmission from infected mothers to infants during pregnancy, birth, or breast-feeding

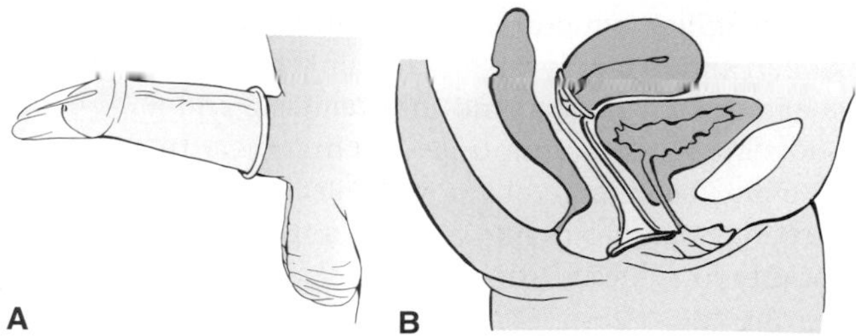

FIGURE 37.4 Applied condoms (**A**) male and (**B**) female.

Pathophysiology and Etiology

Acquired immunodeficiency syndrome is acquired from direct contact with blood or body fluids of an individual infected with HIV or from indirect contact with infected blood or body fluids. When HIV infection occurs, it gradually impairs the ability of infected T4 cells to recognize foreign antigens (e.g., disease pathogens) and stimulate B-cell lymphocytes. While massive numbers of viral particles are being released, infected T4 cells are destroyed by HIV itself and by killer T8-cell lymphocytes that no longer recognize the altered T4 cell's membrane as being "self." Although new T4 cells are produced, the process is never as fast as replication of the virus. Eventually, T4 cells become significantly depleted, and immunodeficiency develops. The infected person ultimately dies from an opportunistic infection.

The rate of progression from HIV infection to AIDS is related to the concentration of virus in the blood. For some, the process may take 10 years or more. Although most people infected with HIV die of their disease, a few are long-term survivors. Some explanations for long-term survival include the following: the infectious HIV is a weak strain, the amount of virus is kept low with stronger-than-normal killer T8 cells, or the combination of drugs used for treatment is effective.

TABLE 37.1 CLASSIFICATION FOR HIV INFECTION

CATEGORY 1	CATEGORY 2	CATEGORY 3
T4 cell count ≥500/mm³	T4 cell count 200–499/mm³	T4 cell count <200/mm³
CATEGORY A	**CATEGORY B**	**CATEGORY C**
HIV positive with one or more of the following: • Asymptomatic • Persistent generalized lymphadenopathy (swollen lymph nodes) • Symptoms formerly known as *AIDS-related complex* (ARC), such as anorexia, weight loss, fever, night sweats, rash, fatigue, lowered resistance to infection, diarrhea	HIV positive with conditions attributed to or complicated by HIV infection such as: • Bacillary angiomatosis • Candidiasis (oral, vulvovaginal) unresponsive to treatment • Cervical dysplasia or carcinoma • Fever or diarrhea for more than 1 month • Hairy leukoplakia • Herpes zoster (at least two episodes) • Idiopathic thrombocytopenic-purpura • Listeriosis • Pelvic inflammatory disease/ tubo-ovarian abscess • Peripheral neuropathy • Toxoplasmosis of the brain • Wasting syndrome	HIV positive with one or more of the following: • Candidiasis (bronchial, tracheal, lungs, or esophagus) • Cervical cancer (invasive) • Coccidiomycosis (disseminated or extrapulmonary) • Cryptococcosis (extrapulmonary) • Cryptosporidiosis for less than 1 month • Cytomegalovirus (other than liver, spleen, or nodes) • Encephalopathy (HIV-related) • Herpes simplex (<1 month) or bronchitis, pneumonitis, esophagitis • Histoplasmosis (disseminated or extrapulmonary) • Isosporiosis (<1 month) • Kaposi's sarcoma • Lymphoma, Burkitt's (or equivalent), immunoblastic (or equivalent), brain (primary) • *Mycobacterium avium* complex or *Mycobacterium kansasii,* disseminated or extrapulmonary • *Mycobacterium tuberculosis,* any site, pulmonary or extrapulmonary • *Mycobacterium,* other species • *Pneumocystis carinii* pneumonia • Pneumonia, recurrent • Progressive multifocal leukoencephalopathy • *Salmonella* septicemia, recurrent

From Centers for Disease Control and Prevention. (1992). 1993 Revised classification system for HIV infection and expanded surveillance case definition for AIDS among adolescents and adults. *Morbidity and Mortality Weekly Report, 41*(51), 961–962.

Prevention Strategies

The transmission of HIV is reduced or eliminated by adhering to the following guidelines:

- Abstain from sexual intercourse.
- Have mutually monogamous sex with an uninfected partner.
- Avoid casual sex with multiple partners.
- Use a condom and spermicide that contains nonoxynol-9 during sexual intercourse.
- Abstain from using IV drugs.
- Use a new needle and syringe each time IV drugs are injected.
- Refrain from donating blood if engaged in high-risk behaviors.
- Bank **autologous blood** (self-donated) or **directed donor blood** (specified blood donors among relatives and friends) when preparing for nonemergency surgical procedures.

Some authorities believe that directed blood is no safer than blood collected from public donors. Those who support this belief say that directed donors may not reveal their high-risk behaviors that put the potential recipient at risk for blood-borne pathogens like HIV.

Nurses and other healthcare workers use Standard Precautions when caring for all clients whose infectious status is unknown. Because postexposure protocols can reduce risk of HIV infection if initiated promptly, nurses must immediately report any needlestick or sharp injury. Infected healthcare workers can continue to practice, but they usually are restricted from performing procedures in which they may exchange blood with clients.

Assessment Findings

At the time of primary HIV infection, one third to more than one half of those infected develop **acute retroviral syndrome** (*viremia*), which often is mistaken for "flu" or some other common illness. Some signs include fever; swollen and tender lymph nodes; pharyngitis; rash about the face, trunk, palms, and soles; muscle and joint pain; headache; nausea; vomiting; and diarrhea. In addition, there may be enlarged liver and spleen, weight loss, and neurologic symptoms like visual changes or cognitive and motor involvement. Admission of risk behaviors for HIV narrows the differential diagnosis. Although viral replication is rapid at this time, antibody tests cannot detect the infection.

Eventually, individuals infected with HIV present with a form of cancer that is atypical for the person's age and health history, or an opportunistic infection. For example, **Kaposi's sarcoma,** a type of connective tissue cancer common among those with AIDS, may be noted (Fig. 37.5). Others who acquire *Pneumocystis* pneumonia (discussed later) have an unproductive cough and shortness of breath. In women, gynecologic problems may be the focus of the chief complaint. Abnormal results of Papanicolaou tests, genital warts, pelvic inflammatory disease, and persistent vaginitis (see Chaps. 56 and 59) also may correlate with HIV infection.

The **enzyme-linked immunosorbent assay** (ELISA) test, an initial HIV screening test, is positive when there are sufficient HIV antibodies or antibodies from other infectious diseases. The test is repeated if results are positive. If results of a second ELISA test are positive, the **Western blot** is performed. A positive result on Western blot confirms the diagnosis, but false-positive and false-negative results on both tests are possible. Written consent must be obtained before an ELISA or Western blot test is performed. Results of the tests require strict confidentiality.

A total T-cell count, T4 and T8 count, and T4/T8 ratio determine status of T lymphocytes. A T4-cell count of less than 500 mm^3 indicates immune suppression; a T4-cell count of 200/mm^3 or less is an indicator of AIDS.

It now is possible to measure a person's viral load, the number of viral particles in the blood. **The p24 antigen test** and **polymerase chain reaction** test measure viral

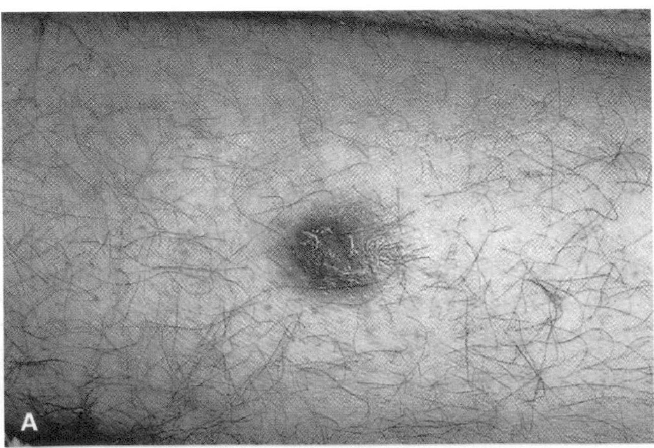

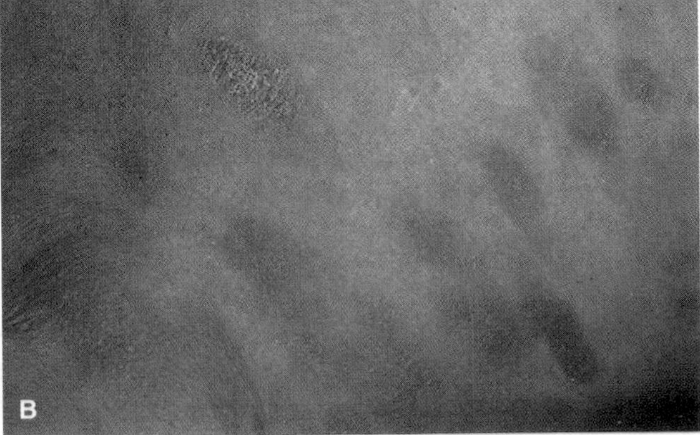

FIGURE 37.5 Kaposi's sarcoma (**A**) single lesion and (**B**) multiple lesions.

loads. They are used to guide drug therapy and follow progression of the disease. Viral load tests and T4-cell counts may be performed every 2 to 3 months once it is determined that a person is HIV positive.

Other general laboratory and diagnostic tests are done when opportunistic infections are involved. Cancer screenings, especially Papanicolaou cervical tests for women (see Chap. 53), are recommended for those infected with HIV. Immunosuppression tends to facilitate development of cancer and accelerate its progression.

Medical Management

People with HIV and AIDS are treated with antiretroviral drugs, adjunct drug therapy to boost the immune response, and supportive care during opportunistic infections. It usually is recommended that clients infected with HIV receive pneumococcal, hepatitis B, and yearly influenza vaccines. Additional medical management includes treating anorexia, diarrhea, and weight loss.

Vaccines that may prevent HIV infection are in clinical trials. Although clients who already are HIV positive cannot benefit from a preventive vaccine, the need to control global spread of HIV is pressing. Currently, one experimental AIDS vaccine, AIDSVAX, has reached Phase III of clinical trials. This phase of testing may last 2 to 10 years and involves human test subjects. AIDSVAX contains only a subunit or part of HIV. The portion used in AIDSVAX is the gp120 protein. It is hoped that the immune system will recognize the foreign gp120 protein, develop memory cells, and speedily destroy the complete virus should it enter the body in the future.

Stop, Think, and Respond ● BOX 37-4

What is the role of the gp120 component of HIV? 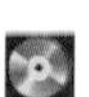

Antiretroviral Drug Therapy

The physician decides when and which antiretroviral drugs to prescribe based on the client's T4-cell and viral load counts, potential compliance, medication side effect profiles, cost, and interactions of each drug. Antiretroviral medications are very expensive—as much as $10,000 or more per year in the United States. Some social agencies and pharmaceutical companies have compassionate need programs that supply antiretroviral drugs to individuals who cannot afford them.

Opinions vary as to when to initiate drug therapy. Development of **drug resistance,** ineffectual response to a prescribed drug because of the survival and duplication of exceptionally virulent mutations (Fig. 37.6), and **drug cross-resistance,** diminished drug response to similar HIV drugs, are common. Because drug resistance limits future treatment options, some physicians believe delaying drug therapy is justified. One guideline is to wait until the client's viral load is greater than 30,000 copies/mL or the T4-cell count is less than 350 mm^3. It is critical that clients with HIV comply with regular appointments for laboratory blood tests.

Drug therapy generally begins with a combination of three antiretroviral drugs: two **reverse transcriptase inhibitors,** drugs that interfere with the virus's ability to make a genetic blueprint, and one **protease inhibitor,** a drug that inhibits the ability of virus particles to leave the host cell (Drug Therapy Table 37.1). Combination therapy, sometimes referred to as a *drug cocktail* or **highly active antiretroviral therapy,** has several benefits:

- The combination of drugs suppresses replication of the virus using different mechanisms.
- The drugs lower the viral load more quickly—sometimes to undetectable levels. Doing so ultimately slows the rate of disease progression, prevents opportunistic infections, and, in turn, lengthens survival.

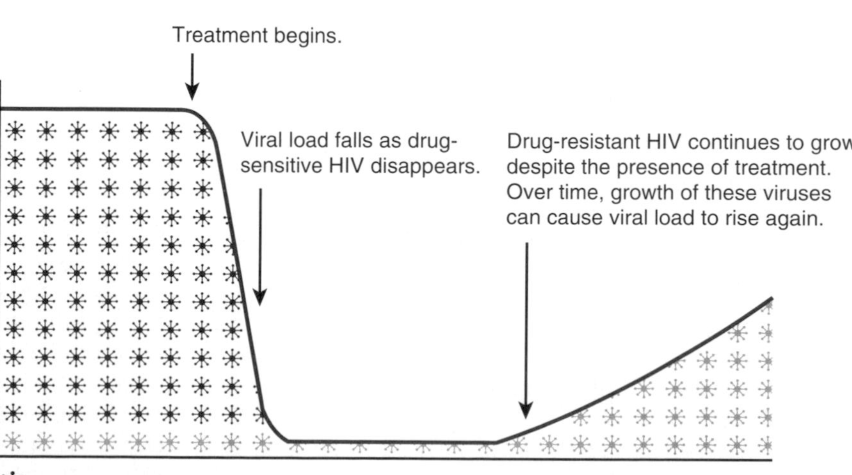

FIGURE 37.6 The development of drug-resistant strains of HIV.

DRUG THERAPY TABLE 37.1 EXAMPLES OF DRUGS USED IN HIV THERAPY

DRUG CATEGORY AND EXAMPLES	SIDE EFFECTS	NURSING CONSIDERATIONS
Reverse Transcriptase Inhibitors		
Nucleoside reverse transcriptase inhibitors (NRTIs)		
zidovudine (AZT, Retrovir)	Anemia, nausea, gastrointestinal pain, diarrhea, myositis, headaches, fever, rash	Monitor T4 cell counts. Administer drug every 4 hours around the clock. Tell client to report extreme fatigue, nausea, vomiting, or rash.
didanosine (ddI, Videx)	Pancreatitis, nausea, vomiting, abdominal pain, hepatotoxicity, bone marrow suppression, insomnia	Administer on an empty stomach, 1 hour before or 2 hours after eating. Advise client to chew tablets thoroughly or crush tablets and dissolve in at least 1 ounce of water.
Nonnucleoside reverse transcriptase inhibitors (NNRTIs)		
nevirapine (Viramune) *Cidofovir (Vistide)*	Rash, hepatotoxicity, headache nausea, vomiting, diarrhea	Use is contraindicated during pregnancy or breast-feeding. Avoid combining with protease inhibitors or oral contraceptives. Monitor hepatic and renal function. Consult physician if severe rash occurs.
efavirenz (Sustiva)	Rash, dizziness, fatigue, unusual dreams, confusion, impaired thinking, amnesia, agitation, hallucinations, hepatotoxicity, false-positive test results for cannabinoids	Control intake of fatty foods, which can elevate drug levels. Assess mental status. Monitor liver function. Warn that drug test results may be falsely positive for marijuana.
Protease Inhibitors		
indinavir (Crixivan)	Nephrolithiasis, gastrointestinal intolerance, headache, blurred vision, dizziness, rash, metallic taste, thrombocytopenia, hyperglycemia, lipodystrophy	Monitor for kidney stones. Increase fluid intake to help prevent formation of kidney stones. Wait 1 hour between administration of indinavir and ddI. Give drug 1 hour before or 2 hours after a meal with skim or low-fat milk. Give hard candies to help mask metallic taste. Check blood glucose levels regularly. Observe for signs of bruising or bleeding. Warn that this drug causes a redistribution of body fat.
saquinavir (Invirase, Fortase)	Headache, weakness, muscle aches, nausea, abdominal discomfort, diarrhea, elevated level of creatinine phosphokinase	Administer with or within 2 hours of a full meal. Protect from injury, which may result from weakness. Report alterations in stool or urine color, which may indicate liver dysfunction.

- Combination therapy diminishes the rate of viral mutations and prolongs drug effectiveness.
- Using two or more drugs simultaneously reduces the chance that the virus will develop resistance or cross-resistance.

The goal of antiretroviral therapy is to bring the viral load to an "undetectable" level. This level is no more than 500 or 50 copies, depending on the sensitivity of the selected viral load test.

Clients who neglect to take antiretroviral drugs as prescribed (i.e., every dose, at its designated time, with or without food as directed) risk development of drug resistance. When drug levels are not adequately maintained, viral replication and mutations increase.

Adjunct Drug Therapy

Other drugs may be used with antiretroviral drug therapy in an overall effort to halt progression of AIDS. One drug is hydroxyurea (Hydrea), usually used to treat cancer. It inhibits an enzyme that functions in DNA synthesis, inhibiting or slowing reproduction of tumor cells. When combined with antiretrovirals, hydroxyurea interferes with viral replication, increasing anti-HIV effects.

The immune system naturally produces interleukin-2 (IL-2), a chemical substance called a *cytokine.* The function of IL-2 is to stimulate production of lymphocytes. The pharmaceutical counterpart of IL-2 is used to increase numbers of T4 helper and natural killer lymphocytes. Natural killer lymphocytes specifically target viral infected cells and cancer cells. Use of IL-2 boosts the body's immune defenses against HIV.

Supportive Care of Opportunistic Infections

Clients with AIDS acquire many infectious disorders, any one of which can cause death. These infectious disorders and their comparative severity are uncommon in populations of relatively healthy people. Management of some common infectious conditions follows.

PNEUMOCYSTIS PNEUMONIA. Clients infected with HIV are at particular risk for acquiring a type of pneumonia caused by an organism called *P. carinii.* The pneumonia may result in respiratory failure. Mechanical ventilation sustains adequate pulmonary function. Aerosol therapy and deep suctioning after instillation of saline often are necessary to clear lungs of thick sputum. To prevent and treat ***Pneumocystis* pneumonia,** trimethoprim-sulfamethoxazole (Bactrim, Septra) is prescribed. Monthly aerosolized pentamidine isethionate (NebuPent) also is effective.

CANDIDIASIS. **Candidiasis** is a yeast infection caused by the *Candida albicans* microorganism. It may develop in the oral, pharyngeal, esophageal, or vaginal cavities or in folds of the skin. It often is called *thrush* when located in the mouth. Inspection of the mouth, throat, or vagina reveals areas of white plaque that may bleed when mobilized with a cotton-tipped swab.

Candidiasis in the mouth and throat can lead to problems with eating and subsequent weight loss. Topical antifungals, such as nystatin (Mycostatin) oral suspension that is swished in the mouth and then swallowed or taken in an alternate lozenge form, are useful for treating oral candidiasis. Clotrimazole (Gyne-Lotrimin, Mycelex) and miconazole (Monistat) cream, vaginal tablets, and suppositories are used to treat vaginitis. Sometimes systemic antifungals like amphotericin B (Fungizone) or fluconazole (Diflucan) are required to control candidiasis.

CYTOMEGALOVIRUS INFECTION. Opportunistic infections caused by the cytomegalovirus (CMV) affect immunosuppressed people such as clients with AIDS. CMV can infect the choroid and retinal layers of the eye, leading to blindness. It also can cause ulcers in the esophagus, colitis and diarrhea, pneumonia, and encephalitis. Foscarnet (Foscavir), cidofovir (Vistide), and ganciclovir (Cytovene) are used in combination to aggressively treat acute CMV infections. Maintenance drug therapy follows to reduce potential for future viral activation.

CRYPTOSPORIDIOSIS. Immunosuppressed clients may develop serious diarrhea as a result of infection with a protozoan called *Cryptosporidium.* The organism is spread by the fecal–oral route from contaminated water, food, or human or animal wastes. Those infected can lose large volumes of fluid per day. This quickly leads to dehydration and electrolyte imbalances. When diarrhea is accompanied by anorexia, nausea, and vomiting, weight is difficult to maintain.

Definitive diagnosis is made by examining the stool for ova and parasites and other cytologic examinations. Antibiotic therapy is then implemented, which may include azithromycin (Zithromax) or clarithromycin (Biaxin), or an antiprotozoal agent such as paromomycin (Humatin).

Management of AIDS-Related Complications

Besides AIDS-related cancers and opportunistic infections, clients may develop **AIDS dementia complex** (ADC), a neurologic condition that causes degeneration of the brain. It primarily affects mood, cognition, and motor functions. Clients exhibit forgetfulness, limited attention span, decreased ability to concentrate, and delusional thinking. Moods range from irritability to euphoria. Possible motor dysfunction is manifested by staggering gait and muscle incoordination, slowing of all movements, or paraplegia, which may be accompanied by incontinence.

Antiretroviral therapy can delay or prevent ADC. Other drugs, currently in clinical trials, slow progression of ADC once it occurs. Antiretroviral therapy may be combined with selegiline (Eldepryl), an anti-Parkinson's drug, to treat motor and cognitive impairments of ADC, and psychiatric drugs to moderate mood and activity levels.

Clients may also develop **distal sensory polyneuropathy** (DSP), characterized by abnormal sensations such as burning and numbness in the feet and later in the hands. Because neuropathy is a side effect of several antiretroviral drugs, it is difficult to determine if the cause is actually destruction of the sensory peripheral nerves or drug therapy. DSP does not respond well to drug therapy. Nevertheless, an effort is made to preserve and promote nerve function using vitamin B_{12} and thiamine supplementation. Neuropathic pain also may be amenable to treatment with tricyclic antidepressants like amitriptyline (Elavil) and nortriptyline (Pamelor) or anticonvulsants such as gabapentin (Neurontin) and carbamazepine (Tegretol).

Nursing Management

The role of the nurse involves health teaching and counseling of high-risk populations. Areas of emphasis include HIV prevention strategies such as sexual abstinence and **safer sex practices,** sexual activities in which body fluids are not exchanged. Encourage diagnostic screening for those whose behaviors place them at risk for HIV infection. Help to interpret results of diagnostic tests and monitor the need for continued follow-up in the months after potential exposure.

For those with an established HIV status, explain the action of each antiretroviral drug and develop a schedule for the client's self-administration. This includes teaching about the need for rigid adherence to the dosage, time, and frequency of drug administration to avoid resistance. Describing side effects of drug therapy is essential, with the admonition to refrain from discontinuing any prescribed drugs without first consulting the physician. Make appointments for laboratory tests for monitoring effects of drug therapy.

An important nursing intervention is referral of HIV-positive clients to support groups and resources for information about new HIV drug development, clinical drug trials, **AIDS drug assistance programs** (state-based programs partially funded by Title II of the Ryan White CARE Act), and progress on vaccine development. See Nursing Care Plan 37-1 for additional nursing management.

Reducing Occupational Risks

Observe Standard Precautions whenever there is a risk of exposure to blood and body fluids. Follow the guidelines for safe handling of needles and sharp instruments. The Occupational Safety and Health Administration (OSHA) also recommends the following when caring for all clients regardless of their infectious status:

- Transport specimens of body fluids in leakproof containers.
- Clean and disinfect utility gloves used for cleaning.
- Remove barrier garments (e.g., face shields, glasses) as soon as possible after leaving a client's room.

If exposed to blood of any client, report the incident to the person in charge of employee health immediately. You will be tested for HIV at regular intervals and treated with antiretrovirals depending on results of tests or potential for infection. While awaiting results of diagnostic tests, follow the same sexual precautions as someone who is diagnosed with AIDS.

Client and Family Teaching

For clients healthy enough to continue as outpatients, develop a teaching plan that includes the following guidelines:

- Follow medication schedule; do not omit or increase dose without physician approval.
- Comply with timing of antiviral medications around meals.
- Eat small, frequent, well-balanced meals; try to maintain or gain weight. Drink plenty of water.
- Check weight weekly. Report progressive weight loss or loss of appetite to the physician.
- Avoid exposure to people with infections, including colds, sore throats, upper respiratory tract infections, and childhood diseases (e.g., mumps, chickenpox), and those recently vaccinated. Avoid crowds.
- Notify physician if signs of infection, such as fever, sore throat, diarrhea, respiratory distress, and cough occur, or if signs of a skin, rectal, vaginal, or oral infection appear.
- Wear gloves and a mask when disposing of animal excreta, such as kitty litter, bird cage liners, and hamster shavings; wash hands thoroughly afterward.
- Wash all food before cooking; do not eat raw meat, fish, or vegetables or food not completely cooked.
- Wash bedding and clothes in hot water and separate from the laundry of others, especially if bedding and clothes are soiled with body secretions.
- Avoid smoking or exposure to secondhand smoke.
- Personal cleanliness is a must. Bathe or shower daily, wash hands before and after preparing food, clean the anal and perineal areas well after each bowel movement, and wash hands after voiding or defecating.
- When possible, avoid dry and dusty areas, excessive humidity, and extreme heat or cold. Wear clothing appropriate to weather and temperature.
- Take frequent rest periods, and space activities to prevent fatigue.
- Do not share IV needles, and do not donate blood.
- Inform healthcare personnel of HIV-positive status.

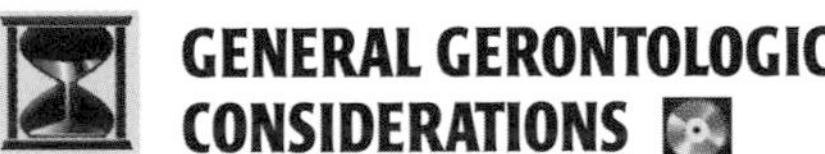

GENERAL GERONTOLOGIC CONSIDERATIONS

According to the CDC, approximately 10% of reported AIDS cases involve those older than 50 years of age.

Stereotyping older adults as asexual may cause the nurse to neglect to question the older adult about sexual matters, resulting in an inaccurate sexual history.

The period between initial infection with HIV and the onset of AIDS-related symptoms is shorter for older adults than others, and death usually occurs earlier in this age group.

Dementia caused by AIDS may be mistaken for other dementias commonly associated with older adults.

Older adults with AIDS may lack an adequate support system and feel lonely, anxious, and isolated.

Older adults in general are less informed about AIDS than younger people. Education campaigns target younger at-risk population and fail to address the possibility or needs of older adults contracting the disease.

Critical Thinking Exercises

1. *What advice would you give adolescents to reduce their risk for becoming infected with HIV?*
2. *A nurse on a medical unit sustains a needlestick injury. What actions should the nurse take? What are the responsibilities of the employing agency?*

NCLEX-STYLE REVIEW QUESTIONS 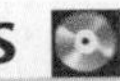

1. A nurse is obtaining a client's consent for receiving blood. The client asks if there is any way that HIV can be acquired from the transfusion. The nurse would be most truthful and accurate in stating:

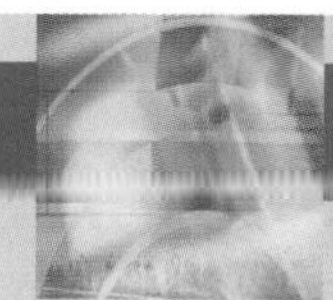

Nursing Care Plan 37-1

THE CLIENT WITH AIDS

Assessment

- *Obtain a thorough history,* including risk factors for HIV infection. List all symptoms, exploring each thoroughly. Determine the client's past and current treatment medications. Inspect oral mucous membranes and all skin surfaces for rashes, skin breakdown, and opportunistic infections such as herpes lesions. Look for Kaposi's sarcoma, which appear as dark purple lesions that may be painful. Examine arms and legs for edema. Auscultate lungs for breath sounds. Question the client about coughing, sputum production, dyspnea, and orthopnea. Palpate lymph nodes and abdomen for organ enlargement. Gather additional data based on the client's complaints or symptoms. Review results of recent laboratory and diagnostic tests.
- *Obtain vital signs and weight.* Question the client about weight loss and weight before he or she became symptomatic. Explore past and current dietary intake. Ask about factors that interfere with eating, such as difficulty swallowing, diarrhea, and oral discomfort.
- *Assess the client's mental status (see Chap. 12) and perform a neurologic assessment (see Chap. 38).* Look for peripheral neuropathies (sensation changes in extremities), which may be side effects of antiretroviral medications. Ask about any visual changes (e.g., floaters, spots, loss of peripheral vision).
- *Evaluate emotional status,* looking for signs of depression or anxiety.
- *Observe for signs of dehydration.* Examine skin and mucous membranes for dryness. Evaluate skin turgor. Note additional findings like decreased urine output, hypotension, and slow filling of hand veins. Look for indications of electrolyte deficit(s) such as excessive thirst, muscle weakness, cramping, nausea, vomiting, cardiac dysrhythmia, shallow respirations, and headache.

Nursing Diagnosis: **Risk for Infection** (opportunistic) related to immunodeficiency

Expected Outcome: Client will experience no secondary infections.

Interventions	*Rationales*
Follow practices of medical and surgical asepsis.	Aseptic practices break the infection cycle by decreasing or eliminating infectious agents, their reservoirs, and vehicles for transmission.
Place client in protective isolation if T4 cell count is ≤ 500 mm^3.	Keeping the immunosuppressed client in a separate environment and using precautions to limit introduction of pathogens in that environment reduce potential for transmission of a nosocomial infection.
Promote hygiene especially before meals and after elimination.	The fecal–oral route is a common mechanism for transfer of endogenous microorganisms from one body site to another, where they can become pathogenic. Handwashing reduces transmission of microorganisms.
Facilitate adequate sleep and nutrition.	Reduces fatigue, stabilizes mood, increases protein synthesis, maintains disease-fighting mechanisms of the immune system, promotes cellular growth and repair, and improves capacity for learning and memory storage.
Prohibit ill visitors and staff from contact with client.	Microorganisms are transferred by one of three routes: airborne, droplet, and contact.

Evaluation of Expected Outcome: Client is free from secondary infections.

***PC: Pneumocystis* Pneumonia**

Expected Outcome: Nurse will manage and minimize pneumonia.

(continued)

Nursing Care Plan 37-1 (Continued)

THE CLIENT WITH AIDS

Interventions	*Rationales*
Auscultate lungs every 4 hours; monitor oxygen saturation at least once per shift.	Diminished or wet lung sounds and arterial oxygen saturation (SpO_2) ≤ 90% indicate poor ventilation and oxygen diffusion.
Assist with measures to clear respiratory secretions such as coughing, pharyngeal suctioning, aerosol treatments, and chest percussion.	Promotes gas exchange.
Give oxygen as medically prescribed if SpO_2 is ≤ 90%.	Keeping SpO_2 above 90% ensures that oxygen in plasma (PaO_2) is between 80 to 100 mm Hg.
Administer prescribed antimicrobials.	Antimicrobials exert either bactericidal or bacteriostatic functions.

Evaluation of Expected Outcome: Nurse ensures management of pneumonia and control of complications.

Nursing Diagnosis: **Risk for Deficient Fluid Volume** related to diarrhea secondary to viremia, opportunistic infection, and side effects of medication

Expected Outcome: Client's fluid intake and output will be balanced.

Interventions	*Rationales*
Keep a record of intake and output, measuring liquid feces.	Provides an objective account of fluid status.
Offer oral fluids every hour while client is awake.	Oral intake increases when the nurse encourages it.
Withhold foods, especially caffeine, that are irritating until bowel function improves.	Fibrous foods increase peristalsis and diarrhea; caffeine is a bowel stimulant and diuretic.
Administer prescribed antidiarrheals.	Antidiarrheals slow peristalsis, adsorbing gastrointestinal irritants and water.
Report evidence of dehydration or electrolyte imbalance.	Parenteral fluids and electrolyte additives are alternate ways to restore fluid and electrolyte balance when the oral route is inadequate.

Evaluation of Expected Outcome: Client's fluid intake and output is 1500 mL/24 hours.

Nursing Diagnosis: **Impaired Oral Mucous Membranes** related to inflammation secondary to opportunistic infections

Expected Outcome: Client's mucous membranes will be pink, moist, and intact.

Interventions	*Rationales*
Provide meticulous oral care after and between meals.	Oral hygiene removes bacteria and yeast from mouth.
Avoid using mouthwashes that contain alcohol.	Irritates inflamed tissue.
Use mouth rinses with warm (not hot) plain water, normal saline solution, or water and hydrogen peroxide.	Warmth increases circulation and promotes healing. Water, saline, and dilute peroxide do not irritate oral tissues.
Use a soft toothbrush or foam swabs for oral care.	Protect gums from injury and infection.

Evaluation of Expected Outcome: Client's mucous membranes are normal.

(continued)

Nursing Care Plan 37-1 (Continued)

THE CLIENT WITH AIDS

Nursing Diagnoses: **Powerlessness** and **Hopelessness** related to poor prognosis

Expected Outcomes: Client will control his or her time, make other personal choices, and develop a realistic perception of the immediate future.

Interventions	*Rationales*
Give client choices whenever possible.	Reaffirms a sense of control.
Help client formulate and achieve short-term goals to enjoy more frequent small successes.	Enhances hope.
Discourage client from abandoning traditional treatment for therapies that lack any evidence of effectiveness.	Desperate clients may turn to unsubstantiated claims of a cure for AIDS.

Evaluation of Expected Outcome: Client makes personal choices that give a sense of control without further damaging health, and realistically perceives his or her future.

1. "With any medical procedure there are risks. You must weigh the risks against the benefits."
2. "The blood supply is screened for HIV antibodies to ensure quality and safety."
3. "Antibody screening will not detect HIV in blood given by those who have not produced significant HIV antibodies."
4. "Transmission of HIV through blood transfusions is very low."

2. A nurse's aide attending respite training at an inpatient hospice center asks the nurse what causes the death in a client with end stage HIV. The nurse is most correct in instructing the nurse's aide that the client infected with HIV ultimately dies from:
1. An opportunistic infection
2. A depleted white blood cell count
3. Deterioration of the brain tissue
4. A massive stroke or heart attack

3. A client with HIV is diagnosed with an oral yeast infection called *Candida albicans.* What type of medication would the nurse expect the physician to prescribe?
1. An antiviral
2. An antiemetic
3. An antifungal
4. An antihistamine

connection

Visit the Connection site at **http://connection.lww.com/go/timbyEssentials** for links to chapter-related resources on the Internet.

References and Suggested Readings

A scourge beyond imagining. (2000, December 18). *U.S. News and World Report, 129*(24), 34.

AIDS Education and Research Trust. (2000; December 20). United States HIV and AIDS Statistics. [On-line.] Available: http://www.avert.org/usastats.htm.

AIDS epidemic update (2003). Joint United Nations Programme on HIV/AIDS, World Health Organization. Available: http://www.unaids.org/en/evenR/world.

Barroso, J. (2002). HIV-related fatigue. *American Journal of Nursing, 102*(5), 83–86.

Bormann, J., & Kelly, A. (1999). HIV and AIDS: Are you biased? *American Journal of Nursing, 99*(9), 38–39.

Centers for Disease Control and Prevention, U.S. Department of Health and Human Services, Public Health Service. (1999). *HIV/AIDS Surveillance Report, 11*(2).

Cochran, A., & Wilson, B. A. (1999). Current management of AIDS and related opportunistic infections. *MEDSURG Nursing, 8*(4), 257–264, 266.

Coyne, P. J., Lyne, M. E., & Watson, A. C. (2002). Symptom management in people with AIDS. *American Journal of Nursing, 102*(9), 48–55.

Daughtry, L. M., Bankston, J. B., & Deschotels, J. M. (2002). HIV meds: Keeping trouble at bay. *RN, 65*(2), 31–35.

Facing facts and AIDS. (2000, July 24). *U.S. News and World Report, 129*(4), 24.

Holzemer, W. L. (2002). HIV and AIDS: The symptom experience. *American Journal of Nursing, 102*(4), 48–52.

Joint United Nations Programme on HIV/AIDS (UNAIDS). (2003). AIDS epidemic update. [On-line.] Available: http://www.unaids.org.

Milone, A. (August 19, 2002). Social security sex. *Advance for Nurses,* 23–24.

Monts, R. L., & Bufalini, M. (2002). HIV & AIDS in rural America. *Community Health Forum,* 17–19.

Muma, D. J., et al. (1999). *HIV manual for health care professionals.* New York: McGraw-Hill.

National Center for Health Statistics, Centers for Disease Control and Prevention. (2001). Mortality data from the National Vital Statistics System. [On-line]. Available: http://www.cdc.gov/nchs.

chapter 38

Introduction to the Nervous System

Words to Know 

acetylcholine
acetylcholinesterase
arachnoid
axon
brain stem
cauda equina
central nervous system
cerebellum
cerebrum
corpus callosum
decerebrate posturing
decorticate posturing
dendrites
dopamine
dura mater
epinephrine
extrapyramidal
flaccidity
medulla oblongata
meninges
midbrain
myelin
neurilemma
neuron
neurotransmitters
norepinephrine
parasympathetic nervous system
peripheral nervous system
pia mater
pons
pyramidal
subarachnoid space
sympathetic nervous system
synapses
ventricles

Learning Objectives

On completion of this chapter, the reader will:

- Name the two anatomic divisions of the nervous system.
- Name the three parts of the brain.
- List the lobes of the cerebrum.
- Describe functions of the spinal cord.
- Discuss the function of the two parts of the autonomic nervous system.
- Describe methods used to assess motor and sensory function.
- List diagnostic procedures performed to detect neurologic disorders.
- Discuss the nursing management of the client undergoing neurologic diagnostic testing.

The nervous system consists of the brain, spinal cord, and peripheral nerves. It is responsible for coordinating body functions and responding to changes in or stimuli from the internal and external environment. Changes in functioning of the nervous system can profoundly affect the entire body.

ANATOMY AND PHYSIOLOGY

The nervous system is divided into two anatomic divisions: the **central nervous system** (CNS) and the **peripheral nervous system** (PNS). The basic structure of the nervous system is the nerve cell or **neuron** (Fig. 38.1). Neurons are either sensory or motor. *Sensory neurons* transmit impulses to the CNS; *motor neurons* transmit impulses from the CNS. A neuron is composed of a cell body, a nucleus, and threadlike projections or fibers called **dendrites.** Dendrites conduct impulses to the cell body and are called *afferent* ("to" or "toward") nerve fibers. An **axon** is a nerve fiber that projects and conducts impulses away from the cell body. It is therefore called an *efferent* ("away from") nerve fiber. The axon usually is larger than the dendrites.

Neurons are separate units and not directly connected to one another. Impulses travel along neurons, moving from one neuron to the next by means of **synapses,** junctions between the axon of one neuron to the dendrite of another. Substances called **neurotransmitters** (or neurohormones) accomplish transmission of an impulse from one neuron to the next (see Chap. 12).

A fatty substance called **myelin** covers some axons in the CNS and PNS. Such axons are called *myelinated,* or white, nerve fibers. A sheath called the **neurilemma** covers the myelin. Myelin serves as an insulating substance for the axon. Axons without myelin are called *unmyelinated,* or gray, nerve fibers.

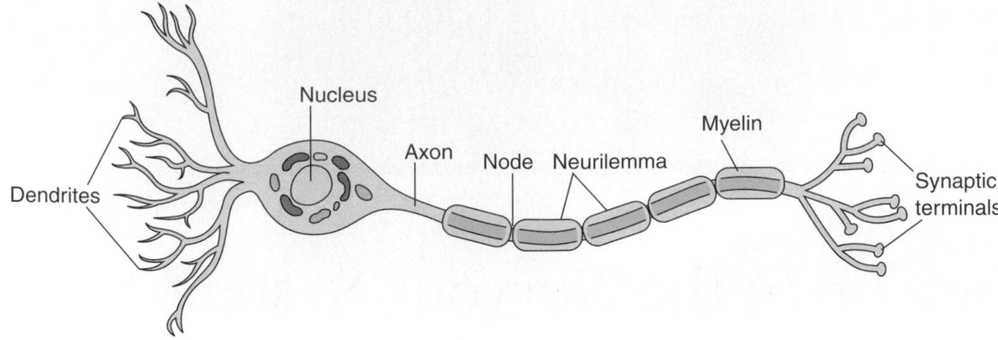

FIGURE 38.1 Neuron. (Adapted from Willis, M. C. [1996]. *Medical terminology: The language of healthcare.* Baltimore: Williams & Wilkins.)

Central Nervous System

The CNS consists of the brain and spinal cord.

Brain

The brain is divided into three parts: the cerebrum, cerebellum, and brain stem. The **cerebrum** consists of two hemispheres connected by the **corpus callosum,** a band of white fibers that acts as a bridge for transmitting impulses between the left and right hemispheres. Each hemisphere has four lobes: frontal, parietal, temporal, and occipital (Fig. 38.2). The cerebral cortex is the surface of the cerebrum. It contains motor neurons, which are responsible for movement, and sensory neurons, which receive impulses from peripheral sensory neurons located throughout the body.

Motor tracts are **pyramidal** or **extrapyramidal.** Pyramidal motor pathways originate in the motor cortex of the cerebrum, cross over at the level of the medulla, and end in the brain stem and spinal cord. Extrapyramidal fibers originate in the motor cortex and project to the cerebellum and basal ganglia. They do not cross over as they connect to motor neurons in the spinal cord.

The **cerebellum,** located behind and below the cerebrum, controls and coordinates muscle movement. The **brain stem** consists of the midbrain, pons, and medulla oblongata. The **midbrain** forms the forward part of the brain stem and connects the pons and cerebellum with the two cerebral hemispheres. The **pons** is located between the midbrain and medulla and connects the two hemispheres of the cerebellum with the brain stem, spinal cord, and cerebrum. The **medulla oblongata** lies below the pons and transmits motor impulses from the brain to the spinal cord and sensory impulses from peripheral sensory neurons to the brain. The medulla contains vital centers concerned with respiration, heartbeat, and vaso-

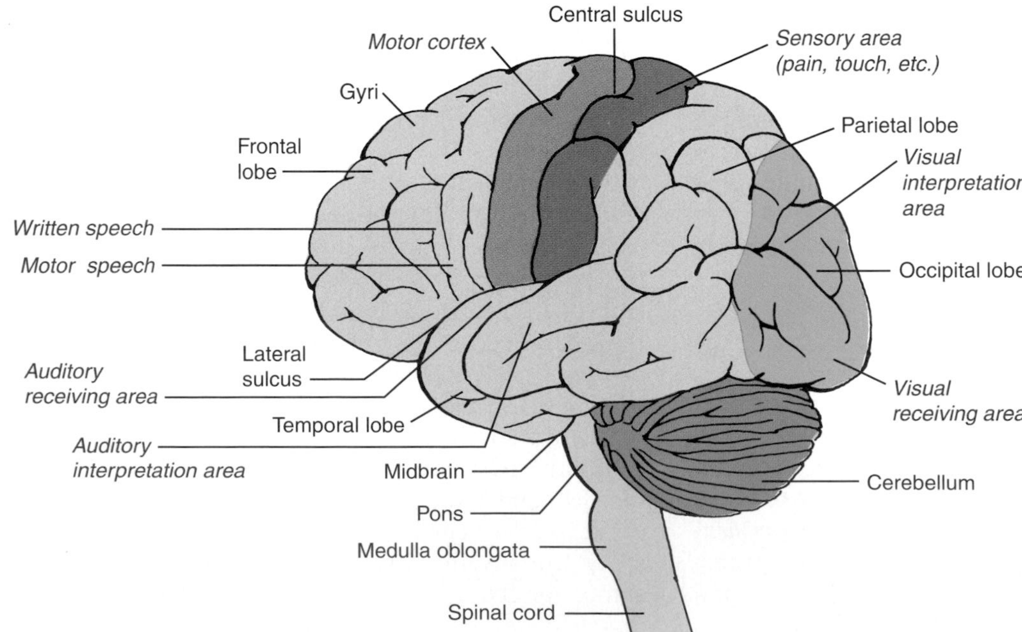

FIGURE 38.2 Structure of the brain. Shaded areas show the region responsible for different functions.

motor activity (the control of smooth muscle activity in blood vessel walls).

The brain is protected by rigid bones of the skull and covered by three membranes or **meninges:** (1) the **dura mater,** the tough, outermost covering; (2) the **arachnoid,** or middle membrane lying directly below the dura; and (3) the **pia mater,** a delicate layer that adheres to the brain and spinal cord. The **subarachnoid space** is between the pia mater and the arachnoid membrane (Fig. 38.3).

Within the brain are four hollow structures called **ventricles,** which manufacture and absorb cerebrospinal fluid (CSF). CSF constantly circulates in the subarachnoid space of the brain and spinal cord. Acting as a cushion, the CSF protects these structures and helps maintain relatively constant intracranial pressure.

Stop, Think, and Respond ● BOX 38-1

Name the three layers of meninges, starting below the skull and proceeding toward the surface of the brain.

Spinal Cord

The spinal cord, covered by meninges, is a direct continuation of the medulla and is surrounded and protected by the *vertebrae* (or vertebral column). The spinal cord ends between the first and second lumbar vertebrae, where it divides into smaller sections called the **cauda equina.**

The spinal cord functions as a passageway for ascending sensory and descending motor neurons. Its two main functions are to provide centers for reflex action and to serve as a pathway for impulses to and from the brain. Sensory fibers enter the posterior (dorsal) portion of the cord. Nerve fibers that transmit motor impulses run outward to the peripheral nerves from the anterior (ventral) portion of the cord.

Peripheral Nervous System

The PNS consists of all nerves outside the CNS.

Cranial Nerves

The 12 pairs of cranial nerves, identified by Roman numerals, are as follows:

- *I*—Olfactory nerve: sense of smell
- *II*—Optic nerve: sight
- *III*—Oculomotor nerve: contraction of iris and eye muscles
- *IV*—Trochlear nerve: eye movement
- *V*—Trigeminal nerve: sensory nerve to face, chewing
- *VI*—Abducens nerve: eye movement
- *VII*—Facial nerve: facial expression, taste, secretions of salivary and lacrimal glands
- *VIII*—Vestibulocochlear (or auditory) nerve: hearing, balance
- *IX*—Glossopharyngeal nerve: taste, sensory fibers of pharynx and tongue, swallowing, secretions of parotid gland
- *X*—Vagus nerve: motor fibers to glands producing digestive enzymes, heart rate, muscles of speech, gastrointestinal motility, respiration, swallowing, coughing, vomiting reflex
- *XI*—Accessory (or spinal accessory) nerve: head and shoulder movement
- *XII*—Hypoglossal nerve: movement of the tongue

Spinal Nerves

There are 31 pairs of spinal nerves: 8 cervical, 12 thoracic, 5 lumbar, 5 sacral, and 1 coccygeal. Spinal nerves have two roots: dorsal and ventral. Dorsal nerve fibers are sensory, and ventral nerve fibers are motor. Peripheral sensory nerve fibers in various areas of the body transmit

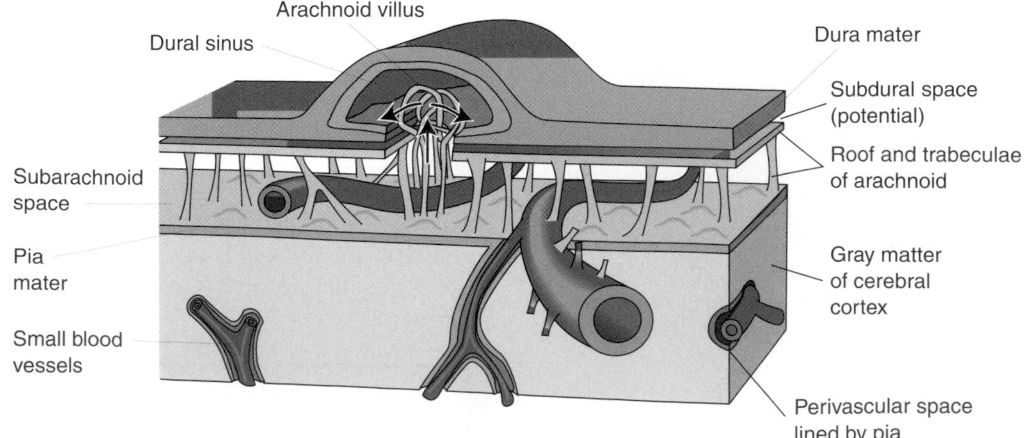

FIGURE 38.3 Schematic diagram of the three connective tissue membranes (pia, arachnoid, and dura) constituting the meninges of the CNS. (From Cormack, D. H. [1987]. *Ham's histology* [9th ed.]. Philadelphia: J. B. Lippincott.)

impulses to the spinal nerves, which then transmit impulses up the spinal cord to the brain. Motor impulses traveling from the brain and down the spinal cord leave by the ventral root and travel to areas of the body. Each spinal nerve root innervates a specific area.

Autonomic Nervous System

The autonomic nervous system consists of the **sympathetic nervous system** and the **parasympathetic nervous system.** It has functions essential to survival. The sympathetic nervous system regulates expenditure of energy. Neurotransmitters of the sympathetic nervous system, collectively known as *catecholamines,* are **epinephrine, norepinephrine,** and **dopamine.** The adrenal medulla produces and secretes epinephrine and norepinephrine. Norepinephrine also is produced at sympathetic nerve endings. Dopamine is a precursor (a substance that precedes another) of norepinephrine. Norepinephrine then becomes epinephrine. Stressful situations such as danger, intense emotion, and severe illness result in the release of catecholamines.

The parasympathetic nervous system works to conserve body energy and is partly responsible for slowing heart rate, digesting food, and eliminating body wastes. **Acetylcholine** is a neurotransmitter released at the nerve endings of parasympathetic nerve fibers, at some nerve endings in the sympathetic nervous system, and at nerve endings of skeletal muscles. Release of acetylcholine allows passage of a nerve impulse from the nerve fiber to the effector organ or structure, where the enzyme **acetylcholinesterase** inactivates acetylcholine.

ASSESSMENT

A neurologic assessment is performed to identify and locate disorders of the nervous system. The scope and extent of the neurologic examination depends on symptoms and probable or actual diagnosis.

History

Explore all symptoms and ask questions to clarify each symptom. The history must include a record of trauma (no matter how slight) to the head or body within the past 6 to 12 months, a drug history, allergy history, and family medical history. Observe the client's speech pattern, mental status, intellectual functioning, reasoning ability, and movement or lack of movement of extremities.

Physical Examination

The physical examination consists of assessment of the cerebral, motor, and sensory areas. Nurses usually assess intellectual function and speech pattern during the history by noting responses to questions. Additional testing of intellectual function includes asking various questions that require mental ability.

Evaluate the client's body posture and any abnormal position of the head, neck, trunk, or extremities. If head trauma has occurred, examine the ears and nose for evidence of bleeding or other drainage. Carefully examine the head for bleeding, swelling, or wounds. Do not move or manipulate the client's head during this part of the assessment, especially if there is a recent history of trauma.

Cranial Nerves

The experienced examiner evaluates all or some of the 12 cranial nerves (Table 38.1).

Motor Function

Assessment of motor function includes muscle movement, size, tone, strength, and coordination. Inspect large muscle areas for evidence of atrophy and assess opposing muscles for equality of size and strength. Ask the client to perform tasks such as pushing the palm or sole against the examiner's palm, picking small and large objects between the thumb and forefinger, grasping objects firmly, and resisting removal of an object from the fist or fingers.

To assess gait, movement, and balance, ask the client to walk away from the examiner, turn, and walk back. Other tests include climbing a small set of stairs, walking and turning abruptly, and walking heel to toe. In the Romberg test, the client stands with feet close together and eyes closed. If the client sways and tends to fall, this is considered a positive Romberg test, indicating a problem with equilibrium. The examiner stands fairly close to the client during this test in case the client loses balance.

Tests that evaluate motor and cerebral function include doing the finger-to-nose test with eyes closed, writing words, and identifying common objects. The choice of tests depends on the original complaints and the findings of diagnostic tests.

Evaluate motor response in the comatose or unconscious client by administering a painful stimulus to determine if the client makes an appropriate response by reaching toward or withdrawing from the stimulus (Fig. 38.4A and B). Those with impaired cerebral function manifest **decorticate posturing** (decorticate rigidity), **decerebrate posturing** (decerebrate rigidity), or **flaccidity** (see Fig. 38.4C–E). Decerebrate posturing is more serious than decorticate posturing; flaccidity is even more ominous.

Stop, Think, and Respond • BOX 38-2

Which type of posturing is evidenced by (A) flexion of the arms, (B) extension of the arms, and (C) no movement of any extremities?

TABLE 38.1 CRANIAL NERVE ASSESSMENT

CRANIAL NERVE	ASSESSMENT TECHNIQUE	NORMAL FINDINGS
I—Olfactory	Ask client to occlude each nostril separately and close the eyes. Present familiar odors, such as vinegar, lemon, coffee, and ammonia.	Client identifies odors correctly.
II—Optic	Help client cover each eye separately; test visual acuity using a Snellen chart (see Chap. 43) or newspaper.	Client names letters or reads words accurately.
	Client and examiner cover an eye, and examiner moves an object from the periphery toward client's nose from superior, inferior, medial, and lateral positions while both fix their gaze straight ahead. Examiner then tests opposite eye. Inspect optic nerve with an ophthalmoscope.	Client and examiner see object at the same time in the visual field. Optic nerve appears round and lighter than surrounding retina.
III—Oculomotor	In a darkened room, shine a bright light in each pupil; ask client to look at a near and far object (see Chap. 43).	Pupil constricts briskly in response to light and dilates when looking far away.
	Ask client to follow an object you move in horizontal, vertical, and oblique directions (see Chap. 43).	Eye movement is coordinated in all directions.
IV—Trochlear	See assessment for motor function of oculomotor nerve.	Eyes move inferiorly and medially.
V—Trigeminal	Observe for jaw symmetry while client opens mouth.	Appearance is symmetrical.
	Instruct client to clamp jaws tightly together.	The muscles contract bilaterally.
	Stroke forehead, cheeks, and jaw with a wisp of cotton, sharp object (e.g., pin), cold and warm objects, and a vibrating tuning fork.	Client shows bilateral sensitivity and correctly identifies sensory experience.
	Touch each cornea with a wisp of cotton.	Client blinks.
	Tap center of chin with a reflex hammer while client slightly opens the mouth.	Jaw closes suddenly and slightly.
VI—Abducens	See assessment for motor function of oculomotor nerve.	Client moves eyes in lateral directions.
VII—Facial	Ask client to wrinkle the forehead, smile, frown, raise eyebrows, look at ceiling, and whistle.	Facial movements are symmetrical.
	Instruct client to close eyelids and resist examiner's efforts to open them.	Both eyes equally resist movements to open them.
	Apply sweet, sour, salty, and bitter flavors to both sides of the anterior tongue.	Client accurately identifies tastes.
VIII—Vestibulocochlear	Test hearing acuity and perform the Rinne and Weber tests with a tuning fork (see Chap. 44).	Client repeats whispered words correctly; sound is lateralized equally and heard longer by air than by bone conduction.
	Have client stand with both feet close together; note for swaying with eyes open and then shut.	Client maintains balance or sways slightly.
IX—Glossopharyngeal	Touch palate with a tongue blade. Ask client to say "ah."	Blade elicits a gag response. Uvula remains in midline.
X—Vagus	Have client say "la, la, la."	Client speaks clearly and distinctly, with no hoarseness.
XI—Spinal-accessory	Instruct client to shrug the shoulders as you apply resistance.	Clients raises shoulders.
XII—Hypoglossal	Tell client to stick out the tongue.	Tongue remains in midline with no lateral deviation.

Sensory Function

Evaluate extremities for sensitivity to heat, cold, touch, and pain. Use various objects such as cotton balls, tubes filled with hot or cold water, and sharp objects (that do not pierce the skin) to check sensation in the extremities.

Level of Consciousness

Depending on the client's symptoms, evaluation of the level of consciousness (LOC) is often necessary. The following classification of LOC applies to altered consciousness from any cause. Differentiating between each level

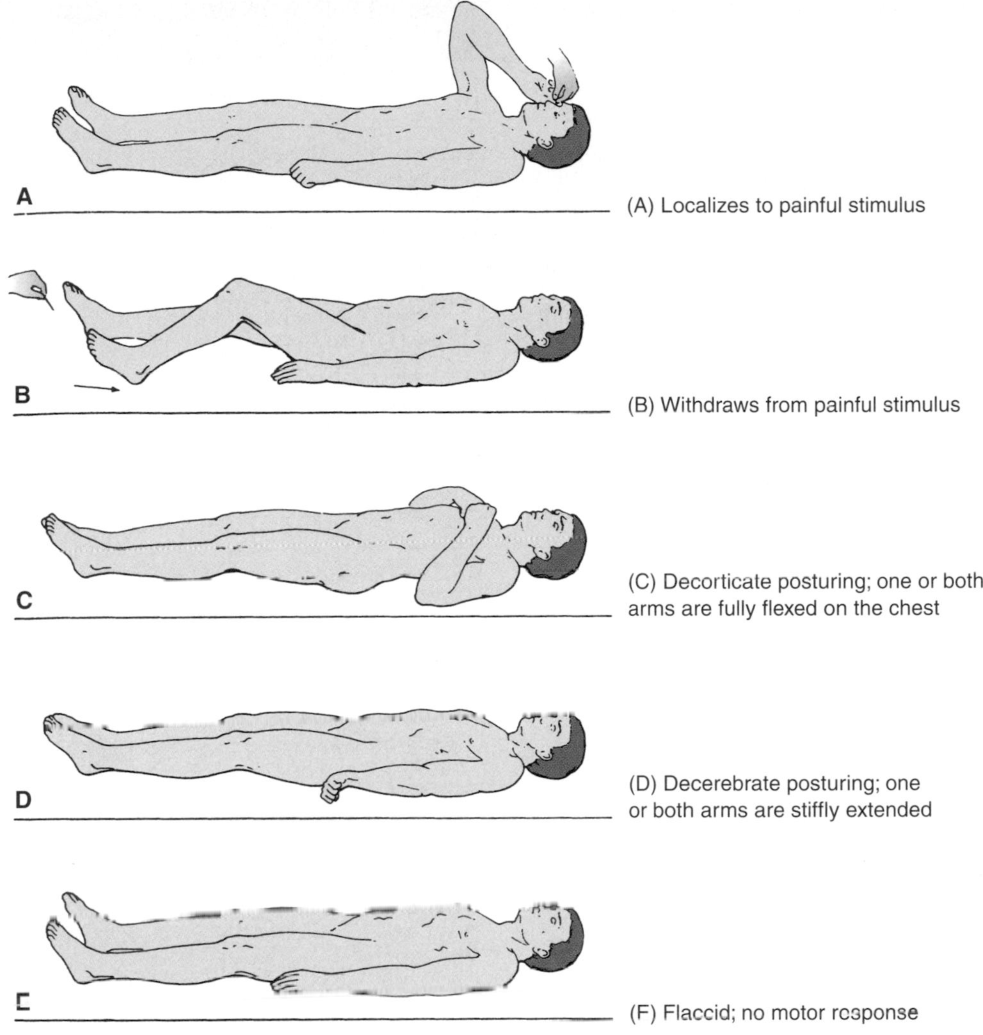

FIGURE 38.4 Responses to pain and posturing.

can be difficult; some clients show characteristics of two or more levels:

- *Conscious:* The client responds immediately, fully, and appropriately to visual, auditory, and other stimulation.
- *Somnolent or lethargic:* The client is drowsy or sleepy at inappropriate times but can be aroused, only to fall asleep again. Responses to questions are delayed or inappropriate. Speech is incoherent. The client responds slowly to verbal commands. He or she responds to painful stimuli.
- *Stuporous:* The client is aroused only by vigorous and continuous stimulation, usually by manipulation or strong auditory or visual stimuli. Stimulation results in one- or two-word answers or in motor activity or purposeful behavior directed toward avoiding further stimulation.
- *Semicomatose:* The client is unresponsive except to superficial, relatively mild painful stimuli to which the client makes some purposeful motor response (movement) to evade stimulation. Spontaneous motion is uncommon, but the client may groan or mutter.
- *Comatose:* The client responds only to very painful stimuli by fragmentary, delayed reflex withdrawal; in deeper stages, he or she loses all responsiveness. There is no spontaneous movement, and the respiratory rate is irregular.

Assess LOC at frequent intervals after injury to the head or neck, cranial surgery, a cerebrovascular accident (acute phase), a ruptured cerebral aneurysm, and other neurologic disorders. Make hourly assessments unless the physician orders otherwise or a change occurs in the client's condition.

The Glasgow Coma Scale (Fig. 38.5) is a measure of the LOC. It consists of three parts: eye opening response, best verbal response, and best motor response. To evaluate responses correctly, several verbal and motor responses are elicited, and the best response is recorded. The eye opening response is determined by talking to the client

The Glasgow Coma Scale is a tool for assessing a client's response to stimuli. A score of 10 or less indicates a need for emergency attention: a score of 7 or less is generally interpreted as coma.

Eye opening response	Spontaneous	4
	To voice	3
	To pain	2
	None	1
Best verbal response	Oriented	5
	Confused	4
	Inappropriate words	3
	Incomprehensible sounds	2
	None	1
Best motor response	Obeys command	6
	Localizes pain	5
	Withdraws (pain)	4
	Flexion (pain)	3
	Extension (pain)	2
	None	1
Total		3 to 15

FIGURE 38.5 Glasgow Coma Scale.

and calling his or her name. If no response is noted (i.e., the eyes do not open spontaneously), a painful stimulus is introduced and the response noted. The verbal response is evaluated by a verbal reply to questions. The motor response is the ability of the client to follow commands, such as "wiggle your toes" or "move your left hand." If there is no response, a painful stimulus is introduced and the response noted. The responses are assigned numbers and the numbers are totaled. A normal response is 15. A score of 7 or less is considered coma. The evaluations are recorded on a graphic sheet; connecting lines show an increase or decrease in the LOC.

The Rancho Los Amigos Scale (Box 38-1) is another tool for assessing LOC. Some rehabilitation centers prefer this scale because it is a more flexible assessment tool for identifying the client's status.

Pupils

The size and equality of the pupils and their reaction to light are an assessment of the third cranial (oculomotor) nerve (see Table 38.1). Pupil size (normal, pinpoint, dilated), equality (equal, unequal in size), and reaction to a bright light (normal, sluggish, no reaction, fixed) are noted (see Chap. 43). When pupils are examined, any abnormal movement or position of one or both eyes is noted.

Unequal pupils (one pupil larger than the other), dilated or pinpoint pupils, and failure of the pupils to respond quickly to light are usually abnormal findings. Any sudden change in pupil size, equality, or reaction to light is an important neurologic finding and is reported to the physician at once.

BOX 38-1 ● Rancho Los Amigos Scales

Level I No response to stimuli. Appears in deep sleep.
Level II Generalized response. First reaction may be to deep pain. Has delayed, inconsistent responses.
Level III Localized response. Inconsistent responses, but reacts in a more specific manner to stimulus. Might follow simple command "squeeze my hand."
Level IV Confused. Agitated. Reacts to own inner confusion, fear, disorientation. Excitable behavior, may be abusive.
Level V Nonagitated. Confused. Inappropriate. Usually disoriented. Follows tasks for 2 to 3 minutes, but easily distracted by environment, frustrated.
Level VI Confused appropriate. Follows simple directions consistently. Memory and attention increasing. Self-care tasks performed without help.
Level VII Automatic appropriate. If physically able, can carry out routine activities. Appears normal. Needs supervision for safety.
Level VIII Purposeful. Alert. Oriented. May have decreased abilities relative to premorbid state.

Neck

The neck is examined for stiffness or abnormal position. Presence of rigidity is checked by moving the head and chin toward the chest. This maneuver should not be performed if a head or neck injury or other body trauma is suspected or known.

Vital Signs

Blood pressure, pulse and respiratory rates, and temperature are closely monitored in clients with a potential or actual neurologic disorder. Temperature often needs to be monitored every hour because CNS disorders can affect the temperature-regulating ability of the hypothalamus. A sudden increase or decrease in any vital sign indicates a change in neurologic status, and the physician is notified immediately.

Diagnostic Tests

Imaging Procedures

Imaging procedures such as computed tomography (CT), magnetic resonance imaging (MRI), positron emission tomography (PET), and single-photon emission computed tomography (SPECT) are used to diagnose neurologic disorders, especially for brain tumors, Alzheimer's disease, intracranial bleeding or hemorrhage, and cerebral infections.

CT scanning uses x-rays and computer analysis to produce three-dimensional views of thin cross-sections, or "slices," of the body. A narrow x-ray beam rotates around the client and results are analyzed by a computer. CT is extremely sensitive to differences in tissue densities, allowing differentiation between intracranial tumors, cysts, edema, and hemorrhage.

An MRI is based on the magnetic behavior of protons in body tissue. This procedure uses radio frequency waves to produce images of tissues of high fat and water content such as soft tissue, veins, arteries, the brain, and spinal cord. Images are produced without contrast dye or radiation.

PET uses radioactive substances to examine metabolic activity of body structures. The client either inhales or is injected with a radioactive substance with positively charged particles that combine with negatively charged particles found normally in the body. Energy emitted when these combine is converted into color-coded images indicating metabolic activity of the organ involved. The radioactive substances are short-lived, resulting in minimal radiation exposure.

SPECT is a noninvasive, three-dimensional imaging tool to detect and measure cerebral blood flow. It also highlights areas of altered metabolism surrounding brain lesions before they are visible on a CT scan or MRI (Hinkle, 2002). The client is injected with a radiopharmaceutical agent that is able to cross the blood-brain barrier. This agent concentrates in areas of highest blood flow within the brain, depicted at the time of scanning. Abnormally bright or dark areas indicate a disease state such as epilepsy or brain tumors.

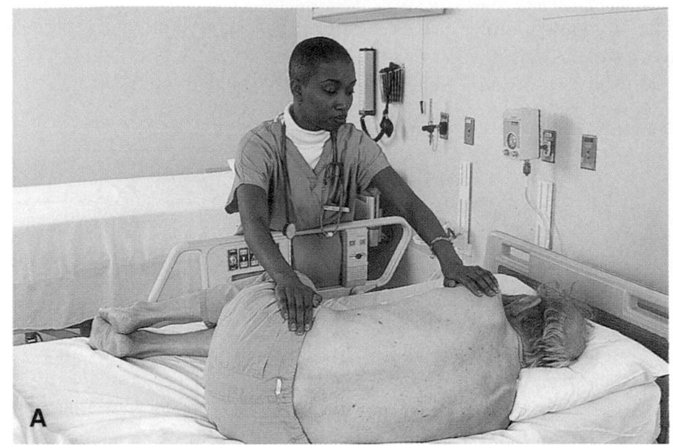

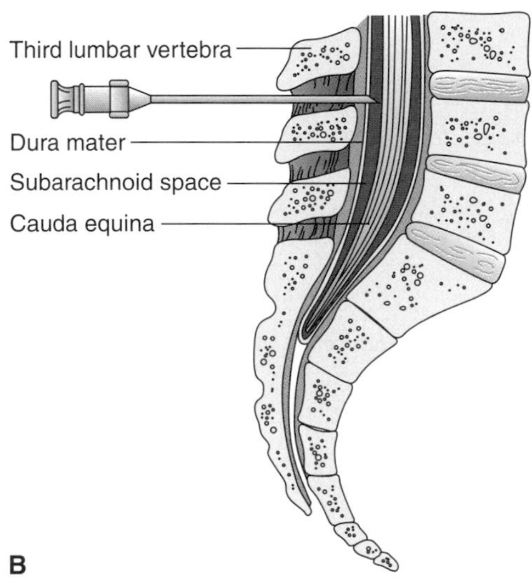

FIGURE 38.6 (**A**) Positioning of the client for lumbar puncture. (**B**) Insertion of the spinal needle into the subarachnoid space. (From Smeltzer, S. C. & Bare, B. G. [2004]. *Brunner & Suddarth's textbook of medical–surgical nursing* [10th ed.]. Philadelphia: Lippincott Williams & Wilkins.)

Lumbar Puncture

Changes in CSF occur in many neurologic disorders. A lumbar puncture (spinal tap) is performed to obtain samples of CSF from the subarachnoid space for laboratory examination and to measure CSF pressure (Fig. 38.6). Bacteriologic tests on specimens of CSF reveal presence of pathogenic microorganisms. Strict aseptic technique is required during the procedure. The CSF normally is clear and colorless with a pressure of 80 to 180 mm H_2O; a pressure over 200 mm H_2O is considered abnormal. A lumbar puncture also is performed to inject a drug into the subarachnoid space (intrathecal injection), to administer a spinal anesthetic, to withdraw CSF for the relief of intracranial pressure, or to inject air, gas, or dye for a neurologic diagnostic procedure.

Contrast Studies

Contrast studies include cerebral angiography, which detects distortion of cerebral arteries and veins, indicating an aneurysm, a tumor, or other vascular abnormality. A radiopaque dye is injected into the right or left carotid artery, the brachial artery, or the femoral artery. A rapid sequence of radiographs is taken as the dye circulates through the cerebral arteries and veins.

For a myelogram, a radiopaque substance is injected into the spinal canal by means of a lumbar puncture. X-rays are taken to demonstrate abnormalities of the spinal canal such as tumors or a ruptured intervertebral disk.

Electroencephalogram

An electroencephalogram (EEG) records electrical impulses generated by the brain. Electrodes are placed on the scalp and electrical activity is recorded on a graph.

Brain Scan

A brain scan identifies tumors, hematomas in or around the brain, cerebral abscesses, cerebral infarctions, or displaced ventricles. A radioactive material is injected before the procedure. The length of this procedure varies from a few minutes to 1 hour. CT scans and MRI are replacing this procedure.

Electromyography

Electromyography (EMG) studies changes in the electrical potential of muscles and the nerves supplying the muscles. Needle electrodes are placed into one or more skeletal muscles and the results recorded on an oscilloscope. This test is useful in determining presence of neuromuscular disorders.

Nerve Conduction Studies

Nerve conduction studies measure the speed with which nerve impulses travel along a peripheral nerve fiber when a specific nerve is electrically stimulated. This test aids diagnosis of nerve injury and compression or neurologic disorders affecting peripheral nerves.

Echoencephalography

An echoencephalogram is an ultrasound examination of the structures of the brain. This procedure is performed to detect abnormalities in the ventricles and the location of intracranial bleeding.

NURSING PROCESS

• The Client Undergoing Neurologic Testing

Assessment

Determine the client's understanding of the diagnostic procedures and answer remaining questions. Check that a consent form is signed and witnessed. Because some contrast media contain iodine, check the client's history for previous allergic reactions to radiographic dyes, iodine, or seafood. Obtain the client's weight, baseline vital signs, and neurologic data such as LOC, pupil response, and muscle strength in all four extremities. Use the assessment findings for comparison when monitoring the client's condition during and after diagnostic testing. Closely observe the client for any mental or physical deviations from baseline assessments.

Diagnosis, Planning, and Interventions

Prepare the client for neurologic diagnostic tests following agency policies. Assist the physician and support the client during a test performed on the nursing unit. During and after the diagnostic test, monitor for adverse consequences and promote recovery after the test. Diagnoses, expected outcomes, and interventions include, but are not limited to, the following.

Deficient Knowledge related to unfamiliarity with diagnostic testing process

Expected Outcome: Client will accurately describe the preparation, procedure, and aftercare that the scheduled diagnostic test involves.

- Clarify the physician's explanation. *Some clients have questions after the physician leaves.*
- Answer client's questions. *Clients have the right to information about their plan of care.*
- Describe procedure to the client as well as what the procedure requires, such as positions to assume or the need to lie still during the procedure. *Decreases anxiety and increases client's trust and confidence in the nurse.*
- Discuss preparation for the diagnostic test, which may include temporarily eliminating CNS depressants, such as barbiturates and minor tranquilizers, and CNS stimulants, such as caffeine, for 24 to 48 hours in the case of an EEG. *Drugs that affect neurologic function sometimes are withheld to ensure that factors other than the client's physiology do not affect test results.*
- Explain that hair will be shampooed before an EEG. *Removing scalp and hair oil ensures that electrodes will remain in place until EEG is completed.*
- Inform client that he or she will be able to shampoo after an EEG. *A second shampoo facilitates removal of paste used to secure electrodes to the scalp.*
- Tell client to expect some discomfort when undergoing a lumbar puncture, myelogram, EMG, or nerve conduction studies. *Without giving the client information about expected discomfort, client may assume that he or she is having an adverse reaction.*

PC: Allergic Reaction to contrast dye

Expected Outcome: The nurse will monitor to detect, manage, and minimize an allergic reaction.

- Report allergy history to the physician. *Helps physician decide to cancel or modify diagnostic test by administering a pretest antihistamine or substituting an alternative dye.*
- Identify allergy information prominently on the client's chart. *Provides a means for communicating information to all healthcare workers.*
- Administer pretest antihistamines according to physician's order. *Antihistamines block histamine receptors and reduce manifestations of an allergic reaction.*
- Monitor client for severe hypotension, tachycardia, profuse diaphoresis, sudden change in LOC, dyspnea, and hives or itching. Notify the physician immediately of any such findings. *The most serious allergic reaction is anaphylaxis.*

PC: Meningeal Irritation or **CNS Changes**

Expected Outcome: The nurse will monitor to detect, manage, and minimize abnormal neurologic changes.

- Observe closely for any neurologic abnormalities such as diminished LOC, weakness, numbness, paralysis in an extremity, unequal or unresponsive pupil reflexes, posturing, and speech disturbance. *Diagnostic tests pose potential risks for neurologic complications, characterized by changes in neurologic functions.*

- Assess for changes in vital signs, restlessness, vomiting, and mental changes in orientation and thought processes. *Rising intracranial pressure affects vital signs, stimulates the vomiting center in the brain, and alters the sensorium and cognition.*
- Report onset of a headache and sudden or severe pain in any area of the body to the physician immediately. *Headache often accompanies increased intracranial pressure; pain of any kind requires further investigation and pain management.*
- Inspect injection sites, especially those made during a lumbar puncture, for signs of a hematoma (collection of blood). *Trauma at an injection site can result in bleeding; bloody drainage also may contain CSF.*
- Position client flat for at least 3 hours or as directed after a lumbar puncture or myelogram. *Keeping the client in a recumbent position provides time for CSF to form and replace what has been lost and reduces potential for a headache.*
- Encourage a liberal fluid intake. *Helps to restore volume of CSF.*
- Keep room dark and quiet after a lumbar puncture or myelogram. *Sensory stimulation tends to magnify discomfort.*
- Administer prescribed analgesic if client develops a headache. *Reduces transmission or perception of pain stimuli.*

Evaluation of Expected Outcomes

Expected outcomes for the client are that he or she understands preparation and performance involved in the neurologic procedure or diagnostic test and aftercare. Gather data concerning the client's allergy history, communicate information appropriately, assess client for allergic symptoms, and implement interventions that control any allergic reaction. Assess client for complications associated with diagnostic tests, use measures to reduce manifestations of complications, and carry out prescribed interventions to relieve discomfort.

GENERAL GERONTOLOGIC CONSIDERATIONS

Diseases more common in older adults (e.g., dementia) often make it difficult to perform a neurologic assessment.

With age, brain weight and number of brain cells decrease. Older adults experience short-term memory loss and a slower reaction time.

Pupillary response is more sluggish in the older adult. When cataracts are present, there may be no pupillary response.

Possibility of drug toxicity always should be considered when an elderly person has a change in mental status.

Older adults who have difficulty following directions during a neurologic examination or diagnostic procedure need brief instructions given one step at a time during the examination or procedure.

Obtain facts necessary for a health history from a family member or friend of an older adult who has difficulty remembering recent or past events, symptoms, drug and medical history, and other facts necessary for a history.

Critical Thinking Exercises

1. *Discuss appropriate nursing assessments when managing the care of clients with neurologic disorders.*
2. *Name two potential complications of neurologic testing procedures. How can the nurse prevent, manage, and minimize them?*

● NCLEX-STYLE REVIEW QUESTIONS 

1. Following a lumbar puncture a client asks to ambulate to the restroom. Which nursing action is most correct?
   1. Explain that the client must lie flat following the procedure and obtain a bedpan.
   2. Provide a bedside commode and assist the client with its use.
   3. Instruct the client to remain still and insert a urinary catheter.
   4. Assist the client to the restroom and wait outside until finished.
2. A client is seen at the neurologist's office stating that she has had chronic dizziness. When asked to assist the physician with a diagnostic Romberg test, which nursing intervention is most appropriate to ensure client safety?
   1. Stand close to the client in case the client should begin to sway.
   2. Advise the client to use a handrail while ambulating to avoid falling.
   3. Provide support as the client performs the neurological test.
   4. Document the results of the testing.
3. An ICU nurse is assessing a client's level of consciousness. She finds notes that the client awakens when his name is called but then quickly drifts off when asked questions. When documenting the client's level of consciousness, the nurse would be most correct to document:
   1. Conscious
   2. Somnolent
   3. Stuporous
   4. Semicomatose

connection—

Visit the Connection site at **http://connection.lww.com/go/timbyEssentials** for links to chapter-related resources on the Internet.

References and Suggested Readings

A quick check of the neurologic system. (1999). *Nursing 1999, 29*(6), Critical Care, 32cc10–32cc11.

Addison, C., & Crawford, B. (1999). Not bad, just misunderstood . . . Glasgow Coma Scale. *Nursing Times, 95*(43), 52–53.

Agostino, P. (2001). Cranial nerve assessment in the unconscious patient. *Nursing Spectrum (New York/New Jersey Metro Edition), 13A*(3), NJ15.

Alverzo, J. P., & Galski, T. (1999). Nurses' assessment of patients' cognitive orientation in a rehabilitation setting. *Rehabilitation Nursing, 24*(1), 7–12, 23, 43.

Cohen, B. J., & Wood, D. L. (1999). *Memmler's the human body in health and disease* (9th ed.). Philadelphia: Lippincott Williams & Wilkins.

Fischer, J. (2001). The history of the Glasgow Coma Scale: Implications for practice. *Critical Care Nursing Quarterly, 23*(4), 52–58.

Fuller, J., & Schaller-Ayers, J. (2000). *Health assessment: A nursing approach* (3rd ed.). Philadelphia: Lippincott Williams & Wilkins.

Hinkle, J. L. (2002). SPECT: A powerful imaging tool. *American Journal of Nursing 102*(3), 24A–G.

Lewis, A. M. (1999). Neurologic emergency! *Nursing 1999, 29*(10), 54–56.

Neatherlin, J. S. (1999). Foundation for practice: Neuroassessment for neuroscience nurses. *Nursing Clinics of North America, 34,* 573–592.

O'Hanlon-Nichols, T. (1999). Neurologic assessment. *American Journal of Nursing, 99*(6), 44–50.

Peters, J. (1999). Dedicated follower of neurological trends . . . neurological assessment. *Nursing Times, 95*(27), 19.

Price, T., Miller, L., & deScossa, M. (2000). The Glasgow Coma Scale in intensive care. *Nursing in Critical Care, 5,* 170–173.

Shpritz, D. W. (1999). Neurodiagnostic studies. *Nursing Clinics of North America, 34,* 593–606.

Watson, R. (2000). Assessing neurological functioning in older people. *Elderly Care, 12*(4), 25–27.

chapter 39

Caring for Clients With Central and Peripheral Nervous System Disorders

Words to Know 

aura
automatisms
bradykinesia
Cheyne-Stokes respirations
choreiform movements
convulsion
Cushing's triad
demyelinating disease
diplopia
epilepsy
fasciculations
foramen magnum
neuralgia
nystagmus
papilledema
parkinsonism
preictal phase
ptosis
seizure
status epilepticus

Learning Objectives

On completion of this chapter, the reader will:

- Discuss nursing care of the client with increased intracranial pressure.
- Describe infectious or inflammatory diseases that affect the central or peripheral nervous system.
- Explain neuromuscular disorders and common related problems.
- Discuss the nursing management of clients with a cranial nerve disorder.
- List the signs and symptoms of Parkinson's disease.
- Discuss therapeutic purposes of drugs commonly prescribed for Parkinson's disease.
- Describe the pathophysiology of seizure disorders.
- Discuss the nursing management of clients with seizure disorders.

Acute central nervous system (CNS) and peripheral nervous system (PNS) disorders are potentially life-threatening. Chronic neurologic disorders, although not imminently fatal, profoundly affect a person's quality of life. When a part of the CNS or PNS is damaged, removed, or destroyed, a permanent neurologic deficit can occur.

INCREASED INTRACRANIAL PRESSURE

Inside the cranium are brain tissue, blood, and cerebrospinal fluid (CSF). If any of these increase significantly without a decrease in either of the other two, intracranial pressure elevates.

Pathophysiology and Etiology

Conditions such as brain tumors, head injury, and infectious and inflammatory disorders of the brain such as encephalitis cause increased intracranial pressure (IICP). As pressure increases, cerebral blood flow decreases, followed by increased $PaCO_2$ (carbon dioxide level in the blood) and decreased blood pH and PaO_2 (oxygen level in the blood). Cerebral edema results, further increasing intracranial pressure (ICP).

If IICP is unrecognized or untreated, contents of the cranium are further compressed. Unrelieved pressure causes brain tissue to herniate or shift from normal locations intracranially and extracranially. The **foramen magnum,** the opening in the lower part of the skull through which the upper part of the spinal cord connects with the brain, provides the only extracranial exit for brain tissue. If the brain stem herniates through the foramen magnum, respiration, heart rate, blood pressure (BP), and functions of descending and ascending nerve fibers are affected. As the condition progresses, vital functions ultimately cease.

Assessment Findings

Signs and Symptoms

Signs and symptoms of IICP (Box 39-1) develop rapidly or slowly. Decreasing level of consciousness (LOC) is one of the earliest signs of IICP. Clients may slip from

BOX 39-1 ● Signs of Increased Intracranial Pressure

- Altered level of consciousness
- Headache
- Vomiting
- Papilledema
- Change in vital signs
- Unequal pupils and abnormal response to light
- Posturing

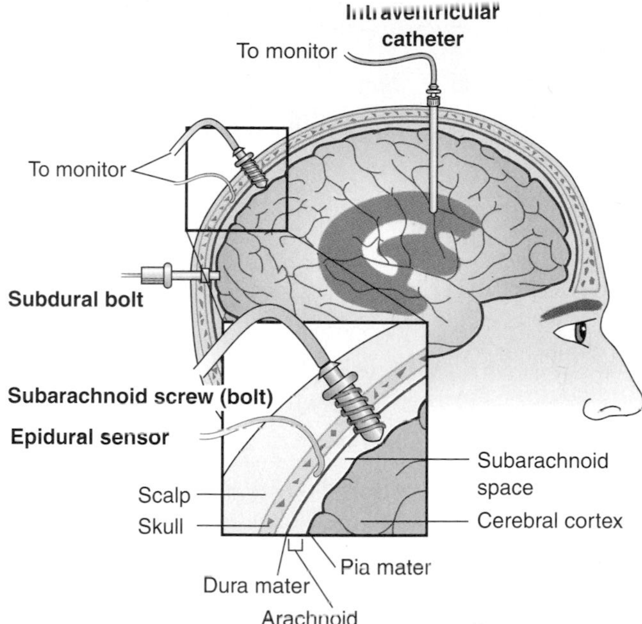

FIGURE 39.1 Technique for monitoring intracranial pressure.

alert and oriented to lethargic, stuporous, semicomatose, and, finally, comatose (see Chap. 38). Confusion, restlessness, and periodic disorientation often accompany decreasing LOC.

Headache is another symptom of IICP. Pain typically is intermittent and increases with activities that elevate ICP, such as coughing, sneezing, or straining at stool. Rest or elevation of the head relieves the pain. A constant headache is a grave sign.

Vomiting associated with a neurologic condition also suggests increasing ICP. Emesis commonly occurs without any forewarning of nausea.

Papilledema (swelling of the optic nerve) is caused by interference with venous drainage from the eyeball and is observed through examination with an ophthalmoscope. Pressure on the oculomotor nerve usually accompanies IICP and affects pupillary response to light. Normal pupil response to strong light is rapid constriction; in IICP, it is sluggish or nonexistent (fixed).

Changes in ICP also influence vital signs. Body temperature may rise or fall depending on the etiology of the IICP or because of its effect on the temperature-regulating center. The pulse increases initially but then decreases, systolic BP rises, and pulse pressure (the difference between the systolic and diastolic measurement) widens—three signs called **Cushing's triad,** occurring late in IICP. The respiratory rate is irregular. Later, **Cheyne-Stokes respirations** occur, consisting of shallow, rapid breathing followed by a period of apnea.

Decorticate or decerebrate posturing (see Chap. 38) develops spontaneously or in response to a painful stimulus when ICP is increased.

Diagnostic Findings

Diagnostic tests that determine the underlying cause of IICP include skull radiography, computed tomography (CT), magnetic resonance imaging (MRI), lumbar puncture, and cerebral angiography.

Medical and Surgical Management

Immediate treatment aims at relieving the cause of IICP. Monitoring devices (Fig. 39.1) are inserted to measure ICP and, in some cases, withdraw CSF. These devices are connected to a transducer and a monitor that display the pressure and a waveform to detect the status of ICP. Normal ICP in the ventricles is 1 to 15 mm Hg. Although ICP varies, a rise of 2 mm Hg from a previous measurement is cause for concern.

Osmotic diuretics such as mannitol (Osmitrol), glycerin (Osmoglyn), or urea (Ureaphil), and corticosteroids such as dexamethasone (Decadron) are given to reduce cerebral edema. Other treatment includes restriction of oral and intravenous (IV) fluids and hyperventilation therapy by means of mechanical ventilation, which produces vasoconstriction of cerebral arteries, followed by decreased cerebral blood volume and reduced ICP. An anticonvulsant may be ordered to prevent seizures, which elevate intracranial pressure.

Depending on the degree and cause of IICP, the physician may order the insertion of an indwelling catheter, a nasogastric tube for gastric decompression or to provide tube feedings, a stool softener to prevent straining at stool, and a histamine antagonist such as famotidine (Pepcid) to prevent stress ulcers. Persistent hyperthermia caused by altered functioning of the hypothalamus requires hypothermic measures such as a cooling blanket if the temperature does not respond to antipyretic drugs.

Emergency surgery is done to remove a blood clot if IICP results from a head injury with bleeding above or below the dura (see Chap 41). Surgery also is performed to relieve pressure caused by a brain tumor.

Nursing Management

Nursing care of the client with IICP is presented in Nursing Care Plan 39-1.

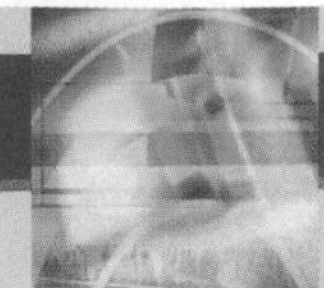

Nursing Care Plan 39-1

THE CLIENT WITH INCREASED INTRACRANIAL PRESSURE (IICP)

Assessment

- Gather from client or a witness, paramedic, or emergency medical technician the history of circumstances surrounding the altered neurologic state. Also gather past medical history, concurrent health problems being treated, current medications, and allergy history.
- Assess level of consciousness (LOC) and vital signs.
- Assist with a head-to-toe physical examination.
- Perform complete neurologic assessments, including the Glasgow Coma Scale (GCS) or Ranchos Los Amigos Scale (see Chap. 38). Repeat these assessments every 30 to 60 minutes.
- Measure current and daily weights and intake and output measurements.
- Study laboratory findings such as serum electrolyte and arterial blood gas levels.
- Evaluate presence of bowel sounds and bowel elimination.
- Note evidence of any seizures.

Nursing Diagnosis: **Ineffective Tissue Perfusion (cerebral)** related to IICP as evidenced by decreased LOC, sluggish pupil response, papilledema, and posturing

Expected Outcome: ICP will be between 1 and 15 mm Hg, and the GCS will be 9 or greater.

Interventions	*Rationales*
Keep head of bed slightly elevated and head in midline (straight). For clients with a basal skull fracture, keep bed flat.	Promotes drainage of venous blood and cerebrospinal fluid from the cranium.
Limit movement, space essential nursing tasks, and reduce or eliminate environmental stimuli (e.g., loud noise, bright lights).	Activities that increase BP, use the Valsalva maneuver, impair blood circulation, or decrease oxygenation raise ICP.
Avoid extreme hip flexion.	Compresses femoral blood vessels and interferes with circulation.
Keep client quiet. Change position with assistance and use a turning sheet. Avoid range-of-motion (ROM) exercises until ICP approaches normal unless ordered otherwise by the physician.	Increases ICP by raising BP. IICP predisposes to cerebral ischemia and cell damage.
Administer reduced fluid volumes at an even rate for 24 hours. Give diuretics and corticosteroids as prescribed; note client's response to therapy.	Decreases volume in the brain. Corticosteroids stabilize cell membranes, which helps prevent fluid shifts from intracellular to extracellular spaces.
Administer prescribed stool softener.	Increases moisture in stool, making stool easy to pass and reducing potential for the Valsalva maneuver.
Ensure that a gastric tube used for decompression or nourishment remains patent.	An obstructed gastric tube can contribute to gastric distention and vomiting. Elevated BP and ICP accompany vomiting.
Administer prescribed medications if vomiting or persistent coughing occur.	Suppressing vomiting and coughing reduces potential for IICP and cerebral ischemia.

Evaluation of Expected Outcome: ICP returns to normal, and cerebral perfusion is restored.

Nursing Diagnoses: **Risk for Ineffective Breathing Pattern** and **Ineffective Airway Clearance** related to diminished LOC and herniation of the brain stem secondary to IICP

Expected Outcomes: (1) Respiratory rate will be sufficient to maintain the SpO_2 above 90% and PO_2 above 80 mm Hg. (2) Airway will be patent.

(continued)

Nursing Care Plan 39-1 (Continued)

THE CLIENT WITH INCREASED INTRACRANIAL PRESSURE (IICP)

Interventions	*Rationales*
Attach pulse oximeter to finger, earlobe, bridge of the nose, or toe.	Measures percentage of oxygen bound to hemoglobin.
Insert oral airway if client is comatose.	Prevents tongue from occluding the natural airway.
Administer prescribed oxygen.	Provides greater percentage of oxygen than in room air.
Suction when necessary to clear tracheal secretions.	Artificial airways increase secretions, reducing volume of air within the airway.

Evaluation of Expected Outcomes: Respirations are normal, airway is free of secretions, and lungs are clear to auscultation.

Nursing Diagnosis: **Risk for Infection** related to impaired skin and tissue integrity secondary to surgery, invasive diagnostic or monitoring procedures, or original head injury

Expected Outcome: Client will be free of infection as evidenced by no fever, no purulent drainage from open areas of skin, and white blood cell count within normal limits.

Interventions	*Rationales*
Keep wounds clean and dry.	Reduces transient pathogens.
Use aseptic technique when handling any part of the intracranial monitoring device or changing a dressing applied after surgery.	Ensures that supplies and equipment are not contaminated with pathogens.
Administer antibiotic therapy, if prescribed.	Inhibits growth of or destroys susceptible microorganisms.

Evaluation of Expected Outcome: Temperature is normal with no sign of infection.

PC: **Hyperglycemia** related to corticosteroid therapy or administration of TPN

Expected Outcome: The nurse will monitor to detect, manage, and minimize elevated blood glucose level.

Interventions	*Rationales*
Assess capillary blood glucose levels three times daily and at bedtime.	Provides reliable measurements of current blood glucose level.
Follow medical orders for administering insulin according to a sliding scale.	Insulin helps lower blood sugar by facilitating its movement into body cells.

Evaluation of Expected Outcome: Blood glucose level is within normal range or lowered with insulin therapy.

PC: **Stress Ulcer** related to hyperacidity secondary to stress response

Expected Outcome: The nurse will monitor to detect, manage, and minimize the development of a peptic ulcer.

Interventions	*Rationales*
Check pH of gastric secretions per shift.	Obtaining a sample of gastric secretions and using chemical strip for pH provides a quick means for monitoring the acidity of the stomach.

(continued)

Nursing Care Plan 39-1 (Continued)

THE CLIENT WITH INCREASED INTRACRANIAL PRESSURE (IICP)

Interventions	Rationales
Report a pH of less than 3.	A pH above 3 helps suppress release of pepsin, which adds to gastric pH created by hydrochloric acid.
Administer prescribed drugs that protect the gastric mucosa, reduce histamine secretion, suppress the release of gastric secretions, or neutralize stomach acids.	Reduces the potential for developing a peptic ulcer.

Nursing Diagnosis: **Self-Care Deficit (total or specify type)** related to diminished LOC as manifested by inability to follow directions and impaired neuromuscular function

Expected Outcome: Client's basic needs will be met.

Interventions	Rationales
Give client complete care, including bathing, oral care, nutrition, and elimination, until ICP is normal and client can resume these activities independently.	The nurse manages needs that a client cannot perform until neurologic function returns.

Evaluation of Expected Outcome: Basic needs are managed.

Nursing Diagnosis: **Impaired Verbal Communication** related to decreased LOC or endotracheal intubation as evidenced by an inability to speak

Expected Outcome: Client will communicate using body language, pantomime, or writing.

Interventions	Rationales
Look for grimacing or moaning.	Sounds of distress are universal.
Correct problems that may be causing discomfort, such as a wrinkled sheet or an object pressing on the skin.	Astute assessment may determine cause of discomfort and facilitate prompt intervention.
Provide paper and pencil or a magic slate if client is alert but intubated.	Written communication is an alternative to oral communication.

Evaluation of Expected Outcome: Client communicates needs to others when conscious. For additional suggestions for nursing management of a client undergoing surgery or who develops a neurologic deficit, see Chapter 42.

Stop, Think, and Respond ● BOX 39-1

What assessment findings suggest that ICP is increasing beyond the compensatory changes that result from autoregulation?

INFECTIOUS AND INFLAMMATORY DISORDERS OF THE NERVOUS SYSTEM

Four neurologic conditions have an infectious or inflammatory cause: meningitis, encephalitis, Guillain-Barré syndrome, and brain abscess (Fig. 39.2). See Chap. 8 for a discussion of meningitis.

● ENCEPHALITIS

Encephalitis is an infectious disease of the CNS characterized by pathologic changes in both the white matter and the gray matter of the spinal cord and brain.

Pathophysiology and Etiology

Bacteria, fungi, or viruses cause encephalitis. The disease can follow a viral infection elsewhere in the body, such as measles, or vaccination. Viruses identified as causing encephalitis include the St. Louis, Western equine, and Eastern equine. Ticks or mosquitoes transmit some viruses.

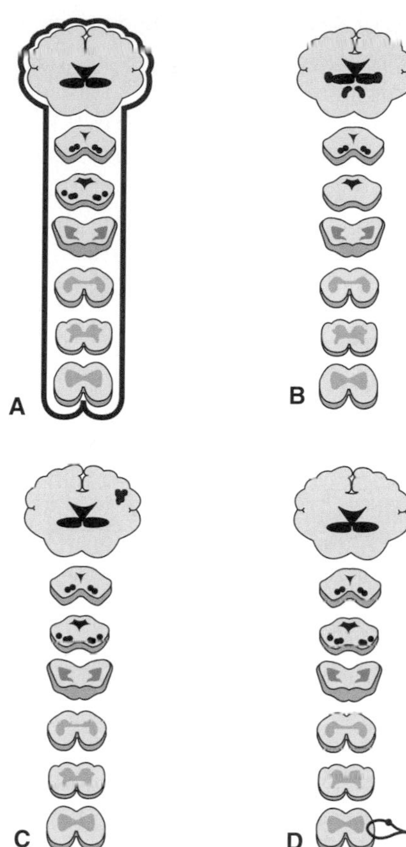

FIGURE 39.2 Sites of infectious and inflammatory disorders. (**A**) Meningitis, (**B**) encephalitis, (**C**) Guillain-Barré syndrome, (**D**) brain abscess.

Severe and diffuse inflammation of the brain occurs. Nerve cell destruction can be extensive. Cerebral edema and neurologic deficits such as paralysis and speech changes, IICP, respiratory failure, seizure disorders, and shock can occur.

Assessment Findings

Sudden fever, severe headache, stiff neck, vomiting, and drowsiness signal onset of viral encephalitis. Other symptoms include tremors, seizures, spastic or flaccid paralysis, irritability, and muscle weakness. Lethargy, delirium, or coma develop. Incontinence and visual disturbances such as photophobia, involuntary eye movements, and double or blurred vision occur.

A lumbar puncture is performed. CSF pressure is elevated, but fluid is clear. In some types of encephalitis, serologic studies show a rise in viral antibodies. Electroencephalography (EEG) reveals slow waveforms.

Medical Management

Because no specific antiviral measure has been developed, treatment is supportive.

Nursing Management

Monitor vital signs and LOC frequently and compare findings with previous assessments. If urinary retention or urinary incontinence develops, consult the physician to discuss whether an indwelling urethral catheter is appropriate. Measure fluid intake and output to detect signs of fluid volume deficit and electrolyte imbalances. Assess bowel elimination to determine if the client needs an enema or a stool softener.

• GUILLAIN-BARRÉ SYNDROME

Guillain-Barré syndrome (acute postinfectious polyneuropathy, polyradiculoneuritis) affects the peripheral nerves and the spinal nerve roots. Most clients begin to recover about 1 month after progression of symptoms ceases. Recovery may be slow and take 1 year or more. Death can occur from complications of immobility, such as pneumonia and infection.

Pathophysiology and Etiology

Although the exact cause is unknown, Guillain-Barré syndrome is believed to be an autoimmune reaction (see Chap. 36) that follows a primary disorder, especially an infectious one. Many clients have a history of a recent viral infection, particularly of the respiratory tract. Others have a history of recent surgery or recent vaccination for a viral disease like influenza. The syndrome also occurs in clients with malignant diseases and lupus erythematosus.

The affected nerves become inflamed and edematous. Myelin is lost. Mild to severe ascending muscle weakness or paralysis develops. Overactivity or underactivity of the sympathetic or parasympathetic nervous system is evidenced by changes in BP and in heart rate and rhythm.

Assessment Findings

Although symptoms vary, weakness, numbness, and tingling in arms and legs often are the first symptoms. Weakness is progressive and moves to upper areas of the body and affects muscles of respiration. Paralysis may follow muscle weakness. If cranial nerve involvement develops, chewing, talking, and swallowing are difficult.

A lumbar puncture reveals elevated CSF protein levels and pressure. Results of electrophysiologic testing show marked slowing in conduction of nerve impulses. Additional neurologic tests are performed to rule out other possible CNS disorders with similar symptoms.

Medical Management

Plasmapheresis, removal of plasma from blood and reinfusion of cellular components with saline, shortens the course of the disease if performed within the first 2 weeks. Otherwise, treatment is primarily supportive. If respiratory muscles are involved, endotracheal intubation and mechanical ventilation are necessary. Difficulty chewing and swallowing necessitate administration of IV fluids, gastric tube feedings, or total parenteral nutrition (TPN).

Nursing Management

Observe the client closely for signs of respiratory distress. Use a spirometer to evaluate the client's ventilation capacity. To assess for pneumonia, check vital signs and lung sounds frequently.

Because immobility incapacitates the client, provide meticulous skin care and change the client's position every 2 hours. Help the client perform passive range-of-motion (ROM) exercises to prevent muscle atrophy.

• BRAIN ABSCESS

A brain abscess is a collection of purulent material in the brain. If untreated, it can be fatal.

Pathophysiology and Etiology

A brain abscess occurs from an infection in nearby structures such as the middle ear, sinuses, or teeth, or from an infection in other organs. A brain abscess can develop after intracranial surgery or head trauma. It can be secondary to such disorders as bacterial endocarditis, bacteremia, and pulmonary or abdominal infections.

A brain abscess produces neurologic changes according to its location. Because it occupies space in the cranium, IICP can develop. Complications include paralysis, mental deterioration, seizure disorder, and visual disturbances.

Assessment Findings

Manifestations of a brain abscess include signs of IICP, fever, headache, and neurologic changes such as paralysis, seizures, muscle weakness, and lethargy.

Laboratory tests show an elevated WBC count. Analysis of CSF obtained by lumbar puncture helps confirm the diagnosis, but this procedure has a risk of herniation of the brain stem. A CT scan, MRI, and skull radiographs are safer techniques for diagnosing and locating the abscess.

Medical and Surgical Management

Antimicrobial therapy begins once the diagnosis is confirmed. A craniotomy, discussed later in this chapter, typically is performed to drain the abscess. Cerebral edema and seizures are treated with drug therapy. Additional treatment includes control of fever, mechanical ventilation, IV fluids, and nutritional support.

Nursing Management

Assess frequently for altered LOC, changes in sensory and motor functions, and signs of IICP. Monitor vital signs frequently. Measure fluid intake and output because overhydration can lead to cerebral edema. Other measures, as discussed in previous sections, are also necessary for clients with a brain abscess.

NEUROMUSCULAR DISORDERS

A neuromuscular disorder involves the nervous system and indirectly affects muscles. Some examples include multiple sclerosis (MS), myasthenia gravis, and amyotrophic lateral sclerosis (ALS)—all of which are chronic and progressively debilitating.

• MULTIPLE SCLEROSIS

Multiple sclerosis is a chronic progressive disease of the central nervous system. Its onset is in young adulthood and early middle age. The highest incidence is between 20 and 40 years of age, and it affects men and women approximately equally. The disease is more common in northern temperate zones than in warm climates.

Pathophysiology and Etiology

The cause is unknown, but MS is considered autoimmune and characterized as a **demyelinating disease** because it causes permanent degeneration and destruction of myelin in the brain and spinal cord. Myelin acts as an insulator, enabling nerve impulses to pass along a nerve fiber. Scar tissue forms after myelin is destroyed, referred to as sclerosis. Loss of myelin and subsequent degeneration and atrophy of nerve axons interrupt transmission of impulses along these fibers (Fig. 39.3). Areas most frequently affected are the optic nerves, cerebrum, brain stem, cerebellum, and the spinal cord (Smeltzer & Bare, 2004).

Many clients experience gradual and continuous worsening of symptoms. A few have the disease in a mild form and do not experience increased severity of symptoms.

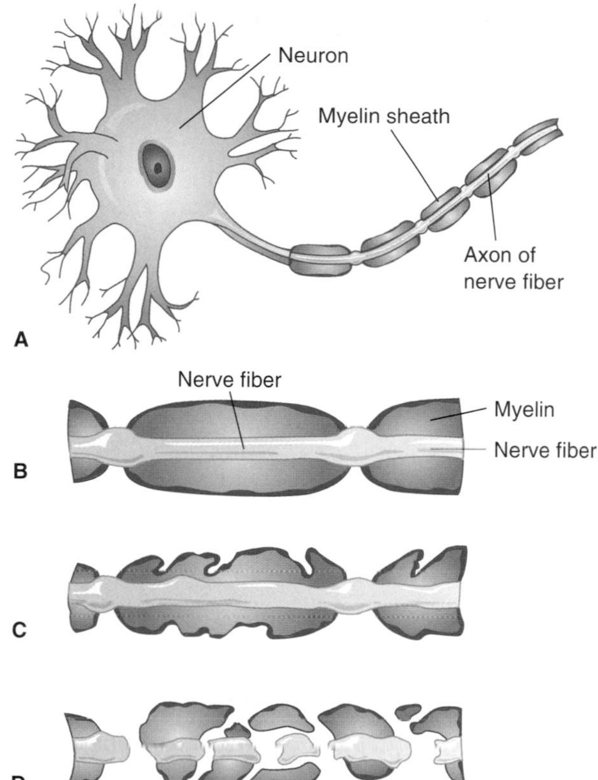

FIGURE 39.3 The process of demyelination. **A** and **B** depict a normal nerve cell and axon with myelin. **C** and **D** show the slow disintegration of myelin, which disrupts axon function. (From Smeltzer, S. C. & Bare, B. G. [2004]. *Brunner & Suddarth's textbook of medical-surgical nursing* [10th ed.]. Philadelphia: Lippincott Williams & Wilkins.)

For some, the symptoms subside during early phases of the illness (remission), and the client seems healthy for several months or even years. With each reappearance (exacerbation), however, the symptoms become more severe and last longer. Infections and emotional upsets precipitate exacerbations. Some people live a long time with MS; survival for 20 years after the diagnosis is not unusual.

As the disease progresses, many complications such as pressure ulcers, cachexia, deformities, and contractures develop. Pneumonia, brought about by limited activity, shallow breathing, and general debility, often is the immediate cause of death.

Assessment Findings

Many clients first dismiss minor symptoms as a result of fatigue or strain. When they no longer can ignore symptoms, clients with MS report blurred vision, **diplopia** (double vision), **nystagmus** (involuntary movement of the eyeball), weakness, clumsiness, and numbness and tingling of an arm or a leg. An intention tremor and slurred, hesitant speech (scanning speech) may develop. Mood swings (emotional lability) are common.

Weakness of an arm or a leg progresses to ataxia (motor incoordination) or paraplegia (paralysis of both legs). Occasional bowel and bladder incontinence leads to total incontinence. Slight visual disturbances end in blindness. The illness impairs intellectual functioning late in its course. Loss of memory, difficulty concentrating, and impaired judgment occur.

Early diagnosis is difficult because symptoms are vague and in some cases temporary. A lumbar puncture and CSF analysis reveal an increased WBC count. Electrophoresis of the CSF, a technique for electrically separating and identifying proteins, demonstrates abnormal immunoglobulin G bands, described as oligoclonal bands. The bands appear separated rather than homogeneous, which is the normal finding. A CT scan and MRI may or may not disclose lesions in the brain's white matter.

Medical Management

There is no cure for MS, nor is there any single treatment that relieves all symptoms. The primary aim of treatment is to keep the client functional as long as possible.

Drugs used to treat symptoms include baclofen (Lioresal) and dantrolene (Dantrium) for muscle spasticity and rigidity, antibiotics for infection, and tranquilizers to alleviate mood swings. Oxybutynin (Ditropan) is used to treat urinary incontinence, and bethanechol (Urecholine) to relieve urine retention. The anti-inflammatory action of corticosteroids relieves symptoms and hastens remissions. Interferon beta-1a (Avonex) is used to treat relapsing forms of MS. It decreases the number of flare-ups and slows the occurrence of some disabilities. Interferon beta-1b (Betaseron) also decreases exacerbations and disability. Both are administered subcutaneously. Glatiramer acetate (Copaxone) blocks damage to the myelin and significantly reduces relapses of MS. It also is administered subcutaneously. More research is being done to develop medications that modify MS.

NURSING PROCESS

● The Client With a Neuromuscular Disorder

Assessment

Perform a thorough neurologic assessment. Evaluate pulmonary function, including respiratory rate, depth, and lung sounds, to determine the client's ability to ventilate. To detect early signs of infection, take the client's temperature regularly. Note the client's ability to chew and swallow effectively and observe for drooling, choking when swallowing liquids, and regurgitating fluids through the nose. Assess muscle strength and coordination as well as the client's response to physical activity. To evaluate fluid status, measure intake and output. Monitor the client's elimination patterns. As data accumulate, analyze trends, using the initial baseline for comparisons. In addition, monitor the client's and caregivers' ability to cope with the progressively debilitating nature of the disorder.

Diagnosis, Planning, and Interventions

Risk for Ineffective Breathing Pattern related to weakening of muscles for respiration

Expected Outcome: Ventilation will be sufficient to maintain the SpO_2 above 90% and PaO_2 above 80 mm Hg.

- Place client in a Fowler's position and support arms on pillows. *Facilitates maximum chest expansion.*
- Eliminate foods that form intestinal gas or promote the expulsion of gas with a rectal tube. *Intestinal gas rises in the abdomen and places pressure on the diaphragm, limiting the volume of air the client can inhale.*
- Encourage client to deep breathe several times an hour. *Increases tidal volumes, fills alveoli with air, and enhances gas exchange.*
- Notify physician immediately if client experiences inadequate ventilation. *Medical interventions may be necessary.*

Risk for Ineffective Airway Clearance related to weak or ineffective cough, **Impaired Swallowing, Risk for Imbalanced Nutrition: Less than Body Requirements,** and **Risk for Aspiration** related to muscular weakness

Expected Outcomes: (1) Airway will be patent. (2) Client will swallow food and fluids without aspiration. (3) Nutritional needs will be met.

- Help client cough and raise respiratory secretions. *Clears the airway.*
- Suction oral cavity and airway. *Helps clear secretions from airway.*
- Offer liquids frequently in small amounts. *Large volumes increase risk for aspiration.*
- Consult with the dietitian on techniques for modifying texture and consistency of foods. *Clients can best swallow smooth foods with texture. Commercial substances are available to thicken liquids to promote swallowing.*
- Provide rest before meals. *Fatigue interferes with attention, coordination, and energy to chew and swallow.*
- Help client to sit upright when eating. *Promotes movement of food from mouth to esophagus and stomach and reduces potential for aspiration.*
- Place food in the posterior of the client's mouth. Flex client's chin toward chest when swallowing to facilitate passage of food into the esophagus. *Facilitates swallowing and diverts food into esophagus rather than airway.*
- Feed client slowly. Wait to place more food in the client's mouth until he or she has swallowed previous bolus. *Decreases risk for airway obstruction or aspiration.*
- Consult with physician about a plan for tube feedings or TPN. *Other nourishment may be necessary if oral nutritional intake is inadequate or dangerous.*

Impaired Physical Mobility, Self-Care Deficit (specify type), and **Risk for Impaired Skin Integrity** related to diminished muscle strength and inactivity

Expected Outcomes: (1) Client will be mobile and use muscles to the maximum extent possible. (2) Basic needs will be met. (3) Skin will remain intact.

- Encourage client to participate in self-care. *Fosters self-image.*
- Provide rest between bathing, shaving, performing oral care, eating, ambulating, toileting, and participating in diversional activities. *Provides time to recover from an activity and builds stamina and endurance.*
- Complete tasks client cannot perform. *Relieves client of further efforts at self-care when he or she is fatigued or weak.*
- Change body position every 2 hours. *Relieves pressure on capillaries that traverse over bony prominences, and reduces potential for skin breakdown.*
- Perform ROM exercises every 8 hours. *Promotes joint flexibility and muscle tone, and supplements or complements musculoskeletal activities the client actively performs.*
- Use a foot board and trochanter rolls to promote a neutral body position. *Keeps body in good alignment and reduces potential for contractures.*
- Consult with a physical or occupational therapist on techniques to facilitate client's independence and self-care. *They are experts in maintaining and regaining functional activities.*
- Use pressure-relieving devices when client is in bed or a wheelchair. *Prevents skin breakdown.*
- Keep bed dry and free of wrinkles. *Moisture softens the epidermis, making it vulnerable to breaking down. Wrinkles create pressure that interferes with blood circulation to cells and tissues.*
- Wash and dry the skin well. *Clean, dry skin decreases risk factors that can alter its integrity.*

Ineffective Coping related to feelings of helplessness secondary to chronic illness

Expected Outcome: Client will cope effectively with situational stressors.

- Suggest joining a support group of people with a similar disorder or subscribing to the support group's newsletter. *Facilitates coping. Clients acquire new coping strategies when others share their problem-solving approaches in person or in written communications.*
- Encourage client to express feelings. *Relieves client's personal emotional burden and fosters support.*
- Provide opportunities in which the client can make choices. *Promotes a feeling of control, which fosters ability to cope.*
- Facilitate client's network of social support, such as with family, neighbors, coworkers, and church members, through personal visits, telephone conversations, cards, and letters. *Decreases burden of coping with an illness as an isolated individual.*
- Provide diversional activities that foster feelings of personal accomplishment. *Helps a client persevere in coping with adversity.*

Risk for Caregiver Role Strain related to unrelenting responsibility for client's care

Expected Outcome: Primary caregiver will cope with long-term care of client

- Listen empathetically while caregiver expresses feelings about caring for client. *Caregiver is likely to feel less guilty if he or she feels comfortable discussing stressors involved with someone other than client or another family member.*
- Help caregiver develop a list of surrogates who may provide regular periods of relief. *The caregiver's dedication will be prolonged if he or she experiences intermittent periods when total responsibility is relieved.*
- Give caregiver permission to meet his or her own needs. *Unless encouraged to do so, caregivers suppress their own needs in deference to those for whom they care.*
- Identify available community resources and offer to facilitate a referral. *The caregiver may be unaware of service organizations whose missions are to provide help and support to clients and caregivers with particular disorders.*

Evaluation of Expected Outcomes

Respirations are of normal rate and depth. The airway is clear, and breathing is effortless. Nutrition is adequate to maintain body weight. The client regains mobility and attends to ADLs with minimal or no assistance. Skin is intact with no evidence of breakdown. The client demonstrates effective coping skills. The caregiver continues his or her responsibilities but implements a plan for periodic relief or assistance.

• MYASTHENIA GRAVIS

Myasthenia gravis is a neuromuscular disorder characterized by severe weakness of one or more groups of skeletal muscles.

Pathophysiology and Etiology

Although its exact cause is unknown, the disease is believed to be autoimmune and to develop when blood cells and thymus gland antibodies destroy nerve ending receptor sites of skeletal muscles. The symptoms develop because acetylcholine cannot stimulate receptors on skeletal muscles (Fig. 39.4). The outcome is extreme muscle weakness.

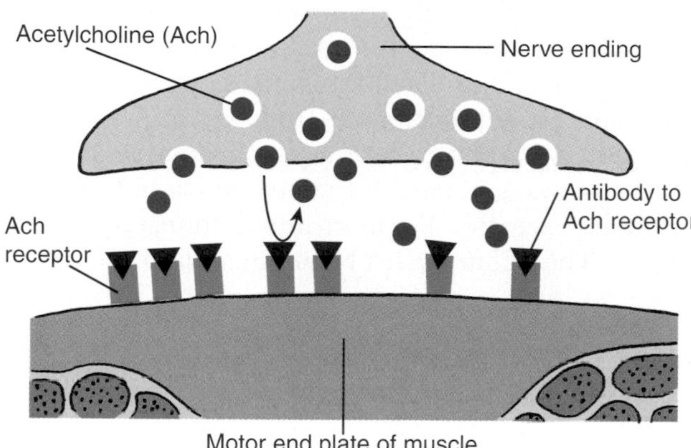

FIGURE 39.4 Inhibition of synaptic transmission of Ach in myasthenia gravis leads to profound muscle weakness. (From Rubin, E. & Farber, J. L. [1999]. *Pathology* [3rd ed.]. Philadelphia: Lippincott Williams & Wilkins.)

Assessment Findings

Muscle weakness varies depending on muscles affected. The most common manifestations are **ptosis** (drooping) of the eyelids (Fig. 39.5), difficulty chewing and swallowing, diplopia, voice weakness, masklike facial expression, and weakness of extremities. The respiratory system also is affected. During a myasthenic crisis, the client experiences increased muscle weakness, respiratory distress, decreased tidal volume, and difficulty talking, swallowing, and chewing.

Diagnostic confirmation is made by IV administration of edrophonium (Tensilon), which relieves symptoms in a few seconds. Chest x-rays may show a tumor of the thymus (thymoma). Electromyography measures the electrical potential of muscles.

Medical and Surgical Management

Treatment involves facilitating normal neurotransmission with administration of an anticholinesterase drug, such as pyridostigmine bromide (Mestinon) or ambenonium chloride (Mytelase). The therapeutic effect prolongs the action of acetylcholine, which sustains muscle contraction. The dose of the drug is adjusted according to the client's response to therapy.

Other treatments include surgical removal of the thymus gland, prednisone, and plasmapheresis for clients who do not respond to other methods of therapy. If myasthenic crisis with severe respiratory distress occurs, the client requires intubation and mechanical ventilation.

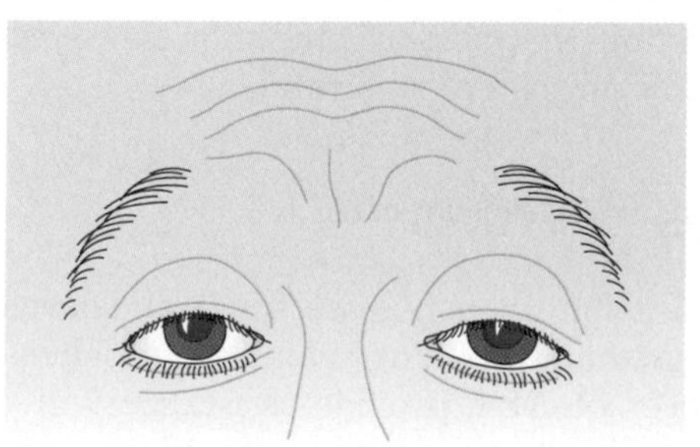

FIGURE 39.5 Ptosis of the eyelids.

Nursing Management

Observe the effects of drug therapy, especially when first initiated or at times of stress. Administer medications at the exact intervals ordered to maintain therapeutic blood levels and prevent symptoms from returning. Observe for signs of drug overdose, such as abdominal cramps, clenched jaws, and muscle rigidity, which indicate that the dose is excessive. For more information, see Nursing Process: The Client With a Neuromuscular Disorder.

● AMYOTROPHIC LATERAL SCLEROSIS

Amyotrophic lateral sclerosis (ALS), also known as *Lou Gehrig's disease,* is a progressive, fatal neurologic disorder. The disease is more common in men than in women.

Pathophysiology and Etiology

The cause of ALS is unknown. The disease is characterized by degeneration of motor neurons of the spinal cord and brain stem, which results in muscle weakness and wasting.

Assessment Findings

Progressive muscle weakness and wasting of arms, legs, and trunk develop. The client experiences episodes of muscle **fasciculations** (twitching). If ALS affects the brain stem, speaking and swallowing become difficult. The client may display periods of inappropriate laughter and crying. Respiratory failure and total paralysis are seen in the terminal stage.

The disorder is difficult to diagnose in the early stages because no specific diagnostic tests are available for this disease. Electromyography validates weakness in the affected muscles.

Medical Management

There is no specific treatment, and death occurs several years after diagnosis in many cases. The client is encouraged to remain active as long as possible. Death usually results from respiratory arrest or overwhelming respiratory infection. Mechanical ventilation is necessary when ALS affects muscles of respiration.

Nursing Management

Perform a comprehensive assessment and develop a plan of care based on the client's identified problems. During early stages of ALS, provide assistance with walking, bathing, shaving, and dressing. As ALS progresses, the client becomes totally dependent on the family or healthcare personnel for care. Teach family members required skills, such as suctioning techniques, how to administer tube feedings, and catheter care. Client and Family Teaching 39-1 provides more information, as does Nursing Process: The Client With a Neuromuscular Disorder. Additional discussion on caring for clients with a neurologic deficit is covered in Chapter 42.

CRANIAL NERVE DISORDERS

● TRIGEMINAL NEURALGIA (TIC DOULOUREUX)

Trigeminal neuralgia is a painful condition that involves the fifth cranial (trigeminal) nerve, which has three major branches: mandibular, maxillary, and ophthalmic (Fig. 39.6). This sensory and motor nerve is important to chewing, facial movement, and sensation.

Pathophysiology and Etiology

The cause of the disorder is unknown. It has been suggested that it is related to compression of the trigeminal nerve root. For reasons not fully understood, the client experiences **neuralgia** (nerve pain) in one or more branches of the trigeminal nerve. The slightest stimulus (e.g., vibration of music, passing breeze, temperature change) over trigger spots (or areas that provoke the pain) can initiate an attack. The forehead over the eyebrow is a common trigger spot when the ophthalmic branch of the nerve is affected.

Assessment Findings

The client describes the pain as sudden, severe, and burning. The pain ends as quickly as it begins, usually lasting a few seconds to several minutes. The cycle repeats many

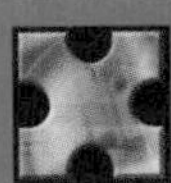

39-1 *Client and Family Teaching* Amyotrophic Lateral Sclerosis

The nurse reviews the following components with the client and family:

- Medication schedule, adverse effects of medications
- Dietary and feeding suggestions
- Agencies that can help with or give home care
- Sources of financial assistance
- Exercises to prevent muscle atrophy
- Positioning and good skin care
- Techniques for preventing skin breakdown

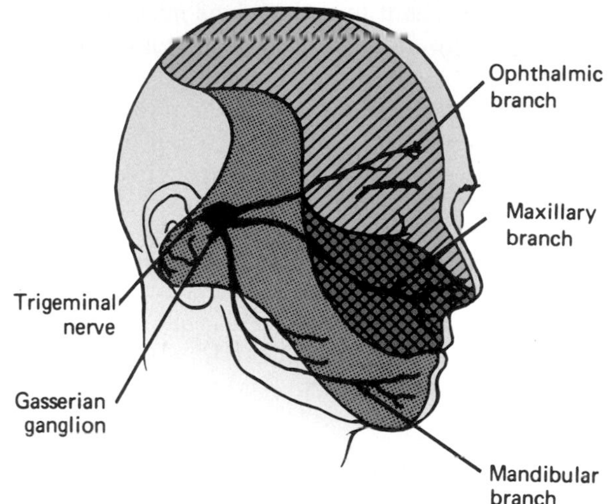

FIGURE 39.6 Areas innervated by the three branches of the trigeminal nerve. These are the areas that become painful in trigeminal neuralgia.

times each day. During a spasm, the face twitches and the eyes tear.

Skull x-rays, MRI, or CT are performed to rule out other pathologies, such as a brain tumor and intracranial bleeding. Ultimately, the diagnosis is based on the symptoms.

Medical Management

Medical treatment is primarily supportive and symptomatic rather than curative. Narcotic analgesics are necessary. Anticonvulsants such as phenytoin (Dilantin) and carbamazepine (Tegretol) are used to reduce pain, but are not always successful. The client is referred to a dentist because correction of dental malocclusion has relieved some cases.

Surgical Management

If medical management is unsatisfactory, surgical intervention is an option. Surgical division of the sensory root of the trigeminal nerve provides permanent relief, but some permanent loss of sensation accompanies this procedure. If the mandibular branch is severed, eating is problematic. The client may bite the tongue without realizing it, food may get caught in the mouth, and the jaw will deviate toward the operative side. Until the client adjusts to the altered sensation, swallowing is difficult.

Nursing Management

Obtain a complete history, then carefully and gently examine the affected area. Ask the client to identify the location, pattern, and events associated with pain and document the information. Inspect the oral cavity for signs of injury. Weigh the client and assess the client's ability to eat food. Ask the client to quantify the severity and intensity of the pain, before and after treatment measures. It is important to instruct the client and family in modifying the environment. Measures such as avoiding drafts and shielding the face from wind and cold are helpful in preventing triggers of pain. If a client is hospitalized, place a sign on the bed stating not to jar the bed or touch the client's face in any way. See Client and Family Teaching 39-2 for more information.

● BELL'S PALSY

Bell's palsy involves the seventh cranial nerve, which is responsible for movement of facial muscles.

Pathophysiology and Etiology

The cause of Bell's palsy is unknown, but a viral link is suspected. Inflammation occurs around the nerve, blocking motor impulses to facial muscles. Inflammation or ischemia resulting from nerve compression leads to impaired nerve function. As a result, there is weakness and paralysis of facial muscles, including the muscles of the eyelids, on one side of the face. Most clients who recover begin to show improvement in a few weeks. Those whose paralysis is permanent fail to show improvement after 3 months or more.

Assessment Findings

Symptoms develop in a few hours or over 1 to 2 days. Facial pain, pain behind the ear, numbness, diminished blink reflex, ptosis of the eyelid, and tearing on the affected side occur. Speaking and chewing become difficult.

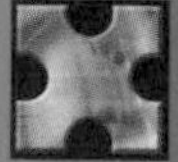

39-2 *Client and Family Teaching* Trigeminal Neuralgia

The nurse instructs the client as follows:

- Inspect the mouth daily for breaks in the mucous membrane.
- Take small sips or bites of food and concentrate on chewing and swallowing if surgery has been performed.
- Chew on the opposite side.
- Avoid eating hot foods.
- Use mouth rinses after eating.
- Keep regular dental appointments because the warning pain of a cavity, abscess, or other dental problem may be mistaken for neuralgia.

There are no specific diagnostic tests for this disorder; diagnosis is based on symptoms and visual examination of the face. In some instances it is necessary to rule out other neurologic problems such as brain tumor and stroke, which have comparable symptoms.

Medical Management

Short-term corticosteroid therapy with prednisone (Deltasone, Meticorten) is prescribed to reduce nerve inflammation and edema. Analgesics are prescribed for pain. Electrotherapy or a facial sling helps to prevent atrophy of the facial muscles on the affected side. Once the diagnosis is confirmed, the client is assured that a more serious problem (e.g., stroke) has not occurred.

Nursing Management

Obtain the client's history, noting any recent illness that suggests a viral infection. Perform a physical examination to determine which side of the face is involved and the appearance of affected structures. Note if the client has any speech impairment and observe the client's ability to chew and swallow food. The client is at risk for an ophthalmic infection because of a diminished blink reflex. Instruct the client to cover the eye with an eye patch to keep the eyelid closed and protect the eye surface from environmental debris. A protective eye shield at night ensures that the client does not scratch or injure the eye during sleep. The client needs to inspect the eye daily for signs of inflammation and infection. Normal saline eye flushes or ophthalmic antibiotic ointment may be ordered. The client will experience loss of sensation in the mouth and paralysis of chewing muscles, manifested by trauma to the cheeks, gums, teeth, or tongue. Scrupulous oral hygiene is essential. Instruct the client in oral hygiene measures, emphasizing the need for inspection of oral mucous membranes, frequent dental exams, and avoidance of very hot food and beverages. Also encourage the client to speak slowly and in short sentences, enabling the client to coordinate use of his or her teeth, tongue, and lips while speaking.

• TEMPOROMANDIBULAR DISORDER

Temporomandibular disorder (TMD) is a cluster of symptoms localized near the jaw.

Pathophysiology and Etiology

Causes of TMD include degenerative arthritis of the mandibular joint, malocclusion of the teeth, bruxism (grinding of the teeth), and dislocation of the jaw during endotracheal intubation.

TMD occurs when the meniscus, or cartilaginous disk, between the condyle (end of the mandible) and the temporal bone are displaced from the fossa (socket) of the temporal bone (Fig. 39.7). Because facial muscles like the masseter and temporalis muscles move this gliding joint, the client has jaw pain from muscle spasms. Nerves and arteries in the area may be compressed. The disorder can be confused with trigeminal neuralgia and migraine headache. The cartilage wears away and affects jaw movement.

Assessment Findings

Symptoms include jaw pain, pronounced muscle spasm, and tenderness of the masseter and temporalis muscles. Headache, tinnitus (ringing in the ears), and ear pain

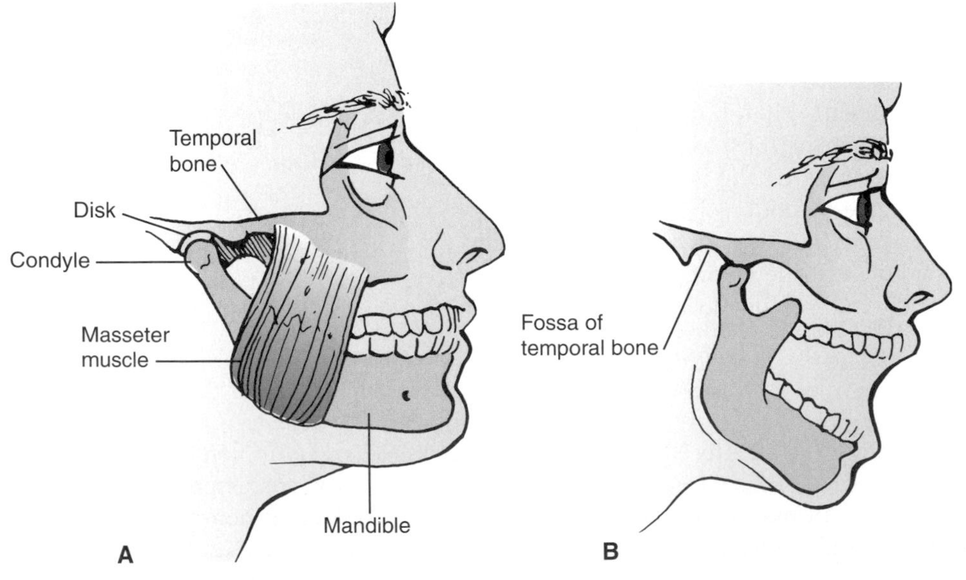

FIGURE 39.7 (**A**) The temporomandibular joint is located between the two bones for which it is named: the temporal bone and mandible. (**B**) The condyle of the mandible, which is covered by a cartilaginous disk, moves forward and backward within the fossa of the temporal bone of the skull, which is located in front of the ear.

accompany localized discomfort. The client experiences clicking or a grating sensation of the jaw when moving the joint, or the jaw can lock, which interferes with opening the mouth. Special dental x-rays often reveal evidence of joint displacement.

Medical and Surgical Management

Treatment is referral to a dentist experienced with managing clients with TMD. Analgesics are prescribed or recommended; the client wears a custom-fitted mouth guard during sleep. Transcutaneous electrical nerve stimulation, injection of a local anesthetic to relieve muscle spasm, and oral irrigations with ice water reduce and relieve discomfort. Reconstructive surgery of the temporomandibular joint is available if conservative treatment is ineffective.

Nursing Management

Clients with TMD are managed at home. Instructions include monitoring the client's weight and ability to consume food. The client should modify the diet to include soft rather than coarse food, which is difficult to chew, and nutritional liquid supplements. The client is also told about pain control methods, including use of a bite guard.

EXTRAPYRAMIDAL DISORDERS

Extrapyramidal disorders originate in the motor cortex and surrounding areas of the cerebellum and basal ganglia. Two common extrapyramidal disorders are Parkinson's disease and Huntington's disease. One of their primary characteristics is abnormal movement.

• PARKINSON'S DISEASE

Parkinson's disease usually begins after 50 years of age. It primarily affects basal ganglia and connections in the substantia nigra and corpus striatum (Fig. 39.8). The term **parkinsonism** describes the cluster of Parkinson's-like symptoms that develop from several etiologies.

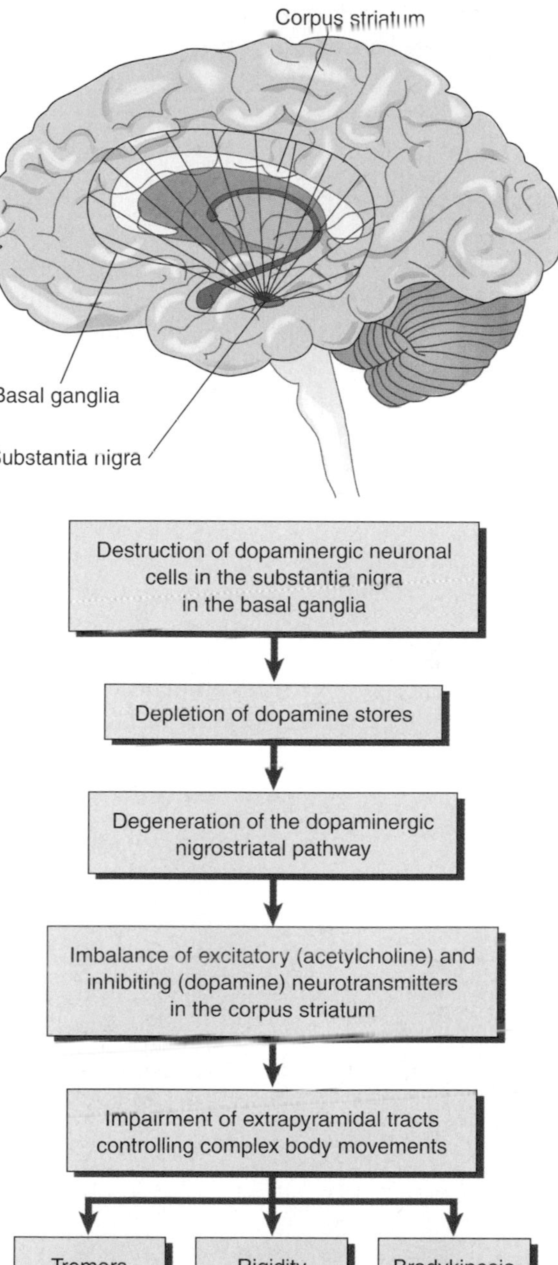

FIGURE 39.8 Nuclei in the substantia nigra protect fibers to the corpus striatum, where the nerve fibers carry dopamine. Loss of dopamine from nerve cells is thought to cause symptoms of Parkinson's disease. (From Smeltzer, S. C. & Bare, B. G. [2004]. *Brunner & Suddarth's textbook of medical–surgical nursing* [10th ed.]. Philadelphia: Lippincott Williams & Wilkins.)

Pathophysiology and Etiology

Parkinson's disease and parkinsonism occur from a depletion of the neurotransmitter dopamine in affected areas of the brain. This upsets the balance between dopamine and acetylcholine, resulting in movement disorders.

In most cases of Parkinson's disease, no cause is found for dopamine depletion. Symptoms of parkinsonism are associated with exposure to environmental toxins such as insecticides and herbicides and self-administration of an illegal synthetic form of heroin known as MPTP, and can occur as a sequela of head injuries and encephalitis. Phenothiazine—a category of antipsychotic drugs—and other antipsychotic drugs used to treat schizophrenia also produce parkinsonism, but symptoms are reversible when the drug is discontinued.

Manifestations of the disorder progress so slowly that years may elapse between the first symptom and diagnosis. Symptoms initially are unilateral, but eventually, whether quickly or slowly, become bilateral.

Assessment Findings

Early signs include stiffness (*rigidity*), and tremors of one or both hands (*pill-rolling*—a rhythmic motion of the thumb against the fingers). The hand tremor is obvious at rest and typically decreases when movement is voluntary, such as picking up an object.

Bradykinesia, slowness in performing spontaneous movements, develops. Clients have a masklike expression, stooped posture, monotonous speech, and difficulty swallowing saliva. Weight loss occurs. A shuffling gait is apparent, and the client has difficulty turning or redirecting forward motion. Arms are rigid while walking (Fig. 39.9).

In late stages, the disease affects the jaw, tongue, and larynx; speech is slurred; and chewing and swallowing become difficult. Rigidity can lead to contractures. Salivation increases, accompanied by drooling. In a small percentage of clients, the eyes roll upward or downward and stay there involuntarily for several hours or even a few days.

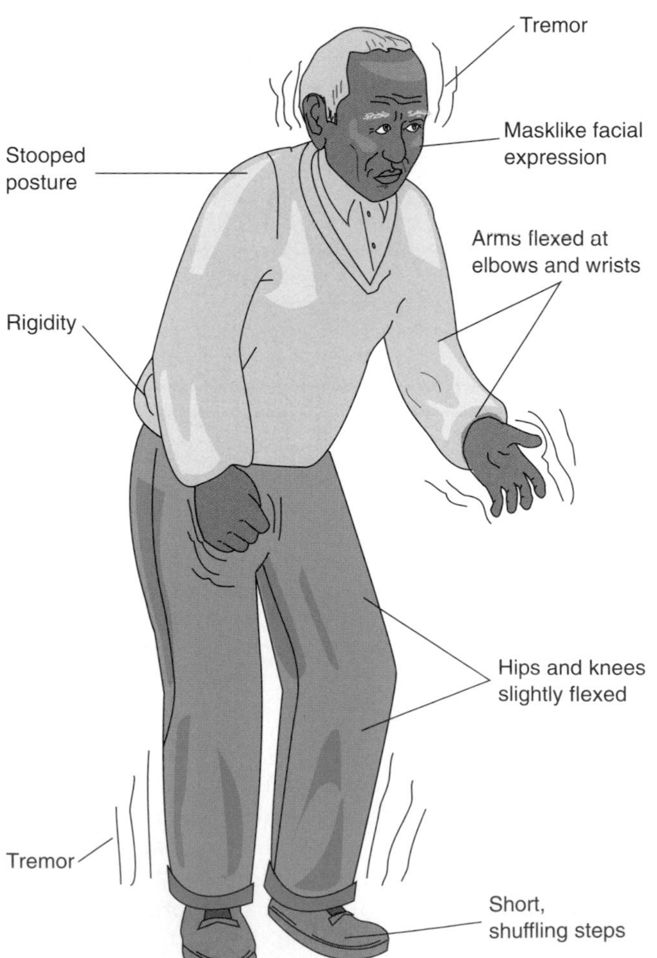

FIGURE 39.9 Typical manifestations of Parkinson's disease.

Diagnosis is based on typical symptoms and a neurologic examination. There are no specific tests for this disorder.

Medical Management

Treatment aims at prolonging independence. Drugs such as selegiline (Eldepryl), which has neuroprotective properties, dopaminergics such as levodopa (Larodopa) or levodopa-carbidopa (Sinemet), amantadine (Symmetrel), dopamine agonists such as bromocriptine (Parlodel), and anticholinergics such as benztropine (Cogentin) are prescribed (Drug Therapy Table 39.1). Their sequence of use is based on the stage of the disorder and the dwindling effectiveness of the medication initially prescribed. Rehabilitation measures, such as physical therapy, occupational therapy, client and family education, and counseling, are used concurrently with drug therapy.

Surgical Management

Surgery (stereotaxic pallidotomy) is performed in selected cases. The procedure destroys part of the thalamus so that excessive muscle contraction is decreased.

There has been limited success with transplantation of dopamine-secreting brain cells from pigs. Outside of the U.S., transplantation may occur from aborted fetuses. Autotransplantation of cells from the client's own adrenal medulla into the brain has been tried as well. Any type of transplantation requires a craniotomy.

Some clients with Parkinson's disease have an implantation of a brain pacemaker (Fig. 39.10). It blocks the tremor with tiny electrical shocks directed at the thalamus and immediately eliminates the tremor in approximately 65% of people in whom it has been used.

Nursing Management

Clients with parkinsonism are admitted to the hospital because of the debilitating effects of the disease. Others are cared for in extended care facilities when they can no longer be managed at home in a chronic state. One of the biggest nursing challenges is managing the client's drug therapy. Levodopa is associated with periods of "breakthrough" in which symptoms are exacerbated when a consistent level is not maintained. Administer drugs closely to the schedule the client previously established at home. Drugs administered for parkinsonism can cause a wide variety of adverse effects, requiring careful observation

Drug Therapy Table 39.1 ANTIPARKINSON AGENTS

DRUG CATEGORY AND EXAMPLES	MECHANISM OF ACTION	SIDE EFFECTS	NURSING CONSIDERATIONS
Monoamine Oxidase B Inhibitor (MAOI)			
selegiline (Eldepryl)	Increases dopaminergic activity Slows Parkinson's disease	Dizziness, light-headedness, confusion, nausea, vomiting, diarrhea, dry mouth, palpitations	Never give narcotic analgesics with an MAOI. Administer twice daily with breakfast and lunch. Use ice chips and sugarless candy for dry mouth.
Dopaminergics			
levodopa (Larodopa, Sinemet)	Dopamine replacement to decrease symptoms	Nausea, vomiting, orthostatic hypotension, dry mouth, constipation, dizziness, cardiac dysrhythmias, sleep disturbance	Do not give with MAOIs. Give with meals. Avoid multivitamins with pyridoxine.
Antiparkinsonism			
amantadine (Symmetrel)	May increase dopamine release to relieve symptoms	Mood changes, drowsiness, blurred vision, insomnia, nausea, orthostatic hypotension, urinary retention	Do not discontinue abruptly to avoid parkinsonian crisis. Report swelling of fingers, ankles, shortness of breath, difficulty urinating, tremors, slurred speech.
Anticholinergics			
benztropine (Cogentin) *trihexphenidyl (Artane)*	Decreases rigidity, akinesia, tremor, and drooling	Dry mouth, constipation, urinary retention, blurred vision, skin rash, flushing, increased temperature, decreased sweating	Decrease or discontinue dosage if dry mouth interferes with eating. Client must use caution in hot weather. Give with meals. Avoid alcohol and sedatives.
Dopamine Agonists			
bromocriptine (Parlodel)	Mimics effects of dopamine; may be effective when levodopa has decreased efficacy	Hallucinations, confusion, dizziness, drowsiness, nausea, vomiting, constipation, hypotension, shortness of breath	Give with food. Taper dosage before discontinuing. Monitor mental status.

of the client. See Nursing Care Plan 39-2 for more discussion of management of the client with an extrapyramidal disorder such as Parkinson's or Huntington's disease.

• HUNTINGTON'S DISEASE

Huntington's disease (Huntington's chorea, hereditary chorea) is a hereditary disorder of the CNS.

Pathophysiology and Etiology

Huntington's chorea is an extrapyramidal disorder transmitted genetically and inherited by both sexes. Basal ganglia and portions of the cerebral cortex degenerate. In early stages, the client can participate in most physical activities. As the disease progresses, hallucinations, delusions, impaired judgment, and increased intensity of abnormal movements develop.

Assessment Findings

Symptoms develop slowly and include mental apathy and emotional disturbances, **choreiform movements** (uncontrollable writhing and twisting of the body), grimacing, difficulty chewing and swallowing, speech difficulty, intellectual decline, and loss of bowel and bladder control. Severe depression is common and can lead to suicide.

Diagnosis is based on symptoms as well as a family history of the disorder. Positron emission tomography shows CNS changes, but there is no specific diagnostic test for the disorder. Genetic testing can predict which offspring will develop the disease.

Medical Management

Treatment is supportive because there is no specific therapy or cure. Tranquilizers and antiparkinson drugs relieve

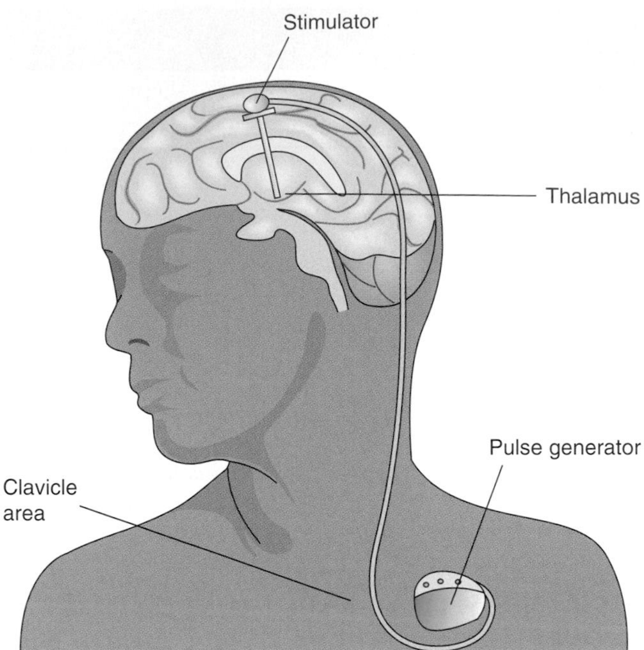

FIGURE 39.10 Deep brain stimulation with the use of a pulse generator. (From Smeltzer, S. C. & Bare, B. G. [2004]. *Brunner & Suddarth's textbook of medical–surgical nursing* [10th ed.]. Philadelphia: Lippincott Williams & Wilkins.)

the choreiform movements in some clients. No drugs are available to halt mental deterioration. Because this disorder is inherited, genetic counseling before pregnancy is advised.

Nursing Management

Nursing management aims at meeting client and family needs, such as preventing complications, as well as encouraging counseling. The stage of the disease determines the scope of nursing care. The client eventually becomes totally dependent on others. Pneumonia, contractures, infections, aspiration of food or fluids, falls, and pressure ulcers are complications. Prevent them by assessing the client frequently and updating the plan of care (see Nursing Care Plan 39-2).

Encourage the client to lead as normal a life as possible. Emphasize the importance of exercise and self-care and explain the medical regimen to the client and family. Demonstrate how to facilitate tasks such as using both hands to hold a drinking glass, using a straw to drink, and wearing slip-on shoes.

SEIZURE DISORDERS

The terms *seizure disorder* and *convulsive disorder* are used interchangeably, but they are not necessarily synonymous. A **seizure** is a brief episode of abnormal electrical activity in the brain. A **convulsion,** one manifestation of a seizure, is characterized by spasmodic contractions of muscles. **Epilepsy** is a chronic recurrent pattern of seizures.

Pathophysiology and Etiology

Seizure disorders are classified as idiopathic (no known cause) or acquired. Causes of acquired seizures include high fever, electrolyte imbalances, uremia, hypoglycemia, hypoxia, brain tumor, and drug withdrawal. Once the cause is removed, seizures cease. Known causes of epilepsy include brain injury at birth, head injuries, and inborn errors of metabolism. In some clients, the cause of epilepsy is never determined.

Seizures represent abnormal motor, sensory, or psychic neural activity. The abnormal neural activity occurs alone or in combination from discharges in one or more specific areas of the cerebral cortex. Each type of seizure disorder is characterized by a specific pattern of events (Box 39-2).

Types of Seizures

Seizures are divided into two general categories: partial and generalized.

Partial Seizures

Partial, or focal, seizures begin in a specific area of the cerebral cortex. They can progress to generalized seizures. Two subcategories of partial seizures are those with elementary (or simple) symptoms and those with complex symptoms. A client who has a partial seizure with elementary symptoms usually does not lose consciousness, and the seizure lasts less than 1 minute. Partial elementary seizures with motor symptoms are accompanied by uncontrolled jerking movements of a body part, such as a finger, mouth, hand, or foot. Partial elementary seizures with sensory symptoms are accompanied by hallucinatory sights, sounds, and odors; mumbling; and use of nonsense words. The terms *jacksonian, focal motor,* and *focal sensory* describe partial elementary seizures.

A client who has a partial seizure with complex symptoms may have several sensory or motor manifestations, which also last less than 1 minute. After the seizure, the client often is confused. Complex partial seizures are manifested by automatic repetitive movements **(automatisms)** that are not appropriate, such as lip smacking and picking at clothing or objects. The terms *psychomotor* and *psychosensory* are used to describe complex partial seizures.

Generalized Seizures

Generalized seizures involve the entire brain. The client loses consciousness, and the seizure may last from sev-

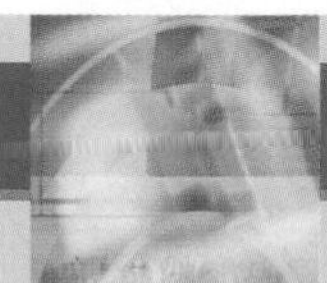

Nursing Care Plan 39-2

THE CLIENT WITH AN EXTRAPYRAMIDAL DISORDER

Assessment

Determine the following:

- Year of diagnosis
- Concurrent medical disorders
- Weight and vital signs
- Any unilateral or bilateral hand tremor
- Gait and balance
- Use of assistive ambulatory devices
- Ability to swallow
- Quality of speech
- Bowel and urinary elimination patterns
- Mental and emotional status
- Drug therapy; time and frequency of medication administration

Nursing Diagnoses: **Impaired Physical Mobility** and **Self-Care Deficit** (specify type) related to muscle rigidity, tremors, choreiform movements, and dementia as evidenced by inability to complete all or some activities of daily living (ADLs)

Expected Outcomes: (1) Client will be physically active. (2) Client will perform self-care to the level at which he or she is capable.

Interventions	*Rationales*
Assist client with walking and physical activities.	Client is at risk for falls and injuries if activities are not assisted or supervised.
Increase type and amount of activity gradually.	Client will have more strength and coordination once response to medications improves.
Minimize fatigue by providing rest periods.	Relieves fatigue and restores stamina and endurance.
Promote involvement in self-care activities within the client's individual capacity.	Promotes dignity and improves self-image.
Allow ample time to perform ADLs.	Given sufficient time, client is more likely to pace himself or herself to complete ADLs semi-independently.
Modify clothing and self-care supplies to promote independence.	Facilitates ability to perform self-care.
Assist client, but only when client cannot perform certain tasks.	Too much assistance cultivates dependence on the nurse.

Evaluation of Expected Outcomes:

- Client is active in his or her immediate environment and uses assistive devices as necessary.
- Client attends to self-care as much as symptoms allow.

Nursing Diagnoses: **Impaired Swallowing** and **Risk for Aspiration**

Expected Outcomes: (1) Client will swallow food and liquids taken in orally. (2) Client's airway will be free of food or liquids.

(continued)

Nursing Care Plan 39-2 (Continued)

THE CLIENT WITH AN EXTRAPYRAMIDAL DISORDER

Interventions	*Rationales*
Place client in a sitting position.	Helps propel food toward the stomach.
Decrease environmental distractions.	Helps client focus attention on chewing and swallowing.
Cut food into small pieces. Incorporate mashed potatoes or other pasty foods.	A large bolus of food is more likely to cause a complete obstruction if aspirated. Foods like mashed potatoes bind in a soft bolus that is swallowed more easily.
Thicken liquids with gelatin, cornstarch, applesauce, mashed bananas, ice cream, or a commercial thickener.	Thickeners provide a consistency that the tongue can easily manipulate against the palate.
Position client's chin on the chest during swallowing.	Decreases potential for food to enter the airway.
Stroke client's throat as he or she swallows or instruct client to swallow several times in a row.	Stimulating swallowing with stroking or repeated swallowing efforts moves food from the oropharynx to the esophagus.

Evaluation of Expected Outcomes:

- Client can swallow food and fluids without choking.
- Client's lungs remain clear of food and liquids.

Nursing Diagnosis: **Impaired Verbal Communication** related to soft voice or inability to articulate words

Expected Outcome: Client will communicate needs, feelings, and ideas.

Interventions	*Rationales*
Reduce environmental noise.	Helps others hear what the client says.
Listen closely to what the client tries to say.	Attention and patience facilitate understanding.
Ask client to speak slowly.	Altering the rate of speech improves clarity.
Anticipate client's needs.	Reduces client's frustration with having to ask for help.

Evaluation of Expected Outcome: Client's verbalizations are heard and understood.

Nursing Diagnosis: **Risk for Loneliness** related to depression and perceived potential for rejection secondary to altered physical appearance or cognitive function

Expected Outcome: Client will maintain social contacts.

Interventions	*Rationales*
Have client identify persons whose company he or she enjoys and activities they share.	Reinforces that the client has a circle of friends.
Encourage client to interact with a few of the designated people for short periods in a place where the client feels secure and comfortable, such as his or her home.	Promotes reestablishing social relationships.
Encourage client to participate in social activities outside the home.	When the client feels more accepted, he or she may extend socialization beyond the home.
Refer client to and encourage joining a support group.	Such groups promote bonding with new acquaintances.

Evaluation of Expected Outcome: Client reestablishes social contacts with previous friends and develops friendships with new acquaintances.

BOX 39-2 ● International Classification of Seizures

I. Partial (Focal) Seizures
- A. Partial seizures (no loss of consciousness)
  1. Motor symptoms
  2. Special sensory symptoms
  3. Autonomic symptoms
  4. Psychic symptoms
- B. Complex partial seizures (with loss of consciousness)
  1. Begins as a partial seizure and progresses to complex partial with loss of consciousness.
  2. Loss of consciousness at onset of seizure

II. Generalized Seizures
- A. Absence seizures
- B. Myoclonic seizures
- C. Clonic seizures
- D. Tonic seizures
- E. Tonic-clonic seizures
- F. Atonic seizures

III. Unclassified Seizures

All seizures that do not fit into other classifications

eral seconds to several minutes. There are three types of generalized seizures.

Absence seizures, formerly referred to as *petit mal seizures,* are more common in children. They are characterized by a brief loss of consciousness, during which physical activity ceases. The person stares blankly, eyelids flutter, lips move, and slight movement of the head, arms, and legs occurs. These seizures typically last a few seconds, and the person seldom falls to the ground. Because of the brief duration and relative lack of prominent movements, these seizures often go unnoticed. People with absence seizures can have them many times a day.

Myoclonic seizures are characterized by sudden, excessive jerking of the arms, legs, or entire body. In some instances, the muscle activity is so severe that the client falls to the ground. These seizures are brief.

Formerly referred to as *grand mal seizures,* tonic-clonic seizures are characterized by a sequence of events. They begin with a **preictal** (or prodromal) **phase,** which is the time immediately before a seizure and consists of vague emotional changes, such as depression, anxiety, and nervousness. This phase lasts for minutes or hours and is followed by an **aura,** a sensation that occurs immediately before the seizure. The aura is sensory (i.e., a hallucinatory odor or sound) or a sensation of weakness or numbness. In clients who experience an aura, the aura almost always is the same.

The aura is followed by the epileptic cry, caused by spasm of the respiratory muscles and muscles of the throat and glottis. This cry immediately precedes loss of consciousness and the ensuing tonic and clonic phases of the seizure. In the tonic phase, muscles contract rigidly; in the clonic phase, muscles alternate between contraction and relaxation, resulting in jerking movements and thrashing of arms and legs. The skin becomes cyanotic, and breathing is spasmodic. Saliva mixes with air, resulting in frothing at the mouth. The jaws are tightly clenched and biting of the tongue and inner cheek occurs. Urinary or fecal incontinence is common. The clonic phase lasts for 1 minute or more, gradually subsides, and is followed by the postictal phase. Manifestations of this phase include headache, fatigue, deep sleep, confusion, nausea, and muscle soreness. Many people fall into a deep sleep for several hours.

Status epilepticus is marked by a series of tonic-clonic seizures in which the client does not regain consciousness between seizures. If this extremely dangerous condition is not terminated, death can occur. Status epilepticus occurs spontaneously in acute neurologic disorders or for no known reason. It can also be precipitated by abrupt discontinuation of anticonvulsant medication.

Other Seizure Types

Atonic (loss of muscle tone) seizures affect muscles. The person loses consciousness briefly and falls to the ground. Recovery is rapid. An akinetic (loss of movement) seizure is similar because muscle tone is lost briefly. The client may or may not fall, and recovery is rapid.

Assessment Findings

The client's motor, sensory, and neurologic functions are normal except at the time of a seizure. Identification of seizure activity and type of seizure often depends on a witness's description of the client's actions during the seizure.

A neurologic examination and EEG are performed. Other laboratory or diagnostic studies, such as a CT scan, MRI, serology, and serum electrolyte levels, are used to confirm the diagnosis and to determine the cause of the seizure disorder. When epilepsy is suspected, a series of EEGs is required if the first results are normal.

Medical Management

Once a diagnosis of a seizure disorder is confirmed, one or more anticonvulsant drugs are used to control the seizures (Drug Therapy Table 39.2). IV barbiturates or diazepam (Valium) are administered to terminate status epilepticus.

Drug therapy controls seizures or reduces their frequency or severity. The dose is adjusted over a period of several weeks. The drug is changed or another drug is added to the regimen to obtain optimum control. Blood levels of some anticonvulsant drugs are monitored for accurate dose adjustment and to prevent toxicity (Table 39.1). Serum levels also identify clients who are not taking the drug as ordered.

DRUG THERAPY TABLE 39.2 AGENTS TO CONTROL SEIZURES

DRUG CATEGORY AND EXAMPLES	MECHANISM OF ACTION	SIDE EFFECTS	NURSING CONSIDERATIONS
Anticonvulsants			
phenytoin (Dilantin)	Stabilizes neuronal membranes Limits spread of seizure activity Controls tonic-clonic seizures	Nystagmus, rash, sedation, gingival hyperplasia, liver toxicity, pancytopenia	Evaluate regular serum levels. Evaluate liver function tests, complete blood count and differential. Assess skin daily. Give oral dose with food. Taper dose gradually; never discontinue abruptly. Instruct client to wear MedicAlert bracelet and have regular dental care.
carbamazepine (Tegretol)	Controls partial seizures with complex symptoms, also tonic-clonic seizures	Dizziness, ataxia, nystagmus, rash, nausea, vomiting, liver toxicity, bone marrow suppression	Same as above
ethosuximide (Zarontin)	Reduces frequency of absence (petit mal) seizures	Drowsiness, rash, headache, nausea and vomiting	Same as above
valproic acid (Depakene, Depakote)	Adjunct treatment for multiple seizure types	Nausea and vomiting, drowsiness, diarrhea, liver toxicity	Avoid alcohol intake. Monitor bruising, bleeding gums. See above nursing considerations.
Barbiturates			
phenobarbital (Luminal)	Anticonvulsant activity	Sedation, rash, hyperactivity, ataxia, respiratory depression	Take oral dose at bedtime. Monitor vital signs, especially respiratory rate. Administer IM dose in deep muscle mass. Taper dosage before drug is discontinued. Periodic laboratory tests are required.
Benzodiazepines			
diazepam (Valium)	Skeletal muscle relaxation; adjunct anticonvulsant treatment	Respiratory depression, hypotension, sedation	Monitor BP, pulse, and respiration. Evaluate liver, kidney function, and blood studies. Taper dose before drug is discontinued. Instruct client to wear Medic Alert bracelet.

TABLE 39.1 ANTICONVULSANT DRUG MONITORING

DRUG	THERAPEUTIC LEVEL	TOXIC LEVEL
Carbamazepine	6–12 μg/mL	>15 μg/mL
Ethosuximide	40–100 μg/mL	>150 μg/mL
Phenobarbital	20–40 μg/mL	>35 μg/mL
Phenytoin	1–2.5 μg/mL	>30 μg/mL
Valproic acid	50–100 μg/mL	>200 μg/mL

(From Fischbach, F. [2002]. Nurses' quick reference to common laboratory and diagnostic tests [3rd ed.]. Philadelphia: Lippincott Williams & Wilkins)

Surgical Management

Seizures caused by brain tumor, brain abscess, or other disorders often require surgical intervention. Surgery for epilepsy is not considered unless the client does not respond to drug therapy and seizures are frequent and severe. The area of the brain with abnormal electrical discharges is identified (mapped). The surgeon must consider if removal of the involved area would result in permanent neurologic dysfunction such as paralysis or loss of speech.

Nursing Management

Obtain a complete history, including drug, allergy, and family history. Question the client regarding events or symptoms before and after the seizure. Acquire a description of the client's seizure(s) from an observer. Obtain information about any past head injury, neurologic infection like meningitis, previous treatment for a seizure disorder, and whether the client takes medication as prescribed.

Note the characteristics of seizures if they occur while under your care. If the client's history is inconclusive and the type of seizure is unknown, it is important to provide a full, detailed description of the seizure (Box 39-3).

The newly diagnosed client with seizures needs information about the specific type of disorder, medications needed to control the seizures, and precautions, if any, to take. In addition, teach the client as follows:

- Take anticonvulsant medication as prescribed.
- Recognize adverse effects of the medication.
- Keep routine follow up visits and laboratory appointments for blood level tests.
- Operate a motor vehicle or perform dangerous tasks only when seizures are controlled for at least 6 months.
- Wear a MedicAlert bracelet, tag, or other medical identification.
- Avoid situations known to trigger seizures, such as repetitively flashing or blinking lights, stress, or lack of sleep.

BOX 39-3 ● Seizure Assessment Data

- Onset—sudden or preceded by an aura
- Duration of seizure
- Behavior immediately before and after
- Type of body movements
- Loss of consciousness, for how long
- Incontinence or not
- Seizure awareness afterward

Clients are at risk for injury during a seizure. Clients with atonic or akinetic seizures may need to wear padded headgear if they experience frequent seizures. Hospitalized clients may require padded side rails. If a client experiences seizure, it is important to assist him or her to the floor and move objects away from the client. Loosening clothing from around the neck facilitates breathing. The client should not be forcibly restrained, because it can increase the potential for injuries such as fractures.

BRAIN TUMORS

A brain tumor is a growth of abnormal cells within the cranium. Brain tumors occur in all age groups. Some types are more common in people younger than 20 years of age; others more frequently affect older people. About 50% of all brain tumors are malignant. A brain tumor, whether malignant or benign, can result in death.

Pathophysiology and Etiology

The cause of brain tumors, which occur in various areas of the brain (Fig. 39.11), remains unknown. A small percentage are congenital, such as hemangioblastomas. Genetic factors are associated with two types of brain tumors, *astrocytoma,* a tumor in the frontal lobe, and *neurofibromatosis.* Other causative factors include viral infection, exposure to radiation, head trauma, and immunosuppression. The brain also is the site of metastatic lesions from primary tumors, especially those of the lung and breast.

Tumors that arise from cerebral tissue, such as malignant gliomas and glioblastomas, and angiomas that involve cerebral blood vessels, expand in the confines of the skull and encroach on brain tissue that is vital for life. Extracerebral tumors, such as meningiomas (tumors of the meninges), press on the brain tissue from without.

Assessment Findings

Because tumors take up space and block the flow and absorption of CSF, symptoms associated with IICP occur. The classic triad of headache, vomiting, and papilledema is common. Headache is most common early in the morning. It becomes increasingly severe and occurs more frequently as the tumor grows. Vomiting occurs without nausea or warning. Seizures also develop. Symptoms of disturbed neurologic function, such as speech difficulty, paralysis, and double vision, may occur depending on the tumor's location.

When the ICP is greatly increased, areas of the brain can herniate. If the brain stem is forced through the foramen magnum, the client is in grave danger because vital centers

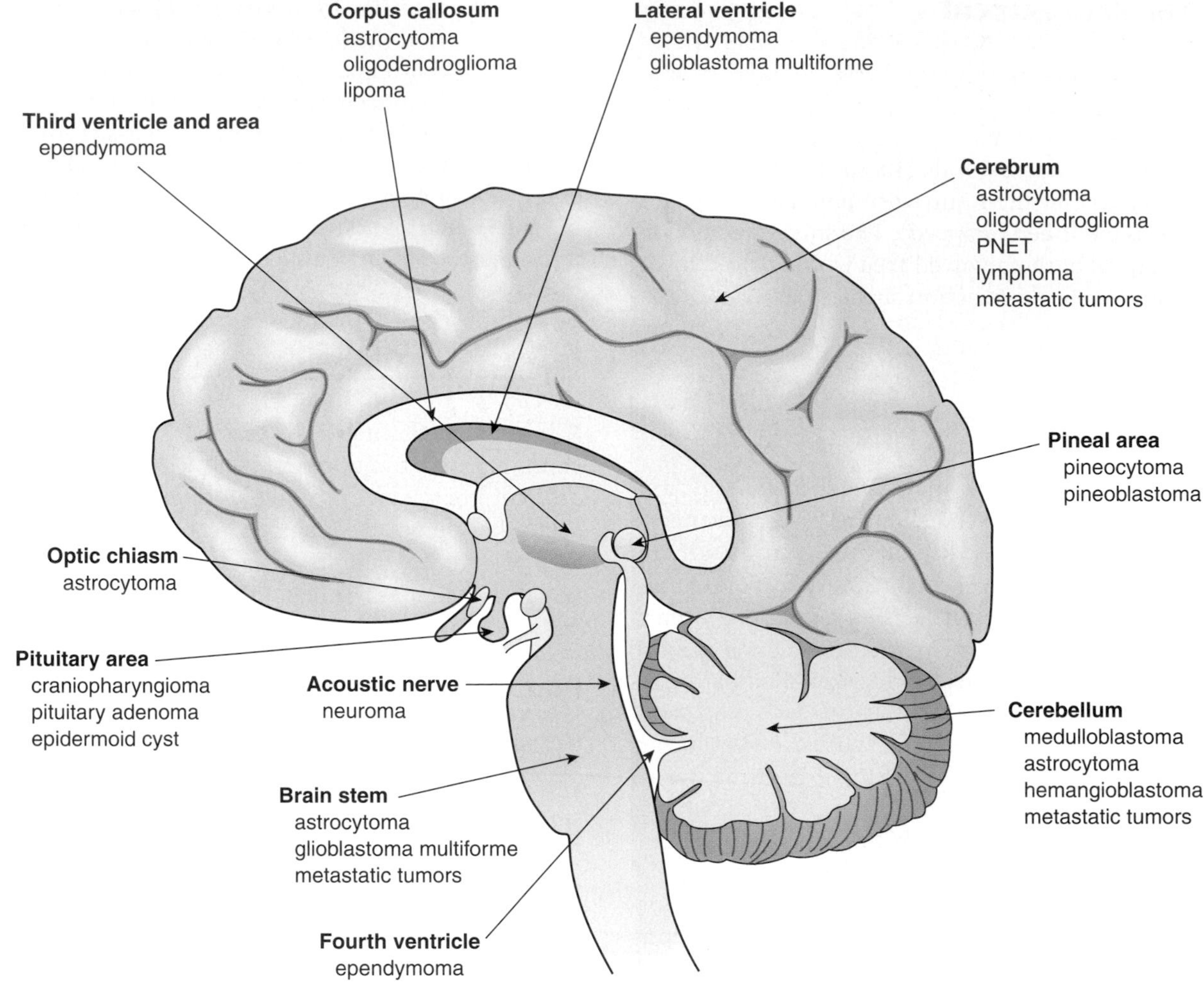

FIGURE 39.11 Common sites for a brain tumor.

that control respiration and heart rate are compressed. Respirations become deeper, labored, and noisy and then slow to only periodic. Unless the condition is relieved, the client dies of respiratory failure and cardiac arrest. Hyperthermia occurs as the temperature-regulating center in the brain is affected. Coma progressively deepens.

Diagnosis is confirmed with CT scan, MRI, brain scan, and cerebral angiography, which reveal the tumor's size and location.

Medical Management

Treatment depends on several factors, including the tumor's location and type (primary or metastatic) and the client's age and physical condition. Brain tumors are treated by surgery, radiation therapy, chemotherapy, or a combination of these methods.

Metastatic tumors and some primary tumors are inoperable, and radiation therapy and chemotherapy are the only treatment choices. Clients who cannot withstand surgery, chemotherapy, or radiation therapy are kept as comfortable and free from pain as possible. Intra-arterial or intrathecal administration of antineoplastic drugs is used to destroy the tumor or slow tumor growth. Symptomatic drug therapy includes corticosteroids and osmotic diuretics to reduce cerebral edema, analgesics, anticonvulsants, and antibiotics.

Complications, such as IICP, paralysis, mental changes, infection, seizures, and prolonged immobility, are treated symptomatically.

Surgical Management

Surgery for an operable brain tumor involves a craniotomy (incision through the skull) or craniectomy (excision of part of the skull). A section of bone (bone flap) is removed to reach the brain (Fig. 39.12). After the tumor is removed, the dura is reapproximated (the cut edges are lined up and sewn together), the bone flap replaced, and the skin sutured. The bone flap is not reinserted when increasing ICP or tumor growth is expected.

The client's postoperative symptoms are determined by the location and function of any damaged or removed brain tissue. Brain tissue does not regenerate.

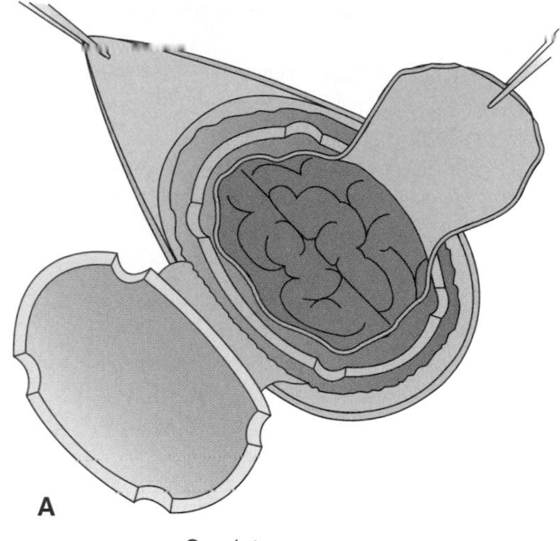

A

Craniotomy

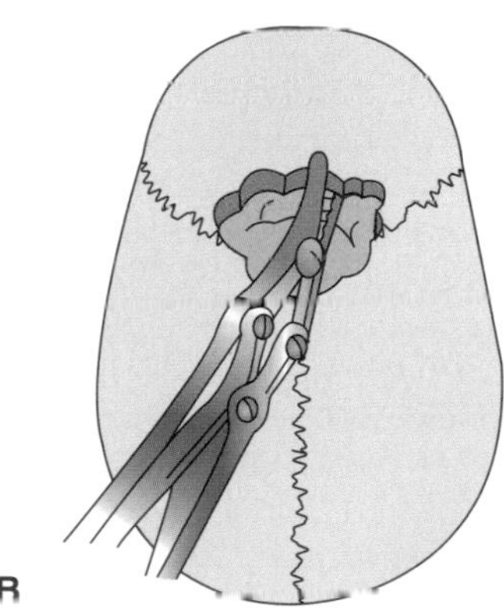

B

Craniectomy

FIGURE 39.12 Neurosurgical techniques. (**A**) Craniotomy, (**B**) craniectomy.

Another method of removing brain tumors uses a laser beam directed at the tumor site. This surgical technique enables the physician to reach tumors that previously were considered inoperable. Radioisotopes also are surgically inserted into the tumor. The cure rate for this procedure, however, is about the same as for external radiation therapy.

Nursing Management

Nursing management depends on the area of the brain affected, tumor type, treatment approach, and the client's signs and symptoms. If the tumor is inoperable or has expanded despite treatment, IICP is a major threat (see Nursing Care Plan 39-1). See Chapter 41 for the care of the client undergoing intracranial surgery. Clients who receive chemotherapy and radiation are supported through the adverse effects associated with antineoplastic drug administration (see Chap. 19). Clarify the client's and family's questions concerning treatment modalities. Direct the client to appropriate professionals to discuss treatment alternatives. Explain hospice care and services to clients with brain tumors that no longer are at a stage where they can be cured.

Before the client is discharged, evaluate the client's and family's immediate and long-term needs. Develop an individualized teaching plan that addresses the medication regimen; appointments for chemotherapy or radiation therapy; adverse effects of chemotherapy or radiation and techniques for managing them; nutritional support; home care considerations; rehabilitation (exercises, physical therapy); and referrals to support services for physical, emotional, and financial assistance.

Help the client express his or her feelings to deal with potential losses. The client needs to have questions answered and clarified and be assured that he or she will not be abandoned and that his or her dignity will be a priority of nursing care. Refer clients in the terminal stage to the local hospice organization.

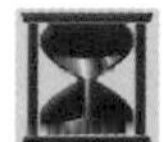

GENERAL GERONTOLOGIC CONSIDERATIONS

Older adults are more susceptible to the complications of prolonged bed rest and immobility. Watch these clients closely for such problems as hypostatic pneumonia, pressure ulcers, contractures, and deformities.

Older adults may not exhibit the typical signs and symptoms of meningitis; rather, they may display a change in mental status, slight to no fever, and no nuchal rigidity or headache.

Mortality rates are high in older adults with meningitis. Contributing factors to death from meningitis are chronic illness and delays in diagnosis (partly because of the atypical signs and symptoms).

Incidence of brain tumor decreases with age. Headache and papilledema are less common symptoms of a brain tumor in the older adult.

Critical Thinking Exercises

1. *When caring for a client with a seizure disorder, what nursing interventions are indicated?*
2. *What information can the nurse provide to a person who recently has been diagnosed with multiple sclerosis?*
3. *What discharge teaching is appropriate when discussing home care with the spouse of a client in the deteriorating stages of Parkinson's disease?*

• NCLEX-STYLE REVIEW QUESTIONS

1. A client diagnosed with Guillain-Barré syndrome is being placed on a medical floor. When selecting the equipment to place in the client's room, the nurse is most correct to include items that facilitate:
   1. Supplemental oxygen
   2. Cardiac monitoring
   3. Nasogastric suction
   4. Intravenous therapy

2. To ensure the safety of a client with Parkinson's disease using a wheeled walker, it is best for the nurse to remind the client to:
    1. Maintain a constant pace of walking.
    2. Keep the walker a full arm's length in front.
    3. Pick up the walker as the client takes steps.
    4. Stand straight with the head up.

connection

Visit the Connection site at **http://connection.lww.com/go/timbyEssentials** for links to chapter-related resources on the Internet.

References and Suggested Readings

Armstrong, T., Hancock, G., & Gilbert, M. (2000). Symptom management of the patient with a brain tumor at the end of life. *Oncology Nursing Forum, 27*(4), 616.

Armstrong, T. S., & Gilbert, M. R. (2000). Metastatic brain tumors: Diagnosis, treatment, and nursing interventions. *Clinical Journal of Oncology Nursing, 4,* 217–225, 231–232.

Backer, J. H. (2000). Stressors, social support, coping, and health dysfunction in individuals with Parkinson's disease. *Journal of Gerontological Nursing, 26*(11), 6–16.

Bensing, K., & Blumenstein, R. (February 4, 2002). Corticosteroids: Management of iatrogenic Cushing's syndrome. *Advance for Nurses,* 18–21.

Buelow, J. M. (2001). Epilepsy management. *Journal of Neuroscience Nursing, 33,* 260–269.

Charles, T., & Swash, M. (2001). Amyotrophic lateral sclerosis: Current understanding. *Journal of Neuroscience Nursing, 33,* 245–253.

Cunning, S. (2000). When the Dx is myasthenia gravis. *RN, 63*(4), 26–31.

Hilton, G. (2000). Cerebral oxygenation in the traumatically brain-injured patient: Are ICP and CPP enough? *Journal of Neuroscience Nursing, 32,* 278–283.

Holland, N. (2000). Multiple sclerosis: New options for care. *Nursing Spectrum (Greater Philadelphia/Tri-State Edition), 9*(18), 15–18.

Lisak, D. (2001). Overview of symptomatic management of multiple sclerosis. *Journal of Neuroscience Nursing, 33,* 224–230.

March, K. (2000). Intracranial pressure monitoring and assessing intracranial compliance in brain injury. *Critical Care Nursing Clinics of North America, 12,* 429–436.

McConnell, E. A. (2001). Clinical do's & don'ts: Preventing transient increases in ICP. *Nursing 2001, 31*(3), 17.

Mosiman, W. (2001). Controlling pain: Taking the sting out of trigeminal neuralgia. *Nursing 2001, 31*(3), 86.

Myers, F. (2000). Meningitis: The fears, the facts. *RN, 63*(11), 52–58.

Parini, S. M. (2001). 8 faces of meningitis: How to tell which type your patient has. *Nursing 2001, 31*(8), 51–53.

Roth, P., & Farls, K. (2000). Pathophysiology of traumatic brain injury. *Critical Care Quarterly, 22*(3), 14–25.

Smeltzer, S. C., & Bare, B. G. (2004). *Brunner & Suddarth's textbook of medical–surgical nursing* (10th ed.). Philadelphia: Lippincott Williams & Wilkins.

Tait, D. (2000). Coping with Bell's palsy. *Nursing Spectrum (Washington, DC/Baltimore Metro Edition), 10*(19), 28.

Wulf, J. A. (2000). Evaluation of seizure observation and documentation. *Journal of Neuroscience Nursing, 32*(1), 27–36.

Yanko, J. R., & Mitcho, K. (2001). Acute management of severe traumatic brain injuries. *Critical Care Nursing Quarterly, 23*(4), 1–23.

chapter 40

Caring for Clients With Cerebrovascular Disorders

Words to Know 

aneurysm
bruit
cephalalgia
cerebral infarction
cerebrovascular accident
collateral circulation
endarterectomy
expressive aphasia
hemianopia
hemiplegia
receptive aphasia
transient ischemic attack

Learning Objectives

On completion of this chapter, the reader will:

- Identify common types of headaches and their characteristics.
- Describe nursing techniques that supplement drug therapy in reducing or relieving headaches.
- Discuss types of cerebrovascular disorders and their usual causes.
- Explain the significance of a transient ischemic attack.
- Discuss medical and surgical techniques used to reduce potential for a cerebrovascular accident.
- Discuss manifestations of a cerebrovascular accident, including those that are unique to right-sided and left-sided infarctions.
- Describe the nursing management of a client with a cerebrovascular accident.
- Describe a cerebral aneurysm and the danger it presents.
- Discuss appropriate nursing interventions when caring for a client with a cerebral aneurysm.

Cerebrovascular disorders are major medical problems that affect adults. Some, such as headaches, can disrupt a client's lifestyle, causing tremendous discomfort and anxiety. Others, such as cerebrovascular accident and transient ischemic attacks, are life-threatening.

HEADACHE

Aching in the head is referred to as **cephalalgia.** It accompanies many disorders such as meningitis, increased intracranial pressure (IICP), brain tumors, and sinusitis. When the duration is relatively brief, a headache is considered transient and benign. Although there are many types of headaches, tension, migraine, and cluster headaches are the most common (Table 40.1). It is possible to experience more than one type of headache.

• TENSION HEADACHE

Tension headache is the most common type of headache, accounting for 90% of all cases.

Pathophysiology and Etiology

Neither the skull nor the brain itself contains sensory nerves. A vast network of sensory and motor nerves, however, are distributed throughout the scalp and facial muscles. During stressful conditions, people tend to contract muscles about the neck, face, and scalp. Those with temporomandibular joint disorder may awaken with a tension headache from clenching the jaw and grinding the teeth during sleep. A tension headache also can develop when a person contracts the neck and facial muscles for prolonged periods, such as looking at a computer screen

TABLE 40.1 FEATURES OF COMMON HEADACHES

FEATURE	CLUSTER HEADACHE	MIGRAINE HEADACHE	TENSION HEADACHE
Client sex	Usually male	Usually female	Equally male/female
Age at onset	20–50 yr	10–40 yr	Any age
Frequency of attacks	1–8/day	1–8/month	Almost daily
Duration of attacks	30 min to 4 hr	4 to 72 hr	Gradual onset, steady
Intensity of pain	Excruciatingly relentless	Moderate to severe	Constant dull ache
Location of pain	Strictly unilateral	Unilateral or bilateral	Bilateral
Nasal congestion	70%	None	None
Droopy, teary eye	Common	Uncommon	Uncommon
Incidence of associated nausea and vomiting	Rare	Common	Rare
Incidence of attacks awakening client from sleep	Common	Rare	Rare
Characteristic behavior	Client cannot remain still during severe attack	Client prefers hibernation	Client prefers hibernation
Family history	7%	90%	Associated with stress
Treatment	Refer to physician	Refer to physician	Refer to physician

or from having limited range of motion from arthritis in the cervical spine. When tensed muscles sensitize *nociceptors,* pain-relaying nerves, in the head, the nociceptors transmit neurochemicals such as prostaglandin and substance P to the brain, which registers the presence and location of discomfort.

Assessment Findings

People who experience tension headaches describe discomfort as pressure or steady constriction on both sides of the head. Symptoms vary from a mild ache to severe, disabling pain. Some correlate onset of the headache with anxiety or emotional conflict. Persistent headache requires tests such as computed tomography (CT) scan, brain scan, head and neck x-rays, and angiography to rule out a brain tumor or intracerebral hemorrhage, cervical spondylitis, or infected sinuses.

Medical Management

Transient tension headaches usually are relieved by rest, a mild analgesic, and stress management techniques like relaxation or imaging (see Chap. 12). Treatment for severe, recurrent tension headaches starts with removing or correcting factors that cause them. If muscle contraction is a reaction to anxiety, counseling and psychotherapy may help clients deal with emotional stressors in healthier ways. Treatment with antidepressants also helps some people who experience tension headaches.

• MIGRAINE HEADACHES

The term *migraine headache* includes several different patterns of headaches that all have a vascular origin. Subcategories include the following:

- *Basilar artery migraine*—dizziness, diplopia, and impaired coordination accompany the headache; it occurs primarily in young women
- *Hemiplegic migraine*—headache and temporary unilateral paralysis occur
- *Ophthalmoplegic migraine*—characterized by head pain, droopy eyelid, double vision, and distortion of visual field
- *Exertional migraine*—brought about by running, lifting, coughing, sneezing, or bending
- *Status migrainosus*—a severe migraine headache and nausea that is sustained for 3 or more days (National Institute of Neurological Disorders and Stroke, 2002)

Migraine headaches are slightly more common in women. Most affected people experience their first episode during childhood to middle age. Often other blood relatives also have migraines. Migraine headaches usually are recurrent and severe. Symptoms usually last for 1 day or more.

Pathophysiology and Etiology

Researchers have targeted a sequence of cofactors for migraine headaches. Changes in particular serotonin receptors promote dilation of cerebral blood vessels and pain intensification from neurochemicals released from the trigeminal nerve. Other possible causes include chemicals in foods that trigger vascular changes, or the headache results from a food-related allergy. Fluctuations in reproductive hormones may also contribute to migraines.

Initially, spasms in arteries in the scalp and neck occur. Platelets that flow through the arteries that supply the brain become trapped in the narrowed passageway. They release serotonin, which alters blood flow. Accessory arteries dilate widely. Subsequently, pain-transmitting neurochemicals are released, which stimulate nociceptors. The outcome is a relentless, excruciating headache.

Assessment Findings

Clients with "classic" migraines experience an *aura,* a sensory phenomenon that precedes the headache by about 10 to 30 minutes. Some have visual disturbances such as flashing lights or wavy lines; some develop weakness or tingling in an extremity; others become confused or have difficulty speaking. For those with the more "common" form of migraine, the prodromal period before the headache is marked by a change in mood, difficulty concentrating, or unusual fatigue. The headache usually starts on one side in the forehead, temple, ear, eye, or jaw, but can involve the entire head before the attack is over. The client describes the pain as "throbbing" or "bursting." Nausea and vomiting, vertigo, sensitivity to light, irritability, and fatigue accompany the headache.

The pattern of headache development and signs and symptoms are typical of migraine headaches. CT scan, angiography, brain scan, and x-rays are used to rule out other disorders.

Medical Management

Rest and drug therapy are mainstays of treatment for migraine headaches. Mild analgesics usually are ineffective. New drugs that affect serotonin levels like methysergide (Sansert) and sumatriptan (Imitrex) are prescribed. Antiemetics also are prescribed if nausea and vomiting become acute during an attack. Some clients learn to shorten or abort migraines with biofeedback techniques (see Chap. 12).

Nursing Management

Reinforce the drug therapy regimen and instruct the client on self-administration of medications. To abort the migraine headache, stress the importance of taking medication as soon as migraine symptoms begin. Encourage the client to lie in bed in a dark room and minimize noise and other stimuli (Client and Family Teaching 40-1).

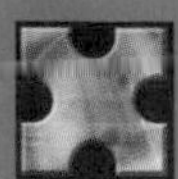

40-1 *Client and Family Teaching*
Migraine Headaches

The nurse includes the following instructions:

- Follow the indications and dosage regimen for medication, and notify the physician of any adverse drug effects.
- Identify and avoid factors that precipitate or intensify an attack.
- Keep a record of the attacks, including activities before the attack, and environmental or emotional circumstances that appear to bring on the attack.
- Lie down in a darkened room, and avoid noise and movement when an attack occurs, if that is possible.

● CLUSTER HEADACHE

The term *cluster* describes episodic headaches in which attacks of head pain last 30 minutes to 2 hours and continually repeat, with brief periods of recovery between attacks. The closely spaced attacks occur over 6 to 8 weeks, with 2 to 10 headaches per day. Each headache quickly escalates in severity, with very little time between the discomfort at onset and the point of maximum pain. Severity tends to diminish when the cycle of episodes begins to terminate. Clients can be headache free from 6 months to 5 years; however, chronic sufferers have attacks much more frequently.

Men and boys experience cluster headaches more commonly than women and girls. In contrast to migraine headaches, family members usually do not have similar headaches.

Pathophysiology and Etiology

The cause of cluster headaches is unknown, but there is a seasonal relationship, suggesting a correlation with physiologic biorhythms. Some suggest that lower-than-normal levels of serotonin may disturb the hypothalamus, which regulates autonomic nervous system activities and biologic responses to circadian rhythms. This theory may explain the mechanism by which serotonin-enhancing drugs help to relieve cluster headaches.

Cluster headaches may be a type of migraine headaches. They can be triggered by vasodilating agents such as nitroglycerin, histamine, and alcoholic beverages. Smoking, which causes vasoconstriction, also is considered a precipitating factor. Tearing and nasal stuffiness accompany cluster headaches, suggesting that acetylcholine, a parasympathetic neurotransmitter, also plays a role in cluster headaches. Thermography (device that measures heat) shows a "cold spot" above the eye, indicating reduced blood flow.

Assessment Findings

A person with a cluster headache has pain on one side of the head, usually behind the eye, accompanied by nasal congestion, *rhinorrhea* (watery discharge from the nose), and tearing and redness of the eye (Fig. 40.1). Pain is so severe that the person cannot lie still; rather, he or she paces or thrashes about. Pain may awaken the person from deep sleep.

Diagnosis is based on history and signs and symptoms that the client discusses and by ruling out other neurovascular causes.

Medical Management

Symptoms are controlled with administration of various drugs such as an ergotamine derivative like dihydroergotamine (Migranal) or methysergide (Sansert). Some respond to corticosteroids, vasoconstricting drugs in the "triptan" group, anticonvulsants, and beta-adrenergic blockers. Inhaled or injected drugs are preferred because they are absorbed more rapidly than those administered orally (Drug Therapy Table 40.1). The client may take a drug daily to prevent development of a headache and take another to abort a headache when it occurs. Oxygen may be used during a headache to reduce the vasodilating compensatory response occurring in the brain. For clients who do not respond to pharmacologic interventions, neurosurgical techniques such as rhizotomy may be the only hope for relief.

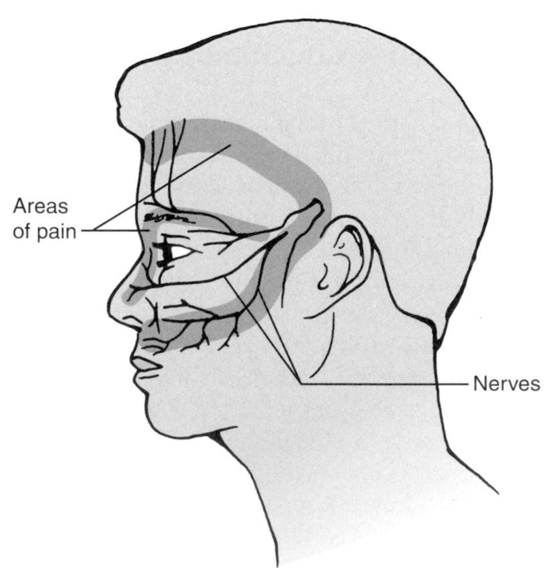

FIGURE 40.1 Affected nerves and areas of pain in cluster headache.

Nursing Management

Ask the client questions about the location, type of pain, and past history of the same type of headache because another disorder or problem may be occurring. Determine if the pain is in one area or over the entire head; factors that appear to bring on, worsen, or relieve the headache; how long the pain lasts; and symptoms such as tearing, nasal congestion, nausea or vomiting, or sensitivity to light.

The client needs instruction about the medication regimen, particularly about daily medications and medications needed to abort the headache. Clients should also record duration and frequency of headaches, any precipitating factors, and any nonpharmacologic relief.

CEREBROVASCULAR DISORDERS

Three million people in the United States each year experience temporary or prolonged deprivation of oxygen to the brain either from a transient ischemic attack (TIA) or cerebrovascular accident (CVA), also known as a *stroke.* A stroke develops in one third of those who experience a TIA. Stroke is the third leading cause of death among U.S. adults.

• TRANSIENT ISCHEMIC ATTACKS

Transient ischemic attacks are sudden, brief attacks of neurologic impairment caused by temporary interruption in cerebral blood flow. Symptoms may disappear within 1 hour or continue for as long as 1 day. When symptoms terminate, the client resumes his or her presymptomatic state. A TIA is a warning that a CVA can occur.

Pathophysiology and Etiology

TIAs result from impaired blood circulation in the brain. Causes include atherosclerosis and arteriosclerosis, cardiac disease, and diabetes (see Chaps. 27, 29, and 52). Circulation is impaired by atherosclerosis (buildup of fatty plaque) in cerebral blood vessels and formation of thrombi and microemboli. The inelastic arterial system affected by arteriosclerosis restricts volume of blood circulating through blood vessels. Dysrhythmias and ineffective heart contraction are catalysts for thrombi that can travel to cerebral vessels. Hypertension associated with some of the previously mentioned etiologies reduces the blood traveling to the brain and increases potential

DRUG THERAPY TABLE 40.1 AGENTS FOR MANAGING HEADACHES

DRUG CATEGORY AND EXAMPLES/ MECHANISM OF ACTION	SIDE EFFECTS	NURSING CONSIDERATIONS
Beta Blockers		
propranolol (Inderal) Prevents vasodilation, drug of choice for prophylaxis	Bradycardia, fatigue, lethargy, depression, GI complaints, orthostatic hypotension	Do not discontinue drug abruptly. Give with food to facilitate absorption. Report difficulty breathing, slow pulse, confusion, depression.
Non-Narcotic Analgesics		
aspirin (Bayer) Analgesic effect early in the attack	Bleeding disorder, GI distress	Monitor for overuse. Give with food to decrease GI upset. Report unusual bleeding.
acetaminophen (Tylenol) Analgesic effect early in the attack	GI, liver, renal effects	Monitor liver and renal function tests. Avoid with use of other over-the-counter preparations.
Nonsteroidal Anti-Inflammatory Drugs (NSAIDs)		
ibuprofen (Advil) *naproxen (Naprosyn)* Analgesic for mild to moderate pain	Headache, dizziness, somnolence, nausea, GI upset, constipation	Better tolerated than ASA. Assess allergy to other NSAIDs. Give with food to reduce GI upset.
Narcotic Analgesics		
codeine For severe headache unrelieved by non-narcotics	Sedation, confusion, constipation	Addictive, use with caution. Report severe nausea, vomiting, palpitations, shortness of breath or difficulty breathing.
meperidine (Demerol) As above	Same as above	Never give to clients taking monoamine oxidase inhibitors. Reassure client that most people who receive opiates for medical reasons do not develop dependency. Avoid alcohol, antihistamines, sedatives, tranquilizers and over-the-counter drugs. Report severe nausea, vomiting, constipation, shortness of breath or difficulty breathing.
butorphanol (Stadol) Relief of severe migraine headache pain (nasal spray)	Sedation, nausea, sweating, vertigo, lethargy, confusion	Very addictive, must be used cautiously. Report severe nausea, vomiting, palpitations, shortness of breath or difficulty breathing, nasal lesions or discomfort.
Ergots		
ergotamine tartrate (Ergostat) Prevents or aborts vascular headaches such as migraine and cluster	Nausea, ergotism: numbness and tingling of fingers and toes, muscle pain and weakness	Administer at first sign of attack. Need to premedicate with antiemetic. Use sparingly to prevent ergotism.
dihydroergotamine (DHE) Rapid control of vascular headaches, parenteral treatment for established headache	Nausea and vomiting, ergotism: numbness, tingling of fingers and toes, muscle pain and weakness	Premedicate with antiemetic. Administer as soon as possible after first sign of attack. Use sparingly to prevent ergotism.
Antiemetics		
promethazine (Phenergan) Controls nausea early in attack	Drowsiness, dizziness, confusion, hypotension, insomnia, vertigo	Give 15–30 min before meperidine or DHE. Avoid alcohol. Avoid sun exposure. Maintain fluid intake. Report sore throat, fever, unusual bleeding, rash, weakness.
prochlorperazine (Compazine) Control of severe nausea and vomiting	Same as above	Same as above.
Other		
sumatriptan (Imitrex) Antimigraine agent for acute attacks	Dizziness, vertigo, weakness, myalgia, blood pressure alterations	Give as soon as possible after first sign of attack. Monitor blood pressure. Report chest pain or pressure, flushing, facial swelling.

GI, gastrointestinal.

for ruptured cerebral vessels from elevated pressure. Smoking and other forms of tobacco use aggravate hypertension. Some medications, such as estrogens used for hormone replacement therapy and oral contraceptives, are thrombogenic. During the ischemic period, motor, sensory, and cognitive functions are temporarily affected.

Assessment Findings

Symptoms of a TIA include temporary light-headedness, confusion, speech disturbances, loss of vision, diplopia, variable changes in consciousness, and numbness, weakness, impaired muscle coordination, or paralysis on one side. Symptoms are short-lived.

A neurologic examination during an attack reveals neurologic deficits. Auscultation of the carotid artery may reveal a **bruit** (abnormal sound caused by blood flowing over the rough surface of one or both carotid arteries). Ultrasound of the carotid artery shows an irregular shape to the artery lining caused by atherosclerotic plaques. A carotid arteriogram shows narrowing of the carotid artery. A CT scan or magnetic resonance imaging (MRI) is used to rule out other neurologic disorders with similar manifestations, such as a brain tumor.

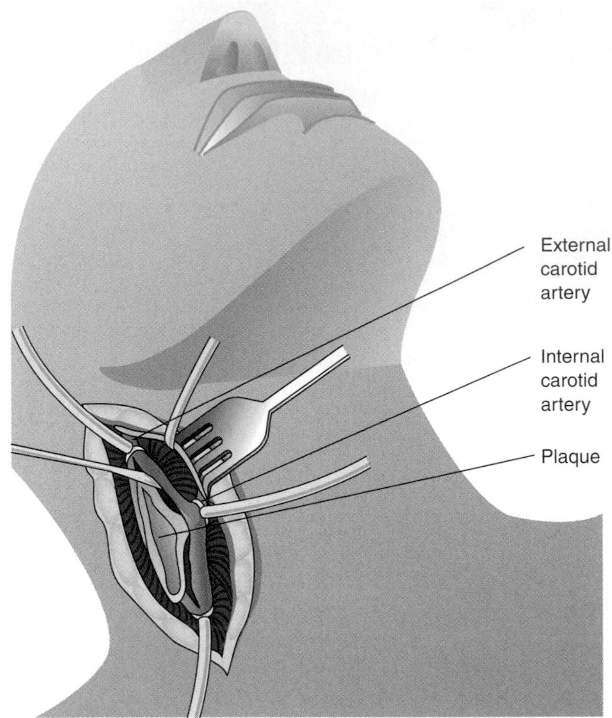

FIGURE 40.2 Plaque is a potential source of emboli in TIAs and CVAs. It is surgically removed from the carotid artery. (From Smeltzer, S. C. & Bare, B. G. [2004]. *Brunner & Suddarth's textbook of medical–surgical nursing* [10th ed.]. Philadelphia: Lippincott Williams & Wilkins.)

Medical and Surgical Management

Antiplatelet and anticoagulant therapy with aspirin, dipyridamole (Persantine), ticlopidine (Ticlid), and warfarin (Coumadin) are prescribed. Hypertension is controlled with drug and diet therapy (see Chap. 29). If narrowing of the carotid artery by atherosclerotic plaques is the cause, a carotid **endarterectomy** (surgical removal of atherosclerotic plaque) is a treatment option (Fig. 40.2). A balloon angioplasty, a procedure similar to a percutaneous transluminal coronary artery angioplasty (see Chap. 27), is performed to dilate the carotid artery and increase blood flow to the brain.

Nursing Management

Obtain a complete history of symptoms and medical, drug, and allergy histories. Weigh the client because obesity, hyperlipidemia, and atherosclerosis are related to cerebrovascular disease. Check the client's capillary blood sugar to help identify hyperglycemia associated with undiagnosed or uncontrolled diabetes mellitus. Measure vital signs and note if blood pressure (BP) is 140/90 mm Hg or greater. Ask the client about smoking habits. Although symptoms of a TIA usually are not permanent, perform a neurologic examination to identify the client's current status and establish a baseline. Document and report even subtle changes.

If the client undergoes carotid artery surgery, perform frequent neurologic checks to detect paralysis, confusion, facial asymmetry, or aphasia. Monitor heart rhythm because dysrhythmias (see Chap. 28) can alter blood flow to the brain as well. It is possible for the neck to swell after surgery, so observe the client closely for difficulty breathing or swallowing and hoarseness. Place an airway at the bedside.

Teach the client to:

- Maintain hydration by drinking the equivalent of eight glasses of fluid a day, unless contraindicated.
- Follow directions for drug therapy, including medications for controlling hypertension and diabetes.
- Monitor for signs of bruising or bleeding if antiplatelet or anticoagulant drugs are prescribed.
- Keep appointments for laboratory tests and medical follow-up to monitor the effectiveness of therapy.
- Report any future instances of sensory or motor impairment, or call 911 for emergency assistance.

● CEREBROVASCULAR ACCIDENT (STROKE)

A **cerebrovascular accident,** or stroke, is a prolonged interruption in flow of blood through one of the arteries supplying the brain (Fig. 40.3). Brain and cerebral nerve

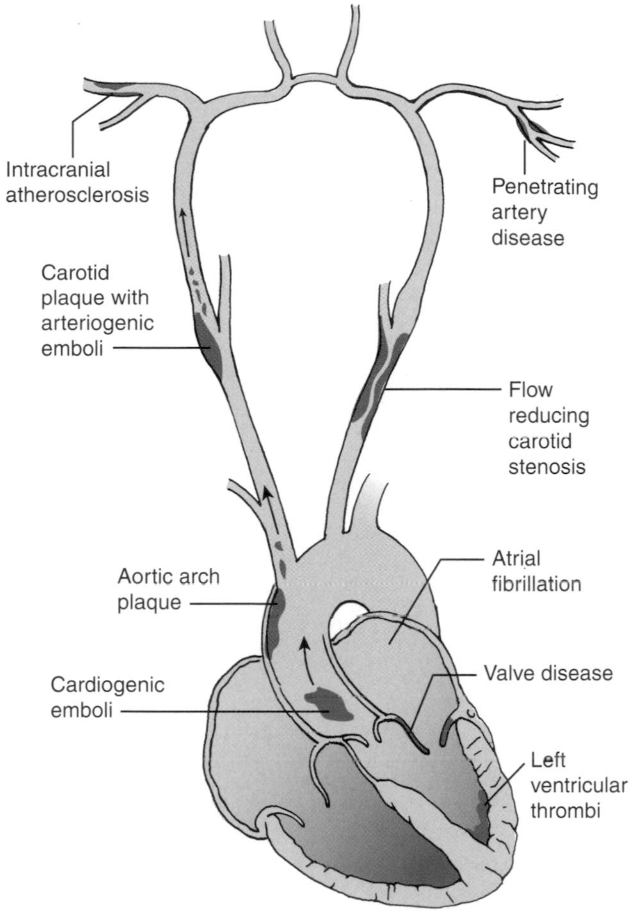

FIGURE 40.3 The most frequent sites of arterial and cardiac abnormalities causing ischemic stroke. (From Albers, G. W., Easton, D., Sacco, R. L., & Teal, P. [1999]. Antithrombotic and thrombotic therapy for ischemic stroke. *Chest, 114* [5], 684S.)

cells are extremely sensitive to lack of oxygen; if the brain is deprived of oxygenated blood for 3 to 7 minutes, both the brain and nerve cells begin to die. Once these cells are destroyed, the outcome is irreversible.

Pathophysiology and Etiology

There are two types of stroke: *ischemic strokes* and *hemorrhagic strokes.* Ischemic strokes occur when a thrombus or embolus obstructs an artery carrying blood to the brain; about 80% of strokes are the ischemic variety. Hemorrhagic strokes occur when a cerebral blood vessel ruptures and blood is released in brain tissue.

Ischemic strokes reduce glucose and oxygen to brain cells. The reduced glucose quickly depletes stores of adenosine triphosphate (ATP), resulting in anaerobic cellular metabolism and accumulation of toxic by-products such as lactic acid. Although some brain cells die from anoxia, lack of oxygen destroys additional brain cells by a secondary mechanism. Oxygen depletion triggers release of glutamate, an excitatory neurotransmitter that activates neuronal receptors known as *N*-methyl-D-aspartate (NMDA) receptors. The receptors allow large amounts of calcium followed by glutamate to enter cells. Once inside brain cells, glutamate literally overexcites them, causing the release of toxic free radicals, which destroy the cells. This secondary assault extends the zone of **cerebral infarction** (death of brain tissue).

When a hemorrhagic stroke occurs, blood leaks from intracerebral arteries. The collection of blood adds volume to intracranial contents, resulting in elevated pressure (see Chap. 39). Hemorrhagic strokes are more common in particular areas of the brain such as the cerebellum, the structure that facilitates balance and coordination, and brain stem, which controls breathing, BP, and heart rate.

Various factors increase the risk for a CVA. Some are controllable and some are uncontrollable (Box 40-1).

Atherosclerosis and arteriosclerosis are major contributors to the formation of thromboemboli and subsequent CVAs. Common causes of cerebral hemorrhage are rupture of cerebral vessels (discussed later in this chapter), hemorrhagic disorders such as leukemia and aplastic anemia, severe hypertension, and brain tumors.

Clinical manifestations are highly variable and depend on the area of the cerebral cortex and the affected hemisphere (Table 40.2), degree of blockage (total, partial), and presence or absence of adequate collateral circulation. **Collateral circulation** is formed by smaller blood vessels branching off from or near larger occluded vessels.

BOX 40-1 ● Risk Factors for Cerebrovascular Accident

UNCONTROLLABLE

Age—Risk of CVA increases with each decade beyond age 55 years.
Sex—Men have a slightly higher risk than women.
Race—African Americans experience more CVAs than do other groups.
Genetics—Those whose blood relatives have had a CVA are at increased risk.

CONTROLLABLE

Hypertension—Forty percent to 90% of clients with CVA have previous hypertension.
Atrial fibrillation—Fifteen percent of those with atrial fibrillation, a dysrhythmia associated with thromboembolic complications, develop a CVA.
Hyperlipidemia—High blood cholesterol and low-density lipoprotein (LDL) levels increase the risk for atherosclerosis and CVA.
Diabetes—Elevated blood glucose level increases triglycerides and accelerates their conversion to LDLs.
History of TIA or CVA—Thirty-five percent of clients who already have had such an episode will have a CVA within 5 years; after one CVA, 42% of men and 24% of women have another.
Smoking—Nicotine is a vasoconstrictor.
Obesity—It contributes to hypertension, hyperlipidemia, and diabetes.
Thrombogenic substances—Stimulants such as herbal products derived from *Ephedra* plants, estrogens, and oral contraceptives increase risk.
Valvular disease or replacement—Thrombi and emboli form and break free from vegetations or valve replacements.

TABLE 40.2 SIGNS AND SYMPTOMS OF RIGHT-SIDED VERSUS LEFT-SIDED HEMIPLEGIA

RIGHT-SIDED HEMIPLEGIA (STROKE ON LEFT SIDE OF BRAIN)	LEFT-SIDED HEMIPLEGIA (STROKE ON RIGHT SIDE OF BRAIN)
Expressive aphasia	Spatial–perceptual defects
Receptive aphasia	Denial; the deficits of the affected side require special safety considerations
Global aphasia	Tendency to distractibility
Intellectual impairment	Impulsive behavior; unaware of deficits
Slow and cautious behavior	Poor judgment
Defects in right visual fields	Defects in left visual fields
Short retention of information	Misjudge distances
Require frequent reminding to complete tasks	Difficulty distinguishing upside-down and right-side-up
Difficulty with new learning	Impairment of short-term memory
Problems with abstract thinking, such as conceptualizing and generalizing	Neglect left side of body; objects and people on left side

Assessment Findings

Signs and Symptoms

In some instances, clients experience one or more TIAs days, weeks, or years before a CVA, or there may be no warning and symptoms develop suddenly. Signs of an impending stroke include numbness or weakness of one side of the face, an arm, or leg; mental confusion; difficulty speaking or understanding; impaired walking or coordination; and severe headache.

Immediately after a large cerebral hemorrhage, the client is unconscious. Breathing is noisy and labored. The cheek on the side of the CVA blows out on exhalation. The eyes deviate toward the affected side of the brain. The pulse is slow, full, and bounding. Initially, BP is elevated. Temperature is elevated during the acute phase and persists for several days. Level of consciousness (LOC) ranges from lethargy and mental confusion to deep coma, which can persist for days or even weeks. The longer the coma, the poorer the prognosis and the less likely that consciousness will return.

A common neurologic result of a CVA in the motor area of the cerebrum is **hemiplegia** (paralysis on one side of the body). Hemiplegia occurs on the side opposite the affected area of the brain because motor nerves cross over at the level of the neck. When the motor area on the right side of the brain incurs a CVA, hemiplegia develops on the left side of the body. There is left-sided hemiplegia when the CVA occurs in the right hemisphere of the brain. Immediately after the CVA, the affected side is flaccid. This progresses to spastic limbs. The arm typically is more severely affected than the leg.

Expressive aphasia, inability to speak, or **receptive aphasia,** inability to understand spoken and written language, can result depending on where the client's speech center is located in the brain. For most, the speech center is in the dominant hemisphere (i.e., if a person is right handed, the speech center is in the left hemisphere). A right-handed person who has a CVA in the left brain usually develops aphasia, and vice versa for a left-handed person.

Clients with a CVA may experience confusion and emotional lability. They also may have **hemianopia** on the affected side, which is blindness for half the field of vision in one or both eyes. This occurs from damage to the visual area of the cerebral cortex or its connections to the brain stem. Any neurological deficit may subside completely, partially, or not at all.

Diagnostic Findings

A CT scan or MRI differentiates a CVA from other disorders, such as a brain tumor or cerebral edema, and shows the size and location of the infarcted area. Transcranial Doppler ultrasonography determines the size of intracranial vessels and the direction of blood flow, and locates the obstructed cerebral vessel. Single-photon emission CT (SPECT) also determines cerebral blood flow. An electroencephalogram reveals reduced electrical activity in the involved area, but is not a specific diagnostic test for a CVA. A lumbar puncture often is performed. If subarachnoid bleeding has occurred, cerebrospinal fluid will be bloody. Cerebral angiography shows displacement or blockage of cerebral vessels.

Medical and Surgical Management

CVAs are prevented by reducing certain risk factors such as hypertension, overweight, cardiac dysrhythmias (especially atrial fibrillation), and high blood cholesterol levels. Prevention measures include prophylactic anticoagulant or antiplatelet therapy (including daily aspirin) in selected people and management of medical disorders, such as diabetes mellitus and cardiovascular disease.

When a CVA occurs, it is a medical emergency. Treatment varies and is directed toward relieving the cause, if known. Tissue plasminogen activator (TPA), a thrombolytic agent, limits neurologic deficits when given within 3 to 6 hours after the onset of the CVA. It is contraindicated in hemorrhagic CVAs, as is anticoagulant therapy. Hypothermia also is used to protect damaged cells by reducing their metabolic need for oxygen.

If atherosclerosis of the carotid artery is the cause, a carotid endarterectomy is considered. A ruptured cerebral aneurysm is treated surgically.

In many cases, treatment is supportive because medical or surgical interventions cannot repair damaged brain tissue. The best treatment available involves an intensive medical program aimed at rehabilitation and the prevention of future CVAs.

Nursing Management

Detailed nursing management for the client with a CVA is discussed in Nursing Care Plan 40-1. Teaching also is essential and focuses on the following points:

- Administer medications as directed and understand the potential side and adverse effects.
- Implement eating and swallowing techniques that reduce the potential for aspiration.
- Perform the Heimlich maneuver to clear the airway if the client cannot speak or breathe after swallowing food.
- Continue follow-up care with the speech pathologist and dietitian.
- Contact community resources such as medical supply companies that rent or sell special care devices such as a hospital bed, bedside commode, walker, or tripod cane.
- Remove throw rugs, clutter, and electrical cords from the client's home environment to reduce the potential for falls.
- Perform regular exercises, change client's position frequently, and apply braces or splints designed to maintain extremities in proper anatomic position.

Stop, Think, and Respond ● BOX 40-1

When a client with an evolving CVA arrives in the emergency department, her speech is difficult to understand, the left side of her face has a drooped appearance, and she cannot move her left arm and leg. Before this client becomes a candidate for TPA, what other information is important to gather?

• CEREBRAL ANEURYSMS

An **aneurysm** is a weakening in the wall of a blood vessel. Most aneurysms occur in arteries, where blood flow is under high pressure. Cerebral aneurysms usually occur in the circle of Willis, a ring of arteries that supply the brain (Fig. 40.4).

Pathophysiology and Etiology

Aneurysms develop at a weakened area in the blood vessel wall. The defect is congenital or secondary to hypertension and atherosclerosis.

An aneurysm can affect cranial nerve function (see Chap. 38) as the aneurysm presses on these structures. For many, there is no prior warning that an aneurysm exists. Berry aneurysms, a type of congenital cerebral aneurysm, can rupture at any time without prior symptoms. Sudden cerebral hemorrhage causes immediate neurologic changes from IICP, interruption of oxygenated blood flow to surrounding cells and tissues, and blood collecting in the subarachnoid space. Occasionally, there is a slow leakage of blood from an aneurysm, and symptoms are less severe.

Assessment Findings

Symptoms include sudden and severe headache, dizziness, nausea, and vomiting, usually followed by a rapid loss of consciousness. If the ruptured aneurysm produces a slow leak, a stiff neck, headache, visual disturbances, and intermittent nausea develop.

Cerebral angiography can reveal an unruptured aneurysm. The procedure is done with caution because added fluid pressure increases risk of rupturing the blood vessel, dislodging plaque-formed emboli, and causing ischemia from vasospasm. A CT scan and MRI are safer for locating the site and determining the amount of blood in the subarachnoid space. A lumbar puncture reveals grossly bloody cerebrospinal fluid when an aneurysm ruptures. The physician may identify the client's status and prognosis based on criteria in the Hunt-Hess classification system (Table 40.3). As the grade increases, the prognosis is less optimistic.

Medical Management

Conservative management is attempted until a decision is made regarding surgical repair of the aneurysm. Some aneurysms are considered inoperable because of anatomic location, and only medical treatment is possible.

Complete bed rest, prevention of rebleeding at the rupture site, and treatment of complications are primary goals. Absolute bed rest in a quiet area, preferably a private room, is essential. Visitors are restricted except for family members. The head of the bed is elevated to reduce ICP and cerebral edema. Hypertension is treated with antihypertensive agents. Anticonvulsants are given to prevent seizures. Tranquilizers or barbiturates are used to keep the conscious client relaxed and quiet. IICP is managed with osmotic diuretics and corticosteroids (see Chap. 39).

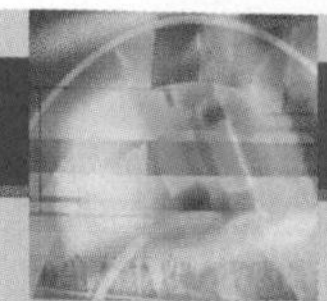

Nursing Care Plan 40-1

THE CLIENT WITH A CEREBROVASCULAR ACCIDENT

Assessment

Determine the following:

- Time symptoms began
- Medical, drug, and allergy history from the family (or client if he or she can report)
- Vital signs and LOC
- Any musculoskeletal weakness or paralysis
- Capacity to speak or understand spoken language
- Changes in visual field
- Ability to swallow
- Any alteration in bladder or bowel control
- Integrity of the skin; evidence of soft tissue injury as a consequence of falling

Nursing Diagnoses: **Impaired Swallowing** related to hemiplegia; **Risk for Aspiration** related to impaired swallowing; **Risk for Deficient Fluid Volume** related to impaired swallowing; **Risk for Imbalanced Nutrition: Less than Body Requirements** related to impaired swallowing

Expected Outcomes: (1) Client will swallow without aspiration. (2) Fluid intake will be at least 2000 mL/24 hours. (3) Client will consume sufficient calories to maintain admission weight.

Interventions	*Rationales*
Elevate client's head for eating or drinking; position client on his or her side at other times.	Sitting and facing food or liquids raises client's awareness and attention; a side-lying position prevents aspiration if vomiting occurs or saliva accumulates in the mouth.
Keep a suction machine at the bedside.	Mechanical suctioning facilitates clearing the airway of saliva, food, and fluids.
Limit distractions (e.g., turn off the television when client eats or drinks).	Increases ability to concentrate and follow nursing instructions.
Use a thickening agent for watery substances; request viscous or pureed food from the dietary department.	The tongue can more easily manipulate thickened liquids against the palate and oral pharynx.
Request small, frequent nourishment from the dietary department rather than three large meals.	Eating small amounts is less tiring, and the client may consume more on a daily basis.
Offer or remind client to load the fork or spoon with a small amount of food.	Small amounts are easier to manage and less likely to cause a complete airway obstruction.
Place thickened liquids or pureed food on the unaffected side of the mouth.	The client can feel and use unaffected side of the mouth for chewing and swallowing.
Lower client's chin to his or her chest when swallowing.	Helps close the laryngopharynx and reduces potential for aspiration.

(continued)

Nursing Care Plan 40-1 (Continued)

THE CLIENT WITH A CEREBROVASCULAR ACCIDENT

Interventions	*Rationales*
Encourage client to swallow several times.	May be necessary to move food to the esophagus.
Check mouth for pocketed food before offering more.	Client may be unaware of food that remains unswallowed.
Instruct client to use the tongue to relocate pocketed food or apply gentle pressure on the cheek to reposition food.	Helps reposition trapped food.

Evaluation of Expected Outcomes: Airway remains patent, and lungs are clear to auscultation.

Nursing Diagnoses: **Total Urinary Incontinence; Bowel Incontinence** or **Risk for Constipation** related to diminished LOC, confusion, and immobility

Expected Outcome: Urinary and bowel elimination will be controlled independently or with minimal assistance.

Interventions	*Rationales*
Maintain a record of bowel elimination.	Data indicates if client requires a stool softener, laxative, suppository, or enema.
Place an elevated seat over the toilet.	Reduces the work of transferring to the toilet seat and back to a wheelchair.
Assist client to the toilet every 2 hours while he or she is awake and after each meal.	Positioning and environmental cues may help stimulate the client to eliminate. The gastrocolic reflex that promotes bowel evacuation is stronger soon after eating.
Dress client in unrestricted clothing that facilitates elimination needs.	Reduces the potential for incontinence.
Avoid negative comments if incontinence occurs; acknowledge client's success when he or she eliminates while on the toilet or commode.	Criticism lowers self-confidence and self-esteem; praise encourages client to continue efforts at controlling elimination.
Apply incontinence garments or place absorbent pads beneath client.	Preserves client's dignity.
Administer prescribed suppository or low-volume enema when necessary.	Increases intestinal contraction, which helps to evacuate the bowel.

Evaluation of Expected Outcome: Bowel and urinary elimination are managed at the highest level the client can achieve.

Nursing Diagnoses: **Self-Care Deficit** related to hemiplegia; **Unilateral Neglect** related to hemianopia; **Impaired Mobility: Physical** related to hemiplegia

Expected Outcomes: (1) Client will resume independent activities of daily living (ADLs). (2) Client will identify and care for paralyzed body parts. (3) Client will use assistive devices to achieve mobility.

(continued)

Nursing Care Plan 40-1 (Continued)

THE CLIENT WITH A CEREBROVASCULAR ACCIDENT

Interventions	*Rationales*
Approach and place objects within client's field of vision.	Client is likely to ignore objects and people that are located in areas where visual field is impaired.
Help reintegrate weak side by reminding client to look at it.	Calling attention to the neglected side of the body helps the client recognize and accept that it exists.
Set realistic goals for self-care.	Unrealistic goals lead to frustration and discouragement.
Consult with an occupational therapist (OT) or physical therapist (PT) regarding modifications in clothing, utensils, and assistive devices.	Therapists have expertise in measures to accommodate for neurologic deficits.
Attach a trapeze above the bed.	Client can use a trapeze with one hand to independently facilitate position changes.
Perform range-of-motion (ROM) exercises at least once each shift.	ROM exercises maintain joint mobility and muscle tone.
Support affected arm in a sling when the client is upright.	An arm sling improves posture and reduces musculoskeletal changes in the shoulder joint.
Position client to avoid contractures (e.g., use a foot board, trochanter roll at the hip, rolled cloth in the paralyzed hand).	Skeletal muscles can become permanently shortened without efforts to maintain normal anatomic position.
Consult the PT about devices to assist ambulation, such as a leg brace and walker.	A brace promotes stability when standing and walking. A walker supports the client and facilitates ambulation.

Evaluation of Expected Outcomes: Client performs ADLs alone or with assistance and learns to use assistive devices.

Nursing Diagnosis: **Impaired Verbal Communication** related to expressive aphasia

Expected Outcome: Client will make needs understood either verbally or nonverbally.

Interventions	*Rationales*
Ask questions requiring a "yes" or "no," and suggest the client respond by nodding the head.	Nodding the head is a form of body language that communicates agreement or disagreement.
Instruct client to speak slowly when attempting to communicate orally.	If unpressured to quickly respond, the client may be able to formulate words and sentences more easily.
Have client point to or write key words or phrases.	Some clients retain ability to read written language although they may not be able to express themselves orally.

Evaluation of Expected Outcome: Client can communicate either orally, in writing, or with techniques that facilitate nonverbal communication.

Mechanical ventilation is necessary to support respirations and provide oxygenation if the client is unconscious. Aminocaproic acid (Amicar) is used to delay lysis (breaking up) of the blood clot because lysis results in rebleeding.

Surgical Management

Surgical repair is attempted after the initial hemorrhage because the danger of further hemorrhage from the weakened aneurysm is great. The operation is not without hazard; manipulation of the small cerebral vessels can result in increased vasospasm or thrombosis and cerebral infarction. The risks of surgery are less serious than dangers of recurrent hemorrhage from the aneurysm. Surgical approaches with a craniotomy include wrapping or clipping the aneurysm in an attempt to control further bleeding (Fig. 40.5).

An alternative to direct repair of the aneurysm by a craniotomy approach is ligation of or application of a clamp

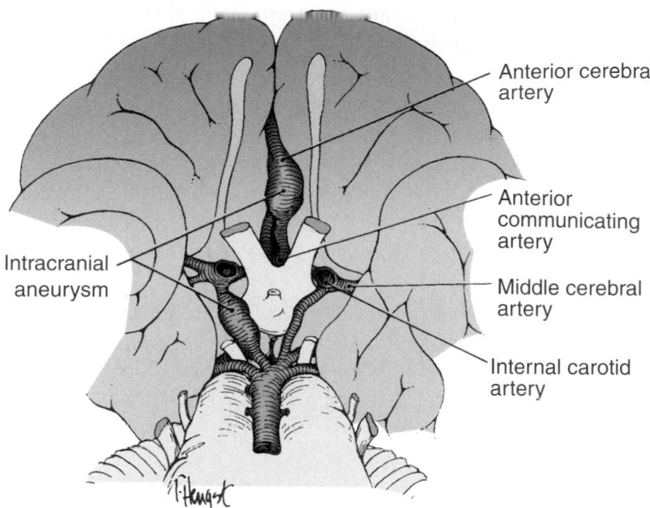

FIGURE 40.4 Intracranial aneurysm within circle of Willis.

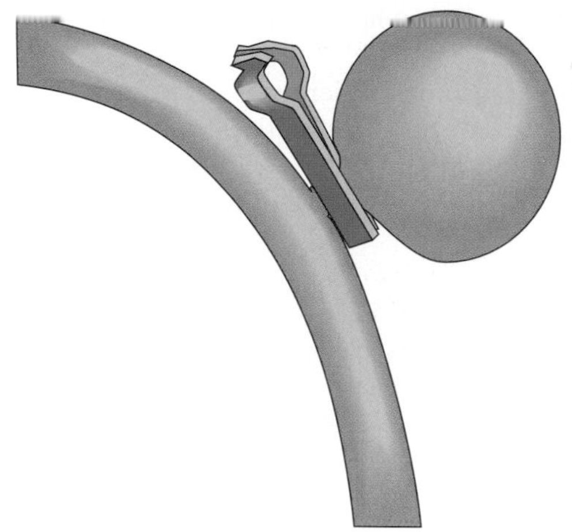

FIGURE 40.5 An aneurysm is clamped to prevent rupture. Wrapping the aneurysm with supportive material is another alternative.

to one of the carotid arteries. This is an extracranial (outside the cranium) procedure because the surgical approach is below the jaw. The purpose of this approach is to obstruct blood flow to the vessel that has an aneurysm, thus reducing the pressure in the aneurysm and preventing rupture or further bleeding. Collateral circulation in the cerebral vessels must be adequate for success.

NURSING PROCESS

● The Client With an Aneurysm

Assessment

Perform a neurologic examination. Measure vital signs frequently. If the client is conscious, ask only essential questions while gathering the client's history, limiting it primarily to the current onset of symptoms. Obtain a more complete history from the family.

TABLE 40.3 THE HUNT-HESS SCALE FOR GRADING A CLIENT WITH A CEREBRAL ANEURYSM

CLASSIFICATION	CLINICAL CRITERIA
Grade I	Alert, oriented, asymptomatic
Grade II	Alert, oriented, headache, stiff neck
Grade III	Lethargic or confused, minor focal deficits such as hemiparesis (weakness on one side)
Grade IV	Stupor, moderate to severe focal deficits such as hemiplegia
Grade V	Comatose, severe neurologic deficits such as posturing (see Chap. 38)

(Adapted from Hickey, J. V. [2002]. *The clinical practice of neurological and neurosurgical nursing* [5th ed.]. Philadelphia: Lippincott Williams & Wilkins.)

Diagnosis, Planning, and Interventions

PC: Increased Intracranial Pressure related to bleeding in the brain

Expected Outcome: The nurse will monitor for, manage, and minimize IICP.

- Use the Glasgow Coma Scale (GCS) to assess neurologic status at least every hour (see Chap. 38). *Provides a systematic assessment tool for documenting neurologic function and identifying early clinical changes.*
- Report neurologic changes as soon as a trend indicates worsening of the client's condition. *Facilitates implementing medically prescribed interventions that will reduce or eliminate more serious complications.*
- Keep client calm and physically still. *Activity or emotional distress elevates BP and ICP, which can contribute to more bleeding.*
- Avoid activities that cause a Valsalva maneuver such as coughing, straining at stool, and rough position changes. *Bearing down raises BP and increases potential for rupture of the aneurysm or increased bleeding if the aneurysm has already ruptured.*
- Follow physician's orders for fluid restrictions and drug therapy for reducing hypertension, potential seizures, restlessness, and anxiety. *Helps to reduce ICP.*
- Elevate client's head or follow physician's order for body position (some prefer that the client remain flat). *Head elevation helps venous blood and cerebrospinal fluid drain from cerebral areas and reduces volume in the cranium.*
- Limit visitors to immediate family; suggest they take turns and stay briefly. *Although visitors' and family members' desire to interact with the client are well intentioned, stimulation can increase ICP or trigger a seizure.*

Self-Care Deficit related to imposed rest and decreased LOC

Expected Outcome: Client's basic needs will be met.

- Perform only those activities of daily living for the client that are absolutely necessary. *Reduces risk for life-threatening complications.*
- Provide rest between necessary nursing tasks. *Prevents overstimulation of the client.*
- Feed client calorie-dense foods in small amounts at frequent intervals. *Client's hunger is managed without requiring a large intake of food at any one time.*

Risk for Ineffective Peripheral Tissue Perfusion and **Risk for Impaired Skin Integrity** related to imposed inactivity

Expected Outcomes: (1) Peripheral circulation will be maintained. (2) Skin will remain intact.

- Apply elastic stockings to lower extremities or use a pneumatic compression device. *Intermittent compression passively moves venous blood toward the heart in a way similar to active skeletal muscle contraction. Elastic stockings support the valves of veins in the lower extremities to prevent venous stasis.*
- Use pressure-relieving pads or a similar type of mattress. *Relieving pressure promotes circulation of oxygenated blood through the capillary to peripheral cells and tissues and facilitates venous blood return.*

Evaluation of Expected Outcomes

ICP is maintained within a safe range. Essential needs for nutrition, hydration, ventilation, and elimination are met. Peripheral circulation is adequate; there are no signs of skin breakdown. For the client who undergoes a craniotomy, refer to Chapter 39.

Discharge teaching depends on the method of treatment and recommendations of the physician. Usually, the nurse instructs clients to avoid heavy lifting, straining at stool, extreme emotional situations, and other work-related activities that could raise BP and increase ICP.

When the client must restrict his or her lifestyle, the changes are likely to cause financial, physical, and social hardships for the client and family. Referrals to a social service worker, counselor, or social service agency are appropriate.

GENERAL GERONTOLOGIC CONSIDERATIONS

Older adults who experience TIAs may ignore the symptoms, thinking that they are part of the normal aging process, because symptoms usually subside shortly.

One major risk factor for stroke is hypertension. At times, the older adult with hypertension may become noncompliant with his or her medication regimen, thus increasing the risk of CVA. Client education is important to foster compliance.

The rehabilitation of the elderly client with a CVA is difficult and subject to more complications than with a younger adult. The family may be unable to provide the care needed in the home setting, and the client may need to go to a rehabilitation center or a nursing home for rehabilitation.

The older adult client is more susceptible to the complications of prolonged bed rest and inactivity. Because the rehabilitation period after a CVA often is prolonged, closely observe the elderly client for problems such as hypostatic pneumonia, pressure ulcers, and contractures.

Older clients with moderate to severe neurologic deficits may place a financial and physical burden on their spouse or children. The nurse must work closely with the family and social service agencies to help the family assume the care of their family member to the extent possible.

Critical Thinking Exercises

1. *What suggestions could you give to someone who has migraine headaches to help reduce their severity?*
2. *When assigned to care for a client with a leaking cerebral aneurysm, what nursing interventions are appropriate for reducing the potential for a serious intracranial bleed?*

● NCLEX-STYLE REVIEW QUESTIONS 

1. A woman arrives at the headache center for an initial evaluation. The client describes flashing lights before the headache begins. The nurse is most correct in documenting the presence of:
    1. A premonition of a migraine headache
    2. An aura prior to a migraine headache
    3. A pupillary response creating the headache
    4. Intense photophobia prior to the headache onset
2. When providing a dietary tray to a client with right hemianopia, it is best for the nurse to:
    1. Place the tray most convenient for staff as the client will need to be assisted.
    2. Place the tray on the right side of the client so that she can feed herself.
    3. Place the tray on the left side of the client so that she can feed herself.
    4. Place the tray directly in front of the client so that she can feed herself.
3. What nursing intervention is most appropriate to decrease the frustration experienced by a client with expressive aphasia?
    1. Use a picture or alphabet board with frequently needed topics.
    2. Ask the client to shake head yes or no to different options.
    3. Offer emotional support by telling the client you know how frustrating this must be.
    4. Arrange for family to be present when attempting to communicate with the client.

connection

Visit the Connection site at **http://connection.lww.com/go/timbyEssentials** for links to chapter-related resources on the Internet.

References and Suggested Readings

Bacoka, J. (2000). Action stat: Aortic dissection—act fast to intervene and prevent stroke, renal failure, or death. *Nursing 2000, 30*(8), 33.

Bostwick, J., & Sneade, M. (2001). Subarachnoid haemorrhage, managing complications. *Nursing Times, 97*(35), 28–29.

Gendreau-Webb, R. (2001). Action stat: Acute ischemic stroke. *Nursing 2001, 31*(9), 120.

Hock, N. H. (1999). Brain attack: The stroke continuum. *Nursing Clinics of North America, 34,* 689–725.

Kunkel, R. S. (2000). Managing primary headache syndromes. *Patient Care, 34*(2), 100–103, 107–110, 115–117+.

Linsey, J. (2000). Implementing a stroke risk assessment program in a community setting. *Journal of Neuroscience Nursing, 32,* 266–271.

Mathers, D. (2001). Kernig's sign . . . Protecting a patient with ruptured cerebral aneurysm. *Nursing 2001, 31*(8), 8.

McGuire, L. (2002). How to treat a migraine. *Nursing 2002, 32*(12), 76.

Mower-Wade, D., Cavanaugh, M. C., & Bush, D. (2001). Protecting a patient with ruptured cerebral aneurysm. *Nursing 2001, 31*(2), 52–58.

National Institute of Neurological Disorders and Stroke. (2002). Headache—hope through research. [On-line.] Available: http://www.ninds.nih.gov/health_and_medical/disorders/headache.htm.

Pfohman, M., & Criddle, L. M. (2001). Epidemiology of intracranial aneurysm and subarachnoid hemorrhage. *Journal of Neuroscience Nursing, 33,* 39–41.

Pope, W., & Morrison, S. R. (2001). Coiled for success: The endovascular treatment of cerebral aneurysms. *Nursing Spectrum (Greater Philadelphia/Tri-State Edition), 10*(6), 26–27.

Pope, W. L. (2002). Cerebral vessel repair with coils and glue . . . Gentler on the mind. *Nursing 2002, 32*(7), 46–49.

Schretzman, D. (2001). Acute ischemic stroke. *Dimensions of Critical Care Nursing, 20*(2), 14–22.

Scott, A. (April 15, 2002). Staving off stroke. *Advance for Nurses,* 24–26.

Vance, D. L. (2001). Treating acute ischemic stroke with intravenous Alteplase. *Critical Care Nurse, 21*(4), 25–35.

Weiss, J. (2001). Assessing and managing the patient with headaches. *Dimensions of Critical Care Nursing, 20*(3), 15–23.

Westergren, A., Karlsson, S., Andersson, P., et al. (2001). Eating difficulties, need for assisted eating, nutritional status and pressure ulcers in patients admitted for stroke rehabilitation. *Journal of Clinical Nursing, 10,* 257–269.

Westergren, A., Ohlsson, O., & Hallberg, I. R. (2001). Eating difficulties, complications and nursing interventions during the first three months after a stroke. *Journal of Advanced Nursing, 35,* 416–426.

Williams, M. P. (2002). How to assess swallowing after a stroke. *Nursing 2002, 32*(8), 32hn5–6.

Willoughby, D. F., Saunders, L., & Privette, A. (2001). The impact of a stroke screening program. *Public Health Nursing, 18,* 418–423.

chapter 41

Caring for Clients With Head and Spinal Cord Trauma

Words to Know 

autonomic dysreflexia
autoregulation
Battle's sign
cerebral hematoma
chemonucleolysis
closed head injury
concussion
contrecoup injury
contusion
coup injury
craniectomy
cranioplasty
craniotomy
diskectomy
epidural hematoma
extramedullary
halo sign
intracerebral hematoma
intramedullary
laminectomy
open head injury
otorrhea
paraplegia
paresthesia
periorbital ecchymosis
poikilothermia
rhinorrhea
spinal fusion
spinal shock
subdural hematoma
tetraplegia
uncal herniation

Learning Objectives

On completion of this chapter, the reader will:

- Differentiate a concussion from a contusion.
- Explain the differences between epidural, subdural, and intracerebral hematomas.
- Discuss the nursing management of a client with a head injury.
- Discuss the nursing management of a client undergoing intracranial surgery.
- Explain spinal shock, listing four symptoms.
- Discuss autonomic dysreflexia and at least five manifestations.
- Describe the nursing management of a client with a spinal cord injury.

Head and spinal cord trauma can result in permanent disability and dysfunction. This chapter discusses head injuries, including lacerations, skull fractures, internal bleeding, and edema of the brain and surrounding tissues. It also discusses spinal disorders caused by trauma and mechanical injury.

HEAD INJURIES

Injury to the head can cause concussions, contusions, hematomas, or skull fracture.

CONCUSSION AND CONTUSION

Pathophysiology and Etiology

A **concussion** results from a blow to the head that jars the brain. It usually is a consequence of falling, striking the head against a hard surface like a windshield, colliding with another person (e.g., between athletes), battering during boxing, or being a victim of violence. A concussion results in diffuse and microscopic injury to the brain. The force of the blow causes temporary neurologic impairment but no serious damage to cerebral tissue. Recovery is complete and usually within a short time. In older adults, however, recovery may take longer.

A **contusion** is more serious than a concussion and leads to gross structural injury to the brain. Contusions result in bruising and sometimes hemorrhage of superficial cerebral tissue. When the head is struck directly, the injury to the brain is called a **coup injury.** Dual bruising can result if the force is strong enough to send the brain ricocheting to the opposite side of the skull, which is called a **contrecoup injury** (Fig. 41.1). Edema develops at the site of or in areas opposite to the injury. A skull fracture can accompany a contusion.

Assessment Findings

With a concussion, the client may experience a brief lapse of consciousness, with temporary disorientation, headache, blurred or double vision, emotional irritability, and dizziness commonly following.

Signs and symptoms of a contusion vary depending on severity of the blow and degree of head velocity. Clients exhibit hypotension, rapid and weak pulse, shallow respirations, loss of consciousness, and pale, clammy skin. While unconscious, they usually respond to strong stimuli, such as pressure applied to base of the nail. On awakening, clients often have temporary *amnesia* (loss of memory) for recent events. Permanent brain damage can impair intellect and gait and cause speech difficulty, seizures, and paralysis.

Skull x-ray is performed to rule out or confirm skull fracture. CT or MRI scans detect bleeding or small hemorrhages in brain tissue, a shift in brain tissue, and edema at the injury site.

Medical Management

For a concussion, the client's activity is temporarily halted until the seriousness of the injury is determined. Mild analgesia (usually acetaminophen) relieves the headache. The client is observed for neurologic complications. For an unstable client with a contusion, the client's vital functions are supported with drug therapy and mechanical ventilation if necessary.

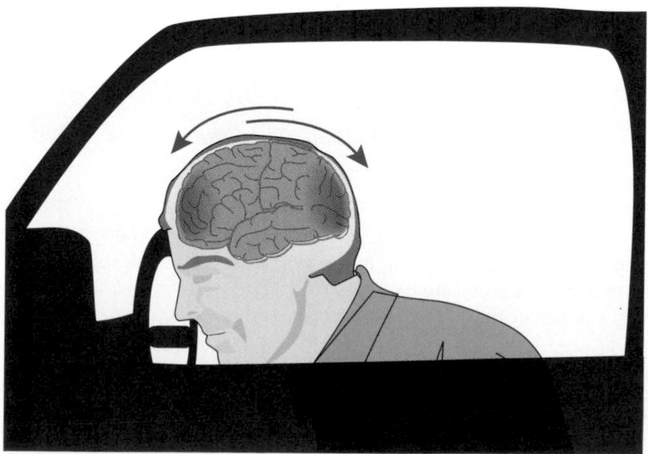

FIGURE 41.1 Coup and contrecoup injuries occur at the point of contact and when the brain rebounds from the opposite direction.

Nursing Management

Perform a neurologic assessment (see Chap. 38). If findings are normal and the client does not require hospitalization, instruct the family to watch the client closely for signs of increased intracranial pressure (IICP), including behavioral alterations, sleepiness, personality changes, vomiting, and speech or gait disturbances (see Chap. 39). Instruct the client and family to contact a physician or return to the emergency department (ED) if any of these symptoms occur. If the client is hospitalized, observe the client closely for changes in level of consciousness (LOC), signs of IICP, neurologic changes, respiratory distress, and changes in vital signs every 1 to 2 hours. If symptoms develop, report them to the physician.

Prevention of health problems is a major component of nursing care. To reduce potential for both minor and life-threatening head injuries, stress:

- Using seat belts for all passengers in automobiles
- Restraining infants in approved car seats located in the rear seats of automobiles
- Wearing protective head gear while riding bicycles or motorcycles and participating in contact sports like hockey, baseball, or softball
- Raising neck restraints on the backs of car seats
- Not driving under the influence of alcohol or drugs

● CEREBRAL HEMATOMAS

A **cerebral hematoma** is bleeding within the skull, which forms an expanding lesion. People at high risk for cerebral hematomas are those receiving anticoagulant therapy or those with an underlying bleeding disorder, such as hemophilia, thrombocytopenia, leukemia, and aplastic anemia (see Chap. 33).

Pathophysiology and Etiology

Most hematomas result from head trauma or cerebral vascular disorders. The types are epidural hematoma, subdural hematoma, and intracerebral hematoma (Fig. 41.2).

An **epidural hematoma** stems from arterial bleeding, usually from the middle meningeal artery, and blood accumulation above the dura. It is characterized by rapidly progressive neurologic deterioration. A **subdural hematoma** results from venous bleeding, with blood gradually accumulating in the space below the dura. Subdural hematomas

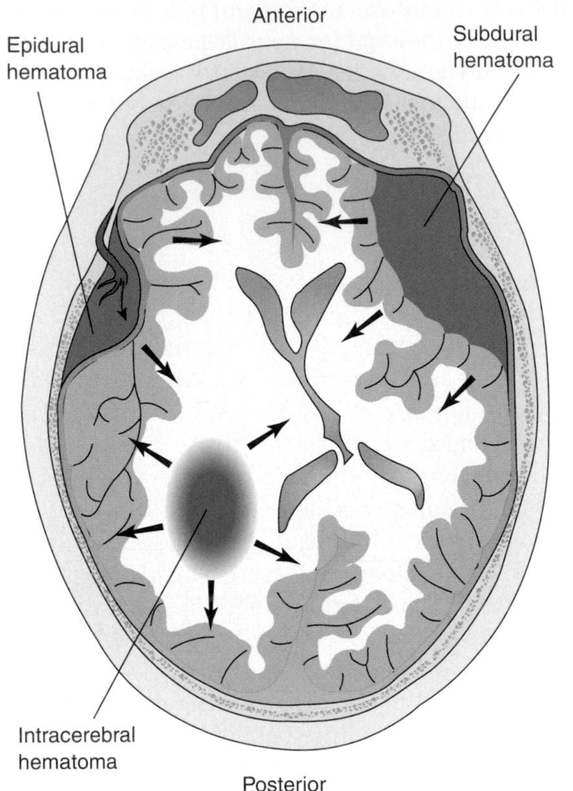

FIGURE 41.2 Location of epidural, subdural, and intracerebral hematomas.

are classified as acute, subacute, and chronic according to the rate of neurologic changes. Symptoms progressively worsen in a client with an acute subdural hematoma within the first 24 hours of the head injury. Clients with subacute and chronic subdural hematomas become symptomatic after 24 hours and up to 1 week later. An **intracerebral hematoma** is bleeding within the brain that results from an open or closed head injury or from a cerebrovascular condition such as a ruptured cerebral aneurysm (see Chap. 40).

Bleeding increases the volume of brain contents and intracranial pressure (ICP), disrupting blood flow and causing the brain to become ischemic and hypoxic. Unrelieved IICP also causes the brain to shift to the lateral side (**uncal herniation**) or herniate downward through the foramen magnum, affecting vital centers for respiration, heart rate, cranial nerve functions, and blood pressure. Death occurs if symptoms are not recognized and bleeding is not stopped.

Assessment Findings

The rapidity and severity of neurologic changes (Table 41.1) depend on the location, rate of bleeding and size of the hematoma, and effectiveness of **autoregulation,** the brain's ability to provide sufficient arterial blood flow despite rising ICP. MRI and CT scans show densities that indicate the location of the hematoma and shifts in cerebral tissue. ICP monitoring (see Chap. 39) provides direct and continuous data for evaluating the extent to which the lesion is expanding or responding to treatment.

Medical Management

The body may wall off and absorb a subdural hematoma with no treatment. Rapid change in LOC and signs of uncontrolled IICP indicate a surgical emergency.

Surgical Management

Surgery consists of drilling holes (*burr holes*) in the skull to relieve pressure, removing the clot, and stopping the bleeding (Fig. 41.3). If the source of bleeding is not located by means of burr holes, more invasive surgery is performed. Epidural hematomas require more prompt intervention because the rate of bleeding is greater from an arterial bleed than from a venous bleed.

Intracranial surgery consists of three possible procedures. A **craniotomy** is a surgical opening of the skull to

TABLE 41.1 DIFFERENCES IN CEREBRAL HEMATOMAS

TYPE	LOCATION	SIGNS AND SYMPTOMS
Epidural	Arterial blood collects between the skull and dura.	Client may be alert after initial unconsciousness, but then becomes increasingly lethargic before lapsing into coma. Common symptoms are headache, ipsilateral (same side as injury) pupil changes, and contralateral (opposite side to injury) hemiparesis (weakness or paralysis).
Subdural	Venous blood collects between the dura and subarachnoid layers.	Deterioration in LOC is progressive. There are ipsilateral pupil changes, decreased extraocular muscle movement, and contralateral hemiparesis, with periodic episodes of memory lapse, confusion, drowsiness, and personality changes.
Intracerebral	Blood collects within the brain.	Client shows classic signs of IICP: headache, vomiting, seizures, posturing, hyperthermia, irregular breathing.

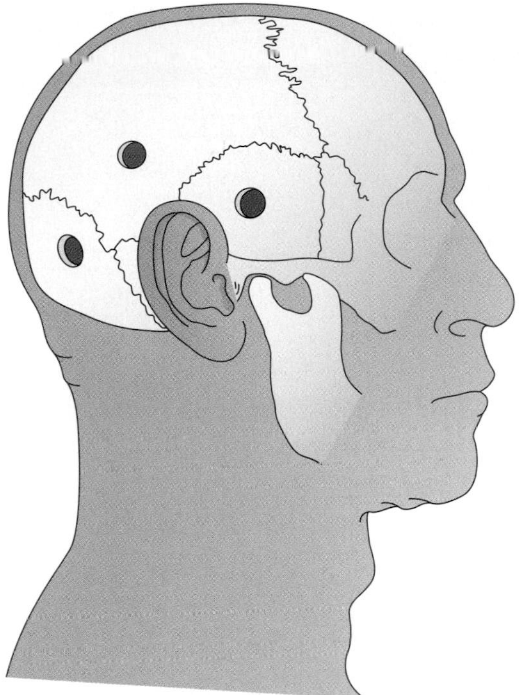

FIGURE 41.3 Neurosurgical procedures may require the use of burr holes to make a bone flap in the skull, aspirate a brain abscess, or evacuate a hematoma. (From Smeltzer, S. C. & Bare, B. G. [2004]. *Brunner & Suddarth's textbook of medical–surgical nursing* [10th ed.]. Philadelphia: Lippincott Williams & Wilkins.)

gain access to structures beneath the cranial bones. It is done to remove a blood clot or tumor, stop intracranial bleeding, or repair damaged brain tissues or blood vessels. A **craniectomy** is removal of a portion of a cranial bone. **Cranioplasty** is the repair of a defect in a cranial bone (see Chap. 39). A metal or plastic plate or wire mesh is used to replace the removed bone or to reinforce a defect in a cranial bone.

In cranial surgery, several burr holes are first made in the skull. A saw cuts a section of bone (bone flap), which is removed to provide a visual field. After surgery is completed, the bone flap usually is replaced. In some instances, such as with an inoperable tumor, the bone flap is not replaced, allowing the tumor to expand and preventing IICP. Complications associated with intracranial surgery include cerebral edema, infection, neurogenic shock (see Chap. 20), fluid and electrolyte imbalances, venous thrombosis (especially in the arms and legs), IICP, seizures, leakage of cerebrospinal fluid (CSF), and stress ulcers and hemorrhage.

Nursing Management

Regard a head injury, no matter how mild it appears, as an emergency. Obtain a history of the injury and perform a neurologic examination, paying particular attention to vital signs, LOC, presence or absence of movement in the arms and legs, and pupil size, equality, and reaction to light. If trauma caused the head injury, examine the head for bleeding, abrasions, and lacerations. Evaluate respiratory status, paying particular attention to the client's ability to maintain adequate oxygenation. Report neurologic changes immediately. See Chapter 39 for nursing care of a client with IICP that is treated medically.

Preoperatively, administer prescribed medications, such as anticonvulsants to reduce risk of seizures before and after surgery, an osmotic diuretic, and corticosteroids. Preoperative sedation usually is omitted. Before surgery, fluids are restricted to avoid intraoperative complications, reduce cerebral edema, and prevent postoperative vomiting. If indicated, insert an indwelling urethral catheter and intravenous (IV) line. To prevent thrombophlebitis and deep vein thrombosis, which may develop from prolonged inactivity during neurosurgery, apply antiembolism stockings. Refer to Nursing Care Plan 41-1 for postoperative care and to Client and Family Teaching 41-1.

Stop, Think, and Respond • BOX 41-1

You are caring for two clients with head injuries. Client A lost consciousness at the time of his head injury. He was alert and oriented on arrival in the ED, but 2 hours later he does not respond even when you press on his nailbeds. Client B has been hospitalized for 1 day. He has not been fully alert since admission and continues to be lethargic. He requires more and more stimulation to give a response. Which client's condition is more serious? Explain your choice.

• SKULL FRACTURES

A skull fracture is a break in the continuity of the cranium. The most common types are simple, depressed, and comminuted fractures (Table 41.2).

Pathophysiology and Etiology

A skull fracture results from a blow to the head. It is associated with an **open head injury,** in which the scalp, bony cranium, and dura mater (outer meningeal layer) are exposed, or it may be a **closed head injury,** in which an intact layer of scalp covers the fractured skull.

Open head injuries create a potential for infection because they expose internal brain structures to the environment. They are less likely to produce rapid IICP because the opening gives the brain some room to expand as pressure increases.

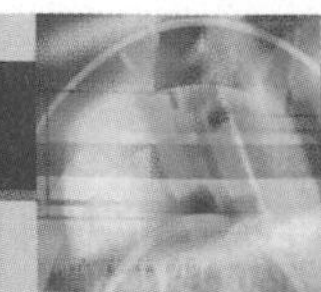

Nursing Care Plan 41-1

CARE OF THE CLIENT UNDERGOING INTRACRANIAL SURGERY

Assessment

- Assess vital signs, LOC, verbal response, and understanding of oral communication.
- Determine type and level of discomfort (e.g., headache, sensitivity to light).
- Assess level of pain tolerance using a scale of 0 to 10.
- Evaluate orientation to person, place, and time.
- Check cognitive function by determining ability to follow simple instructions or perform basic mathematical calculations.
- Check pupil size, equality, and response to light. Look for changes in visual field, blurred vision, or diplopia.
- Assess symmetry in facial appearance.
- Test mobility and strength in all four extremities.
- If client is unconscious, look for restlessness.
- Check appropriateness of mood.
- Ask about nausea, and look for evidence of vomiting.
- Monitor seizure activity and status of corneal blink and gag reflexes.
- Monitor urine production, and evaluate the sensation of thirst.

Nursing Diagnosis: **Risk for Ineffective Breathing Pattern** related to depressive effects of anesthesia and compression of medulla secondary to edema of the brain

Expected Outcome: Breathing will be sufficient to maintain an SpO_2 of at least 90% and a PaO_2 of at least 80 mm Hg.

Interventions	*Rationales*
Monitor SpO_2 with a pulse oximeter.	SpO_2 of at least 90% indicates PaO_2 is at least 80 mm Hg.
Maintain a patent airway by keeping the head erect and in midline, inserting an oral or nasopharyngeal airway if necessary, and suctioning secretions.	Neck flexion or rotation can compromise the diameter of the natural airway; an oral or pharyngeal airway prevents the tongue from obstructing the airway; suction removes secretions that reduce air exchange.
Encourage client to deep breathe at least 10 times each hour or to use a bedside spirometer.	Gas exchange depends on moving atmospheric air to the level of the alveoli and exhaling to remove CO_2.
Avoid administering narcotic analgesia.	Narcotics depress respirations.
Elevate head of the bed.	Lowers abdominal organs away from diaphragm, improving inspired volume and reducing intracranial swelling.

Evaluation of Expected Outcome: Client's airway is patent, and respirations are normal.

PC: **Seizures**

Expected Outcome: The nurse will monitor to detect, manage, and minimize seizure activity.

(continued)

Nursing Care Plan 41-1 (Continued)

CARE OF THE CLIENT UNDERGOING INTRACRANIAL SURGERY

Interventions	*Rationales*
Observe client for changes in consciousness and involuntary muscle contraction.	Seizures are categorized as generalized or partial; manifestations vary (see Chap. 39).
Pad side rails; keep the bed in low position.	Padding reduces potential for trauma.
Stay with the client if a seizure occurs; protect him or her from injury, suction secretions, and promote adequate ventilation.	Serious injury is less likely if a client falls from a bed in low position.
Administer prescribed anticonvulsants.	During a seizure, a client cannot protect himself or herself. Secretions accumulate, increasing the risk for aspiration. Contraction of the diaphragm and intercostal muscles can lead to hypoxia.

Evaluation of Expected Outcome: The nurse detects seizures and implements interventions to minimize their consequences.

Nursing Diagnosis: **Risk for Hyperthermia** related to hypothalamic dysfunction or infection

Expected Outcome: Client will maintain body temperature within normal range.

Interventions	*Rationales*
Measure body temperature every 4 hours.	Provides early indications of changes in client's thermoregulation.
Help client maintain an adequate oral fluid intake.	Perspiration assists with heat loss through evaporation.
Remove heavy blankets if client develops a fever. Place client on an electrical cooling blanket to reduce fever.	Blankets trap body heat and interfere with convection. A cooling blanket reduces body temperature through conduction.
Administer prescribed antipyretic when fever does not respond to heat reduction methods.	Antipyretics lower set-point for body temperature in the hypothalamus.

Evaluation of Expected Outcome: Temperature does not exceed 99.8°F.

Nursing Diagnosis: **Disturbed Thought Processes** related to cognitive deficits secondary to structural changes in brain tissue and physiology

Expected Outcome: Client will be oriented to person, place, and time.

Interventions	*Rationales*
Orient client at frequent intervals.	Until cognition and sensorium return to normal, client may not recall his or her location and reasons for medical care.
Provide environmental clues such as a calendar with large numbers.	Helps reorient the client to time.
Investigate contributing causes of disorientation and restlessness (e.g., full bladder, pain) and intervene as appropriate.	Clients may sense that they are uncomfortable but be unable to identify specifics of distress.
Share current events, and turn on newsworthy television or radio programs.	Sensory stimulation and communication tend to elevate cognitive functions.
Repeat explanations or answers to questions as needed.	Repetition reinforces information and promotes storage of memory.

Evaluation of Expected Outcome: Client is oriented to person, place, and time.

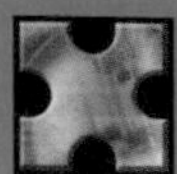

41-1 *Client and Family Teaching* Care After Intracranial Surgery

If the client is discharged directly home, the nurse must provide the following verbal and written instructions:

- Signs of intracranial bleeding and infection (expect swelling around the eye and below the incision)
- Purposes for prescribed medications (e.g., anticonvulsants, anti-inflammatory drugs, drugs to control gastric acidity), schedule for administration, and side effects to report
- Expected sensory changes such as hearing a "clicking" sound around the bone flap, which will disappear as healing takes place; headaches also are common, but the client must notify the surgeon if a mild analgesic like acetaminophen (Tylenol) fails to relieve them
- Care for the surgical site as directed by the physician; some recommendations include keep the incision clean, avoid scrubbing it, secure remaining hair away from the incision, resume shampooing the hair when the staples or sutures are removed, and wear a hat when outside to avoid sunburn until hair growth resumes
- Safety precautions to maintain at home, including ambulating only with assistance and ensuring well-lit and clutter-free rooms; driving privileges are temporarily restricted until the risk for seizures has been eliminated
- Exercises that promote strength and endurance
- Techniques to ensure bowel and bladder elimination
- Feeding or nutritional suggestions
- Follow-up appointments for measuring anticonvulsant blood levels, electroencephalograms, and continued medical care and evaluation

Basilar skull fractures are located at the skull base. Trauma in this location is especially dangerous because it can cause edema of the brain near the origin of the spinal cord (*foramen magnum*), interfere with circulation of CSF, injure nerves that pass into the spinal cord, or create a pathway for infection between the brain and middle ear, which can result in meningitis.

TABLE 41.2 TYPES OF SKULL FRACTURES

TYPE	DESCRIPTION
Simple	Linear crack without any displacement of the pieces
Depressed	Broken bone pushed inward toward the brain
Comminuted	Bone splintered into fragments

Assessment Findings

Simple skull fractures produce few, if any, symptoms and heal without complications. The client may complain of a localized headache. A bump, bruise, or laceration may be visible on the scalp.

Symptoms depend on the area of the brain that is injured. For example, a large bone fragment pressing on the motor area can cause hemiparesis. In any type of skull fracture, shock can develop from injury to the skull or some other area of the body.

Because basilar skull fractures tend to tear the dura, **rhinorrhea,** leaking of CSF from the nose, or **otorrhea,** leakage of CSF from the ear, may occur. In some cases **periorbital ecchymosis,** referred to as *raccoon eyes,* or bruising of the mastoid process behind the ear, called **Battle's sign,** can be present (Fig. 41.4). Conjunctival hemorrhages can occur as well. Injury to brain tissue may result in seizures. Epilepsy can develop as a sequela of head injury.

Skull x-rays, CT scan, or MRI show brain tissue injuries such as a fracture line or embedded skull fragments (compound skull fracture), cerebral edema, or a subdural or epidural hematoma.

Medical and Surgical Management

Simple skull fractures require bed rest and close observation for signs of IICP. If the scalp is lacerated, the wound is cleaned, debrided, and sutured.

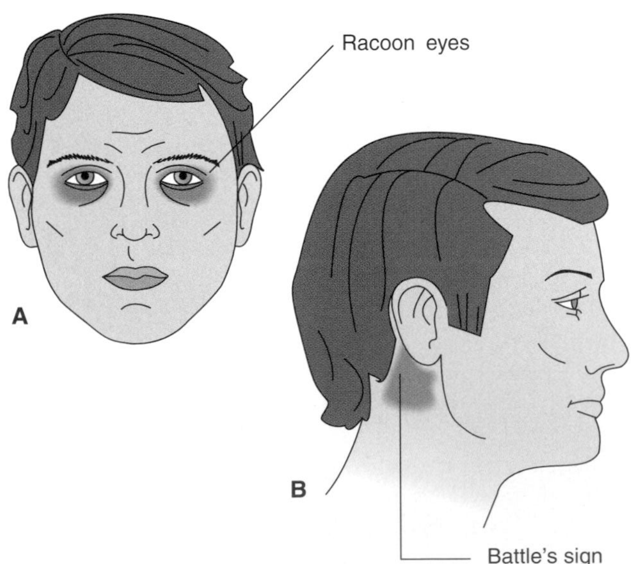

FIGURE 41.4 (**A**) Periorbital ecchymosis, called *racoon eyes,* and (**B**) periauricular ecchymosis, called *Battle's sign.*

Depressed skull fractures require a craniotomy to remove bone fragments and control bleeding, elevation of the depressed fracture, and repair of damaged tissues. A piece of mesh is inserted to replace bone fragments that are removed. Additional treatment includes antibiotics to control infection, an osmotic diuretic or corticosteroids to prevent or treat cerebral edema, and an anticonvulsant to prevent or treat seizures.

Nursing Management

Most clients are hospitalized for at least 24 hours after a significant head injury. Examine the client to identify signs of head trauma and test drainage from the nose or ear (Nursing Guidelines 41-1). To detect any CSF drainage, look for a **halo sign** (Fig. 41.5). If drainage is present, allow it to flow freely onto porous gauze and avoid tightly plugging the orifice.

Perform neurologic assessments, which include an hourly evaluation of LOC and of pupil, motor, and sensory status, even if the injury appears mild. It is possible for a hematoma to accompany a skull fracture. Obtain vital signs every 15 to 30 minutes and prepare for the possibility of seizures. See Chapter 39 for additional nursing care.

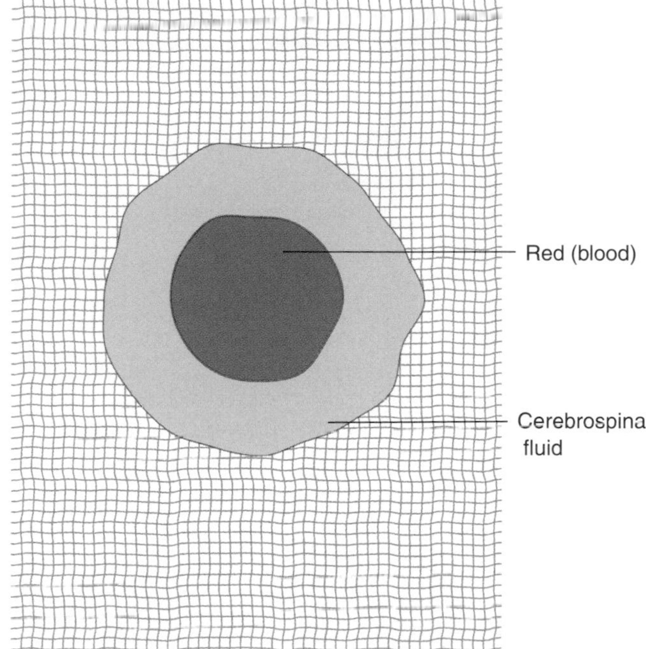

FIGURE 41.5 Halo sign. Clear drainage that separates from bloody drainage suggests the presence of cerebrospinal fluid.

SPINAL CORD INJURIES

Spinal cord trauma is serious and sometimes fatal. The cervical and lumbar vertebrae are the most common sites of injury. Correct emergency management at the time of injury is crucial because moving the client incorrectly can permanently damage the spinal cord.

NURSING GUIDELINES 41-1

Detecting Cerebrospinal Fluid in Drainage

Method #1

1. Wet a Dextrostick or Testape strip with drainage from the nose or ear.
2. Observe if the color change indicates the presence of glucose.
3. Use method #2 if the test is positive, because blood also contains glucose and can result in false results.

Method #2

1. Collect droplets of drainage on a white absorbent pad.
2. Observe the wet area after a few minutes for a halo sign.
3. Note if a yellow ring encircles a central ring that is red: the red ring indicates blood; the yellow ring suggests CSF.

Pathophysiology and Etiology

Common causes of spinal cord injury include accidents and violence. Vehicular accidents are the leader, followed by violence, falls, sports, and miscellaneous injuries. Trauma to the back can fracture or collapse one or more vertebrae, causing a portion of bone to injure the spinal cord and interfere with the transmission of nerve impulses (Fig. 41.6). Even with no fracture, edema may lead to cord compression, which may permanently damage the cord.

Spinal cord injury also can lead to bleeding within the cord. Because the blood has no place to drain, it forms a hematoma that occupies space and compresses the nerve roots. Injury to the cord also can completely or partially sever spinal cord nerve fibers. With such an injury, the client experiences various consequences of motor and sensory dysfunction below the site of the injury (Table 41.3).

Tetraplegia (a term that replaces *quadriplegia*) results in paralysis of all extremities when there is a high cervical spine injury. **Paraplegia,** paralysis of both legs, occurs with injuries at the thoracic level. When the tracts of the spinal nerves are severed, no effective nerve regeneration occurs. Muscle spasms occur spontaneously, but are not evidence that the client is regaining motor function. Many paraplegics return home, live independently, and, in some instances, resume work. Tetraplegics may return home but require extensive physical care.

Respiratory arrest and spinal shock are immediate complications of spinal cord injury. Long-term complications include autonomic dysreflexia, pressure ulcers, contractures, respiratory and urinary tract infections, calcium loss from bones, and renal calculus formation.

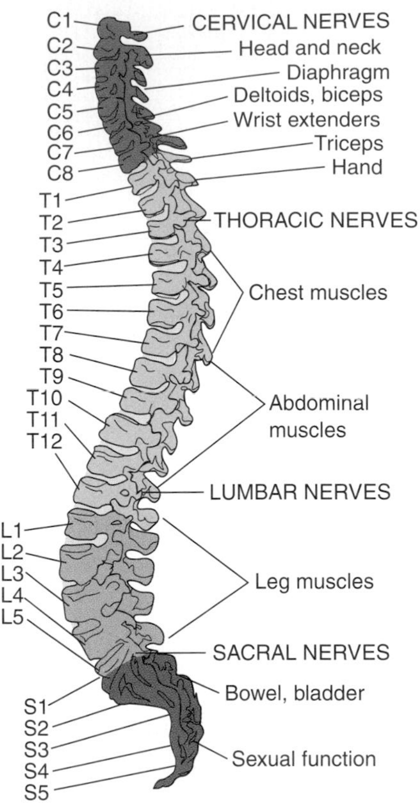

FIGURE 41.6 Structures affected by spinal nerves.

Spinal Shock (Areflexia)

Spinal shock is loss of sympathetic reflex activity below the level of injury within 30 to 60 minutes of a spinal injury. It is characterized by immediate loss of all cord functions below the point of injury. Other manifestations include pronounced hypotension, bradycardia, and warm, dry skin. If the level of injury is in the cervical or upper thoracic region, respiratory failure can occur. Bowel and bladder distention develops. The client does not perspire below the level of injury, impairing temperature control. The client manifests **poikilothermia,** body temperature of the environment. Spinal shock may persist for 1 week to months until the body adjusts to damage imposed by the injury. Until then, vital functions require medical support.

Autonomic Dysreflexia (Hyperreflexia)

Autonomic dysreflexia is an exaggerated sympathetic nervous system response among those with a spinal cord injury above T6. It can occur suddenly at any time after spinal shock subsides. Box 41-1 lists factors that precipitate autonomic dysreflexia. Characteristics of this acute emergency are severe hypertension, slow heart rate, pounding headache, nausea, blurred vision, flushed skin, sweating, goosebumps (erection of pilomotor muscles in the skin), nasal stuffiness, and anxiety. Uncontrolled autonomic dysreflexia can lead to seizures, stroke, and death. Prevention is the best treatment, but additional measures such as administering antihypertensive drug therapy with nifedipine (Procardia), nitroglycerin ointment, phentolamine (Regitine), hydralazine (Apresoline), or diazoxide (Hyperstat); raising the client's head; and relieving the precipitating cause are necessary once it develops.

Assessment Findings

The degree and location of the injury determine immediate symptoms. There is pain in the affected area, diffi-

TABLE 41.3 CONSEQUENCES OF SPINAL CORD INJURIES

LEVEL OF INJURY	COMMON MOTOR EFFECTS	COMMON SENSORY EFFECTS
C1, C2, C3	Paralysis below neck; impaired breathing; bowel and bladder incontinence; sexual dysfunction	No sensation below neck
C4, C5	Shoulder elevation possible; ventilation support required	No sensation below clavicle
C6, C7, C8	Some elbow, upper arm, and wrist movement; can do diaphragmatic breathing	Some sensation in arms and thumb; sensation in chest impaired
T1–T6	Paralysis below waist; control of hands; abdominal breathing	No sensation below midchest
T7–T12	Varying degrees of trunk and abdominal control	Varying degrees of sensation below waist
L1–L2	Hip adduction impaired	No sensation below lower abdomen; some sensation in inner thighs
L3–L5	Knee and ankle movement impaired	No sensation below upper thighs
S1–S5	Varying degrees of bowel/bladder control and sexual function	No sensation in perineum

C, cervical; T, thoracic; L, lumbar; S, sacral.

BOX 41-1 ● Common Causes of Autonomic Dysreflexia

- Full bladder
- Abdominal distention
- Impacted feces
- Skin pressure or breakdown
- Overstretched muscles
- Sexual intercourse
- Labor and delivery
- Sunburn below the cord injury
- Infected ingrown toenail
- Exposure to hot or cold environmental temperature
- Taking over-the-counter decongestants

culty breathing, numbness, and paralysis. If the injury is high in the cervical region, respiratory failure and death occur because the diaphragm is paralyzed. When the cord is completely severed, the client permanently loses function below the level of the injury. He or she maintains some function if damage to the cord is minimal.

A neurologic examination reveals the level of spinal cord injury. X-rays, myelography, MRI, and CT scan show evidence of fracture or compression of one or more vertebrae, edema, or a hematoma.

Medical Management

Initially, the head and back are immobilized mechanically with a cervical collar and back support. An IV line is inserted to provide access to a vein if shock develops. Vital signs are stabilized. Corticosteroids may be given to reduce spinal cord edema.

After the client is stabilized, the injured portion of the spine is further immobilized using a cast or brace or surgical intervention. Traction with weights and pulleys is applied to provide correct vertebral alignment and increase space between vertebrae. Additional weight is added over the next few days to increase space between vertebrae and move them into correct alignment. A turning frame is used to change the client's position without altering the alignment of the spine (Fig. 41.7).

Surgical Management

Depending on the extent of the injury, it may be necessary surgically to remove bone fragments, repair dislocated vertebrae, and stabilize the spine. The vertebrae are fused with bone obtained from the iliac crest or stabilized with a steel rod. External immobilization with a brace or cast often is necessary.

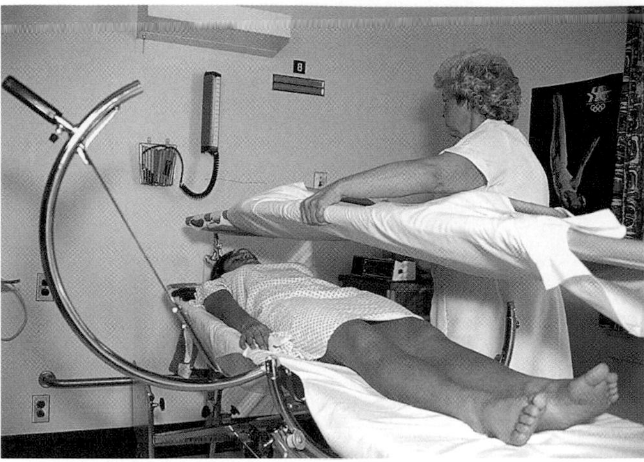

FIGURE 41.7 The nurse frequently turns a client on the Stryker frame to relieve pressure. (From Smeltzer, S. C. & Bare, B. G. [2000]. *Brunner & Suddarth's textbook of medical–surgical nursing* [9th ed.]. Philadelphia: Lippincott Williams & Wilkins.)

NURSING PROCESS

● Care of the Client With Spinal Trauma

Assessment

When the client arrives in the ED, obtain information about the injury and treatment given at the scene from family, witnesses, or those who transported the client to the hospital. Perform a neurologic assessment, taking care to document findings on a flow sheet to provide a database. Assess vital signs, with attention to respiratory status. During the acute phase, repeat neurologic assessments frequently. Determine if the client has movement and sensation below the level of injury, look to see if neurologic damage is worsening, and observe for signs of respiratory distress and spinal shock.

Diagnosis, Planning, and Interventions

Keep the client's body and head aligned and limit all movement. If directed by the physician, insert a urinary retention catheter. Assist with immobilization of the injured spine (Fig. 41.8). Burr holes in the skull are required for inserting the pointed ends of traction tongs or the halo traction apparatus. When applying traction, check that weights hang free. Instruct others on the nursing team never to lift or remove weights or increase or decrease the amount of prescribed weight. The use of external stabilizing devices like the halo vest facilitates early discharge from the acute care facility. To ensure the client's safety and prevent complications, see Nursing Guidelines 41-2. Besides monitoring for and intervening in cases of spinal shock and autonomic dysreflexia, the nurse's role may include the following.

Ineffective Breathing Pattern, Ineffective Airway Clearance, and **Risk for Impaired Gas Exchange**

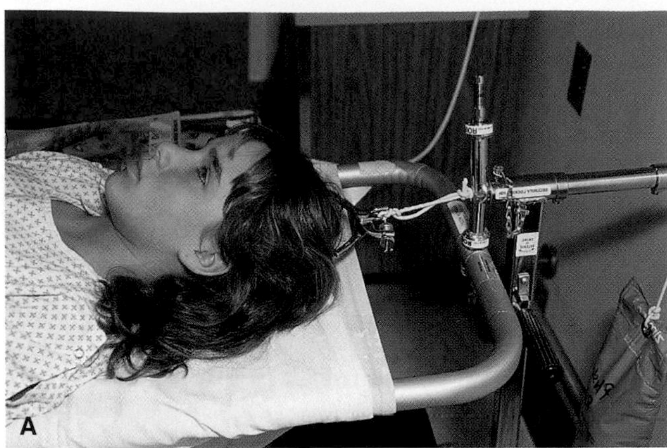

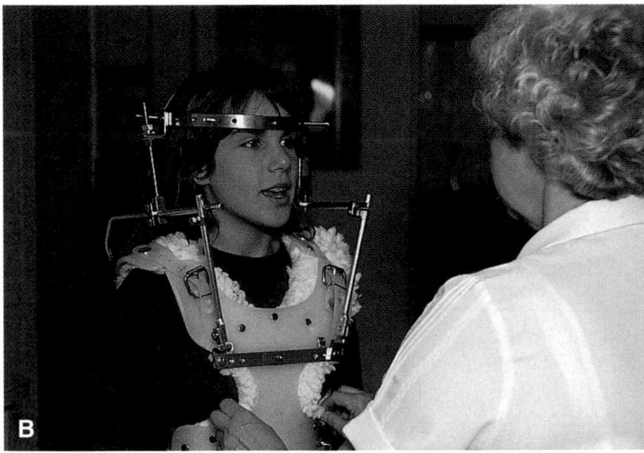

FIGURE 41.8 (**A**) Traction for cervical fractures may be applied with tongs. (**B**) A halo vest may be used to maintain alignment in cervical injuries. (From Smeltzer, S. C. & Bare, B. G. [2000]. *Brunner & Suddarth's textbook of medical–surgical nursing* [9th ed.]. Philadelphia: Lippincott Williams & Wilkins.)

related to paralysis of respiratory, chest, and abdominal muscles

Expected Outcomes: (1) Client will breathe independently at a rate of 16 to 20 breaths/minute. (2) The airway will be free of secretions. (3) The client's blood oxygen saturation (SpO_2) will be 90% or higher.

- Maintain a patent airway. *A patent airway maximizes passage of air in and out of the lungs.*
- Be prepared for endotracheal intubation and mechanical ventilation if respiratory failure occurs. *An endotracheal tube provides an airway from the nose or mouth to an area above the mainstem bronchi. Mechanical ventilation provides a means to regulate respiratory rate, volume of air, and percentage of oxygen when a client cannot breathe independently.*
- Suction airway to remove secretions. *A client with spinal trauma may not be able to cough effectively. An artificial airway increases production of respiratory secretions.*
- Administer oxygen as prescribed. *To prevent hypoxemia, the client may require more oxygen than available in room air.*

NURSING GUIDELINES 41-2

Instructing Clients in Halo Vest Management

Teach client as follows:

- Turn your whole body rather than trying to turn your head; you will not be able to look down.
- Do not drive a car.
- Walk only on level surfaces until you become accustomed to the vest; avoid stairs, curbs, and uneven terrain unless assistance is available.
- Take care getting in and out of vehicles to avoid bumping the halo and loosening the pins.
- Use a mirror to inspect the pin sites and as a guide while cleaning them.
- Clean the pin sites two to three times a day with cotton-tipped applicators saturated with hydrogen peroxide; remove loose crusts.
- Use a clean applicator after making a full circle around the pin site.
- Clip the hair that grows around the pin sites.
- Report pain, redness, drainage from pin sites, fever, or neck tingling or pain to the physician.
- Never independently adjust the vest if it becomes tight or loose; consult the physician.
- Pad the vest if it causes pressure or friction.
- Take sponge baths to maintain hygiene; seek assistance for areas you cannot reach such as around the anus.
- Use a dry shampoo or consult physician on how to shampoo hair without wetting the vest.
- Use pillows for support and comfort when sleeping.
- Wear loose-fitting clothing with wide necklines for ease in dressing.
- Wear shoes with flat heels that are easy to slip on and off.

PC: Neuropathic Pain related to irritated nerve root and soft tissue injury

Expected Outcome: The nurse will monitor to detect, manage, and minimize neuropathic pain.

- Administer prescribed analgesia intravenously. *Avoids administration of injections into tissues where absorption is compromised.*
- Assist physician with nerve block procedures if analgesia is ineffective. *A nerve block is a form of regional anesthesia in which an anesthetic agent is injected close to the nerve transmitting pain impulses.*

Impaired Physical Mobility and **Risk for Disuse Syndrome** related to loss of motor function

Expected Outcome: (1) Client's ability to be mobile will be maintained. (2) Client will use assistive devices to move and perform activities of daily living. (3) Client will not experience complications associated with inactivity and immobility.

- Position client to avoid joint contractures and foot drop. *Prevents permanent changes to the musculoskeletal system. Inactivity causes joints to assume a position of flexion.*
- Help client perform exercises identified by the physical therapist. *Maintains joint flexibility and reduces muscle atrophy and atony. For exercises to be effective, clients must perform them several times a day.*
- Apply leg braces when ambulation is possible. *Braces support joints, allowing client to ambulate independently or with a walker or crutches.*
- Maintain skin integrity by changing client's position at least every 2 hours, using pressure-relieving devices, massaging bony prominences, and keeping skin clean and dry. *Position changes and pressure-relieving devices ensure that capillary pressure stays above 32 mm Hg, thus providing oxygenated blood to cells for their continued survival. Massage increases blood flow to temporarily deprived areas. Keeping skin clean and dry prevents maceration and decreases the potential for bacterial growth.*
- Facilitate urine elimination and keep bowel evacuated. *Urinary retention and stasis may contribute to autonomic dysreflexia and formation of renal calculi. Infrequent bowel evacuation leads to constipation and impaction.*
- Keep client hydrated. *Reduces potential for formation of thrombi and renal calculi.*
- Provide oral or enteral nutrition. *Provides nutrients and elements necessary for energy and to sustain cellular growth and repair.*

Evaluation of Expected Outcomes

Breathing is adequate to maintain oxygenation. Pain is relieved or reduced to a tolerable level. The client regains mobility using minimal assistive devices. Complications from inactivity are prevented or reduced. The client and family demonstrate understanding of postdischarge home care.

SPINAL NERVE ROOT COMPRESSION

There are two basic types of spinal nerve root compression: **intramedullary** lesions that involve the spinal cord and **extramedullary** lesions that involve the tissues surrounding the spinal cord. The most common site of nerve root compression is at the level of the three lower lumbar disks, but nerve root compression also occurs in the cervical spine.

Pathophysiology and Etiology

Pressure on spinal nerve roots results from trauma, herniated intervertebral disks, and tumors of the spinal cord and surrounding structures (Fig. 41.9). Stress caused by poor body mechanics, age, or disease weakens an area in the vertebra, causing the spongy center of the vertebrae, the *nucleus pulposus,* to swell and herniate. Commonly called a *slipped disk,* the displacement puts pressure on nearby nerves.

Pain along the distribution of the nerve root is common. Actions that increase pressure intensify pain. Weakness and changes in sensation occur. Symptoms intensify with increasing nerve root compression.

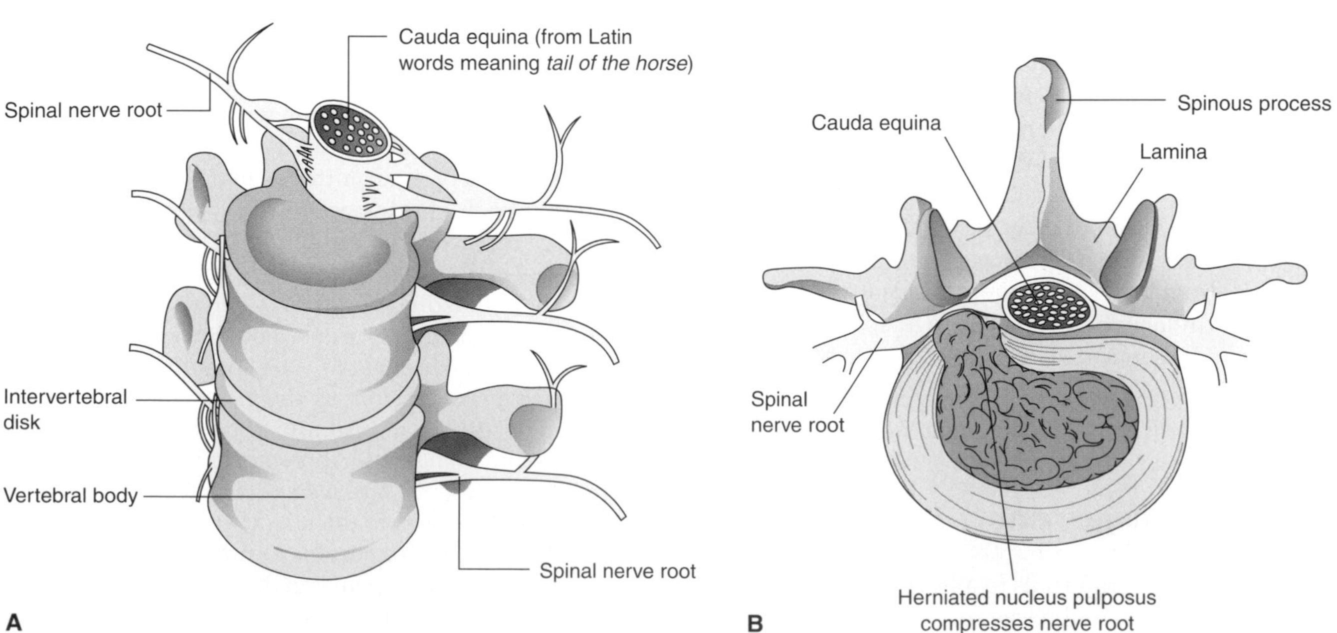

FIGURE 41.9 (**A**) Normal lumbar spine vertebrae, intervertebral disks, and spinal nerve root. (**B**) Ruptured vertebral disk. (From Smeltzer, S. C. & Bare, B. G. [2000]. *Brunner & Suddarth's textbook of medical–surgical nursing* [9th ed.]. Philadelphia: Lippincott Williams & Wilkins.)

Assessment Findings

Symptoms, depending on the cause of compression and level involved, usually include weakness, paralysis, pain, and **paresthesia** (numbness, tingling). When a herniated disk in the lumbar region compresses the sciatic nerve, the client describes feeling pain down the buttocks and into the posterior thigh and leg. Physical examination reveals weakness or paralysis of the extremity innervated by the compressed nerve. If a nerve in the lumbar or sacral area is affected, the client experiences pain when lying supine and lifting the leg without bending the knee. Pain increases when straining, coughing, or lifting a heavy object. Walking and sitting become difficult. Spinal x-ray, CT, MRI, myelography, and electromyography show displacement or herniation of an intervertebral disk, a tumor, or bleeding around the nerve root.

Medical Management

When a client has a herniated intervertebral disk, conservative therapy is tried first. Metastatic spinal cord tumors also are treated conservatively because removal is not feasible. A herniated cervical disk is treated by immobilizing the cervical spine with a cervical collar or brace. When inflammation subsides, the client wears the collar or brace intermittently when walking or sitting. Bed rest with a firm mattress and bed board is used for clients with a lumbar herniated disk.

Skin traction, which can be applied in the home, decreases severe muscle spasm as well as increasing the distance between adjacent vertebrae, keeping the vertebrae correctly aligned, and, in many instances, relieving pain for an extended period.

Hot moist packs treat muscle spasm. Skeletal muscle relaxants, such as carisoprodol (Soma) and chlorzoxazone (Paraflex), help clients with a herniated intervertebral disk. Diazepam (Valium), a tranquilizer with skeletal muscle-relaxing action, is used to reduce anxiety associated with pain of a herniated disk and to relax the skeletal muscle. Drugs such as aspirin, phenylbutazone (Butazolidine), and corticosteroids treat inflammation. Reducing inflammation and muscle spasm helps ease pain, but additional analgesics are given to control pain. Clients with an inoperable spinal cord tumor are given analgesics to maintain comfort.

Surgical Management

If conservative therapy fails to relieve symptoms of a herniated disk with spinal nerve root compression, surgery is considered. Procedures for relieving spinal nerve root compression include the following:

- **Diskectomy**—removal of the ruptured disk
- **Laminectomy**—removal of the posterior arch of a vertebra to expose the spinal cord. The surgeon can remove whatever lesion is causing compression: a herniated disk, tumor, blood clot, bone spur, or broken bone fragment.
- Diskectomy with **spinal fusion**—removal of ruptured disk followed by grafting a piece of bone taken from another area, such as the iliac crest, onto the vertebra to fuse the vertebral spinous process. Bone also may be obtained from a bone bank.
- **Chemonucleolysis**—injection of the enzyme chymopapain into the nucleus pulposus to shrink or dissolve the disc, which then relieves pressure on spinal nerve roots

Spinal fusion stabilizes the vertebrae weakened by degenerative joint changes, such as osteoarthritis, and by laminectomy. It results in a firm union; the client loses mobility and must become accustomed to a permanent area of stiffness. When part of the lumbar spine is fused, the client usually does not feel the stiffness after a short time because motion increases in the joints above the fusion. Motion is more limited when the area of fusion is in the cervical spine. Spinal fusion also is performed for spinal cord tumors and fractures and dislocations of the spine.

Nursing Management

Perform a neurologic examination and note any limitation of motion and the type of movement that causes pain. For nursing responsibilities unique to various types of spinal surgery, see Nursing Guidelines 41-3. For clients being treated conservatively, use a firm mattress or apply a bedboard because a firm surface supports the spine and promotes alignment. Maintain the client on bed rest, placing him or her in Williams' position with the knees and head slightly elevated to relieve lumbosacral pain. Apply halo vest traction. For intermittent pelvic or cervical skin traction, attach skin device to the client, support the weights, and lower the client gently to avoid a sudden and strong pull. Remind the client to roll from side to side without twisting the spine. When the client gets out of bed, reinforce use of proper body mechanics. Advise clients with cervical nerve root compression to avoid extreme hyperextension of the neck and side-to-side rotation of the head. Administer prescribed muscle relaxants and analgesics. Apply moist heat for no longer than 20 minutes, but repeat several times a day.

Periodically evaluate the client's response to conservative therapy. It is important to note the activities and positions that increase pain and the gain or loss in motion or sensation since the previous observation. It is important to note a change in symptoms when the client is removed from traction.

NURSING GUIDELINES 41-3

Nursing Care After Specific Spinal Surgeries

Postcervical Diskectomy

- Keep a cervical collar in place at all times; do not remove without a physician's order.
- Instruct client to keep the neck straight in midline position until healing occurs.
- Support client's head, neck, and upper shoulders when moving from a lying to sitting to standing position or when getting into and out of a chair.
- Observe for Horner's syndrome, a complication following anterior cervical diskectomy from cervical sympathetic nerve damage. Manifestations are lid ptosis (drooping), constricted pupil, regression of eye in the orbit, and lack of perspiration on one side of the face.

Postlumbar Laminectomy or Diskectomy With Spinal Fusion

- Logroll when turning client every 2 hours; maintain alignment at all times.

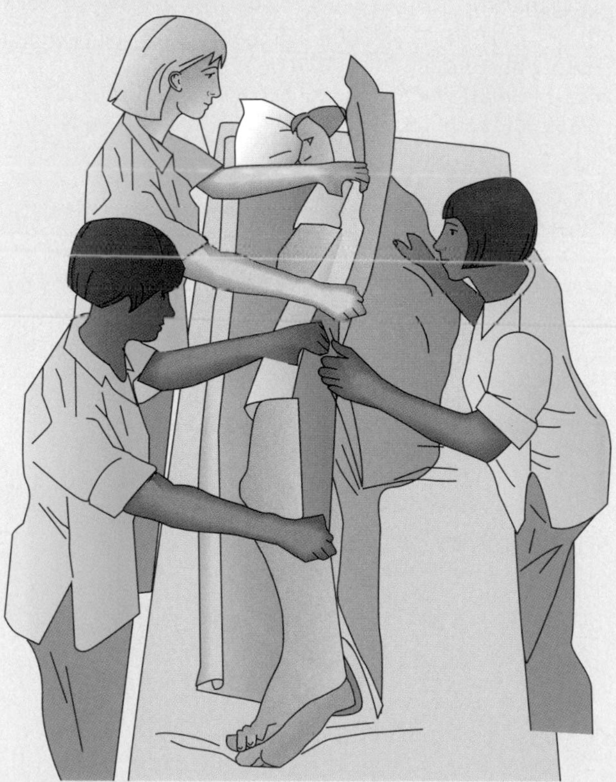

- Caution client to avoid turning self.
- Teach client to avoid twisting or jerking the back; sitting during the first week and prolonged sitting thereafter (client should use a straight-backed chair and not slump); bending from the waist (client should bend from the knees and hips).

Nursing interventions after spinal surgery are as follows:

- Monitor vital signs.
- Assist client to perform hourly deep breathing exercises while awake but avoid forced coughing because it increases pressure within the spinal canal.
- Examine dressing for CSF leakage or bleeding.
- Assess neurovascular status (color, temperature, mobility, sensation) in extremities below the area of surgery, which may result from edema or hemorrhage at the operative site.
- Report an inability to void or an output of less than 240 mL in 8 hours.
- Use a fracture bed pan.

GENERAL GERONTOLOGIC CONSIDERATIONS 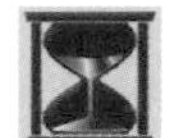

Older adults often respond less favorably to therapies for a neurologic deficit.

Older adults tend to drink less water and, therefore, may incur a chronic fluid volume deficit. Encourage a fluid intake of 1500 to 2000 mL/day (if physical condition permits).

Critical Thinking Exercises

1. *A man involved in a motor vehicle accident is brought to the ED. You are told that he was not wearing a seat belt and struck his head on the steering wheel. What neurologic assessments would you make? Why?*
2. *You are caring for a paraplegic client. What signs and symptoms suggest that the client is experiencing autonomic dysreflexia? What nursing measures are appropriate?*

NCLEX-STYLE REVIEW QUESTIONS 

1. A nurse on a medical flight crew is assessing an alert but lethargic client with a possible closed head injury. The nurse is correct in giving priority attention to which of the following for data relating to the client's neurologic status?
    1. Temperature and blood pressure.
    2. Respiratory rate and breathing effort.
    3. Level of consciousness and pupillary responses.
    4. Peripheral vision and cranial nerve function.
2. The nurse in the emergency department is obtaining a history from the wife of a client just admitted. Which statement by the wife characterizes the progression of disease symptoms in epidural hematoma?
    1. "My husband had a headache all day. He rested in bed with the lights out."
    2. "I noticed that he was confused and then collapsed in the kitchen. It happened so fast."
    3. "I have noticed that he has become increasingly more forgetful over the past week."
    4. "His coordination was poor this morning, but he still drove to the hospital."

3. A nurse in a rehabilitation setting is caring for a client with minimal damage to the lumbar region of the spinal cord. In developing the plan of care, which of the following will be a priority for nursing management?
1. Total paralysis from the neck down
2. Symptoms of autonomic dysreflexia
3. Assistance needed with ambulation
4. Assistance needed with feeding

connection

Visit the Connection site at **http://connection.lww.com/go/timbyEssentials** for links to chapter-related resources on the Internet.

References and Suggested Readings

Barker, E., & Saulino, M. F. (2002). First-ever guidelines for spinal cord injuries. *RN, 65*(10), 32–37.

Bond, C. (2002). Traumatic brain injury: Help for the family. *RN, 65*(11), 61–66.

Bryant, G. A. (2000). When spinal cord injury affects the bowel. *RN, 63*(2), 26–30.

Calhoun, K. H. (2000). In consultation. Evaluating patients with nasal fracture: When to suspect more serious injury. *Journal of Critical Illness, 15,* 528.

Carrigan, T. D., Walker, E., & Barnes, S. (2000). Domestic violence: The shaken adult syndrome. *Journal of Accident and Emergency Medicine, 17,* 138–139.

Danis, D. (2001). Clinical decisions. Interdisciplinary practice: Spinal cord injury. *International Journal of Trauma Nursing,* 7(2), 64–66.

Guin, P. R. (2001). Advances in spinal cord injury care. *Critical Care Nursing Clinics of North America, 13,* 399–409.

Hedger, A. (2002). Spinal cord injury. *Nursing 2000, 32*(12), 96.

Herbert, C. (2001). Use of morphine for pain after intracranial surgery. *Professional Nurse, 16,* 1029–1033.

Hilton, G. (2001). Emergency. Acute head injury: Distinguishing subdural from epidural hematoma. *American Journal of Nursing, 101*(9), 51–52.

Inamasu, J., Hori, S., Aoki, K., et al. (2000). CT scans essential after posttraumatic loss of consciousness. *American Journal of Emergency Medicine, 18,* 810–811.

Karlet, M. C. (2001). Acute management of the patient with spinal cord injury. *International Journal of Trauma Nursing,* 7(2), 43–48.

Kavchak-Keyes, M. A. (2000). Autonomic dysreflexia. *Rehabilitation Nursing, 25*(1), 31–35.

McIlvoy, L., Meyer, K., & Vitaz, T. (2000). Use of an acute spinal cord injury clinical pathway. *Critical Care Clinics of North America, 12,* 521–530.

Perduta-Fulginiti, S. (April 1, 2002). When your client has SCI. *Advance for Nurses,* 30–32.

Robinson, R., & Peacock, J. E. (2000). Law and the emergency nurse. Just "sleeping it off." *Journal of Emergency Nursing, 26,* 249–250.

Roth, P., & Farls, K. (2000). Pathophysiology of traumatic brain injury. *Critical Care Nursing Quarterly, 23*(3), 14–25.

Slade, J. (2002). Understanding brain death criteria. *Nursing 2002, 32*(12), 68–69.

chapter 42

Caring for Clients With Neurologic Deficits

Words to Know

neurologic deficit

Learning Objectives

On completion of this chapter, the reader will:

- Define *neurologic deficit.*
- Describe the phases of a neurologic deficit.
- Give the primary aims of medical treatment of a neurologic deficit.
- Name members of the healthcare team involved with management of a client with a neurologic deficit.
- Describe nursing management of a client with a neurologic deficit.

A **neurologic deficit** is when one or more functions of the central and peripheral nervous systems are decreased, impaired, or absent. Examples include paralysis, muscle weakness, impaired speech, inability to recognize objects, abnormal gait or difficulty walking, impaired memory, impaired swallowing, or abnormal bowel and bladder elimination. Clients with a neurologic deficit face many problems. Often, the deficit affects more than one body system. The client may be unable to walk, talk, do simple tasks like feeding, or recognize family members.

Many members of the healthcare team are involved with the complex management of the client with a temporary or permanent neurologic deficit: the physician, nurse, nursing assistant, social worker, physical therapist, occupational therapist, speech therapist, prosthetist, psychotherapist, dietitian, pharmacist, and vocational counselor. With intensive therapy and a coordinated approach by all team members, many clients can return to normal or near-normal function or successfully adapt to changes in function.

PHASES OF A NEUROLOGIC DEFICIT

Neurologic deficits are divided into three phases: acute, recovery, and chronic. Not all clients experience all three phases. Some clients have deficits that begin with an acute phase and move into a recovery phase or into a lifelong chronic phase.

ACUTE PHASE

The acute phase follows a sudden neurologic event, such as a cerebrovascular accident (CVA) or a head or spinal cord injury. During the acute phase, the client usually is critically ill, with many signs and symptoms such as altered level of consciousness (LOC), hypertension or hypotension, fever, difficulty breathing, or paralysis.

Medical and Surgical Management

During the acute phase, the goal is to stabilize the client and prevent further neurologic damage. The client with a CVA may require management of hypertension or hypotension through drug therapy or respiratory support through mechanical ventilation. Clients with a head or spinal cord injury may require surgical intervention to stabilize the injured area or remove bone fragments, blood clots, or foreign objects. Sometimes, surgery is postponed until the client is stabilized and the acute phase has passed. For others, surgery is performed during the acute phase as a lifesaving measure.

Nursing Management

Perform frequent and thorough neurologic assessments to evaluate the client's status, need for additional medical or surgical interventions, and response to treatment. Use the Glasgow Coma Scale (see Chap. 38) or other neurologic assessment tools like the Mini-Mental Status Examination (see Chap. 12) to record observations. When significant changes occur, immediately report them to the physician. Assess vital signs as often as necessary and maintain the blood pressure (BP) to ensure adequate cerebral oxygenation. Measure intake and output and observe for signs of electrolyte imbalances and dehydration. Report a urinary output of less than 500 mL/day or urinary or bowel incontinence.

Beginning basic rehabilitation during the acute phase is an important nursing function. Measures such as position changes and prevention of skin breakdown and contractures are essential aspects of care during the early phase of rehabilitation. The nursing goal is to prevent complications that may interfere with the client's potential to recover function. (See this chapter's Nursing Process section for additional nursing management.)

TABLE 42.1 DOMAINS OF NEUROLOGIC IMPAIRMENT

DOMAIN	DESCRIPTION
Motor	A single deficit, or combination of deficits, involving the face, arms, and legs, which affects speech, swallowing, muscle tone and strength, gait, coordination, and ability to use objects for their intended purpose
Sensory	Altered sensation (e.g., numbness, tingling, exaggerated sensation), or altered perception (e.g., inability to identify objects by touch, loss of writing ability)
Vision	Loss of vision in one eye or in the temporal or nasal fields; blindness
Language	Disturbances in comprehension, naming, repeating, clarity of speech, reading
Cognition	Changes in memory, attention, orientation, calculation, and construction
Affect	Altered mood, lability of mood

• RECOVERY PHASE

The recovery phase begins when the client's condition is stabilized. It starts several days or weeks after the initial event and lasts weeks or months.

Medical and Surgical Management

Medical management during the recovery phase aims at keeping the client stable and preventing or treating complications, such as pneumonia, and further neurologic impairment.

Nursing Management

During recovery, work with team members to plan a rehabilitation program in several domains according to client's abilities and limitations (Table 42.1). Various assessment tools can help identify a client's level of functioning and potential for improvement with a rehabilitation program. One example is the Barthel Index (Table 42.2).

Rehabilitation is designed to meet the client's immediate and long-term needs. Environmental changes may be necessary to help the client adapt to disability and fully use any remaining functions. Although deficits can be temporary, a prolonged period and enrollment in a rehabilitation program often are necessary before a client regains partial or full function. Devices that help a client walk, eat, groom, and perform other motor skills are recommended or devised to suit particular needs. Flotation pads for wheelchairs, walkers, sheepskin boots, and range-of-motion (ROM) exercises are examples of the many appliances and procedures used in rehabilitation. (See this chapter's Nursing Process section for additional nursing management.)

• CHRONIC PHASE

For some clients (e.g., those with multiple sclerosis or Alzheimer's disease), a neurologic deficit results in a prolonged or lifelong chronic phase. In this phase, the client shows little or no improvement, remains stationary, or progressively worsens. Physical and psychological rehabilitation continues in the chronic phase to prevent complications such as pressure ulcers and muscle contractures.

Medical and Surgical Management

Medical management continues throughout the chronic phase and uses a wide range of therapies and treatments, such as control of BP, physical therapy, dietary management, and treatment of complications related to disuse and immobility. In some cases, surgery is performed to correct deformities or problems that have developed. Examples include muscle and skin grafts to close a pressure ulcer,

TABLE 42.2 MODIFIED BARTHEL INDEX

ITEM	UNABLE TO PERFORM TASK	SUBSTANTIAL HELP REQUIRED	MODERATE HELP REQUIRED	MINIMAL HELP REQUIRED	FULLY INDEPENDENT
Personal hygiene	0	1	3	4	5
Bathing self	0	1	3	4	5
Feeding	0	2	5	8	10
Toilet	0	2	5	8	10
Stair climbing	0	2	5	8	10
Dressing	0	2	5	8	10
Bowel control	0	2	5	8	10
Bladder control	0	2	5	8	10
Ambulation	0	3	8	12	15
or wheelchair*	0	1	3	4	5
Chair/bed transfer	0	3	8	12	15

*Score only if client is unable to ambulate and is trained in wheelchair management.

DEPENDENCY NEEDS

Categories	MBI Total Scores	Dependency Level	Hours of Help Required per Week (Maximum)
1	0–24	Total	27.0
2	25–49	Severe	23.5
3	50–74	Moderate	20.0
4	75–90	Mild	13.0
5	91–99	Minimal	<10.0

surgery to correct a contracture deformity, or removal of a kidney stone (a complication of prolonged immobility).

Stop, Think, and Respond ? ● BOX 42-1

You are caring for a client with a head injury who is being transferred to an extended care facility for rehabilitation. What information is important to include to help nurses at the new facility plan the client's care?

Nursing Management

Clients in the chronic phase often are admitted to a hospital for treatment of complications. They also are transferred to a skilled nursing facility or long-term care facility when family members no longer can manage their care, or when the disease has progressively worsened so that skilled care is mandatory. Nursing management focuses on preventing physical and psychological complications. Therapy in a rehabilitation center may include retraining in skills such as using the telephone, handling money, shopping, using public transportation, maintaining a household, and vocational training.

PSYCHOSOCIAL ISSUES AND HOME MANAGEMENT

Overview

Leaving the inpatient setting, where daily, intensive support of the healthcare team is readily available, and returning home with life-altering changes is frightening. The client and family need support to adapt to a new lifestyle. Although many clients recover sufficiently to assume responsibility for some aspects of their own care, others do not. The burden of care often falls on the spouse, who may have physical problems as well, or adult children, who may not be available or willing to share this responsibility.

Financial resources are strained during a lengthy hospitalization, which may continue after discharge. Adapting the home to accommodate a wheelchair or special bed can be costly. Wide doorways, ramps instead of stairs, and special fixtures in the bathroom for bathing and toileting are examples of changes that often are necessary. The client may have been the major wage earner. Some clients can enter training programs that allow them to find employment outside the home, whereas others learn skills that enable them to be employed at home. Others, because of age or extreme physical disability, cannot be gainfully employed.

Nursing Management

Listen and be alert to subtle hints about the client's and family's adaptation to the client's change in functional status. Ask direct questions to identify problems and needs. Evaluate the client's ability to perform self-care, resume his or her role in the family, and call on a support system. Assess available facilities, family support system, physical aids required, and amount of assistance the client requires with activities of daily living. Encourage the family to help plan for the client's return home, to ask questions about care, and to seek assistance from agencies that can provide emotional, physical, and financial support.

Coping

Address each client individually. Offer reassurance and emotional support and display empathetic understanding of the multiple problems the client is facing. Many clients have difficulty coping with their disability. Provide encouragement and praise throughout rehabilitation and show personal interest and pleasure in each accomplishment, no matter how small, to help clients accept what they cannot or never will be able to do.

Give clients time to talk about their problems, fears, and concerns. Once needs are identified, encourage the client to set attainable goals, which may help maintain independence as long as possible. Work with the client and family to develop solutions and possible alternatives.

At times, improvement is slow and barely noticeable. A client often has difficulty coping. Discouragement, depression, withdrawal, and anger are not unusual. Suggest available support groups.

Socialization

As soon as clients respond to those around them, encourage socialization with others. It can be limited to health team members and family. Encourage family to talk to the client, discuss current events, and motivate the client to respond. Those with speech difficulties tend to become withdrawn and depressed. Encourage visitors to include the client in their conversations, and ask the client questions. Family members need patience when trying to understand what a client with aphasia is trying to communicate.

Occupational and recreational therapies are part of the rehabilitation program and require a team effort. In the beginning, occupational therapy is designed to help strengthen muscles that are under voluntary control. Later, certain tasks are learned or relearned to help client interact with others.

Family Processes

The family faces many disruptions because of permanent disability of a family member. Lifestyles are altered, financial resources strained, conflicts arise, and people must accept new responsibilities. Allow the family time to deal with and accept changes, and provide opportunities to talk and openly express their anger, fears, guilt, and helplessness. The following suggestions may help the family adjust to present and future changes:

- Include family in the client's rehabilitation.
- Give encouragement and praise when a family member helps with part of home care.
- Explain the purpose of each segment of rehabilitation (e.g., ROM exercises, positioning).
- When the family wants responsibility for procedures to be performed at home, teach each procedure or task slowly and give the family time to practice under supervision.
- Prepare a list of public or private agencies that assist with home care, transportation, and financial and emotional support.

Client and Family Teaching

Develop a teaching plan for home care management incorporating therapies prescribed by the physician and other members of the team. Begin teaching long before discharge to allow sufficient time to learn and understand home care management. The individualized teaching plan includes discussion of one or more of the topics presented in Client and Family Teaching 42-1.

NURSING PROCESS

● The Client With a Neurologic Deficit

Assessment

Obtain a thorough history (including drugs and allergies) from client or family. Assess vital signs and level of comfort. Weigh client for future comparisons. Perform a general neurologic assessment and use a standardized assessment tool (see Table 42.2) to note the extent of neurologic deficits related to swallowing, vision, weakness or paralysis of extremities, speech, and understanding of language. Ask about any seizures and for a description of those that occurred. Evaluate airway, breathing, circulation, and LOC. Inspect skin, auscultate the abdomen for bowel sounds, palpate bladder for distention, and determine client's ability to control bowel and bladder. Explore the client's emotional and mental status such as stability of mood, evidence of depression, and motivation for rehabilitation.

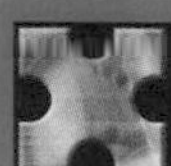

42-1 Client and Family Teaching
Home Care for the Client With a Neurologic Deficit

A teaching plan for the client and family addresses the following key areas and points:

Skin Care

- Explain that the client may not feel discomfort caused by a beginning pressure ulcer.
- Demonstrate how to inspect and care for the skin.
- Recommend a change in position at least every 2 hours to relieve pressure on bony prominences.
- Tell the client to contact a healthcare provider immediately if skin is reddened, warm, or disrupted.

Body Alignment

- Explain the importance of good body alignment.
- Demonstrate how to put joints through a full ROM. Explain that the client must perform ROM exercises several times per day.
- Demonstrate how the client can use various devices, such as rolled blankets or pillows, to support or align areas of the body, such as the back, hips, and legs. Explain the use of a footboard or other device to prevent footdrop.

Nutrition and Fluids

- Discuss the importance of a high fluid intake to prevent urinary tract complications. Recommend taking fluids frequently.
- Discuss the importance of a balanced diet in maintaining optimal health.
- Emphasize that the client may better tolerate small meals and between-meal snacks than three large meals.
- Explain that the client who must be fed needs time to chew the food and take fluids.

Bowel and Bladder

- Stress the importance of continuing a bowel and bladder training program.
- Demonstrate clean rather than sterile technique for irrigating, changing, or inserting catheters at home.
- Advise inspecting the urine for cloudiness (which may indicate a urinary tract infection).
- Recommend contacting the physician if chills and fever occur or if the urine is bloody, cloudy, or has an offensive odor.
- Describe skin care of the genitalia and perineum. Emphasize and demonstrate the special care to be given to the anal area and the genitalia after defecation. If an external urinary sheath is used for the male client, demonstrate its application and how to clean the penis daily to remove urine and dried secretions.

Activity

- Stress the importance of social contacts, hobbies, and changes in the daily routine to relieve boredom.
- Emphasize the importance of avoiding fatigue and exposure to infection.
- Discuss the importance of having the client take deep breaths every 1 or 2 hours while awake and to cough to raise secretions.

Therapies, Community Services, and Equipment

- Discuss the importance of working with the therapists and of following their advice.
- Make the client and family aware of services available for home care.
- Discuss and list the specific types of equipment that will be necessary for home care.
- Provide the names of agencies or retail stores from which the equipment may be purchased, rented, or borrowed.
- Recommend a consultation with a social service worker regarding financial assistance or the availability of loan closets that allow people who need certain types of equipment to borrow these materials.

Diagnosis, Planning, and Interventions

Risk for Impaired Skin or Tissue Integrity related to immobility, incontinence, or other factors (specify)
Expected Outcome: Skin will remain intact and free from infection.

- Inspect pressure points daily; keep skin clean and dry at all times. *Identifies problems. Clean, dry skin reduces bacteria and moisture that promotes their reproduction.*
- Massage bony prominences that blanch when pressure is relieved. *Increases circulation to tissues, bringing oxygen and removing carbon dioxide and cellular wastes. Massage is contraindicated if skin is already impaired, as evidenced by areas that remain reddened with relief of pressure.*
- Use a flotation mattress, sheepskin pads, and other devices to relieve pressure when client is lying and sitting. *The integument becomes impaired when capillary pressure falls below 32 mm Hg* (Fig. 42.1).

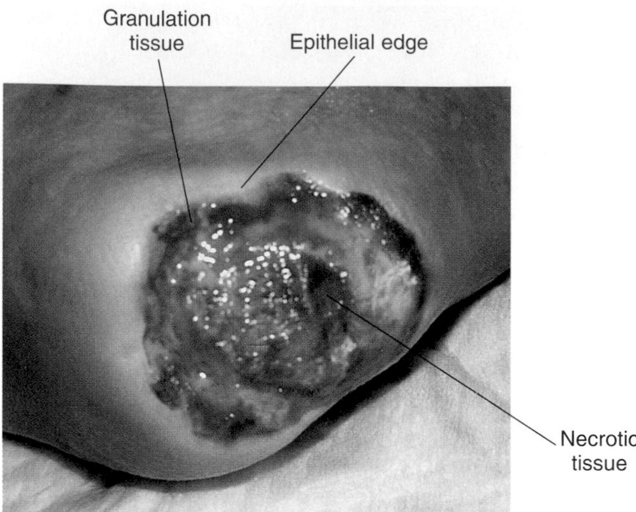

FIGURE 42.1 Pressure ulcer of the elbow in a client with a cerebrovascular accident cared for at home. This client was admitted to the hospital for treatment of multiple pressure ulcers.

- Change client's position every 2 hours. *Relieves pressure over bony prominences and maintains sufficient capillary pressure to keep integument intact.*

Risk for Disuse Syndrome related to musculoskeletal inactivity and neuromuscular impairment

Expected Outcome: Client will maintain ROM in all joints.

- Keep extremities aligned with pillows, trochanter rolls, and splints. *Facilitates functional use of limbs.*
- Perform passive ROM exercises with the weak or paralyzed extremity. *Maintains joint flexibility and prevents permanent contractures (Fig. 42.2).*
- Prevent footdrop with a footboard. *Positions foot and ankle to prevent plantar flexion.*
- Remove and reapply elastic stockings at least twice a day. *Elastic stockings support vein walls, reduce hemostasis, and decrease potential for thrombophlebitis.*

Total Urinary Incontinence or **Urinary Retention** related to effects of disease or injury to the nervous system or spinal cord nerves, loss of bladder tone

Expected Outcome: Client will void, bladder will empty with no urinary retention, or both.

- Use indwelling catheter or intermittent catheterization. *Some neurologic deficits are permanent; urinary elimination and continence may require a catheter.*
- Measure intake and output when client has an indwelling urethral catheter and takes fluids poorly and when first removing an indwelling urethral catheter. *Helps identify whether fluid volume is within normal expectations.*
- Palpate the lower abdomen for bladder distention; notify physician if client cannot void. *The bladder is not palpable unless it becomes distended. The urge to void occurs when the bladder contains 150 to 300 mL; urination needs to occur several times a day to avoid overdistention.*

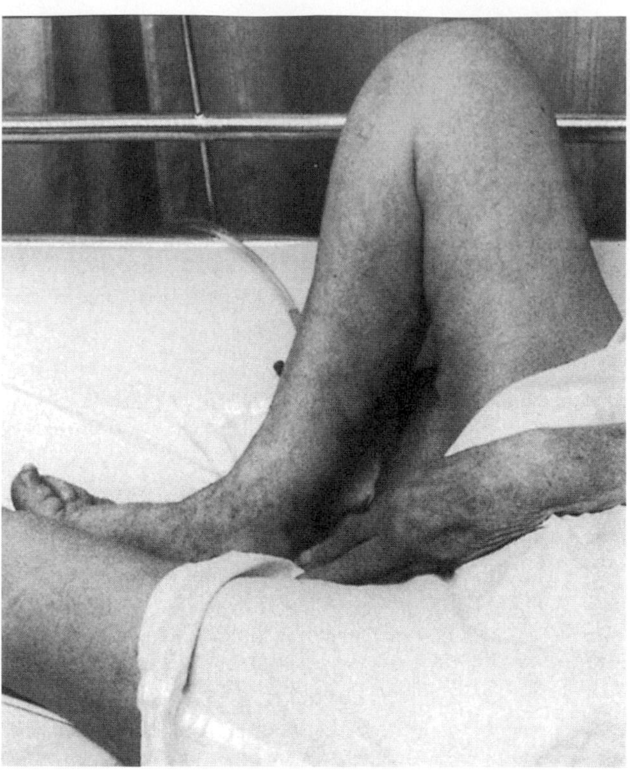

FIGURE 42.2 Contracture of the right leg in a client cared for at home after a cerebrovascular accident. (Photograph by D. Atkinson)

- Have client use incontinence pads or absorbent underwear. *Wicks urine away and keeps bedding dry.*
- Institute a bladder training program as soon as possible (see Chap. 59). *Bladder training promotes urinary continence.*

Impaired Physical Mobility related to muscle weakness and paralysis

Expected Outcome: Client will tolerate increased physical mobility as demonstrated by use of devices for mobility and remain free of contractures.

- Perform active or passive ROM exercises on the affected and unaffected extremities or encourage client to perform ROM exercises independently (Figs. 42.3 and 42.4). *Prevents contractures and muscle atrophy.*
- Regularly position clients with paraplegia or tetraplegia in an upright posture. *Helps client take in the immediate environment and promotes circulation.*
- Apply abdominal binder and elastic stockings before client gets up. *Decreases pooling of blood in distal areas and prevents dizziness and faintness.*
- Suggest using parallel bars or a walker. *Clients can learn to support body weight and move forward with a variety of ambulatory aids.*

Risk for Sexual Dysfunction related to disturbance or loss of nerve function to genitalia

Expected Outcome: Client will explore sexual alternatives.

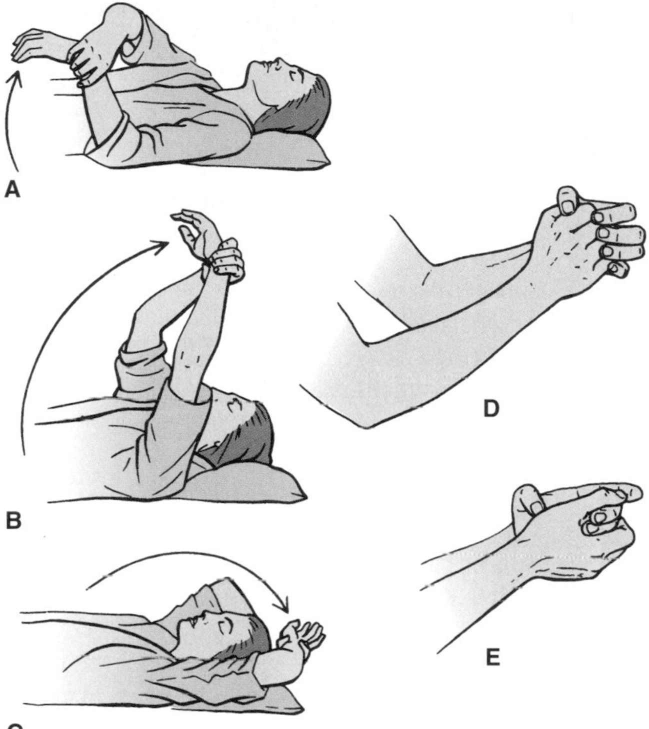

FIGURE 42.3 Exercises of the affected hand and arm that hemiplegic clients can learn to do themselves. (**A–C**) The affected arm is grasped at the wrist by the unaffected hand and is raised over the head. (**D** and **E**) The unaffected hand is slipped into the spastic hand, and each finger is extended slowly in turn.

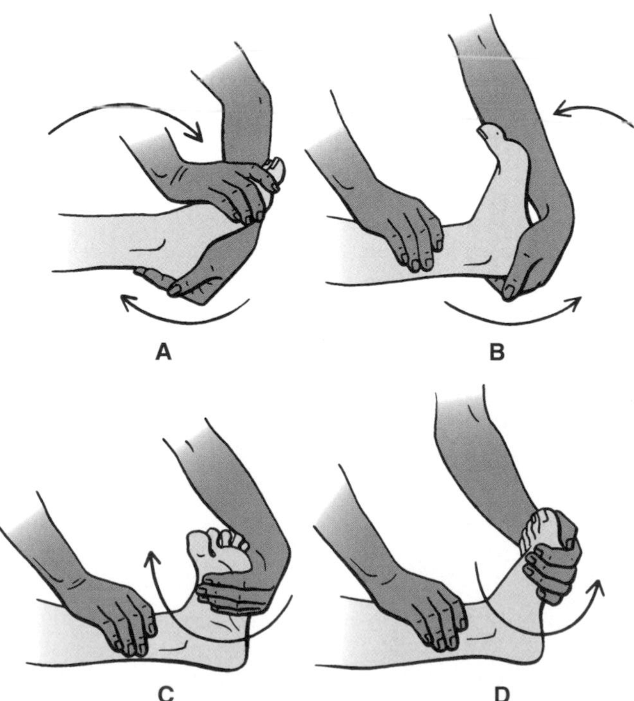

FIGURE 42.4 Range-of-motion exercises for the affected foot in hemiplegia. The motions should be conducted slowly and smoothly, with a momentary pause when spasticity causes resistance. As soon as the client has movement, these exercises can be done actively rather than passively.

- Be alert to subtle references to sexual dysfunction or problems. *Most clients are hesitant to discuss sexuality openly and frankly.*
- Allow client time to talk or ask questions. *Most clients refrain from sexual discussions if they sense the nurse is unreceptive or pressed for time.*
- Convey acceptance; recommend that client and sexual partner speak with a physician or sexual therapist. *May provide alternatives to former sexual activities.*
- Explain to paralyzed men that spontaneous erections may occur when bladder is full. *Spontaneous erections are unpredictable and sometimes circumstantially inconvenient.*
- Offer information about penile implants (see Chap. 55). *Penile implants provide temporary or permanent penile erection, facilitating vaginal penetration during intercourse.*
- Inform paralyzed men that ejaculation is rare, reducing potential for fathering children. *Clients with paraplegia or tetraplegia have the right to information about their potential for fertility.*
- Suggest that having intercourse on a water bed may facilitate sexual activity. *The buoyancy of a water bed promotes pelvic movement.*
- Share that some couples use mutual masturbation or electronic vibrators during sexual activity. *Orgasmic arousal can be achieved using alternatives.*
- Instruct female clients that they are still fertile and may need contraception if pregnancy is undesired. *Motor paralysis does not affect ovulation.*

Risk for Situational Low Self-Esteem related to effects of disability on perception of self-worth

Expected Outcome: Client will maintain positive self-regard, accept changes in body function, express feelings about disability, and participate in rehabilitation.

- Assess for signs of negative responses, such as refusal to discuss loss, lack of participation in care, and increased isolation. *Nonverbal cues provide more reliable feedback about self-regard.*
- Convey respect and hope; encourage verbalization of feelings. *Remaining nonjudgmental and giving the client an opportunity to express feelings help relieve stressors.*
- Help client identify positive attributes and strengths from past experiences. *Focusing on successes rather than failures decreases feelings of helplessness and hopelessness.*
- Identify ways to support client's independence and role in the family. *Helping client maintain his or her previous level of functioning maintains self-esteem.*

Evaluation of Expected Outcomes

Expected outcomes vary, depending on the original goals and nursing diagnoses. The client has no evidence of skin breakdown. Complications associated with inactivity and immobility do not develop. The client works through the grieving process and accepts altered abilities. Defecation and urinary elimination are managed. The client is physically active, as demonstrated by use of trapeze, wheelchair, and other methods for mobility. The client continues sexual activities or learns about sexual alternatives. The client participates in decision-making regarding daily activities, social outlets, vocational options, and applicable therapies.

GENERAL GERONTOLOGIC CONSIDERATIONS

Older adults with a neurologic deficit may lack an adequate support system once they are discharged from the hospital. Involve social services and other agencies to assist clients and caregivers with rehabilitation.

Functional problems that accompany aging may complicate recovery for a client with a neurologic deficit. For example, an age-related delay in the relaxation of the internal bladder sphincter can make bladder training more difficult.

Older adults cannot perform activities or answer as quickly as younger adults. Therefore, they may become frustrated, irritable, or depressed when they cannot respond quickly. To prevent frustration and depression, allow extra time for older adults to answer questions, perform activities, and so forth.

Regularly palpate the bladder of an older adult for distention. A behavior change or irritability may be the only sign of urinary retention in older adults with a neurologic deficit.

Critical Thinking Exercises

1. *Discuss methods to help clients achieve success in a bowel and bladder training program.*
2. *A client had a CVA 6 months ago and is paralyzed on his right side. He cannot speak and shows signs of mental changes. He now appears agitated and is making motions with his left hand to various areas of his body, mainly his abdomen. What assessments could you make to determine the possible cause of his agitation?*
3. *A 22-year-old client had a spinal cord injury at T11 and is paraplegic. During a conference, team members mention his depression and withdrawal. What other members of the healthcare team and services may be helpful in this client's care?*

• NCLEX-STYLE REVIEW QUESTIONS 

1. A client is in the skilled rehabilitation setting during the early phase of rehabilitation. When devising the client's nursing plan of care, which long-term goal would be most appropriate?
   1. The client will maintain adequate nutritional status.
   2. The client will exhibit no skin breakdown or contractures.
   3. The client will exhibit no signs of clinical depression.
   4. The client will function using all extremities.
2. A home care nurse is teaching a client and family about coping with a recent disability. They have identified several needs. Which of the following interventions would be most important for the nurse to address first?
   1. Identify for the client and family solutions to their stated needs.
   2. Encourage outside assistance from community agencies and resources.
   3. Assist the client and family to identify solutions and attainable goals.
   4. Call the physician and ask for suggestions on solving the needs.

connection

Visit the Connection site at **http://connection.lww.com/go/timbyEssentials** for links to chapter-related resources on the Internet.

References and Suggested Readings

Booth, J., Davidson, I., Winstanley, J., et al. (2001). Observing washing and dressing of stroke patients: Nursing intervention compared with occupational therapists. What is the difference? *Journal of Advanced Nursing, 33,* 98–105.

Hickey, J. V. (2002). *The clinical practice of neurological and neurosurgical nursing* (5th ed.). Philadelphia: Lippincott Williams & Wilkins.

Hobart, J. C., & Thompson, A. J. (2001). The five item Barthel Index. *Journal of Neurology, Neurosurgery, and Psychiatry, 71,* 258–261.

Thorn, S. (2000). Neurological rehabilitation nursing: A review of the research. *Journal of Advanced Nursing, 31,* 1029–1038.

Timby, B. K. (2005). *Fundamental skills and concepts in patient care* (8th ed.). Philadelphia: Lippincott Williams & Wilkins.

chapter 43

Caring for Clients With Eye Disorders

Words to Know 

accommodation	*keratoplasty*
astigmatism	*myopia*
cataract	*near point*
central vision	*nystagmus*
conjunctivitis	*ophthalmoscopy*
corneal transplantation	*photophobia*
corneal trephine	*presbyopia*
diplopia	*proptosis*
emmetropia	*ptosis*
endophthalmitis	*refraction*
enucleation	*retinal detachment*
glaucoma	*tonometry*
hordeolum	*trabeculoplasty*
hyperopia	*visual acuity*
intraocular lens implant	*visual field examination*
iridectomy	*visually impaired*
keratitis	

Learning Objectives

On completion of this chapter, the reader will:

- Describe the basic anatomy and physiology of the eyes.
- Explain different types of refractive errors.
- Differentiate between the terms *blindness* and *visually impaired.*
- Identify appropriate nursing interventions for a blind client.
- Discuss the nursing management of clients with eye trauma.
- Describe the technique for instilling ophthalmic medications.
- Explain how different infectious and inflammatory eye disorders are acquired.
- Specify visual changes that result from delayed or unsuccessful treatment of macular degeneration.
- Differentiate between open-angle and angle-closure glaucoma.
- Distinguish categories and mechanisms of actions of medications used to control intraocular pressure.
- Identify a category of drugs contraindicated in clients with glaucoma.
- Name activities clients with glaucoma should avoid because they elevate intraocular pressure.
- Describe methods for improving vision after a cataract is removed.
- Discuss postoperative measures that help prevent complications after a cataract extraction.
- Give classic symptoms associated with a retinal detachment.
- Discuss the care and cleaning of an eye prosthesis.

This chapter presents the structure and function of the eyes. It also discusses the most important disorders that can affect the eyes, as well as accompanying treatment and nursing care measures.

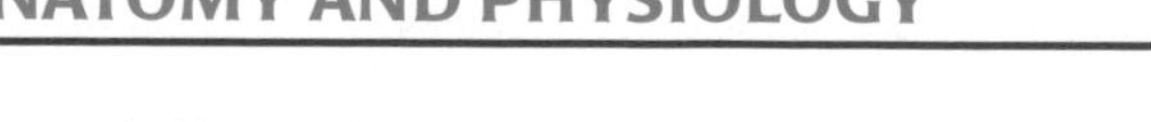

ANATOMY AND PHYSIOLOGY

The *eyeballs* are globes located in a protective bony cavity or *orbit* of the skull. Frontal, maxillary, zygomatic, sphenoid, ethmoid, lacrimal, and palatine bones form the walls of the orbit. Fat and muscle protect posterior, superior, inferior, and lateral aspects of each eyeball.

Muscles that permit movement include the superior and inferior rectus (move eye up and down), the medial and lateral rectus (move eye toward nose and temple), and the superior and inferior oblique muscles (move eye to left and right). Six cranial nerves innervate the eye, ocular muscles, and lacrimal apparatus: the optic, oculomotor, trochlear, trigeminal, abducens, and facial cranial nerves.

Extraocular Structures

The eyelids, eyelashes, and tears protect the anterior or exposed surface of the eye. The upper and lower eyelids are folds of skin that meet at an angle referred to as the *canthus.* The outer or lateral canthus is the outer angle, and the inner or medial canthus is at the inner aspect of the eye. The line between the lateral and medial canthus usually is horizontal. Children with Down syndrome have a line that slants upward and outward. People of Asian descent have an epicanthal fold, which is a fold of skin that covers the inner canthus.

Eyelids protect against foreign bodies and adjust the amount of light entering the eye. Eyelashes trap foreign debris. Periodic blinking clears dust and particles from the surface of the eyes. Eyelids also spread tears over the surface of the eye and have multiple glands, including sebaceous, sweat, and accessory lacrimal glands. They are lined with a sensitive, transparent mucous membrane called *conjunctiva.* This membrane extends from the lid margins and meets the *cornea* (the transparent domelike structure that covers most of the anterior portion of the eyeball) at the *limbus,* the outermost edge of the iris. The lacrimal *caruncle* is a small, reddish elevation on the conjunctiva located at the inner canthus.

Tears, composed of water, sodium chloride, and lysozyme, an antibacterial enzyme, are produced by *lacrimal (tear) glands* found beneath the bony orbital ridge. The *lacrimal apparatus* includes the lacrimal glands, *punctum, lacrimal canals, lacrimal sac,* and *nasolacrimal ducts.* Tears flow across the eyes, continually bathing and lubricating the surface. Tears drain through the punctum into the lacrimal canals and lacrimal sac to nasolacrimal ducts, tiny openings at the junction of the upper and lower lids, and then into the nose (Fig. 43.1).

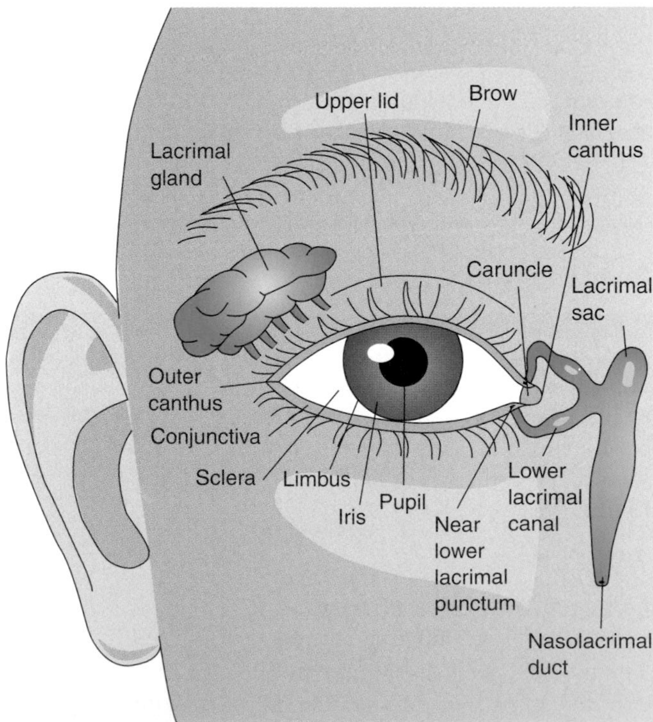

FIGURE 43.1 External structures of the eye and position of the lacrimal structures. (From Smeltzer, S. C. & Bare, B. G. [2004]. *Brunner & Suddarth's textbook of medical–surgical nursing* [10th ed.]. Philadelphia: Lippincott Williams & Wilkins.)

Intraocular Structures

Three layers form intraocular structures. The first layer is the *sclera,* commonly referred to as the "white of the eye." It is composed of tough connective tissue. The sclera protects structures in the eye. It connects directly to the cornea, anterior chamber, iris, and pupil.

The middle layer is the *uvea,* or vascular coat of the eye, located immediately under the sclera. The uvea includes the *choroid* (contains blood vessels and darkly pigmented cells that prevent light from scattering inside the eye) and the *iris* (the highly vascular, pigmented portion of the eye surrounding the pupil). The *pupil* is an opening that dilates and constricts in response to light. *Aqueous humor* is a nutrient-rich liquid that nourishes eye structures. Ciliary muscles help change the shape of the lens when adjusting to near or far vision. The *anterior chamber,* behind the cornea, is filled with clear aqueous humor, providing nourishment to the cornea. The lens lies behind the pupil and iris.

The *posterior chamber* is a small space behind the lens. Aqueous fluid flows from the posterior chamber to the anterior chamber. It then drains into the *canal of Schlemm.*

Vitreous humor is thick, gelatinous material that maintains the spherical shape of the eyeball and placement of the retina (Fig. 43.2). The *retina,* the innermost layer of the eye, is composed of a pigmented outer layer and an inner neurosensory layer. Light stimulates this neurosensory layer, which contains nerve cells called *rods* and *cones.* Rods function in night or dim light and assist in distinguishing black and white. Cones function in bright light and are sensitive to color. Nerve cells of the retina extend from the optic nerve.

The *macula lutea,* or the "yellow spot," is composed of cones and allows for detailed vision. It is in the center of the retina. The *fovea centralis* is at the center of the macula. The blood vessels are displaced from the fovea centralis, allowing light to pass to the cones. Density of cones decreases away from the fovea centralis, as the number of rods increases in the periphery of the retina. The *optic disc,* the anterior surface of the optic nerve, is easily distinguished from the macula because of the vasculature that radiates from the optic disc. No blood vessels radiate directly from the macula (Fig. 43.3). The macula is the area of the eye that provides **central vision,** the ability to discriminate letters, words, and details of any image. If the macula degenerates or is damaged, only the ability to see movement and gross objects in the peripheral fields of vision remains.

Visual Function

The primary function of the eyeball is to "transform light energy into nerve signals that can be transmitted to the

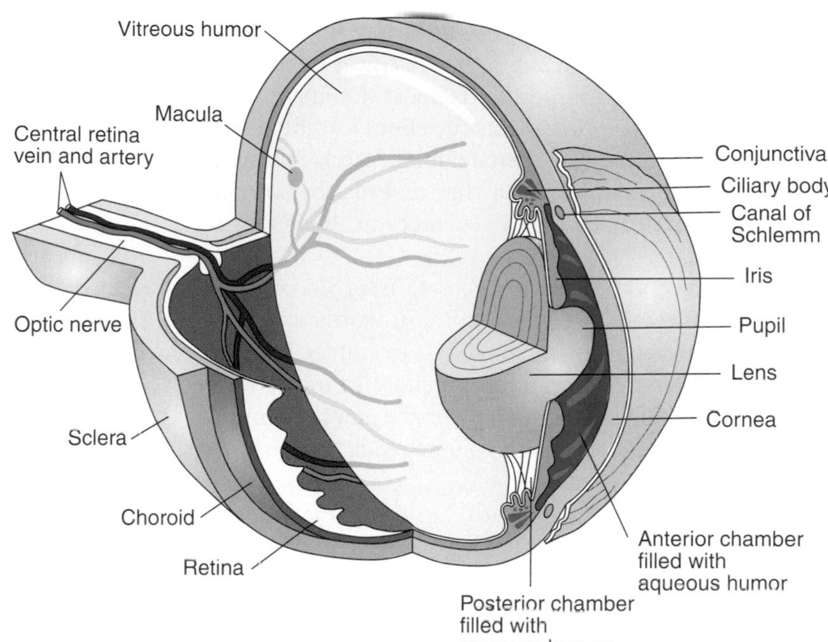

FIGURE 43.2 Three-dimensional cross-section of the eye. (From Smeltzer, S. C. & Bare, B. G. [2004]. *Brunner & Suddarth's textbook of medical–surgical nursing* [10th ed.]. Philadelphia: Lippincott Williams & Wilkins.)

cerebral cortex for interpretation" (Porth, 2002, p. 1242). Every object reflects light. For a person to see it clearly, reflected light must pass through the intraocular structures—the cornea, anterior chamber, pupil, lens, and vitreous humor. These structures cause **refraction,** which means that light rays bend and change speed. The lens focuses light into an upside-down and reversed image on the retina. Rods and cones in the retina send nerve impulses by way of the optic nerve and optic tract to the visual cortex of the occipital lobe. This is where the image is interpreted.

The lens is more convex on the posterior side and can change shape, a process known as **accommodation.** The ciliary muscles contract or relax to focus an image onto the retina, allowing one to clearly see distant or near objects. For viewing distant objects, ciliary muscles relax and the lens flattens. The opposite occurs to view objects that are closer. The closest point a person can clearly focus on an object is called the **near point.** Aging results in loss of lens elasticity and makes use of reading glasses for near vision necessary. When the lens becomes opaque, as when a cataract forms, light is blocked from reaching the macula and the visual image becomes blurred or cloudy.

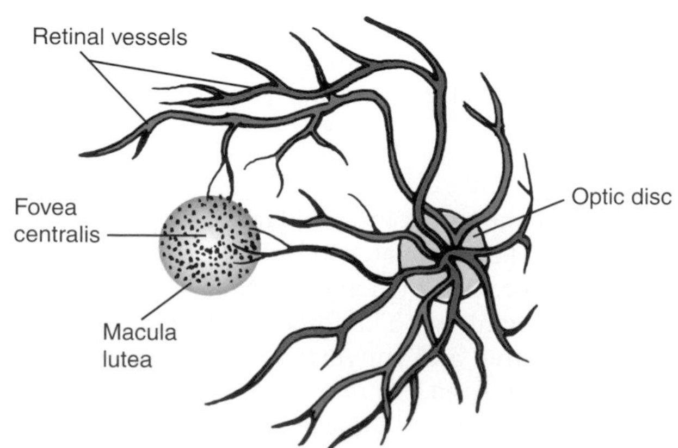

FIGURE 43.3 Structures of the optic disc, including the macular region.

ASSESSMENT

The ophthalmic assessment provides information about a client's eye health. Nurses usually examine the client's external eye appearance, pupil responses, and eye movements, as well as obtain information about the client's ophthalmic condition. For more complex examinations, nurses need additional education or training. Ongoing eye examinations and treatment require the care of specialists, such as ophthalmologists and optometrists.

Visual Screening Tests

The *Snellen eye chart* is a simple screening tool for determining **visual acuity,** the ability to see far images clearly. With the chart 20 feet away, the examiner asks the client to identify letters of decreasing size. Results are expressed as a fraction that compares the client's vision with standard norms. If a client has 20/20 vision, it means that he or she sees letters at 20 feet that others see clearly and accurately at 20 feet; a client with 20/40 vision sees letters at 20 feet that most others can read at 40 feet, and so on.

If the client cannot identify even the largest letters on the chart, the examiner asks him or her to count the number of fingers that the examiner holds up. If the finger count is inaccurate, the examiner tests the client's ability to distinguish light from dark. Visual acuity also is measured with a computerized refractor that records the strength and type of lenses necessary to correct the client's visual problem.

A *Jaeger chart* or *Rosenbaum Pocket Vision Screener* evaluates near vision. These charts contain words, numbers, and letters in various print sizes. The examiner instructs the client to hold the chart approximately 14 inches away and read the smallest print that he or she can see comfortably. The size of the print the client reads indicates the quality of his or her near vision.

Color vision is assessed with *Ishihara polychromatic plates*. The client receives a series of cards on which the pattern of a number is embedded in a circle of colored dots. The numbers are in colors that color-blind individuals commonly cannot see. Clients with normal vision readily identify the numbers.

Stop, Think, and Respond • BOX 43-1

A client asks you what 20/200 visual acuity means. What is the best explanation?

Nursing Assessment

The objective of obtaining a history is to identify specific problems the client is experiencing and possible causes. Box 43-1 lists questions that nurses may ask when taking an ocular history. Gather information related to eye problems: past and current ability to see; any discomfort, pain, or other symptoms; how long the client has experienced problems; any treatments and medications; and other illnesses that may affect eye health. It is important to include questions about previous eye trauma.

After the interview, inspect the eyes for symmetry. Also observe lid margins for signs of inflammation, exudate, or loss of eyelashes. Determine the pupil size, and their change and response to light. Normal pupils are round, of equal size, and constrict simultaneously when stimulated. Check the extraocular muscles by asking client to keep his or her head still while following an object moved up, down, left, and right. Other observations include looking for **ptosis,** which is a drooping upper eyelid; **proptosis,** which is an extended or protruded upper eyelid that delays closing or remains partially open; and **nystagmus,** which is uncontrolled oscillating movement of the eyeball.

BOX 43-1 • Questions to Ask During an Eye Assessment

- Are you having any problems with your eyes?
- Do you have any problems with your vision? Do you wear glasses or contact lenses?
- Have you experienced blurred, double, or distorted vision?
- Do you have any pain? Is it sharp or dull? Is it worse when you blink?
- Do you have any itching or feeling that something is in your eye?
- Is there any discharge? What does it look like?
- Are both eyes affected?
- How long have you had this problem?
- Has this happened before?
- What have you done to treat the problem?
- Does anything make the problem better or worse?
- What medications have you used to treat the eye problem?
- Do you have any other diseases or conditions?
- What medications are you taking?
- Have you ever had eye surgery? What? When?
- Do any family members have any eye conditions?
- Do you have any problems with seasonal conjunctivitis (inflammation of the conjunctiva) associated with hay fever?

Diagnostic Studies

Ophthalmoscopy

Direct **ophthalmoscopy** examines the fundus or interior of the eye. It is done with a direct ophthalmoscope, an instrument that illuminates the internal surface of the eyes and allows the examiner to see the lens, retina, retinal blood vessels, and optic disc under magnification.

Indirect ophthalmoscopy uses an instrument that produces a bright, intense light. The ophthalmologist uses this instrument in conjunction with an ophthalmoscope to see larger areas of the retina, although no magnification is involved.

Retinoscopy

Use of a *retinoscope* and trial lenses determines the focusing power of each eye. A retinoscope is a hand-held instrument producing a line of light. The light appears distorted in the eyes of clients with refractive errors. Trial lenses of varying refractive powers are then placed in front of the eye until the light streak does not deviate in any direction.

Tonometry

Tonometry measures intraocular pressure (IOP). It is done by using a tonometer to indent or flatten the surface of the eye. The principle is that a soft eye indents more than a hard eye. The force that produces indentation is measured and converted to a pressure reading. Normal IOP is 10 to 21 mm Hg. High readings indicate high IOP; low readings indicate low pressure (Smeltzer & Bare, 2004).

There are various methods for performing tonometry. Two methods require a topical anesthetic solution to be instilled in the lower conjunctival sac. Anesthesia begins almost immediately and lasts a few minutes. The client does not feel the tonometer while the eye is anesthetized. A *noncontact* tonometer, although less accurate, blows a puff of air against the cornea, and no local anesthetic is required.

Visual Field Examination

A **visual field examination** measures peripheral vision and detects gaps in the visual field. The client fixes his or her gaze on a stationary point straight ahead. A light or white object is moved from a point on the side, where it cannot be seen, toward the center. The client indicates at which point he or she sees the stimulus without directly looking at it. Certain disorders, such as glaucoma, stroke, brain tumor, or retinal detachment, are associated with changes in the visual field.

Slit-Lamp Examination

A *slit lamp* is a binocular microscope that magnifies the surface of the eye. A beam of light, narrowed to a slit, is directed at the cornea, facilitating examination of structures and fluid in the anterior segment of the eye. This examination identifies disorders such as corneal abrasions, iritis, conjunctivitis, and cataracts.

Retinal Angiography

Retinal angiography detects vascular changes and blood flow through retinal vessels. Sodium fluorescein, a water-soluble dye, is injected into a peripheral vein. The examiner uses a special camera to photograph the appearance and distribution of the dye in the retinal arteries, capillaries, and veins at 1-second intervals. The photographs provide a record of vascular filling and emptying defects. Many conditions affect retinal circulation, such as diabetes mellitus, hypertension, drug toxicity, tumors, and acquired immunodeficiency syndrome. Intravenous fluorescein causes skin to yellow slightly for 6 to 8 hours. The urine also turns bright yellow, but the color becomes less noticeable over the following 24 to 36 hours as the dye is excreted.

Ultrasonography

Ultrasonography is used when pathologic changes such as an opaque lens, cloudy cornea, or bloody vitreous make it difficult to look directly at the posterior of the eye. Using sound waves, the contour and shape of contents in the eye are imaged and recorded. After instillation of anesthetic ophthalmic drops, an ultrasound probe is placed on the cornea and a recording is made on an oscilloscope. This technique is helpful in detecting eye lesions and measuring for an intraocular lens implant before extracting a cataract.

Retinal Imaging

A new ophthalmologic screening tool uses a *retinal imaging* system to produce a high-resolution image of almost the entire retina without having to dilate the pupil. The Panoramic 200 Non-mydriatic Scanning Laser Ophthalmoscope (Optos, Dunfermline, Scotland) can detect retinal disorders such as diabetic retinopathy, and provides an excellent baseline screening test (Scerra, 2000).

IMPAIRED VISION

• REFRACTIVE ERRORS

Emmetropia, or normal vision, means that light rays are bent to focus images precisely on the retina. In refractive errors, vision is impaired because light rays are not sharply focused on the retina (Fig. 43.4). Refractive errors include myopia, hyperopia, presbyopia, and astigmatism. Refractive errors are inherited or occur as a result of surgical treatment of disorders of the cornea or lens. Presbyopia occurs because of degenerative changes.

Pathophysiology and Etiology

Myopia is nearsightedness, causing people to hold things close to their eyes to see them clearly. It occurs in people with elongated eyeballs. Light rays focus in the vitreous humor before they reach the retina. Myopic persons cannot focus sharply on a distant object. **Hyperopia,** farsightedness, occurs in people with shortened eyeballs. Light rays focus at a theoretical point behind the retina. Clients with hyperopia can see things better at a distance.

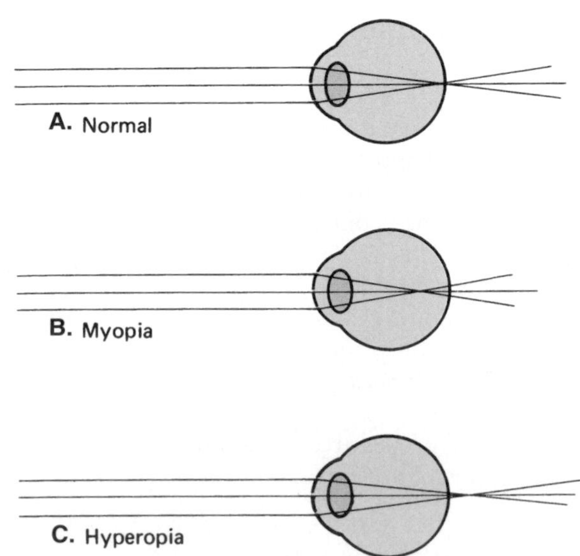

FIGURE 43.4 Ocular focusing of parallel light rays.

Presbyopia occurs with aging and creates difficulty with seeing things at close range. Clients experiencing presbyopia hold reading material or handwork at a distance to see it more clearly. It is caused by gradual loss of elasticity of the lens, leading to decreased ability to accommodate, or focus, for near vision. Presbyopia occurs gradually.

Astigmatism is visual distortion resulting from unequal curvatures in the shape of the cornea. Parallel rays do not focus perfectly on the retina, but instead are bent at different angles and not focused at a single point. Many people have both astigmatism and myopia or hyperopia.

Assessment Findings

People with refractive errors experience blurred vision. Some seek help for recurrent headaches caused by straining to see clearly.

Refractive errors are detected with the Snellen and Jaeger charts. During retinoscopy, the vision of myopes improves when concave trial lenses correct the focusing power of the eyes. Hyperopes experience improvement when convex lenses are used. The amount of power needed to improve visual acuity indicates the degree of refractive error. The refractive error is not always the same in both eyes.

Medical Management

Refractive errors usually are corrected with eyeglasses or contact lenses, which bend light rays to compensate for the refractive error. People with recurrent eye infections, low tear production, or severe allergic reactions may have trouble wearing contact lenses.

Surgical Management

Incisional radial keratotomy (RK) is a surgical procedure to correct refractive disorders. Under local anesthesia, the cornea is reshaped by making incisions. The eye surgeon makes incisions to make a flatter cornea for myopic clients and a more cone-shaped cornea for hyperopic clients. This enables light rays to converge directly at the back of the retina. This procedure has complications, including infection and increased glare from microscarring of the cornea. Some clients report worse vision after surgery. When successful, clients no longer need to wear corrective lenses.

Two newer procedures are similar but use laser to achieve the desired results:

- *Laser-assisted in situ keratomileusis (LASIK)*—The eye surgeon uses a surgical instrument to create a corneal flap, which is gently folded back to expose the inner cornea. A cool-beam laser then resculpts the cornea and the flap is returned to its original position.
- *Photorefractive keratectomy (PRK)*—This procedure involves the removal of the epithelial layer (top surface) of the cornea, exposing the inner cornea. This allows a computer-assisted laser to resculpt the curvature of the eye.

Both procedures potentially provide complete correction of refractive errors, but can result in overcorrection or undercorrection. Other complications include decentered ablation, dry eye syndrome, epithelial abrasion, or infection. With LASIK, complications include wrinkles in the flap, debris under the flap, a displaced flap, or infection or inflammation of the flap.

Nursing Management

Nurses in pediatric offices, industrial sites, community school systems, and public health clinics perform screening examinations and refer clients to eye specialists. They are instrumental in teaching clients how to care for corrective lenses and remove and clean contact lenses. Nurses provide preoperative and postoperative care and teach clients about postoperative care at home. Nursing Guidelines 43-1 provides some postoperative teaching points for clients having LASIK or PRK.

● BLINDNESS

Blindness is a legal term for visual acuity of 20/200 or less even with corrective lenses. The term **visually impaired** is used to describe visual acuity between 20/70 and 20/200 in the better eye with use of glasses. Many who are considered blind perceive light and motion. People with severe loss of visual field also are referred to as blind. Blindness can be congenital or caused by injury, a high fever that damages the optic nerve, or disorders such as cataracts, glaucoma, retinal detachment, macular degeneration, and tumors. See Chapter 8 for further discussion of impaired vision.

Medical Management

Vision is improved to its maximum extent with corrective lenses. Clients who are severely visually impaired or blind are referred to a rehabilitation center or other resource for supportive services. Blind or nearly blind clients are taught skills for independent living, how to use a cane for mobility, and how to read and write Braille, a system that uses raised dots to form letters of the alphabet and numbers. Some individuals use trained guide dogs.

NURSING GUIDELINES 43-1

Postoperative Teaching for Clients Having LASIK or PRK Surgery

LASIK

- Stitches are not needed—the corneal flap remains in place through natural eye pressure.
- Antibiotic eyedrops are ordered for up to 1 week to prevent infection.
- The client may resume normal activity within 3 days but must avoid strenuous exercise for 1 week.
- Avoid rubbing eyes for about 1 week.
- Healing occurs within 1 week, but it may take 1 to 3 months for vision to fully stabilize.
- Clients may initially experience discomfort for 5 to 6 hours after the procedure. They may use nonsteroidal anti-inflammatory drugs for relief.

PRK

- Antibiotic and anti-inflammatory eye medications are ordered for 2 to 5 days after surgery.
- Clear contact lenses are placed on each eye for 2 to 5 days to prevent infection.
- The epithelial layer begins to regenerate in 2 to 5 days, but complete healing takes 3 to 4 months.
- Avoid rubbing eyes for at least several weeks.
- Avoid strenuous exercise for 1 week.
- Clients may require pain medication for 1 to 2 days after surgery because of pain fibers located on the surface of the cornea.

NURSING PROCESS

The Client Who Is Blind

Assessment

In addition to assessing the degree of the client's impairment, ask questions about how the client is coping with his or her visual problems. Grief is a normal response to being newly blind or having severely compromised vision. Anger or sadness is a typical reaction as clients face disability. Help and support clients during depression. It is therapeutic to acknowledge grief rather than attempt to cheer clients. Another helpful approach is to express confidence that the client has inner resources to deal with adversity.

Diagnosis, Planning, and Interventions

One of the nurse's most important roles is to help a visually impaired client achieve independence. Whether the condition is temporary because both eyes are patched, or permanent, the following measures are appropriate:

- Introduce yourself each time you enter the room because many voices sound similar.
- Call client by name during group conversations because the blind client cannot see to whom questions or comments are directed.
- Speak before touching client.
- Tell client when you are leaving the room.

In addition, care of a client who is blind or whose vision is severely impaired includes, but is not limited to, the following:

Disturbed Sensory Perception: Visual related to impaired vision

Expected Outcome: Client will independently complete activities of daily living (ADLs).

- Ask client's preference for where to store hygiene articles and other objects needed for self-care. *Promotes client's control over environment.*
- Keep personal care items in the same location at all times. *Provides client with ability to locate toiletries easily.*
- Move food items from tray to a larger surface area. *Facilitates locating food and eating.*
- At mealtimes, describe where food is on the plate using the positions on the face of a clock. *Assists the client to identify location of food.*
- Offer to open containers, butter bread, and so forth. *Allowing client a choice facilitates independence.*

Risk for Injury related to compromised vision

Expected Outcome: The client will remain free of trauma.

- Orient client to physical environment. *Assists the client to remain familiar with environment and avoid injury.*
- Indicate location of the signal cord for obtaining nursing assistance. *Facilitates client's ability to get help.*
- Keep doors fully open rather than ajar. *Helps maintain a safe environment.*
- Help client feel where door to bathroom is located. *Promotes independence and prevents injury.*
- Remove chairs or objects in the client's walking pathway. *Maintains a safe environment.*
- Instruct client to grasp your elbow and walk slightly behind and to side when ambulating. *Helps client feel secure and ensures safety.*

Situational Low Self-Esteem related to impaired adjustment to loss of vision

Expected Outcome: Client will redevelop a positive self-image.

- Call attention to tasks client successfully performs without assistance if client focuses on self-pity. *Promotes positive feelings about ability to care for self.*
- Help client clarify activities that are essential and then develop a plan for mastering each one. *Reduces frustration and systematically helps client achieve short-term goals.*
- Review progress to nurture self-confidence, self-reliance, and improved self-image. *Promotes a positive self-image.*

Deficient Diversional Activity related to transition from sighted to nonsighted

Expected Outcome: Client will develop interests in activities that contribute to enjoyment and enrichment of life.

- Refer partially sighted client to public library where large-print editions of books and magazines are available, as well as "talking books" (recordings of printed books). *Diversional activities must be tailored to the client's abilities.*
- Suggest that the partially sighted client use a magnifying lens to read. *Enables client to enhance sight.*
- Contact or refer clients who can read Braille to special agencies for books, Braille typewriters, and other assistive devices. *Assists client to reach maximum potential.*
- Inform client about availability of optical scanners that use synthesized voice. *Scanners make it possible for the client to "read" printed materials.*
- Tell client that telephone companies exempt visually impaired customers from directory assistance charges and offer a "talking" yellow pages information service. *Providing clients with information about available resources assists them to achieve more independence.*
- Instruct client that laws prohibit exclusion of patrons with guide dogs from public restaurants, public transportation, schools, and places for entertainment. *Possessing accurate knowledge assists clients to make informed decisions.*

Evaluation of Expected Outcomes

The client can perform self-care activities. He or she remains free of injury and demonstrates an ability to arrange for outside support to meet needs. The client expresses more positive feelings about ability to meet needs independently. The client begins to access resources that provide diversional activities and support.

● EYE TRAUMA

Trauma or injury to the eye and surrounding structures can result in decreased or total loss of vision.

Pathophysiology and Etiology

Children and adults are subject to eye injuries from wind, sun, chemical sprays, direct blows to the eye, lacerations, and penetrating objects. Cell and tissue injury causes inflammation. Secondary infections may follow the initial injury. When trauma involves the cornea, scar tissue may affect refraction of light. If the capsule that contains the lens is damaged, aqueous fluid and vitreous penetrate the lens, causing it to become an opaque cataract. Penetrating trauma can lead to **endophthalmitis,** a condition in which all three layers of the eye and the vitreous are inflamed; removal of the eye may be necessary.

Assessment Findings

The injured eye is painful or described as feeling "gritty." There is tearing, and the client usually tries to relieve discomfort by squeezing the eyelids closed. The effort helps to control eye movement and reduces light entering the eye. Vision may be blurred. If the bony orbit is fractured, the eyes may appear asymmetric and the client has **diplopia** (double vision).

A blow to or near the eye results in swelling and bleeding into soft tissues with ultimate discoloration (black eye). Hemorrhage may be observed in the subconjunctival tissue. The eye may appear to recede into the orbit, with a change in normal size or shape of the iris or pupil. Adjacent lid structures may be lacerated, bloody, and swollen. Shining a penlight obliquely across the eye detects an obvious or obscured foreign body. Sometimes the upper lid must be everted to detect an object trapped beneath (Fig. 43.5). If treatment is delayed, purulent drainage may be in the conjunctival sac.

Staining the eye surface with fluorescein dye identifies a minute foreign body or abrasion to the cornea. A slit-lamp examination provides magnification and light to visualize structures in the anterior and posterior segments. Radiography and computed tomography help find

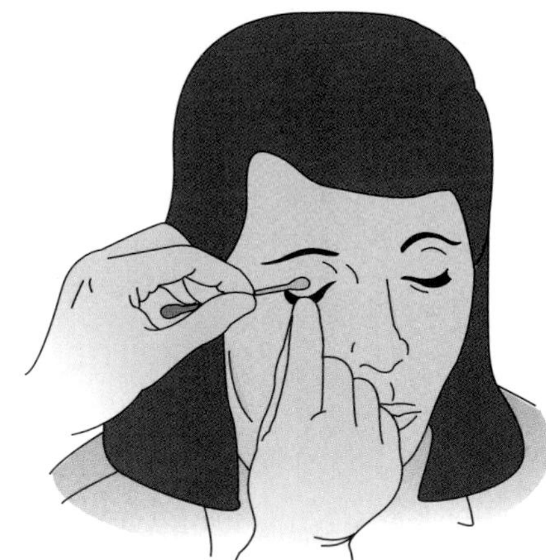

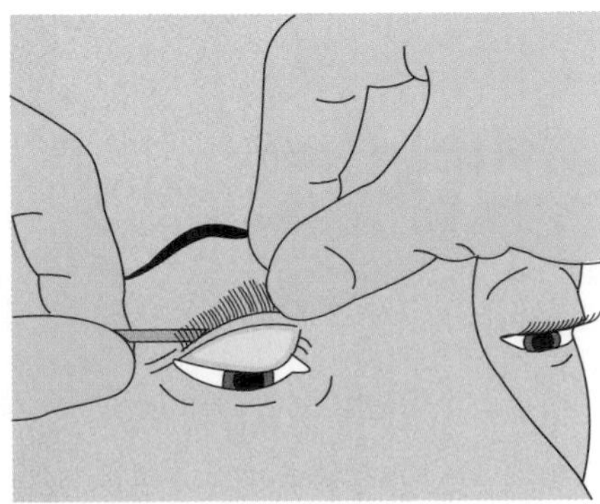

FIGURE 43.5 To evert the eyelid, the client looks down, and the eyelash is grasped and pulled up as a cotton-tipped applicator is pressed gently above the eyelid fold. The eyelid resumes its normal position when the client looks upward or the eyelash is pulled gently forward.

a penetrating foreign body. A radiograph confirms an orbital fracture.

Medical and Surgical Management

After emergency first aid, the eye is anesthetized to ease examination. Antibiotic ointment or drops are instilled, and the eye is patched. Clients with blunt trauma are hospitalized to reduce danger of intraocular complications. To repair a laceration of the eyelid, the physician injects a local anesthetic and lid margins are approximated with sutures. A cut on the eyeball, especially the cornea, is serious and requires immediate treatment. Surgery is performed if internal eye structures are damaged.

Nursing Management

If trauma does not involve gross injury, gently inspect the eye. Darken the room and direct a penlight at the eye to inspect for presence of a foreign body. If none is found, evert the lower lid, instruct the client to look up, and inspect the inferior conjunctival sac using direct vision or magnification. If this fails to locate a foreign body, evert the upper lid and direct the client to look down. If possible, perform a gross vision assessment.

To prevent eye trauma, recommend use of glasses with shatter-resistant lenses or safety goggles while working with substances that can injure the eyes. When eye trauma occurs, obtain a brief history of the type or cause of injury from the client or a family member. If eye pain is severe, or if the client cannot or is unwilling to permit an initial examination, loosely patch both eyes and refer the client immediately for medical treatment. If a foreign body is present, pressure on the eye may push the object into the tissues of the eyeball.

It is important to reduce a client's pain. Irrigating eyes, dimming lights, closing and patching both eyes, or initially applying cool compresses or ice packs help to decrease pain. Anesthetic eyedrops are administered according to physician's orders. If the client experienced a chemical injury, flushing eyes with running water is crucial to neutralize chemical effects and prevent tissue ulceration. Flushing generally takes 10 to 15 minutes. To prevent secondary infection, scrupulous handwashing is needed. Administer antibiotic ointment or drops per orders, and change eye dressings as indicated, using aseptic technique.

The following instructions are for home care and instilling eye medications:

- Wash hands thoroughly.
- Wipe lids and lashes in a direction away from nose with a moistened, soft gauze pad, paper tissue, or cotton ball. Use a separate item for each wipe.
- Pull the tissue near cheek downward, forming a sac in the lower lid.
- Tilt head slightly backward and toward eye in which medication is to be instilled.
- Do not allow the tip of container to touch eye.
- Instill prescribed number of drops into conjunctival pocket, or apply a thin ribbon of ointment directly into the conjunctival pocket, beginning at inner corner and moving outward.
- Close eye gently.
- Wipe away excess medication.
- Secure dressing to face with tape and use an eye shield for additional protection, especially at night.
- Do not rub eye, and visit an ophthalmologist or return to emergency department if it is not completely comfortable within a short time.
- Keep all follow-up visits to check condition of eye and surrounding structures.

> **Stop, Think, and Respond • BOX 43-2**
>
> *You are accompanying a group of 10-year-olds on a field trip. One of the boys runs into a tree branch and immediately starts crying and holding his eye, stating that something is stuck in it. What action should you take?*

INFECTIOUS AND INFLAMMATORY EYE DISORDERS

• CONJUNCTIVITIS

Conjunctivitis is inflammation of the conjunctiva. It commonly is called *pinkeye* because hemorrhage of the subconjunctival blood vessels causes pink appearance. Some forms are highly contagious. See Chap. 8 for further discussion.

• KERATITIS AND CORNEAL ULCER

Keratitis is an inflammation of the cornea. A corneal ulcer is an erosion in the corneal tissue.

Pathophysiology and Etiology

Corneal trauma (e.g., wearing hard contact lenses for an extended period) and infectious agents (e.g., bacteria, fungi, viruses) cause keratitis. Secondary infections are common once the epithelium is damaged. Most clients experience severe pain because of the abundance of nerve endings in the cornea. Inflammation and disruption of the tissue interfere with transparency and smoothness of the cornea, temporarily impairing vision. When and if scar tissue forms, visual impairment is permanent. The degree of visual change depends on size and density of corneal scar tissue.

Assessment Findings

Keratitis is associated with localized pain or sensation that a foreign body is present. Blinking increases the discomfort. **Photophobia** (sensitivity to light), blurred vision, tearing, purulent discharge, and redness develop.

In addition to flashlight illumination and slit-lamp examination, fluorescein drops or strips provide evidence of corneal tissue erosion.

Medical and Surgical Management

Treatment begins promptly to avoid permanent loss of vision. Keratitis is treated with topical anesthetics, mydriatics, and local and systemic antibiotics. Dark glasses are recommended to relieve photophobia. Treatment in early stages of a corneal ulcer is the same as for keratitis. Once corneal scar tissue has formed, the only treatment is **corneal transplantation (keratoplasty).**

Nursing Management

Remove exudate that harbors microbes and instill antibiotic eye medication. Follow aseptic principles to avoid transferring microorganisms to injured corneal tissues. Advise clients who wear contact lenses to stop wearing them temporarily.

• HORDEOLUM (STY)

A **hordeolum** or sty is inflammation and infection of the Zeis or Moll gland, a type of oil gland at the edge of the eyelid. See Chapter 8 for further discussion.

• CHALAZION

A *chalazion* is a cyst of one or more meibomian glands, a type of sebaceous gland in the inner surface of the eyelid at the junction of the conjunctiva and lid margin.

Pathophysiology and Etiology

A chalazion forms when the meibomian gland becomes obstructed and release of sebaceous secretions is blocked. Consequently, the meibomian gland becomes inflamed and enlarged.

Assessment Findings

A chalazion appears similar to a sty, but swelling in the upper or lower eyelid is not tender. As the chalazion matures, it feels hard. Enlargement within the eyelid causes clients to feel self-conscious about their appearance and affects their visual acuity.

If a chalazion grows large enough to obscure the pupil or compress corneal tissue, distortion of vision is similar to that caused by astigmatism.

Medical and Surgical Management

Treatment of a chalazion is not necessary if the cyst is small and does not interfere with vision. Warm soaks and massage of the surrounding area are prescribed to promote spontaneous drainage. If the cyst is firm, becomes infected, or interferes with closure of the eyelid, it is surgically excised.

Nursing Management

Prepare the client for examination and treatment by a physician. Give instructions on methods for carrying out treatment measures. Some points to include when teaching clients with infectious and inflammatory eye disorders are as follows:

- Comply with full course of prescribed drugs to achieve satisfactory results.
- Wash hands thoroughly before cleaning eyelids, instilling eyedrops, or applying eye ointment.
- Do not rub eyes, and keep hands away from eyes.
- Use a separate washcloth or towel if disorder is infectious.
- Do not use nonprescription eye products during or after treatment unless approved by physician.
- Eliminate use of eye cosmetics or use hypoallergenic products and replace them frequently to avoid harboring microorganisms.
- Keep all follow-up appointments.

MACULAR DEGENERATION •

Macular degeneration is the breakdown of or damage to the macula, the point on the retina where light rays converge for the most acute visual perception. The disorder usually occurs in both eyes, but vision in one eye tends to deteriorate more rapidly.

Pathophysiology and Etiology

Macular degeneration is more common in aging adults. The underlying problem seems to stem from an opening between one of the membranous layers of the retina and the choroid. Serous fluid seeps into the separation, like a blister, and elevates an area of the retina. One or more blood vessels grow into the defect and produce a subretinal hemorrhage. After the bleed, scar tissue forms. Damage almost always is confined to the macular area.

Assessment Findings

Blurred or distorted vision is the first symptom of macular degeneration. Other symptoms include color vision disturbance (colors become dim), difficulty reading and doing close work, and distortion of objects (especially those with lines). When the macula becomes irreparably damaged, clients compare their vision to a target in which the bull's-eye area of the image is absent (Fig. 43.6). The peripheral field, or side vision, is unaffected, but the client cannot see images by looking at them directly.

Fluorescein angiography shows pooling of the dye in the blister area.

Medical Management

A laser procedure called *photocoagulation* is done to seal the serous leak and destroy encroachment of blood vessels in the area. It must be done early to prevent progression of the disorder. For many clients, diagnosis is made too late and laser treatment no longer is an option. The client is then provided with suggestions for coping with the visual impairment. Aids, such as magnifying glasses, may be of value, and high-intensity reading lamps have helped some people. The ophthalmologist may refer the client to a specialized center for evaluation and selection of assistive devices.

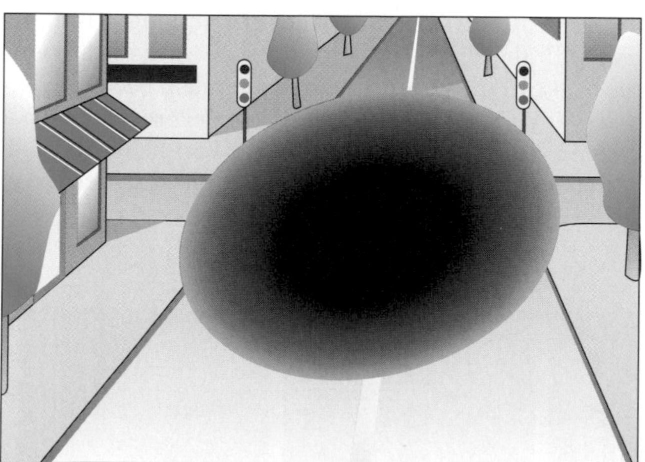

FIGURE 43.6 Visual loss associated with macular degeneration. (From Smeltzer, S. C. & Bare, B. G. [2004]. *Brunner & Suddarth's textbook of medical–surgical nursing* [10th ed.]. Philadelphia: Lippincott Williams & Wilkins.)

Some studies have found that foods containing carotenoids are beneficial in preventing progression of macular degeneration and vision loss. Dietary supplements of vitamins C, E, beta-carotene, and zinc also have beneficial effects. Other procedures such as porphyrin-laser photodynamic therapy (PDT) are showing promise in closing abnormal blood vessels behind the retina, as well as antiangiogenic drug therapy, which prevents new blood vessels from growing (Finger, 2003).

Nursing Management

Help the client cope with loss of vision. For additional nursing management of the client with permanent visual impairment, review information that accompanies the previous discussion of blindness.

GLAUCOMA

Glaucoma, the second most common cause of blindness in the United States, is caused by an imbalance between production and drainage of aqueous fluid. When the drainage system is obstructed, the anterior chamber becomes congested with fluid and IOP rises.

Glaucoma is classified as either open-angle or angle-closure. *Open-angle glaucoma,* formerly called *chronic* or *simple glaucoma,* is the most common form. Its onset is slow, and the client may not experience noticeable symptoms for several years. *Angle-closure glaucoma* is less common, but acute angle closure requires immediate recognition and treatment to prevent blindness.

Pathophysiology and Etiology

Glaucoma occurs congenitally; secondary to other eye disorders such as ocular trauma, ophthalmic infections, and cataract surgery; or as a primary disease among adults older than 40 years of age. It is more prevalent among those who have a family history of the disorder. Incidence is higher among African Americans, who are four to eight times more likely to develop blindness from glaucoma than are other ethnic groups.

Open-angle glaucoma occurs when structures in the drainage system (i.e., trabecular meshwork and canal of Schlemm) degenerate and the exit channels for aqueous fluid become blocked. As the IOP rises, it causes edema of the cornea, atrophy of nerve fibers in the peripheral areas of the retina, and degeneration of the optic nerve.

Angle-closure glaucoma occurs among people who have an anatomically narrow angle at the junction where the iris meets the cornea (Fig. 43.7). This deviation makes them vulnerable to angle closure when nearby structures protrude into the anterior chamber and occlude the drainage pathway. For example, an attack can be precipitated when the iris thickens in response to a mydriatic drug, by pupil dilation while sitting in the dark, or when the lens enlarges with age and bulges forward. A delay in treatment may result in partial or total loss of vision in the affected eye.

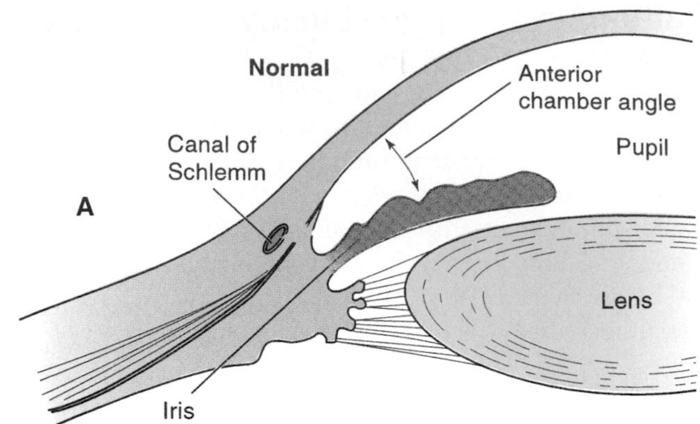

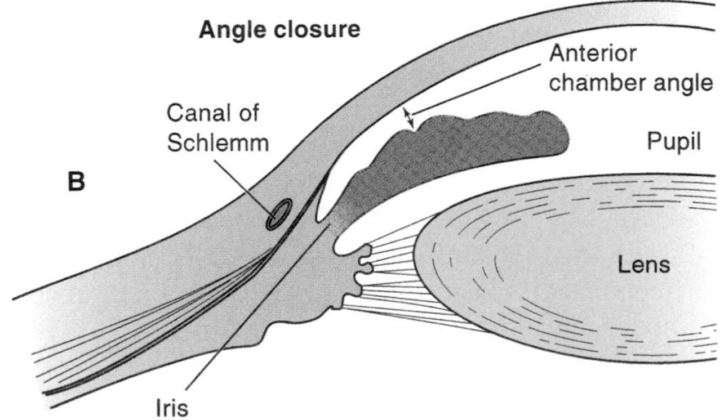

FIGURE 43.7 In the normal eye (**A**), the pathway to the canal of Schlemm is wide and unobstructed. In angle-closure glaucoma (**B**), the movement of fluid is impaired because of the narrowed approach to the canal of Schlemm.

Assessment Findings

Many clients experience no symptoms with open-angle glaucoma and the condition may not be discovered until a routine ophthalmologic examination. When symptoms do occur, they often are ignored because they are not dramatic. Clients may complain of eye discomfort, occasional and temporary blurred vision, the appearance of halos around lights, reduced peripheral vision, and the feeling that their eyeglass prescription needs to be changed (Fig. 43.8). Clients with acute angle-closure glaucoma become symptomatic quite suddenly. The eyes are rock hard, painful, and sightless. Nausea and vomiting may occur. The conjunctiva is red; the cornea becomes cloudy and commonly is described as appearing "steamy." The attack is self-limiting, but with each subsequent attack, vision is more impaired.

The optic disc, when visualized directly with an ophthalmoscope or with retinal angiographic photographs, shows a cupping effect (widening and deepening of the optic disc). When the anterior chamber of the eye of a client with angle-closure glaucoma is inspected with a penlight or slit lamp, the angle between the iris and cornea is found to be narrow. Tonometry reveals elevated IOP and reduced aqueous outflow. The visual field examination demonstrates a loss of peripheral vision.

Medical Management

Clients with either type of glaucoma are treated initially with medications (Drug Therapy Table 43.1). In an acute attack of angle-closure glaucoma, analgesics are given to relieve pain, and the client is kept at complete rest.

Surgical Management

When compliance is poor (e.g., client fails to instill eyedrops as directed) or drug therapy no longer is effective, or if the client develops severe adverse reactions to the medication, more aggressive treatment becomes necessary to preserve vision. One of several procedures that create accessory drainage channels can be performed. These procedures include laser or surgical **iridectomy,** laser **trabeculoplasty,** and **corneal trephine.**

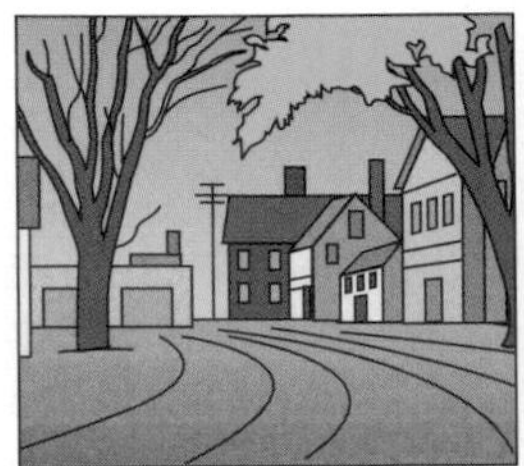
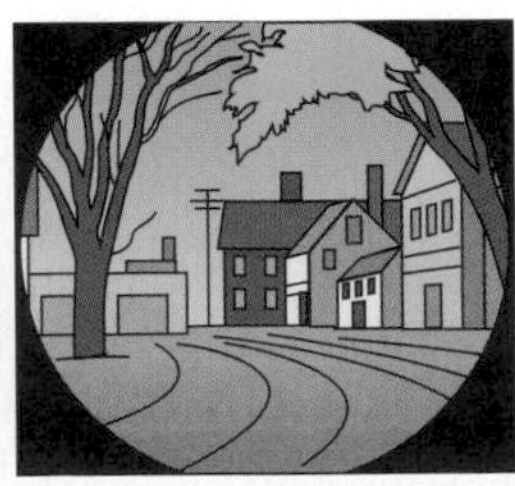
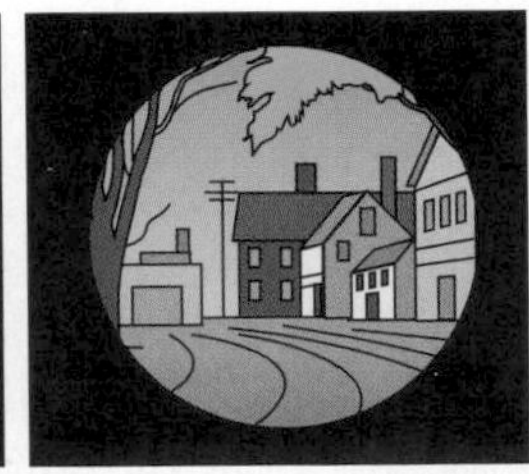
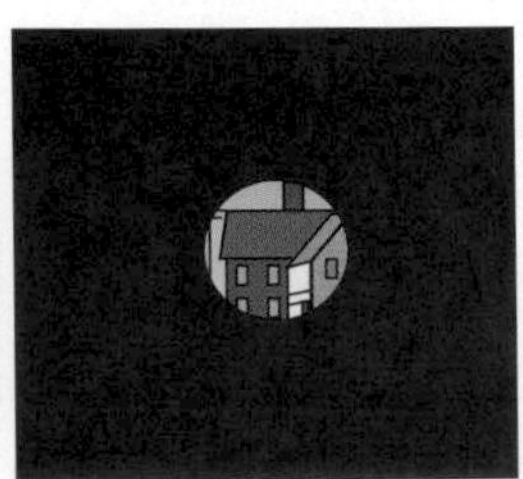

FIGURE 43.8 Gradual loss of vision from glaucoma.

Drug Therapy Table 43.1 MEDICATIONS USED IN MANAGING GLAUCOMA

DRUG CATEGORY AND EXAMPLES	MECHANISM OF ACTION	SIDE EFFECTS	NURSING CONSIDERATIONS
Cholinergics (Miotics)			
pilocarpine (Pilocar), carbachol (Miostat)	Increases aqueous fluid outflow by contracting the ciliary muscle and causing miosis (constriction of the pupil) and opening of trabecular meshwork	Periorbital pain, blurry vision, difficulty seeing in the dark	Warn clients about diminished vision in dimly lit areas.
Adrenergic Agonists			
dipivefrin (Propine), epinephrine (Epirin)	Reduces production of aqueous humor and increases outflow	Eye redness and burning; can have systemic effects, including palpitations, elevated blood pressure, tremor, headaches, and anxiety	Teach clients punctal occlusion to limit systemic effects.
Beta-Adrenergic Blockers			
betaxolol (Betoptic), timolol (Timoptic)	Decreases aqueous humor production	Can have systemic effects, including bradycardia, exacerbation of pulmonary disease, and hypotension	Contraindicated in clients with asthma, chronic obstructive pulmonary disease, second- or third-degree heart block, bradycardia, or cardiac failure; teach patients punctal occlusion to limit systemic effects.
Alpha-Adrenergic Agonists			
apraclonidine (Iopidine), brimonidine (Alphagan)	Decreases aqueous humor production	Eye redness, dry mouth and nasal passages	Teach clients punctal occlusion to limit systemic effects.
Carbonic Anhydrase Inhibitors			
acetazolamide (Diamox), methazolamide (Neptazane), dorzolamide (TruSopt)	Decreases aqueous humor production	Oral medications (acetazolamide and methazolamide) associated with serious side effects, including anaphylactic reactions, electrolyte loss, depression, lethargy, gastrointestinal upset, impotence, and weight loss; topical form (dorzolamide) side effects include topical allergy	Do not administer to clients with sulfa allergies; monitor electrolyte levels.
Prostaglandin Analogs			
latanoprost (Xalatan)	Increases uveoscleral outflow	Darkening of the iris, conjunctival redness, possible rash	Instruct clients to report any side effects.

Laser iridectomy, in which holes are burned into the iris to increase areas for drainage, is performed first. If this procedure is unsuccessful, it is followed by a standard surgical iridectomy in which a section of the iris is removed. Either a peripheral or sector iridectomy is used (Fig. 43.9). A laser trabeculoplasty is an alternative to a surgical iridectomy. In this procedure, the laser beam is directed at the trabecular network, which lies near the canal of Schlemm, creating multiple openings for drainage. A corneal trephine is similar to a trabeculoplasty in that it produces a small hole at the junction of the cornea and sclera to provide an outlet for aqueous fluid. The opening is then covered by a flap of the conjunctiva.

Nursing Management

Determine the client's history of symptoms, if the client is already on medication, medications that are prescribed, and whether the client is adhering to the prescribed medication schedule. It also is important to ask when the client was first diagnosed with glaucoma.

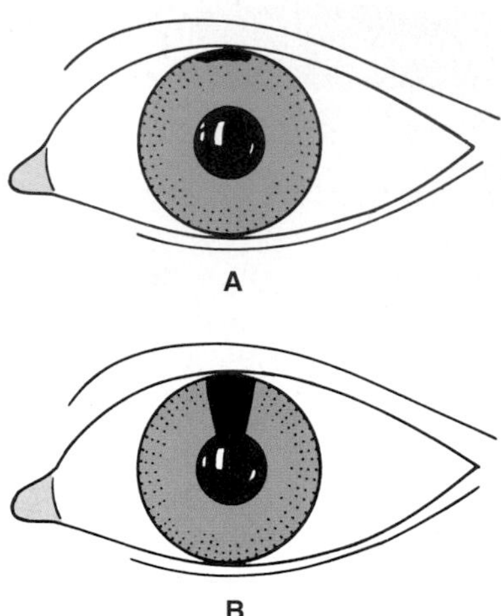

FIGURE 43.9 (**A**) Appearance of the eye after peripheral iridectomy. (**B**) Appearance of eye after keyhole (sector) iridectomy.

Acute angle-closure glaucoma is an emergency. Refer the client for medical treatment immediately because vision can be permanently lost in 1 to 2 days. Severe pain requires analgesics. To promote the maximum effect from analgesic drug therapy, it is essential to limit sensory stimulation, such as loud noise, activity, and movement. Inform the physician immediately if the client states that the pain is worse despite treatment. Mydriatics (drugs that dilate the pupil) must never be administered to clients with glaucoma. Consult the physician if drugs with anticholinergic properties, such as atropine sulfate, are prescribed because dilation of the pupil can further obstruct drainage of aqueous fluid, raise IOP, and damage remaining vision.

Because glaucoma tends to run in families, advise adults to be examined regularly. Early diagnosis and treatment can prevent loss of vision. Clients already diagnosed with glaucoma are encouraged to maintain close follow-up and comply with the medication regimen. Explain drug instillation techniques. Besides eyedrops, some clients insert an *ocular therapeutic system* under the upper lid, which is a small, thin film containing eye medication. The film, replaced weekly, continuously releases medication and eliminates the need for frequent eyedrop instillation.

If a client cannot remember when to take the medication, recommend a watch with a timer. For the client who does not understand the chronic and progressive nature of the disease, it is important to stress that glaucoma has no cure but can be controlled, and that blindness caused by glaucoma usually is preventable.

Other general instructions include the following:

- Obtain assistance from a family member, relative, or friend if you have trouble instilling eyedrops.
- Avoid drugs that contain atropine. Check with physician or pharmacist before using any nonprescription drug; preparations for cold or allergy symptoms may contain an atropine-like drug.
- Maintain regular bowel habits; straining at stool can raise IOP.
- Avoid heavy lifting and emotional upsets (especially crying) because they increase IOP.
- Limit activities that strain or tire eyes.
- Keep an extra supply of prescribed drugs on hand for vacations, holidays, or in case some is lost or spilled.
- Seek medical attention immediately if pain or a visual disturbance occurs.
- Tell all physicians that you have this disorder and the treatment prescribed by the ophthalmologist.
- Carry identification stating that you have glaucoma in case of illness or injury.

Stop, Think, and Respond ● BOX 43-3

What is appropriate advice for a person with a family history of glaucoma?

CATARACTS

A **cataract** is a condition in which the lens of the eye becomes opaque. One or both eyes may be affected.

Pathophysiology and Etiology

Cataracts occur as a result of the aging process or are congenitally acquired, caused by injury to the lens, or secondary to other eye diseases. When cataracts occur in response to injury, they usually develop quickly. Most cataracts result from degenerative changes associated with aging and develop slowly. A high incidence of cataracts occurs among people with diabetes and those with a family history. Prolonged exposure to ultraviolet rays (e.g., sunlight, tanning lamps), radiation, or certain drugs (e.g., corticosteroids) are associated with cataract formation. In all cases, vision decreases because light no longer has a transparent pathway to the retina.

Assessment Findings

One of the earliest symptoms is seeing a halo around lights. Other symptoms include difficulty reading, changes in color vision, glaring of objects in bright light, and distortion of objects. As the cataract worsens, visual acuity is severely reduced and the client can read only the largest letter on a Snellen chart, count fingers, and distinguish movement. On inspection, a white or gray spot is visible behind the pupil (Fig. 43.10).

Under ophthalmoscopic and slit-lamp examination, the lens is in varying stages of opacity. Some lenses are so cloudy that the examiner cannot see through the cataract

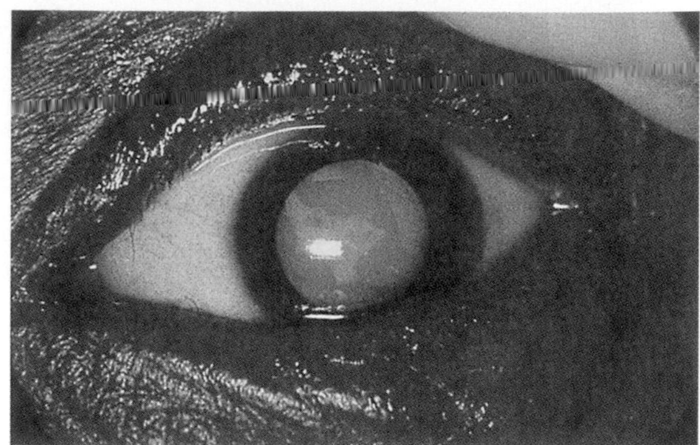

FIGURE 43.10 A cataract is a cloudy or opaque lens that appears gray or milky. (From Rubin, E. & Farber, J. L. [1999]. *Pathology* [3rd ed.]. Philadelphia: Lippincott Williams & Wilkins.)

to the posterior eye. Tonometry determines whether the cataract is raising the IOP.

Surgical Management

Cataracts must be surgically removed. Surgery usually is done under local anesthesia. A tranquilizer is given before and during surgery to relax the client.

The lens is removed by *intracapsular extraction* (removal of the lens within its capsule) or *extracapsular extraction* (removal of the lens, leaving the posterior portion of its capsule in position).

Phacoemulsification uses ultrasound to break the lens into minute particles that are then removed by aspiration. This technique may accompany the extracapsular method. When used, a smaller incision is required. Most clients return to full activity sooner than after other methods.

After surgery, vision is restored with one of three methods: corrective eyeglasses, a contact lens, or an **intraocular lens** (IOL) **implant.** When cataract eyeglasses are prescribed, the correcting lens for the *aphakic eye* (the eye without a lens) causes the client to see objects about one third larger than normal. These lenses also distort peripheral vision, and the client must learn to turn his or her head to see objects that are not in the center of vision. If only one lens is removed, the client must use one eye or the other to avoid seeing a distorted image. A coating usually is applied to the eyeglasses so that only the aphakic eye with a corrective lens is used.

A contact lens also can restore vision after cataract extraction. Advantages are that peripheral vision is not lost and objects appear about their actual size. A disadvantage is that the lens must be removed at night, cleaned, and reinserted daily, which can be difficult for an older client.

A third method for improving vision is insertion of an IOL at the time of cataract surgery, most commonly behind the iris (Fig. 43.11). Candidates for IOLs are clients older than 60 years of age and at risk for experiencing difficulty with a contact lens or cataract glasses. Ultrasonography is done before surgery to determine size and prescription of the IOL. When implanted, vision is blurred for a week or more. Reading glasses are required for optimum vision.

Complications after cataract surgery include infection, loss of vitreous, intraocular hemorrhage, retinal detachment, clouding of the lens capsule, and displacement of the IOL implant. Loss of vitreous is serious because the vitreous body does not regenerate. Its loss, as well as hemorrhage, seriously damages the eye.

Nursing Management

If outpatient surgery is planned, explain and provide a written list of preoperative preparations. The nurse is responsible for providing preoperative and postoperative care of the surgical client as well as discharge instructions (Nursing Care Plan 43-1). Help the client to follow

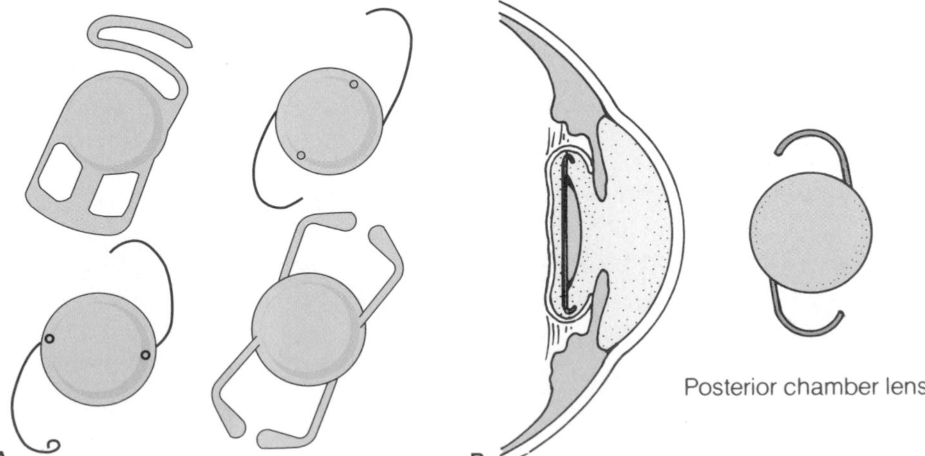

FIGURE 43.11 (**A**) Intraocular implants are designed to be held in place by various wing-like attachments that center and support the lens. (**B**) The intraocular lens implant is placed in the lens capsule after cataract extraction.

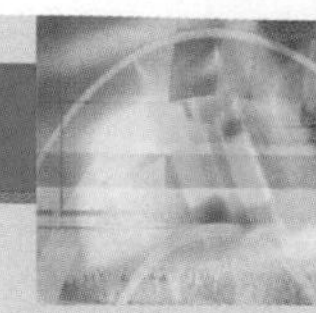

Nursing Care Plan 43-1

POSTOPERATIVE MANAGEMENT OF THE CLIENT UNDERGOING EYE SURGERY

Assessment

Clients having eye surgery require the usual preoperative care. Frequently, they have surgery in ambulatory care settings, so preoperative assessments may be done before the day of surgery. Obtain preoperative vital signs to have a baseline for postoperative monitoring.

Depending on the type of surgery, it is important to ask the client about medications. Check to ensure that instructions about withholding any medications before surgery were followed. Examples include the following:

- Anticoagulation therapy withheld as ordered. For example, if the client takes warfarin (Coumadin), a prothrombin time of 1.5 is the desired level before surgery.
- Aspirin withheld for 5 to 7 days.
- Nonsteroidal anti-inflammatory drugs (NSAIDs) withheld for 3 to 5 days.

In addition, check the preoperative orders and administer eyedrops as ordered.

PC: **Ophthalmic Hemorrhage** or **Increased Intraocular Pressure** (IOP)

Expected Outcome: Bleeding and IOP will be managed and minimized.

Interventions	*Rationales*
Report sudden or intense pain immediately.	Pain may indicate hemorrhage or increased IOP, which may require emergency surgery.
Instruct client to avoid coughing, vomiting, straining at stool, bending forward, or lifting anything heavier than 5 lb.	Prevents the IOP from rising.

Evaluation of Expected Outcome: Client experiences no complications.

Nursing Diagnosis: **Pain** related to surgery.

Expected Outcome: Client will experience little or no pain or discomfort.

Interventions	*Rationales*
Acknowledge client's discomfort and administer prescribed analgesic that is appropriate for the level of pain.	Acknowledging and treating client's pain provide validation and pain relief.
Keep room lights dim. Provide dark glasses if light causes discomfort.	Reduces eye sensitivity to light.
If allowed, instruct client to gently use a clean, moist washcloth to remove eye discharge.	Promotes increased comfort.

Evaluation of Expected Outcome: Client reports little or no pain.

Nursing Diagnosis: **Risk for Infection** related to impaired tissue integrity.

Expected Outcome: Incised tissue will heal without evidence of infection.

(continued)

Nursing Care Plan 43-1 (Continued)

POSTOPERATIVE MANAGEMENT OF THE CLIENT UNDERGOING EYE SURGERY

Interventions	*Rationales*
Perform conscientious handwashing before an eye assessment or treatment procedure.	Reduces or prevents the transmission of microorganisms.
Follow principles of asepsis when cleaning the eye or applying a new dressing.	Asepsis prevents infection of operative site.
Keep the tips of all medication applicators clean.	Prevents contamination of equipment and infection of the operative site.

Evaluation of Expected Outcome: Incision heals without evidence of redness, swelling, or unusual drainage.

Nursing Diagnosis: **Risk for Injury** related to compromised vision

Expected Outcome: Client's safety will be maintained.

Interventions	*Rationales*
While client is hospitalized, raise side rails and identify location of the signal device.	Provides client with security and orients the client as to how to get needed assistance.
Encourage client to use a dim light or nightlight in the room after sundown.	Provides a light source and prevents injury.
Reorient confused client. Ask family member to sit at bedside if confusion persists.	Provides client with a sense of where he or she is and where things are. Visual compromise can cause confusion. Having someone stay promotes safety.
Apply a shield over the patched eye.	Provides additional protection and prevents client from rubbing or accidentally poking eye.
Assist client to ambulate; ensure the pathway is clear.	Maintains client's safety.

Evaluation of Expected Outcome: Client remains free of injury.

these postoperative measures to prevent complications and keep IOP from rising:

- Tell the client to avoid coughing or sneezing.
- Give antiemetics if nausea occurs.
- Patch both eyes and give dilating drugs to keep the client from squinting.
- Tell the client to avoid lying on the operative side, bending, and lifting.
- Administer stool softeners to prevent straining.

Positioning depends on the type of cataract surgery performed. If an air bubble is instilled in the eye to occupy the space where the lens is removed, the client may have the head elevated slightly and is not permitted to lie flat because this would push the iris toward the anterior chamber and obstruct flow of aqueous fluid. Intense pain in the eye or near the brow is an indication of intraocular hemorrhage or rising IOP, and is reported immediately.

RETINAL DETACHMENT

In **retinal detachment,** the sensory layer is separated from the pigmented layer of the retina.

Pathophysiology and Etiology

Retinal separation is associated with a hole or tear in the retina caused by stretching or degenerative changes (Fig. 43.12). Retinal detachment may follow a sudden blow, penetrating injury, or eye surgery. Tumors, hemorrhage in front of or behind retina, and loss of vitreous fluid are

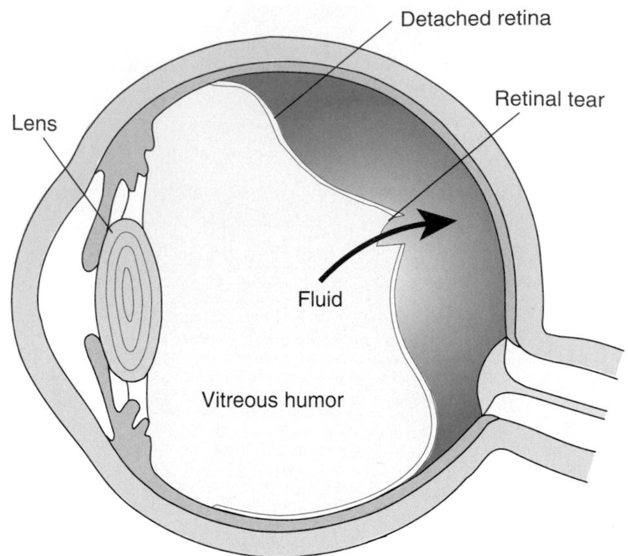

FIGURE 43.12 Retinal detachment. (From Smeltzer, S. C. & Bare, B. G. [2004]. *Brunner & Suddarth's textbook of medical–surgical nursing* [10th ed.]. Philadelphia: Lippincott Williams & Wilkins.)

particularly likely to lead to retinal detachment. This condition may also be a complication of other disorders, such as advanced diabetic changes in the retina. In many instances, the cause of retinal detachment is unknown. Retinal separation is more common after 40 years of age.

Separation of the two layers of the retina deprives the sensory layer of its blood supply. Vision is lost in the affected area because the sensory layer no longer receives visual stimuli. Vitreous fluid moves between separated layers of the retina, holding layers apart and causing further separation.

Assessment Findings

Many clients notice definite gaps in their vision or blind spots. They describe the sensation that a curtain is being drawn over their field of vision and often see flashes of light. Seeing spots or moving particles, called *floaters,* is common. Complete loss of vision may occur in the affected eye. The condition is not painful, but clients usually are extremely apprehensive. When the retina is inspected with an ophthalmoscope, tissue appears gray in the detached area.

Medical Management

In a few select cases, an office procedure called *pneumatic retinopexy* is performed. Before the procedure, the client must recline for about 16 hours to allow the separated retina to fall back toward the choroid. Then, 0.5 to 1 mL of gas is injected intraocularly into the posterior area of the eye. The gas compresses the retina and holds it in place. To ensure success from the procedure, the client must again assume a restricted position, sometimes up to 8 hours each day for 3 weeks. If pneumatic retinopexy is not appropriate, the physician usually recommends prompt admission to the hospital for surgery.

Surgical Management

Surgical interventions for retinal reattachment include cryosurgery, electrodiathermy, laser reattachment, and scleral buckling. The amount of sight regained depends on the extent of detachment and success of the surgery.

Cryosurgery involves application of a supercooled probe to the sclera. The sclera, choroid, and retina then adhere to one another as a result of scar tissue formation.

With *electrodiathermy,* an electrode needle is inserted into the sclera so that the fluid that has collected underneath the retina can escape. The retina ultimately adheres to the choroid. This method seldom is used.

Laser reattachment involves focusing a laser beam on the damaged area of the retina and causing a small burn. Exudate that forms between the retina and choroid results in adhesion of the retina to the choroid. Laser therapy can be used only when the retinal separation involves a small area.

Scleral buckling is a surgical procedure that shortens the sclera, thus allowing contact between the choroid and retina (Fig. 43.13). A section of the sclera is exposed, opened, and retracted from the choroid. A laser beam or cryosurgery probe is then used to produce adhesion of the retina and choroid. A small silicone patch is placed between the sclera and choroid, and the sclera is pulled over the patch and sutured. The inward displacement of

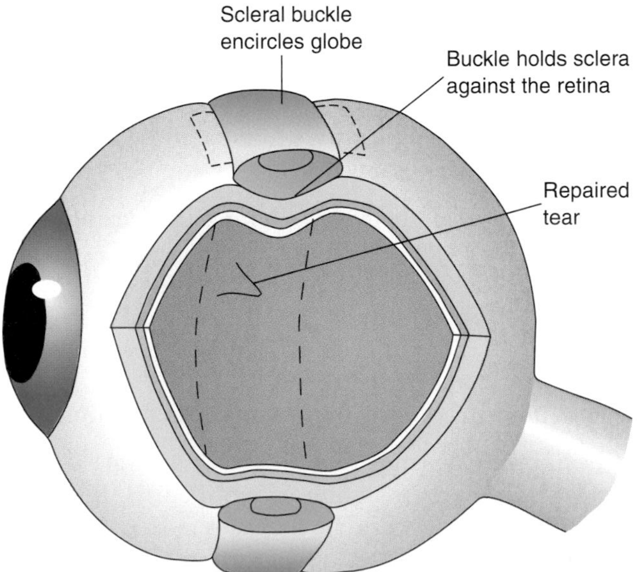

FIGURE 43.13 Scleral buckle. (From Smeltzer, S. C. & Bare, B. G. [2004]. *Brunner & Suddarth's textbook of medical–surgical nursing* [10th ed.]. Philadelphia: Lippincott Williams & Wilkins.)

the choroid allows for reattachment of the retina to the choroid.

Before surgery, the client is on complete bed rest with the affected eye dependent until surgery is performed. Sedation may be ordered. Eyes are patched and covered with an eye shield. Mydriatic eyedrops are instilled to dilate the pupil and facilitate further examination of the retina.

Nursing Management

Anyone with sudden loss of vision is referred immediately for examination by a physician. If surgery is performed, the client usually is kept on complete bed rest for several days with the head immobilized. The client is not turned or moved without orders. If an air bubble is instilled to promote contact between the retina and choroid, the client is positioned with face parallel to the floor so that the bubble floats to the posterior of the eye. If floaters are still seen after the eye heals, tell the client that they eventually become absorbed or settle to the inferior floor of the eye, out of the line of vision. For additional postoperative nursing management, see Nursing Care Plan 43-1.

ENUCLEATION

Enucleation is the surgical removal of an eye. It is necessary when the eye is destroyed by injury or disease, a malignant tumor develops (rare), or to relieve pain if the eye is severely damaged and sightless. Sometimes only the contents of the eyeball are removed and the sclera is left in place. Other times, the entire eyeball is removed as well as tissues in the bony orbit.

Medical and Surgical Management

When enucleation is performed, a metal or plastic ball is buried in the capsule of connective tissue from which the eyeball is removed (Fig. 43.14). A pressure dressing is applied to control hemorrhage, a complication of enucleation. After tissues have healed, a shell-shaped prosthesis is placed over the buried ball. The shell is painted to match the client's remaining eye. The shell is the only portion that is removed for cleaning.

Nursing Management

Observe the client after surgery for signs and symptoms of bleeding or infection. The client usually is allowed out of bed the day after surgery. When healing is complete, in about 2 to 4 weeks, teach the client how to insert and remove the prosthetic shell. The prosthesis typically is removed before going to bed and inserted the next morning. Instruct the client to hold the head over a soft surface, such as a bed or padded table, when removing or inserting the prosthesis to avoid damage if he or she drops the prosthetic eye. The client should clean the shell after removal and keep it in a safe place where it will not become scratched or broken.

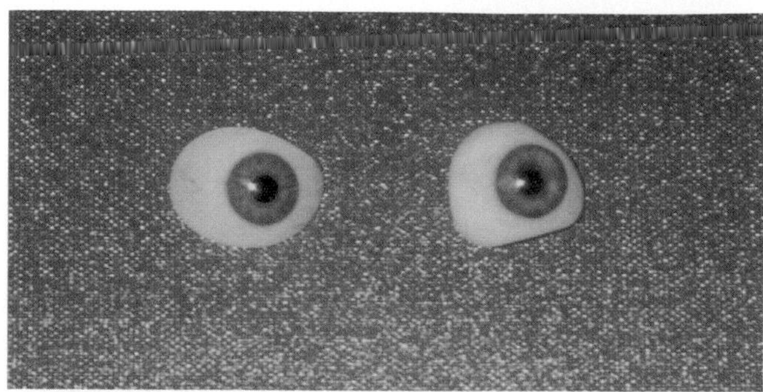

FIGURE 43.14 Eye prostheses. (**Left**) Anophthalmic ocular prosthesis. (**Right**) Scleral shell. (From Smeltzer, S. C. & Bare, B. G. [2004]. *Brunner & Suddarth's textbook of medical-surgical nursing* [10th ed.]. Philadelphia: Lippincott Williams & Wilkins.)

GENERAL GERONTOLOGIC CONSIDERATIONS

Older adults need to use their glasses or contact lenses when explanations are provided about test procedures.

Teaching aids with large-sized letters are helpful for older clients who are experiencing lens changes associated with aging.

Visual changes can result in accidents and injuries. Assisting older adults with visual deficits with ADLs is essential.

To ensure safety of older adults with visual impairments, the room should be kept dimly lit at night. Objects, chairs, and footstools are placed away from areas where the client walks, and assistance is given whenever the client is out of bed.

Visual impairment curtails favorite activities such as reading, watching television, and engaging in hobbies or other forms of recreation, resulting in depression and withdrawal.

Critical Thinking Exercises

1. *If a client reports having difficulty seeing, what additional data are important to obtain?*
2. *Discuss preventive measures for transmitting an infectious eye disorder.*
3. *Explain the preoperative and postoperative management of a client undergoing a cataract extraction.*

● NCLEX-STYLE REVIEW QUESTIONS

1. A 5-year-old who attends day care is rubbing his eye, which is pinkish-red with excessive tearing. The child's mother brings the child to the physician's office, and

conjunctivitis is diagnosed. The nurse advises the child's mother to use a separate tissue for each eye when wiping away excess drainage to:
   1. Prevent injury and trauma to the unaffected eye
   2. Prevent cross-contamination of microorganisms to the unaffected eye
   3. Allow the mother to observe the color and amount of drainage for each eye
   4. Allow the mother to assess whether a foreign body has been washed free

2. A teenage girl comes to the clinic and reports that over the past few months she has had repeated eye infections. What assessment information is most important for the nurse to ask about?
   1. The amount of sleep the girl is getting per night
   2. Whether the girl is sharing eye makeup
   3. The brand of makeup the girl is using
   4. If the girl has a history of excessive tearing

3. A nurse is teaching a hospitalized client with an eye condition home care instructions for the instillation of eyedrops. Which action by the client alerts the nurse to the need for further instruction?
   1. The client wipes excess medication using a different tissue for each eye.
   2. The client touches the tip of the medication dropper to the eyeball.
   3. The client applies eyedrops into the lower lid.
   4. The client washes his hands prior to putting in drops.

connection

Visit the Connection site at **http://connection.lww.com/go/timbyEssentials** for links to chapter-related resources on the Internet.

References and Suggested Readings

Barnie, D. C. (2002). Restoring vision in older patients. *RN, 65*(1), 30–35.

Bullock, B. A. & Henze, R. L. (2000). *Focus on pathophysiology.* Philadelphia: Lippincott Williams & Wilkins.

Finger, P. (2003). Macular degeneration network. [On-line.] Available: http://www.eyccarefoundation.org.

Kobel-Lamento, H. (December 9, 2002). Lasers in surgery. *Advance for Nurses,* 17–19.

Metules, T. J. (2001). Protect your eyes! *RN, 64*(10), 69–71.

Porth, C. M. (2002). *Pathophysiology: Concepts of altered health states* (6th ed.). Philadelphia: Lippincott Williams & Wilkins.

Scerra, C. (2000). Retinal imaging system works with pupil dilation. *Ophthalmology Times.* [On-line.] Available: http://www.findarticles.com/cf_0/m0VEY/18_25/65197577/pl/article.jhtml.

Smeltzer, S. C., & Bare, B. G. (2004). *Brunner & Suddarth's textbook of medical–surgical nursing* (10th ed.). Philadelphia: Lippincott Williams & Wilkins.

Smith, S. E. (2000). Time to manage seasonal ocular allergies. *Journal of Ophthalmic Nursing and Technology, 19*(2), 68–73.

chapter 44

Caring for Clients With Ear Disorders

Words to Know 

acoustic neuroma
audiometry
caloric stimulation test
cochlear implant
conductive hearing loss
decibels
electronystagmography
Ménière's disease
nystagmus
otitis externa
otitis media
otosclerosis
otoscope
ototoxicity
presbycusis
Rinne test
Romberg test
sensorineural hearing loss
sign language
speech reading
stapedectomy
tinnitus
tuning fork
Weber test

Learning Objectives

On completion of this chapter, the reader will:

- Describe the anatomy and physiology of the ear.
- List types of hearing impairment and acuity levels for each.
- Name techniques that clients with impaired hearing use to communicate with others.
- Give examples of support services available for the hearing impaired.
- Discuss the role of the nurse in caring for clients with a hearing loss.
- Name conditions that involve the external ear.
- Discuss methods for preventing or treating disorders of the external ear.
- Name conditions that affect the middle ear.
- Describe nursing interventions appropriate for managing the care of a client with ear surgery.
- Explain the pathophysiology of Ménière's disease.
- Discuss the nursing management of clients with Ménière's disease.

Ear disorders occur throughout the life cycle. Many ear disorders result in hearing loss, a common sensory deficit among older adults. Hearing aids compensate for some but not all forms of hearing loss.

ANATOMY AND PHYSIOLOGY

The ear (Fig. 44.1) is divided into three areas: the outer, middle, and inner sections. Sound is perceived because of a chain reaction involving all three areas of the ear. The inner ear also helps maintain balance.

Outer Ear

The outer ear, or *auricle,* consists of the *pinna,* the fleshy external projection of the ear, and the *external acoustic meatus,* a 1-inch canal that extends to the *tympanic membrane,* or eardrum. The outer ear collects sound waves and directs them inward. The external acoustic meatus contains the glands that produce *cerumen,* a waxy substance that lubricates the ear canal, protects the eardrum, and helps prevent external ear infections. Chewing and talking help to move cerumen to the outer area of the external acoustic meatus, where it is easily washed away.

Middle Ear

The middle ear is a small, air-filled cavity in the temporal bone. The *eustachian tube* extends from the floor of the middle ear to the pharynx and is lined with mucous membrane. It equalizes air pressure in the middle ear. A chain of three small bones, the *malleus,* the *incus,* and the *stapes,* stretches across the middle ear cavity from the tympanic membrane to the *oval window.* They move when struck by sound waves transmitted from the outer ear. When these bones are set in motion, the very flexible footplate of the stapes strikes the oval window, agitating fluid in the inner ear.

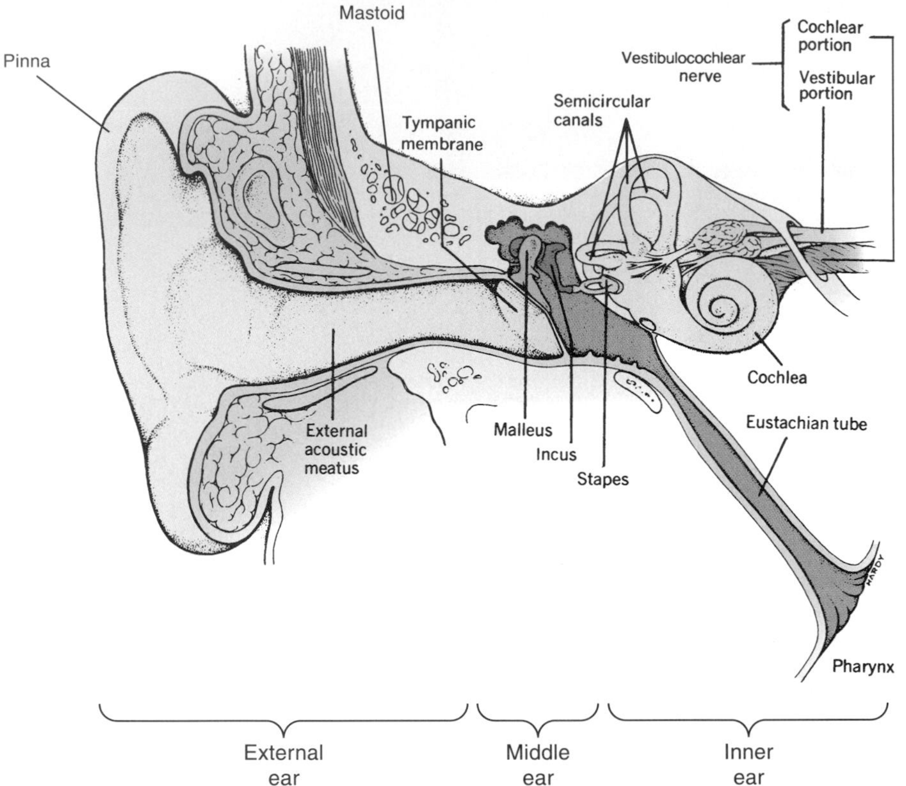

FIGURE 44.1 Diagram of the ear, showing the external, middle, and internal subdivisions.

Inner Ear

The inner ear, or *labyrinth,* consists of a series of cavities and canals containing fluid. It contains the *cochlea,* which provides for hearing, and the *semicircular canals,* which promote balance, and the *vestibulocochlear nerve (cranial nerve VIII).*

Fluid motion created by the vibrating stapes excites the nerve endings in the sensitive sound receptors of the *organ of Corti* located in the cochlea. The impulses are converted to nerve impulses and transmitted along the cochlear nerve to the brain, where sound is perceived.

Nerve receptors for balance are found both in the vestibule and semicircular canals. They transmit information about motion through the vestibular nerve, which joins with the cochlear nerve to form the eighth cranial nerve, the vestibulocochlear nerve (formally called the *auditory* or *acoustic nerve*).

ASSESSMENT

Although family practice physicians assess and treat many ear disorders, they refer some clients to *otolaryngologists,* physicians who specialize in diagnosis and treatment of ear, nose, and throat disorders. An *audiologist* is a paraprofessional with special training in performing hearing tests, measuring hearing loss, and recommending methods for improving the perception of sound. Box 44-1 outlines the nursing assessment.

Basic Auditory Acuity Tests

A general method used to assess a client's gross auditory acuity is referred to as the *whisper test.* The examiner covers the untested ear with his or her palm and stands 1 to 2 feet from the client's uncovered ear. He or she whispers a number or a phrase and asks the client to repeat it. The examiner whispers several numbers to ensure valid test results. Another technique is to sit beside the client and bring a ticking watch toward the ear. The client should perceive the sound at the same time as the nurse, who is assumed to have normal hearing.

Otoscopic Examination

An otoscopic examination involves inspecting the external acoustic canal and tympanic membrane using an **otoscope,** a handheld instrument with a light, lens, and optional speculum for inserting into the client's ear (Fig. 44.2). If normal, the canal appears smooth and empty. The normal tympanic membrane is intact, looks pearly gray, and transmits light. Excessive cerumen interferes with inspection.

BOX 44-1 • Nursing Assessment of the Ear and Basic Hearing Acuity

- Obtain client's appraisal of his or her hearing, including whether the client experiences tinnitus.
- Observe for actions that suggest a hearing problem such as leaning forward, turning the head, or cupping a hand to the ear to hear better.
- Document the use of a hearing aid.
- Ask client about allergies, a history of upper respiratory and middle ear infections, high fevers, or exposure to loud sounds, because all these can cause hearing loss.
- Inspect external ear for signs of infection, such as swelling, redness, drainage, or evidence of trauma.
- Shine a penlight into the ear to grossly inspect the ear canal; straighten the ear canal by gently pulling the ear up and back for an adult and downward and backward for small children.
- Palpate the areas in front of and behind the ear lobe for tenderness and swelling.
- Perform a basic hearing acuity test.

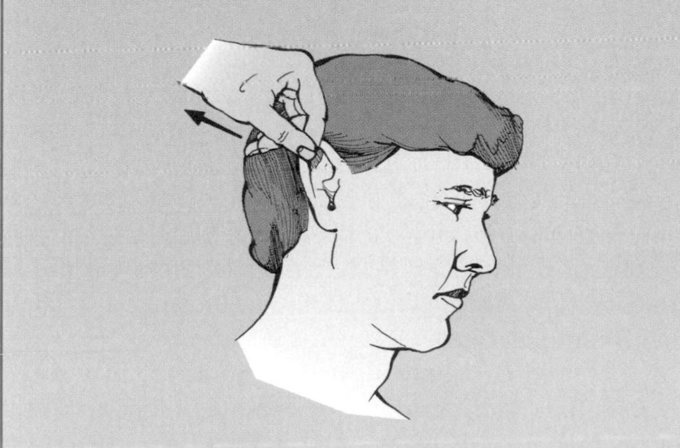

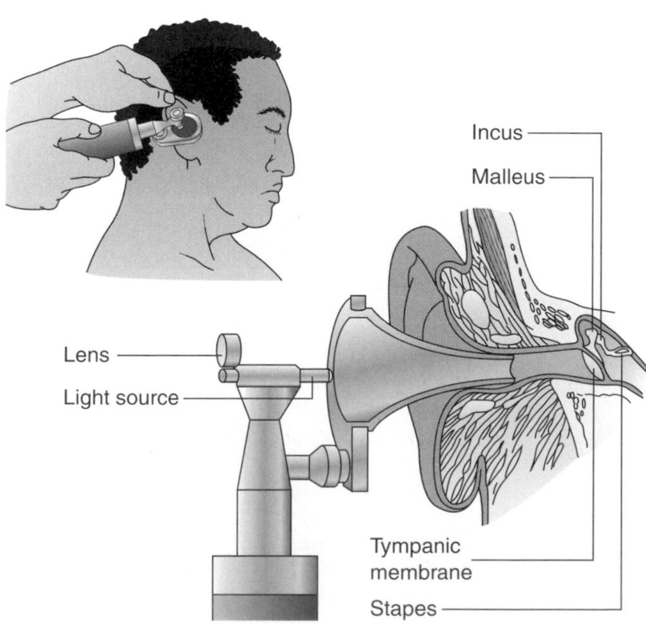

FIGURE 44.2 Technique for using the otoscope.

Tuning Fork Tests

A **tuning fork** is an instrument that produces sound in the same range as human speech. It is used to screen for conductive or sensorineural hearing loss. **Conductive hearing loss** involves interference in transmission of sound waves to the inner ear. **Sensorineural hearing loss** results from nerve impairment.

The **Rinne test** involves striking the tuning fork, placing it on the mastoid process behind the ear, and holding it there until client indicates the sound has stopped. Immediately after that, the still vibrating tuning fork is held beside the ear and the client again says when the sound stops. Normally, air conduction beside the ear measures twice as long as by bone conduction through the mastoid.

The **Weber test** is performed by striking the tuning fork and placing its stem in the midline of the client's skull or center of the forehead. A person with normal hearing perceives sound equally well in both ears. If the sound is lateralized to one ear, it suggests a conduction hearing loss in that ear or a sensorineural loss in the opposite ear.

Romberg Test

The **Romberg test** evaluates a person's ability to sustain balance. The client stands with feet together and both arms extended, and closes his or her eyes. Swaying, losing balance, or arm drifting are abnormal responses. Because central nervous system lesions cause similar abnormal results, additional testing is needed to confirm an inner ear dysfunction.

Diagnostic Studies

Audiometry

Audiometry is done by an audiologist to measure hearing acuity precisely. During the test, controlled intensities of sound, measured in **decibels** (dB), are projected to one ear at a time through a headset. The client indicates when sound is heard. The lowest level of sound that normal individuals can first perceive is 20 dB; painful sounds occur at 120 dB. Hearing acuity is determined by measuring the intensity at which a person first perceives sound.

Caloric Stimulation Test

A **caloric stimulation test** assesses vestibular reflexes of the inner ear that control balance. Warm (40°C) or cool (25°C) water or air is instilled into the external meatus of each ear separately. The fluid alters the temperature of the temporal bone and creates convection currents in the fluid of the inner ear that simulate movement of the head. **Nystagmus,** a quivering movement of the eyes, is the expected response. Slight dizziness also may be experienced. A diminished response in one eye is significant for an inner ear disorder such as Ménière's disease (discussed later).

Electronystagmography

Electronystagmography is a more precise method for evaluating vestibular function, the mechanisms that facilitate maintaining balance. It is performed in conjunction with caloric stimulation. When fluid is instilled within the ear, a machine records duration and velocity of eye movements with electrodes attached superiorly, inferiorly, and laterally about the eyes.

HEARING IMPAIRMENT

Hearing impairment is described as mild, moderate, severe, or profound, depending on intensity of sound required for a person to hear it (Table 44.1). Diminished hearing results from a conductive loss, sensorineural loss, or both. Conductive hearing loss occurs from conditions such as an accumulation of cerumen in the external acoustic meatus or failure of the tiny ear bones to vibrate. Sensorineural hearing loss occurs secondary to atherosclerosis, a tumor of the vestibulocochlear nerve, infections, or drug toxicity. Clients with a hearing impairment often have **tinnitus,** buzzing, whistling, or ringing noises in one or both ears. Box 44-2 elaborates on causes of conductive and sensorineural hearing loss. Hearing loss also can result from repeated exposure to excessive noise, such as live concerts, high volumes from stereos or headphones, or loud work environment (machinery or jackhammers).

Hearing loss seriously impairs the ability to protect oneself and communicate with others. Age at which hearing loss occurs plus severity of impairment has extensive consequences. Hearing loss during the first 3 years of life, the most critical period for learning to make sounds, affects language acquisition at the word, phrase, and sentence levels. If uncorrected, hearing deficits can lead to depression and social isolation.

Medical Management

Besides treating the cause of hearing loss, medical management includes recommendations for a hearing aid, a battery-operated device that fits in the external ear and amplifies sound. Clients with a conductive hearing loss benefit more from a hearing aid because the structures that convert sound into energy and facilitate perception of sound in the brain continue to function.

Some clients with hearing deficits learn **sign language,** a method for communication that uses a hand-spelled alphabet and word symbols, and **speech reading,** also called *lip reading.*

Many technologic devices promote communication. Some television programs are transmitted using closed-caption inserts. Some theaters provide headsets that amplify actors' voices to individual patrons. Telephones can be adapted with a hearing amplifier that increases sound from incoming callers. Another device is a telecommunication device for the deaf (TDD), which is a combination special typewriter and telephone used to call someone else with a TDD. Computer modems also facilitate communication.

Other products allow the hearing impaired to perceive (rather than hear) sound. For example, light-activated alarms in smoke detectors, alarm clocks, doorbells, and telephones flash a light when sound is produced. Hearing dogs, like guide dogs for the blind, are specially trained to warn their owners when certain sounds occur.

Surgical Management

Sensorineural hearing loss usually is irreversible. It is somewhat improved with a **cochlear implant,** a device

TABLE 44.1 HEARING ACUITY

HEARING RANGE	DECIBELS (DB)	WITHOUT A HEARING AID	WITH A HEARING AID
Normal	20–120	Can hear faint to painful sounds	Unnecessary
Mild impairment	40–120	Cannot hear unvoiced consonants such as "s" and "f"	Helpful, but not necessarily worth the expense
Moderate impairment	60–120	Cannot hear conversational volume unless others talk loudly	Beneficial for restoring ability to hear normal conversations
Severe impairment	70–120	Misses most conversational content	Amplifies 40-dB sounds to 75 dB, but also amplifies nonspeech and background noise
Profound impairment	90–120	Depends heavily on speech reading	Helps hearing vowels, but amplified speech and background noise are painful
Total deafness	120	Hears only painfully loud sounds or vibrations created by loud sounds	Not useful for understanding speech

BOX 44-2 ● Common Causes of Conductive and Sensorineural Hearing Loss

CONDUCTIVE HEARING LOSS
- External ear conditions
  - Impacted ear wax or foreign body
  - Otitis externa
- Middle ear conditions
  - Trauma
  - Otitis media
  - Otosclerosis
  - Tumors

SENSORINEURAL HEARING LOSS
- Trauma
  - Head injury
  - Noise
- Central nervous system infections (e.g., meningitis)
- Degenerative conditions
  - **Presbycusis** (impairment of hearing in old age)
- Vascular
  - Atherosclerosis
- Ototoxic drugs
- Tumors
- Ménière's disease

MIXED CONDUCTIVE AND SENSORINEURAL HEARING LOSS
- Middle ear conditions
- Temporal bone fractures

(Adapted from Porth, C. M. [2002]. *Pathophysiology: Concepts of altered health states* [6th ed., p. 1298]. Philadelphia: Lippincott Williams & Wilkins.)

surgically placed in the inner ear and connected to a receiver in the bone behind the ear (Fig. 44.3). Even with a cochlear implant, clients frequently have difficulty understanding and learning speech.

Nursing Management

Observe for signs of hearing impairment and assess gross hearing using techniques described earlier. Also determine clarity of the client's speech. Refer a client for diagnosis and subsequent treatment of a hearing impairment and speech therapy. Many people deny that their hearing is impaired and consider it a sign of aging and deterioration. If the client fears that wearing a hearing aid is a stigma, describe various types of hearing aids that are available, some of which fit almost unnoticeably in the ear (Fig. 44.4). Also stress the importance of avoiding the purchase of a hearing aid from a mail-order catalogue or a company salesman.

If a hearing impairment exists, obtain information about its severity and methods used to understand speech of others. When a client hears poorly, determine the communication method the client prefers: speech reading, signing, writing, or typing. Suggestions for oral communication are listed in Nursing Guidelines 44-1. If the client uses a hearing aid, safeguard the instrument, assist the client with its insertion, and help maintain its function.

Use illustrations, pamphlets, and written directions to aid teaching and include a family member. Ask the client to repeat information and demonstrate technical skills. Initiate a referral to a community agency to evaluate if and how well the client is performing self-care after discharge.

Stop, Think, and Respond ● BOX 44-1

What recommendations can you make for someone to prevent injury to the ears or hearing loss?

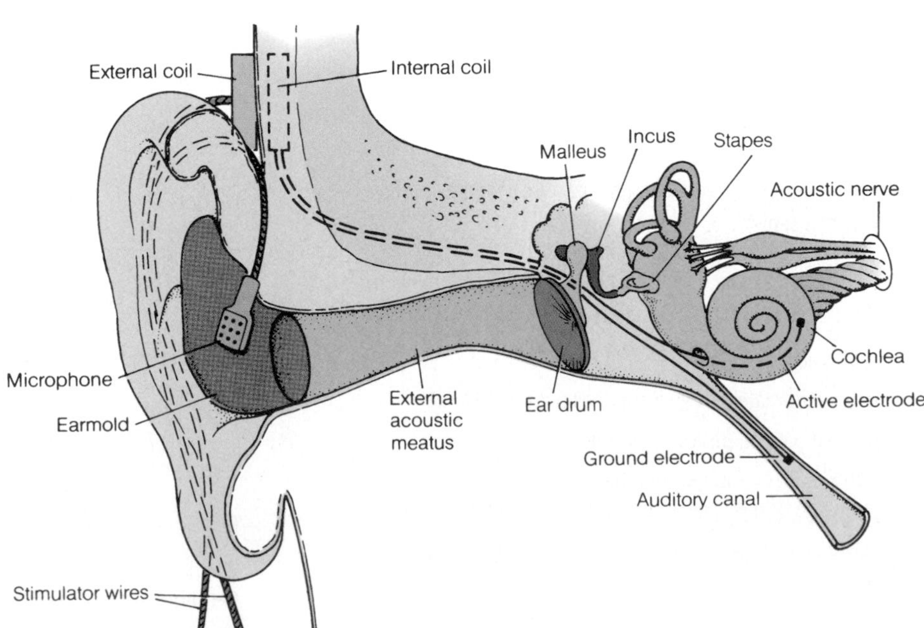

FIGURE 44.3 With a cochlear implant, sound is passed from the external transmitter to the inner coil by magnetic conduction and is then carried over an electrode to the cochlea.

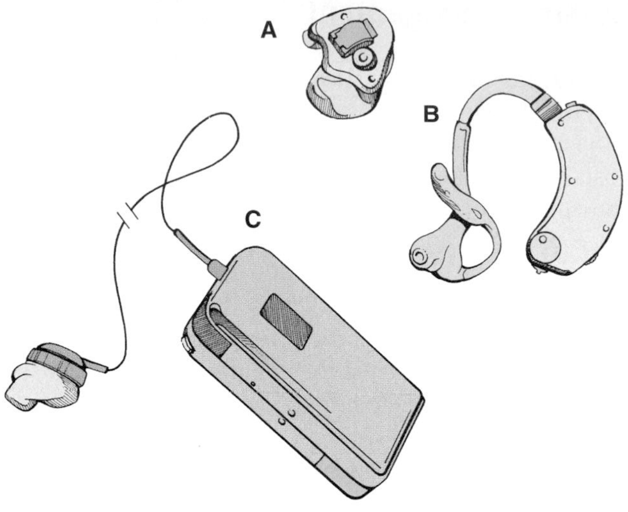

FIGURE 44.4 Examples of hearing aids: (**A**) in-the-ear, (**B**) behind-the-ear, and (**C**) body aid.

DISORDERS OF THE EXTERNAL EAR

Various disorders such as impacted cerumen, injury from foreign objects, or otitis externa affect the external acoustic meatus. If these disorders are not treated carefully and adequately, they may spread to the middle ear.

NURSING GUIDELINES 44-1

Communicating With People Who Have a Hearing Loss

- Eliminate background noise as much as possible.
- Stand or sit on the side of the client's better ear.
- Ensure that there is adequate light.
- Get the client's attention.
- Face the client.
- Speak clearly and at a normal pace without exaggerating pronunciations.
- Do not shout, but avoid dropping conversational volume at the end of a sentence.
- Promote a clear image of your mouth; do not chew gum or cover your mouth.
- Use gestures and facial expressions to enhance what is being said orally.
- Rephrase whatever the client does not understand.
- Remain patient, positive, and relaxed.
- Provide paper and pencil if the client communicates by sign language or has speech that is difficult to understand.
- Use a support person who can communicate by signing.

(Adapted from Trychin, S. [1993]. *Communication issues related to hearing loss.* Bethesda, MD: Self Help for the Hard of Hearing People, Inc.)

● FOREIGN OBJECTS

Foreign objects find their way into the ear either by accident or deliberate insertion. Sharp objects can scratch the skin or cause blunt penetration of the eardrum. Insect stings cause local inflammation.

The client describes discomfort, diminished hearing, feeling movement, or hearing a buzzing sound. On gross inspection, there is evidence of abrasion from trauma or an insect, or an object is seen. Inspection with a penlight or otoscope reveals swelling and redness in the auditory canal.

Mineral oil is instilled into the ear to smother an insect. Solid objects are removed with a small forceps.

Instruct clients to clean ears with a face cloth rather than inserting objects into the ears. A hat with earflaps or a scarf is recommended when venturing into the woods or other areas with a high insect population.

● OTITIS EXTERNA

Otitis externa is an inflammation of the tissue in the outer ear. Inflammation usually is caused by an overgrowth of pathogens. Microorganisms tend to follow trauma to the lining of the ear, or their growth is supported by retained moisture from swimming. Another possibility is that a hair follicle is infected, causing a furuncle or abscess to develop.

Tissue in the external ear looks red. It may be difficult to see the tympanic membrane because of swelling. Clients describe discomfort that increases with manipulation during examination. Hearing is reduced because of swelling. In severe infections, a fever develops and lymph nodes behind the ear enlarge.

Otoscopic examination reveals diffuse or confined inflammation, swelling, and pus. A culture of drainage identifies the specific pathogen. Treatment includes warm soaks, analgesics, and antibiotic ear medication.

Instruct the client to carry out the medical treatment and provide health teaching to prevent recurrence. Advise swimmers to wear soft plastic ear plugs to prevent trapping water in the ear. If chewing produces or potentiates discomfort, encourage the client to temporarily eat soft foods or consume nourishing liquids. Advise the client to avoid use of nonprescription remedies unless approved by physician and to contact physician if symptoms are not relieved in a few days.

DISORDERS OF THE MIDDLE EAR

● OTITIS MEDIA

Otitis media is an inflammation or infection in the middle ear. Clients may have acute or chronic forms of either serous otitis media, also known as secretory or nonsuppurative otitis media, or the purulent or suppurative type. Although otitis media is more common among young children, adults can and do develop middle ear infections. See Chapter 8 or more information.

● OTOSCLEROSIS

Otosclerosis is the bony overgrowth of the stapes and a common cause of hearing impairment among adults. Fixation of the stapes occurs gradually.

Pathophysiology and Etiology

The underlying cause of otosclerosis is unknown. The condition, more common in women than in men, usually becomes apparent in the second and third decades of life. It seems to be accelerated during pregnancy. Most clients have a family history of the disease, which indicates a possible hereditary relationship.

Otosclerosis interferes with the vibration of the stapes and transmission of sound to the inner ear. Although hearing loss in otosclerosis is of the conductive type, when and if progression of the disease involving the cochlea of the inner ear occurs, a mixed type of hearing loss develops.

Assessment Findings

A progressive, bilateral loss of hearing is the most characteristic symptom. The client notices the hearing loss when it begins to interfere with the ability to follow conversation. There is particular difficulty hearing others when they speak in soft, low tones, but hearing is adequate when sound is loud enough. Tinnitus appears as loss of hearing progresses, especially noticeable at night.

The eardrum appears pinkish-orange from structural changes in the middle ear. When the Rinne test is performed, sound is heard best when the tuning fork is applied behind the ear. The sound lateralizes to the more affected ear when the Weber test is performed.

Audiometric tests reveal the type and severity of hearing loss. A computed tomography (CT) scan demonstrates the location and extent of excessive bone growth.

Medical and Surgical Management

Although otosclerosis has no cure, a hearing aid helps. The level of restored hearing depends greatly on severity of the sensorineural involvement. The outcome is best if the hearing loss is purely conductive. If surgical treatment is selected, a **stapedectomy** is performed on the ear most affected. All or part of the stapes is removed and a prosthesis is inserted that can vibrate the oval window (Fig. 44.5). Once the stapes is freed or replaced, the client experiences an immediate, dramatic improvement in hearing. Hearing temporarily diminishes after surgery because of swelling, but eventually returns. Complications include dislodgment of the prosthesis and continued hearing loss, infection, dizziness, and facial nerve damage. Depending on the outcome of surgery, the procedure may be repeated for the opposite ear.

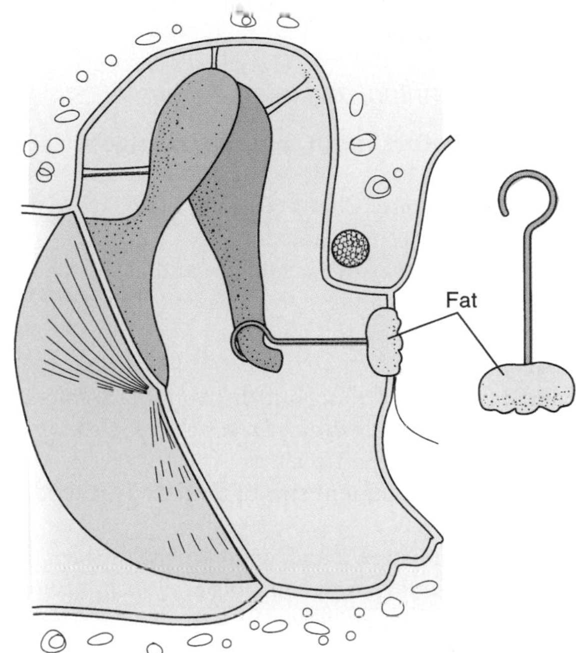

FIGURE 44.5 A wire prosthetic stapes is positioned in the middle ear.

Nursing Management

Use selected alternatives for communicating with the client as identified earlier in Nursing Guidelines 44-1, and provide the preoperative client with an explanation of what to expect in the immediate postoperative period. Tell the client that activity is restricted for 24 hours or more after surgery and that hearing may be temporarily the same as or worse than before surgery.

After surgery, position the client on the nonoperative side. Take care to prevent dislodgment of the prosthesis as a result of coughing, sneezing, or vomiting. Nausea and dizziness are common problems. Assess facial nerve function by checking symmetry when the client smiles or frowns.

NURSING PROCESS

● The Client Recovering From Stapedectomy

Assessment

After the client returns from surgery, nursing assessments include taking vital signs and monitoring for complications, drainage from the affected ear, and level of discomfort. It is important that the nurse report any elevation in temperature.

Diagnosis, Planning, and Interventions

Impaired Comfort (pain, nausea, vertigo) related to tissue disruption

Expected Outcome: Client will experience relief of discomfort to at least a tolerable level.

- Administer prescribed analgesic and assess again in 30 minutes. *Determines effectiveness of pain medication.*
- Give an antiemetic for nausea or vomiting. *Promotes relief of nausea.*
- Validate client's feelings of discomfort. *Promotes the nurse–client relationship and reassures the client that his or her needs are important.*
- Provide small, frequent sips of fluid or light food. *Prevents nausea.*
- Limit head movement and avoid jarring the bed. *Movement aggravates vertigo. Limiting movement minimizes pain, dizziness, and nausea.*

Risk for Infection related to impaired tissue integrity secondary to the surgical incision

Expected Outcome: Client will remain free of a secondary infection.

- Adhere strictly to aseptic principles when changing a dressing or cleaning the ear. *Reduces introduction and transmission of microorganisms and protects client from exposure to pathogens.*
- Administer prescribed antibiotics. *Promotes consistent blood level needed to treat or prevent infection.*
- Instruct client to keep his or her hands away from the dressing or packing. *Maintains integrity of the dressings and prevents contamination from opportunistic infections.*
- Keep external ear and surrounding skin meticulously clean and free of purulent drainage. *Promotes healing and prevents infection through reduction of microorganisms.*

Risk for Injury related to vertigo

Expected Outcome: Client will be free of injury.

- Encourage client to use the side rails and handrails for support when preparing to ambulate. *Prevents client from falling or causing injury to the affected ear.*
- Walk with the client who is dizzy. *Promotes client's safety and reduces chance for injury.*

Evaluation of Expected Outcomes

The client remains comfortable, as evidenced by minimal complaints of pain and no complaints of nausea or vertigo. He or she has no signs or symptoms of infection. The client experiences mild vertigo but maintains safety.

Discuss the prescribed medical regimen and restrictions with client or a family member. Include one or more of the following in a teaching plan:

- Avoid blowing nose because this can dislodge the prosthesis.
- Avoid high altitudes or flying.
- Do not lift heavy objects, strain when defecating, or bend over at the waist; these activities increase pressure in middle ear.
- Do not get water in the ear. Avoid swimming, showering, and washing hair until approved by the physician.
- Follow physician's instructions for keeping ear clean.
- Stay away from people with respiratory infections. If a head cold occurs, contact physician immediately.
- Notify physician immediately if severe pain, excessive drainage, a sudden loss of hearing, or fever occurs.
- Adhere to restriction of activities recommended by physician until told otherwise.

DISORDERS OF THE INNER EAR

● MÉNIÈRE'S DISEASE

Ménière's disease is a term given to the episodic symptoms created by fluctuations in production or reabsorption of fluid in the inner ear. This ear disease is analogous to glaucoma of the eye—there is too much circulating fluid (Smeltzer & Bare, 2004).

Pathophysiology and Etiology

The cause of excessive fluid production is unknown. There appears to be malabsorption of fluid in the endolymphatic sac, although some clients may have a blockage in the endolymphatic duct.

Several theories attempt to explain Ménière's disease. These include abnormal hormonal and neurochemical influences that affect blood flow to the labyrinth, electrolyte disturbances, allergic reactions, and autoimmune responses. A last theory suggests that abnormally high levels of metabolites (e.g., glucose, insulin, triglycerides, cholesterol) destroy the microvasculature of the inner ear (Porth, 2002).

Ménière's disease typically is unilateral, appears during middle age, and occurs equally in men and women. It causes a triad of hearing loss, vertigo, and tinnitus (Porth, 2002). When fluid accumulates, it dilates the cochlear duct, diminishing hearing. It also affects equilibrium as the vestibular system is damaged, and tinnitus occurs. At times, the client is symptom free except for permanent, residual hearing loss as the number of attacks increase. Occasionally, clients recover spontaneously.

Assessment Findings

The client periodically experiences severe vertigo, tinnitus, and progressive hearing loss. Nausea and vomiting accompany vertigo. Nystagmus of the eyes may occur, caused by an imbalance in vestibular control of eye movements (Porth, 2002). Some clients experience preattack symptoms of headache and a full feeling in the ear.

An attack lasts from a few minutes to weeks and can occur with alarming suddenness. Some clients are reluctant to leave their homes for fear they will have an attack in public. Continued employment becomes impossible for some clients.

A caloric stimulation test and electronystagmography demonstrate a difference in eye movement response. A CT scan or magnetic resonance imaging (MRI) rules out other possible causes of the symptoms, such as a tumor that involves the vestibulocochlear nerve. Audiometry identifies the type and magnitude of the hearing deficit.

Medical and Surgical Management

Treatment aims at reducing fluid production in the inner ear, facilitating its drainage, and treating symptoms that accompany the attack. A low-sodium diet lessens edema. Smoking is contraindicated to prevent vasoconstriction, which interferes with fluid drainage. Treatment of the allergy or avoidance of the allergen is recommended. Bed rest may be necessary during acute attacks. Specific drug therapy may include the following:

- Meclizine (Antivert)—an antihistamine often prescribed because it suppresses the vestibular system
- Diazepam (Valium) or other tranquilizers—may be ordered for acute episodes to help control vertigo; these are used only for short-term therapy because of the addictive potential
- Promethazine (Phenergan)—an antiemetic to help control the nausea and vomiting; has an antihistamine effect
- Hydrochlorothiazide or other diuretics—may decrease the fluid in the endolymphatic system and relieve symptoms (Smeltzer & Bare, 2004)

If clients are extremely incapacitated, surgery becomes an option. Surgeries range from decompression of the endolymphatic sac to insertion of intraotologic catheters to vestibular nerve section.

Nursing Management

Obtain a history of symptoms, their duration, and complete medical, drug, and allergy histories. Assess gross hearing and perform the Weber and Rinne tests.

The client with Ménière's disease requires emotional support because of the unpredictability of the attacks and resulting impairments. During an attack, administer prescribed drugs, limit movement, and promote the client's safety. Assist the client with activities of daily living because the least amount of motion can produce severe vertigo.

Be available, empathic, and responsive to the client. Trust and confidence develop when the client does not feel abandoned or required to convince caregivers of the necessity for attention. Clients are comforted when the nurse acknowledges that dealing with temporary or permanent hearing loss is a challenge.

If a low-sodium diet is recommended, the dietitian provides a list of foods to avoid or a specific diet to follow. If an allergy is suspected as the cause of the disorder, advise the client to take prescribed antihistamines as directed and to avoid known allergens. If a hearing aid is recommended, refer the client to an audiologist for instructions on its use and care.

Stop, Think, and Respond ● BOX 44-2

A nurse admits a client with Ménière's disease who is having an acute episode. After assessing the client, the nurse selects ***Risk for Deficient Fluid Volume*** *as the best nursing diagnosis. Complete the diagnostic statement with expected outcomes.*

● OTOTOXICITY

Ototoxicity describes the detrimental effect of certain medications on the eighth cranial nerve or hearing structures. Signs and symptoms of ototoxicity include tinnitus and sensorineural hearing loss. Vestibular toxicity includes signs and symptoms of light-headedness, vertigo, nausea, and vomiting. Drugs associated with ototoxicity include salicylates, loop diuretics, quinidine, quinine, and aminoglycosides. Box 44-3 lists selected ototoxic medications. It is important that nurses are knowledgeable about the ototoxic effects of certain medications, and that they carefully monitor dosage and frequency of administration, as well as assessing clients for changes in hearing.

● ACOUSTIC NEUROMA

An **acoustic neuroma** is a benign Schwann cell tumor that progressively enlarges and adversely affects cranial nerve VIII (the vestibular and cochlear nerves). Most acoustic tumors arise in the auditory canal and extend into the cerebellar region, pressing on the brain stem.

Pathophysiology and Etiology

The cause of acoustic neuroma is unknown. Men and women are equally affected. The tumor usually is unilateral. Hearing loss occurs secondary to compression of the cochlear nerve or interference with blood supply to the nerve and cochlea.

BOX 44-3 ● Selected Ototoxic Substances

DIURETICS
ethacrynic acid
furosemide
acetazolamide

CHEMOTHERAPEUTIC AGENTS
cisplatin
nitrogen mustard

ANTIMALARIALS
quinine
chloroquine

ANTI-INFLAMMATORY AGENTS
salicylates (aspirin)
indomethacin

CHEMICALS
alcohol
arsenic

AMINOGLYCOSIDE ANTIBIOTICS
amikacin
gentamicin
kanamycin
netilmicin
neomycin
streptomycin
tobramycin

OTHER ANTIBIOTICS
erythromycin
minocycline
polymyxin B
vancomycin

METALS
gold
mercury
lead

Assessment Findings

Signs and symptoms vary according to size and location of the tumor. The client may exhibit or experience hearing loss (usually gradual), impaired facial movement, altered facial sensation, tinnitus, vertigo with or without balance disturbance, or all these problems. Generally the problems are unilateral.

Initial audiometric studies reveal significant differences in hearing and the presence of tinnitus and vertigo. MRI with contrast agents determines the location and extent of the tumor. Cerebrospinal fluid (CSF) studies demonstrate increased pressure and presence of proteins.

Medical and Surgical Management

Surgical removal of the tumor is the usual treatment. Acoustic neuromas do not respond well to chemotherapy or radiation therapy. The challenge of this surgical procedure is to remove the tumor and retain facial nerve function. Usually hearing loss already has occurred, so destruction of the hearing mechanism that occurs with the surgical approach is not a consideration. If the client has little or no hearing loss, however, the suboccipital or middle cranial fossa approach is used, with close monitoring of cranial nerve VIII function.

Complications of acoustic neuroma excision include facial nerve paralysis, CSF leak, meningitis, cerebral edema, and increased intracranial pressure.

Nursing Management

Assessment of a client with acoustic neuroma includes evaluating hearing function, observing client's facial movements, and testing for facial sensation. If the client has hearing deficits, refer to Nursing Guidelines 44-1 for measures to communicate with people with a hearing loss. For clients with vertigo, protect the client from injury.

After surgery, implement the aforementioned measures and monitor client for signs of increased intracranial pressure, including restlessness, confusion, or unresponsiveness, pupillary changes, bradycardia, hypertension, and respiratory changes. Maintain strict asepsis to prevent transmission of microorganisms. Clients are at risk for wound infection and meningitis.

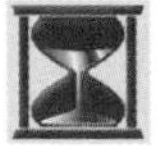

GENERAL GERONTOLOGIC CONSIDERATIONS

Older clients form drier cerumen and experience an increased incidence of impaction in the external acoustic meatus.

Hearing loss is common as adults age. Options in the style of prescribed hearing aid are limited by the client's ability to care for and maintain it.

The older adult with a hearing impairment may become disoriented and confused in strange surroundings. Frequent contact and reorientation prevent confusion.

Critical Thinking Exercises

1. *Describe techniques that promote communication when interacting with clients who have a hearing deficit.*
2. *What cues can a nurse observe in an older client who has possible hearing loss?*

● NCLEX-STYLE REVIEW QUESTIONS

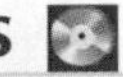

1. The nurse is revising the history of a client with suspected ototoxicity. The client's symptoms include ringing in the ears and hearing loss. Which of the following questions would be most important?
   1. "Are you taking aspirin?"
   2. "Have you been swimming in nonchlorinated water?"
   3. "Is there a family history of this condition?"
   4. "Have you had a cold or runny nose?"

2. A client comes to the clinic for a routine check up. The nurse notes that the client exhibits signs of hearing loss. As the nurse assesses the client's ability to hear, she informs the client that a tuning fork will be placed on the center of the head. Which test is the nurse performing?

1. Romberg
2. Weber
3. Rinne
4. Caloric stimulation

connection

Visit the Connection site at **http://connection.lww.com/go/timbyEssentials** for links to chapter-related resources on the Internet.

References and Suggested Readings

Aschenbrenner, D. S., Cleveland, L. H., & Venable, S. J. (2002). *Drug therapy in nursing.* Philadelphia: Lippincott Williams & Wilkins.

Bullock, B. A., & Henze, R. L. (2000). *Focus on pathophysiology.* Philadelphia: Lippincott Williams & Wilkins.

Grossan, M. (2000). Safe, effective techniques for cerumen removal. *Geriatrics, 55,* 83–86.

Hearing loss: What to do when sound fades. (2001). *Mayo Clinic Women's Health Source, 5*(10), 6.

McConnell, E. A. (2002). *How to converse with a hearing-impaired patient. Nursing 2002, 32*(8), 20.

Porth, C. M. (2002). *Pathophysiology: Concepts of altered health states* (6th ed.). Philadelphia: Lippincott Williams & Wilkins.

Smeltzer, S. C., & Bare, B. G. (2004). *Brunner & Suddarth's textbook of medical–surgical nursing* (10th ed.). Philadelphia: Lippincott Williams & Wilkins.

Stock, S. (January 21, 2002). When silence isn't golden. *Advance for Nurses,* 24–25.

chapter 45

Introduction to the Gastrointestinal System and Accessory Structures

Words to Know 

barium enema
barium swallow
cholangiography
cholecystography
colonoscopy
endoscopic retrograde cholangiopancreatography
enteroclysis
esophagogastroduodenoscopy
flexible sigmoidoscopy
gallbladder series
lower gastrointestinal series
panendoscopy
percutaneous liver biopsy
peristalsis
proctosigmoidoscopy
PY test
radionuclide imaging
ultrasonography
upper gastrointestinal series

Learning Objectives

On completion of this chapter, the reader will:

- Identify major organs and structures of the gastrointestinal system.
- Discuss important information to ascertain about gastrointestinal health.
- List facts in the client's history that provide pertinent data about the present illness.
- Discuss physical assessments that provide information about the functioning of the gastrointestinal tract and accessory organs.
- Describe common diagnostic tests performed on clients with gastrointestinal disorders.
- Explain nursing management of clients undergoing diagnostic testing for a gastrointestinal disorder.

The gastrointestinal (GI) system (Fig. 45.1) is arbitrarily divided into two sections. The upper GI tract begins at the mouth and ends at the jejunum. The lower GI tract begins at the ileum and ends at the anus. Accessory structures include the peritoneum, liver, gallbladder, and pancreas. Primary functions of the GI tract are digestion and distribution of food.

ANATOMY AND PHYSIOLOGY

Mouth

Food normally enters the GI system at the mouth, where it is chewed (masticated) before being swallowed. Food that contains starch undergoes partial digestion when it mixes with the enzyme *salivary amylase,* which the *salivary glands* secrete (Table 45.1).

Esophagus

The *esophagus* begins at the base of the pharynx and ends at the opening between the esophagus and stomach. Layers of muscle tissue surround the esophagus, consisting of striated muscle tissue in the proximal esophagus, striated and smooth muscle in the mid-esophagus, and smooth muscle in the lower esophagus. Coordinated movement of these muscle layers, referred to as **peristalsis,** propels food into the stomach. An *upper esophageal sphincter* or *hypopharyngeal sphincter* prevents food or fluids from re-entering the pharynx.

Stomach

The stomach temporarily holds ingested food and prepares it by mechanical and chemical action to pass in semiliquid form into the small intestine. The opening between

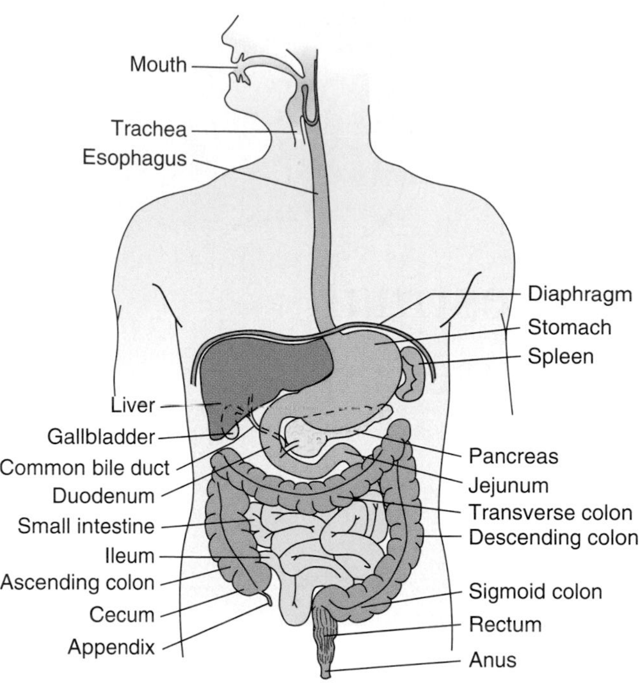

FIGURE 45.1 Organs of the gastrointestinal tract.

the esophagus and stomach is called the *lower esophageal sphincter* or *cardiac sphincter*. The opening between the stomach and duodenum is called the *pyloric sphincter*. Both sphincters are circular bands of muscle fibers. When contracted, these sphincters keep contents in the stomach. When the pyloric sphincter relaxes, stomach contents flow to the duodenum.

Gastric secretions that contain digestive enzymes are released continuously but increase when food is eaten. Gastric secretions are acidic because they contain hydrochloric acid (HCl). Contractions of the stomach mix food with gastric secretions and move the mixture of semiliquid food called *chyme* to the small intestine by peristalsis. Time required for the stomach to empty depends on the amount and composition of food. Fats, for example, delay stomach emptying.

Small Intestine

The small intestine is divided into three portions. The *duodenum,* approximately 10 inches long, is the first region of the small intestine and the site where bile and pancreatic enzymes enter. These secretions continue to promote chemical breakdown of food and transform chyme to an alkaline state. Peristalsis mechanically propels the mixture, which is semiliquid at this point, into the *jejunum* and *ileum,* the other two regions of the small intestine. They have a combined length of approximately 23 feet.

The primary function of the small intestine is to absorb nutrients from chyme, which occurs at different sites in the small intestine. When a part of the small intestine is diseased or removed surgically, absorption in that area is diminished or lost altogether.

The *ileocecal valve* lies at the distal end of the small intestine and regulates flow of intestinal contents, which are liquid at this point, into the large intestine. It also prevents reflux of bacteria from the large intestine, preserving the relative sterility of the small intestine.

Large Intestine

The large intestine, approximately 4 to 5 feet long and 2 inches in diameter, receives waste from the small intestine and propels waste toward the *anus,* the opening from the body for elimination. The large intestine absorbs water, some electrolytes, and bile acids. The cecum, colon, rec-

TABLE 45.1 SELECTED DIGESTIVE ENZYMES/SECRETIONS

LOCATION	ENZYME	SUBSTANCE THE ENZYME ACTS ON	PRODUCTS OF ENZYMATIC ACTION
Salivary glands	Salivary amylase	Starch	Smaller carbohydrates
Stomach	Pepsin	Proteins	Polypeptides (process activated by HCl)
	Gastric lipase	Triglycerides (lipids)	Glycerides and fatty acids
	HCl	Proteins	Smaller polypeptides
Pancreas	Trypsin	Proteins and polypeptides	Smaller polypeptides, amino acids
	Nuclease	Nucleic acids	Nucleotides (base + sugar + phosphate)
	Pancreatic amylase	Starch	Smaller carbohydrates
	Pancreatic lipase	Lipids, especially triglycerides	Glycerides, free fatty acids, glycerol
Small intestine	Peptidases	Peptides	Amino acids
	Lactase, maltase, sucrase	Disaccharides	Monosaccharides
	Intestinal lipase	Fats	Glycerides, fatty acids, glycerol
Liver	Bile	Fats	Glycerides, fatty acids, glycerol

HCl, hydrochloric acid.

tum, and anal canal make up the structures of the large intestine through which fecal material passes.

The *cecum* is a pouchlike structure at the beginning of the large intestine. The *appendix,* a narrow blind tube at the tip of the cecum, has no known function in humans.

The colon is divided into *ascending, transverse, descending,* and *sigmoid* colons and *rectum.* In the colon, unabsorbed material becomes fecal matter, composed of water, food residue, microorganisms, digestive secretions, and mucus. Water is reabsorbed by means of diffusion across the intestinal membrane as the mixture moves through the colon. When the mixture reaches the descending and sigmoid colon, the portion of the bowel adjacent to the rectum, it is a formed mass. The rectum holds and retains fecal matter through contraction of the internal and external anal sphincters. As fecal mass accumulates, it distends the rectal wall, creating the urge to defecate. When the external anal sphincter relaxes, fecal matter is expelled through the anus.

If any portion of the large intestine becomes diseased or is surgically removed, its absorptive function is diminished or lost. This may result in the passage of loose stools and potential fluid and electrolyte imbalance. Passage of liquid stool, which contains many bile salts, makes the client especially vulnerable to skin breakdown in the perianal area. If stool remains in the large intestine too long, constipation results. The client may then strain to evacuate hard, solid stool, which can disrupt skin integrity.

Accessory Structures

The three accessory digestive organs are the liver, gallbladder, and pancreas. Although not an accessory structure itself, the peritoneum encloses the abdominal organs.

Peritoneum

The *peritoneum,* a membrane lining the inner abdomen, encloses the viscera and serous fluid that it secretes. It allows abdominal organs to move about without creating friction. Walls of the digestive organs normally prevent gastric and intestinal contents from escaping into the peritoneal cavity. Any perforation that allows material to seep out of the digestive tract is serious because microorganisms and enzymes can cause a severe inflammation and infection of the surrounding tissue. This condition is known as *peritonitis.*

Liver

The *liver,* the largest glandular organ in the body, weighs between 1 and 1.5 kg (2 to 3 pounds). It is located in the right upper abdomen just under the diaphragm, which separates the liver from the right lung. The liver is involved in many vital, complex metabolic activities. It forms and releases bile; processes vitamins, proteins, fats, and carbohydrates; stores glycogen; contributes to blood coagulation, metabolizes and biotransforms many chemicals (including drugs), bacteria, and foreign matter; and forms antibodies and immunizing substances (gamma globulin). See Chapter 49 for more information.

Gallbladder

The *gallbladder,* attached to the mid-portion of the undersurface of the liver, has a thin wall and holds approximately 60 mL of bile. The liver forms approximately 1 L of bile each day. When bile reaches the gallbladder from the common hepatic duct, water and minerals are absorbed from the bile to form a more concentrated product. Gallbladder contraction, triggered by ingested food (especially fats), causes bile to be released first through the cystic duct and then the common bile duct into the duodenum, where it aids in absorption of fats, fat-soluble vitamins, iron, and calcium. Bile also activates the pancreas to release its digestive enzymes and an alkaline fluid that neutralizes stomach acids that reach the duodenum.

Pancreas

The *pancreas* is both an *exocrine gland,* one that releases secretions into a duct or channel, and an *endocrine gland,* one that releases substances directly into the bloodstream. As an endocrine organ, it produces the hormones insulin and glucagon (see Chap. 52). As an exocrine organ, it produces various protein-, fat-, and carbohydrate-digesting enzymes. At the appropriate time for digestion, pancreatic enzymes are released in inactive forms and transported to the duodenum, where they are activated.

ASSESSMENT

Many conditions disrupt normal function of the GI system. In addition to disorders of the GI tract and accessory organs, disorders involving other organ systems can affect GI function. As a result, the client with a GI disorder may experience a wide variety of health problems involving disturbances of ingestion, digestion, absorption, and elimination. Accurate recording of the client's health history and physical assessment findings help the healthcare team diagnose and treat GI disorders.

History

The history includes the chief complaint; a focus assessment of current nutritional, metabolic, and elimination patterns; and past history. Gather information about why the client has sought treatment and current symptoms. This includes how long the symptoms have been present and what appears to cause or be related to them. Note which types of food produce distress, and when symptoms are most likely. Also determine what measures, if any, the client uses to relieve symptoms, and effects of these measures.

During GI assessment, the focus is on nutritional, metabolic, and elimination patterns, including quality of the client's appetite; problems associated with chewing or swallowing; what and how much the client eats each day; discomfort before, during, or after food consumption; nutritional supplements, if any, that the client uses (e.g., vitamins, herbs, home remedies); weight gain or loss; and bowel elimination patterns (usual consistency and color of stools, visible blood, stool frequency, effort or pain with passage of stool).

After obtaining a current health history, obtain a history of all past medical and surgical disorders and their treatment. Compile a family history of illnesses and causes of death. Family history of digestive disorders is especially important because several, such as colorectal cancer, have a hereditary link. Also explore the client's work history to evaluate possibility of exposure to environmental toxic wastes or radioactive materials.

Obtain a complete allergy history, including adverse reactions to foods, because food allergies can cause various GI symptoms. The medication history includes prescription and nonprescription drugs, especially those affecting GI function. For each drug, list the name, dose, frequency, and reason for taking.

Stop, Think, and Respond ● BOX 45-1

A client says that she has been experiencing nausea and occasional vomiting for several days. What questions should you ask to gain more information? 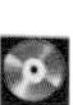

Physical Examination

General Appearance

Assess the client's overall physical condition and measure weight, height, and vital signs. Evaluate general appearance with regard to age and body size and assess hygiene, energy, breathing pattern, emotional attitude, and mental status to the degree that they may affect the client's general appearance.

Skin

Using natural sunlight or bright artificial light, inspect skin for any abnormal color, such as a yellowish tint indicating jaundice. In very dark-skinned clients, inspect the hard palate, gums, conjunctiva, and surrounding tissues for discoloration. If skin appears jaundiced, inspect the sclera to see if it is yellow. Also look for other abnormalities, such as *spider angiomas* (superficial red discolorations consisting of blood vessels that assume a spider-shaped pattern), distended abdominal veins ("caput medusae"), and scars. Assess for dryness of the oral mucosa and skin turgor, which may be poor in clients who are dehydrated as a result of fluid losses from the GI tract.

Mouth

Examine the lips for sores, cracks, lesions, or other abnormalities. Using a tongue blade and a flashlight, inspect the mouth for inflammation, sores, swellings, or discolorations. Assessment of the quality of oral care is essential and includes evaluating for missing teeth and partial plates, bridges, or dentures. If the client has dentures, ask if they fit well and whether the client can eat regular food. If the client can eat only soft foods, communicate this information to the physician and dietary department.

Abdomen

Ask the client to lie supine for an abdominal examination. Abdominal areas typically are described in quadrants (right upper, right lower, left upper, and left lower), with the umbilicus as the center point for both horizontal and vertical divisions. Inspect the abdomen's contour, noting if it is flat, round, concave, or distended, as well as effort associated with breathing. Distention may cause dyspnea as a result of upward pressure on the diaphragm.

Abdominal auscultation is done before palpation because palpation disrupts normal bowel sounds. Using a stethoscope, listen over each quadrant for bowel sounds, which sound like gurgles. Describe the location, pitch quality, and frequency, which usually is every 5 to 30 seconds. Listening for a full 5 minutes over each quadrant is important to confirm absence of bowel sounds. Measurement of abdominal girth is done at the widest point (usually at the umbilicus). Using a pen, mark the measurement location on the abdomen to ensure that additional examiners use the same reference point.

Next is abdominal palpation to determine if it is soft or firm and to detect masses and areas of pain or tenderness. If the client reports tenderness, probe the lower liver margin. An enlarged liver may be felt below the right lower rib cage. Pain or discomfort in this area may suggest a liver disorder, gallbladder or intestinal disease, or a pancreatic disorder. Percuss the abdomen to elicit changes in sounds from dullness over an area with a solid mass, such as the liver, to resonance over less dense structures or those filled with air.

Anus

Examine the anal area for external hemorrhoids, skin tags, or fissures (small tears in the anal opening). Inspect the skin surrounding the anus for breaks, lesions, rash, inflammation, and drainage. If and when stool passes, examine its characteristics. Shape, color, and consistency of stool usually are helpful in differential diagnosis of GI disorders. Foods and medications alter the color of stool (Table 45.2).

TABLE 45.2 FOODS AND MEDICATIONS THAT ALTER STOOL COLOR

ALTERING SUBSTANCE	COLOR
Meat protein	Dark brown
Spinach	Green
Carrots and beets	Red
Cocoa	Dark red or brown
Senna	Yellow
Bismuth, iron, licorice, and charcoal	Black
Barium	Milky white

(From Smeltzer, S. C. & Bare, B. G. [2004]. *Brunner & Suddarth's textbook of medical–surgical nursing* [10th ed., p. 946]. Philadelphia: Lippincott Williams & Wilkins.)

Diagnostic Tests

Radiographic Studies

X-ray studies are used to identify the location and structural appearance of organs or other space-occupying masses (air, fluid, tumors, foreign objects) in the abdomen, chest, or GI system. These studies involve use of radiopaque contrast media. *Fluoroscopy* may be used to observe the shape and contour of empty organs and how these hollow structures fill with and evacuate radiopaque dye (contrast medium).

BARIUM SWALLOW OR UPPER GASTROINTESTINAL SERIES. Sometimes the terms *barium swallow* and *upper GI series* are used interchangeably. Strictly speaking, a **barium swallow** is fluoroscopic observation of the client actually swallowing a flavored barium solution and its progress down the esophagus. Barium swallow facilitates identification of structural abnormalities of the esophagus as well as swallowing discoordination and oral aspiration. An **upper gastrointestinal series** also includes radiographic observation of barium moving into the stomach and the first part of the small intestine.

Structural abnormalities in the esophagus include tumors, strictures, varices, and hiatal hernia. Structural abnormalities below the esophagus include gastric tumors, peptic ulcers, and numerous gastric disorders (see Chaps. 46 and 47). The examination may take as little as 20 minutes if only a barium swallow is performed. If stomach filling and emptying need to be observed, the test may take approximately 1 hour.

For several days before the procedure, the client is on a low-residue diet. Usually, he or she takes nothing by mouth (NPO) for 8 to 12 hours before the test. A laxative may be given to clean out the GI tract. Smoking stimulates gastric motility, so the client is asked not to smoke the day of the procedure. With rare exceptions (e.g., anticonvulsants, insulin), all medications are withheld.

Barium is very constipating. Once any test using barium is over, the client needs to drink fluids liberally to dilute barium and promote its elimination from the GI tract. Stools will appear white, streaky, or clay colored from the barium. Wait to obtain stool specimens until the client has fully excreted the barium. A laxative may help with evacuation. Failure to have a bowel movement within a reasonable time must be reported to the physician because retained barium may cause a blockage.

SMALL BOWEL SERIES. A small bowel series is fluoroscopy of the small intestine after ingestion of a contrast medium. It is used to identify tumors, inflammation, or obstruction in the jejunum or ileum. It is performed like an upper GI series, but the client must swallow more barium for the small intestine to be well visualized. If an obstruction or *fistula* (a leaking channel between two structures) is suspected, a water-soluble contrast medium such as methylglucamine diatrizoate (Gastrografin) is substituted for the barium. The test takes 5 to 6 hours, which is when the contrast medium reaches the lower portion of the small intestine.

ENTEROCLYSIS. Also known as a *small bowel enema*, **enteroclysis** requires nasal or oral placement of a flexible feeding tube. The tip is positioned in the proximal jejunum. This study uses two contrast media. First, 500 to 1000 mL of a thin barium suspension is infused through the tube, followed by methylcellulose. The two contrast media fill in and pass through the intestinal loops. The examiner observes the intestine continuously by fluoroscopy and takes periodic x-rays of various sections of the small intestine. Even with normal motility, this process can take up to 6 hours (Smeltzer & Bare, 2004). If sedation is administered to ensure the client's comfort, he or she requires monitoring accordingly. Risk for aspiration of contrast media is increased if the client vomits while under sedation. Positioning of the client on his or her side and availability of a suction apparatus are critical.

BARIUM ENEMA OR LOWER GASTROINTESTINAL SERIES. A **barium enema** or **lower gastrointestinal series** is used to identify polyps, tumors, inflammation, strictures, and other abnormalities of the colon. The radiographic technologist rectally instills 1 to 1.5 L of barium solution. He or she observes the rectum, sigmoid colon, and descending colon fluoroscopically during filling. To facilitate this process, the examiner directs the client to make multiple position changes. The client must retain the barium during this test, which may take up to 30 minutes.

During the test, the client may experience abdominal cramping and a strong urge to defecate. Reassure the client that most people can retain instilled barium throughout the test. X-rays are taken again after the client expels the barium. In some cases, air is instilled to compress the barium residue against the wall of the lower intestine to aid in detecting mucosal defects. Stool specimens are not collected until the barium is expelled completely.

Twenty-four to 72 hours before the barium enema, the client follows certain restrictions and procedures to reduce formation of stool and remove residual stool:

- Low-residue diet 1 to 2 days before the test
- Clear liquid diet the evening before the test
- A laxative the evening before the test
- NPO after midnight
- Cleansing enemas the morning of the test (if not contraindicated by inflammation or active bleeding)

Fluids are not restricted, and the client usually does not have to withhold oral medications. The client may have up to three cleansing enemas (or until the evacuated solution appears clear) before the procedure. After the examination is complete, the client may resume eating. Encourage the client to rest and drink fluids liberally. Also monitor the passage of stool and inform the client that feces will appear white until barium is completely eliminated.

ORAL CHOLECYSTOGRAPHY OR GALLBLADDER SERIES. Oral **cholecystography** or **gallbladder series** identifies stones in the gallbladder or common bile duct and tumors or other obstructions. The test also determines the ability of the gallbladder to concentrate and store a dyelike, iodine-based, radiopaque contrast medium. After dye is absorbed, it goes to the liver, is excreted into the bile, and passes into the gallbladder, making it radiographically visible. X-rays of the gallbladder should be performed before other GI examinations in which barium is used because residual barium tends to obscure the image of the gallbladder and its ducts.

To prepare for this test the client swallows six dye tablets—one every 5 minutes after the evening meal with a total of 250 mL of water or more. Instruct the client that he or she may not eat or drink until the test is complete. If tablets cause nausea and vomiting, notify the physician so that more tablets can be administered or the test rescheduled. Once initial x-rays are obtained, a fatty test meal is given and additional x-rays taken to determine the gallbladder's ability to empty.

CHOLANGIOGRAPHY. **Cholangiography** determines the patency of the ducts from the liver and gallbladder. It is used when the gallbladder is not distinctly visualized with an oral cholecystogram, vomiting interferes with retention of oral dye, or the status of the ductal system needs to be determined during or after surgery.

The dye for cholangiography usually is instilled intravenously (IV). Other routes include infusion through a T-tube surgically placed in the common bile duct, a cannula advanced through the skin at a site below the rib margin, or an endoscope inserted through the upper GI tract into the sphincter of Oddi (where the common bile duct empties into the duodenum).

The client must sign a consent form. Ask if the client is allergic to iodine or shellfish. Administer a cleansing enema if ordered. The client may need to restrict food and fluids for several hours before the examination. Inform the client that he or she may experience a warm sensation and nausea when dye is instilled. After the procedure, the client may eat and drink. Encourage the client to drink liberally to promote dye excretion.

RADIONUCLIDE IMAGING. **Radionuclide imaging** detects lesions of the liver or pancreas and assists in evaluating gastric emptying. A radionuclide is a radioactive natural or synthetic element, such as technetium. Once the radionuclide is injected IV or ingested orally, the radiologist may examine a body organ by passing the radionuclide imaging scanner over the structure. This test demonstrates the size of the organ, as well as defects or lesions such as tumors. Specialized radionuclide studies are done to identify sites of bleeding or inflammation in the GI tract. Radionuclides have rather short half-lives, lasting a few hours to days, during which they emit radiation, usually less than with diagnostic x-rays.

Pretest measures include weighing the client to calculate radionuclide dose and determining pregnancy and lactation. Breast milk may be pumped and discarded so that the nursing child remains safe from radioactivity. The test is contraindicated in pregnant women.

COMPUTED TOMOGRAPHY. Computed tomography (CT) scanning may be performed to detect structural abnormalities of the GI tract. These tests help detect metastatic lesions that might not be apparent on regular GI x-rays. Oral barium sulfate or IV calcium phosphate may be given to provide contrast for the hollow GI organs examined by CT scan. The client is NPO for 6 to 8 hours before the CT test. Before the test, the bowel may be cleaned to reduce stool and gas. Drugs may be administered to decrease peristalsis or improve gastric motility.

Nonradiographic Studies

MAGNETIC RESONANCE IMAGING. Magnetic resonance imaging (MRI) uses magnetic energy rather than radiation to visualize soft tissue structures, particularly when CT scanning is inadequate. Oral contrast agents are used to enhance evaluation of GI disorders, such as abscesses or bleeding.

The client is NPO for 6 to 8 hours before the MRI. He or she must remove metal objects, credit cards, wristwatch, jewelry, and the like. IV fluids must be infused by gravity during MRI because changes in electrical charges during the test can affect mechanical infusers or pumps. The nurse informs clients that the scanner, a narrow, tunnel-like machine that will enclose them during the test, makes loud repetitive noises while the test is in progress. Clients who tend to be claustrophobic (fear enclosed spaces) may need sedation because it is imperative that they lie still and not panic during the test.

ULTRASONOGRAPHY. In **ultrasonography** (also called *ultrasound*), high-frequency sound waves are directed through the body, where they bounce off nearby structures, such as the liver and pancreas. Returning sound waves are then interpreted and recorded electronically. Ultrasonography, which shows size and location of organs and outlines structures and abnormalities, helps detect cholecystitis, cholelithiasis, and some disorders of the biliary system. It may be useful in detecting changes caused by appendicitis. Although the client can drink water before ultrasonography, discourage drinking through a straw, smoking, or chewing gum, because the client may swallow air and distort sound wave transmission.

PERCUTANEOUS LIVER BIOPSY. In **percutaneous liver biopsy,** the physician obtains a small core of liver tissue by placing a needle through the client's lateral abdominal wall directly into the liver. Tissue is then examined microscopically to detect abnormalities, which may include malignant changes, infectious or inflammatory processes, liver damage ("cirrhosis"), and signs of rejection in clients who have a liver transplant.

The client must have coagulation studies before the procedure. A major complication after liver biopsy is bleeding. Ultrasound or CT scanning is performed before or during the biopsy to identify an appropriate site for placement of the biopsy needle. The client usually receives a sedative and anesthetic.

If assisting with a percutaneous liver biopsy, ensure that biopsy equipment is assembled and in order. Assist the client to a supine position with a rolled towel beneath the right lower ribs. Before the physician inserts the needle, instruct the client to take a deep breath and hold it to keep the liver as near to the abdominal wall as possible. After specimen cells are obtained, they are placed in a preservative. Make sure that the specimen container is labeled and delivered to the laboratory (Nursing Guidelines 45-1).

GASTROINTESTINAL ENDOSCOPY. Gastrointestinal endoscopy is the direct visual examination of the lumen of the GI tract. It facilitates evaluation of the appearance and integrity of the GI mucosa and detects lesions. It provides access for therapeutic procedures. GI endoscopy is performed using a flexible fiberoptic endoscope. Diagnostic uses include obtaining biopsies of the mucosa, obtaining samples of fluids found in the GI tract, and injecting dyes for radiographic purposes. Therapeutic uses include inserting tubes and drains, electrocautery, and injecting medications. GI endoscopy (Box 45-1) procedures include **proctosigmoidoscopy, esophagogastroduodenoscopy** (EGD) (Fig. 45.2), small bowel enteroscopy, peritoneoscopy, **colonoscopy, flexible sigmoidoscopy, panendoscopy,** and **endoscopic retrograde cholangiopancreatography** (ERCP).

Before an endoscopic procedure, the client follows dietary and fluid restrictions and bowel preparation procedures if the examination involves the lower GI structures. For the client undergoing an EGD, it is necessary for the client to spray or gargle with a local anesthetic. For an EGD and a colonoscopy, the client receives an anxiolytic agent [e.g., midazolam (Versed)] before the procedure to provide sedation and relieve anxiety.

During an endoscopic procedure, monitor respirations and vital signs. Assessing the client's level of pain

NURSING GUIDELINES 45-1

Client Care After Liver Biopsy

- Assist client to roll on right side after procedure, placing a small pillow under the costal margin.
- Instruct client to remain in this position for several hours to prevent the release of blood, bile, or both.
- Ask client to avoid coughing or straining while immobilized.
- Take vital signs every 15 minutes for the first hour, then every 30 minutes for the next 2 hours, or until client is stable. Changes in vital signs may indicate bleeding.
- Teach client to avoid heavy lifting or strenuous activity postprocedure.

BOX 45-1 ● Common Gastrointestinal Endoscopic Procedures

ESOPHAGOGASTRODUODENOSCOPY (EGD)
Examination of the esophagus, stomach, and duodenum through an endoscope advanced orally to inspect, treat, or obtain specimens from any one or all of the upper GI structures.

COLONOSCOPY
Examination of the entire large intestine with a flexible fiberoptic colonoscope. The colonoscope is advanced anally from the rectum to the cecum, allowing visualization of the rectum, sigmoid, and descending colon. The distal portion of the small intestine, the terminal ileum, may be inspected as well. Air may be instilled to promote visualization within the folds of the intestinal mucosa. Clients are sedated briefly (and monitored accordingly) with IV medication during the procedure.

PROCTOSIGMOIDOSCOPY
Examination of the rectum and sigmoid colon using a rigid endoscope inserted anally about 10 inches. To facilitate examination, the client must lie in a knee chest position. The test is brief and no sedation is needed.

ENDOSCOPIC RETROGRADE CHOLANGIOPANCREATOGRAPHY (ERCP)
Combined endoscopic and radiographic examination using radiopaque contrast medium instilled in the biliary tree to visualize the biliary and pancreatic ducts.

PERITONEOSCOPY
Examination of GI structures through an endoscope inserted percutaneously through a small incision in the abdominal wall with the patient receiving a local, spinal, or general anesthetic. Also called *laparoscopy*.

SMALL BOWEL ENTEROSCOPY
Endoscopic examination and visualization of the lumen of the small bowel.

PANENDOSCOPY
Examination of both the upper and lower GI tracts.

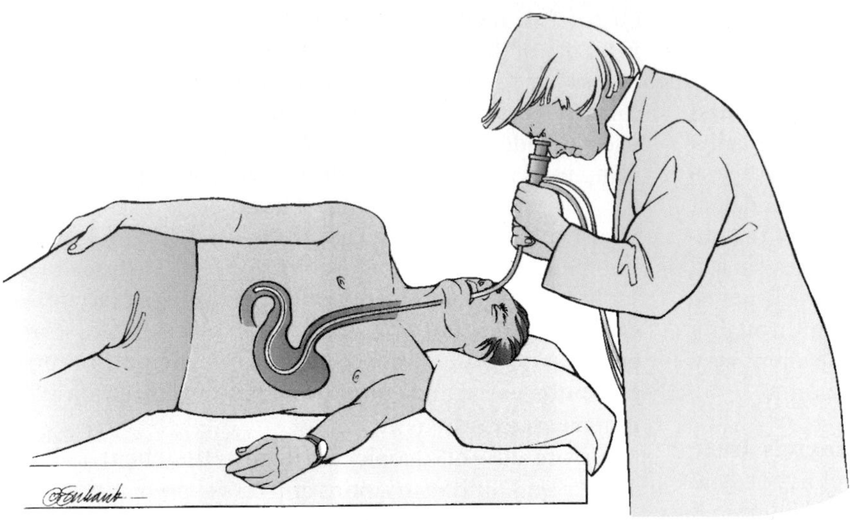

FIGURE 45.2 Esophagogastroduodenoscopy. (From Smeltzer, S. C. & Bare, B. G. [2004]. *Brunner & Suddarth's textbook of medical–surgical nursing* [10th ed.]. Philadelphia: Lippincott Williams & Wilkins.)

and discomfort during the procedure is important, as is medicating the client as indicated. After the test, monitor the client for complications, especially signs of perforation. These include fever, abdominal distention, abdominal or chest pain, vomiting blood, or bright red rectal bleeding. Offer the client food and fluids, unless the procedure was an EGD. After an EGD, the client may not have food or fluids until the gag reflex returns. Once the gag reflex is present, the nurse may introduce clear fluids and advance diet to regular foods and fluids according to client's tolerance. The client may complain of a sore throat after EGD. When the client's gag reflex returns, the nurse may offer saline gargles, ice chips, or cool drinks.

New procedures are evolving that may eventually replace colonoscopy and other endoscopic procedures. One involves swallowing a "capsule" that videotapes the GI tract as it makes its way through the system. Another, called "virtual colonoscopy," combines CT scanning with computer graphics. The physician is able to see more of the colon and view it from various angles. Clinical studies are in process to determine if these tests are as accurate as endocsopic procedures.

LABORATORY TESTS. Depending on the suspected or confirmed diagnosis, various blood and urine tests are ordered. Laboratory tests may include a complete blood count, urinalysis, serum bilirubin, cholesterol, serum ammonia level, prothrombin time, protein electrophoresis, and enzymes, such as amylase, lipase, aspartate aminotransferase, and lactic acid dehydrogenase. Common tumor marker blood studies include carcinoembryonic antigen and alpha-fetoprotein. Tests specific to the GI system are described in the following sections.

Gastric Analysis. Analysis of gastric fluids assists in determining problems with the secretory activity of the gastric mucosa. It also evaluates gastric retention in clients with partial or complete pyloric or duodenal obstruction. For 8 to 12 hours before the test, the client is NPO. A small nasogastric tube is inserted into the stomach. Gastric contents are aspirated every 15 minutes for at least 1 hour and analyzed for acidity (pH), volume, and cytology if indicated.

PY Test. The **PY test** uses ^{14}C-urea capsules to detect *Helicobacter pylori,* the bacteria associated with peptic ulcer disease. This test is simple and straightforward (Fig. 45.3). The client takes a ^{14}C-urea capsule, waits approximately 10 minutes, and blows up a balloon. Air in the balloon is then transferred to a special vial for analysis. If gastric urease, an enzyme not normally present in human cells, is identified in the balloon air, the client most likely has *H. pylori* infection. This breath analysis is 90% accurate.

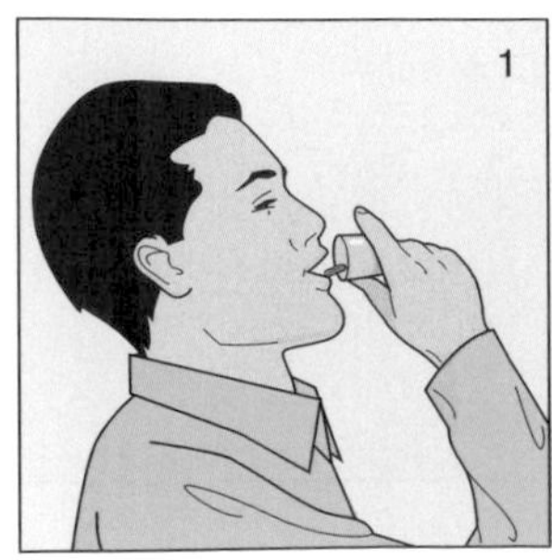

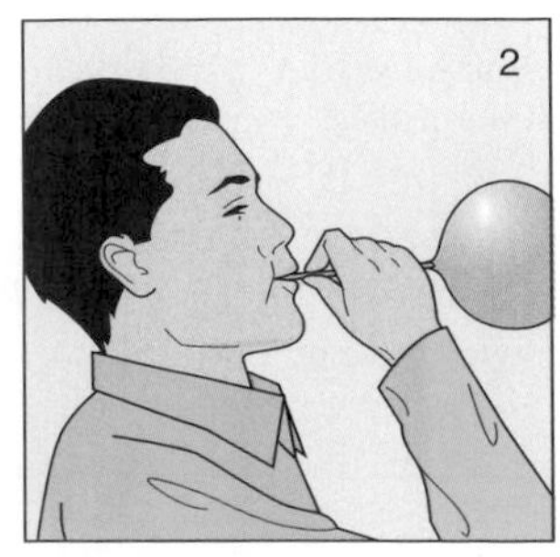

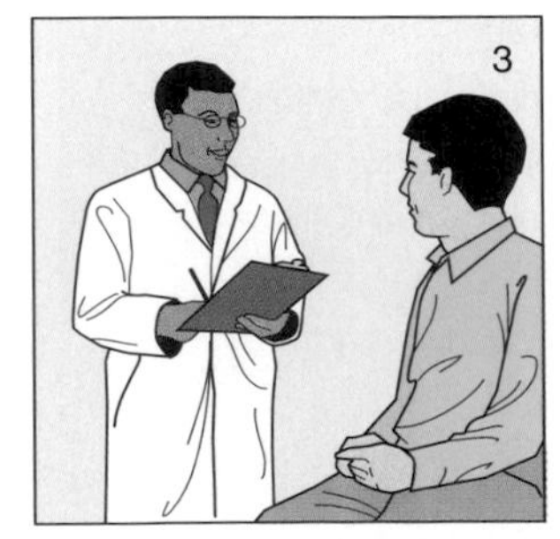

FIGURE 45.3 The breath test that indicates *Helicobacter pylori* is performed in three easy steps: (1) the client takes a ^{14}C-urea capsule and waits about 10 minutes. (2) The client blows up a balloon. (3) The client waits while the air in the balloon is analyzed for gastric urease.

Clients having this test must avoid antibiotics or bismuth for 1 month, proton pump inhibitors and sucralfate for 2 weeks, and food and fluids for 6 hours before the test. To ensure accurate test results, advise the client not to handle or chew the test capsule but instead to swallow it intact.

Hydrogen Breath Testing. This test involves collecting a breath sample before and at intervals after ingestion of a carbohydrate solution. The two major gases in expired air are hydrogen and carbon dioxide. Elevated hydrogen levels in the expired breath sample indicate carbohydrate malabsorption. The type of solution used for the test depends on the suspected type of malabsorption. Lactose malabsorption (lactose intolerance) is a common disorder investigated using this technique.

Stool Analysis. Stool specimens are collected to identify white blood cells (indicating inflammation), red blood cells (indicating GI blood loss), and fat (indicating malabsorption). They also are collected to identify infection. Routine cultures may reveal bacterial infections (e.g., *Salmonella, Shigella, Campylobacter*). Placement of the specimen in a specific preservative to detect parasites and their ova allows diagnosis of parasitic infections (e.g., *Giardia, Cryptosporidium*).

Stool specimens that require examination for microorganisms should be fresh and warm for analysis. Only a small amount of stool needs to be collected; it always should be placed in a covered container. Eating red meat or other foods containing peroxidase within the previous 3 days may produce a false-positive result in some tests used for detecting occult blood.

NURSING PROCESS

● Diagnostic Testing for a Gastrointestinal Disorder

Assessment

Interview the client to determine past familiarity with the test or similar procedure. Ask the client to discuss previous experiences or current expectations. If the client is responsible for self-preparation before the test, review those preparations. Explore any data on prior hypersensitivity or allergy to test preparations. In particular, ask about reactions to radionuclide or iodine-based contrast medium (dye) signaled by allergy to seafood. In some situations, the nurse labels an allergic client's chart and applies a special band or tag to the client's identification bracelet.

Take vital signs and weigh the client if required before the procedure. Encourage the client to empty the bladder before some tests. Recording other essential baseline data is important for later comparison and identification of serious reportable changes or complications (e.g., rectal bleeding). Record the client's informed consent. The client and family members need teaching and reassurance about the test's purpose and procedure. They also need to know care measures needed after the test.

Diagnosis, Planning, and Interventions

Anxiety related to lack of knowledge of test procedure or possible test findings

Expected Outcomes: (1) Client will demonstrate knowledge of the test procedure. (2) Client will express feelings of relief from anxiety.

- Review test preparations. *Ensures that the client understands and carries out preparations as required.*
- Provide printed directions. *Reinforces verbal instructions.*
- Encourage client to express fears. *Assists in alleviating fear and clarifying misconceptions.*
- Discuss client's perceptions of the test and explain what to expect during and after. *Provides opportunity to reinforce knowledge and clarify expectations for the test.*
- Respect client's individuality and remain nonjudgmental and supportive. *Makes client more likely to ask questions without fear of ridicule.*

Risk for Deficient Fluid Volume related to fluid restriction or loss associated with diarrhea or vomiting

Expected Outcome: Client will maintain fluid volume balance as evidenced by normal findings on intake and output records.

- Weigh client and monitor color and amount of urine. *Provides a baseline for client's response to tests, fluid loss related to diarrhea or vomiting, or both.*
- Monitor pulse rate and blood pressure. *Changes may indicate dehydration.*
- Report dizziness and confusion. *May indicate dehydration.*
- Administer oral fluids as soon as possible. *Replaces fluid loss.*
- When testing is complete, monitor intake and output and encourage liberal intake. *Ensures that client is taking in adequate fluids.*

Risk for Constipation related to barium retention

Expected Outcome: Client achieves regular bowel elimination pattern within 2 to 3 days.

- Encourage client to drink at least 2000 mL of fluid per 24 hours after tests using barium. *Provides sufficient fluid to facilitate evacuation of stool.*
- Administer post-test laxative or enema if ordered. *Promotes faster evacuation of barium.*
- Monitor stool passage, observing stool for barium. *Stools with barium appear light-colored or white-streaked.*
- Report diminished or hyperactive bowel sounds. *May indicate barium retention.*

Evaluation of Expected Outcomes

The client reports minimal anxiety, maintains adequate fluid balance, and evacuates all barium. Normal bowel elimination resumes, as evidenced by one bowel movement of soft-formed brown stool per day.

GENERAL GERONTOLOGIC CONSIDERATIONS

Fluid balance for clients, especially older adults, may be precarious, given fluid restrictions and multiple enemas or laxatives required for GI tests.

Older adults are at higher risk for dehydration when undergoing a lower GI series or endoscopic examinations of the bowel than are younger people because they tend to have fewer physiologic reserves to compensate for fluid loss. A history of vomiting or diarrhea or diuretic therapy may compound potential for fluid deficit.

The older adult usually has less control of the rectal sphincter than a younger adult because of age-related changes in innervation, a diminished awareness of the filling reflex, and decreased muscle tone.

To detect fluid volume deficit, weigh client and observe color and amount of urine.

Explain the diagnostic examination to the older adult in simple language, allowing ample time to answer questions. Repeated explanations and assurances may be necessary to ease the older adult's anxiety.

After the diagnostic test, the older adult may experience dizziness or confusion from the stress of the examination or enduring 6 to 8 hours without food or fluids. Provide nourishment as soon as possible after the examination, and give assistance with ambulation when necessary.

Critical Thinking Exercise

1. *A client is preparing for an EGD. This includes withholding food and fluids for 6 to 12 hours and receiving a sedative before the test. In addition, the nurse will spray the client's throat with a local anesthetic or the client will gargle with the local anesthetic. What precautions does the nurse take before the client goes for the EGD?*

• NCLEX-STYLE REVIEW QUESTIONS

1. A nurse is teaching a group of clients with stomach disorders about anatomy and physiology. Which portion of the small intestine would the nurse identify as the entry point of bile and pancreatic enzymes?
   1. Jejunum
   2. Ileum
   3. Sigmoid
   4. Duodenum
2. The nurse is assessing a client's abdominal region. Which assessment sequence is most correct?
   1. Auscultation, palpation, inspection
   2. Inspection, palpation, auscultation
   3. Inspection, auscultation, palpation
   4. Palpation, auscultation, inspection
3. A client is returning from an esophagogastroduodenoscopy (EGD). Which nursing assessment is the highest priority?
   1. Intake and output
   2. Gag reflex
   3. Bowel sounds
   4. Urinary function

connection

Visit the Connection site at **http://connection.lww.com/go/timbyEssentials** for links to chapter-related resources on the Internet.

References and Suggested Readings

Ahmed, D. S. (2000). Hidden factors in occult blood testing. *American Journal of Nursing, 100*(12), 25.

Bickley, L. S. (2003). *Bates' guide to physical examination and history taking* (8th ed.). Philadelphia: Lippincott Williams & Wilkins.

Bullock, B. A., & Henze, R. L. (2000). *Focus on pathophysiology*. Philadelphia: Lippincott Williams & Wilkins.

Chartrand, S. (May 5, 2003). 'Virtual' colonoscopy wins patients. *The New York Times*. [On-line.] Available: wysiwyg://3/http://www.nytimes.com/2003.

Mehta, M. (2003). Assessing the abdomen. *Nursing 2003, 33*(5), 54–55.

Smeltzer, S. C., & Bare, B. G. (2004). *Brunner & Suddarth's textbook of medical–surgical nursing* (10th ed.). Philadelphia: Lippincott Williams & Wilkins.

chapter 46

Caring for Clients With Disorders of the Upper Gastrointestinal Tract

Words to Know 

anorexia
dumping syndrome
dyspepsia
esophagitis
fundoplication
gastrectomy
gastric decompression
gastritis
gastroesophageal reflux disease (GERD)
gastrostomy
hiatal hernia (diaphragmatic hernia)
jejunostomy
nasoenteric intubation
nasogastric intubation
odynophagia
orogastric intubation
peptic ulcer
percutaneous endoscopic gastrostomy (PEG)
pyrosis

Learning Objectives

On completion of this chapter, the reader will:

- Discuss assessment findings and treatment of disorders that affect eating, disorders of the esophagus, and gastric disorders.
- Describe nursing management of a client with a nasogastric or gastrointestinal tube or gastrostomy.
- List suggestions for relieving upper gastrointestinal discomfort.
- Discuss the nursing management of clients undergoing gastric surgery.

Digestion begins in the mouth and continues in the stomach and small intestine, with food traveling through the esophagus in between. The nurse is responsible for managing the care of clients with disorders affecting the upper gastrointestinal (GI) tract (see Fig. 45.1).

DISORDERS THAT AFFECT EATING

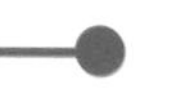

• ANOREXIA

Simple **anorexia,** or lack of appetite, is a common symptom of many diseases. Prolonged anorexia may lead to serious consequences, such as malnutrition.

Pathophysiology and Etiology

The appetite center, which stimulates or suppresses appetite, is located in the hypothalamus. Pleasant or noxious food odors, effects of drugs, emotional stress, fear, psychological problems, or illnesses may affect appetite.

Brief periods of anorexia are not life-threatening but can cause temporary malnutrition. During periods of reduced food consumption, most people have sufficient reserves of stored glycogen, which provide energy through *glycogenolysis,* conversion of glycogen to glucose. Hormones such as glucagon, glucocorticoid hormones from the adrenal cortex, and thyroid hormones stimulate the liver to carry out *gluconeogenesis,* which depends on use of stores of fat-soluble vitamins. Selective reabsorption by the kidneys can temporarily maintain electrolyte balance.

Assessment Findings

Hunger usually is absent, and clients describe having no desire for food. Some clients state that they feel nauseous when they smell food or even think about eating. Some eat a small amount only because they feel they should. Amounts of weight loss vary, depending on how long anorexia and reduced food intake last. Eventually the client may show signs of *hypovitaminosis* (vitamin deficiency). The body does not store any water-soluble vitamins (B vitamins, including folic acid and vitamin C) except for B_{12}. Deficiencies in these vitamins may be seen in more acute phases of illness. The body does store fat-soluble vitamins (A, D, E, and K) but requires fat absorption to do so. Chronic illnesses and those that directly affect fat absorption (e.g., cystic fibrosis, pancreatitis, liver disease) result in deficiency of fat-soluble vitamins.

Depending on the chronicity of anorexia, hemoglobin level and blood cell counts may be reduced. Red blood cells (RBCs) may become abnormally enlarged. Serum albumin, electrolyte, and protein levels may be low, with accompanying cardiac dysrhythmias. For example, an elevated U wave on an electrocardiogram may indicate potassium deficiency.

Medical and Surgical Management

Management depends on the cause. Short-term anorexia (less than 1 week) usually requires no medical intervention. Persistent anorexia may require various approaches, such as a high-calorie diet, high-calorie supplemental feedings, tube feedings, and total parenteral nutrition (TPN). Psychological support, psychiatric treatment, or both may be essential for a client whose anorexia is linked with *anorexia nervosa,* a psychiatric disorder, instead of a defined organic disease (see Chap. 16).

Nursing Management

To maintain sufficient nutrition and sustain normal body weight, the client must eat an adequate quantity of food. In assisting the client to meet this goal, monitor weight daily. Also obtain a complete medical and allergy (drugs and food) history from the client or a family member and compile a dietary history, including a description of the client's eating patterns and food preferences. For more information, see Nursing Guidelines 46-1.

NURSING GUIDELINES 46-1

Managing Care of the Client With Anorexia

- Provide foods that the client likes during meals.
- Offer nourishing beverages (egg nog, milk shakes, and commercial concentrates such as Ensure or Instant Breakfast) as between-meal snacks.
- If the client is hospitalized or in another healthcare facility, encourage family members to bring favorite foods that can be refrigerated or reheated.
- Conduct a daily caloric count if necessary to determine total caloric intake and the amount of vitamins, minerals, fats, proteins, and carbohydrates in the client's diet.
- Keep serving sizes and containers small to avoid overwhelming the client.
- Serve and keep hot foods hot and cold foods cold.
- Encourage eating in the company of others.
- Formulate a nutritional plan with the client and dietitian that promotes weight gain (approximately 600 calories per meal).
- If necessary, arrange for supplementation based on documented deficiencies in the client's intake.
- Consult the physician and dietitian in cases of prolonged anorexia.

• NAUSEA AND VOMITING

Nausea and vomiting are common and often coexisting problems. If these symptoms are prolonged, weakness, weight loss, nutritional deficiency, dehydration, and electrolyte and acid-base imbalances may result.

Pathophysiology and Etiology

Some common causes of nausea and vomiting are drugs, infections and inflammatory conditions of the GI tract, intestinal obstruction, systemic infections, lesions of the central nervous system, food poisoning, emotional stress, early pregnancy, and uremia. Nausea usually precedes vomiting and results from distention of the duodenum. Increased salivation and peripheral vasoconstriction, which causes cold, clammy skin and tachycardia, accompany nausea. The vomiting center, located in the medulla, is sensitive to parasympathetic neurotransmitters released in response to gastric irritation. The Valsalva maneuver, which accompanies forceful expulsion of stomach contents, causes dizziness, hypotension, and bradycardia.

Assessment Findings

The client describes an unpleasant feeling, identified as nausea, usually associated with loss of appetite and refusal to eat. When a client vomits, he or she may retch while evacuating stomach contents. The process occurs once or several times in succession.

The client who experiences excessive fluid loss (dehydration) with vomiting may complain of excessive thirst and report decreased or no urine production. Eyes and oral mucosa appear dry or dull, and poor skin turgor reflects fluid loss.

The client's history may include ingestion of noxious substances, such as excessive amounts of alcohol, contaminated food, or drugs that can cause GI side effects. Exposure to other people with similar symptoms suggests a bacterial or viral cause.

When vomiting is secondary to intestinal obstruction, the abdomen is distended, tender, and firm to touch. Bowel sounds may be absent or hypoactive.

Prolonged vomiting may lead to low levels of serum sodium and chloride. Bicarbonate levels may rise to compensate for loss of chloride and accumulation of metabolic acids. A high hematocrit value is secondary to hemoconcentration that accompanies dehydration.

Medical and Surgical Management

In some instances nausea and vomiting are short-lived and do not require medical intervention, but in others intravenous (IV) fluids, electrolyte replacement, and drug therapy are necessary. To eliminate the cause, various interventions, ranging from stopping a drug to surgical intervention for intestinal obstruction, are needed. Symptomatic relief may be achieved by administering an antiemetic agent (Drug Therapy Table 46.1), providing IV fluid and electrolyte replacement, and temporarily restricting food intake until the cause of vomiting is eliminated.

DRUG THERAPY TABLE 46.1 ANTIEMETIC MEDICATIONS

DRUG CATEGORY AND EXAMPLES/ MECHANISM OF ACTION	SIDE EFFECTS	NURSING CONSIDERATIONS
Serotonin Receptor Antagonist		
ondanestron *(Zofran)* Blocks receptors for $5HT_3$, which affects the neural pathways involved in nausea and vomiting	Headache, dizziness (low blood pressure), myalgia (muscle aches and pains), malaise, fatigue, drowsiness	Review client's allergy history before administering medication. Provide oral drug form q8h around the clock for 1 to 2 days after chemotherapy or radiation to prevent nausea and vomiting. Caution client about side effects that may make activities such as driving a car or operating other machinery hazardous.
Phenothiazine		
prochlorperazine *(Compazine)* Inhibits the CTZ and vomiting center in the brain	Drowsiness, hypotension, changes in heart rhythms, photophobia, blurred vision, dry mouth, discolored urine	Tell client that this drug is for short-term control of nausea and vomiting and should be used exactly as directed. Explain side effects and advise client not to save any medicine for a later date or give any to any one else. Monitor older clients because effects of drug may lead more rapidly to dehydration than in younger clients.
Antihistamines		
hydroxyzine *(Atarax, Vistaril)* Blocks H_1 receptors, decreasing stimulation of the CTZ and vomiting center	Drowsiness, tremor, dry mouth, hypersensitivity reaction (includes difficulty breathing), tremors, loss of coordination, sore muscles, or muscle spasms	Take full health history to help determine underlying cause of nausea and vomiting. Give by deep intramuscular injection in volume prescribed to control vomiting. Report breathing problems, tremors, muscle problems and incoordination.
promethazine *(Anergan, Phenergan)* Blocks H_1 receptors, decreasing stimulation of the CTZ and vomiting center	Dizziness, drowsiness, poor coordination, confusion, restlessness, excitation, epigastric distress, thickened bronchial secretions, urinary frequency, dysuria	Take drug and health history. Because this drug interacts with several others, review potential for drug interactions; for example, do not administer medication if client is taking monoamine oxidase inhibitor. Do not give to a client with a lower respiratory tract disorder. Advise client to avoid drinking alcohol when taking this medication.
dimenhydrinate *(Dramamine)* Inhibits vestibular stimulation in the ear, thereby relieving motion sickness	Drowsiness, confusion, nervousness, restlessness, headache, dizziness, vertigo, tingling, heaviness and weakness of hands, epigastric discomfort, low blood pressure, nasal stuffiness, chest tightness, rash, photosensitivity	Advise client not to take if pregnant or lactating. Review client history for glaucoma, peptic ulcer, bronchial asthma, heart problems because drug may pose a danger. Urge client to avoid alcohol because serious sedation could result. Advise client to report breathing problems, tremors, loss of coordination, visual disturbances or hallucinations, and irregular heartbeat.

CTZ, chemoreceptor trigger zone.

Nursing Management

Obtain a complete medical, dietary, drug, and allergy history. In addition, compile a list of symptoms that occurred before and along with nausea and vomiting, how long the problem has existed, and frequency, color, and amount of vomited material. Because the cause may be unknown, list foods and where the client ate in the past 24 hours. In addition, assess general appearance, weight, and vital signs. Documenting intake and output and monitoring for signs of fluid volume deficit are additional essential assessment requirements.

Offer clear fluids in small amounts to help the client to develop tolerance and determine if he or she can advance the diet. Recommend commercial over-the-counter beverages such as Gatorade, which replace fluids and electrolytes. Inform the physician if urine output is below 500 mL/day or serum electrolyte levels are abnormal. These findings indicate severe dehydration and need for IV replacement fluids. Monitor the client's weight daily to determine trends in weight loss or gain. Assess skin turgor and mucous membranes for any signs of dehydration.

When the client tolerates clear fluids, advance diet to full liquids, then to soft, bland foods, such as creamed soups, crackers, or toast. Collaborate with a dietitian to provide nutritional foods. The dietitian can help create a plan that assists the client to increase caloric intake with foods that he or she can tolerate. Discourage caffeinated or carbonated beverages, which may decrease appetite and lead to early satiety.

• CANCER OF THE ORAL CAVITY

Cancer cells undergo changes in structure and appearance. They multiply, eventually forming a colony of abnormal and dysfunctional cells (see Chap. 19). When cancer affects the oral cavity, cells in the lips, mouth, or pharynx undergo malignant changes. When cancers of the oral cavity are detected early, the rate of cure is fairly good.

Pathophysiology and Etiology

Development of oral cancers is linked with smoking, chewing tobacco, and drinking alcohol in excess. Lip cancer is associated with pipe smoking and prolonged exposure to wind and sun. As cancer cells in the oral cavity increase, the mass may distort a client's appearance; exert pressure on surrounding tissue, making it difficult to masticate (chew); cause local pain; or produce *dysphagia* (difficulty swallowing). The most common oral cancer is squamous cell carcinoma. Malignant growths usually occur on lips, sides of tongue, or floor of the mouth. If not treated, cancerous growths may extend into nearby tissue, such as the middle ear or nasal sinuses; infiltrate regional lymph nodes; or invade large blood vessels, such as the carotid arteries, near the oral cavity. Serious hemorrhage ("carotid blowout") and death may result when cancer cells invade an artery that becomes ulcerated or when necrosis follows radiation therapy.

Assessment Findings

The early stage of oral cancer is characteristically asymptomatic. The client may notice a lesion, lump, or other abnormality of the lips or mouth. Other changes, such as pain, soreness, and bleeding, follow. If a lesion is on the tongue, the client experiences difficulty eating or tasting food. Pain and numbness also follow. Dentists and oral hygienists may be the first to notice changes in mouth tissues, such as *leukoplakia,* a white patch on the tongue or inner cheek that may be cancerous. A biopsy discloses malignant cells, confirming the diagnosis of oral cancer.

Medical and Surgical Management

Treatment depends on location and type of tumor, extent (or stage) of involvement, and client's physical condition. In cases of hemorrhage, transfusions are given to replace lost blood. Ligation of the bleeding vessel usually is necessary. Drugs such as antianxiety agents are prescribed to relieve client's apprehension.

Surgical treatment of most oral cancers includes tumor excision alone or with follow-up radiation therapy. Chemotherapy usually is not beneficial for primary tumors. Surgical excision may result in complete cure, if done early. A neck dissection is performed if cancer has spread to lymph nodes near the jaw or below the ears. Cancer of the tongue usually involves radical surgery to remove part or all of the tongue. Excision of the tumor from parts of the jaw or palate is disfiguring.

For clients with advanced disease, treatment is palliative only. Chemotherapy or radiation therapy is used to relieve pain and temporarily decrease tumor size. A tracheostomy and tube feedings are instituted to maintain an adequate airway and provide nourishment.

Nursing Management

General nursing management of the client with oral cancer is much the same as for any client with cancer (see Chap. 19). The focus is on maintaining a patent airway, promoting adequate fluid and food intake, and supporting communication that the tumor or treatment may impair.

Nurses collaborate with speech pathologists to address communication problems. They must be patient when the client chooses to communicate by speaking and clarify or repeat what he or she says if speech is not understandable. Nurses may substitute written forms for communicating if speech is impaired. They also offer the client pencil and paper, a Magic Slate, or an alphabet board, or suggest that the client use hand signals.

When the client returns from the operating room after oral surgery, he or she should be positioned flat, either on the abdomen or side, with head turned to the side to facilitate drainage from the mouth. After recovery from the anesthetic, the client is positioned with the head of the bed elevated, to make it easier for client to breathe deeply and cough up secretions. It also controls edema in the operative area.

After oral surgery, there should be equipment for suctioning and administration of oxygen. If the client does not have a tracheostomy, a tracheostomy tray must be nearby for emergency use because respiratory distress or airway obstruction requires immediate attention. If the client has a tracheostomy, suction secretions from the cannula and clean it on a regular basis.

Do not irrigate the client's mouth until the client is awake and alert. When mouth irrigation is carried out, turn the client's head to the side to allow solution to run in gently and flow out into an emesis basin. Instill only a small amount of solution and wait for fluid to drain before administering more. In addition, suction the mouth as necessary to remove secretions, blood, or irrigating solution.

The client must not receive oral liquids or foods until a written order exists. Observe the client's ability to swallow small amounts of liquid. In cases of coughing or other difficulty, suction the liquid from the mouth immediately.

The client may receive prescribed antiemetics for nausea or vomiting. If the client has a gastric tube, the nurse checks it for patency. Clients should not use a straw because it causes the client to swallow air, which can distend the stomach.

The client's emotional response to radical oral surgery is a real and difficult problem. Extensive surgery of the mouth and adjacent structures is not only disfiguring but incapacitating. It interferes with communication, eating, and control of saliva. Many clients and families cannot grasp all the ensuing effects. The first time family members or clients see the effects of surgery, it is traumatic. Promote effective coping and therapeutic grieving at this time. Responses may range from crying or extreme sadness and avoiding contact with others to refusing to talk about the surgery or changes in appearance. Allowing the client time to mourn, accept, and adjust to losses is essential. The client needs opportunities to express feelings. Observe severely depressed clients closely. Clients who are suicidal need psychological evaluation and counseling. Provide time for family members to express fears, ask questions, and grieve. It may help to refer clients and family members to support groups and counselors.

Nutritional management is a particular challenge when caring for clients with oral cancer. If the client can take oral nourishment, a nutritional consultation may be necessary to modify diet according to client's ability to chew and swallow. Because oral tissues are sensitive, the client should avoid hot and cold liquids and spicy foods. Consult with the physician about prescribing a topical anesthetic mouthwash containing lidocaine (Xylocaine), which numbs tissues, or a systemic analgesic to relieve pain. Providing nourishment by a route other than the mouth may be necessary.

Stop, Think, and Respond ● BOX 46-1

A client comes to the clinic with complaints of difficulty chewing and swallowing. What questions should you ask?

Gastrointestinal Intubation for Feedings or Medications

At some time during the care of the client with oral cancer, as well as when caring for others with GI disorders, the nurse may have to perform GI intubation, which is the insertion and management of GI tubes. GI intubation is done to provide nutrition, medications, or both; perform **gastric decompression,** removal of gas and fluids from the stomach; lavage the stomach to remove ingested toxins; diagnose GI disorders, a process that may include aspiration of gastric contents for analysis; treat GI obstruction; or apply pressure to a GI bleed. Examples of different types of GI intubation include **nasogastric intubation** (tube passes through nose into stomach via esophagus), **orogastric intubation** (tube passes through mouth into stomach), **nasoenteric intubation** (tube passes through the nose, esophagus, and stomach to the small intestine), **gastrostomy** (tube enters stomach through a surgically created opening into the abdominal wall), and **jejunostomy** (tube enters jejunum or small intestine through a surgically created opening into the abdominal wall). See Table 46.1.

The nasal route is the preferred route for passing a tube when the client's nose is intact and free from injury. The type of tube selected depends on the reason for placing the tube (Box 46-1). In general, smaller tubes are used for feeding because they tend to be more easily tolerated by clients; larger tubes are used for decompression because they allow for evacuation of large pieces of debris or blood clots from the upper GI tract.

Before beginning a tube feeding, determine why the client requires it, such as to improve nutritional and hydration status for chronic illness. Evaluating renal function and checking for any digestive issues are essential, as is assessing previous stool patterns, present weight, and any vomiting.

When a client is receiving tube feedings, medications, or both (Table 46.2), the nurse's role is to ensure that lungs remain free of liquid substances, the client does not

TABLE 46.1 NASOGASTRIC, NASOENTERIC, AND FEEDING TUBES

TUBE TYPE	LENGTH	SIZE (FRENCH)	LUMEN	OTHER CHARACTERISTICS
Nasogastric Tubes				
Levin (plastic or rubber)	125 cm	14–18	Single	Circular markings serve as guidelines for insertion.
Gastric Salem sump (plastic)	120 cm	12–18	Double	Smaller lumen acts as a vent.
Moss	90 cm	12–16	Triple	Tube contains both a gastric decompression lumen and a duodenal lumen for postoperative feedings.
Sengstaken-Blakemore (rubber)			Triple	Two lumens are used to inflate the gastric and esophageal balloons.
Nasoenteric Decompression Tubes				
Miller-Abbott (rubber)	300 cm	12–18	Double	One lumen uses tungsten or air for balloon inflation.
Harris	180 cm	14, 16	Single	Tip is tungsten weighted.
Cantor (rubber)	300 cm	16	Single	Bag is tungsten weighted.
Baker (plastic)	270 cm	16	Double	One lumen is used for balloon inflation.
Nasoenteric Feeding Tubes				
Dobhoff or Keofeed II (polyurethane or silicone rubber)	160–175 cm	8–12	Single	Tip is tungsten weighted, radiopaque.

BOX 46-1 ● Uses of Gastrointestinal (GI) Tubes

Gastrointestinal tubes come in several types, depending on their uses. Among common GI tubes used for decompression are the Levin tube and the Salem sump. Narrower, more flexible tubes, such as Keofeed, Dobhoff gastrostomy, jejunostomy, and others, are made of polyurethane or silicone and are used for administering liquid nourishment.

Feeding tubes are longer than Levin tubes and terminate in the upper, small intestine. Their advantages include ease of insertion, more comfort for the client, reduced potential for vomiting and aspiration because the formula is instilled below the pylorus, and extended use because they may remain in the same nostril for up to 4 weeks. Their disadvantage is that distal location is difficult to assess without a chest or abdominal radiograph.

FEEDING METHODS

Liquid nourishment is administered by bolus, intermittent, cyclic, or continuous methods. Depending on institutional policy and individual feeding orders, the feeding tube is flushed with water at various intervals to ensure patency. Many tube feeding formulas are available to suit a client's different nutritional needs. Nursing observation of tolerance of the feeding is essential to determine which tube and formula are best for the client.

Bolus tube feedings

- Allow introduction of 250 to 400 mL formula through the tube in a short period (usually 15–30 minutes)
- Administered by syringe or gravity flow system attached to the distal end of the feeding tube

Intermittent tube feedings

- Allow delivery of between 250 and 400 mL formula over 30 to 60 minutes
- Delivered by gravity flow system or an electronic feeding pump

Continuous tube feedings

- Allow formula to be administered at lower rates—usually 1.5 mL/minute over a longer time (usually 12–24 hours)
- Delivered by gravity flow system or an electronic feeding pump

Cyclic tube feedings

- Allow formula to be administered continuously for 8 to 12 hours during sleep followed by a 12- to 16-hour pause
- Ensure adequate nutrition during weaning from tube to oral feeding
- Alternated with oral food intake until client can take most nutrition orally

acquire an infection, and intake and output are appropriate for the client's age and size. Additional objectives include providing adequate nutrition, promoting appropriate stool patterns (amount, consistency, and frequency), and preserving intact skin and nasal mucosa. Mucous membranes tend to dry from mouth breathing and restricted oral fluids. It is important to keep them moist. Frequent mouth care relieves discomfort from dryness and unpleasant tastes and odors. Ice chips and analgesic throat lozenges, gargles, or sprays may help if client's mouth and throat are sore. Providing mouth care after removal of the tube is an important nursing intervention, as is informing the client that a sore throat (aftereffect of intubation) may persist for several days.

The client is at risk not only for dry mouth but also fluid volume deficit resulting from insufficient fluid

TABLE 46.2 MEDICATION ADMINISTRATION BY WAY OF FEEDING TUBE

TYPE	PREPARATION
Liquid	None
Simple compressed tablets	Crushed and dissolved in water
Buccal or sublingual tablets	Give as intended
Enteric-coated tablets	Cannot be crushed; change in form required
Time-release tablets	Some can be opened; cannot be crushed because doing so may release too much drug too quickly (overdose); check with pharmacist

intake. Be aware of the client's normal fluid needs and whether formula alone can meet them. Observation for signs and symptoms of dehydration is very important.

While ensuring adequate hydration, also protect the client from infections that stem from microbes in the tube-feeding formula. Signs and symptoms of infection include diarrhea, fever, or abnormal white blood cell count. Interventions to prevent infection include washing hands before handling equipment; keeping feeding formula refrigerated or unopened until it is ready for use; warming bolus, intermittent, or cyclic feeding formula to room temperature just before administering; hanging continuous formula-feeding containers with only the volume for 4 to 6 hours; flushing tubing with water before adding more formula and after giving a bolus or intermittent feeding or medications; discarding any premixed formula after 24 hours; thoroughly cleaning and drying all equipment used for bolus feedings (i.e., syringe, feeding adapters, tubing, containers) after each use; and replacing infusion container and tubing used for a continuous tube feeding every 24 hours or as directed by agency policy.

Before each intermittent feeding or every 4 to 8 hours for continuous feedings, aspirate and measure residual content. If it measures more than 100 mL or 10% to 20% of the hourly amount for a continuous feeding, the feeding needs to be delayed. Re-administer the residual amount so that the client does not lose nutrients and digestive enzymes.

Before and after medications or intermittent feedings, administer 15 to 30 mL of water. This is done every 4 to 6 hours for continuous feedings.

Clients need to be in semi-Fowler's position during feedings and for 30 to 60 minutes after intermittent feedings. It is essential that the nurse checks tube placement prior to feedings to prevent aspiration. If the client vomits or you suspect aspiration, stop the feeding.

Gastrointestinal Intubation for Decompression

The larger GI tube is used to relieve abdominal distention caused by problems after surgery, episodes of acute upper GI bleeding, or symptoms associated with intestinal obstruction, or for diagnostic purposes. It is inserted by following the same procedure as is used for insertion of a feeding tube.

Some tubes, such as a gastric sump tube, have a double lumen, one of which serves as a vent, allowing a small amount of air to be drawn in when the tube is connected to suction. Sump tubes decrease the possibility of the stomach wall adhering to and obstructing the tube openings during gastric decompression. A common problem associated with vented tubes is leakage from the vent lumen. The nurse may prevent this by keeping the vent above the level of the client's stomach. Newer gastric sump tubes have a one-way antireflux valve that allows air to enter but prevents gastric contents from escaping. In many cases, decompression tubes are connected to a source of suction, which is discussed in Nursing Guidelines 46-2.

NURSING GUIDELINES 46-2

Managing the Care of a Client Needing GI Suction and Decompression

- Locate the suction source, usually a wall outlet or portable machine.
- Adjust the suction level on the wall outlet or portable machine to provide the amount and frequency of suction specified by the physician.
- Select intermittent high, low, or continuous suction when using a Salem sump tube; select low intermittent suction when using a Levin tube because the single lumen may adhere to the lining of the stomach during continuous suction. (If the tube is used only to obtain specimens for diagnostic purposes, manual suction may be achieved by attaching a syringe to the end of the tube and drawing back on the plunger.)
- Insert the gastric decompression tube in accord with accepted standards and connect it to the suction.

Maintain Safe Suction

- Observe the amount and quality of the gastric contents being suctioned and the client's response.
- Monitor the procedure frequently because abdominal or gastric distention caused by suction failure may have serious consequences, such as strain on surgical sutures or vomiting around the tube.
- Check equipment frequently to make sure it is operating properly. If the suction is not operating satisfactorily, obtain another suction machine.

Maintain Tube Patency

- If the decompression tube is occluded, irrigate or replace it.
- First review the client's chart. The physician may order irrigation on an as-needed basis.
- When irrigating the tube, use normal saline solution to prevent disturbance of electrolyte balance. Also use a large syringe to instill the irrigant into the distal end of the tube.
- After the fluid is instilled, remove it by gently pulling back on the plunger.
- Document the amount of solution used and the amount of fluid returned on the client's intake and output record.

Ensure Client Comfort

- Provide ice chips sparingly because water pulls electrolytes into the gastric secretions, which are then removed by suction, increasing the risk for an electrolyte disturbance.

Gastrostomy Tubes for Long-Term Feeding

A client with a gastrostomy has a transabdominal opening into the stomach that provides long-term access for administering fluids and liquid nourishment. Creating a gastrostomy is a relatively minor procedure performed surgically or endoscopically.

GENERAL CONSIDERATIONS. Surgical placement of a gastrostomy involves laparotomy and surgical creation of an external stoma through which a gastrostomy tube is placed. When a **percutaneous endoscopic gastrostomy** (PEG) is performed, an endoscope is introduced orally and advanced into the stomach so that the physician can see the correct location for the tube. This location also is identified on the external abdominal surface before an incision is made (see Fig. 46.1). Endoscopic placement is preferred to surgical laparotomy unless the client has ascites, is morbidly obese, or has had previous gastric surgery. If the client's condition eventually improves, the gastrostomy tube is removed and the opening closes over time.

Gastric feedings are given by bolus, intermittent, cyclic, or continuous methods, using techniques described before. Intermittent, cyclic, or continuous feedings simulate normal passage of food into the small intestine and usually are well tolerated.

Gastrostomy feeding devices may be skin-level devices (known as *buttons*) or tubes. Some have a double lumen to allow infusion of two different fluids at once, such as medications and feeding formula, without interruption. Most gastrostomy tubes have an external bumper and a firm internal bumper or an inflatable balloon. That makes it difficult to dislodge accidentally.

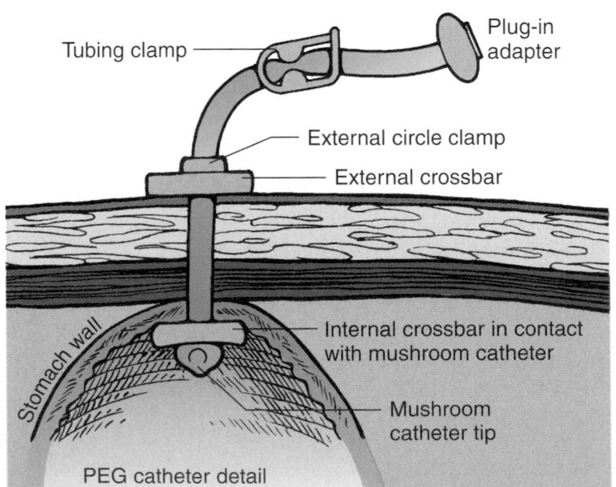

FIGURE 46.1 Detail of abdomen and PEG tube, showing catheter fixation. (From Smeltzer, S. C., & Bare, B. G. [2004]. *Brunner & Suddarth's textbook of medical–surgical nursing* [10th ed.]. Philadelphia: Lippincott Williams & Wilkins.)

NURSING MANAGEMENT. Before insertion of a PEG tube, weigh the client, assess vital signs, and auscultate bowel sounds. Determine the client's perception of the procedure, clarifying information, and checking that proper consent forms are signed and in order. Prepare the client's skin and conduct other ordered preprocedural activities, such as inserting an IV line and administering sedatives.

Monitor vital signs (i.e., respiratory rate, oxygen saturation, heart rate and rhythm) throughout and after the procedure. Monitor and document the client's tolerance of the procedure. Observe the stoma and surrounding skin for signs of infection and check dressings frequently for evidence of bleeding and drainage.

Examine the appearance and volume of drainage from the gastrostomy tube during the first 24 hours when the tube may be temporarily attached to gravity drainage. Auscultate bowel sounds and palpate the abdomen lightly for signs of distention and tenderness and inspect the oral mucosa for excessive dryness. Note the client's tolerance of the formula when tube feedings begin, reporting abdominal distention, vomiting, fever, and severe pain to the physician. Also monitor characteristics and pattern of bowel elimination and trends in daily weight.

If the gastrostomy tube is accidentally removed, it needs to be replaced. Clients with recently placed gastrostomy devices (less than 2 weeks) do not have a well-established tract and are at high risk for inadvertent replacement into the peritoneum instead of the stomach. If fluids are administered into this device, resulting peritonitis may be life-threatening. Notify the physician immediately and take steps to ensure proper placement of the replacement device. For clients with well-established tracts, maintain patency of the tract by inserting a clean catheter (i.e., Foley) and inflating the balloon to hold the catheter in place. The diameter of the replacement device should be the same as that of the device that was removed. Notify the physician so a new feeding device can be inserted. It is safe to administer gastric feedings through a catheter until it is replaced.

DISORDERS OF THE ESOPHAGUS

Various disorders can affect the esophagus. Examples include gastroesophageal reflux disease (GERD), hiatal hernia, and cancer. Esophageal varices, which result from hypertension in the portal venous system, are discussed in Chapter 49.

• GASTROESOPHAGEAL REFLUX DISEASE

Gastroesophageal reflux disease (GERD) is a common disorder that develops when gastric contents flow upward into the esophagus. Adults and children normally have some degree of reflux, especially after eating. GERD is considered a disease process only when it is excessive or causes undesirable symptoms, such as pain or respiratory distress.

Pathophysiology and Etiology

GERD results from an inability of the lower esophageal sphincter (LES; also called *cardiac sphincter*) to close fully, allowing stomach contents to flow freely into the esophagus. Obesity and pregnancy increase susceptibility to GERD because of the upward pressure that increased abdominal girth associated with these conditions places on the diaphragm.

Assessment Findings

Common symptoms associated with GERD are epigastric pain or discomfort (**dyspepsia**), burning sensation in the esophagus (**pyrosis**), and regurgitation. Other symptoms include difficulty swallowing (dysphagia), painful swallowing (**odynophagia**), inflammation of the lining of the esophagus (**esophagitis**), aspiration pneumonia, and respiratory distress. Clients with esophagitis related to GERD may experience bleeding from the lining of the esophagus, manifested by vomited blood (*hematemesis*) or tarry stools (*melena*). Sometimes *occult* (hidden) *bleeding* for long periods produces iron-deficiency anemia. Because the esophagus is anatomically close to the heart, clients with epigastric pain may think they are having a heart attack. A myocardial infarction must be ruled out. Severe esophagitis can lead to scarring and stricture formation.

Barium swallow findings show inflammation or stricture formation from chronic esophagitis. Upper endoscopy with biopsy confirms esophagitis. Tests of stool may show positive findings of blood. Twenty-four–hour esophageal monitoring allows for observation of the frequency of reflux episodes and associated symptoms. Bronchoscopy with analysis of fluids found in the lungs and nuclear medicine scans test for aspiration.

Medical and Surgical Management

Medications used to control esophageal reflux are discussed in Drug Therapy Table 46.2. The surgical procedure performed for GERD is **fundoplication,** a procedure that tightens the LES by wrapping the gastric fundus around the lower esophagus and suturing it into place. It may be performed using laparoscopic technique, endoscopic technique, or open laparotomy. Esophageal strictures may be managed by endoscopic dilatation. Clients can be taught self-dilatation using a tapered flexible dilator in the home setting.

Nursing Management

Educate the client with GERD about diet and lifestyle changes to reduce reflux symptoms. This includes avoiding foods and beverages that lower pressure in the LES (e.g., alcohol, peppermint, licorice, caffeine, high-fat foods), which may control mild symptoms. Additional measures include losing weight, avoiding tight-fitting garments, elevating head of the bed, stopping smoking, and avoiding food and drink for several hours before bedtime. Teach the client about medications to control reflux. Also teach about the importance of controlling severe GERD to prevent possible complications, such as esophageal stricture formation and esophageal cancer. Closely observe for postoperative abdominal distention and nausea because many clients cannot belch or vomit after fundoplication.

Stop, Think, and Respond ● BOX 46-2

You are assigned to care for a client with GERD. After lunch, the client tells you that he needs to take a nap. What should you advise?

● HIATAL HERNIA

A **hiatal** or **diaphragmatic hernia** is a protrusion of part of the stomach into the lower portion of the thorax. There are two types of hiatal hernias (Fig. 46.2):

- *Axial or sliding*—The junction of the stomach and esophagus and part of the stomach slide in and out through the weakened portion of the diaphragm.
- *Paraesophageal*—The fundus is displaced upward, with greater curvature of the stomach going through the diaphragm next to the gastroesophageal junction.

Pathophysiology and Etiology

A hiatal hernia results from a defect in the diaphragm at the point where the esophagus passes through it. It is particularly common in women. There is congenital muscle weakness or weakness resulting from trauma. Factors that increase intra-abdominal pressure also contribute to potential for hiatal hernia and include multiple pregnancies, obesity, and loss of muscle strength and tone that occurs with aging. When the upper portion of the stomach slips from its usual position and becomes trapped, gastroesophageal reflux occurs.

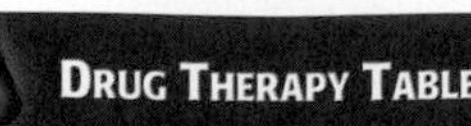

DRUG THERAPY TABLE 46.2 MEDICATIONS USED TO TREAT PROBLEMS IN THE UPPER GI TRACT

DRUG CATEGORY AND EXAMPLES	MECHANISM OF ACTION	SIDE EFFECTS	NURSING CONSIDERATIONS
Antacids			
calcium carbonate (Tums)	Neutralize gastric acid to relieve heartburn and sour stomach	Constipation, hypercalcemia, hypophosphatemia	Avoid using in large amounts for a prolonged time. These drugs may be used as calcium supplements.
aluminum hydroxide (AlternaGEL)		Constipation, indigestion	Do not administer to clients on a sodium-restricted diet. Do not administer with tetracycline.
aluminum hydroxide with magnesium hydroxide (Gaviscon, Maalox, Mylanta)		Hypermagnesemia, hypophosphatemia	Observe for central nervous system depression and other symptoms of hypermagnesemia, especially in clients with renal failure.
Histamine-2 Antagonists			
cimetidine (Tagamet)	Suppress gastric acid by blocking H_2 receptors	Blood abnormalities (agranulocytosis, neutropenia, thrombocytopenia), diarrhea, dizziness, sleepiness, headache, confusion, increased plasma creatinine level, cardiac rhythm disturbances, erectile dysfunction (reversible), rash	Give drug with meals and at bedtime. Urge client to report sore throat, fever, unusual bruising/bleeding, or dizziness.
ranitidine (Zantac)		Headache, GI disturbance, insomnia, nausea/vomiting, rash, blood abnormalities, erectile dysfunction	Give drug with meals and at bedtime. Encourage regular checkups. Urge client to report sore throat, fever, unusual bruising/bleeding, dizziness, severe headache, or muscle/joint pain.
famotidine (Pepcid)		Headache, dizziness, diarrhea, constipation, muscle cramps, erectile dysfunction	Give drug with meals and at bedtime. Encourage regular checkups. Advise client to report sore throat, fever, unusual bruising/bleeding, dizziness, severe headache, or muscle/joint pain.
Antiulcer Agents			
sucralfate (Carafate)	Protect ulcers from acid and pepsin	Dizziness, insomnia, vertigo, constipation, GI discomfort, dry mouth, rash, back pain	Give drug to client with an empty stomach 1 hour before or 2 hours after meals and at bedtime. Do not administer concurrently with an antacid or H_2 antagonist. Advise client to report severe gastric pain.
Proton Pump Inhibitors			
omeprazole (Prilosec)	Suppress gastric acid by blocking enzymes associated with the final step of acid production	Headache, fatigue, dizziness, depression, abdominal pain, cramps, gas, nausea, diarrhea, flulike symptoms, rash, arthralgia	Give before meals to prevent upset stomach. Instruct client to swallow capsule whole without breaking, opening, or crushing contents. Caution client not to drive car or operate machinery if side effects are severe.

(continued)

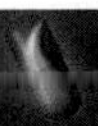

Drug Therapy Table 46.2 MEDICATIONS USED TO TREAT PROBLEMS IN THE UPPER GI TRACT (Continued)

DRUG CATEGORY AND EXAMPLES	MECHANISM OF ACTION	SIDE EFFECTS	NURSING CONSIDERATIONS
lansoprazole (Prevacid)		Diarrhea, abdominal pain, nausea/vomiting, constipation, dry mouth, headache, dizziness, vertigo, insomnia, upper respiratory symptoms (reversible), rash	Give drug before meals. Arrange for client to be medically monitored while taking drug. Advise client to report worsening symptoms, severe headache, fever, or chills.
GI Motility Agents			
metoclopramide (Reglan)	Stimulate upper GI tract and gastric emptying without stimulating release of gastric acid	Restlessness, drowsiness, fatigue, extrapyrimidal symptoms, parkinsonism-like reactions, nausea, diarrhea	Instruct client not to use alcohol or sleeping pills because resulting sedation may be dangerous. Advise client to report severe depression, diarrhea, and involuntary tremors or tics of the face, eyes, arms, and legs.
cisapride (Propulsid)		Headache, abdominal pain, diarrhea, constipation, nausea/vomiting, serious cardiac dysrhythmias from potential drug interactions, runny nose	Assess medication history and for gallbladder disease, GI bleeding or obstruction, pregnancy, or lactation. Give 15 minutes before each meal and at bedtime. Instruct client not to use alcohol or sleeping pills because resulting sedation may be dangerous.
bethenechol (Urecholine)		Abdominal discomfort, salivation, nausea/vomiting, sweating, flushing	Administer on an empty stomach. Monitor bowel function, especially in older adults.
Anticholinergics			
atropine sulfate (Atropine)	Relax smooth muscles of GI tract and inhibit gastric secretions	Blurred vision, dilated pupils, cycloplegia, dizziness, nervousness, insomnia, dry mouth, increased intraocular pressure, palpitations, heart rhythm changes, life-threatening paralytic ileus, urinary retention, intolerance to heat	Assess for health conditions that may contraindicate therapy. Give 30 minutes before meals. Be sure client has adequate fluid intake. Keep room temperature cool but comfortable. Tell client to report eye pain, abnormal heartbeats, difficulty swallowing, or breathing problems.
dicyclomine HCl (Bentyl)		Constipation, dry mouth, blurred vision, sensitivity to light, difficulty urinating, irregular heartbeat, intolerance to heat	Ensure adequate fluids. Keep room temperature stable to prevent problems resulting from heat intolerance. Tell client to report eye pain, abnormal heartbeats, difficulty swallowing, breathing problems, and so forth. Assess for health conditions that contraindicate therapy (glaucoma, bronchial asthma).
propantheline bromide (Pro-Banthine [Can])		Constipation, dry mouth, blurred vision, sensitivity to light, difficulty urinating, irregular heartbeat, intolerance to heat	

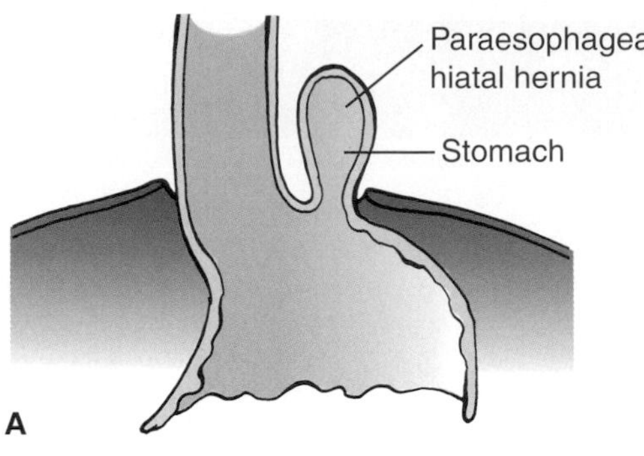

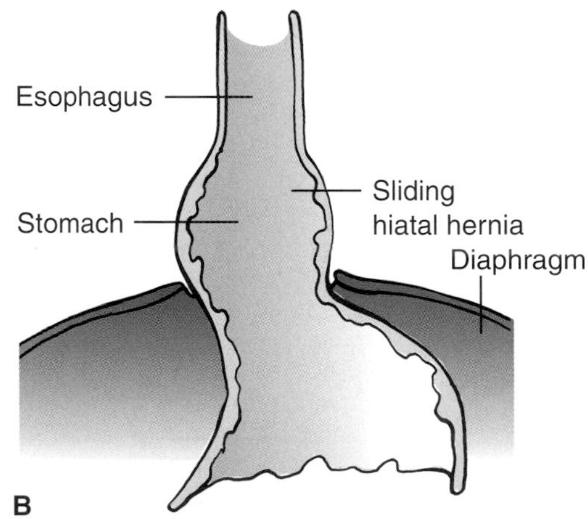

FIGURE 46.2 (**A**) Paraesophageal hiatal hernia. (**B**) Sliding hiatal hernia.

Assessment Findings

The client describes having heartburn, belching, and a feeling of substernal or epigastric pressure or pain after eating and when lying down. He or she may report increased symptoms when bending at the waist. If scars form, swallowing becomes difficult. As food distends the esophagus, the client may vomit. Reflux does not usually accompany gastroesophageal hernias, because the gastroesophageal sphincter remains intact. Sliding hernias, however, are associated with reflux. A barium swallow confirms the diagnosis by outlining the abnormal positioning of the stomach. An esophagoscopy shows the extent of irritation and scarring in the esophagus.

Medical and Surgical Management

Medical management of hiatal hernia is the same as that of GERD. The narrowed esophagus is stretched endoscopically, but the procedure may need to be repeated often. Clients who do not respond to a rigid medical regimen are treated surgically, which involves restoring the stomach to its proper position and repairing the diaphragmatic defect.

Nursing Management

Ask the client about his or her appetite, particularly changes, difficulty swallowing, and problems after meals, such as discomfort, bloating, regurgitation, and belching. If the client indicates that he or she has pain after meals, ask if pain follows every meal or certain foods, if other things (e.g., a particular position) seem to aggravate it, and if pain is a burning sensation or associated with stomach fullness or pressure. Determine if the client has lost weight. Finding out if the client has tried antacids or other over-the-counter medications to relieve symptoms also is important. Weigh the client and check for signs of malnutrition and dehydration. When completing the history, ask about past infections, exposure to irritants, and alcohol and tobacco use.

For clients who undergo thoracic surgery to repair a hiatal hernia, nursing care is the same as for a client who had chest surgery. Regardless of the surgical approach, postoperative care will likely involve intubation for gastric decompression to prevent stomach distention and avoid pressure on the surgical repair (see Nursing Guidelines 46-2). When managing nonsurgical care of clients with hiatal hernia or other esophageal disorders, encourage the client to eat frequent, small, well-balanced meals, eat slowly and chew food thoroughly, avoid foods that cause discomfort, and avoid alcohol or tobacco products. The client should remain upright for at least 2 hours after meals to prevent reflux and avoid eating before bedtime. Teach the client to avoid activities that may involve the Valsalva maneuver (e.g., lifting heavy objects, straining for bowel movements) because it increases intra-abdominal pressure and may cause the stomach to wedge above the diaphragm. Also instruct the client to take medications as prescribed.

• CANCER OF THE ESOPHAGUS

Esophageal cancer is a serious condition. Clients usually do not experience symptoms until the disease interferes with swallowing and passage of food, leading to weight loss.

Pathophysiology and Etiology

Esophageal cancer affects men more often than women. Clients usually are diagnosed in the fourth or fifth decade of life. The tumor usually is a squamous cell carcinoma, but some are classified as adenocarcinomas. A strong correlation exists among esophageal cancer, alcohol abuse, and cigarette smoking. As cancer advances, the mass occupies space and interferes with swallowing. If the tumor grows unchecked, it obstructs passage of food into the stomach, causing possible aspiration. The tumor may ulcerate, leading to occult or frank blood loss.

Assessment Findings

Symptoms develop slowly, beginning with vague discomfort and difficulty swallowing some foods. Weight loss accompanies progressive dysphagia. Later, solid foods are almost impossible to swallow, and the client resorts to consuming liquids only. He or she may regurgitate food and liquids. The tumor also may hemorrhage, resulting in hemoptysis. When swallowing difficulty is pronounced, the cancer may have invaded surrounding tissues and lymphatics. Expansion of the tumor causes back pain and respiratory distress. Pain is a late symptom. The client also exhibits weight loss and weakness.

A barium swallow shows a filling defect caused by a space-occupying mass. A biopsy of tissue removed during esophagoscopy reveals malignant cells. A bronchoscopy may be done to determine if cancer cells have affected the trachea.

Medical and Surgical Management

Clients who are not candidates for surgery are treated with palliative measures and, possibly, endoscopic laser surgery to destroy some of the tumor. Esophageal dilatation may be used to enlarge the obstructed area. A prosthesis (stent placement) may be inserted at the tumor site to widen the narrowed area or when a fistula forms at the tumor site.

When surgery is a curative option, the type depends on tumor location, extent of the lesion, and evidence of metastasis. If the tumor is in the lower third of the esophagus, the surgeon removes the affected area and attaches the remaining two thirds to the stomach. If the tumor is in the upper two thirds of the esophagus, the surgeon removes the affected area and replaces that portion of esophagus with a section of jejunum or colon.

Nursing Management

A major goal is adequate or improved nutrition and eventually stable weight. Encourage small, frequent meals. If the client has difficulty swallowing, ensure that the client receives soft foods or high-calorie, high-protein semiliquid foods. The client needs to refrain from consuming foods that contain significant air or gas, such as soufflés and carbonated drinks. To reduce bloating, the client should avoid drinking from straws or narrow-necked bottles to reduce volume of air trapped in the esophagus or stomach. The client should receive liquid supplements between meals.

Nutritional needs of the client with inoperable cancer of the esophagus are met with nasogastric or gastrostomy tube feedings or TPN. Nursing management involves caring for skin at the tube insertion site, preventing infection, administering nourishment, maintaining tube patency, and preparing the client or family for self-care or home care after discharge. (See the earlier sections on GI intubation and gastrostomy.)

Clients who return from esophageal or gastric surgery need to be turned and perform deep breathing and coughing every 2 hours. They also must know how to support the surgical incision for coughing and deep breathing. The nurse may use an incentive spirometer to motivate the client. The client must ambulate to mobilize secretions, increase depth of respiration, and promote expulsion of intestinal gas.

To avoid gastric distention, the client should not have oral nourishment until bowel sounds resume and are active. Provide oral liquids, when allowed, to thin secretions. To minimize dyspnea, give frequent, small meals and do not allow the client to lie down immediately after eating.

Explain the reasons for treatment and instruct the client and family to adhere to the therapeutic regimen, follow the dietary modifications, and attend medical follow-up appointments regularly. The client should inform the physician immediately of worsening symptoms, steady weight loss, difficulty swallowing soft foods, abnormal bleeding, or other new problems.

GASTRIC DISORDERS

• GASTRITIS

Gastritis is inflammation of the stomach lining (gastric mucosa). It may be acute or chronic.

Pathophysiology and Etiology

Causes of gastritis include dietary indiscretions; reflux of duodenal contents; use of aspirin, steroids, nonsteroidal anti-inflammatory drugs (NSAIDs), alcohol, or caffeine; cigarette smoking; ingestion of poisons or corrosive substances; food allergies; infection; and gastric ischemia secondary to vasoconstriction caused by a stress response. Gastric secretions are highly acidic. *Parietal cells* in the stomach increase acid production (hydrochloric acid) in response to seeing, smelling, and eating food. The parasympathetic vagus nerve releases histamine and acetylcholine, chemicals that also stimulate parietal cells. An increasing level of acid triggers conversion of pepsinogen to pepsin, creating a chemical mixture strong enough to digest the stomach wall. Because mucus protectively coats the stomach lining, pepsin normally has little effect.

When irritating substances reduce or penetrate the mucous layer, submucosal layers of the stomach can become inflamed. The client experiences epigastric discomfort, often described as *heartburn*. Mucus-producing cells usually heal and regenerate in 3 to 5 days. Chronic irritation leads to ulceration.

Assessment Findings

Usually the client complains of epigastric fullness, pressure, pain, anorexia, nausea, and vomiting. When a bacterial or viral infection causes the gastritis, the client may experience vomiting, diarrhea, fever, and abdominal pain. Drugs, poisons, toxic substances, and corrosives can cause gastric bleeding. Clients may see blood in emesis or note a darkening of stool color. Chronic gastritis may have no symptoms or symptoms similar to mild indigestion.

A complete blood count may reveal anemia from chronic blood loss. Stool testing for occult blood often detects RBCs. Gastroscopy may be performed to visualize the mucosa and obtain specimens, which are examined for pathogens or cellular abnormalities.

Medical and Surgical Management

Treatment depends on cause and symptoms. Ingestion of poisons requires emergency treatment. In acute cases, eating is restricted and IV fluids are given to correct dehydration and electrolyte imbalances, particularly with severe vomiting. Antiemetics are prescribed to control nausea and vomiting, and antibiotics may be prescribed to inhibit or destroy infection.

Usual treatment of chronic gastritis is avoidance of irritating substances, such as alcohol and NSAIDs. Some clients may wish to avoid spicy foods, high-fat foods, and caffeine, if these items aggravate their symptoms. Various drugs, such as antacids, histamine-2 antagonists, and proton pump inhibitors may be prescribed.

Nursing Management

Monitor the client's symptoms and evaluate the client's response to dietary modifications and prescribed medications. Observe color and characteristics of vomitus or stool. Teach about diet, drug therapy, and the need for continued medical follow-up. For complications such as ulcer formation, refer to the section on Nursing Management of peptic ulcer disease.

● PEPTIC ULCER DISEASE

A **peptic ulcer** is a circumscribed loss of tissue in an area of the GI tract that is in contact with hydrochloric acid and pepsin. Most peptic ulcers occur in the duodenum, but may develop at the lower end of the esophagus or in the stomach. Men are affected more frequently by peptic ulcer disease (PUD) than women are. The highest incidence occurs during middle life, but the condition can occur at any age.

Pathophysiology and Etiology

PUD occurs when the normal balance between factors that promote mucosal injury (gastric acid, pepsin, bile acid, ingested substances) and factors that protect the mucosa (intact epithelium, mucus, and bicarbonate secretion) is disrupted. The single greatest risk factor for development of PUD is infection with *Helicobacter pylori*. *H. pylori*, a gram-negative microorganism, is present in the gastric or duodenal mucosa of 80% to 90% of clients with PUD. The bacteria, which shelter themselves in the bicarbonate-rich mucus, are a factor in chronic gastritis and PUD. It appears that *H. pylori* secrete an enzyme that theoretically depletes gastric mucus, making it more vulnerable to injury.

Family history is thought to be an additional risk factor for development of PUD. A genetic component may exist, as there is a high incidence among first-degree relatives. Another explanation is the clustering of infection with *H. pylori* in families. Other risk factors include chronic use of NSAIDs, cigarette smoking, alcohol ingestion, and physiologic stress.

Ulcers develop when there is prolonged hyperacidity or chronic reduction in mucus. Once gastric acid has penetrated the mucosal layer, the acid begins to digest the stomach wall (Fig. 46.3). Histamine, released from injured cells, triggers hypersecretion of more hydrochloric acid and pepsin. The body responds with the inflammatory process. Capillary permeability is increased; the mucosa swells and bleeds easily.

Because food dilutes stomach acid, clients with PUD experience more discomfort when the stomach is empty. Unless controlled, the erosion can lead to obstruction from scar formation or penetrate the entire thickness of the stomach wall, spilling gastric contents into the peritoneal cavity, possibly accompanied by hemorrhage.

Aging and chronic stomach inflammation lead to atrophy of the glandular epithelium of the stomach. Chronic gastric inflammation causes parietal cells to secrete less hydrochloric acid, resulting in *hypochlorhydria* (reduced gastric acidity) or *achlorhydria* (absence of hydrochloric acid). The gastric mucosa produces intrinsic factor, required for absorption of vitamin B_{12}. Chronic gastric inflammation inhibits production of intrinsic factor,

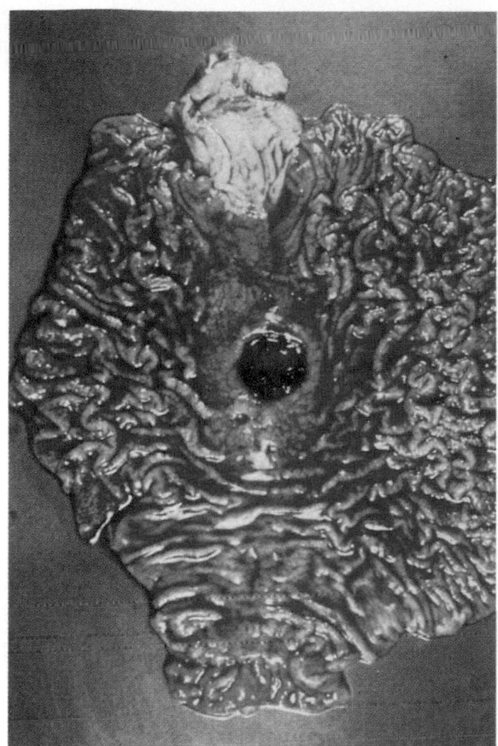

FIGURE 46.3 Gastric ulcer. (From Rubin, E., & Farber, J. L. [1999]. *Pathology* [3rd ed.]. Philadelphia: Lippincott Williams & Wilkins.)

leading to poor absorption of this essential nutrient. The client is at high risk for pernicious anemia.

Assessment Findings

Most clients with PUD have abdominal pain, usually confined to the epigastrium. Clients describe pain as a "burning" sensation. They often complain of pain that disturbs sleep and occurs 1 to several hours after meals. Eating food may relieve pain. Back pain suggests that the ulcer is irritating the pancreas. Approximately 20% of clients may have bleeding as the first sign of the ulcer. Hemorrhage, hematemesis, or melena may occur. Protracted vomiting, secondary to scarring and resultant obstruction, is seen among those who ignored earlier symptoms.

Diagnosis is suggested by history and confirmed by results of an upper GI series or esophagogastroduodenoscopy. To differentiate between benign and malignant ulcers, a gastric washing or biopsy for cytologic analysis may be done. The hemoglobin level and RBC count are low from chronic blood loss. Vomiting alters electrolyte levels.

Medical and Surgical Management

Effectiveness of dietary therapy in treating PUD is unknown. Foods known to increase acid production include milk and milk products, alcohol, caffeinated beverages, and decaffeinated coffee. Clients are provided with small, frequent meals and instructed to avoid eating foods that are particularly irritating.

In the presence of *H. pylori,* eradication therapy is initiated, which includes a combination of antibiotics (e.g., tetracycline), metronidazole (Flagyl), and bismuth salts. Treatment may also include histamine (H_2) antagonists, proton pump inhibitors, cytoprotective agents, and antacids. The following list provides examples of drugs used to treat PUD:

- *Antibiotics:* Tetracycline, amoxicillin, and clarithromycin exert bactericidal effects to eradicate *H. pylori.*
- *Amebicides:* Metronidazole (Flagyl) assists in the eradication of *H. pylori.*
- *Bismuth salts:* Bismuth salicylate (Pepto-Bismol) suppresses *H. pylori* and assists in healing mucosal lesions.
- *Antacids:* These drugs initially buffer stomach acid. They are not absorbed from the GI tract and therefore do not produce alkalosis, even when given in large doses.
- *Histamine (H_2) antagonists:* Cimetidine (Tagamet), famotidine (Pepcid), nizatidine (Axid), and ranitidine (Zantac) block H_2 receptors and decrease acid secretion in the stomach.
- *Cytoprotective agents:* Sucralfate (Carafate) forms a seal over the ulcer, protecting it from irritation. Misoprostol (Cytotec), a synthetic prostaglandin, sustains the mucosal layer, especially among clients who require large doses or long-term treatment with aspirin or NSAIDs.
- *Proton pump inhibitors:* Omeprazole (Prilosec), lansoprazole (Prevacid), esomeprazole (Nexium), rabeprazole (Aciphex), and pantoprazole (Protonix) block the final step in acid production at the surface of parietal cells.

Clients who have obstruction from edema and inflammation will have a gastric tube inserted. Treatment of hemorrhage includes complete rest, blood transfusions, and gastric lavage with saline solution. Iced saline solution no longer is used because it can cause hypothermia. Nothing is given by mouth, and IV fluids are administered until the bleeding stops. Clients with recurrent ulcers, severe hemorrhage, unrelieved obstruction, perforation, or malignant changes may need surgery as described in Table 46.3.

Clients having a total **gastrectomy** (removal of the stomach) require vitamin B_{12} injections or intranasal vitamin B_{12} for life because, without the stomach, the intrinsic factor necessary for absorption of vitamin B_{12} no longer is produced.

When clients begin to take food after a gastrojejunostomy, they may develop **dumping syndrome,** which

TABLE 46.3 SURGICAL PROCEDURES TO TREAT PEPTIC ULCER DISEASE

PROCEDURE	DEPICTION
Vagotomy—a branch of the vagus nerve is cut to reduce gastric acid secretion. ***Pyloroplasty***—the pylorus is repaired or reconstructed to expand the stomach outlet narrowed by scarring or improve gastric motility and emptying.	Left vagus nerve Right vagus nerve Pylorus Vagotomy/Pyloroplasty
Antrectomy—The antrum (lower portion of the stomach, including the pylorus) is removed to eliminate a benign ulcer in the lesser curvature of the stomach if the ulcer has not healed after 12 weeks of medical treatment or is recurring. ***Gastroduodenostomy (Billroth I)***—Part of the stomach is removed, while the remaining portion is connected to the duodenum. Usually, a vagotomy also is performed. This procedure is done to remove an ulcerated area in the stomach that is prone to hemorrhage, perforation, and obstruction.	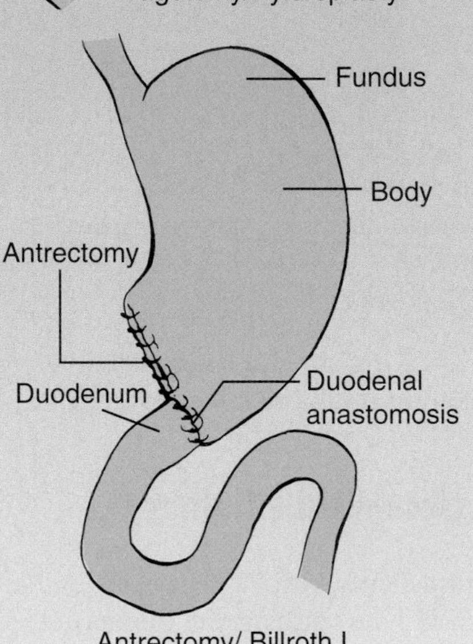 Antrectomy/ Billroth I
Gastroduodenostomy (Billroth II)—Same as Billroth I, except the remaining portion is connected to the jejunum in cases of extensive duodenal inflammation or perforation. ***Total gastrectomy***—The entire stomach is removed and the esophagus is joined to the jejunum to remove an ulcer high in the stomach near the gastroesophageal junction. It is performed to treat a gastric malignancy.	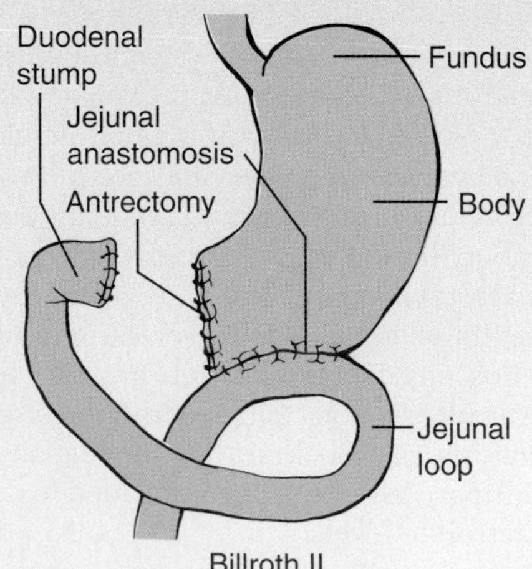 Billroth II

produces weakness, dizziness, sweating, palpitations, abdominal cramps, and diarrhea. This results from rapid emptying (dumping) of large amounts of hypertonic chyme (a liquid mass of partly digested food) into the jejunum. This concentrated solution in the gut draws fluid from the circulating blood into the intestine, causing hypovolemia. The drop in blood pressure can produce syncope. As the syndrome progresses, the sudden appearance of carbohydrates in the jejunum stimulates the pancreas to secrete excessive amounts of insulin, which in turn causes hypoglycemia.

Nursing Management

Explore each symptom of PUD in depth. If pain occurs, determine its type, onset in relation to eating food, location, and duration. A dietary history includes information about foods that cause distress, amount of food eaten at each meal, and whether eating food relieves pain.

For a client to continue eating, it may be necessary to modify ingredients, temperature or consistency of foods, and portions. Clients need nutritional supplements. If the client is receiving tube feedings, it is necessary to re-instill the gastric residual because of partially digested nutrients and essential electrolytes.

In addition, note the client's bowel patterns and stool characteristics. Also evaluate the client's emotional status and response to activity. Monitor the nonsurgical client closely for medical complications, which includes assessing vital signs and fluid status. Refer to Nursing Guidelines 46-3 for assessment of gastric pH. For a discussion of appropriate nursing management of a surgical client, refer to the Nursing Management section that accompanies the discussion of cancer of the stomach.

NURSING GUIDELINES 46-3

Assessing the pH of Aspirated Fluid

Purpose: To evaluate the effectiveness of antacid or histamine-2 antagonist therapy in peptic ulcer disease by aspirating stomach fluid and testing gastric pH. Desired pH range is 3 to 5.

- Obtain a pH test kit.
- Put on gloves.
- Verify that the distal tip of the client's nasogastric tube is in the stomach and has not migrated to the intestine.
- Use a separate syringe for withdrawing the test specimen because antacid residue or irrigating solution in the nasogastric tube will falsely raise the gastric pH.
- Connect the syringe to the tube.
- Instill a small amount of air to clear fluid from the gastric tube just before aspirating.
- Aspirate a small amount of fluid.
- Drop a sample of the gastric fluid onto a pH color indicator strip.
- Compare the color on the test strip with the color guide supplied in the test kit.
- Record the findings.

NURSING PROCESS

● The Client With a Gastric Disorder

Assessment

Ask about current symptoms, looking for specific information about such symptoms as indigestion, fullness, heartburn, nausea, and vomiting. How long has the client had these symptoms? Does the client experience problems before or after eating or with certain foods? Do situations such as stress make the problems worse? Does anything relieve the problem? Having the client provide a record of dietary intake for the last 72 hours is useful. Ask about previous gastric problems and treatments/surgery. In addition, assess for signs of abdominal discomfort/pain, malnutrition, and dehydration.

Diagnosis, Planning, and Interventions

Risk for Deficient Fluid Volume related to vomiting, diarrhea, bleeding, or all these factors

Expected Outcome: Client will maintain adequate fluid balance.

- Assist client to set a goal for minimum oral liquid intake during waking hours. *Involving the client in planning helps to meet his or her needs.*
- Provide fluids with calories and electrolytes hourly. Offer different choices. *Frequent fluid intake maintains fluid balance. Various choices prevent monotony.*
- Monitor fluid intake and output. *Indicates trends in fluid balance and early signs of dehydration.*

Deficient Knowledge about dietary management and gastric disorder

Expected Outcome: Client will demonstrate knowledge of dietary management as evidenced by appropriate choices of foods and fluids.

- Review client's fluid and nutritional needs. *Understanding of fluid and nutritional needs promotes better compliance and intake.*
- Provide a list of foods and substances to avoid. *May help prevent gastric irritation.*
- Review medications with client, including reasons for medications, schedule, and side effects and their management. *Promotes better compliance and outcomes.*

Evaluation of Expected Outcomes

Fluid intake is 2000 mL/24 hours, with a urine output of 1850 mL/24 hours. Nutritional intake is adequate as evidenced by maintenance of preillness weight. The client adheres to medical regimen as evidenced by appropriate choice of foods and fluids and compliance with medication schedule.

• CANCER OF THE STOMACH

Pathophysiology and Etiology

Cancer of the stomach is characterized by an enlarged mass or ulcerating lesion that expands or penetrates several tissue layers. Stomach malignancies are most common among natives of Japan, African Americans, and Latinos. Heredity and chronic inflammation of the stomach appear to be contributing factors. Although a single etiology has not been identified, *achlorhydria* (absence of free hydrochloric acid in the stomach), which may promote bacterial growth, and chronic ingestion of toxins such as food preserved with nitrates or cooked over charcoal, are linked to stomach cancer. When gram-negative microorganisms proliferate in the stomach, they produce a high level of nitrate reductase, which converts gastric nitrates to nitrites. These eventually become nitrosamines—known carcinogens. Stomach cancer often spreads to lymph nodes and metastasizes to the spleen, liver, pancreas, or colon.

Assessment Findings

Early symptoms are vague. As the tumor enlarges, symptoms include a prolonged feeling of fullness after eating, anorexia, weight loss, and anemia. Stool usually contains occult blood. Pain is a late symptom. A barium swallow or computed tomography (CT) scan and a tissue biopsy obtained by gastroscopy or open laparotomy confirm the diagnosis. Gastric analysis may show no free hydrochloric acid. CT scanning or ultrasonography determines the depth of the cancer.

Medical and Surgical Management

A subtotal (partial) or total gastrectomy is the only curative approach. The type and extent of surgery usually depend on tumor location, symptoms, and metastasis. A subtotal gastrectomy preserves more normal digestion. Surgery may not achieve a complete cure, but it may control bleeding or relieve obstruction at the cardiac or pyloric junction. Chemotherapy with drugs such as 5-fluorouracil (5-FU) or doxorubicin (Adriamycin) and palliative radiation also may be used.

Nursing Management

The nurse's role in management of gastric cancer includes teaching the public, especially susceptible ethnic groups or clients with a family history of stomach cancer, how to change dietary habits. The nurse also may instruct high-risk groups, such as those who have had vagotomy or take medications to reduce hydrochloric acid formation, on early warning signs of cancer and the value of frequent health assessments. Nursing roles in managing clients undergoing surgery for gastric cancer are extensive. See Nursing Care Plan 46-1 and Client and Family Teaching 46-1.

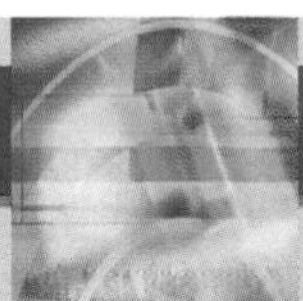

Nursing Care Plan 46-1

THE CLIENT UNDERGOING GASTRIC SURGERY

Preoperative Assessment

In addition to performing assessments for the client with a GI disorder:

- Obtain a complete health, drug, tobacco, and allergy history.
- Ask approximately how long symptoms have lasted, whether eating is normal, and how much weight, if any, the client has lost.
- Assess bowel sounds for presence and quality.
- Ask about food intolerance and current dietary management.
- Determine bowel elimination patterns and stool characteristics.
- Assess understanding of diagnostic tests, scheduled surgery, and preparations for surgery.

Nursing Diagnosis: **Anxiety** related to test results, diagnosis, and surgical procedure

Expected Outcome: Anxiety will be mild as evidenced by a calm demeanor, appropriate questions, and expressions of fear.

(continued)

Nursing Care Plan 46-1 (Continued)

THE CLIENT UNDERGOING GASTRIC SURGERY

Interventions	Rationales
Provide time for client to verbalize fears and express needs related to diagnosis and surgery.	Being present and supportive encourages communication.
Allow client to express his or her personal reaction to the threat to well-being.	Expressing feelings without being judged can help reduce fears.
Explain tests, procedures, and surgery, using nonmedical speech and allowing time for questions.	Education helps to increase coping skills.
Keep client informed of progress and explain delays or changes in plans.	Adequate explanations make clients feel more secure and less anxious.
If surgery is emergent (such as in GI hemorrhage), provide explanations to family members and anticipate questions and concerns that client will have after surgery.	Family members will have decreased anxiety and thus appear less anxious and better able to provide support when seeing client after surgery.

Evaluation of Expected Outcome: Client is less anxious, expressing fears and questions about diagnosis and surgery.

Postoperative Assessment: When the client returns from surgery:

- Assess vital signs.
- Review chart about type of surgery performed and client's progress during surgery and in the postanesthesia recovery unit.
- Inspect surgical dressing for drainage and tubes or catheters for placement, patency, and type of drainage.
- Carefully observe nasogastric tube drainage for bleeding. Although the nasogastric tube may contain a small amount of dark blood when the client first returns from the operating room, drainage should promptly return to the yellow-green of normal gastric secretions.
- Inspect IV site and note current rate and progress of fluid infusion.
- Document fluid intake and output as well as level of consciousness and comfort.
- Closely monitor client for change in vital signs, especially fluctuations in blood pressure (BP may increase initially in response to shock), increased pulse rate, and elevated temperature; extreme restlessness; difficulty breathing (increased respiratory rate, cyanosis); severe pain, especially after an analgesic is given or in an area other than the operative site; abdominal distention or rigidity; excessive or absent nasogastric output; urinary output less than 35 mL/hour if catheterized or failure to void within 8 hours of surgery; failure to pass flatus or stool more than 48 hours after surgery; profuse diaphoresis; excessive bloody drainage from the nasogastric tube, surgical drains, or surgical dressing; separation of the surgical wound edges; and unusual color or odor of drainage.

Nursing Diagnosis: **Imbalanced Nutrition: Less than Body Requirements** related to poor nutritional intake before surgery and changed GI system after surgery

Expected Outcome: Client will achieve optimal caloric intake to maintain weight.

Interventions	Rationales
Assess client for changes in physiologic status that will interfere with nutrition.	Malnutrition contributes to poor recovery from surgery.
Administer total parenteral nutrition (TPN) as ordered.	Provides adequate calories, nutrition, and fluid replacement and supports metabolic needs.
Administer nasogastric feedings as ordered (see section in this chapter).	Provides adequate calories, nutrition, and fluid replacement and support metabolic needs.

(continued)

Nursing Care Plan 46-1 (Continued)

THE CLIENT UNDERGOING GASTRIC SURGERY

Interventions	*Rationales*
When bowel sounds return, advance oral diet as ordered and tolerated. Encourage small, frequent meals.	Provides opportunity for client to eat and adjust. Small, frequent meals prevent fullness and nausea.
Monitor food intake.	Identifies trends in client's nutritional status.
Weigh client twice a week.	Determines weight loss, gain, or maintenance.
Report laboratory values such as low blood cell and hemoglobin counts and decreased iron, serum protein, transferrin, or ferritin level.	Such findings may indicate malnutrition.

Evaluation of Expected Outcome: Client attains optimal nutrition as evidenced by reasonable weight and tolerance of six small meals of soft foods and liquids.

PC: **Dumping syndrome**

Expected Outcome: The nurse will minimize and manage problems associated with dumping syndrome.

Interventions	*Rationales*
Offer small, frequent feedings low in simple sugars.	Delays entry of foods into the jejunum, allowing time for dilution and absorption.
Withhold oral fluids at meals. Provide fluids 1 hour after meals.	Avoids rapid emptying of food from the stomach.
Encourage client to lie down for about 30 minutes after a meal.	Helps food to remain longer in the stomach.
Maintain bed rest if dizziness and weakness occur.	Decreases other symptoms, such as nausea, vomiting, and palpitations.

Evaluation of Expected Outcome: Client does not have any signs or symptoms of dumping syndrome and follows dietary restrictions.

GENERAL GERONTOLOGIC CONSIDERATIONS

Severe and prolonged episodes of vomiting can be especially serious for older adults whose nutritional and fluid intake may be marginal; more profound electrolyte imbalances and severe dehydration can result.

Anorexia and weight loss are common in the older adult and can result from ill-fitting dentures or dysphagia (caused by oropharyngeal dysphagia), or may be a manifestation of depression.

Oropharyngeal dysphagia occurs in approximately 50% of institutionalized older adults and is manifested by difficulty swallowing, drooling or leakage of fluids from the mouth, and coughing or choking while eating or drinking.

With age, salivary glands become less active and the numbers of taste buds are reduced, contributing to anorexia in the older adult.

Consider food preferences, economic status, and inability of the older adult to chew because of tooth loss or ill-fitting dentures when modifying a diet.

The older adult has a diminished gag reflex. This places the elderly client at greater risk for aspiration.

As individuals age, the gastric mucosa becomes thinner, predisposing older adults to superficial gastritis and gastric ulcers.

Older adults are more prone to developing gastritis, gastric bleeding, and gastric ulcers because many regularly take drugs to treat osteoarthritis (e.g., aspirin or NSAIDs) or vascular or cardiac conditions (e.g., anticoagulant medications).

Incidence of hiatal hernia increases with age. Approximately 60% of individuals older than 70 years of age develop hiatal hernia. Hiatal hernia is more likely to develop in older women than in older men.

The older adult is at increased risk for pernicious anemia because a degeneration of the gastric mucosa results in a loss of parietal cells. The loss of parietal cells decreases the production of the intrinsic factor and absorption of vitamin B_{12}, leading to pernicious anemia.

Critical Thinking Exercises

1. *An older adult is admitted to a healthcare facility because of unexplained weight loss. What assessments are appropriate?*
2. *A man is diagnosed with a peptic ulcer. He tells you that he had an ulcer many years ago, and that he watched his diet*

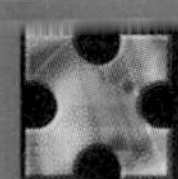

46-1 *Client and Family Teaching* The Client With Stomach Cancer

The type and extent of teaching depends on the surgery that is performed. If tube or gastrostomy feedings, tracheostomy care, and suction techniques will continue after discharge, the nurse involves the client and a family member in practicing these procedures while the client is still hospitalized. He or she identifies where medical supplies can be purchased and offers a referral for home care from a local community agency. Other points to instruct the client and family about in the discharge teaching plan include the following:

- Adhere to the diet (e.g., foods to eat or avoid) recommended by the physician. Also adhere to the dietary, fluid, and positional modifications to avoid the dumping syndrome.
- Take medications exactly as prescribed. Follow the directions on the label, paying particular attention to when you should take the drug (e.g., before, after, or with food or meals).
- Monitor weight weekly. Report any significant weight loss to the physician.
- Keep appointments for periodic medical follow-up.

carefully and used antacids, and eventually the symptoms subsided. He asks if he should start doing this again. What should you advise him?

• NCLEX-STYLE REVIEW QUESTIONS 

1. A client is transferring from the operating room to the recovery room following oral surgery. The assigned nurse is most correct to position the client:
   1. Flat, with the head turned to facilitate drainage
   2. Semi-Fowler's, with the head tilted to the operative side
   3. Trendelenburg, with the head down to decrease bruising
   4. Fowler's, with the head bent forward to facilitate drainage
2. A client is ordered intermittent tube feedings every 4 hours. The nurse aspirates the stomach contents and notes 35 mL of residual. Which is the next appropriate nursing action?
   1. Re-administer the residual amount obtained.
   2. Discard the residual contents.
   3. Flush the tube with sterile water.
   4. Clamp the tube and recheck for residual in 1 hour.
3. During preoperative teaching of a client scheduled for a gastrectomy, which medication will the nurse instruct the client that he will need for life?
   1. Penicillin
   2. Protonix
   3. Coumadin
   4. Vitamin B_{12}

connection

Visit the Connection site at **http://connection.lww.com/go/timbyEssentials** for links to chapter-related resources on the Internet.

References and Suggested Readings

Bowers, S. (1999). Nutrition support for malnourished, acutely ill adults. *MedSurg Nursing, 8*(3), 145–166.

Bullock, B. A., & Henze, R. L. (2000). *Focus on pathophysiology.* Philadelphia: Lippincott Williams & Wilkins.

Galvin, T. J. (2001). Dysphagia: Going down and staying down. *American Journal of Nursing, 101*(1), 37–42.

Holmes, S. L. (September 10, 2001). GERD: A primer reference for nurses. *Advance for Nurses,* 15–18.

Noble, K. (2003). Name that tube. *Nursing 2003, 33*(3), 56–62.

Resto, M. A. (2000). Gastroesophageal reflux disease. *American Journal of Nursing, 100*(9), 24D, F, H.

Smeltzer, S. C., & Bare, B. G. (2004). *Brunner & Suddarth's textbook of medical–surgical nursing* (10th ed.). Philadelphia: Lippincott Williams & Wilkins.

Warner, E., Addison, C., Markus, I., et al. (August 5, 2002). Gastric bypass surgery. *Advance for Nurses,* 23–25.

chapter 47

Caring for Clients With Disorders of the Lower Gastrointestinal Tract

Words to Know 

abdominoperineal resection
appendectomy
appendicitis
colectomy
Crohn's disease
diverticula
diverticulitis
diverticulosis
fissure
fistula
fistulectomy
fistulotomy
hemorrhoidectomy
hemorrhoids
hernia
hernioplasty
herniorrhaphy
inflammatory bowel disease
irritable bowel syndrome
paralytic ileus
peritonitis
pilonidal sinus
segmental resection
short bowel syndrome
skip lesions
spastic colon
toxic megacolon
ulcerative colitis
ulcerative proctitis

Learning Objectives

On completion of this chapter, the reader will:

- List factors that contribute to constipation and diarrhea.
- Explain symptoms of irritable bowel syndrome.
- Contrast Crohn's disease and ulcerative colitis.
- Describe features of appendicitis and peritonitis.
- Describe the nurse's role as related to tubes for intestinal decompression.
- Differentiate diverticulosis and diverticulitis.
- Identify factors that contribute to formation of an abdominal hernia.
- Discuss nursing management for a client with constipation, diarrhea, inflammatory bowel disease, acute abdominal inflammatory disorders, intestinal obstruction, or surgical repair of a hernia.
- Describe warning signs of colorectal cancer.
- List common problems that accompany anorectal disorders.

The lower gastrointestinal (GI) tract includes the small and large intestines from the duodenum to anus (see Fig. 45.1). Material that moves down the lower GI tract consists of food residues, microorganisms, digestive secretions, and mucus. The mixture of these substances composes feces. Disorders of the lower GI tract usually affect movement of feces toward the anus, absorption of water and electrolytes, and elimination of dietary wastes.

ALTERED BOWEL ELIMINATION

Normal bowel patterns range from three bowel movements per day to three bowel movements per week. In differentiating normal from abnormal, consistency of stools and comfort with which a person passes them are more reliable indicators than is the frequency of bowel elimination. The type and amount of food a person consumes greatly affect stool consistency. High-fiber diets, those containing whole grains, fresh fruits, and uncooked vegetables, form an increased residual of cellulose, an insoluble, indigestible product, in the bowel. Cellulose absorbs water. Cellulose and water increase and soften fecal volume, speeding the passage of feces through the lower GI tract.

Lower GI system disorders usually present as changes in bowel elimination. The most common problems are constipation and diarrhea. Irritable bowel syndrome is a motility problem in which constipation and diarrhea are alternately present. The following sections address these conditions.

• CONSTIPATION AND DIARRHEA

Pathophysiology and Etiology

Under normal conditions, fecal matter collects in the rectum and presses on the internal anal sphincter, creating an urge to defecate (eliminate stool). Peristalsis and distention of the colon provide the signal to release stool. The gastrocolic reflex, most active after the first meal of the day, accelerates peristalsis.

With constipation, the stool is dry, compact, and difficult and painful to pass. Clients with insufficient fiber and water intake are prone to constipation. Other causes include ignoring the urge to defecate, emotional stress, inactivity, or use of drugs that slow peristalsis. Anatomic disorders of the colon, rectum, and anus, including strictures and anal stenosis, may predispose a client to constipation. Impaired GI motility in conditions such as hypothyroidism or musculoskeletal disorders also can lead to chronic constipation. It also can result from chronic use of laxatives ("cathartic colon"), because they can cause loss of normal colonic motility and intestinal tone. Whatever the cause, low volume and dry stools are propelled through the lower GI tract more slowly. When stool is stationary in the large intestine, more moisture is absorbed from the residue, causing the retained stool to become dryer and harder.

Diarrhea is the frequent passage of liquid and semiliquid stool, resulting from increased peristalsis that moves fecal material through the GI tract more rapidly than normal. This rapid speed causes cramping and decreases time for water to be absorbed from the stool in the large intestine, resulting in very soft or liquid stool. Other problems include dehydration, electrolyte imbalances, and vitamin deficiencies. Causes of diarrhea include intestinal bacterial or viral infections, lactose or food intolerance, food allergies, intestinal diseases, rapid addition of fiber, overuse of laxatives, and effects of some drugs or tube feedings. Infections most frequently cause diarrhea. Clients usually report being around others with diarrhea, foreign travel, or drinking impure water. Diarrhea also may result from metabolic disorders such as inflammatory bowel disease. Surgical resection of large portions of the bowel can cause diarrhea (short bowel syndrome).

Assessment Findings

Clients with constipation have infrequent or irregular bowel movements and report feeling bloated. The abdomen may be tympanic or distended; bowel sounds may be hypoactive. Clients experience rectal fullness, pressure, and pain with attempted elimination efforts. Passed stool is hard and dry and may stretch and tear rectal tissue, resulting in rectal bleeding. Upon examination, the stool feels like small hard rocks. A thorough history and physical examination determine the underlying cause, the need for further diagnostic testing, and treatment. Abdominal x-rays help determine the extent of constipation. If a structural abnormality or motility disorder is suspected, the physician may order a barium enema and motility studies.

Clients with diarrhea have watery and frequent stools, with blood and mucus in severe cases. The client feels urgency and abdominal discomfort. Bowel sounds are hyperactive. Skin around the anus may be excoriated from contact with fecal material and digestive products (e.g., gastric acid, bile salts). Fever may be present. Infectious diarrhea usually has a sudden onset with accompanying malaise. Stool cultures identify bacterial infections as a cause. Ova and parasites from stool specimens are analyzed. Blood tests are needed to identify amebic infections. Nurses test stools for blood and observe stool for overt signs of bleeding. Chronic inflammation or alterations in the mucosal layer of the large intestine are identified by colonoscopy, upper GI series with small bowel follow-through, or both.

Medical and Surgical Management

The best relief for constipation is treating the cause. The physician prescribes an enema or laxative in oral or suppository form, followed by prophylactic administration of a stool softener. Dietary management is also promoted.

Treatment of diarrhea that is mild or of short duration involves resting the bowel by limiting intake to clear liquids for one or two meals, with gradual advancement to a regular diet. For persistent diarrhea or for very young, elderly, or debilitated clients, medical treatment may include one or more of the following:

- Administration of an antidiarrheal agent, such as diphenoxylate hydrochloride with atropine sulfate (Lomotil), loperamide hydrochloride (Imodium), or a combination product such as kaolin and pectin (Kaopectate)
- Fluid and electrolyte replacement either orally or intravenously
- Dietary adjustments, involving elimination of foods that cause diarrhea
- Total parenteral nutrition (TPN) for severe and prolonged diarrhea unrelieved or aggravated by oral fluids and food

Chronic diarrhea depletes the bowel of helpful organisms and allows yeasts and fungi to thrive unchecked. To recolonize the bowel, capsules or granules containing *Lactobacillus acidophilus* (Bacid or Lactinex) are prescribed. These agents are referred to as probiotics.

Nursing Management

In addition to completing assessments for a client with a GI disorder (see Chapter 45), obtain a complete health, dietary, allergy, and drug history, including the pattern of laxative and enema use and any newly prescribed drugs such as antibiotics. Obtain a description of the bowel elimination pattern, asking about frequency, overall appearance and consistency of stool, blood in stool, pain, and any effort needed to pass stool if the client is constipated. In discussing bowel elimination, determine the client's definition of constipation and diarrhea. Observe the client's emotional status, because anxiety affects bowel motility.

For a client who reports diarrhea, ask about recent constipation, because diarrhea can result from an impacted fecal mass. Inquire about the onset of diarrhea in relation to the possibility of eating tainted foods. Asking the client about recent foreign travel is also important. Drinking unsanitary water or consuming uncooked food washed with contaminated water may transmit intestinal pathogens.

Auscultate the abdomen for bowel sounds and palpate for distention and masses. For the client with constipation, inspect the stool or gently insert a lubricated, gloved finger in the anal canal to assess characteristics of unpassed stool. Inspect the anal area for redness or other tissue changes. For clients with diarrhea, monitor characteristics and frequency of stools and measure the volume of liquid stools to assess fluid loss. Also assess for signs of dehydration, electrolyte imbalance, and metabolic acidosis. Baseline data collection includes daily weights and periodic vital signs. Immediately report the sudden onset of acute abdominal pain to the physician.

Examples of nursing diagnoses for clients with constipation or diarrhea include the following:

- Constipation related to immobility or inadequate fluid intake
- Diarrhea related to an enteric infection
- Pain related to rectal distention, difficulty passing stool, or anal tears
- Risk for Deficient Fluid Volume related to frequent passage of watery stools and inadequate fluid intake
- Risk for Impaired Skin Integrity related to mechanical and chemical trauma to the rectum

Major goals for clients with constipation or diarrhea are restoring normal bowel function, relieving rectal discomfort and anxiety, and helping the client understand how to maintain normal bowel function. When the alteration in bowel elimination is related to dietary habits, provide a list of dietary modifications (Box 47-1). Maintaining fluid intake is essential; eight or more glasses of water and fruit juice promote regularity. Daily exercise stimulates bowel motility. Instruct the client about use of medications to treat constipation or diarrhea, with caution not to overuse laxatives or enemas. Clients with underlying GI disorders must consult with a physician before taking any over-the-counter medications to treat constipation or diarrhea.

BOX 47-1 ● Dietary Modifications for Common Intestinal Problems

HIGH-FIBER DIET TO MANAGE CONSTIPATION

Adding fiber to the diet relieves constipation by adding bulk and moisture to the stool. The following foods increase dietary fiber:

- Bran and whole grains (100% bran, rolled oats, granola, wheat germ, brown rice, cornmeal)
- Legumes (dried peas, beans, lentils; split peas; black-eyed peas; pinto, kidney, navy beans; red or yellow lentils)
- Seeds and nuts (sesame, sunflower, poppy, crunchy peanut butter, popcorn)
- Fruits: raw (apples with skin, pears, oranges, melons, berries) and dried (prunes, dates, raisins)
- Vegetables: raw (sprouts, spinach, carrots, peppers, broccoli, cabbage) and steamed (peas, potatoes with skin)

LOW-RESIDUE DIET TO MANAGE DIARRHEA

Reintroducing food after a bout of diarrhea usually calls for a low-residue diet to reduce the volume of stool. The following foods may be used to manage diarrhea:

- Dairy products (all forms of milk, yogurt, pudding, cottage cheese) unless client is lactose intolerant
- Meat and meat substitutes (baked, steamed, roasted or pressure-cooked poultry without skin; tuna or salmon; poached or boiled eggs)
- Fruits and vegetables (strained, cooked, steamed without skins or seeds, applesauce, bananas)
- Grains (products made with refined flour such as white bread or soda crackers)

● IRRITABLE BOWEL SYNDROME

Irritable bowel syndrome (IBS), or **spastic colon,** is a paroxysmal motility disorder that affects the colon. It is a cluster of symptoms that occur despite absence of a disease process. Persons with IBS experience alternating periods of constipation and diarrhea. One or the other elimination pattern predominates. Women are affected more often than men.

Pathophysiology and Etiology

Fluctuating intestinal motility is the underlying factor that produces symptoms (Fig. 47.1). The autonomic nervous system affects motor function in the GI tract, and neuron stimulation and inhibition influence bowel motility. When a parasympathetic neurotransmitter (e.g., acetylcholine) is released, intestinal motility increases and diarrhea results. An opposite effect occurs when smooth muscle of the gut responds to sympathetic neurotransmission. IBS appears to intensify with stress.

The cause of IBS is unknown, although some factors are associated with it: heredity; psychological stress or illness; a diet high in rich, stimulating, or irritating foods; alcohol consumption; smoking (Smeltzer & Bare, 2004); and intolerance of lactose and other sugars (Porth, 2002). Some people with IBS have no precipitating factors.

Assessment Findings

Most clients with IBS describe having chronic constipation with sporadic bouts of diarrhea. Most clients expe-

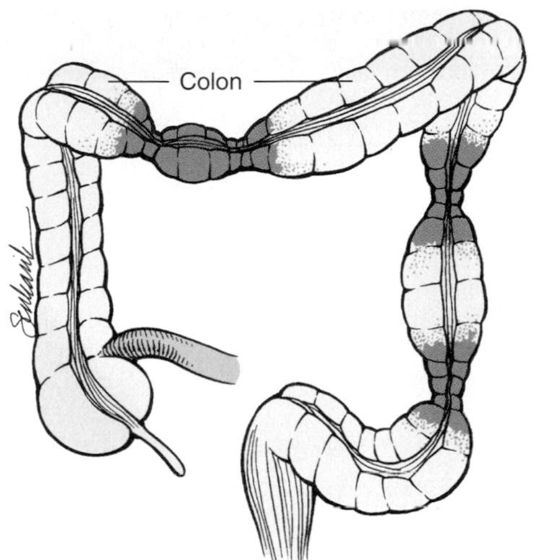

FIGURE 47.1 In irritable bowel syndrome, the spastic contractions of the bowel are visible in x-ray contrast studies. (From Smeltzer, S. C., & Bare, B. G. [2004]. *Brunner & Suddarth's textbook of medical–surgical nursing* [10th ed.]. Philadelphia: Lippincott Williams & Wilkins.)

rience various degrees of abdominal pain that defecation may relieve. Many clients suffer with belching and flatulence (intestinal gas). Symptoms usually do not awaken clients. Some with IBS report anxiety, insecurity, depression, or anger.

Weight usually remains stable. When diarrhea occurs, malabsorption of nutrients does not accompany it. Stools, although frequent, are loose, low volume, and may contain mucus. Blood usually is not found in the stool because the bowel is not locally inflamed.

Radiographic and endoscopic tests rule out other disorders with similar symptoms, such as peptic ulcer disease, colorectal cancer, diverticulosis, or inflammatory bowel disease.

Medical and Surgical Management

Dietary changes reduce flatulence and abdominal discomfort. By trial and error, the client eliminates foods that cause discomfort or intestinal gas, such as beans or cabbage. A high-fiber diet or a bulk-forming agent, such as products containing psyllium (e.g., Metamucil), is prescribed to regulate bowel elimination. Fiber draws water into constipated stool and adds bulk to watery stool. An anticholinergic, such as dicyclomine (Bentyl), has an antispasmodic effect if taken before meals. Either a prescription or nonprescription antidiarrheal is used for temporary relief from diarrhea.

Nursing Management

Clients with IBS are not hospitalized. Nurses are involved in their care during diagnostic testing, follow-up visits, or hospitalization for a concurrent problem. During these encounters, gather a database of symptoms, help manage problems associated with constipation and diarrhea, explain therapeutic treatments, evaluate the client's understanding of the regimen for self-care, and monitor response to therapy.

Stop, Think, and Respond ● BOX 47-1

A neighbor confides that she has IBS. She wonders if you can provide her with any tips about managing her condition. What is your best response?

INFLAMMATORY BOWEL DISEASE

Inflammatory bowel disease (IBD) is a chronic illness characterized by exacerbations and remissions. Ulcerative colitis and Crohn's disease collectively comprise IBD. These distinct disorders are grouped together because of similar symptoms and treatments. Their characteristics are summarized in Table 47.1. Presenting symptoms and results of diagnostic procedures are similar, making differential diagnosis difficult. Unlike IBS, IBD does not resolve without medical intervention.

• CROHN'S DISEASE

Crohn's disease, a chronic inflammatory condition, can occur in any portion of the GI tract, but predominantly affects the terminal portion of the ileum. Onset occurs in young adulthood.

Pathophysiology and Etiology

Inflammation in Crohn's disease extends transmurally through all layers of the bowel, but the submucosal layer is most involved. Hyperemia (increased blood supply), edema, and ulcerations characterize affected areas. Endoscopic examination shows inflamed areas alternating with healthy tissue. Inflamed areas occur randomly, a phenomenon described as **skip lesions.** The bowel is described as having a "cobblestone" appearance because of deep ulcerations that form among the edematous tissue (Fig. 47.2).

Because Crohn's disease is a transmural inflammatory process, inflammation can extend beyond the lining of the bowel. Inflammatory channels containing blood, mucus, pus, or stool may develop, referred to as a **fistula.** Fistulae may form a channel between the bowel and skin surface (enterocutaneous fistulae). Common sites are perianal and perilabial sites. Inflammation also may extend between the bowel and other pelvic organs (e.g., vagina),

TABLE 47.1 CHARACTERISTICS OF INFLAMMATORY BOWEL DISEASE

CHARACTERISTICS	CROHN'S DISEASE	ULCERATIVE COLITIS
Onset of symptoms	Gradual	Abrupt
Location	Diffuse	Localized
Distribution	Can occur at any location in the GI tract, most commonly found in the ileum	Rectum to cecum
Type of lesion	Patchy, positioned between areas of normal tissue, and referred to as *skip lesions*	Continuous from rectum to cecum, without areas of healthy tissue
Extent of inflammation	May extend through all bowel layers; may be visible in the large intestine or invisible if located in the higher GI tract	Limited to mucosal lining
Blood in stool	Occult	Visible
Weight loss	Common	Less common
Perianal disease	Typical (fistula formation, abscesses)	Atypical
Extraintestinal symptoms (joint pain, skin lesions, inflammatory conditions of the eyes)	Common	Less common but can occur
Biopsy findings	Signs of chronic inflammation; granulomas	Signs of chronic inflammation; granulomas rare
Carcinogenesis	Rare	Common
Surgery	Does not relieve chronicity	Curative

between the bowel and bladder, or between loops of bowel. Fistulae also may form between the rectum and vagina in women, evidenced by passage of stool from the vagina. Chronic inflammation in Crohn's disease can lead to scarring and stricture formation and eventual obstruction.

The cause of Crohn's disease is unknown. Incidence is increased among family members, suggesting a genetic predisposition. Other factors include allergic and autoimmune responses triggered by diet or infectious microbial antigens. Recurrent attacks may result from an exaggerated immune response, explaining the chronic nature of the disease. The role of stress in Crohn's disease is not defined. Stress may influence the client's ability to cope with symptoms. Many clients with IBD also may have IBS.

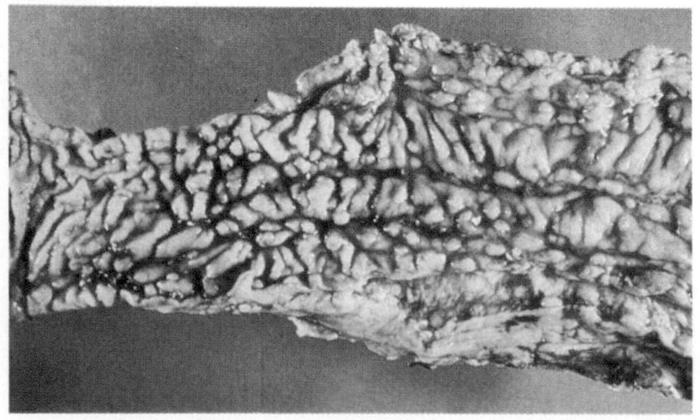

FIGURE 47.2 Crohn's disease. (From Rubin, E., & Farber, J. L. [1999]. *Pathology* [3rd ed.]. Philadelphia: Lippincott Williams & Wilkins.)

Assessment Findings

Usually, onset is gradual, and the course of the disease varies. Most clients have abdominal pain, distention, and tenderness in the lower abdominal quadrants, especially on the right side. Pain may occur with eating. The client may have a history of chronic diarrhea and fatigue. Growth failure is common in children and adolescents. Fever may be present. As Crohn's disease progresses, anorexia, weight loss, dehydration, and signs of nutritional deficiencies occur. Symptoms gradually increase in some clients, whereas acute exacerbations alternate with remissions in other clients.

The systemic nature of this disease is evidenced by symptoms outside the GI tract. They include arthritis, arthralgias, skin lesions, inflammation in the eyes (uveitis, conjunctivitis, and iritis), and disorders of the liver and gallbladder. Usually, those conditions are not present when bowel disease is under control.

During physical examination, palpation may reveal an abdominal mass. Inspection of the perineum and perianal areas may reveal scars from previous fissures, skin tags, or evidence of fistulae or perianal abscesses.

Stool cultures are negative, but occult blood and white blood cells (WBCs) often are found in the stool. Blood studies indicate anemia from chronic blood loss and nutritional deficiencies. The WBC count and erythrocyte sedimentation rate may be elevated, confirming an inflammatory disorder. Serum protein and albumin levels may be low because of malnutrition. Low serum levels of fat-soluble vitamins also reflect the client's malnourished state.

These laboratory findings do not confirm IBD because they also are associated with other disorders. Abnormal serum electrolyte levels and a disturbed acid-base balance may accompany severe diarrhea. Specific blood tests identify certain antibodies common to those with Crohn's disease and those with ulcerative colitis. These tests do not confirm IBD because some may not test positive for the antibodies, and others who do not have IBD may test positive. They are an important adjunct to other diagnostic tests.

A barium enema may show inflammation in the large intestine, but confirmation of the diagnosis requires endoscopic examination (colonoscopy or sigmoidoscopy). This shows mucosal abnormalities (e.g., skip lesions, ulcerations, cobblestone appearance). Biopsies taken during colonoscopy or sigmoidoscopy are examined for evidence of chronic inflammation and possible granuloma, which is an aggregate of inflammatory cells. It confirms diagnosis of Crohn's disease. Absence of a granuloma does not rule out Crohn's disease. Clients with Crohn's disease are vulnerable to intestinal perforation during barium enema and endoscopy because of poor bowel wall integrity.

Medical Management

Treatment is supportive. A high-fiber diet is indicated when it is desirable to add bulk to loose stools. A low-fiber diet is indicated in cases of severe inflammation or stricture. A high-calorie and high-protein diet helps replace nutritional losses from chronic diarrhea. The client may need nutritional supplements, depending on the area of the bowel affected. Clients who experience lactose intolerance need to avoid lactose-rich foods.

Some clients need an elemental diet formula, such as Tolerex, Vivonex, or Peptamen. These reduce proteins, fats, and carbohydrates to an easily absorbed form and effectively induce remission in Crohn's disease without medications. Clients are not allowed to eat or drink normally while on the elemental diet, making it unacceptable for many. Elemental formulas are not very palatable. Some may need to be administered through a nasogastric tube. Success with elemental diet therapy requires extensive education and client motivation. Newly introduced polymeric diets (Modulen, Nestle, U.S.A.) may induce remission and are more palatable. TPN may become necessary to provide intestinal rest. IV fluids, electrolytes, and whole blood are given to correct anemia and restore fluid and electrolyte balance.

Drug therapy involves supplementary vitamins, iron, antidiarrheal drugs, anti-inflammatory corticosteroids and 5-acetylsalicylic acid (5-ASA) medications, immune modulating agents, and antibiotics (Drug Therapy Table 47.1). Antidiarrheal agents, such as diphenoxylate (Lomotil) and loperamide (Imodium), are used sparingly and only when clients do not have an infection. Decreasing motility in cases of infection predisposes clients with IBD to **toxic megacolon,** a complication discussed in the section on ulcerative colitis.

Considered first-line treatment for IBD, 5-ASA drugs contain salicylate, which is bonded to a carrying agent that allows the drug to be absorbed in the intestine. These drugs work by decreasing the inflammatory response. The 5-ASA medications include sulfasalazine (Azulfidine), olsalazine (Dipentum), and mesalamine (Asacol, Pentasa). Mesalamine also is available in enema or suppository form (Rowasa) and may be used to treat distal disease. Folic acid is recommended for clients taking sulfasalazine, which interferes with absorption of this nutrient. Corticosteroids (prednisone) are used during acute exacerbations of symptoms and when 5-ASA drugs cannot control the symptoms. Hydrocortisone is available in enema form (Cortenema) and is effective in controlling distal disease without posing a high risk for systemic side effects.

Failure to maintain remission requires an immune-modulating agent such as mercaptopurine (6-MP) or azathioprine (Imuran). These agents often allow clients to discontinue corticosteroids without exacerbating symptoms. Other immune modulators are cyclosporine (Sandimmune), tacrolimus (Prograf), and methotrexate (MTX). Antibiotics such as metronidazole (Flagyl) and ciprofloxacin (Cipro) are effective adjuncts to treating Crohn's disease, especially related fistulas.

Infliximab (Remicade) achieves and maintains remission in many clients with Crohn's disease. It fits into a new classification of medications known as biologic agents. Infliximab is an antibody that interferes with the inflammatory process early in the immune response. It is given IV over 2 hours in an outpatient or inpatient setting. Repeat infusions may help to sustain remission.

Surgical Management

Surgical treatment is reserved for complications such as intestinal obstruction, perforation, or fistula formation. The need for surgical intervention is common in Crohn's disease. More than 75% of clients with Crohn's disease require surgery within 20 years of the onset of symptoms, and 90% require surgery within 30 years. Unlike surgical treatment for ulcerative colitis, removing the inflamed portion of the intestine does not alter disease progression or recurrence. Many clients who undergo surgery for Crohn's disease require additional surgery within a few years.

Surgical removal of a large amount of intestine results in the loss of absorptive surface, called **short bowel syndrome.** Massive bowel resection results in dependence on TPN, possibly for life. Removal of the colon requires

DRUG THERAPY TABLE 47.1 AGENTS FOR DISORDERS OF THE LOWER GI TRACT

DRUG CATEGORY AND EXAMPLES	SIDE EFFECTS	NURSING CONSIDERATIONS
Antidiarrheals		
bismuth subsalicylate (Pepto-Bismol)	Constipation, dark discoloration of oral mucous membranes and stools	Do not administer to clients who are allergic to aspirin or salicylates.
kaolin and pectin (Kaopectate)	Constipation, abdominal pain	This drug may interfere with absorption of nutrients and other drugs.
diphenoxylate with atropine sulfate (Lomotil)	Sedation, dizziness, dry mouth, paralytic ileus, constipation	Monitor closely for proper bowel function. Advise client not to drive or operate dangerous machinery while taking this drug.
loperamide (Imodium)	CNS depression, abdominal pain and distention, nausea, vomiting, constipation	If necessary and prescribed, administer naloxone to counteract CNS depression from overdosage. Avoid prolonged use.
Laxatives, Cathartics, and Bulk-Forming Agents		
bisacodyl (Dulcolax)	Abdominal cramps, nausea, vomiting, rectal irritation (from suppository form)	Advise client that prolonged use creates dependence. Do not administer within 1 hour of milk or antacids.
magnesium preparations (milk of magnesia, magnesium citrate, magnesium oxide)	Abdominal cramps, diarrhea, nausea, vomiting	Monitor serum magnesium levels and avoid prolonged use. Explain that these drugs may interfere with absorption of histamine-2 antagonists, phenytoin, steroids, and some antibiotics.
mineral oil *polyethylene glycol-electrolyte (GoLYTELY, Colyte)*	Leakage of oil from rectum, diarrhea, abdominal cramps	Mineral oil may cause lipid pneumonitis if aspirated. Do not administer to clients who are vomiting and therefore at risk for aspiration. Prolonged use in high doses may result in poor absorption of fat-soluble vitamins. Monitor serum levels of these vitamins.
psyllium (Metamucil, Citrucel)	Nausea, vomiting, abdominal distention and cramps Nausea, vomiting, diarrhea, intestinal gas, abdominal cramps	Administer for bowel evacuation prior to GI testing. Explain that large amounts may be administered. Compliance may be difficult. Do not give if client has intestinal obstruction or fecal impaction. Some forms require reconstitution with water.
Anti-inflammatory 5-Acetylsalicylic Acid Medications		
sulfasalazine (Azulfidine), olsalazine (Dipentum), mesalamine (Pentasa, Asacol, Rowasa)	Headache, diarrhea, abdominal pain and cramps, malaise, hair loss, rash, harmless orange discoloration of urine, bone marrow suppression, photosensitivity, decreased sperm motility (sulfasalazine)	These drugs are contraindicated in clients allergic to salicylates. Continued GI symptoms may indicate an exacerbation of the disease and should be reported to the physician. Routine blood tests to monitor for bone marrow suppression are indicated. Encourage application of sunscreen to prevent skin damage (sulfasalazine). Decreased sperm motility is reversible with discontinuing sulfasalazine. Clients taking Asacol may report passing the tablets whole in the stool, which is not harmful. They should notify the physician if this occurs repeatedly.
Anti-inflammatory Corticosteroids		
prednisone, methylprednisolone (Medrol)	Cushingoid appearance, hypertension, acne, water retention,	Monitor closely for side effects, especially with long-term use.

(continued)

Drug Therapy Table 47.1 AGENTS FOR DISORDERS OF THE LOWER GI TRACT (Continued)

DRUG CATEGORY AND EXAMPLES	SIDE EFFECTS	NURSING CONSIDERATIONS
	weight gain, hair loss, increased appetite, hypokalemia, gastric irritation, ulcer formation, adrenal suppression, decreased resistance to infection, complications associated with prolonged use (osteoporosis, development of cataracts, growth retardation, peptic ulceration, hyperglycemia)	Administer with food to decrease gastric irritation. Encourage low-sodium diet to minimize water retention. Clients with diabetes may have increased insulin needs; monitor blood glucose levels. Abrupt withdrawal may precipitate addisonian crisis, which may be fatal. Caution clients that drug should be weaned. Monitor blood pressure. Monitor linear growth in children. Instruct clients taking prednisone to wear a bracelet or necklace that states they are taking prednisone and may need additional corticosteroids during a medical crisis. Clients taking corticosteroids may not have a normal immune response to infection. Monitor closely for signs of infection, prevent exposure through universal precautions, and encourage consultation with physician regarding routine immunizations. Encourage regular physical examinations to monitor for long-term side effects. Clients should consider a calcium supplement to help prevent osteoporosis.
Immune-Modulating Agents		
mercaptopurine, 6-MP (Purinethol), azathioprine (Imuran)	Bone marrow suppression, increased vulnerability to infection, rash, arthralgias, hepatic dysfunction, nausea, vomiting, diarrhea, pancreatitis, hair loss, development of neoplasms	Encourage client to undergo routine blood tests used to screen for bone marrow suppression and hepatic dysfunction. Clients taking these agents may not have a normal immune response to infection. Monitor closely for signs of infection, prevent exposure through standard precautions, and encourage client to consult the physician before routine immunizations. Drugs may be teratogenic: women of childbearing age should consult their physician before considering pregnancy. Sexually active females should use appropriate birth control. Drugs may be toxic to infants when transmitted through breast milk.
Biologic Agents		
infliximab (Remicade)	Infusion-related reactions: pruritus, rash, chest pain, hypotension, hypertension, dyspnea; other potential side effects: headache, nausea, vomiting, fatigue, fever, autoantibody, lupus-like syndrome, lymphoproliferative disorders, increased susceptibility to infection	Drug is currently approved for a single dose in moderate to severely active Crohn's disease and is being investigated for multidose use to maintain remission in both Crohn's disease and ulcerative colitis. Clients often are given acetaminophen (Tylenol) and diphenhydramine (Benadryl) before the infusion to minimize side effects. Clients with a history of previous infusion reaction may be pretreated with prednisone. Drug is administered intravenously over 2 hours: monitor client for infusion reaction every ½ hour during the infusion. Should a reaction develop, discontinue the infusion and notify the ordering physician. Instruct client to continue routine medications unless otherwise directed by physician. Encourage client to undergo routine medical follow-up care. Clients taking this medication may not have a normal immune response to infection. Monitor closely for signs of infection, prevent exposure through universal precautions, and encourage client to consult physician before routine immunizations. Safety during pregnancy and breast-feeding has not been established.

CNS, central nervous system.

a permanent ileostomy because the disease tends to recur in any rectal pouch (see Chap. 48).

Nursing Management

A health history helps determine onset, duration, and nature of the client's GI problems. Medical, drug, allergy, and diet histories also are important. Nursing care focuses on monitoring the client for complications, managing fluid and nutrition replacement, supporting the client emotionally, and teaching about diet and medications.

Determine the average number of stools the client passes each day and their appearance. Provide regular skin care to avoid breakdown. In addition, ask the client about weight loss and whether any foods increase the frequency of bowel movements or cause discomfort. The client will require assistance to maintain adequate nutritional intake. Monitor the client's intake and collaborate with the dietitian to replace uneaten food with something more acceptable.

Physical examination includes auscultating and lightly palpating the abdomen and inspecting the rectal area. Take vital signs, weigh the client, and measure and document intake and output. Advise the client to report whenever a bowel movement occurs so it can be inspected and a sample sent to the laboratory for occult blood and other analysis.

● ULCERATIVE COLITIS

In **ulcerative colitis,** chronic inflammation usually is limited to the mucosal and submucosal layers of the colon. It is most common in young and middle-aged adults but can occur at any age. Some clients experience prolonged remission, whereas others experience mild to severe (and potentially life-threatening) exacerbations of symptoms.

Pathophysiology and Etiology

Although the exact cause is unknown, multiple factors appear to trigger ulcerative colitis, including genetic predisposition, infection, allergy, and abnormal immune response. Clients with ulcerative colitis often have other coexisting immune-related disorders such as ankylosing spondylitis and other extraintestinal manifestations.

Inflammation usually begins in the rectum and extends proximally and continuously. Healthy tissue does not appear between inflamed areas, as in Crohn's disease. When inflammation remains confined to the most distal area of the large intestine, the client has **ulcerative proctitis.** When inflammation extends beyond the sigmoid colon, the client has ulcerative colitis.

The lining of the colon tends to bleed easily. Ulceration may extend to the muscular layer of the bowel wall. Superficial abscesses form in depressions in the mucosa. Poor integrity of the bowel wall may lead to *toxic megacolon,* a complication in which the colon dilates and becomes atonic (lacks motility). The thin bowel wall is vulnerable to perforation under these conditions, leading to peritonitis, septicemia, and need for emergency surgical repair.

Assessment Findings

The onset of the disease usually is abrupt. The client experiences severe diarrhea and expels blood and mucus along with fecal matter. Cramps accompany diarrhea. Eating precipitates cramping and diarrhea, resulting in anorexia and fatigue. The urge to defecate may come so suddenly and with such urgency that the client is incontinent. Some clients experience incontinence during sleep. Despite intense tenesmus, the client may expel very little stool.

Laboratory findings are similar to those described in the section on Crohn's disease. Barium enema reveals evidence of inflammation. Definitive diagnosis requires proctosigmoidoscopy or colonoscopy with biopsy. Endoscopic examination and biopsy of the lining of the colon reveals characteristic inflammatory lesions. Biopsies of the intestinal mucosa reveal evidence of chronic inflammation. These diagnostic studies usually are withheld in cases of toxic megacolon because of the high risk for perforation.

Medical and Surgical Management

Medical treatment aims toward achieving and maintaining remission. The diet is modified to increase caloric and nutritional content. The client is instructed temporarily to refrain from eating foods associated with discomfort. If all foods cause discomfort, symptoms are likely from the disease itself and not food. The client may be given TPN and intermittent lipid infusions to rest the bowel. The use of an elemental diet, as described with Crohn's disease, has not proved effective for ulcerative colitis.

Blood transfusions and iron are given to correct anemia. The client also may need parenteral fluids and electrolytes. Because frequent bowel movements interfere with absorption of nutrients, supplementary vitamins are prescribed.

Medications used to treat Crohn's disease also are used to treat ulcerative colitis (see section on Crohn's Disease and Drug Therapy Table 47.1). Corticosteroids, given orally, IV, or rectally, are used if other measures are not effective. Corticosteroids are tapered and discontinued according to the client's response. When tapering corticosteroids without exacerbating the disease becomes impossible, immunomodulating agents (azathioprine, 6-mercaptopurine) are used to decrease the immune response and allow tapering. Goals of therapy are to induce and retain remission, allow the client to be as healthy as possible when contemplating elective surgery, or both.

Surgery is necessary when the disease does not respond to medical treatment or with complications such as dysplastic tissue (a precancerous condition), perforated colon, or hemorrhage. Removal of the colon under elective, nonemergent circumstances offers the client the best possible outcome and is the definitive cure. Current standard treatment is ileoanal pull-through and anastomosis (see Chap. 48), which typically is done in two stages, several weeks apart. In the first stage, the colon is removed, and a rectal "pouch" is created from a section of the ileum. Rectal mucosa is removed to create a temporary ileostomy. In the second stage, the surgeon closes the ileostomy and connects the intestine to the rectum, allowing the client to defecate normally. When an emergency colectomy is performed (i.e., for toxic megacolon or perforation), an anastomosis (rejoining of the bowel) may be impossible, necessitating creation of a permanent ileostomy.

Nursing Management

Obtain a health history to identify the nature of the abdominal pain, number and frequency of stools, anorexia, and weight loss. Ask the client about dietary patterns, including daily amounts of alcohol and caffeine. Auscultate the abdomen for bowel sounds and their characteristics and palpate the abdomen to determine any pain or tenderness.

Compile a comprehensive database and conduct frequent focused assessments to identify early changes in the symptoms, which may herald rapidly progressing complications. Until the disease is confirmed, preparing clients for diagnostic tests is necessary. Question diagnostic protocols for harsh laxatives and cleansing enemas when the client is experiencing severe diarrhea because bowel irritation and stimulation tend to aggravate symptoms.

Once diagnosis is confirmed, the physician orders drug and fluid therapy. If antispasmodics and opiates are prescribed, administer them cautiously because they may trigger development of toxic megacolon. Report any sudden onset of abdominal distention, severe pain, or fever in a client with acute ulcerative colitis. In addition, observe the client receiving steroids for subtle changes because these drugs mask inflammatory symptoms accompanying complications. Dosage and frequency of steroids gradually are tapered when clients no longer need them. Teach the client about the disease and measures for self-care as soon as he or she is well enough to learn (Client and Family Teaching 47-1).

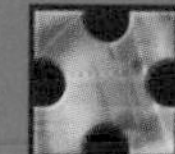

47-1 *Client and Family Teaching* Inflammatory Bowel Disease

The nurse should include the following topics in the plan for teaching the client and family about IBD:

- Special dietary modifications and the importance of complying with them
- Name, purpose, dosage, and adverse effects of prescribed drugs
- Use of medications to control symptoms rather than cure the disease
- Importance of keeping all follow-up physician and laboratory appointments so potentially dangerous complications of disease and side effects of medications can be monitored
- Techniques for rectal hygiene and skin care
- Signs to report immediately to the physician such as more frequent bowel movements, extreme fatigue, severe abdominal pain, visible blood in the stool, adverse drug effects, or weight loss
- Recommendations for regular medical checkups, even when symptoms subside, because clients with ulcerative colitis have an increased risk for the development of colon cancer

Clients who are discharged and need high levels of care, such as enteral feeding or TPN, require extensive teaching specific to their home care needs. Central venous catheter care and maintenance of TPN are a few examples of these special learning needs. The nurse thoroughly covers all technical procedures for the client or significant other to perform and allows time for the client or caregiver to perform them with nursing supervision before discharge. The nurse makes a referral to a home care agency to provide continuity of care and to ease the transition from acute care to home care.

ACUTE ABDOMINAL INFLAMMATORY DISORDERS

● APPENDICITIS

Appendicitis is inflammation of a narrow, blind protrusion called the *vermiform appendix* at the tip of the cecum in the right lower quadrant (RLQ) of the abdomen (Fig. 47.3). Appendicitis is most common in teens and

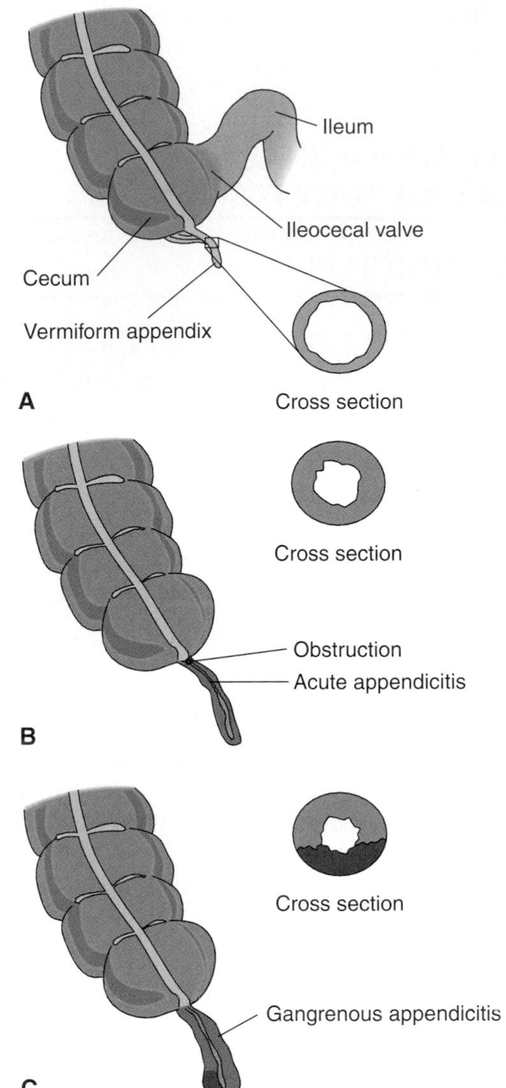

FIGURE 47.3 (**A**) Normal appendix. (**B**) Acute appendicitis resulting from obstruction (note the narrowing in the cross section). (**C**) Appendicitis and gangrene.

young adults. It is difficult to diagnose at its onset because initial symptoms resemble a host of other disorders such as gastroenteritis, Crohn's disease, ovarian cyst, tubal pregnancy, and inflammation of the kidney or ureter.

Pathophysiology and Etiology

Inflammation begins when the opening of the appendix narrows or becomes obstructed. Obstruction may result from a hard mass of feces, called a *fecalith,* a foreign body, local edema, or a tumor. The blockage interferes with drainage of secretions from the appendix, which accumulate in the confined space. The appendix enlarges and distends, and the swelling compresses surrounding blood vessels. Locally damaged cells are easily infected with bacteria from within the intestinal lumen. Unless inflammation resolves, the appendix can become gangrenous or rupture, spilling bacteria throughout the peritoneal cavity.

Assessment Findings

An attack of abdominal pain is the most frequent symptom. At first, pain is generalized throughout the abdomen or around the umbilicus. Later, pain localizes in the RLQ at McBurney's point, an area midway between the umbilicus and the right iliac crest. Often the pain is worse when manual pressure near the region is suddenly released, a condition called *rebound tenderness.* Fever, nausea, and vomiting may be present. The abdomen is tense, and the client usually flexes the right hip to relieve discomfort.

A WBC count reveals moderate leukocytosis, with a differential count of an ever-increasing number of immature neutrophils, indicating progression of the inflammatory condition. A computed tomography (CT) scan or abdominal ultrasound shows enlargement at the cecum.

Medical and Surgical Management

Antibiotics are given, and the client is restricted from eating or drinking while a decision is made about surgery. IV fluids are prescribed to meet the client's fluid needs. Analgesics may be withheld initially to avoid masking symptoms that may affect the diagnosis. If symptoms worsen, the surgeon performs an **appendectomy** to remove the appendix before it spontaneously ruptures. The appendix has no known function in the body. Its removal results in cure with no physiologic changes.

Nursing Management

Assess vital signs and the client's pain to detect early changes in symptoms. If ordered, administer IV fluid therapy and observe the client's response to antibiotics. When analgesics are withheld, be empathetic and facilitate comfort with positioning, imagery, and distraction.

When surgery is indicated, preparing the client quickly is important to avoid delay that may cause surgical complications. Soon after surgery, if no complications occur, the client ambulates and tries light nourishment. Convalescence may be rapid, although progress depends on the client's age, general physical condition, and extent of complications. A healthy young adult usually can return to normal activities soon. Clients need to avoid heavy lifting or unusual exertion for several months.

Stop, Think, and Respond ● BOX 47-2

An older adult client presents with vague symptoms of lower abdominal pain, nausea, and one episode of vomiting. In the initial assessment, what is an important question to ask?

● PERITONITIS

Pathophysiology and Etiology

In **peritonitis,** the peritoneum, a serous sac lining the abdominal cavity, becomes inflamed. Peritonitis may be caused by perforation of a peptic ulcer, the bowel, or the appendix; abdominal trauma; IBD; ruptured ectopic pregnancy; or infection introduced during peritoneal dialysis, a procedure used to treat kidney failure.

Spillage of chemical contents and bacteria inflames the peritoneum, leading to localized abscess formation or generalized inflammation. Vascular fluid shifts to the abdomen, lowering blood pressure and producing hypovolemic shock or septic shock. If the condition is not treated promptly or adequately, death may follow.

Assessment Findings

Symptoms include severe abdominal pain, distention, tenderness, nausea, and vomiting. Temperature rises as infection becomes established. The client avoids moving the abdomen when breathing because movement increases pain. He or she may draw the knees up toward the abdomen to lessen pain. Lack of bowel motility typically accompanies peritonitis. The abdomen feels rigid and boardlike as it distends with gas and intestinal contents. Bowel sounds typically are absent. The pulse rate is elevated, and respirations are rapid and shallow. If peritonitis is unresolved, severe weakness, hypotension, and a drop in body temperature occur as the client nears death.

The results of a WBC count show marked leukocytosis. Abdominal radiographs reveal free air and fluid in the peritoneum. A CT scan or ultrasonography identifies structural changes in abdominal organs.

Medical and Surgical Management

A nasogastric tube relieves abdominal distention by suctioning the accumulated gas and stagnant upper GI fluids. IV fluids and electrolytes replace substances relocated in the peritoneal cavity and lost through vomiting and drainage from gastric intubation. Large doses of antibiotics are prescribed for infection. Analgesics such as meperidine (Demerol) or IV morphine sulfate are ordered to relieve pain and promote rest. The perforation is surgically closed so that intestinal contents can no longer escape.

Nursing Management

Monitor the acutely ill client while completing preparations for diagnostic tests or surgery. Administer analgesics and infuse IV fluids with secondary administrations of antibiotics. If ordered, pass a nasogastric tube and connect it to suction (see Chap. 46). The client may need a urinary retention catheter. Assess circulatory status by taking vital signs frequently and monitoring central venous and pulmonary artery pressures.

For the client who has had surgery, assess vital signs, fluid balance, the incision, dressing, and drains. Assessing pain level is important, as is medicating according to the medical orders. For clients who have prolonged recovery time, TPN may be initiated.

Clients are fearful of the emergent nature of the peritonitis and subsequent surgery. Provide frequent explanations and emotional support. Clients also need monitoring for continued abdominal infection. If the client experiences abdominal distention, fever, changes in level of consciousness, or deviations in vital signs, notify the physician quickly.

● INTESTINAL OBSTRUCTION

Intestinal obstruction occurs when a blockage interferes with normal progression of intestinal contents through the intestinal tract. Causes are classified as mechanical or nonmechanical (adynamic) and as partial or complete. Severity depends on the region of the bowel affected, degree to which the lumen is obstructed, and degree to which blood circulation to the intestine is impeded (Smeltzer & Bare, 2004). An intestinal obstruction is extremely dangerous and may be fatal if not treated promptly.

Pathophysiology and Etiology

Mechanical obstructions result from narrowing of the bowel lumen with or without a space-occupying mass. A mass may include a tumor, *adhesions* (fibrous bands that constrict tissue), incarcerated or strangulated hernias, or impacted feces or barium (Table 47.2).

The intestine can become adynamic (lacking peristalsis, referred to as **paralytic ileus**) from an absence of normal nerve stimulation to intestinal muscle fibers. Paralytic ileus is common 12 to 36 hours after abdominal surgery. It also can result from inflammatory conditions (e.g., peritonitis), electrolyte disturbances (e.g., hypokalemia), or adverse drug effects (e.g., narcotics, cholinergic blockers).

When intestinal contents cannot move freely, the portion above the obstruction distends, whereas the portion below the obstruction is empty. If the obstruction is complete, no gases or feces are expelled rectally. Both forward and reverse peristalsis becomes forceful in an attempt to clear the obstruction. Stasis of the accumulating volume and the violent muscular peristaltic contractions potentiate risk for intestinal rupture.

Locally, the increased pressure pushes electrolyte-rich fluid from the intestine and capillaries into the peritoneal cavity. Failure of the mucosa to reabsorb secretions contributes to water and electrolyte imbalances and shock.

TABLE 47.2 MECHANICAL CAUSES OF OBSTRUCTION

CAUSE AND COURSE OF EVENTS	APPEARANCE
Adhesions—Loops of intestine adhere to areas that heal slowly or scar after abdominal surgery. The adhesions cause the intestinal loop to kink 3 to 4 days later.	
Hernia—The intestine protrudes through a weakened area in the abdominal muscle or wall. Intestinal flow and blood flow to the area may be completely obstructed.	
Tumor—A tumor in the intestinal wall extends into the intestinal lumen; or a tumor outside the intestine causes pressure on the intestinal wall. The lumen becomes partially obstructed; if the tumor is not removed, complete obstruction results.	

Increasing pressure on the bowel from severe distention and edema impairs circulation and leads to necrosis and eventually gangrene of a portion of the bowel. Perforation of the gangrenous bowel, which results from pressure against weakened tissue, causes intestinal contents to seep into the peritoneal cavity, resulting in peritonitis.

Small bowel obstruction and large bowel obstruction are similar in terms of development and resulting pathophysiology. Dehydration occurs more slowly with large intestine obstruction, because the colon can absorb the fluid contents and distend to a considerably greater size.

Assessment Findings

Nausea and abdominal distention are common. When obstruction occurs high in the GI tract, the client usually vomits whatever contents are in the stomach and small intestine. The emesis appears to contain bile or fecal material. If obstruction is lower in the GI tract, vomiting may not occur. The client may have one or two bowel movements soon after the intestine is obstructed because he or she is expelling material already past the obstruction. The client may experience severe intermittent cramps. Sudden, sustained pain; abdominal distention; and fever are symptoms of perforation.

In a nonmechanical obstruction, peristalsis is absent. In a mechanical obstruction, the bowel sounds usually are high-pitched above the obstructed area. Pulse and respiratory rates are elevated. Blood pressure falls, and urine output decreases if shock develops.

Clinical symptoms associated with large bowel obstruction occur more slowly. Constipation may be the only symptom for many days. Eventually the client experiences abdominal distention. It is possible to see loops of bowel outlined through the abdominal wall, and the client complains of lower abdominal cramps and pain. Fecal vomiting also may occur. The client can have symptoms of shock.

A radiographic study of the abdomen shows air and fluid collecting in a segment of the intestine. A barium enema (used when risk of perforation is low) pinpoints the location of the obstruction. Tests of serum electrolytes may indicate low levels of sodium, potassium, and chloride. Metabolic alkalosis is evidenced by arterial blood gas results. A complete blood count (CBC) shows an increased WBC count in instances of infection. The hematocrit level is elevated if dehydration develops.

Medical and Surgical Management

During diagnostic tests, the client is medically supported. The client has nothing by mouth (NPO). IV fluids with electrolytes are administered to correct fluid and electrolyte imbalances, and antibiotics are ordered to treat infection.

To relieve intestinal distention, cramping, and vomiting and to reduce potential for intestinal rupture with peritonitis, intestinal decompression is begun. Intestinal decompression is accomplished by suctioning large amounts of accumulated secretions and gas through a nasogastric tube or longer intestinal tube, which may or may not be weighted. Nasogastric tubes are used when obstruction is partial or located high in the small intestine.

Before surgery, decompression alone may be sufficient to relieve a nonmechanical obstruction or symptoms in clients who are undergoing surgery for mechanical obstruction. In some cases, mechanical obstructions are treated during colonoscopy by removing obstructing polyps or destroying benign tumors with laser therapy or electrocautery. Most mechanical obstructions, however, require surgery. A section of the obstructed bowel is removed and then the proximal and distal sections are reconnected (bowel resection and anastomosis). A temporary or permanent ostomy (see Chap. 48) may be performed in some cases.

Nursing Management

In addition to assessments performed on the client with a GI disorder, obtain complete medical, drug, and allergy histories, assess fluid intake and output, and take vital signs. Document all symptoms and obtain detailed information about each. For example, if vomiting has occurred, gather information regarding its onset, amount, and color. If an intestinal tube has been inserted, monitor its progress (Nursing Guidelines 47-1).

The care of a client with an intestinal obstruction involves managing pain, maintaining fluid balance to prevent deficits related to fluid shifts and losses from vomiting, and helping the client deal with fear related to severe, possibly life-threatening symptoms and an unstable condition. Manage pain by maintaining the patency of the decompression tube and administering a prescribed narcotic analgesic as long as blood pressure and respiratory rate indicate that doing so is safe. Maintain uninterrupted infusion of IV fluids and shorten the siege of vomiting by maintaining intestinal decompression, even though intestinal fluid is lost in the suctioning. It is crucial to monitor urinary output hourly and to report output below 50 mL/hour, a finding that may indicate that the client is going into shock.

NURSING GUIDELINES 47-1

Managing Care of a Client With an Intestinal Tube

Preparations

- Auscultate and examine abdomen for bowel sounds, distention, and tenderness.
- To provide a baseline for reference, measure abdominal girth, placing a measuring tape around the largest diameter of the abdomen.
- Mark the measuring location on skin (with an indelible marker) to facilitate consistency when obtaining future comparison measurements.
- Assemble all equipment the physician will need. If a weighted double-lumen tube is selected, label the tip of the adapter leading to the lumen through which tungsten gel is instilled to avoid confusing which lumen to use for suction.

Tube Advancement

- After the physician inserts the tube, ambulate the client, if possible, to facilitate tube passage through the pylorus. When a radiographic image indicates that the tube has advanced beyond the stomach, position the client as follows:
  - On right side for 2 hours
  - On back in a Fowler's position for 2 hours
  - On left side for 2 hours
- Observe lines or numbers on the tube periodically to evaluate tube's progressive movement and approximate anatomic location.
- Advance tube several inches at specified intervals as directed to avoid tension as it descends into the intestine.
- Stabilize or tape tube to the nose after an x-ray verifies that the tube has reached the obstruction. Coil excess length, securing it to the bedding or the client's hospital gown.
- Attach proximal end to suction.
- Prepare x-ray to be performed daily to evaluate progress toward relieving the obstruction.

Removal

- Remove tube once the obstruction is relieved or another treatment replaces intubation.
- Disconnect tube from suction.
- If removing a weighted tube, withdraw tungsten gel by aspirating it with a 10-mL syringe. Remove tungsten gel in the other types of tubes after the tube is withdrawn.
- Withdraw 6 to 10 inches of tube between 10-minute pauses. When the tube is in the esophagus, as determined by 18 inches of length remaining in the client, flush tube with a small amount of air to remove debris.
- Clamp tube to prevent secretions from being deposited in the client's upper airway and instruct client to hold breath while tube exits the esophagus.
- If removing a Cantor-like or Harris-like tube, grasp the bag of tungsten gel with a forceps and withdraw it from the client's mouth when it reaches the oropharynx.
- Once the tungsten gel is removed from bag, remove tube from the client's nose. Provide nasal and oral hygiene immediately afterward.

DIVERTICULAR DISORDERS

Diverticula are sacs or pouches caused by herniation of the mucosa through a weakened portion of the muscular coat of the intestine or other structure (Fig. 47.4). They can appear anywhere in the GI tract (see Chap. 46).

• DIVERTICULOSIS AND DIVERTICULITIS

Asymptomatic diverticula are called **diverticulosis.** When they become inflamed, the term **diverticulitis** is used. Diverticula are common in the colon, especially in the sigmoid area in people older than 50 years of age.

Pathophysiology and Etiology

Incidence of diverticula is higher in individuals with a low intake of dietary fiber. There also may be a congenital predisposition. It is thought that most diverticula result from weakness in the muscular coat associated with aging.

Diverticula become inflamed when fecal material is trapped in one or more blind pouches. Inflammation causes swelling of the tissue in the area. If localized swelling involves several diverticula in one area, the edema may be severe enough to cause an intestinal obstruction. Abscesses form when inflamed tissue becomes infected with bacteria present in the bowel. The swollen tissue

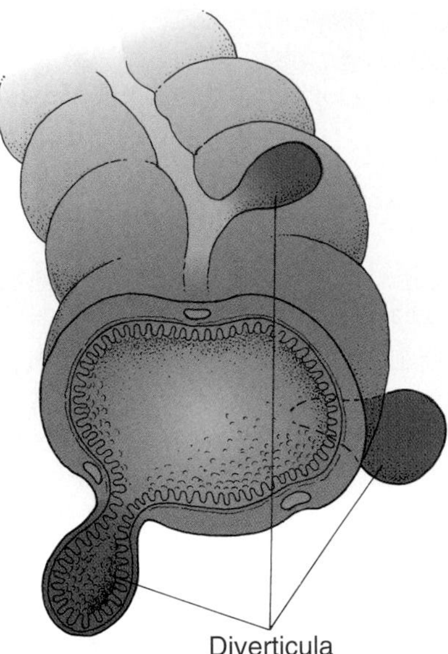

FIGURE 47.4 Intestinal diverticula, particularly common in the sigmoid colon of older adults, usually do not cause symptoms except for occasional rectal bleeding. They may become inflamed and infected from fecal matter that becomes lodged in the pouchlike herniations.

has the potential to rupture into the peritoneal cavity or form a fistular connection with an adjacent organ such as the bladder.

Assessment Findings

Constipation alternating with diarrhea, flatulence, pain and tenderness in the left lower quadrant, fever, and rectal bleeding may occur. A palpable mass may be felt in the lower abdomen. When diverticula bleed, stools appear maroon and are described as resembling "currant jelly."

A barium enema shows an irregular mucosal wall. A colonoscopy identifies the areas of inflammation. A CT scan may be used as an alternative to a barium enema or colonoscopy because both require an aggressive bowel preparation that is contraindicated when the large intestine is acutely inflamed. Risk for perforation is increased. A CBC shows leukocytosis. A stool specimen may reveal occult blood.

Medical and Surgical Management

Diverticula noted during routine examination require no treatment if asymptomatic. Avoiding foods that contain seeds of any kind is recommended. A high-fiber diet supplemented with bran or a bulk-forming agent (e.g., Metamucil) helps to avoid constipation.

When symptoms occur, the diet is temporarily adjusted to low-residue foods. If inflammation is severe and accompanied by pain and local tenderness, the client is maintained on IV fluids for several days with no oral intake. As inflammation subsides under antibiotic therapy, oral fluids and food are reintroduced.

If diverticulitis does not respond to medical treatment, or if complications such as perforation, intestinal obstruction, or severe bleeding occur, surgery is necessary. The portion of colon that contains the diverticula is removed, and continuity of the bowel is reestablished by joining the remaining portions of the colon. Depending on the location and extent of the disease and whether there is intestinal obstruction, a temporary colostomy may be necessary (see Chap. 48). The continuity of the bowel is restored, and the colostomy is closed 3 to 6 weeks later.

Nursing Management

Obtain a history of symptoms, diet, drug use, and allergies and ask questions regarding pain, bowel elimination, and diet habits. Take vital signs to establish a baseline and to determine if the client is febrile. Examine the abdomen for pain, tenderness, and masses.

Explain the underlying pathology and rationale for treatment. Because dietary compliance reduces the potential for recurrences, consulting the dietitian for teaching is useful. If surgery is necessary, prepare the client before surgery and manage postoperative care. A dietary consult or a list of foods to eat or avoid is necessary. Include the following points in the teaching plan:

- Follow the diet recommended by the physician, which will probably reduce pain and discomfort.
- Bran adds bulk to the diet. Unprocessed bran can be sprinkled over cereal or added to fruit juice.
- Avoid the use of laxatives or enemas except when recommended by the physician.
- Avoid constipation. Do not suppress the urge to defecate.
- Drink at least 8 to 10 large glasses of fluid each day.
- Take prescribed medications as directed, even if symptoms improve.
- Exercise regularly if the current lifestyle is somewhat inactive.
- If severe pain or blood in the stool occurs, see a physician immediately.

ABDOMINAL HERNIA

Although **hernia** refers to protrusion of any organ from the cavity that normally confines it, the term most commonly describes protrusion of the intestine through a defect in the abdominal wall. Certain areas in the abdominal wall are weaker than other areas and more vulnerable to development of a hernia. They include the inguinal ring, the point on the abdominal wall where the inguinal canal begins; the femoral ring at the abdominal opening of the femoral canal; and the umbilicus.

If protruding structures can be replaced in the abdominal cavity, it is a *reducible hernia.* Placing the client in a supine position and applying manual pressure over the area may reduce the hernia. An *irreducible* or *incarcerated hernia* is one in which the intestine cannot be replaced in the abdominal cavity because of edema of the protruding segment and constriction of the muscle opening through which it emerged. If the process continues without treatment, the blood supply to the trapped segment of bowel can be cut off, leading to gangrene. This development is referred to as a *strangulated hernia.*

Pathophysiology and Etiology

Common abdominal hernias are *inguinal, umbilical, femoral,* and *incisional* (Box 47-2). Inguinal hernias are the most common type and are more prevalent in men than women. Umbilical and femoral hernias are more frequent among women than men.

A hernia develops when intra-abdominal pressure increases, such as lifting something heavy, having a bowel movement, or coughing or sneezing forcefully. When pressure increases, a segment of intestine moves into a weak area of abdominal muscle. In areas that are naturally predisposed to weakness, the abdominal wall may be thin or stretched from an inadequate amount of collagen. Such a condition may be present at birth or develop as a result of aging, abdominal surgery, or obesity.

At first, the abdominal wall defect is small. As the hernia persists and organs continue to protrude, the defect grows larger. Eventually the bowel is trapped in the weakened pouch. If blood supply to the bowel is compromised, it becomes gangrenous.

BOX 47-2 ● Types of Hernias

Inguinal—Protrusion of the hernial sac contains the intestine at the inguinal opening.
Direct—Hernia extends through inguinal ring; it follows spermatic cord in males and round ligament in females.
Indirect—Protrusion follows the posterior inguinal wall; it often descends into the scrotum in males.
Umbilical—Hernia occurs in the umbilical region, through which the hernial sac protrudes. This type occurs in children when the umbilical orifice fails to close shortly after birth. It may occur in obese adults who have prolonged abdominal distention.
Femoral—Intestines descend through the femoral ring where the femoral artery passes into the femoral canal, below the inguinal ligament. Incidence of strangulation is high.
Incisional—This type occurs through the scar of a surgical incision when healing is impaired. Careful surgical technique, particularly prevention of wound infection, can prevent incisional hernias. Obese, older, or malnourished clients are prone to the development of incisional hernias.

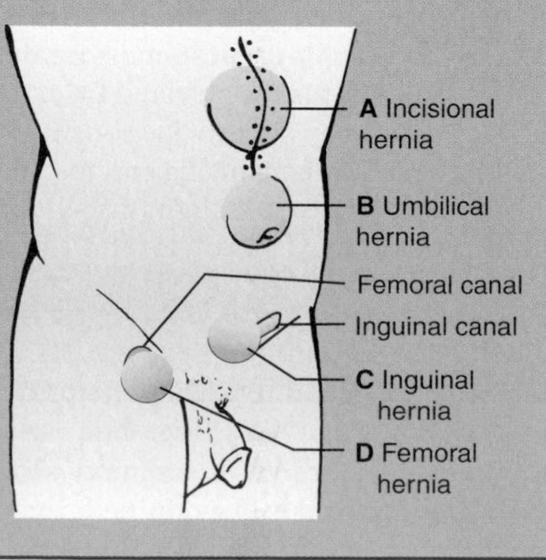

Assessment Findings

A hernia initially causes swelling on the abdomen with no other symptoms. When the client coughs or bears down, the protrusion is more obvious. Sometimes swelling is painful, but the pain subsides when the hernia is reduced. Incarcerated hernias cause severe pain, and if not treated, may become strangulated. Severe pressure on the loop of intestine protruding outside the abdominal cavity causes intestinal obstruction.

Medical and Surgical Management

Hernias tend to enlarge, leading to serious complications. Surgery is the only method of elimination. Some clients, either because they are unwilling to have or are not candidates for surgery, may wear a truss, an apparatus that presses over the hernia and prevents protrusion of the bowel. The client also may lie supine while manual pressure is applied over the protruding area to reduce the hernia periodically. Some clients learn to do this themselves.

A **herniorrhaphy,** surgical repair of a hernia, is the recommended treatment. When a herniorrhaphy is performed, protruding intestine is repositioned in the abdominal cavity and the abdominal wall defect is repaired. Herniorrhaphy is performed under local, spinal, or general anesthesia. Some types of hernias can be treated using a laparoscopic approach. When a hernia is neglected for many years, tissues in the area weaken, and postoperative healing may be impaired. Obese people who delay surgical repair for a long time are prone to recurrence of the hernia, despite surgical repair. For these cases, the surgeon also may perform a **hernioplasty.** The weakened area is reinforced with wire, fascia, or mesh. The obese client usually is advised to lose weight before surgery to lessen possibility of recurrence.

Strangulation is an acute emergency. Unless surgery is performed promptly, blood flow to the intestine is impaired. If necrosis occurs, the gangrenous part of the intestine must be excised and portions of the intestine reconnected.

Nursing Management

If the client is managing herniation with a truss and not undergoing surgery, nursing care centers primarily on teaching. Educate the client about ways to avoid constipation, control a cough, and perform proper body mechanics. The client needs to know the signs of incarceration and strangulation of the hernia. Teach the client how to wear a truss and observe for and treat skin irritation from friction caused by continuous rubbing. Advise the client to keep the skin clean and dry or to use cornstarch to absorb moisture. Explain that compression from a truss may produce localized edema from interference with lymphatic and venous blood flow.

When surgery is scheduled, prepare the client and manage postoperative care. Assessment of clients undergoing surgery includes obtaining a complete medical and drug history because malnutrition, diabetes, or concurrent use of corticosteroids or antimetabolite cancer drugs can affect wound healing. Obtain the client's allergy history, especially to seasonal inhalants (i.e., ragweed pollen), and smoking history, because sneezing and coughing can increase intra-abdominal pressure after surgery and place the client at risk for weakening the surgical repair. Before surgery, take vital signs, auscultate the lungs to identify infectious or respiratory risk factors, and document the client's weight and duration of the hernia. Assess the client's urinary and bowel patterns to determine if the client has any preexisting problems affecting elimination. After surgery, inspect the scrotum of male clients because it is common for edema to follow surgical repair.

Hernia repairs are performed mainly on an outpatient basis. Teach measures to the client and significant others who will provide care after discharge. Reinforce verbal instructions with written instructions about signs and symptoms of possible complications (i.e., bleeding, infection) and the need to report these symptoms to the physician. Instructions include techniques for avoiding constipation and straining to have a bowel movement. Include instructions to avoid strenuous exertion and heavy lifting until the physician determines that the client can safely undertake such activities. For clients who perform heavy physical labor, it is essential to explore how they may modify the manner in which they perform their jobs, take an extended sick leave, or apply for a temporary leave of absence. Explain to those whose work is sedentary or light that they usually can return to full employment with few activity restrictions within a few weeks.

CANCER OF THE COLON AND RECTUM

Intestinal malignancies may develop anywhere in the lower GI tract. Approximately 75% of cases develop in the lower sigmoid colon and rectum. Colorectal cancer ranks second among causes of cancer deaths in the United States. Incidence of the disease increases with age. The American Cancer Society recommends annual fecal occult blood testing and colonoscopy every 10 years for colorectal cancer screening in individuals older than 50 years of age. Screening may be done for younger clients who have risk factors, such as a family history of colorectal cancer or ulcerative colitis.

Pathophysiology and Etiology

Many malignant colorectal tumors develop from benign adenomas in the mucosal and submucosal intestinal layers. It is believed that genetic, environmental, and lifestyle factors spark transformation from a benign to a cancerous state. Catalysts seem to include chronic bowel inflammation, as in ulcerative colitis, and a lifetime pattern of eating low-fiber, high-fat foods.

Having a blood relative with this disease is a high-risk factor. Genetic testing may be carried out to identify some types of familial colon cancer. At some point, normal cells undergo mutation, which affects their proliferation and growth pattern. The malignant cells reproduce rapidly and eventually proceed to invade the muscle wall.

Although malignant growth remains in situ (confined to its site of origin), it may change the shape of the stool, compressing it or making it appear pencil-like as it passes by the protruding mass. Untreated, the cancer extends to other organs by way of the mesentery lymph nodes or portal vein leading to the liver.

Assessment Findings

The chief characteristic of cancer of the colon is a change in bowel habits, such as alternating constipation and diarrhea. Occult or frank blood may be present in the stool. Sometimes a client may feel dull, vague abdominal discomfort. Pain is a late sign of cancer. On physical assessment, the abdomen feels distended, and a mass may be palpated in the abdomen or rectum.

Genetic screening may detect chromosomal markers for particular types of colon cancer. An elevated carcinoembryonic antigen (CEA) test result suggests a tumor. Unfortunately, a CEA test is not effective in identifying colorectal cancer in its earliest, most treatable stages. Unless malignant growths are elevated from the mucosal wall, a barium enema may not provide conclusive evidence either. A tissue sample taken during proctosigmoidoscopy or colonoscopy may detect malignant cells in the area of the biopsy. A CBC may show a low erythrocyte count from chronic blood loss.

Medical and Surgical Management

When polyps are discovered during endoscopic examination, they are removed and examined. Even if polyps are benign, the client continues to undergo periodic endoscopic examinations to identify recurrent polyps for early malignant changes. An exception to this rule is the finding of juvenile polyps in young children. These benign growths do not tend to recur. Primary treatment of colorectal cancer is surgical, but sometimes treatment involves a combination of surgery, radiation therapy, and chemotherapy.

An encapsulated colorectal tumor may be removed without taking away surrounding healthy tissue. This type of tumor, however, may call for partial or complete surgical removal of the colon (**colectomy**). Occasionally, the tumor causes a partial or complete bowel obstruction. If the tumor is in the colon and upper third of the rectum, a **segmental resection** is performed. In this procedure, the surgeon removes the cancerous portion of colon and rejoins the remaining portions of the GI tract to restore normal intestinal continuity.

Cancers in the lower third of the rectum are treated with an **abdominoperineal resection**—wide excision of the rectum and creation of a sigmoid colostomy. Surgical procedures used to treat cancers in the middle third of the rectum vary. A low resection with a temporary colostomy usually is attempted to preserve the anal sphincter. Radiation therapy is indicated in many cases of colon cancer, whereas chemotherapy usually is reserved for those with evidence of lymphatic infiltration or metastasis. If the cancer metastasizes, a colostomy may be performed to relieve an intestinal obstruction. In some cases, the obstruction is relieved or bleeding is controlled with laser surgery.

Nursing Management

Advise and prepare clients for routine colorectal screening. Follow standard guidelines for collecting stool specimens and sending them to the laboratory for analysis (Box 47-3). Advise anyone who is asymptomatic but whose stool test results are positive for blood to undergo a colonoscopy, the next step in cancer detection. Nursing management of the client with a colostomy is discussed in Chapter 48.

BOX 47-3 • Testing Stool for Occult Blood

Seven to 10 days before and throughout the test, the nurse:

- Tells the client not to drink alcohol or take aspirin, NSAIDs, vitamin C, or iron preparations
- Checks with physician if anticoagulants, steroids, colchicines (used to treat gout), or cimetidine (for peptic ulcer treatment) have been prescribed

Two days before and throughout the test, the nurse:

- Advises client to consume a high-fiber diet and to avoid red meat, substituting with poultry and fish
- Informs client to avoid turnips, cauliflower, broccoli, cantaloupe, horseradish, and parsnips

During the test, the nurse or client:

- Collects stool within a toilet liner or bedpan
- Uses an applicator stick and removes a sample from the center of the stool
- Applies a thin smear of stool onto the test area supplied with the screening kit
- Takes care to cover the entire space
- Places two drops of developer solution onto the test area
- Waits precisely 60 seconds
- Observes for a blue color, indicating a positive reaction (for more valid results, test samples from several stools over 3 to 6 days)

ANORECTAL DISORDERS

Clients with anorectal disorders usually experience localized pain and bleeding, and thus seek medical attention. They also may have problems with perianal itching, tenderness, and swelling. They may delay defecation secondary to pain and other discomfort.

• HEMORRHOIDS

Hemorrhoids are dilated veins outside or inside the anal sphincter (Fig. 47.5). Thrombosed hemorrhoids are veins that contain clots.

Pathophysiology and Etiology

Chronic straining to have a bowel movement or frequent defecation with chronic diarrhea likely weakens tissue supporting the veins. Clients whose work requires prolonged sitting are at increased risk for development of hemorrhoids. Pregnancy, prolonged labor, portal hypertension, or other intra-abdominal conditions that interfere with venous blood return can cause or aggravate the condition. Veins near the anal sphincter probably are displaced downward from their natural location as the result of a loss of supporting tissue. Without adequate connective tissue and smooth muscle support, veins dilate and fill with blood. Dry stool passes by the engorged hemorrhoids, stretches and irritates the mucosa, and gives rise to the local symptoms of burning, itching, and pain. Passing dry, hard stool causes the hemorrhoids to bleed.

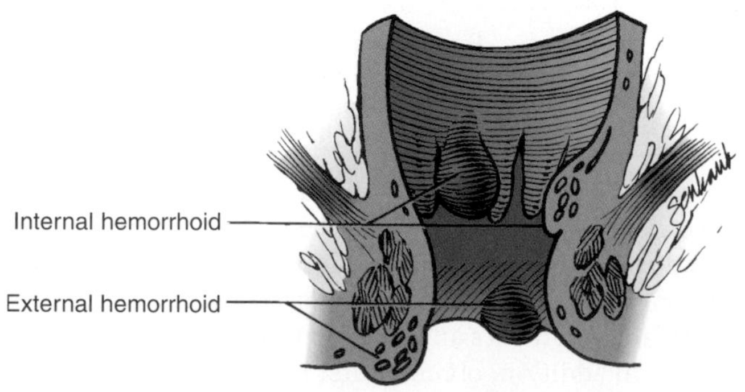

FIGURE 47.5 Internal and external hemorrhoids. (From Smeltzer, S. C., & Bare, B. G. [2004]. *Brunner & Suddarth's textbook of medical–surgical nursing* [10th ed.]. Philadelphia: Lippincott Williams & Wilkins.)

Assessment Findings

External hemorrhoids may cause few symptoms or produce pain, itching, and soreness of the anal area. They appear as small, reddish-blue lumps at the edge of the anus. Thrombosed external hemorrhoids are painful but seldom cause bleeding.

Internal hemorrhoids cause bleeding but are less likely to cause pain, unless they protrude through the anus. The amount of bleeding varies from an occasional drop or two of blood on toilet tissue or underwear to chronic loss of blood, leading to anemia. Internal hemorrhoids usually protrude each time the client defecates but retract after defecation. As the masses enlarge, they remain outside the sphincter.

An anoscope, an instrument for examining the anal canal, or a proctosigmoidoscope allows visualization of internal hemorrhoids. A colonoscopy rules out colorectal cancer, which has similar symptoms.

Medical Management

Small external hemorrhoids may disappear without treatment, or the client may obtain relief through symptomatic treatment. The physician may recommend warm soaks, an ointment that contains a local anesthetic for relief of pain and itching, topical astringent pads to relieve swelling, a diet that corrects or prevents constipation, and a stool softener. In some cases, the hemorrhoid is ligated (tied off) with a rubber band. Infrared photocoagulation, in which protein and water in hemorrhoidal tissue is destroyed, is an alternative to traditional surgery.

Surgical Management

A **hemorrhoidectomy,** surgical removal of hemorrhoids, may be necessary in chronic and severe cases. The procedure is performed using conventional surgery or laser surgery, the client receives a local anesthetic or regional nerve block. Internal packing of lubricated gauze, external gauze dressing, or a perineal pad is applied to absorb blood. A T-binder holds the absorbent material in place.

Nursing Management

Obtain a complete history, including drug and allergy histories. Because bleeding accompanies many colorectal disorders, ask the client to describe the bleeding as well as other related symptoms. Determine if there is a history of constipation or alternating diarrhea and constipation, and if the client uses any prescription or nonprescription drugs. In addition, obtain a diet history, paying particular attention to the type of foods (especially fiber) included in the diet.

Health teaching is focused on self-management. Review the physician's home care instructions, demonstrate wound care to the client or responsible caregiver, and provide an opportunity for returning the demonstration. Recommend dietary modifications and offer a list of high-fiber foods. Instruct about stool softeners as indicated, emphasize the importance of an active lifestyle and increased fluid intake, and caution against the prolonged use of laxatives.

● ANORECTAL ABSCESS, ANAL FISSURE, AND ANAL FISTULA

An anorectal abscess is an infection with a collection of pus in an area between the internal and external sphincters. An anal **fissure** (fissure in ano) is a linear tear in the anal canal tissue. An anal fistula (fistula in ano) is a tract that forms in the anal canal.

Pathophysiology and Etiology

An anorectal abscess is common among clients with Crohn's disease. Infections also are transmitted from others through anal intercourse or foreign bodies inserted in the rectum. The source of infection may be microorganisms harbored in the intestine itself.

Usually, infectious microorganisms invade anal crypts, small tubular cavities in the anal skin and rectal mucosa. A purulent exudate collects, and pressure causes pain and swelling. The abscess eventually may develop into a fistulous tract.

Constipation is the leading cause of anal fissures. Other factors that may lead to formation of a slitlike tear include eversion of the anus during vaginal delivery and trauma to the anus, such as during anal intercourse or through insertion of foreign bodies or medical instruments. When the anal canal is excessively stretched, the skin rips apart, exposing underlying tissue.

When healing of an anorectal abscess is inadequate, an inflamed tunnel develops, connecting the area of the original abscess with perianal skin (Fig. 47.6). Purulent material drains from the opening.

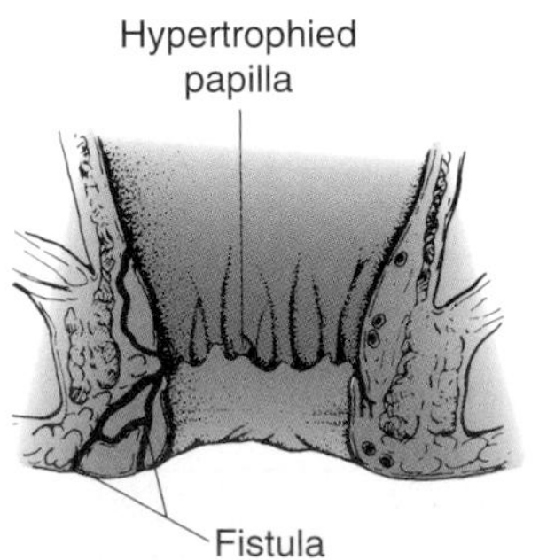

FIGURE 47.6 Anal fistula.

Assessment Findings

Clients with an anorectal abscess experience pain aggravated by walking and sitting or other activities that increase intra-abdominal pressure such as coughing, sneezing, and straining to have a bowel movement. A swollen mass is evident in the anus. Fever and abdominal pain develop if the abscess extends into deeper tissues. Foul-smelling drainage may leak from the anus if the abscess spontaneously ruptures. A culture of anal drainage reveals the infectious microorganism.

Clients with an anal fissure experience severe pain and bleeding on defecation. Clients are reluctant to defecate because of the pain and experience constipation if they did not already have it. The torn area may be visible when the anus is inspected visually or via anoscopy.

Clients with an anal fistula also have pain with defecation. The fistula opening appears red, and pus leaks from the external opening of the fistula or can be expressed if the area is compressed. If the fistula is superficial, it feels cordlike on palpation.

Medical and Surgical Management

Treatment for anorectal abscess, fissure, or fistula includes analgesics; sitz baths; anesthetic creams, ointments, or suppositories; and prevention of constipation. Antibiotic therapy is ordered to treat gonorrheal, staphylococcal, streptococcal, or other drug-sensitive bacteria. Treatment of underlying Crohn's disease may allow for resolution of a fistula without surgery. Incision and drainage are used to remove infected material. Deeper excision may be needed for removal of a fistulous tract or a fissure.

Most simple low-lying fistulae can be managed by **fistulotomy.** This procedure involves incising the fistula along with partial sphincter division and is used for those fistulae that arise from relatively normal surrounding tissue. Another surgical procedure, referred to as **fistulectomy,** involves excision of the fistulous tract. This type usually is the recommended surgery.

Nursing Management

To limit the spread of infectious microorganisms, instruct the client to practice scrupulous handwashing after each bowel movement, to use separate hygiene articles, to cleanse the bathtub after each use, and to use a condom if having anal intercourse. In addition, include the following the plan of care:

- Teach the client how to insert a suppository.
- Instruct the client in how to take a sitz bath.
- Discuss strategies to relieve constipation.

Refer to Nursing Care Plan 47-1 for more information.

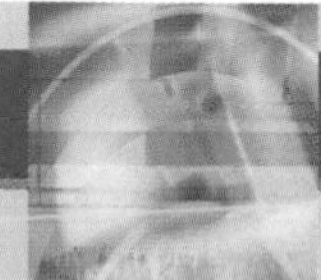

Nursing Care Plan 47-1

THE CLIENT WITH AN ANORECTAL CONDITION

Assessment

Include the following questions in the health history:

- Do you have any burning, itching, or pain in the anorectal area? If so, when do these symptoms occur—with defecation? How long do they last? Do you have any other discomfort, such as abdominal cramps?
- Is any blood in the stool or on the toilet tissue when you wipe the rectum? How much? Is the blood bright or dark red?
- Is there mucus or pus from the rectal area?
- What is your stool pattern?
- Do you use laxatives? If so, how often?
- What is your typical diet?
- Do you exercise regularly? If so, what is the exercise?
- Do you sit or stand for long periods?

Nursing Diagnosis: **Risk for Constipation** related to fear of painful elimination

Expected Outcome: Client identifies measures that prevent or treat constipation.

(continued)

Nursing Care Plan 47-1 (Continued)

THE CLIENT WITH AN ANORECTAL CONDITION

Interventions	*Rationales*
Instruct client, unless contraindicated, to increase intake of water to 2 L/day.	Prevents hard, dry stools and eases defecation.
Provide a list of high-fiber foods.	Promotes bulk of stool and prevents constipation.
Instruct client in use of laxatives or stool softeners as ordered.	Prolonged use of these measures is not encouraged; they should be used only as indicated.
Teach the client to heed the urge to have a bowel movement.	Prevents constipation.

Evaluation of Expected Outcome: Client practices measures that prevent constipation, as evidenced by increased fluid and fiber intake and passage of soft, formed stools.

Nursing Diagnosis: **Acute Pain** related to surgical procedure

Expected Outcome: Client will report that pain management regimen relieves his or her pain.

Interventions	*Rationales*
Administer pain medications as ordered.	Promotes ongoing pain relief.
Encourage client to rest in a comfortable position that removes pressure from surgical site, or to use a flotation device.	Relieves pressure and decreases pain at the surgical site.
Apply ice and analgesic ointments as indicated.	Promotes pain relief.
Use warm compresses or sitz baths three to four times daily as indicated.	Warmth through compresses or baths relaxes rectal sphincter spasm and soothes irritated tissues.

Evaluation of Expected Outcome: Client states that positioning and use of sitz baths relieve pain.

Nursing Diagnosis: **Risk for Ineffective Therapeutic Regimen Management** related to deficient knowledge

Expected Outcome: Client will demonstrate ability to manage therapeutic regimens.

Interventions	*Rationales*
Instruct client to cleanse perianal area with warm water and to dry with cotton wipes.	Prevents infection and irritation.
Teach client how to do sitz baths at home, using warm water, three to four times each day.	Promotes healing, decreases skin irritation, and relieves rectal spasms.
Instruct client to take a sitz bath after each bowel movement.	Helps keep the perianal area clean.
Encourage client to follow diet and medication instructions.	Promotes compliance with therapeutic regimen and prevents complications.
Encourage moderate exercise.	Promotes healing and normal stool patterns.

Evaluation of Expected Outcome: (1) Incision heals without complications. (2) Client has no signs of infection and eats a diet high in fiber. (3) Vital signs are normal. (4) Stools are soft-formed and regular.

• PILONIDAL SINUS

Pilonidal means "a nest of hair." A **pilonidal sinus** is an infection in the hair follicles in the sacrococcygeal area above the anus (Fig. 47.7). Other local infections, such as osteomyelitis and furuncles of the skin, also have common presenting signs and symptoms and must be ruled out. The terms *pilonidal sinus* and *pilonidal cyst* are both used to describe the condition.

Pathophysiology and Etiology

The condition typically occurs after puberty. People who have a deep intergluteal cleft and those who have abundant hair in the perianal and lower back regions are predisposed to the condition. Inadequate personal hygiene, obesity, and trauma to the area also contribute to its development.

A sinus or cyst begins to form when skin deep in the cleft softens as a result of being chronically moist. Stiff hairs then irritate and pierce the soft, macerated skin, becoming embedded in it. The irritation inflames the tissues. Infection readily follows because the break in the skin allows microorganisms to enter. Several channels may lead from the sinus to the skin.

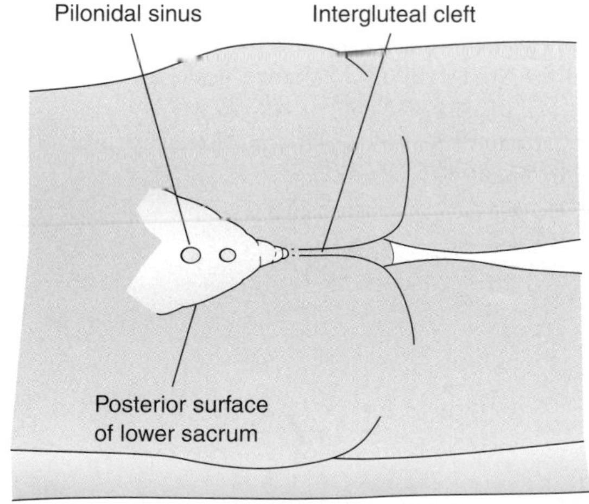

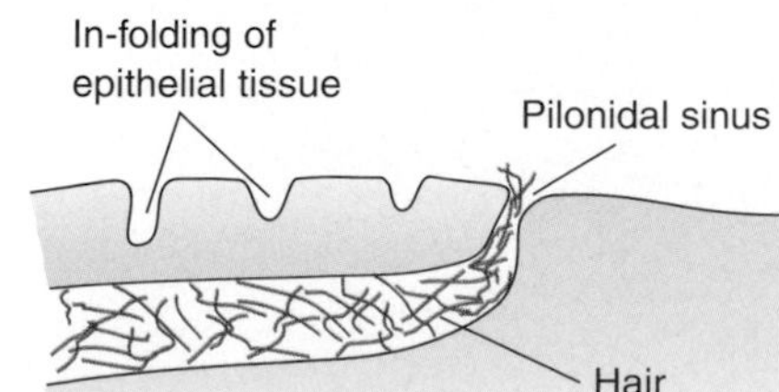

FIGURE 47.7 (**A**) Pilonidal sinus on lower sacrum about 5 cm (2 in) above the anus in the intergluteal cleft. (**B**) Note: hair particles emerge from the sinus tract, and localized indentations (pits) can appear on the skin near the sinus openings. (From Smeltzer, S. C., & Bare, B. G. [2004]. *Brunner & Suddarth's textbook of medical–surgical nursing* [10th ed.]. Philadelphia: Lippincott Williams & Wilkins.)

Assessment Findings

Pain and swelling at the base of the spine and purulent drainage occur. On inspection, the sinus opening may be located in the gluteal fold. Dilated pits of hair follicles in the sinus are a unique characteristic.

Medical and Surgical Management

The abscess is drained, and tissue is incised. The sinus and all its connecting channels are laid open, and purulent material and hair are removed. Packing is inserted into the cavity, and the wound heals by secondary intention. In some cases, the wound edges are approximated. Healing by primary intention sometimes allows purulent material to reform and collect, causing another abscess. Because infection is localized, systemic antibiotics usually are not prescribed.

Nursing Management

Teach the client how to minimize discomfort and facilitate postoperative bowel elimination. As appropriate, instruct a family member in the procedures for removing the packing, cleaning the incised tissue, and redressing the area. See Nursing Care Plan 47-1 for additional nursing management.

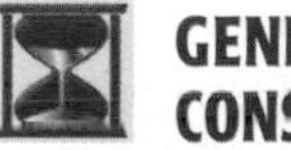

GENERAL GERONTOLOGIC CONSIDERATIONS

Constipation is a common problem in older adults and often results from inadequate intake of dietary fiber, lack of exercise, and decreased fluid intake.

Encourage older adults to schedule regular health examinations, including screenings for colorectal cancer, because its incidence increases with age.

The gastric mucosa (mucous lining of the stomach) atrophies with age, resulting in decreased production of gastric acids.

With age, peristaltic action of the GI tract decreases; therefore, risk for constipation in the older adult increases.

Constipation can occur in an older adult who feels rushed when defecating or cannot get to the toilet in time.

An older adult with prolonged constipation or constipation that shifts to diarrhea must be checked for a fecal impaction. Liquid feces may ooze around the impacted feces, giving the appearance of diarrhea.

Older adults with appendicitis may not display the type of acute pain that younger adults with the condition experience. Severe pain may be absent, minimal, or referred in the older adult, causing a delay in diagnosis and a greater incidence of complications.

Critical Thinking Exercises

1. *The admitting department notifies the nursing unit to expect a client with ulcerative colitis. Based on the characteristics of*

the disease process, what assessments are essential to obtain at the time of admission?

2. *As you assist an older adult with using a bedpan, you notice blood on the toilet tissue. What other data are appropriate to gather at this time?*

● NCLEX-STYLE REVIEW QUESTIONS 

1. A client who recently had a total hip replacement is experiencing abdominal pain and constipation. The last bowel movement 5 days ago was a small amount of hard, dry, and difficult-to-pass stool. Which nursing action is most appropriate first?
   1. Instruct the client on exercise, fluids, and a high-fiber diet.
   2. Offer to obtain an order for a stool softener with a mild laxative.
   3. Remove the stool digitally with a gloved, lubricated finger.
   4. Provide prune juice with snacks and meals daily.
2. A client with acute diarrhea is NPO for 3 days to rest the bowel and slow peristalsis. Following this period, which of the following dietary choices would the nurse encourage when assisting the client with meal planning?
   1. Turkey and rice
   2. Hamburger and French fries
   3. Spaghetti and meatballs
   4. Macaroni and cheese
3. The physician orders dicyclomine (Bentyl) for a client with irritable bowel syndrome. When assessing the effectiveness of the medication, which client statement best indicates that dicyclomine has been effective?
   1. "I have not had any diarrhea over the past 4 hours."
   2. "I have not been passing gas and belching as much."
   3. "I have not had sudden abdominal cramping as before."
   4. "My stools have been thicker in consistency."

connection

Visit the Connection site at **http://connection.lww.com/go/timbyEssentials** for links to chapter-related resources on the Internet.

References and Suggested Readings

Ahmed, D. S. (2000). Hidden factors in occult blood testing. *American Journal of Nursing, 100*(12), 25.

Heitkemper, M., & Jarrett, M. (2001). Irritable bowel syndrome. *American Journal of Nursing, 101*(1), 26–32.

Holmes, S. (January 7, 2002). Caring for the patient with Crohn's disease. *Advance for Nurses,* 15–17.

Noble, K. (2003). Name that tube. *Nursing 2003, 33*(3), 56–62.

Porth, C. M. (2002). *Pathophysiology: Concepts of altered health states* (6th ed.). Philadelphia: Lippincott Williams & Wilkins.

Rayhorn, N. (2002). An in-depth look at inflammatory bowel disease. *Nursing 2002, 32*(7), 37–43.

Sargent, C., & Murphy, D. (2003). What you need to know about colorectal cancer. *Nursing 2003, 33*(2), 36–41.

Smeltzer, S. C., & Bare, B. G. (2004). *Brunner & Suddarth's textbook of medical–surgical nursing* (10th ed.). Philadelphia: Lippincott Williams & Wilkins.

U.S. Preventive Services Task Force. (2002). Screening for colorectal cancer: Recommendations and rationale. *American Journal of Nursing, 102*(9), 107–114.

Veronesi, J. F. (2003). Defense gone awry: Inflammatory bowel disease. *RN, 66*(5), 38–45.

Zimmerman, P. G. (2002). Triaging lower abdominal pain. *RN, 65*(12), 52–57.

chapter 48

Caring for Clients With an Ileostomy or Colostomy

Words to Know 

abdominoperineal resection
appliance
colostomy
continent ileostomy (Kock pouch)
double-barrel colostomy
effluent
enterostomal therapist
ileoanal reservoir (anastomosis)
ileostomy
loop colostomy
ostomate
ostomy
segmental resection
single-barrel colostomy
stoma

Learning Objectives

On completion of this chapter, the reader will:

- Differentiate between ileostomy and colostomy.
- Discuss preoperative nursing care of a client undergoing ostomy surgery.
- List complications associated with ostomy surgery.
- Discuss postoperative nursing management of a client with an ileostomy.
- Describe the components used to apply and collect stool from an intestinal ostomy.
- Summarize how to change an ostomy appliance.
- Explain how stool is released from a continent ileostomy.
- Describe the two-part procedure needed to create an ileoanal reservoir.
- Discuss various types of colostomies.
- Explain ways that clients with descending or sigmoid colostomies may regulate bowel elimination.

Ostomy refers to an opening between an internal body structure and the skin. The most common intestinal ostomies are the **ileostomy,** an opening from the distal small intestine, and the **colostomy,** an opening from the colon (Table 48.1). Fecal material exits through a **stoma,** an opening on the exterior abdominal surface. Most ostomies are created in response to an inflammatory bowel disorder that fails to respond to medical treatment or complications such as rupture of a portion of intestine, irreversible obstruction, compromised blood supply to the intestine, or cancerous tumor. Whether an ostomy is temporary or permanent, clients need individual plans of care that include surgical preparation, recovery, and teaching for self-care.

ILEOSTOMY

For a conventional ileostomy, the entire colon and rectum (total colectomy) are removed. The terminal end of the ileum is brought through the right lower quadrant of the abdomen slightly below the umbilicus, near the outer border of the rectus muscle (Fig. 48.1). The cut end is everted and sutured to the skin, which creates a stoma. When an ileostomy is done, the stoma continually releases stool and gas. Fecal material discharged from an ileostomy is liquid or mushy and contains digestive enzymes.

• THE OSTOMY APPLIANCE

The stoma promotes healing and provides a smooth peristomal area that permits immediate postoperative application of an **appliance,** the collection device worn over a stoma. Clients with an ileostomy always wear an appliance that requires frequent emptying. Various appliances can meet the individual needs of the **ostomate** (client with an ostomy). All consist of one-piece or two-piece devices with a pouch for collecting feces and a faceplate, or disk, attached to the abdomen with an opening through which the stoma protrudes (Fig. 48.2). The faceplate adheres to skin with self-adhesive backing or another

TABLE 48.1 TYPES OF INTESTINAL OSTOMIES

TYPE	STOMA LOCATION	FECAL CONSISTENCY	FECAL CONTROL
Conventional ileostomy	Lower abdomen	Liquid	Never
Continent ileostomy	Lower abdomen	Liquid	By siphoning
Ascending colostomy	Middle right abdomen	Semiliquid	Never
Transverse colostomy	Center of the abdomen below the belt line	Semiliquid	Never
Descending colostomy	Middle left abdomen	Soft	Sometimes
Sigmoid colostomy	Lower left abdomen	Formed	Usually

bonding substance such as an adhesive powder, paste, or wafer. Karaya gum is a common component in ostomy supplies. It becomes gelatinous when in contact with moisture and is used in place of an adhesive. Karaya gum protects skin and promotes adhesion of the ostomy appliance. Karaya gum rings are used around the stoma. They are pulled or pushed into any shape and are ideal for correcting problems created by an ill-fitting appliance. Unlike rings made of rigid material, a karaya gum ring fits snugly around the stoma without injuring it.

A disposable or temporary appliance is preferred in the immediate postoperative phase, because the size of the stoma changes over time as a result of swelling from the procedure. The size of the stoma may change rapidly and differ from one appliance change to the next. After the stoma heals and reaches its final size and shape, a permanent (reusable) appliance is fitted.

Reusable equipment consists of a sturdier pouch with a custom-sized faceplate and "O" ring. The pouch is designed to fasten into position when pressed over the ring, much like snapping a lid on a plastic margarine tub. The pouch has a clamp at the bottom, which can be released when the pouch needs to be emptied. The pouch may be fastened to a belt for more security. The belt supports the weight of liquid fecal material and prevents the faceplate from being pulled away from the abdominal skin. Foam rubber, gauze, or flannel padding is placed under a belt if the belt cuts into the flesh. The client requires two sets of permanent appliances so one can be cleaned periodically. Disposable equipment may be appropriate for some clients. Disposable bags, faceplates, and attachment rings are replaced with new ones with each change of the ostomy appliance (usually daily with bathing).

• PREOPERATIVE PERIOD

Surgical Management

Before surgery, the physician explains the purpose for the surgical procedure along with benefits and risks. He or she describes the appearance and function of the stoma, where it will be placed, and its required care. The site is marked to ensure that it is away from bony prominences, skin creases, and scars; is within the rectus abdominis

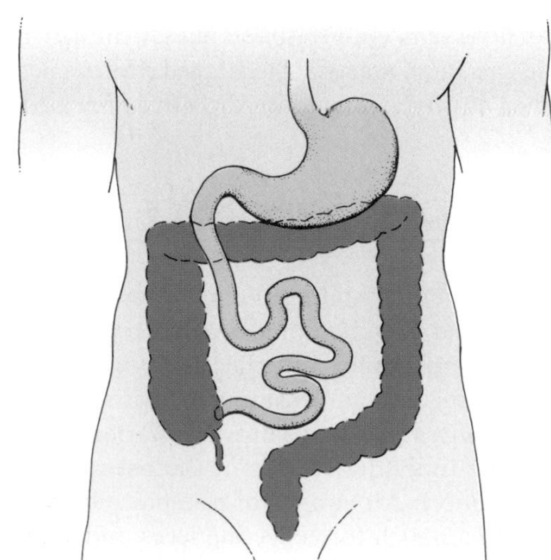

FIGURE 48.1 An ileostomy.

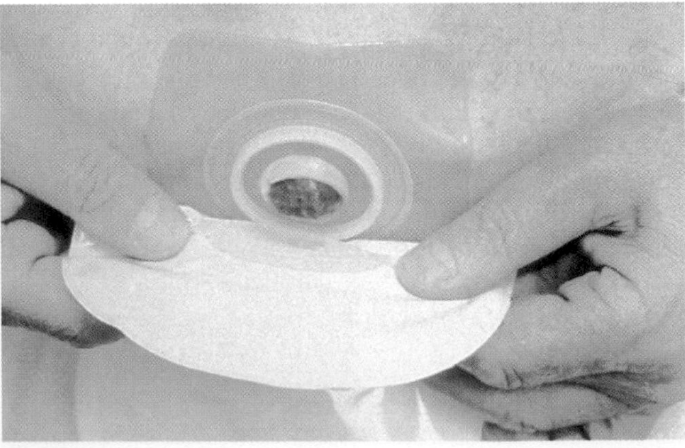

FIGURE 48.2 The ostomy appliance. (From Smeltzer, S. C., & Bare, B. G. [2000]. *Brunner & Suddarth's textbook of medical-surgical nursing* [9th ed.]. Philadelphia: Lippincott Williams & Wilkins.)

muscle; is unobstructed; and is visible to the client. Clients benefit from preoperative interactions with an enterostomal therapy nurse (also known as an **enterostomal therapist**). This nurse assists with marking placement of the stoma and collaborates with the surgeon regarding placement and the client's educational needs.

The physician identifies potential risks from the total colectomy, such as possible bladder and sexual dysfunction secondary to parasympathetic nerve injury. Sexual dysfunction in men after a total colectomy is unusual but does occur in some clients undergoing this procedure. If such dysfunction persists after a colectomy, operative and nonoperative options are available to facilitate erection. Young male clients may wish to collect and store sperm for later use if they plan to have children. A colectomy may slightly diminish fertility in women; however, this procedure does not preclude the ability to achieve a full-term pregnancy with a normal vaginal delivery.

Cleansing of the bowel before surgery is carried out using dietary restrictions in combination with laxative or lavage agents (e.g., GoLYTELY, NuLytely, Colyte), depending on the client's condition (i.e., presence or absence of obstruction) and according to the surgeon's preference. Opinions vary regarding the need for antibiotic prophylaxis. Most surgeons order a combination of intravenous (IV) antibiotics (i.e., a third-generation cephalosporin and metronidazole) before surgery and continue administration after surgery.

Whenever possible, prednisone should be tapered and discontinued before surgery to avoid negative effects of the drug on tissue healing. Immunosuppressive agents such as azathioprine, 6-mercaptopurine, and cyclosporine should be discontinued 3 to 4 weeks before surgery to prevent negative effects on tissue healing. Aspirin-containing compounds are discontinued at least 1 week before surgery to minimize the risk of bleeding. Blood samples are taken before surgery, and the client's blood is typed and crossmatched for replacement of losses that occur during surgery.

Nursing Management

Obtain complete medical, allergy, diet, and drug histories. Ask the client if he or she has been taking corticosteroids—if so, monitor the client closely for signs and symptoms of adrenal insufficiency such as weakness, lethargy, hypotension, nausea, and vomiting as dosages are tapered. Inspect the skin over the abdomen, auscultate bowel sounds, and get the client's vital signs and weight. Check preoperative laboratory test results to determine if blood cell counts and serum electrolyte levels are within normal ranges. Ask the client about preoperative preparations, such as dietary modifications and antibiotic therapy. Implement the medical orders for cleansing the bowel, inserting a nasogastric tube, and preparing the client for surgery.

Referral to community and professional resources before surgery may positively affect the client's postoperative quality of life. Resources for education and support include the medical and surgical teams and the lay public (e.g., the Crohn's and Colitis Foundation of America, the United Ostomy Association).

Provide an overview of preoperative procedures, using explanations the client understands. Allow time for the client to ask questions and express fears. Assess previous positive coping skills and assist client to access them again. Encourage the client to discuss feelings about the stoma. Inform the client that an assigned staff nurse will be there when the client first views and touches the stoma. If the client expresses interest, provide a list of appropriate community resources.

• POSTOPERATIVE PERIOD

Surgical Management

The rectum is packed with gauze during surgery to absorb drainage and promote gradual healing. The rectal pack usually is removed in 5 to 7 days. Irrigations may be ordered to promote healing. A nasogastric tube is used for gastrointestinal (GI) decompression until normal bowel motility resumes. Fluid, electrolyte, and nutritional balances are maintained with IV fluids until oral nourishment is possible. Within several days, the nasogastric tube is removed and oral feedings begin. Antibiotic therapy continues. Analgesics are prescribed for pain relief. Wound healing is monitored, and complications that develop are managed.

Possible postoperative complications include intestinal obstruction; bleeding; and impaired blood supply to, stenosis of, or prolapse or excessive protrusion of the stoma. Intestinal obstruction, a serious complication, may result from a twisted, strangulated, or incarcerated segment of the remaining intestine or a bolus of poorly chewed or inadequately digested food. When a collection of food causes obstruction, the physician may attempt to correct the problem by irrigating the stoma. If the bowel is twisted or strangulated, surgical intervention is necessary.

Prolapse or protrusion of the ileostomy is fairly common. If it is moderate (1 or 2 inches), no treatment is required. A severe prolapse of the stoma is a serious complication, however. If edema occurs, it may cause an obstruction and restrict stomal blood supply. Stomal necrosis results if the prolapse is not promptly and skillfully managed. Once the stoma prolapses, recurrence is likely.

NURSING PROCESS

● The Client Recovering From Ileostomy Surgery

Assessment

Review the medical record for information regarding the type of surgery and any problems during or immediately after surgery. Postoperative assessments include obtaining vital signs; inspecting the dressing and stoma for bleeding and signs of infection (Table 48.2); monitoring rate and progress of fluid and blood infusions; checking function of gastric suction; measuring intake and output; and inspecting the collection appliance, special drains, packing, or tubes. The nurse records all immediate postoperative findings to provide a database. For a step-by-step discussion of how to replace an ostomy appliance, see Nursing Guidelines 48-1.

Teach the client and another family member about managing the ostomy, adopting dietary modifications, recognizing how drug therapy affects bowel elimination, and adjusting to various surgery-related changes, such as possible sexual dysfunction (Box 48-1). Additional aspects to include in the teaching plan are discussed in Client and Family Teaching 48-1.

Diagnosis, Planning, and Interventions

Risk for Impaired Skin Integrity related to effects of fecal material and adhesives on the skin

Expected Outcome: Client will maintain intact peristomal skin.

- Demonstrate safe, gentle removal of the pouch. *Prevents skin irritation.*
- Gently cleanse the peristomal area with warm water and mild soap. *Minimizes skin irritation and abrasions.*
- Teach client to apply a skin barrier, such as a wafer, gel, paste, or powder. *Protects peristomal skin from digestive enzymes and bacteria.*

Risk for Infection related to fecal contamination of the surgical wound

Expected Outcome: Client's wound is free from infection.

- Apply dressing securely, covering the surgical wound completely. *Protects the incision from contact with fecal material.*
- Change ostomy pouch when it is loose and leaking. *Minimizes risk of fecal drainage entering the incision.*
- When drainage leaks near the incision, wipe it away from the incision and change dressing if soiled at all. *These measures keep fecal drainage away from incision, ensuring that dressing always is clean.*
- Observe for signs of wound infection: wound drainage, abdominal pain, and elevated temperature. *These signs indicate possible wound infection.*

Bowel Incontinence related to loss of sphincter control and change in intestinal motility

Expected Outcome: Client will not experience leaking from appliance or soiling with fecal material.

- Instruct the client how to prepare the drainage pouch for a secure fit around stoma, leaving an extra $\frac{1}{8}$ inch in the appliance opening. (Use a gauge for measuring, provided by the manufacturer.) *Provides room for stoma clearance and potential swelling.*
- Press adhesive faceplate around stoma for about 30 seconds. *Ensures secure attachment of the pouch to the peristomal skin.*
- Demonstrate frequent emptying of the pouch. *Prevents tension on pouch and skin from weight of drainage.*
- Use the following measures to avoid leaking:
  - Press adhesive faceplate from the stomal edge outward. *Prevents the formation of wrinkles.*
  - Ask client to remain inactive for 5 minutes. *Allows time for body heat to strengthen adhesive bond.*
  - Allow a small amount of air to be trapped in the pouch. *Liquid feces will then drain to bottom of pouch, placing less tension on it.*

TABLE 48.2 CHARACTERISTICS OF HEALTHY AND UNHEALTHY STOMAS

CHARACTERISTICS	HEALTHY STOMA	UNHEALTHY STOMA
Color	Bright pink or red	Dusky blue or black
Size	Comparable in diameter to the intestine from which it has been formed; may be somewhat large after surgery because of edema	Larger or smaller in comparison to size after resolution of postoperative edema
Opening	Patent, unobstructed	Tight or narrow
Surface	Moist, shiny with an overlying layer of mucus; may bleed slightly when being cleansed	Dull, dry; excessive bleeding
Length	Protrudes from or is just flush with the skin	Protrudes beyond 2 inches from the skin or retracts beneath it
Sensation	Painless	Peristomal burning
Function	Regular passage of feces	Sparse or absent elimination of feces

NURSING GUIDELINES 48-1

Changing an Ostomy Appliance

Assemble clean gloves, scissors, ostomy belt, stoma gauge, faceplate, pouch, adhesive or protectant (e.g., Karaya paste), and cleaning materials such as gauze pads, water, or adhesive solvent.

- Wash hands and put on gloves.
- Empty pouch when it is one-third full.
- Change the faceplate only when needed, that is, if it becomes loose or tight or client experiences discomfort. If the faceplate is changed too frequently, skin around stoma may become raw and excoriated secondary to removal of protective layers of epithelium with the faceplate.
- If the ostomy appliance is being replaced routinely, schedule the change when the gastrocolic reflex is less active. For many clients, this time is early in the morning, before eating, or 2 or 3 hours after mealtime.
- Gently ease the faceplate from the skin. If the faceplate was applied with adhesive, roll the adhesive from the skin and appliance. If it does not roll off, use a small amount of solvent, which chemically loosens the adhesive bond. Because some solvents irritate the skin, apply solvent sparingly between the body and faceplate using a sprayer, medicine dropper, or gauze pad. Avoid rubbing, which may further irritate skin. Clean the area with soap and water and pat dry after a solvent has been used.
- Inform the client that the most common causes of discomfort are reactions to the adhesive or solvent used to remove it or irritation from leaking fecal drainage. The client may experience stinging, tingling, or itching immediately after an appliance change, which quickly subsides. If a sensation is prolonged or intensified, remove the appliance regardless of whether it has been on for 1 hour or several days. When using a new adhesive product, remember to patch test it first on nonirritated skin at the inner aspect of client's forearm.
- After removing the faceplate and pouch, protect the peristomal area from drainage by placing a tissue cuff around the stoma or using a receptacle such as a small paper cup to collect the drainage. Use a soapy washcloth to clean the skin around the stoma and wipe the soap from the skin. Pat the area or allow it to air dry.
- Inspect the stoma and skin carefully. If excoriation is observed, use a temporary appliance or hydrocolloid dressing, such as DuoDERM or Tegasorb, to cover the excoriated skin to promote moist healing.
- Create an even surface for reapplying the pouch by filling irregular hollows in the peristomal skin with karaya paste before replacing the faceplate.
- Measure the circumference of the stoma and cut a comparable hole in the faceplate, allowing $\frac{1}{8}$-inch margin to account for potential swelling in a new stoma.
- Secure the pouch to the faceplate. Be sure to smooth out ridges or openings in the closure. Also be sure to seal the pouch.
- Peel the backing from the faceplate.
- Affix the faceplate to the skin.

BOX 48-1 ● Sexual Modifications for Ostomates

- Always practice good hygiene. Bathe and apply a fresh pouch before having sex.
- Disguise the pouch by enclosing it within a purse-string cloth cover.
- When anticipating sexual activity, avoid eating or drinking substances that activate the bowel or create a lot of gas.
- Fashion a cummerbund with a pocket or fold into which the pouch can be held.
- Remove the belt and temporarily secure the pouch to the skin with tape.
- If accidents happen, cultivate a sense of humor that may similarly relieve the anxiety of the sexual partner as well.
- Consult with members of a local ostomy group who also may provide support and counseling regarding sexual matters.

- Make several pinhole-sized punctures at the upper edge of the pouch. *Allows excess gas to escape and decreases tension on the pouch.*

Risk for Deficient Fluid Volume related to decreased appetite, vomiting, or increased loss of fluids and electrolytes from ileostomy

Expected Outcome: Client maintains adequate fluid and electrolyte balance.

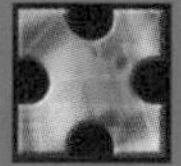

48-1 *Client and Family Teaching* Postoperative Ileostomy Care

The nurse discusses the following issues with the client and his or her family:

- Restrict oral intake only with medical supervision.
- Eat slowly and chew food well with the mouth closed to help lessen the development of gas.
- Avoid foods that cause discomfort, excessive gas, or loose stools.
- Drink extra fluids, especially in warm weather.
- Dilate the stoma if the volume of stool decreases for some unexplained reason. To do this, cut the nail on the index or little finger, cover the finger with a finger cot, lubricate it thoroughly, and then insert the finger gently into the stoma for a few minutes.
- Clean the pouch thoroughly to prevent odors.
- Use an internal odor-absorbing substance or one that can be added to the pouch to control lingering or stubborn odors.
- Use an old or disposable pouch when medications or offending foods that cause disagreeable odors are excreted.
- Slip a plastic cover over the pouch to act as a second barrier against escaping odors.
- Check with a physician before self-administering any drug, especially a laxative or antidiarrheal agent.

- Assess fluid balance. *Determines any deficits.*
- Examine serum and urine test results for sodium and potassium levels. *Indicates imbalances or other potential problems (e.g., acidosis, cardiac dysrhythmias).*
- Observe skin turgor and appearance of tongue. *Poor skin turgor and dry tongue indicate fluid deficits.*

Ineffective Coping related to disturbed body image and altered bowel function

Expected Outcome: Client will cope effectively with body changes.

- Ensure privacy when teaching and providing ileostomy care. *Allows client to get used to changes without fear of embarrassment in front of others.*
- Help client set realistic goals and identify personal skills and knowledge. *Allows the client to make decisions and move toward independence.*
- Use empathetic communication, allowing time for client to express fears and concerns. *A supportive environment promotes coping.*
- Refer client to support networks, such as ostomy groups or other ostomates. *Helps client problem solve and increase coping skills.*

Evaluation of Expected Outcomes

Peristomal skin is not reddened, there is no evidence of edema or drainage, and the client does not complain of burning sensations. The incision heals without infection. Stool is contained in the ostomy pouch. The client maintains adequate fluid balance as evidenced by balanced intake and output, good skin turgor, moist tongue and mucous membranes, and normal serum and urine sodium and potassium levels. He or she also demonstrates coping skills as evidenced by interest in self-care, ability to seek assistance, and ability to maintain relationships.

CONTINENT ILEOSTOMY (KOCK POUCH)

A **continent ileostomy** or **Kock pouch** provides an internal reservoir for storage of GI **effluent** (discharged fecal material or liquid feces). The reservoir stores this effluent for several hours until the client removes it with a catheter, which eliminates need for an external appliance.

Surgical Management

After removing the diseased portion of the ileum, the surgeon forms a reservoir with a portion of the terminal ileum and creates a nipple valve by telescoping the distal ileal segment into the reservoir. The surgeon then forms a permanent external stoma and anchors it to the abdominal wall (Fig. 48.3).

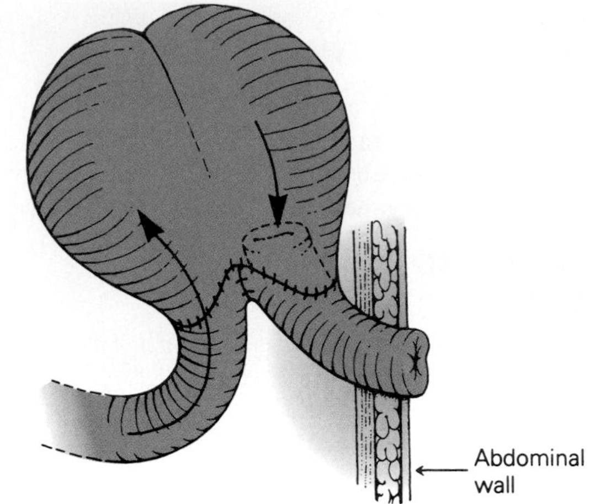

FIGURE 48.3 Continent ileostomy.

During the operation, a temporary catheter is inserted through the nipple valve and sutured in place so that its end protrudes from the external stoma. Gauze is packed in the perineal area from which the lower intestine was removed with gauze. Packing remains in place for about 1 week.

Nursing Management

Reinforce the perineal packing, as needed, during the postoperative period. Check the abdominal dressing for drainage and connect the stomal catheter, if ordered, to low, intermittent suction to empty the reservoir continuously, preventing tension on healing suture lines. Check the ileal catheter frequently for signs of obstruction: lack of fecal drainage, the client's complaint of feeling full in the area of the ileal pouch, or leakage of liquid stool around the catheter. Note the color and amount of drainage, observe the size and color of the stoma, and administer either routine or as-needed irrigations of the ileal catheter with small amounts of normal saline solution if the catheter appears to be obstructed, according to physician's orders. Keep the skin clean around the stoma, change gauze dressing over the stoma when it becomes wet with mucus or serosanguinous drainage, and change the dressing every 6 to 8 hours as drainage decreases.

Monitor ileal output carefully during the entire postoperative period. As GI function resumes, the initial amount of ileal drainage usually is high. If excessive fluids and electrolytes are lost, parenteral fluid and electrolyte replacement is necessary. When ileal drainage stabilizes, about 10 to 14 days after surgery, the physician removes the ileal catheter. The reservoir then holds the accumulating effluent until the nurse or client siphons it. Initially the reservoir is emptied every 2 to 4 hours. As the capacity of the reservoir increases (usually in about 6 months), the client or caregiver performs the procedure three or four times daily.

Include the following information in the teaching plan:

- To care for stoma and catheter, assemble a clean catheter, lubricant, basin, tissues, irrigating syringe and solution, and gauze dressing.
- Sit on or beside the toilet or on the side of the bed.
- Warm catheter to body temperature and lubricate the tip. Insert it about 2 inches into stomal opening.
- Expect resistance when the catheter reaches the nipple valve (about 2 inches), which controls the retention of waste matter. Gently push the catheter a little further into the ileal pouch. At the same time, exhale, cough, or bear down as if to pass stool until fecal material begins to drain.
- Direct the external end of the catheter into a basin or the toilet about 12 inches below the stoma.
- Allow 5 to 10 minutes for drainage to cease; then remove the catheter, clean it with soapy water, and store it in a sealable plastic bag until needed again.
- Wash the area around the stoma and pat the skin dry.
- Place an absorbent pad or dressing over the stoma.

For additional nursing management, refer to the discussion that addresses similar problems experienced by a client with an ileoanal reservoir. For tips on how to manage an obstructed catheter, see Box 48-2.

ILEOANAL RESERVOIR

The **ileoanal reservoir** (also called an ileoanal **anastomosis**; Fig. 48.4) is a procedure that maintains bowel continence. It is performed on clients with chronic ulcerative colitis or whose disease does not affect the anorectal sphincter. The client can control bowel elimination, as opposed to a conventional ileostomy procedure with total colectomy. It also preserves innervation to male genitalia. The client is unlikely to experience bladder dysfunction, erectile dysfunction, or infertility.

BOX 48-2 ● Unblocking the Catheter in a Continent Ileostomy

If the catheter used to drain fecal matter or mucus from the internal reservoir becomes obstructed, suggest the following measures:

- Bear down as if to have a bowel movement.
- Rotate the catheter tip inside the stoma.
- Milk the catheter.
- If these are not successful, remove the catheter, rinse it, and try again.
- Notify the physician if these efforts do not result in any drainage.
- Never wait longer than 6 hours without obtaining drainage.

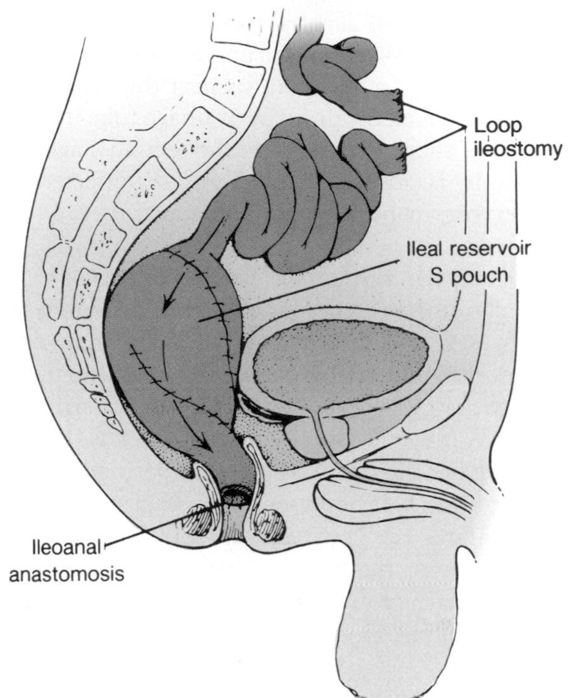

FIGURE 48.4 An ileoanal anastomosis joins a section of ileum to create an ileal reservoir. The distal end of the ileum is sutured above the anus. Intestinal effluent is temporarily discharged through the proximal stoma of a loop ileostomy until the second stage of surgery is performed.

Surgical Management

An ileoanal anastomosis is done in two stages. First, the surgeon creates a temporary ileostomy, removes a large length of diseased colon down to the terminal section of the rectum above the anal sphincter, joins several distal loops of healthy ileum to form a pouch for holding stool, and connects the ileal reservoir to the anal cuff. After this stage, clients experience an almost continuous discharge of mucus from the anus and a frequent discharge of fecal material from the ileostomy. The client cannot control the frequent watery discharge.

The second stage is done 2 or 3 months later. At this time, the surgeon closes the temporary ileostomy and reunites the two sections of ileum, which is called an *anastomosis.* This establishes a normal flow of fecal material through the ileum to the reservoir. Fecal material, which is stored in the ileal reservoir, is then expelled from the anus. Control is achieved as edema subsides and the anal sphincter becomes stronger.

Nursing Management

The preoperative assessment of a client having an ileoanal reservoir (both stages) is essentially the same as for the client with an ileostomy. The postoperative assessment after the first stage of ileoanal reservoir surgery includes making the same observations and assessments as those for an ileostomy. In addition, inspect the anal area for drainage and check the drain or drainage tube in the presacral area if there is one. After the second stage, when the ileostomy is closed and the ileum is connected to the anal reservoir, inspect the anal area and operative sites for drainage.

The postoperative plan of nursing care involves measures pertaining to general surgery and related client problems, such as risk for deficient fluid volume, risk for bowel incontinence, and impaired perianal skin integrity (refer to Nursing Process: The Client Recovering From Ileostomy Surgery). To reduce risk for bowel incontinence, instruct the client to perform perineal exercises four to six times a day to re-establish anal sphincter control and enlarge the ileoanal reservoir. These exercises involve tightening the anus as if trying to prevent a bowel movement and holding the contraction for a count of 10 before relaxing. Urge the client to do this exercise for 10 repetitions.

Keeping the perianal area clean is especially important. After first-stage ileoanal surgery, teach the client to use a squirt bottle to clean the perianal area and avoid skin irritation. After second-stage repair, instruct the client to cleanse the anus with warm, soapy water to remove mucus, stool, or both. The client also must dry the area well.

Teach the client and family the following:

- Continue with perineal strengthening exercises daily.
- Apply protective ointments or creams as recommended by the physician.
- Inspect anal area daily using a hand-held mirror. Contact the physician if the anal area becomes sore or skin changes (e.g. ulceration, bleeding) are apparent.
- Use a thin sanitary shield or disposable, lined underwear to absorb fecal drainage until anal sphincter control is achieved.

COLOSTOMY

A colostomy is an opening in the large bowel created by bringing a section of the large intestine out to the abdomen and fashioning a stoma. A cancerous lesion, an ulcerative inflammatory process, multiple polyposis (condition of numerous polyps), and traumatic injury to the bowel are indications for a colostomy.

Types

A temporary or permanent colostomy may be created in the ascending, transverse, descending, or sigmoid areas of the colon (Fig. 48.5). Consistency of fecal material ranges

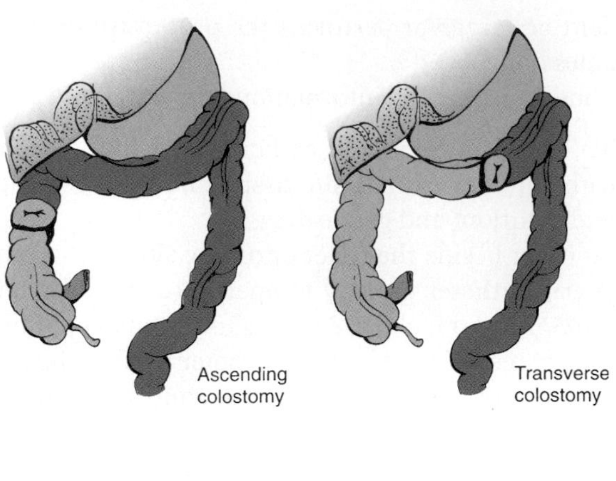

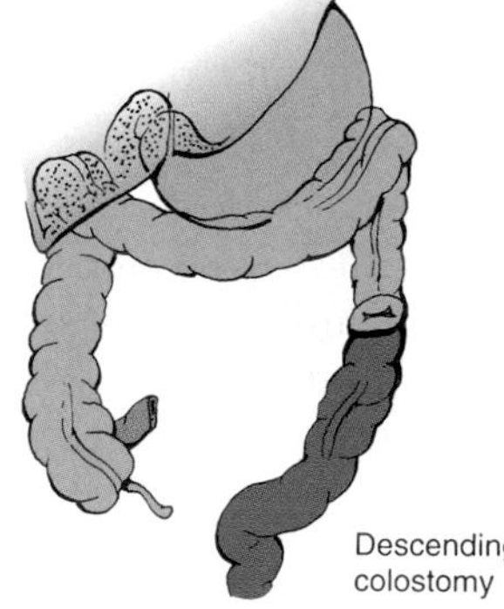

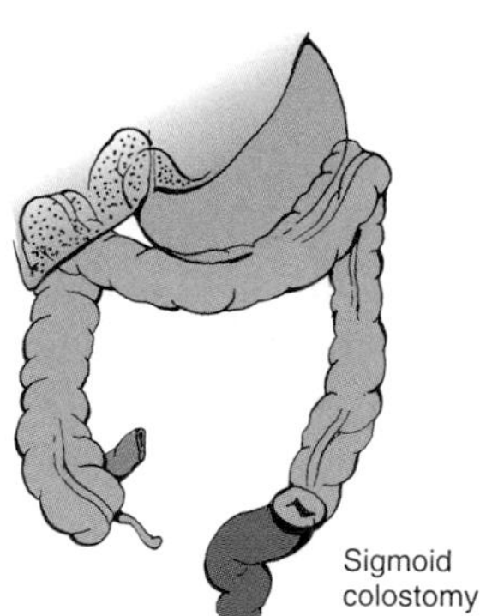

FIGURE 48.5 Various colostomies.

from semiliquid to formed depending on the intestinal area from which the colostomy is formed (see Table 48.1). Regular irrigations may control a sigmoid colostomy, and sometimes a descending colostomy, thus eliminating the need for the client to constantly wear an appliance.

The stoma may be found anywhere from the lower right, center, to middle or lower left positions on the abdomen. The terms *single-barrel, double-barrel,* and *loop* are used to describe the appearance of the colostomy.

Surgical Management

The term **single-barrel colostomy** indicates the ostomy has a single stoma through which fecal matter passes. The colon is cut above the diseased area, and the healthy end is brought through the abdominal wall to form the matured stoma. The diseased portion of the bowel is removed, with the remaining distal end closed for later reconnection (**segmental resection**). For tumors in the lower third of the sigmoid, that portion, the rectum, and anus may be surgically removed through a perineal incision in a procedure referred to as an **abdominoperineal resection.** After performing this procedure, the surgeon leaves a drain or pack in the perineal area for about 1 week. Then it is removed and irrigations of the perineal wound may be ordered.

A **double-barrel colostomy,** performed most often in the transverse section of the large intestine, contains both a proximal and distal stoma. Each stoma is everted and sutured in place. The proximal stoma expels fecal material. The distal stoma leads from the lower portion of the cut bowel to the anus. Because fecal drainage is diverted, the distal portion of the bowel does not pass feces. The distal stoma and the anus may expel mucus. When a double-barrel colostomy is done, the physician is asked to identify the distal and proximal stomas. A diagram is provided in the medical record, and the nurse may duplicate it on the nursing care plan, which helps when assessing bowel function and if irrigations are required. Irrigation (Nursing Guidelines 48-2) may be ordered for both the proximal and distal portions of the bowel, or for the proximal portion only.

A double-barrel colostomy often is temporary and performed to rest a portion of the bowel to treat a disorder such as acute diverticulitis, chronic constipation, or inflammatory bowel disease. The interval before re-establishing continuity of the bowel may be 16 months or longer. When the diseased portion of the bowel is removed or healed, the bowel is reconnected and functions normally. In the meantime, the stoma may need irrigation (Box 48-3) or other methods for regulating bowel elimination (Box 48-4).

Stop, Think, and Respond ● BOX 48-1

A client calls the doctor's office 4 months after a double-barrel colostomy. He tells the triage nurse that the stool is more liquid than usual and that he is emptying the pouch every 4 hours. What questions does the triage nurse need to ask?

A **loop colostomy** indicates that a loop of bowel has been lifted through the abdomen and is supported in place with a glass rod or plastic butterfly device. About 24 to 72 hours after surgery, the anterior wall of the loop is opened at the client's bedside or in a treatment room, either by incising the bowel or using a cautery machine to form the stoma. The posterior wall of the bowel is left intact, resulting in a proximal and distal opening to the bowel.

By delaying opening of the intestinal loop, the incision begins to heal without danger of contamination. Opening the bowel does not cause any discomfort because the bowel lacks pain receptors. When a loop colostomy is opened, the bed and client's clothing are well protected. Preparing the client for the pungent odor of cauterized tissue, which subsides shortly, and the initial gush of fecal material is important. A temporary ostomy pouch initially receives the flow of liquid feces.

Nursing Management

Preoperative nursing management is similar to that for clients having an ileostomy. Because a colostomy may be performed for cancer of the colon or rectum, however, the client may be more anxious about the procedure. Postoperative cancer treatment options also may serve to increase the client's anxiety.

After the client returns from surgery, assessments include taking vital signs, checking dressings, and monitoring nasogastric tubes and IV infusions. Review the client's chart for type of colostomy and location of the stoma(s). If an abdominoperineal resection was done,

NURSING GUIDELINES 48-2

Standard Colostomy Irrigation

Colostomy irrigation begins on the fourth or fifth postoperative day. Standard irrigation is a scheduled irrigation, using 500 to 1500 mL tepid water. Check physician orders. Try to use colostomy irrigation equipment that the client will use at home.

- Ask client to sit on a toilet seat or chair near the toilet.
- Prepare irrigation, purging air from the tubing.
- Place irrigation sheath over the stoma, directing sheath into toilet.
- Lubricate distal end of the catheter.
- Hang container of irrigant so that the bottom of the solution bag is about 12 inches above the stoma.
- Gently insert catheter tip into the stoma and advance it 2 to 3 inches.
- If there is resistance, remove catheter, release tubing clamp, and gently reinsert the catheter while solution is flowing.
- Allow irrigant to flow slowly and gradually into stoma.
- If client complains of cramping, clamp the tubing and ask the client to take a few deep breaths.
- Once cramping subsides, continue irrigation.
- If water escapes from the stoma during the irrigation, clamp tubing until it stops. If a catheter tip is used instead of a cone, introduce catheter further into the stoma, but no more than 6 inches.
- When prescribed amount of solution is instilled, remove catheter. The client may remain sitting or walk around (clamp the distal end of the irrigation sheath). Complete drainage usually takes 30 minutes.
- If irrigant fails to return properly, gently massage lower abdomen or have client take several deep breaths and relax or reposition his or her body. Notify physician if these measures do not work.
- Document the procedure, including the amount of irrigant used, appearance of returns, and client's response.

BOX 48-3 ● Alternatives to Standard Irrigation

If the client has a double-barrel colostomy, irrigate the proximal stoma in the same manner as a single-barrel colostomy. To irrigate the distal stoma, try the following:

- Have the client sit on a toilet or a bedpan because the irrigation fluid and a small amount of mucus will leave by way of the anus. During the immediate postoperative period, necrotic tissue also may be expelled.
- Use a bulb syringe, short catheter, container of solution, plastic sheath or apron, and an emesis basin as another technique for irrigation. This method calls for several instillations of 250 to 500 mL solution at a time, sometimes twice a day. Some clients have found this method effective for controlling spillage for 24 hours or more. It may be used as an alternate choice when the standard method cannot be used.

check the drain or packing in the perineal area and note the characteristics of the drainage.

Monitor vital signs every 4 hours or as ordered. Take the client's temperature by a route other than rectal. Report a sudden elevation in temperature over 38.3°C (101°F) or an increase in pain and abdominal tenderness or distention to the physician immediately. Check the surgical dressing frequently in the early postoperative period and observe the characteristics of the stoma. Monitor urine output and the volume of suctioned gastric secretions. If urine output is markedly decreased or less than 500 mL/day, inform the physician immediately.

Perform standard postsurgical measures to maintain the airway and relieve pain and anxiety. Perform nasogastric decompression as ordered (see Chap. 46) and monitor fluid and electrolyte status. Measure fluids lost through decompression and replace them by administering additional IV fluids. An indwelling catheter may be used to relieve abdominal pressure and prevent urine retention during the first few days after surgery.

Teach the client how to care for the colostomy by demonstrating the irrigating procedure and, if possible, outlining nonirrigation methods for keeping the ostomy patent and establishing a regular pattern of bowel elimination. The time between use of these methods and eventual regularity is unique to each client.

Demonstrate skin and stoma care and appliance application and removal. After demonstrating one aspect of care, the client returns the demonstration. Add other material when the client feels self-confident. Reinforce verbal information and demonstrated skills with printed material that may be available from ostomy associations or the enterostomal therapy nurse. Arrange a dietary consultation to discuss nutrition and food modifications. Include the following points in the teaching plan:

- Changes in size and color of the stoma vary with activity and emotional status. Anger or extreme annoyance may cause the stoma to turn red or purple. Small beads of blood may ooze from the surface. Fright may cause the stoma to blanch. These reactions are normal and insignificant as long as tissues revert to normal when the cause is alleviated.
- Eat a regular diet, but avoid gas-forming foods to control intestinal gas.
- In most cases, increasing fiber in the diet and drinking extra water correct constipation.
- Diarrhea may be related to diet. Characteristics of diarrhea include both increased stool output and liquid nature of the stool. One or two loose stools per day does not necessarily indicate a problem. Eliminating food items that result in diarrhea may help to control the problem. If diarrhea persists for more than 2 days, the client should contact the physician.
- Eat slowly with the mouth closed and chew food well to decrease gas that results chiefly from swallowing air rather than from digestion.
- With the exception of tight clothing, no adjustments are necessary in clothing worn. Clients who require firm support (e.g., those who wear girdles, have back problems, wear braces) may find a stoma shield helpful in preventing irritation or undue pressure on the stoma.
- Check body weight weekly. Contact the physician if there is a sudden weight loss or gain.
- Perform irrigations at approximately the same time each day. The best time to irrigate is after a meal because food in the digestive tract stimulates peristalsis and defecation.
- The schedule for irrigations gradually progresses to every other day, every third day, or even twice a week. If constipation occurs, contact the physician regarding a change in the irrigation schedule.
- Do not restrict travel or activities outside the home. Changes in stool pattern may be normal when daily routine is altered. Preassembled kits that contain all materials needed for irrigation and changes of the colostomy appliance are available.

BOX 48-4 ● Regulating Bowel Elimination Without Irrigating

Some ostomates learn to regulate bowel elimination without irrigating frequently. The following tips may be encouraging to new ostomates, who may be able to establish regular elimination patterns.

- Insert a suppository, such as glycerin or bisacodyl (Dulcolax), into the stoma. The suppository should be recommended by the physician. Up to 7 days or more of daily use may be needed before a regular elimination pattern is established. Initially movements may occur three or four times daily, but each day movements should decrease until only one or two movements occur daily.

Other methods to stimulate bowel elimination and a regular schedule include:

- Drinking prune or fruit juice
- Eating fiber-rich foods and dried fruits and performing mild exercise
- Using a stool softener, mineral oil, or milk of magnesia if recommended by the physician

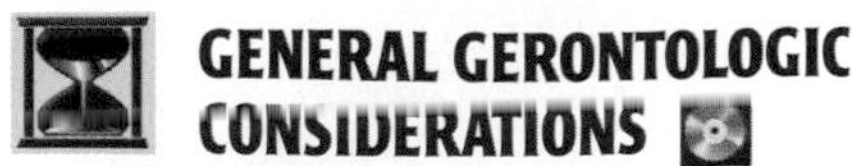

GENERAL GERONTOLOGIC CONSIDERATIONS

Teach ostomy care as appropriate for the client's age and prior understanding. Presenting the material in brief sessions is best. Supplement the instructions with illustrations and written directions.

Teach a family member or another responsible person how to perform ostomy care in case the client cannot temporarily assume responsibility for this task. Always provide the telephone number of an individual to contact (i.e., the enterostomal therapist) if problems occur after discharge.

Older adult ostomates with chronic disorders such as poor vision and arthritis may encounter difficulty in changing the appliance, performing skin care, irrigating the colostomy stoma, and caring for the permanent appliance. Consult with an enterostomal therapist about which equipment may best meet the client's needs. If the older adult will be permanently unable to assume care for an ostomy, healthcare professionals need to arrange for daily care. Depending on the situation, a family member, visiting nurse, or home healthcare nurse needs to assume this responsibility. In some instances, transfer to a skilled nursing facility or nursing home may be necessary.

Ostomates are particularly vulnerable to emotional distress, including loss of self-esteem, poor body image, and increased anxiety. Actively listen to expressed concerns and fears over adjusting to and caring for the ostomy and rejection from family and friends. Some clients benefit from professional psychological support in coping with a new body image. Sexuality issues surface during puberty and continue throughout the client's adulthood. Never assume that an older adult is not concerned about the effects of the ostomy on sexuality. Provide an opportunity to discuss sexual concerns. Support groups are available.

Critical Thinking Exercises

1. *In what ways does the care of a 20-year-old client with an ileostomy differ from that of a 60-year-old client with a colostomy?*
2. *A client with an ileostomy is disturbed by the need to empty liquid stool from his appliance so frequently. He intends to reduce his intake of fluids. What information is important to give this client?*
3. *What recommendations are appropriate for the client with a colostomy who has been experiencing an unusual amount of intestinal gas?*

● NCLEX-STYLE REVIEW QUESTIONS

1. Which question by a new postsurgical ostomy client best indicates a readiness for teaching?
    1. "Did you show my daughter how to care for the ostomy?"
    2. "Will you sit with me while I view the ostomy?"
    3. "How long will I need to have this ostomy?"
    4. "Do you think I'll be able to care for the ostomy?"
2. To prevent skin breakdown around the ostomy site, the nurse would include which of the following in the plan of care?
    1. Place a skin barrier such as a wafer, gel, or paste around the ostomy site.
    2. Change the ostomy appliance three times a day for cleanliness.
    3. Place paper tape around the periphery of the appliance.
    4. Apply alcohol to clean the skin around the stoma site.
3. A client has perineal packing following surgical creation of a Kock pouch. Upon assessment, the nurse notes serosanguinous drainage on the postoperative dressing. Which nursing action is most appropriate?
    1. Remove the perineal packing and repack.
    2. Call the physician to report the findings.
    3. Reinforce the perineal dressing and document.
    4. Continue to monitor the dressing for changes.

connection—

Visit the Connection site at **http://connection.lww.com/go/timbyEssentials** for links to chapter-related resources on the Internet.

References and Suggested Readings

Ball, E. M. (2000). Part two: A teaching guide for continent ostomy. *RN, 63*(12), 35–38.

Banks, N., & Razor, B. (2003). Preoperative stoma site assessment and marking. *American Journal of Nursing, 103*(3), 64A–64D.

Bryant, D., & Fleischer, I. (2000). Changing an OSTOMY appliance. *Nursing 2000, 30*(11), 51–55.

Cartwright, B. A., & Gillen, P. B. (2002). What's wrong with this patient? *RN, 65*(7), 37–40.

Thompson, J. (2000). Part one: A practical ostomy guide. *RN, 63*(11), 61–66.

Young, M. (2000). Caring for patients with coloanal reservoirs for rectal cancer. *MEDSURG Nursing, 9,* 193–197.

c h a p t e r 49

Caring for Clients With Disorders of the Liver, Gallbladder, or Pancreas

Words to Know 

alpha-fetoprotein
ascites
balloon tamponade
biliary colic
caput medusae
cholecystitis
choledocholithiasis
cholelithiasis
cholestasis
cirrhosis
Cullen's sign
esophageal varices
hepatic encephalopathy
hepatic lobectomy
hepatitis
hepatorenal syndrome
injection sclerotherapy
laparoscopic cholecystectomy
lithotripsy
open cholecystectomy
pancreatectomy (partial, total)
pancreatitis
portal hypertension
radical pancreato-duodenectomy (Whipple procedure)
steatorrhea
T-tube
Turner's sign

Learning Objectives

On completion of this chapter, the reader will:

- List common findings manifested by clients with cirrhosis.
- Discuss common complications of cirrhosis.
- Identify modes of transmission of viral hepatitis.
- Describe nursing measures after liver biopsy.
- Discuss nursing management for clients with a medically or surgically treated liver disorder.
- Identify factors that contribute to, signs and symptoms of, and medical treatments for cholecystitis.
- Name techniques of gallbladder removal.
- Discuss nursing management for clients with a T-tube.
- Summarize the nursing management of clients undergoing medical or surgical treatment of a gallbladder disorder.
- Describe treatment and nursing management of pancreatitis.
- Describe treatment of pancreatic carcinoma.
- Explain nursing management of clients undergoing pancreatic surgery.

The liver, gallbladder, and pancreas play important roles in digestion. They also are responsible for many other physiologic activities (see Chap. 45). Their poor function impairs the digestive process and the client's overall nutritional status.

DISORDERS OF THE LIVER

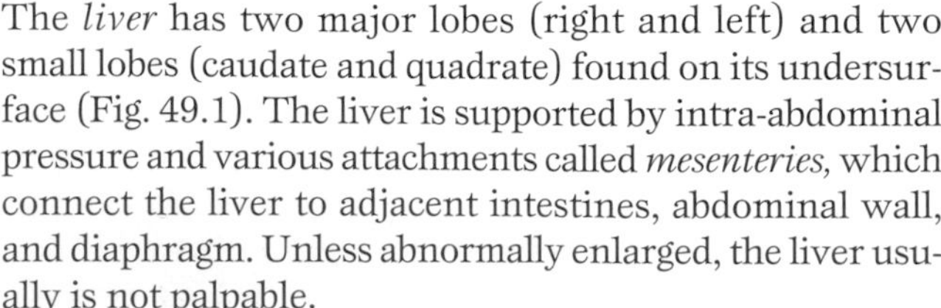

The *liver* has two major lobes (right and left) and two small lobes (caudate and quadrate) found on its undersurface (Fig. 49.1). The liver is supported by intra-abdominal pressure and various attachments called *mesenteries,* which connect the liver to adjacent intestines, abdominal wall, and diaphragm. Unless abnormally enlarged, the liver usually is not palpable.

The liver has various functions (Box 49-1) and a rich blood supply. It receives arterial blood from the hepatic artery, an indirect branch of the aorta. The portal vein transports blood from the intestinal tract to the liver. After blood circulates in the liver, the hepatic veins collect the blood and transport it to the inferior vena cava and then back to the heart (Fig. 49.2).

Microscopically, the liver's internal structure includes smaller branches of the hepatic artery, the hepatic and portal veins, the lymphatics, and the bile ducts. Cellular constituents of the liver are the hepatic parenchymal cells, which perform most of the liver's metabolic functions, and the Kupffer cells, which engage in the liver's immunologic, detoxifying, and blood-filtering actions.

• JAUNDICE (ICTERUS)

Jaundice, also called *icterus,* is a greenish-yellow discoloration of tissue. It is a sign of disease but is not itself a unique disease. Jaundice accompanies many diseases

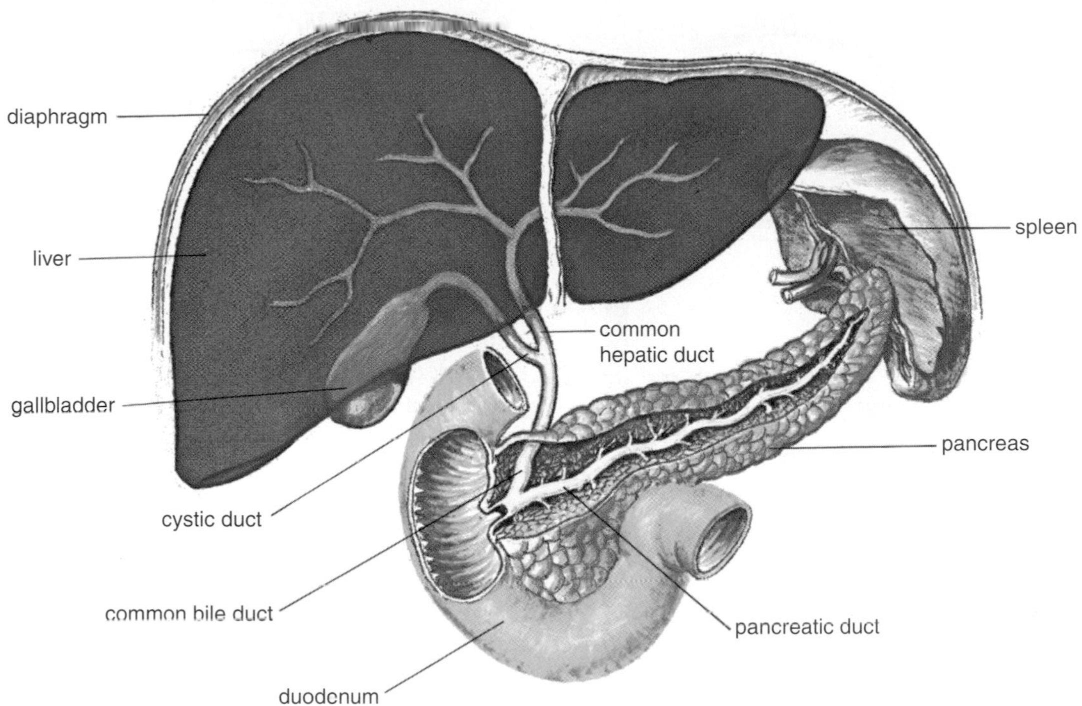

FIGURE 49.1 The liver and biliary system. (From Smeltzer, S. C. & Bare, B. G. [2004]. *Brunner & Suddarth's textbook of medical-surgical nursing* [10th ed.]. Philadelphia: Lippincott Williams & Wilkins.)

that directly or indirectly affect the liver and is probably the most common sign of a liver disorder.

Jaundice results from an abnormally high concentration of the pigment *bilirubin* in the blood. Normally, total bilirubin concentration ranges from 0.2 to 1.3 mg/dL. If the serum bilirubin level exceeds 2.5 mg/dL, jaundice is visible, notably on skin, oral mucous membranes, and (especially) sclera.

Bilirubin is produced in the liver, spleen, and bone marrow. It also results from hemoglobin metabolism and is a byproduct of hemolysis (red blood cell [RBC] destruction). The reticuloendothelial system also produces bilirubin. The liver removes bilirubin from the body, excreting it in *bile,* of which bilirubin is the major pigment. Thus, serum contains a normal amount of bilirubin. Serum bilirubin levels increase when (1) there is excessive destruction of RBCs or (2) the liver cannot excrete bilirubin normally.

There are two forms of bilirubin. *Indirect* or *unconjugated bilirubin* binds with protein as it circulates in blood. This form normally circulates in the blood; when its level is elevated, the usual cause is increased hemolysis. The other form of bilirubin is *direct* or *conjugated bilirubin,* which circulates freely in the blood until reaching the liver. The liver conjugates direct bilirubin with glucuronide. The conjugated bilirubin is excreted in the bile. As bile enters the bile ducts and moves into the intestine, bacterial enzymes transform direct bilirubin into *urobilinogen.* Some urobilinogen is changed into *urobilin,* the brown pigment of stool; some is excreted in urine; and some is carried back to the liver by the bloodstream for re-excretion in the bile.

There is no direct test for indirect bilirubin levels. They are calculated by subtracting direct bilirubin levels from total bilirubin levels. For example, if the total bilirubin level is 1.0 mg/dL and the conjugated bilirubin level is 0.1 mg/dL, then the indirect bilirubin level is 0.9 mg/dL.

There are three forms of jaundice: (1) *hemolytic jaundice,* caused by excess destroyed RBCs (see Chap. 33); (2) *hepatocellular jaundice,* caused by liver disease; and (3) *obstructive jaundice,* caused by a block in the passage

BOX 49-1 ● Functions of the Liver

- Metabolizes glucose
- Regulates blood glucose concentration
- Converts glucose to glycogen to glucose to maintain normal glucose levels
- Synthesizes amino acids from the breakdown of protein or from lactate that muscles produce during exercise to form glucose (*gluconeogenesis*)
- Converts ammonia (byproduct of gluconeogenesis) into urea
- Metabolizes proteins and fats
- Stores vitamins A, B_{12}, D, and some B-complex vitamins, as well as iron and copper
- Metabolizes drugs, chemicals, bacteria, and other foreign elements
- Forms and excretes bile
- Excretes bilirubin
- Synthesizes factors needed for blood coagulation (e.g., prothrombin, fibrinogen)

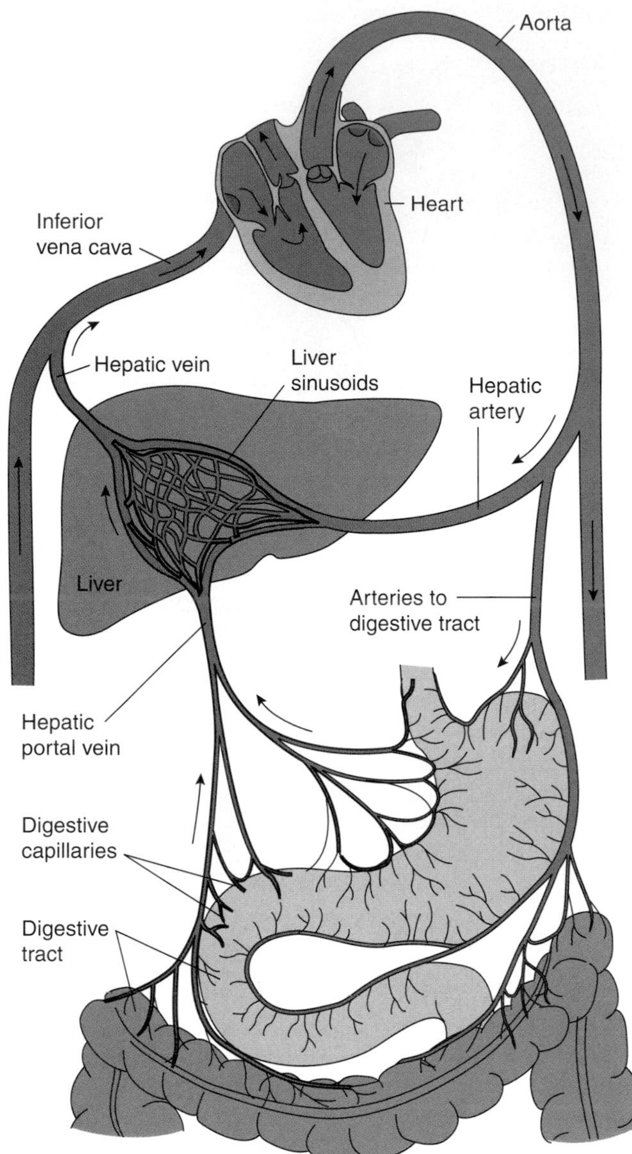

FIGURE 49.2 Hepatic blood supply and circulation.

of bile between the liver and intestinal tract (Table 49.1). Because unconjugated and conjugated bilirubin are distinct and can be differentiated, they are important in the differential diagnosis of diseases that produce jaundice.

● CIRRHOSIS

Cirrhosis is a degenerative liver disorder caused by generalized cellular damage.

Pathophysiology and Etiology

Once liver cells are irreversibly damaged, nonfunctional fibrous connective scar tissue replaces them, leading to considerable anatomic distortion and partial or complete occlusion of blood channels in the liver. The liver cannot carry out its many functions, which leads to disturbances in digestion and metabolism, defects in blood coagulation, fluid and electrolyte imbalances, and impaired ability to metabolize hormones and detoxify chemicals. Because bile begins to drain into the intestine, the client experiences fat malabsorption and an inability to absorb fat-soluble vitamins (A, D, E, and K). Portal hypertension, esophageal varices, ascites, and hepatic encephalopathy are complications of advanced cirrhosis (see later discussion).

There are several types of cirrhosis. *Alcoholic* or *Laënnec's cirrhosis,* the most common type, results from chronic alcohol intake and is associated with poor nutrition. It can follow chronic poisoning with certain chemicals (e.g., carbon tetrachloride, a cleaning agent) or ingestion of hepatotoxic drugs (e.g., acetaminophen). Alcoholic cirrhosis is characterized by necrotic liver cells, which gradually are replaced by scar tissue. Eventually the amount of scar tissue exceeds functional liver tissue. The liver takes on a characteristic "hobnail" appearance, in which there are islands of normal tissue, regenerating tissue, and scar tissue. The disease develops over a long period of 30 years or more.

Postnecrotic cirrhosis results from destruction of liver cells secondary to infection (e.g., hepatitis), metabolic liver disease, or exposure to hepatotoxins or industrial chemicals.

In *biliary cirrhosis,* scarring occurs around the bile ducts in the liver. The cause usually is related to chronic biliary obstruction and infection.

The prognosis for clients with cirrhosis is based on bilirubin and albumin levels, ascites (serous fluid in the

TABLE 49.1 TYPES OF JAUNDICE

TYPE	DESCRIPTION	CHANGES IN BILIRUBIN LEVELS
Hemolytic	Hemolytic processes (e.g., multiple blood transfusions, pernicious anemia, sickle cell anemia) cause an overproduction of bilirubin.	Elevated unconjugated bilirubin levels
Hepatocellular	Liver cells damaged by viral infections, medications, or chemical toxicity cannot clear bilirubin from the blood.	Elevated conjugated and unconjugated bilirubin levels
Obstructive	Gallstones, inflammation, or tumors obstruct the bile duct, causing reabsorption of bile into the blood.	Elevated conjugated bilirubin levels

peritoneal cavity), neurologic involvement, and nutritional status.

Assessment Findings

Signs and Symptoms

Signs and symptoms of cirrhosis increase in severity as the disease progresses (Box 49-2). Clinical manifestations are categorized as compensated and decompensated. *Compensated cirrhosis* is less severe, and signs and symptoms are more vague. As the disease progresses, it is referred to as *decompensated cirrhosis.* Signs and symptoms are very pronounced and indicate liver failure.

The client's history often correlates with factors that predispose to cirrhosis, such as chronic alcohol use, hepatitis, and exposure to toxins. Typical symptoms are chronic fatigue, anorexia, dyspepsia, nausea, vomiting, and diarrhea or constipation, with weight loss. Many clients report passing clay-colored or whitish stools as a result of no bile in the gastrointestinal (GI) tract. They also may report dark or "tea-colored" urine from increased concentrations of urobilin. Abdominal discomfort and shortness of breath are common complaints as a result of organ compression from the enlarged liver. Many clients mention nosebleeds, bleeding from gums, or easy bruising. Skin may itch (pruritus) from accumulated bile salts.

A client with cirrhosis has an enlarged liver and sometimes an enlarged spleen, causing the abdomen to appear distended. The skin, sclera, or oral mucous membranes are jaundiced. Edema may be present in the legs and feet. Veins over the abdomen may be dilated (**caput medusae**). Because the dysfunctional liver cannot fully metabolize estrogen, men may present with *gynecomastia* (enlarged breasts) and testicular atrophy. *Palmar erythema* (bright pink palms) and *cutaneous spider angiomata* (tiny, spider-like blood vessels) may be visible. These findings also are related to an inability to inactivate estrogen.

Diagnostic Findings

A liver biopsy, which reveals hepatic fibrosis, is the most conclusive diagnostic procedure. The biopsy is obtained percutaneously with mild sedation on the nursing unit or through a surgical incision. It also can be performed in the radiology department with ultrasound or computed tomography (CT) to identify appropriate placement of the trochar or biopsy needle.

Certain blood tests provide information about liver function (Box 49-3). Prolonged prothrombin time (PT) and low platelet count place the client at high risk for hemorrhage. The client may receive intravenous (IV) administration of vitamin K or infusions of platelets before liver biopsy to reduce risk of bleeding. Other tests used to examine the liver include CT, magnetic resonance imaging (MRI), and radioisotope liver scan, all of which may demonstrate the liver's enlarged size, nodular configuration, and distorted blood flow.

Medical and Surgical Management

No specific cure for cirrhosis exists. The goal is to prevent further deterioration by treating underlying causes preserving remaining liver function. Vitamins and nutritional supplements promote healing of liver cells. Improved nutritional status helps the client feel better. Malnutrition is treated with enteral or parenteral feedings. Because of

BOX 49-2 ● Clinical Manifestations of Cirrhosis

COMPENSATED
Intermittent mild fever
Vascular spiders
Palmar erythema (reddened palms)
Unexplained epistaxis
Ankle edema
Vague morning indigestion
Flatulent dyspepsia
Abdominal pain
Firm, enlarged liver
Splenomegaly

DECOMPENSATED
Ascites
Jaundice
Weakness
Muscle wasting
Weight loss
Continuous mild fever
Clubbing of fingers
Purpura (due to decreased platelet count)
Spontaneous bruising
Epistaxis
Hypotension
Sparse body hair
White nails
Gonadal atrophy

BOX 49-3 ● Common Blood Test Findings in Cirrhosis

Blood studies of clients with cirrhosis are likely to show:

- Increased unconjugated and conjugated bilirubin levels
- Increased enzyme levels of AST (SGOT), ALT (SGPT), and GGT
- Low RBC count—cells appear large
- Decreased leukocytes and thrombocytes
- Low fibrinogen level
- Prolonged PT
- Decreased platelet count
- Low serum albumin level
- Increased globulin level
- Hypokalemia

ALT, alanine transaminase; AST, aspartate phosphatase; GGT, gamma glutamyltransferase; PT, prothrombin time; RBC, red blood cell; SGOT, serum glutamic-oxaloacetic transaminase; SGPT, serum glutamic-pyruvic transaminase.

impaired absorption of the fat-soluble vitamins, clients take supplements. Vitamin K is used to correct coagulopathy, which results from prolonged PT and partial thromboplastin time (PTT). Vitamin B complex, vitamin C, and iron also may be prescribed. IV albumin may be given if hypoproteinemia is severe. The client *must not* consume alcohol.

Protein intake is restricted in clients with advanced liver disease because it increases ammonia in the intestine, precipitating hepatic encephalopathy (see Complications of Cirrhosis, later). Lactulose is administered to detoxify ammonium and to act as an osmotic agent, drawing water into the bowel, which causes diarrhea in some clients. Antacids may be used to reduce gastric disturbances and decrease the potential for GI bleeding. Potassium-sparing antidiuretics such as spironolactone are used to treat ascites (see Complications of Cirrhosis, later).

Transfusions of platelets may be necessary to correct thrombocytopenia (low platelet count). Packed RBCs may be administered in cases of anemia or blood loss. Cholestyramine may be prescribed to bind bile salts and relieve pruritus. Additional measures to relieve pruritus include skin care and routine cleansing with a nondrying agent. Skin is patted dry, and moisturizing lotion is applied immediately after bathing. Ursodeoxycholic acid (Actigall) may be used to promote bile flow from the liver. Sodium intake is carefully regulated and often restricted because of potential water retention, which can lead to edema, circulatory congestion, and heart failure. Fluid intake also may be restricted. Liver transplantation is an option for treating liver failure as well as chronic liver disease.

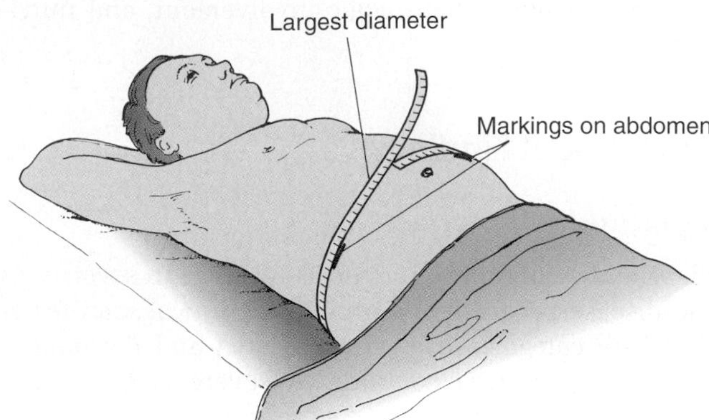

FIGURE 49.3 To measure abdominal girth, place a tape measure around the largest diameter of the abdomen. Make guide marks on the skin so that future measurements are obtained from the same site.

Nursing Management

If the client has active alcoholism, monitor vital signs closely. A rise in blood pressure (BP), pulse, and temperature correlates with alcohol withdrawal; the nurse must recognize and treat these appropriately along with the other presenting symptoms (see Chap. 17).

Weigh the client daily and keep an accurate record of intake and output. If the abdomen appears enlarged, measure it according to a set routine (Fig. 49.3). Because of anorexia that accompanies severe cirrhosis, the client may better tolerate frequent, small, semisolid or liquid meals rather than three full meals a day.

Evaluate the client's response to drug therapy, because the liver cannot metabolize many substances. Report any change in mental status or signs of GI bleeding immediately because they indicate secondary complications.

Provide educational information specific to the liver disorder. Refer the client to the American Liver Foundation (or a similar organization) for information about available support groups. Emphasize the need for abstinence from alcohol and all nonprescription drugs unless approved by the physician. Contact social services about referrals to alcohol or drug cessation programs. Additional teaching depends on the type and cause of the disorder and the physician's prescribed or recommended home care. For additional nursing management, see Nursing Care Plan 49-1 and Client and Family Teaching 49-1.

Complications of Cirrhosis

Portal Hypertension

The portal system consists of gastric veins from the stomach, the mesenteric vein from the intestines, the splenic vein from the spleen and pancreas, and the portal vein. All drain into and through the liver and out the hepatic veins into the inferior vena cava.

In the scarred cirrhotic liver, intrahepatic veins may be compressed. Blood backs up into the portal system, which is the venous pathway through the liver. This congestion and increased fluid pressure are called **portal hypertension.** As the normal pathway for blood is obstructed, collateral veins become distended and engorged with blood (Fig. 49.4). These distended collateral vessels develop primarily in the esophagus (esophageal varices) and rectum (hemorrhoids) and on the abdominal surface (caput medusae).

Methods of treating portal hypertension aim to reduce fluid accumulation and venous pressure. Sodium is restricted. A diuretic, usually an aldosterone antagonist such as spironolactone (Aldactone), is prescribed (Drug Therapy Table 49.1). Diuretics such as furosemide (Lasix) also may be given to promote urinary excretion of excess fluids. These diuretics must be administered with caution, because long-term use can cause sodium depletion. Administration of a beta-adrenergic blocker, such as propranolol (Inderal), reduces BP and lowers pressure in the portal system.

A *surgical shunt* may be created, which uses a graft to decompress the portal system by diverting blood flow

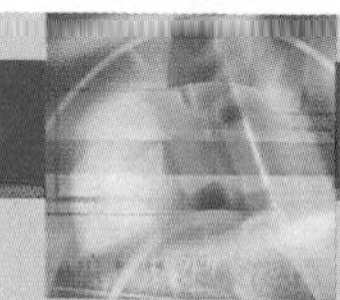

Nursing Care Plan 49-1

THE CLIENT WITH A LIVER DISORDER

Assessment

- Obtain complete diet, drug, and allergy histories and a history of symptoms from client or family. Depending on the circumstances, in-depth questioning may be necessary. Contributing factors may include exposure to toxic chemicals, history of hepatitis, or long-term alcohol abuse.
- Pay special attention to ventilation, abdominal size, weight, and any jaundice or other symptoms of liver disease.
- Analyze food intake and fluid records.
- Review laboratory and diagnostic studies and the physician's progress notes daily to assess client's response to therapy.

Nursing Diagnosis: **Fatigue** related to malnutrition and liver disease

Expected Outcome: Client will report improved energy and adhere to plan to conserve energy.

Interventions	*Rationales*
Assess client's ability to perform activities of daily living and pattern of fatigue.	Provides a baseline for comparison and helps nurse and client to target ways to conserve energy.
Assist client to set small, short-term goals that will be easy to achieve.	Helps the client accomplish tasks without being overwhelmed or exhausted.
Encourage the client to limit demands on his or her time.	Helps the client set priorities and balance demands with available energy.
Offer a high-protein (if client does not have severe liver disease) and high-calorie diet.	Inadequate nutrition contributes to fatigue.
Encourage client to rest frequently.	Inadequate sleep contributes to fatigue.

Evaluation of Expected Outcome: Client participates in appropriate activities, gradually increases activities, and reports feeling stronger and more energetic.

Nursing Diagnosis: **Ineffective Breathing Pattern** related to ascites and liver enlargement

Expected Outcome: Client will breathe without effort.

Interventions	*Rationales*
Assess respiratory pattern, noting what causes and relieves dyspnea.	Assessing the cause of dyspnea helps the nurse provide relief measures and improve client's ventilatory efforts.
Place client in an upright or semi-Fowler's position.	Facilitates lung expansion by reducing pressure on the diaphragm.
Schedule rest periods before and after activity.	Reduces metabolic and oxygen requirements.
Provide supplemental oxygen if client is short of breath.	Decreases dyspnea by reducing central drive mediated by chemoreceptors in the carotid bodies.

Evaluation of Expected Outcome: Client reports decreased shortness of breath and improved comfort with breathing.

Nursing Diagnosis: **Excess Fluid Volume** related to peripheral edema, ascites, and sodium retention

Expected Outcome: Client will maintain fluid balance.

(continued)

Nursing Care Plan 49-1 (Continued)

THE CLIENT WITH A LIVER DISORDER

Interventions	Rationales
Assess location and extent of edema. Measure and record abdominal girth daily.	Helps locate changes in peripheral edema and ascites.
Monitor weight daily.	Reflects changes in body fluid volume.
Restrict sodium and fluid intake as ordered.	Reduces peripheral edema and ascites.
Administer prescribed diuretics and potassium.	Promotes fluid excretion through the kidneys to maintain fluid and electrolyte balance.
Monitor serum albumin levels. Administer protein supplements as ordered.	Low albumin levels can cause severe peripheral edema because of impaired movement of fluid from interstitial spaces to intravascular spaces.
Maintain IV infusion rates carefully.	Prevents inadvertent infusion of excess fluid volumes.
Encourage client to turn at least every 2 hours when in bed.	Edematous tissue is vulnerable to ischemia and pressure ulcers.

Evaluation of Expected Outcome: Client maintains fluid balance, as evidenced by stable BP, adequate urine output, and decreased peripheral edema and ascites.

Nursing Diagnosis: **Ineffective Protection** related to risk for impaired blood coagulation, bleeding from portal hypertension, and infection

Expected Outcome: Client will not demonstrate evidence of new bleeding or infection.

Interventions	Rationales
Carefully monitor vital signs.	Changes may indicate onset of bleeding or infection.
Notify physician promptly when client has signs of infection: fever, chills, or drainage.	Prompt treatment reduces risk of morbidity and mortality.
Monitor bleeding times, clotting studies, and platelet counts.	Abnormal results indicate increased risk for bleeding.
Teach client to avoid aspirin or nonsteroidal anti-inflammatory drugs and to use electric razors and soft toothbrushes.	These drugs can cause GI bleeding, and aspirin interferes with platelet function. Electric razors and soft toothbrushes can minimize unnecessary trauma.
Practice aseptic measures and teach family members to do so.	Reduces the risk of infection.
Observe stools for color and consistency. Test stool for occult blood.	Tests detect blood in stool.
Note any complaints of anxiety, epigastric fullness, weakness, and restlessness.	These findings may indicate bleeding and early shock.
Monitor for ecchymosis, epistaxis, petechiae, and bleeding from gums.	These findings indicate altered clotting mechanisms.
Monitor client carefully during blood transfusions.	Helps detect transfusion reaction.
Administer vitamin K as ordered.	Promotes clotting.

Evaluation of Expected Outcome: Client does not exhibit any new signs of bleeding or infection. Vital signs are stable, and laboratory values are normal.

Nursing Diagnosis: **Impaired Skin Integrity** related to pruritus, jaundice, bleeding tendencies, and edema

Expected Outcome: Skin will remain intact.

(continued)

Nursing Care Plan 49-1 (Continued)

THE CLIENT WITH A LIVER DISORDER

Interventions	Rationales
Provide frequent skin care, avoiding drying soaps and alcohol-based lotions.	Removes waste products deposited in skin and prevents drying.
Encourage client to keep fingernails short and smooth.	Prevents excoriation and infection from scratches.
Turn client at least every 2 hours, massaging bony prominences with emollients.	Mobilizes edema and improves circulation.
Use nonallergenic bed linens; instruct family to avoid harsh detergents.	Decreases skin irritation.

Evaluation of Expected Outcome: Skin remains intact with no evidence of pressure ulcers.

PC: **Hepatic Encephalopathy**

Expected Outcome: The nurse will minimize and manage problems associated with hepatic encephalopathy.

Interventions	Rationales
Assess cognitive and neurologic status at least every 8 hours.	Provides a means by which to determine changes.
Restrict dietary protein as ordered.	Protein is a source of ammonia, contributing to encephalopathy.
Give small, frequent feedings high in carbohydrates.	Provides energy and spares protein breakdown.
Restrict medications that increase encephalopathy.	Sedatives, hypnotics, and opioids may precipitate hepatic encephalopathy and increase confusion.
Monitor laboratory results, especially ammonia levels.	Increased ammonia levels indicate hepatic encephalopathy, which can lead to coma.
Administer medications that reduce serum ammonia levels, such as lactulose.	Reduced serum ammonia levels are a key goal.
Report any new or sudden increase in mental confusion.	Indicates increased hepatic encephalopathy and possible coma, requiring immediate medical intervention.
Orient client to name, place, time, and date as needed.	Reinforces reality and provides the client with cues about the world.
If hepatic coma develops, monitor respiratory status and initiate measures to prevent complications.	Clients in hepatic coma are at increased risk for pneumonia and infection.

Evaluation of Expected Outcome: Client remains free from injury.

into the systemic circulation. There is a high incidence of complications and shunt failure. An alternative, nonsurgical method of shunt placement is a *transjugular intrahepatic portosystemic shunt* (*TIPS*), which involves creation of a tract from the hepatic to the portal vein. In TIPS, a cannula with an expandable stent is inserted in the portovenous system through the jugular vein. The stent serves as the intrahepatic shunt between the hepatic vein and portal circulation to relieve portal hypertension. TIPS may be carried out using conscious sedation or anesthesia.

Esophageal Varices

Dilated, bulging esophageal veins are referred to as **esophageal varices,** which overfill as a result of portal hypertension. They are vulnerable to bleeding because they lie superficially in the mucosa, contain little protective elastic tissue, and are easily traumatized by rough food or chemical irritation.

Esophageal bleeding is a cardinal sign of esophageal varices. It may be slight but chronic, or massive and rapid, leading to a life-threatening medical emergency. Once

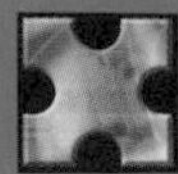

49-1 *Client and Family Teaching* The Client With Cirrhosis

The following topics are appropriate for a teaching plan:

- Follow the diet recommended by the physician.
- Consult a dietitian if you require a special diet (i.e., a low-sodium diet to prevent edema and ascites). Many metabolic liver disorders require highly specialized diets and necessitate extensive teaching from nursing and nutritional staff. Some diets require routine monitoring and home care.
- Avoid situations that could further damage the liver, such as drinking alcohol, taking tranquilizers, or inhaling chemicals such as benzene or vinyl chloride, which are toxic.
- Rest frequently, especially if activity causes fatigue.
- Avoid exposure to people with known infections.
- Continue skin care.
- Avoid nonprescription drugs (especially aspirin and products that contain it because they contribute to bleeding problems) unless approved by the physician.
- Contact the physician immediately about vomiting of blood, tarry stools, extreme fatigue, yellow skin, light-colored stools, or dark urine.

bleeding begins, clotting disorders common to liver damage occur. Barium swallow or esophagoscopy confirm the diagnosis of esophageal varices.

Measures to treat portal hypertension reduce the potential for bleeding varices. A soft diet and elimination of alcohol, aspirin, and other locally irritating substances may prevent varices. Antitussives and stool softeners are prescribed when the client is symptomatic, to reduce coughing or straining, which increases vascular pressure.

Esophageal varices also are treated with injection sclerotherapy or variceal banding. In **injection sclerotherapy,** the physician passes an endoscope orally to locate the varix (single vein). A thin needle is passed through the endoscope into the varix and a sclerosing agent (sodium tetradecyl, sodium morrhuate) is injected to solidify and stop circulation to the varix.

In *variceal banding* (*variceal band ligation*), another endoscopic procedure, the physician uses a device with small rubber bands at the end of the endoscope. After locating the varix, the physician places a rubber band over it. The band restricts blood flow to the varix, which sloughs off after a few days. Persistent portal hypertension allows varices to form again, making it necessary to repeat sclerotherapy or banding procedures regularly.

Acute hemorrhage from esophageal varices is life-threatening. Resuscitative measures include administration of IV fluids and blood products. IV octreotide (Sandostatin) is started as soon as possible, which reduces pressure in the portal venous system. If bleeding is too rapid to permit endoscopy, **balloon tamponade** with a Sengstaken-Blakemore tube may be used to compress the varices and stem the flow of blood (Fig. 49.5). This method usually allows only temporary relief from hemorrhage, necessitating endoscopy with sclerotherapy or banding after the client's condition stabilizes.

Ascites

Ascites is collection of fluid in the peritoneal cavity. Portal hypertension is a major underlying factor in the development of ascites. It leads to a cascade of events, called the **hepatorenal syndrome,** that ultimately alter fluid distribution and interfere with fluid excretion.

Increased pressure in the portal system forces serum proteins into the peritoneal cavity. The proteins draw plasma from the circulating blood by osmosis. Kidneys respond to decreases in blood volume and renal BP by initiating the rennin–angiotensin–aldosterone system (see Chap. 29). In response, the body conserves sodium ions, further contributing to fluid retention. Low renal blood volume also may suppress antidiuretic hormone, causing water to be reabsorbed rather than eliminated as urine. These combined factors promote fluid accumulation in the abdomen. Ascites is visible as extensive and massive abdominal swelling.

Abdominal paracentesis removes ascitic fluid. Abdominal fluid is rapidly removed by careful introduction of a needle through the abdominal wall, allowing the fluid to drain. This usually eases severe discomfort caused by distention and relieves breathing difficulty secondary to a high volume of abdominal fluid pressing on the diaphragm and lungs. Up to 6 to 8 L of fluid may be removed over 60 to 90 minutes. IV albumin is simultaneously infused to pull fluid back into the vascular space. Monitoring of BP and urine output is crucial to evaluate effects of fluid shifts. Diuretic therapy is prescribed if the circulatory volume is excessive.

Additional treatment includes maintenance diuretic therapy and a sodium-restricted diet. The potassium-sparing diuretic spironolactone (Aldactone) may be chosen because it specifically antagonizes the hormone aldosterone. Reversing the effects of aldosterone causes excretion of sodium and water, retention of potassium, and reduction of ascitic fluid.

If ascites repeatedly develops despite conservative treatment, the physician may surgically insert an internal catheter to redirect the ascitic fluid back into the vascular space. See the section on portal hypertension for more information.

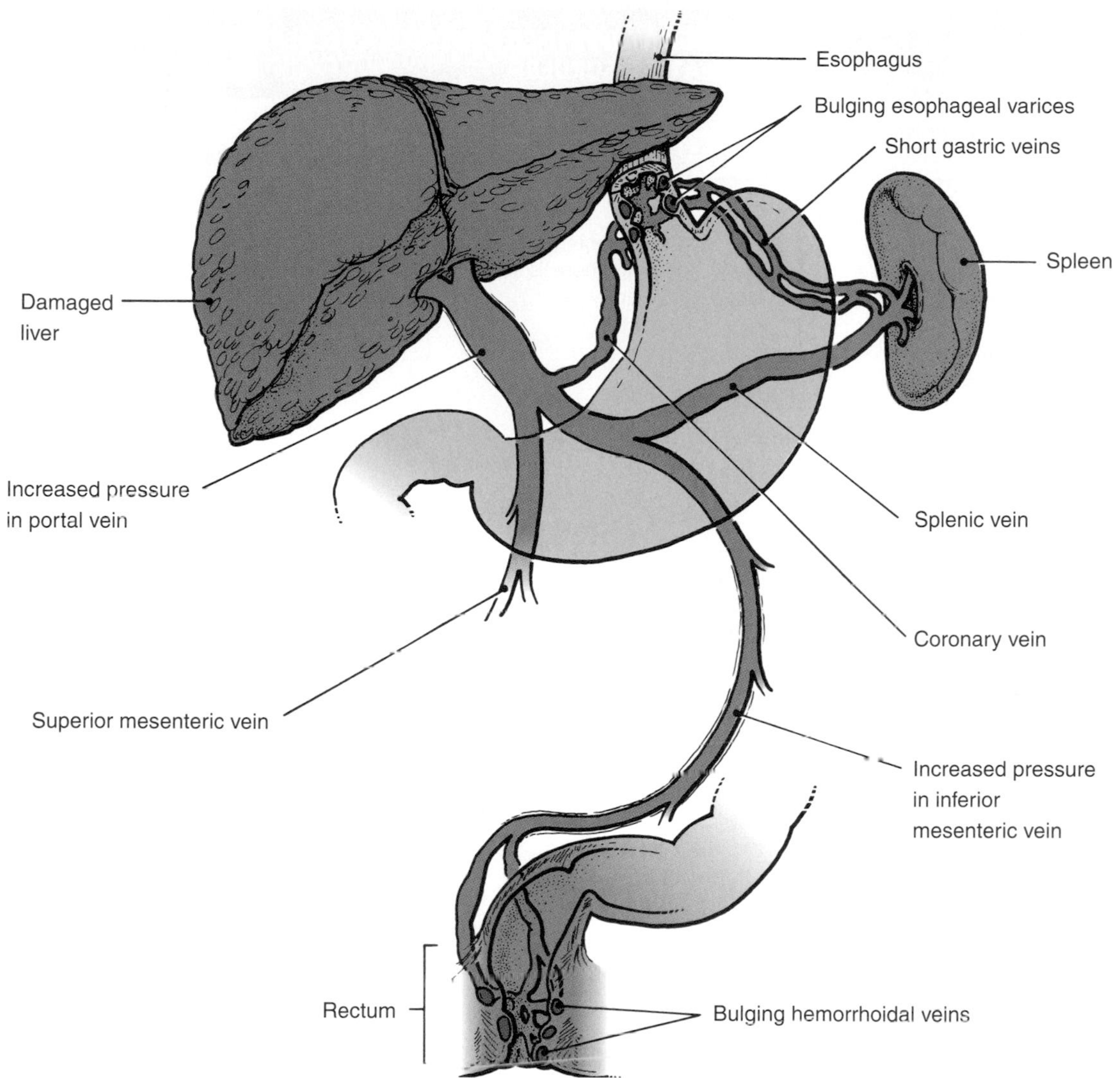

FIGURE 49.4 In portal hypertension, collateral vessels become dilated

Hepatic Encephalopathy

Hepatic encephalopathy is a central nervous system (CNS) manifestation of liver failure, leading to coma and death. It is related to increased serum ammonia level. Ammonia forms in the intestine by bacterial action on ingested proteins. The liver normally detoxifies ammonia by converting it to urea, which the kidneys then excrete in urine. A failing liver, as in advanced cirrhosis, cannot break down ammonia, causing it to accumulate in the blood. Ammonia can cross the blood-brain barrier and enter brain cells, where it interferes with brain metabolism, cell membrane pump mechanisms, and neurotransmission.

Indications of CNS effects include disorientation, confusion, personality changes, memory loss, a flapping tremor called *asterixis,* a positive Babinski reflex, sulfurous breath odor, and lethargy to deep coma. Symptoms usually worsen after the client eats a high-protein meal or has active GI bleeding because both dietary protein and digested blood cells increase ammonia volume in the intestine. Electroencephalography may show abnormal waveforms.

Treatment includes eliminating dietary protein, removing residual protein (such as blood if the client had a recent GI hemorrhage), and depleting intestinal microorganisms with drugs, laxatives, and enema therapy. Antibiotics, such as neomycin or kanamycin (Kantrex), which are poorly absorbed from the GI tract, are prescribed to destroy intestinal microorganisms and thereby decrease ammonia production. The administration of lactulose (Cephulac) reduces the serum ammonia concentration. In the colon, lactulose splits into lactic acid and acetic acid, attracts ammonia from the blood, and forms a compound that can be eliminated in the feces. Levodopa (L-dopa) is a precursor of dopamine that restores normal neurotransmission

Drug Therapy Table 49.1 SELECTED MEDICATIONS USED FOR LIVER, GALLBLADDER, AND PANCREATIC DISORDERS

DRUG CATEGORY AND EXAMPLES/ MECHANISM OF ACTION	SIDE EFFECTS	NURSING CONSIDERATIONS
For Liver Disorders		
Procoagulant vitamin K (Aquamephyton, Mephyton, Konakion) Promotes blood coagulation in bleeding conditions resulting from liver disease	Dizziness, transient hypotension, rapid and weak pulse, diaphoresis, flushing, skin rash, anaphylaxis	Instruct client not to take additional vitamin supplements unless specifically directed to do so by the physician. Assess adequacy of therapy by measuring prothrombin time.
Aminoglycoside antibiotic kanamycin (Kantrex) Decreases intestinal bacteria, thereby decreasing serum ammonia level	Diarrhea, cramping, ototoxicity, nephrotoxicity	Administer orally to decrease intestinal bacteria and serum ammonia levels. Note that discoloration does not indicate the loss of potency. Assess adequacy of therapy by measuring serum ammonia levels.
Laxative and ammonia reduction agent lactulose (Cephulac, Chronulac, Constilac, Duphalac, Heptalac, Portalac) Degrades intestinal bacteria	Diarrhea, cramping, abdominal distention, flatulence, nausea, vomiting, belching, hypernatremia	Because acidic stools excoriate the perianal area, perform careful cleansing after bowel movements to maintain skin integrity. Monitor serum sodium level for hypernatremia. Assess adequacy of therapy by measuring serum ammonia levels.
Bile acid sequestrant cholestyramine (Questran) Reduces pruritus by binding bile salts for excretion in feces	Headache, anxiety, vertigo, dizziness, insomnia, fatigue, tinnitus, constipation, hematuria, dysuria, skin rash, muscle and joint pain	Give all other drugs at least 1 hour before or 4 hours after cholestyramine because drug interferes with absorption of fat-soluble vitamins (A, D, E, and K), as well as many other drugs. Mix powder with liquid. Taking the medication in its dry form causes esophageal irritation and severe constipation.
Potassium-sparing diuretic cironolactone (Aldactone, Spirotone) Promotes excretion of sodium and water, particularly in cases of ascites	Headache, drowsiness, lethargy, confusion, ataxia, diarrhea, gastric bleeding, cramping, vomiting, urticaria, skin eruptions, hyperkalemia, dehydration, hirsutism, agranulocytosis	To enhance absorption, give with meals. Protect drug from light. Monitor serum electrolytes, intake and output, weight. Administer in the morning to prevent nocturia. Avoid potassium supplements and salt substitutes.
Immune agents interferon alfa-2b, recombinant (Intron A) Promotes virus-fighting capacities	Dizziness, confusion, paresthesia, lethargy, depression, insomnia, anxiety, fatigue, amnesia, malaise, hypotension, chest pain, anorexia, nausea, diarrhea, abdominal pain, dyspepsia, constipation, stomatitis, gingivitis, transient impotence, gynecomastia, leukopenia, anemia, thrombocytopenia, dyspnea, cough, rash, pruritus, alopecia, dermatitis, flulike symptoms (fever, fatigue, chills, headache, muscle aches), back pain, diaphoresis	Administer intramuscularly or subcutaneously for chronic hepatitis. Administer at bedtime to minimize daytime drowsiness. Monitor for flulike symptoms. Monitor blood studies for hematologic side effects. Explain to the client the increased risk for infection when taking this drug. Advise avoiding contact with those who have an acute illness and those who have recently received oral polio vaccine. The client should not receive vaccines prepared with live virus, unless specifically instructed to do so by the physician.
Immunosuppressives cyclosporine (Sandimmune) Prevent rejection of transplanted organ	Tremor, headache, seizures, confusion, paresthesia, hypertension, gum hyperplasia, nausea, vomiting, diarrhea, nephrotoxicity, hepatotoxicity, anemia, leukopenia, thrombocytopenia, hemolytic anemia, acne, flushing, infection, hirsutism, anaphylaxis, gynecomastia	Administer from a glass container or dropper to minimize adherence of the drug to container walls. Monitor cyclosporine blood levels to ensure that the client's level is within therapeutic range. Monitor renal function, blood urea nitrogen (BUN) and creatinine levels. Monitor liver enzyme levels for hepatotoxicity.

(*continued*)

DRUG THERAPY TABLE 49.1 SELECTED MEDICATIONS USED FOR LIVER, GALLBLADDER, AND PANCREATIC DISORDERS (Continued)

DRUG CATEGORY AND EXAMPLES/ MECHANISM OF ACTION	SIDE EFFECTS	NURSING CONSIDERATIONS
		Because the client is at increased risk for infection when taking this drug, advise against contact with those who have an acute illness and those who have recently received oral polio vaccine. The client should not receive vaccines prepared with live virus, unless specifically instructed to do so by the physician.
tacrolimus (Prograf, FK506) Prevent rejection of transplanted organ	Headache, tremor, insomnia, paresthesia, hypertension, peripheral edema, diarrhea, nausea, constipation, abnormal liver function test, anorexia, abdominal pain, abnormal renal function, elevated creatinine or BUN levels, oliguria, hyperkalemia, hypokalemia, hyperglycemia, hypomagnesemia, anemia, leukocytosis, thrombocytopenia, pleural effusion, dyspnea, atelectasis, pruritus, rash, back pain, ascites, anaphylaxis	Monitor for neurotoxicity and nephrotoxicity, especially in clients who receive high doses, or who have renal dysfunction. Monitor serum magnesium and electrolyte levels and blood glucose levels. Monitor liver enzymes. Inform client of an increased risk for infection when taking this drug. The client should avoid contact with those who have an acute illness and those who have recently received oral polio vaccine. The client should not receive vaccines prepared with live virus, unless specifically instructed to do so by the physician.
For Gallbladder Disease		
Gallstone-dissolving agents chenodiol—also called chenodeoxycholic acid (Cheodiol, Chenix) Suppresses hepatic synthesis of cholesterol and cholic acid	Diarrhea, cramping, heartburn, constipation, nausea, anorexia, epigastric distress, elevated liver enzymes, possible hepatotoxicity	Administer orally to dissolve gallstones; may require long-term therapy for effectiveness. Monitor the client's liver enzyme levels. Avoid administering during pregnancy.
ursodiol (Actigall) Suppresses hepatic synthesis of cholesterol and inhibits intestinal absorption of cholesterol	Headache, fatigue, anxiety, depression, sleep disorders, rhinitis, nausea, vomiting, dyspepsia, metallic taste, abdominal pain, biliary pain, diarrhea, constipation, flatulence, cough, pruritus, rash, dry skin, urticaria, alopecia, myalgia, back pain	Administer orally to dissolve cholesterol-related gallstones; may require long-term therapy for effectiveness and may be helpful in promoting bile flow in liver disease. Monitor the client's liver enzyme levels.
For Pancreatic Disorders		
Pancreatic enzymes pancreatin (Creon, Boglan, Panazyme, Donnazyme, Entozyme) pancrelipase (Pancrease, Cotazym, Creon 10 and Creon 20, Protilase, Ultrase, Viokase, Zymase) Promote digestion and fat, protein, and carbohydrate absorption	Anorexia, nausea, diarrhea, allergic reactions, perianal irritation	Administer with meals and with snacks. Monitor stool consistency. Open capsules and sprinkle onto a small quantity of soft food. Do not crush or chew enteric-coated preparations. Expect dosage to vary with degree of malabsorption, amount of fat in diet, size of the meal and enzyme activity of individual preparations (300 mg pancrelipase/17 g dietary fat). Cautious use in history of allergy to pork products or enzymes.

in the brain. Supportive measures include administering IV fluids containing electrolytes and multivitamins or total parenteral nutrition (TPN).

The prognosis for clients with hepatic encephalopathy is grim. Only a few survive without a liver transplant.

● HEPATITIS

Hepatitis is inflammation of the liver. The disease may be acute or chronic.

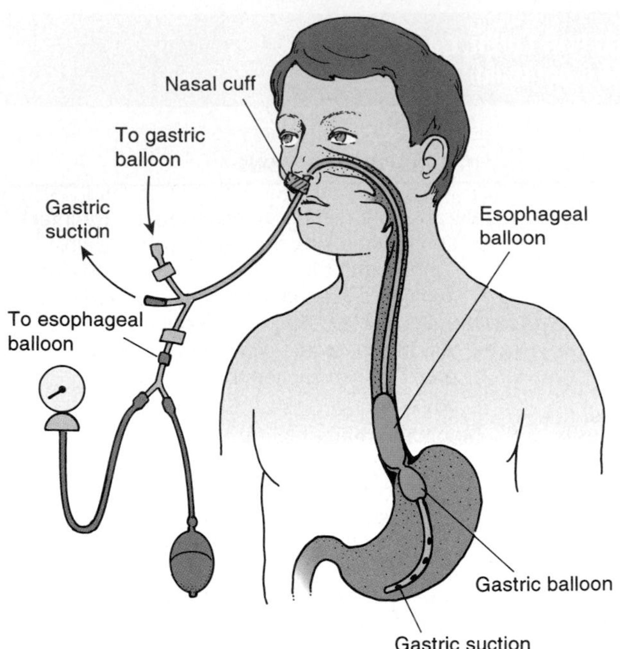

FIGURE 49.5 The Sengstaken-Blakemore tube has three separate openings: one lumen inflates the gastric balloon, another inflates the esophageal balloon, and the third one is used to aspirate blood from the stomach.

Pathophysiology and Etiology

The liver may become inflamed shortly after exposure to hepatotoxic chemicals or drugs, after lengthy alcohol abuse, or by invasion with an infectious microorganism. The most common cause of hepatitis is a viral infection, which is the focus of this discussion. The letters A, B, C, D, and E identify the viruses that infect the liver (Table 49.2). Modes of transmission and incubation periods differentiate each virus.

Once the virus invades the *hepatocytes* (liver cells), it alters their structure. An immune reaction ensues, in which infected cells become inflamed and dysfunctional. The active disease process affects uptake, conjugation, and excretion of bilirubin.

Most people recover from acute infection, but a few suffer from chronic active hepatitis and subsequent liver damage. In chronic persistent hepatitis (most common with hepatitis B, C, and D), liver damage does not worsen, but it does not improve, and the liver remains enlarged. Some clients may develop cirrhosis. Others deteriorate rapidly with liver failure and die unless liver transplantation is performed. Invasion of the transplanted liver by the virus is common, but it usually takes years before the newly transplanted liver develops cirrhosis.

Hepatitis B and C commonly are associated with hepatocellular carcinoma. Routine monitoring (e.g., blood test for alpha-fetoprotein and ultrasound) should be carried out for clients with chronic forms of these diseases.

A sixth viral type is hepatitis G, considered to be non-A, non-B, and non-C. It occurs 14 to 145 days after a blood transfusion. It cannot be identified as can the other types, and thus is designated type G. It is similar to hepatitis C.

Other types of hepatitis include:

- *Autoimmune hepatitis*—results from an abnormal immune system response. Treatment consists of the administration of corticosteroids and immune-modulating agents (azathioprine or 6-mercaptopurine) (see Drug Therapy Table 47.1). Without treatment, many of these clients will die or require a liver transplant.
- *Toxic hepatitis*—develops when certain chemicals toxic to the liver (e.g., chloroform, phosphorus, carbon tetrachloride) cause liver necrosis. Treatment includes removing the toxin and treating symptoms. If liver damage is severe and prolonged, prognosis is not good without a liver transplant.
- *Drug-induced hepatitis*—occurs when a drug reaction damages the liver. This form of hepatitis can be severe and fatal. Examples of drugs causing a severe reaction are anesthetic agents, antidepressants, or anticonvulsants. High-dose corticosteroids are administered to treat the reaction. Liver transplantation may be necessary.

Assessment Findings

Signs and symptoms of the various forms of hepatitis sometimes are indistinguishable. Three phases of all forms of hepatitis are as follows:

1. *Preicteric phase:* nausea; vomiting; anorexia; fever; malaise; arthralgia; headache; right upper quadrant (RUQ) discomfort; enlargement of the spleen, liver, and lymph nodes; weight loss; rash; and urticaria
2. *Icteric phase:* jaundice, pruritus, clay-colored or light stools, dark urine, fatigue, anorexia, and RUQ discomfort; symptoms of the preicteric phase may continue
3. *Posticteric phase:* liver enlargement, malaise, and fatigue; other symptoms subside

Not all clients with hepatitis experience all the listed symptoms, and severity of any one symptom may vary. Even though symptoms are categorized, not all clients with hepatitis necessarily develop jaundice.

Serologic analysis can detect specific viral antibodies. Ribonucleic acid (RNA) testing may be performed to identify the virus itself. Test results may take up to 1 week. The white blood cell count may be elevated. Evidence of **cholestasis** (ineffective bile drainage) is seen with elevated bilirubin levels. Hepatic aminotransferase (alanine

TABLE 49.2 FORMS OF VIRAL HEPATITIS

TYPE	CAUSE	MODE OF TRANSMISSION	INCUBATION	SIGNS AND SYMPTOMS	OUTCOME
Hepatitis A (previously called *infectious hepatitis*)	Hepatitis A virus (HAV)	Oral route from feces and saliva of infected persons; water, food, and equipment contaminated with HAV	3–5 weeks	May occur with or without symptoms; flu-like illness Preicteric phase: headache, malaise, fatigue, anorexia, fever Icteric phase: dark urine, jaundice, tender liver	Usually mild with full recovery; fatality rate <1%; no carrier state or increased risk of chronic hepatitis, cirrhosis, or hepatic cancer
Hepatitis B (previously called *serum hepatitis*)	Hepatitis B virus (HBV)	Infected blood or plasma; needles, syringes, surgical or dental equipment contaminated with infected blood; also sexually transmitted through vaginal secretions and semen of carriers or those actively infected	2–5 months	Arthralgias, rash; may occur without symptoms	May be severe; fatality rate 1% to 10%; carrier state possible; increased risk of chronic hepatitis, cirrhosis, and hepatic cancer; some infected people become carriers
Hepatitis C (previously called *non-A, non-B hepatitis–NANB*)	Hepatitis C virus (HCV)	Infected blood or blood products; sexual contact	2–20 weeks	Similar to HBV, although less severe and without jaundice	Frequent occurrence of chronic carrier state and chronic liver disease; increased risk of hepatic cancer
Hepatitis D (also called *delta hepatitis*)	Hepatitis D virus (HDV)	Same as HBV; cannot infect alone; occurs as dual infection with HBV	2–5 months	Similar to HBV	Similar to HBV with greater likelihood of carrier state, chronic active hepatitis, and cirrhosis
Hepatitis E	Hepatitis E virus (HEV)	Fecal–oral routes; low risk of person–person contact; found more in countries with poor sanitation and water quality	2–9 weeks	Similar to HAV—very severe in pregnant women	Similar to HAV—very severe in pregnant women

aminotransferase [ALT] and aspartate aminotransferase [AST]) levels rise during the incubation period and begin to fall once symptoms appear. Chronic disease may result in persistent elevation of the transaminases. A prolonged PT or PTT reflects poor synthetic liver function. Additional indicators of poor synthetic function include low blood glucose and serum albumin levels. Liver biopsy and histologic examination of the specimen evaluate any inflammation, fibrosis, and cirrhosis.

Medical and Surgical Management

Treatment is symptomatic and includes bed rest, a balanced diet of small feedings at intervals, and IV fluid administration if the client is extremely ill or has poor fluid intake. Vitamins, especially fat-soluble vitamins, are necessary regardless of oral intake because they are poorly absorbed. Antiemetics are given to relieve vomiting, but usually drug therapy is avoided until the liver recovers.

Recombinant interferon alfa-2b (Intron A, Roferon) may be given to clients with chronic hepatitis B, C, and D to force the virus into remission. It frequently is administered in combination with ribavirin (Rebetol), a synthetic antiviral. The combination therapy increases the likelihood of a sustained virus-free response (more than 6 months). Ribavirin may cause birth defects, so clients of childbearing age need to be counseled about using strict birth control methods while taking this drug (Chene & Decker, 2001).

For clients with chronic disease who do not respond to medical treatment, a liver transplantation may be done. This involves total removal of the diseased liver and transplantation of a healthy liver in the same location. Immunosuppressant agents are given for transplantation to succeed and include cyclosporine, tacrolimus, serolimus, corticosteroids, and azathioprine. The goal is to find immunosuppressive agents that effectively reduce rejection of transplanted organs and cause the fewest side effects.

Nursing Management

Practice preventive techniques to control spread of hepatitis viruses and teach the family and general public how to reduce risk of infection (Nursing Guidelines 49-1). Nursing care in the early stages focuses on maintaining physical rest, supporting nutritional intake, and preventing complications. Before discharge, teach self-care measures to promote health and avoid transmitting infection to others. The client must avoid alcohol and drugs that can further damage the liver. For clients who develop chronic active or persistent hepatitis and require liver transplants, see Nursing Management in the following section.

Stop, Think, and Respond ● BOX 49-1

You are assigned to a client who is recovering from abdominal surgery. She tells you that the client in the next room has chronic hepatitis, and she is afraid she will catch it. Which answer would best help this client?

NURSING GUIDELINES 49-1

Techniques for Preventing Viral Hepatitis

*Preventing Hepatitis A**

- Receive hepatitis A virus (HAV) vaccine, especially when considered at high risk (healthcare workers, day-care workers, foreign travel).
- Obtain immune globulin (IG) injection if exposed (in household or sexual contacts with infected individuals) to hepatitis without previous immunization.
- Observe Standard Precautions. Wear gloves if hands come into contact with body fluids; wear gown and face shield if body fluids may be splashed.
- Require child care staff to wear gloves during diaper changes and to perform adequate handwashing.
- Perform conscientious handwashing after removing gloves.
- Screen food handlers.
- Avoid eating from public salad bars and buffets that do not have sneeze guards or other hygienic devices and practices to prevent food contamination.
- Use liquid soap dispensers and hand dryers in public restrooms rather than bar soap and cloth towels.
- Avoid placing fingers and hand-held objects in mouth.
- Do not share cigarettes, eating utensils, or beverage containers.
- Avoid eating raw seafood or seafood harvested from possibly polluted water.
- Use a pocket mask when giving pulmonary resuscitation.
- Drink bottled water in underdeveloped countries. Avoid ice unless it was made from bottled water.

Preventing Hepatitis B†

- Receive hepatitis B virus (HBV) vaccine, especially if in a high-risk category (dialysis, blood dyscrasias, IV drug abuser, homosexual, healthcare worker, school teacher).
- Adhere to American Academy of Pediatrics guidelines for immunization.
- Obtain hepatitis B immune globulin (HBIG) if exposed to HBV and not previously vaccinated within 24 hours but no later than 7 days after blood contact.
- Observe Standard Precautions (wear gloves if hands may come into contact with body fluids; wear gown and face shield if body fluids may be splashed).
- Do not recap needles.
- Dispose of needles and other sharp objects in a puncture-resistant container.
- Use a condom when engaging in sexual intercourse.
- Do not share razors, fingernail tools, toothbrushes, or any personal care item that may come into contact with blood or body fluids.
- If contemplating surgery, investigate the possibility of donating and storing your own blood for later use.
- Wear a mouth shield when giving mouth-to-mouth resuscitation.

*Prevention of hepatitis A also prevents hepatitis E; no vaccine or postexposure treatment is available for hepatitis E.

†Prevention of hepatitis B also prevents hepatitis C and D; no vaccine or postexposure treatment is available for hepatitis C or D.

- *"Don't worry, dear. That kind of hepatitis can only be transmitted sexually."*
- *"There are many kinds of hepatitis—do you know which kind she has?"*
- *"Hospital staff always use precautions to prevent any possibility of transmission of infectious diseases to other clients."*
- *"There is no problem—that client is not a carrier of the disease."*

• TUMORS OF THE LIVER

A tumor of the liver is an abnormal mass of cells in the liver. Liver tumors may be benign or malignant (see Chap. 19). If malignant, the tumor may be a primary lesion (classified as a *hepatoma*) or a metastasis.

Pathophysiology and Etiology

Primary malignancies (hepatomas) are rare but appear to have increased incidence in people with previous hepatitis B or D viral infections or cirrhosis, especially those with the postnecrotic form. The most common liver malignancy is a metastatic lesion from the breast, lung, or GI tract. Causes of benign liver tumors are tuberculosis and fungal and parasitic infections. Oral contraceptives and anabolic steroids also have been implicated in the development of benign hepatic lesions.

Tumor cells grow at an accelerated rate. They function in a disorganized manner and eventually impair the liver's physiologic activities. They may obstruct bile flow, leading to jaundice, liver failure, portal hypertension, and ascites.

Assessment Findings

Symptoms can be vague and confused with those of cirrhosis. Jaundice is common. Once the tumor is sufficiently large, the client may report pain in the RUQ. Weight loss and debilitation are common. The client usually experiences bleeding tendencies. Eventually, the abdomen becomes distended from liver enlargement and related ascites.

Alpha-fetoprotein, a serum protein normally produced during fetal development, is a marker indicating a primary malignant liver tumor. Total bilirubin and serum enzyme (ALT, AST, alkaline phosphatase) levels are elevated. A liver scan, ultrasonography, MRI, or CT scan identifies the tumor and its location. A biopsy, performed to identify the specific type of tumor cells, also can define and disclose damage to adjacent liver tissue.

Medical and Surgical Management

If the tumor is confined to a single lobe of the liver, a **hepatic lobectomy** may be attempted to remove primary malignant or benign tumors. Metastatic tumors usually are considered inoperable because they often are scattered throughout the liver. Frequency of metastasis and poor survival rate usually eliminate liver transplantation as an option. Sometimes biliary ducts obstructed by disease are bypassed with percutaneous biliary or transhepatic drainage. A catheter is inserted under fluoroscopy through the abdominal wall, past the obstruction, into the duodenum. This procedure relieves the pressure and pain caused by bile buildup and decreases jaundice and pruritus. In some cases *cryosurgery* or *cryoablation* is used. This technique uses liquid nitrogen at −196°C to destroy tumors. Two or three freeze-and-thaw cycles are administered through probes inserted with open laparotomy. Effectiveness of this procedure is still being evaluated (Smeltzer & Bare, 2004).

For malignancies, short-term improvement may be achieved with IV chemotherapy or infusions directly into the hepatic artery or peritoneum. Doxorubicin hydrochloride (Adriamycin) and 5-fluorouracil (5-FU) are common choices for drug therapy. Results from chemotherapy tend to be transient. Radiation therapy may be administered to reduce pain and discomfort.

Nursing Management

Determine if the client will be undergoing a lobectomy or a liver transplantation. Postoperative assessments include checking vital signs and the function of drains and tubes. Observe for potential complications (hemorrhage, shock, infection, rejection in cases of transplant, electrolyte imbalances, and hepatic coma). Observe the client with cirrhosis for signs of alcohol withdrawal. Standard postsurgical assessments include evaluating breathing patterns, airway patency, and pain.

In terminal stages of the disease, keep the client as comfortable as possible by administering analgesics, supporting ventilation compromised by ascites, and reducing discomfort from pruritus. When the liver fails and coma develops, institute safety measures and continue performing total care. While the client is alert, provide support for the client and family as both begin grieving their potential losses. As appropriate, make referrals for hospice care. Additional nursing management depends on symptoms and treatment.

Teaching includes the following points:

- Follow the diet recommended by the physician.
- Plan rest periods during the day.
- Avoid heavy lifting.

- Take medications exactly as prescribed. Follow directions on the label, particularly with regard to taking the drug before, after, or with food or meals.
- Record weight weekly or as recommended by the physician. Report significant weight gain or loss to the physician.
- Contact the physician about significant increase in abdominal size, fever, nausea, vomiting, vomiting of blood (bright red, coffee ground), tarry stools, difficulty concentrating or changes in level of consciousness, jaundice, or swelling of the ankles.
- Make and keep appointments for periodic follow-up office visits.

DISORDERS OF THE GALLBLADDER

Several disorders affect the *biliary system* (Box 49-4), which refers to the *gallbladder* and *bile ducts,* which carry bile (Fig. 49.6). These disorders impair the drainage of bile into the duodenum.

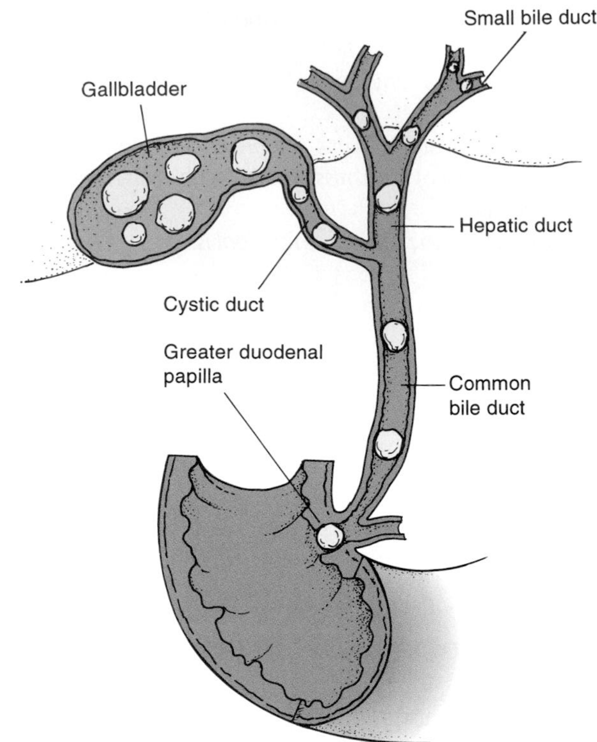

FIGURE 49.6 Gallstones may form in many locations within the biliary tree.

● CHOLELITHIASIS AND CHOLECYSTITIS

Cholelithiasis denotes stones that form in the gallbladder. Gallstone formation represents the most common abnormality of the biliary system. If stones are located in the common bile duct, the condition is referred to as **choledocholithiasis.** Formation of stones often leads to **cholecystitis,** an inflammation or infection of the gallbladder, which may be chronic or acute.

Pathophysiology and Etiology

Cholelithiasis and cholecystitis usually coexist. Their incidence increases progressively with age. Gallstones are more frequent in women than men, particularly those who are middle-aged or have a history of multiple pregnancies, diabetes, and obesity. Causes of cholelithiasis remain unestablished; bile stasis, diet, and infection are suspected. Formation of pigmented stones is associated with hemolytic anemia, which increases free bilirubin (see Chap. 33). Cholesterol-type stones are linked to a high-fat diet or predisposition to hypercholesterolemia.

Symptoms tend to develop when one or more gallstones partially or totally impair passage of bile, causing the gallbladder to become inflamed, swollen, and distended with bile. Each time the person eats fatty foods, *cholecystokinin,* a hormone secreted by the small intestine, stimulates the gallbladder to send bile for its digestion. The gallbladder responds by contracting forcefully. Discomfort results from a combination of the inflammation and contractile spasms. Digestion problems result from reduced or absent bile. If the swelling and distended volume remain unrelieved, the gallbladder can become necrotic or rupture, leading to peritonitis.

BOX 49-4 ● Terms Related to the Biliary System

Cholecystitis: inflammation of the gallbladder
Cholelithiasis: the presence of calculi in the gallbladder
Cholecystectomy: removal of the gallbladder
Cholecystostomy: opening and drainage of the gallbladder
Choledochotomy: opening into the common duct
Choledocholithiasis: stones in the common duct
Choledocholithotomy: incision of common bile duct for removal of stones
Choledochoduodenostomy: anastomosis of common duct to duodenum
Choledochojejunostomy: anastomosis of common duct to jejunum
Lithotripsy: disintegration of gallstones by shock waves
Laparoscopic cholecystectomy: removal of gallbladder through endoscopic procedure
Laser cholecystectomy: removal of gallbladder using laser rather than scalpel and traditional surgical instruments

Assessment Findings

Initially, clients experience belching, nausea, and RUQ discomfort, with pain or cramps after high-fat meals. Symptoms become acute when a stone blocks bile flow from the gallbladder. With acute cholecystitis, clients usually are very sick with fever, vomiting, tenderness over the liver, and severe pain called **biliary colic.** Pain may radiate to the back and shoulders. The gallbladder may be so swollen that it becomes palpable. Slight jaundice may be noted. Urine appears dark brown; the stools may be light-colored.

Various tests are performed to rule out other disorders with similar symptoms. Eventually, stones and structural changes in the gallbladder are imaged by means of *cholecystography* (gallbladder imaging), ultrasonography, CT scan, or radionuclide imaging. Percutaneous transhepatic cholangiography distinguishes jaundice caused by liver disease from jaundice caused by gallbladder disease. Endoscopic retrograde cholangiopancreatography (ERCP) locates stones in the common bile duct. Magnetic resonance cholangiopancreatography is a noninvasive technique that uses MRI to detect gallstones and gallbladder disorders.

Clients with jaundice have elevated bilirubin levels. Leukocytosis findings correlate with inflammation. Serum liver enzymes may be elevated. The PT may be prolonged as a result of interference with absorption of vitamin K.

Medical and Surgical Management

When the gallbladder is acutely inflamed, the client takes nothing by mouth. Instead, a nasogastric tube is inserted, and antibiotics and parenteral fluids are prescribed until inflammation subsides. Treatment of mild or chronic cholecystitis involves a low-fat diet. To relieve pain and discomfort, analgesics, anticholinergics, and even nitroglycerin are prescribed. Fat-soluble vitamins may be ordered to compensate for their reduced absorption. A bile binding resin, such as cholestyramine (Questran), is prescribed to relieve pruritus.

Clients who are a surgical risk and whose gallstones appear radiolucent on diagnostic studies receive oral bile acids, either chenodeoxycholic acid (chenodiol, Chenix, or CDCA) or ursodeoxycholic acid (ursodiol, Actigall, or UDCA), in an attempt to dissolve the gallstones. These drugs, which may take between 6 and 12 months to be effective, are only moderately successful. Success rate is greatest when stones are small, but the rate of recurrence within 5 years is high.

Dissolving stones by direct contact may be attempted by instilling a solvent, methyl-tert-butyl ether, into the gallbladder or common bile duct through a percutaneously placed catheter. If successful, the stones clear in hours or a few days. The rate for recurrence is unknown at this time.

Lithotripsy, a nonsurgical procedure using shock waves generated by a machine called a *lithotriptor,* may be used to break up some types of gallstones. Shock waves are directed at the gallbladder while the anesthetized client lies in a specially designed water tank. After shock waves fragment gallstones, endoscopy or direct contact dissolution removes fragments.

Stones in the common bile duct can be removed by performing a *sphincterotomy* (opening of the sphincter of Oddi where the common bile duct joins the duodenum) using an endoscope. The stone is snared or retrieved using a basket-like attachment on the endoscope. Other nonsurgical techniques for removing gallstones are pictured in Figure 49.7.

Laparoscopic cholecystectomy is the treatment of choice for about 80% of clients with gallbladder disease.

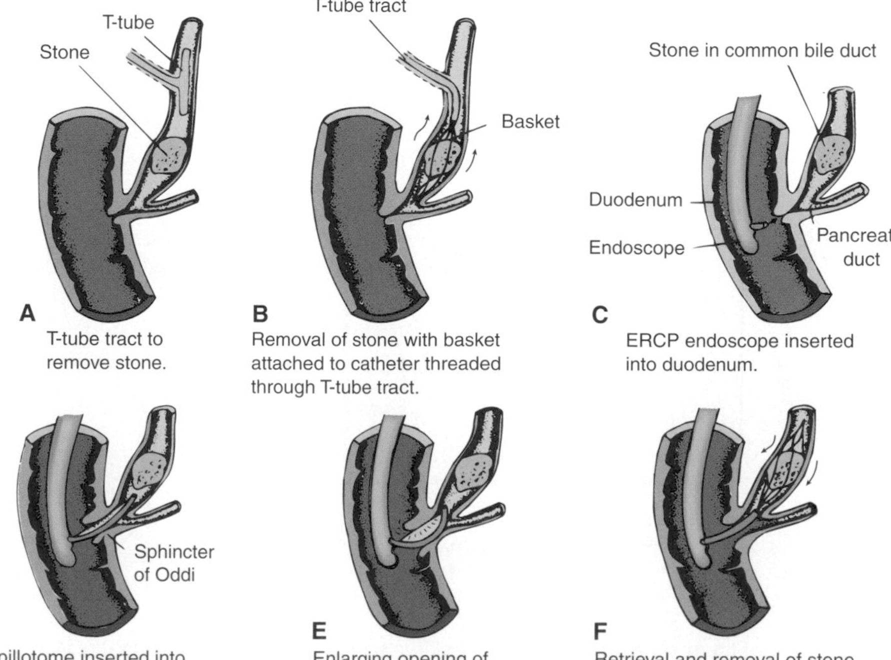

FIGURE 49.7 Nonsurgical techniques for removing gallstones. (From Smeltzer, S. C. & Bare, B. G. [2004]. *Brunner & Suddarth's textbook of medical–surgical nursing* [10th ed.]. Philadelphia: Lippincott Williams & Wilkins.)

It requires general anesthesia, but the surgery is performed with an endoscope inserted in one of three or four small puncture sites in the abdomen (Fig. 49.8). After inflating the abdomen with carbon dioxide to displace abdominal structures and provide a better view, the surgeon drains the gallbladder, dissects the vessels and ducts, and then grasps and removes the gallbladder. Next, the surgeon staples the puncture sites closed and covers incisions with a light dressing.

Most clients return home in the evening or the morning after the procedure. Although a nasogastric tube may have been inserted during surgery, it is removed before the client is awake and alert. Mild analgesics are administered to relieve minor discomfort. The client may eat food once effects of anesthesia subside. A prolonged recovery period usually is unnecessary. Most clients resume normal activities within 1 week.

When the gallbladder is extremely distended and fragile from inflammation and infection or contains unusually large or multiple stones, its removal through a small abdominal opening may be impossible or dangerous. In these cases, the surgeon performs an **open cholecystectomy,** which involves a laparotomy (abdominal incision). A *Penrose drain,* a wide, flat rubber tube, or a *vacuum drain,* a plastic tube connected to a bulb or other collecting device, is inserted in the wound to remove serosanguineous fluid. After surgery, clients experience a lengthy period of gastric decompression and acute postoperative pain and about 1 week of hospitalization. A 6-week recovery period follows after discharge.

During cholecystectomy, a *choledochotomy,* surgical opening and exploration of the common bile duct, may be performed. A **T-tube** (a tube used to drain bile) usually is inserted while the surgical wound heals (Fig. 49.9). The T-tube is brought through the abdomen near the incision and connected to gravity drainage. Bile salts such as dehydrocholic acid (Decholin) may be prescribed to promote drainage.

Nursing Management

During an attack of biliary colic, ensure that the client rests. Monitor the client's ability to digest a bland liquid diet. Administer prescribed antispasmodics or analgesics. If gastric decompression is required, insert a nasogastric tube and connect it to suction (see Chap. 46). If lithotripsy or another procedure is initiated to remove stones, close

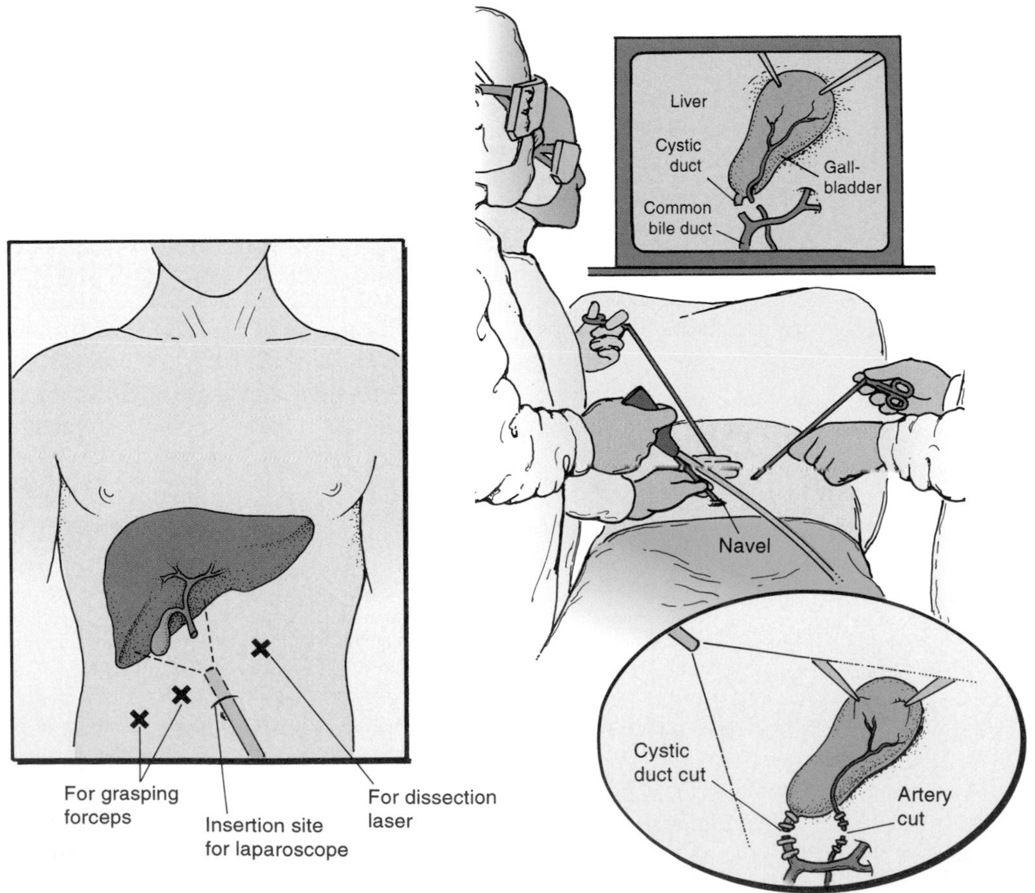

FIGURE 49.8 In laparoscopic cholecystectomy, the abdominal organs are viewed on a television monitor while the gallbladder is removed.

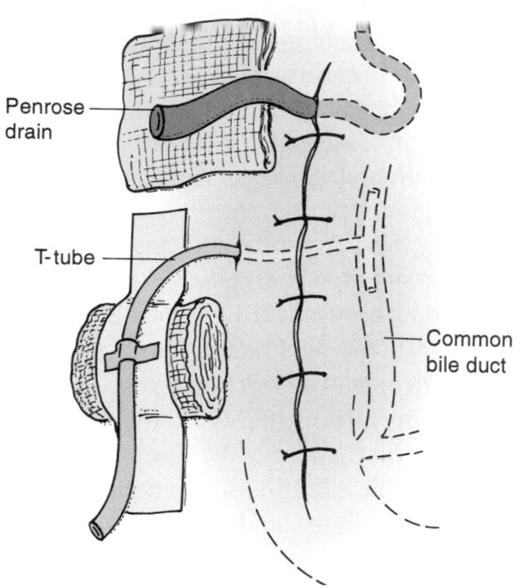

FIGURE 49.9 After an open cholecystectomy, a wound drain removes exudates from the area formerly occupied by the gallbladder and a T-tube diverts bile, which the liver is still forming.

observation of the client after the procedure for increased pain, shock, or signs of internal bleeding is important.

Same-Day Surgery

When outpatient or laparoscopic surgery is scheduled, instruct the client on presurgical procedures, laboratory tests, and the consent form. On the day of surgery, complete preoperative skin preparation, insert an IV line, and administer sedation. After the client recovers from anesthesia and before discharge, provide intensive instruction to the client and accompanying caregiver regarding self-care. Give written instructions for reference. In accord with agency policy, perform follow-up measures, such as telephoning the client the day after surgery to inquire about recovery progress.

Cholecystectomy

Ask the client to describe symptoms experienced before admission such as type and location of pain or discomfort. Ask whether and which specific foods cause pain or discomfort and discuss other problems, such as nausea, vomiting, or abdominal cramping. Inspect skin and sclera for jaundice and palpate the abdomen for tenderness. Routine presurgical and postsurgical assessments are necessary when the client returns from surgery.

If a T-tube is in place after an open cholecystectomy, monitor and record the drainage and maintain tube patency by keeping the collector below the level of the incision. This prevents bile from flowing back into the duct. A physician's order is necessary to clamp a T-tube. As healing occurs, the physician may direct that the T-tube be clamped temporarily before a meal and reopened later after eating.

Change dressings frequently as needed. Apply protectants such as zinc oxide or petrolatum to skin around drainage tubes. Observe sclerae for jaundice. Report abdominal pain, nausea, vomiting, bile drainage around T-tube, or clay-colored stools.

Measure bile drainage every 8 hours or according to agency policy. If more than 500 mL of bile drains within 24 hours or if drainage is significantly reduced, notify the physician. Preventing tension on the tubing is important because it may be dislodged internally. A return of normal color to stool and urine indicates that bile is being deposited normally in the GI tract.

Client and Family Teaching

Diet and drug regimens are among the many aspects of care for clients with gallbladder disease. The client should meet with a dietitian and needs a complete list of foods to avoid. He or she also needs to know how to read food product labels to determine their fat content.

When applicable, explain the purpose of drug therapy, schedule to follow for its administration, and potential side effects. Inform the client to continue the medication even if symptoms disappear, and that frequent monitoring of the effect of drug therapy is necessary. Reinforce the importance of notifying the physician immediately of severe pain, jaundice, or fever or if the color of the stools or urine changes.

DISORDERS OF THE PANCREAS

The pancreas is in the upper abdomen. Disorders of the pancreas can affect both exocrine and endocrine functions.

• PANCREATITIS

Pancreatitis, inflammation of the pancreas, may be acute or chronic with a long history of relapse and recurrences.

ACUTE PANCREATITIS

Acute pancreatitis ranges from mild to severe and can be fatal. Characteristics of the mild form are inflammation and edema of the pancreas. Although the client is very ill, pancreatic function usually returns to normal within 6 months. In the severe form, more generalized and complete enzymatic digestion of the pancreas occurs. Tissue becomes necrotic, and the client develops many local and systemic complications.

Pathophysiology and Etiology

Primarily, the pancreas becomes inflamed when the organ's own enzymes—especially trypsin—cause the pancreas to digest itself (*autodigestion*). Autodigestion develops when there is reflux of bile and duodenal contents into the pancreatic duct, activating exocrine enzymes that the pancreas produces. Swelling of the opening to the pancreatic duct impairs or even obstructs release of bicarbonate, which neutralizes chyme as it enters the small intestine. It also obstructs release of the enzymes trypsin, which digests proteins; amylase, which digests carbohydrates; and lipase, which digests fats. As enzymes accumulate in the gland, they begin to digest pancreatic tissue itself. Destruction of the pancreas leads to impairment of endocrine functions.

Causes of acute pancreatitis vary widely. Known causes include structural abnormalities, abdominal trauma, infections, metabolic disorders (e.g., hyperlipidemia, hypercalcemia), vascular abnormalities, inflammatory bowel disease, hereditary factors, ingestion of alcohol or certain other drugs, or refeeding after prolonged fasting or anorexia. Sometimes, acute pancreatitis develops without any predisposing factors or other identifiable causes.

Complications from severe acute pancreatitis are serious and sometimes fatal. Hyperglycemia results from an imbalance of glucagon, insulin, and somatostatin. Necrosis and hemorrhage of the gland, peritonitis, severe fluid and electrolyte imbalance, shock, pleural effusion, acute respiratory distress syndrome, and blood coagulation problems ensue. When lipase digests fatty tissue around the pancreas, calcium binds with released fatty acids. In rare cases, this reduces the level of circulating calcium to a dangerous degree, resulting in tetany and convulsions. Pancreatic cysts and abscesses also can develop.

Assessment Findings

The most common complaint of clients with pancreatitis is severe mid- to upper-abdominal pain, radiating to both sides and straight to the back. Nausea, vomiting, and flatulence usually are present. The client may describe stools as being frothy and foul-smelling, a sign of **steatorrhea,** increased fat in the stool, from poor fat digestion. Symptoms, which worsen after the client eats fatty foods or drinks alcohol, are relieved when the client sits up and leans forward or curls into a fetal position.

Physical examination may reveal jaundice. Bowel sounds are diminished or absent with accompanying distention, and the abdomen is tender to palpation. The client may be hypotensive, indicating hypovolemia and shock caused by release of large amounts of protein-rich fluid into the tissues and peritoneal cavity. A bluish-gray discoloration to the skin about the umbilicus (**Cullen's sign**) or on the flanks (**Turner's sign**) indicate the injured pancreas is releasing blood. The client may be feverish and tachycardic. Breathing is shallow from severe pain. Chvostek's sign (facial twitching when the skin over the facial nerve is tapped) and Trousseau's sign (spasms of the fingers when a blood pressure cuff is inflated) indicate low calcium levels.

Elevated serum and urine amylase, lipase, and liver enzyme levels accompany significant pancreatitis. If the common bile duct is obstructed, the bilirubin level is above normal. Blood glucose levels and white blood cell counts can be elevated. Serum electrolyte levels (calcium, potassium, and magnesium) are low. Pancreatic edema and necrosis appear on CT scan with vascular enhancement. Various endoscopic examinations and ultrasound assist the differential diagnosis and determine any pancreatic cysts, abscesses, and pseudocysts (fibrous capsules filled with fluid, blood, enzymes, pus, and tissue debris).

Medical and Surgical Management

Medical treatment concentrates on relieving pain, reducing pancreatic secretions, restoring fluid and electrolyte losses, and preventing or treating systemic complications such as respiratory distress syndrome, acute (renal) tubular necrosis, and bleeding abnormalities. The client usually is NPO, and a nasogastric tube is inserted and connected to suction. This relieves nausea, distention, and vomiting and reduces stimulation of the pancreas by gastric contents that otherwise may enter the duodenum. Along with general fluid therapy for hydration purposes, IV albumin may be given to pull fluid trapped in the peritoneum back into circulation. Administration of diuretics is necessary if circulating fluid is excessive.

Atropine or other anticholinergics reduce the activity of the vagus nerve, which stimulates the pancreas. IV antibiotic therapy prevents localized abscesses or treats systemic sepsis. If pseudocysts develop, they are located by CT scan and drained by percutaneous needle aspiration. Improvement, if it is forthcoming, usually occurs in about 1 week. A clear liquid diet is prescribed initially, with slow progression to a low-fat diet. Alcohol, caffeine, and pepper, which are digestive stimulants, are withheld. If pancreatic exocrine function is impaired, pancreatic enzyme replacement therapy is administered with meals to promote digestion.

In severe cases, surgical management involves opening the abdomen to debride necrotic tissue. Every 2 to 3 days, the process is repeated to prevent spread of infection. Multiple sump drains, inserted into the cavity to remove debris, are attached to continuous irrigation (Fig. 49.10). If acute cholecystitis or obstruction of the common duct is thought to be a coincidental or inciting factor, drainage and simple stone removal may be necessary.

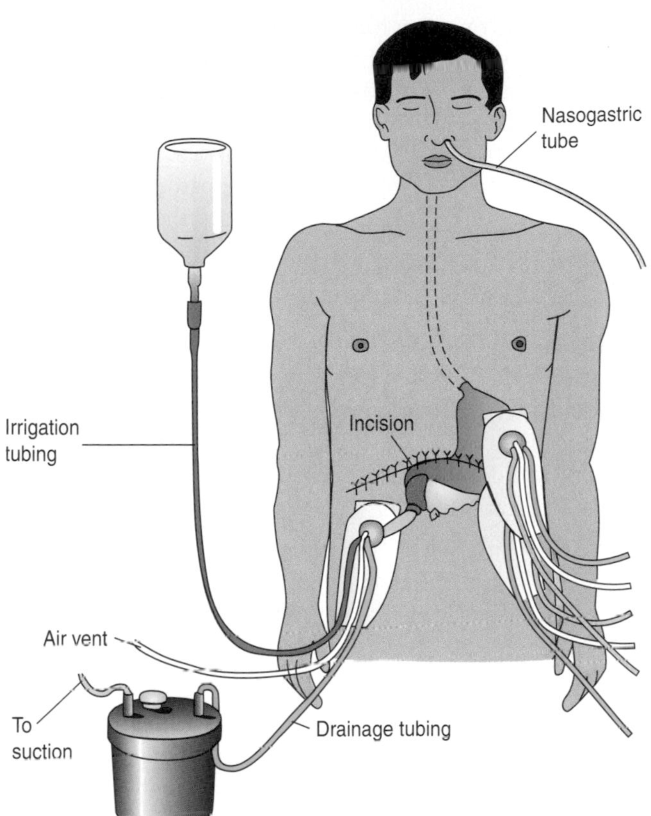

FIGURE 49.10 Multiple sump tubes are used after pancreatic surgery. Triple-lumen tubes consist of ports that provide tubing for irrigation, air venting, and drainage. (From Smeltzer, S. C. & Bare, B. G. [2004]. *Brunner & Suddarth's textbook of medical-surgical nursing* [10th ed.]. Philadelphia: Lippincott Williams & Wilkins.)

Nursing Management

Nursing management involves monitoring the client for life-threatening changes and alcohol withdrawal if substance abuse is part of the client history and performing prescribed treatment measures. Insert a nasogastric tube, maintain its patency, and infuse IV fluids. If gastric decompression is prolonged, the client can receive jejunal feedings of a low-fat formula or TPN. Monitor blood glucose levels closely. Clients with acute pancreatitis require frequent administrations of analgesics. Most clients with acute pancreatitis are severely ill. Continuously monitor intake and output, especially urine volume. If the physician inserts a pulmonary artery or central venous catheter, monitor pressure measurements. Cardiac monitoring is continuous because electrolyte imbalances can produce dysrhythmias. Continue to perform other assessments, including vital signs, lung sounds, serum electrolyte values, and observe for bleeding tendencies. If the client develops severe respiratory problems, he or she may require intubation and mechanical ventilation. Report any sudden change in the client's general condition or symptoms (i.e., pain or abdominal distention) to the physician immediately. When surgery is performed, infuse irrigation solution and ensure that suction is functioning effectively. Provide skin care if pancreatic drainage leaks from sump drain sites.

CHRONIC PANCREATITIS

Pathophysiology and Etiology

Chronic pancreatitis is prolonged and progressive inflammation of the pancreas. In most cases, alcohol is the cause. Alcohol can lead to edema of the duodenum and decrease the tone of the sphincter of Oddi. Consequently, duodenal contents can move into the pancreatic duct. Other causes include hereditary predisposition, hyperparathyroidism, hypertriglyceridemia, autoimmune pancreatitis, trauma, and anatomic abnormalities. In 20% of cases, the cause is not identifiable. With chronicity, the gland undergoes fibrotic scarring from recurring inflammation. The pancreas hardens, and exocrine and endocrine functions are partly or completely lost as pancreatic tissue is destroyed.

Assessment Findings

In chronic pancreatitis, the client has severe to persistent pain, weight loss, and digestive disturbances, such as flatulence, vomiting, and diarrhea. If pseudocysts form, they put pressure on adjacent organs or rupture. If secondary diabetes develops, the client may experience increased appetite, thirst, and urination. A firm mass may be palpated in the upper left quadrant. Urine may be dark; stools may be light-colored and foul-smelling. Fatty streaks appear in the stool. With loss of plasma proteins from the blood, peripheral edema and ascites develop.

Abnormal laboratory findings are the same for chronic pancreatitis as for acute disease. CT scans, MRI, ultrasound, and endoscopic retrograde studies of the pancreas show diagnostic results similar to those in clients with acute pancreatitis. Results of a glucose tolerance test show impaired ability to metabolize carbohydrates because of malfunctioning endocrine cells in the islets of Langerhans.

Medical and Surgical Management

Treatment depends on the cause and whether the pancreatic duct is obstructed. If the duct is not obstructed, treatment consists of abstinence from alcohol; a clear liquid to bland, fat-free diet; and correction of associated biliary tract disease or hyperparathyroidism. The client who adheres to treatment may have good results.

Drug therapy with meperidine (Demerol) is ordered in deference to morphine sulfate (morphine causes spasm of the sphincter of Oddi). Narcotics are used cautiously. The focus is on management of pain using nonopioid methods. Treatment for insulin and digestive enzyme deficiencies includes diet, insulin, and pancreatic enzyme replacement therapy. Such therapy uses pancreatic enzymes, such as pancreatin (Creon, Panazyme, Donnazyme, Entozyme) or pancrelipase (Pancrease, Cotazym, Creon 10 and Creon 20, Protilase, Ultrase, Viokase, Zymase, Pancrecarb), which help digest and absorb fats, proteins, and carbohydrates.

When surgery is part of treatment, some or all of the pancreas (**partial** or **total pancreatectomy**) may be removed. If there is scarring, with stricture and stenosis of portions of the pancreatic duct, various surgical measures are done to try to reconstitute the duct. A pancreaticojejunostomy (joining of the pancreatic duct to the jejunum) can relieve ductal obstruction. Pancreatic autotransplantation is a recent surgical development. It involves excision and relocation of the pancreas. During this procedure, innervation is severed, effectively treating pain symptoms. Although exocrine function is lost, necessitating enzyme replacement, endocrine function and normal insulin production are preserved.

NURSING PROCESS

The Client With Pancreatitis

Assessment

Initial assessment includes a history of symptoms the client experienced before admission as well as a complete medical history. Ask about the frequency and amount of alcohol ingestion and determine when the client had his or her last drink as a method of evaluating if or how soon withdrawal symptoms may occur. Involve family members in compiling assessment data (if possible), especially if the client's condition is serious. During the interview, obtain a description of pain with respect to location, type, severity, and circumstances that aggravate or relieve it. Gently palpate the abdomen, especially the epigastric area, for pain, tenderness, distention, or rigidity.

Include an immediate evaluation of vital signs because shock often is an outstanding symptom of acute pancreatitis. Describe the client's general appearance and inspect the skin for Cullen's and Turner's signs. Periodically weigh the client. Instruct the client to save stool for inspection or laboratory testing. Initiate blood glucose testing.

Diagnosis, Planning, and Interventions

Administer prescribed analgesics. The client may exhibit or develop tolerance as a result of cross-addiction to alcohol or chronic use of analgesics. Monitor for signs of alcohol withdrawal, which may develop within the first 24 hours of admission. Implement measures to manage nutrition and blood glucose levels and administer insulin as indicated. Provide therapeutic skin care to prevent breakdown from frequent, loose stools. If surgery is planned, manage preoperative and postoperative care. Diabetic and diet teaching begin before the client is discharged from the hospital (Client and Family Teaching 49-2). Provide referrals to a community substance abuse rehabilitation program if appropriate.

Pain related to distention, edema, and irritation of the inflamed pancreas

Expected Outcome: Client will report reduced pain.

- Administer analgesics as ordered. *Prompt administration of analgesics provides a therapeutic level of analgesia and promotes pain relief.*
- Withhold oral feedings. *Doing so limits the reflux of bile and duodenal contents into the pancreatic duct, preventing activation of the exocrine enzymes produced by the pancreas.*
- Instruct client to remain on bed rest. *Bed rest reduces metabolic rate and thus decreases secretion of pancreatic and gastric enzymes.*
- Report unrelieved pain or sudden increased intensity of pain. *Increased pain stimulates secretion of pancreatic enzymes. Sudden increased pain may indicate pancreatic rupture.*
- Administer anticholinergic medications as ordered. *They reduce gastric and pancreatic secretions.*
- Maintain continuous nasogastric drainage. *Drainage removes gastric contents and prevents gastric secretions from entering the duodenum.*

Ineffective Breathing Pattern related to severe pain and pancreatic distention, edema, and inflammation

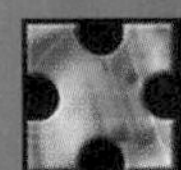

49-2 *Client and Family Teaching* Pancreatitis

Most clients with pancreatitis require a prolonged recovery period. The following instructions are usual:

- Follow the written instructions for a bland, low-fat, calorie-controlled diet.
- Eat four or more small meals daily.
- Take prescribed medications, including enzyme replacements, as directed.
- If alcohol abuse is known to cause acute or chronic pancreatitis, avoid all alcoholic beverages. Strongly consider self-referral to Alcoholics Anonymous or a medical treatment center. Urge the family to attend Al-Anon meetings. (If insulin administration is necessary because of diabetes mellitus, see Chap. 52.)

Expected Outcome: Client will maintain adequate lung function as evidenced by improved breathing patterns and clear lungs.

- Position client with head of bed elevated or in semi-Fowler's position. *These measures reduce pressure on the diaphragm from abdominal distention and promote lung expansion.*
- Reposition client at least every 2 hours. *Repositioning prevents atelectasis and pooling of respiratory secretions.*
- Monitor pulse oximetry. Report episodes of desaturation to physician. *Pulse oximetry helps show changes in respiratory status and promotes early interventions.*
- Encourage client to deep breathe and cough every 2 hours. *Deep breathing and coughing clear the airway and reduce atelectasis.*

Deficient Fluid Volume related to vomiting, decreased fluid intake, fever, diaphoresis, and fluid shifts

Expected Outcome: Client will be adequately hydrated as evidenced by sufficient urine output and normal BP and skin turgor.

- Monitor intake and output at least every 8 hours. *This record can show if fluid loss is excessive.*
- Monitor serum electrolytes and BUN levels. *Findings might indicate a need for fluid and electrolyte replacements.*
- Administer IV fluids and electrolytes as ordered. *Replacing fluids and electrolytes restores fluid balance.*
- Administer plasma, albumin, and blood products as ordered. *Clients with severe pancreatitis lose large amounts of blood and plasma, which decreases effective circulating blood volume.*

Diarrhea related to impaired fat and protein digestion

Expected Outcome: Client experiences decreased diarrhea.

- Monitor number and characteristics of stools. *Such monitoring provides a baseline for determining fluid and electrolyte loss from stools.*
- Maintain low-fat diet if client is allowed food. *Decreased fat intake reduces the amount that the client cannot properly digest.*
- Administer antidiarrheal medications if ordered. *They assist in decreasing diarrhea and, in turn, reduce fluid and electrolyte losses.*

Risk for Injury related to alcohol withdrawal

Expected Outcome: Client remains uninjured with stable vital signs and no seizures.

- Monitor client for signs of CNS stimulation, such as agitation or belligerence. Observe for signs of hand tremors and emotional lability. *Such findings may indicate that the depressant effects of alcohol are wearing off.*
- Report if client's heart rate is over 100 beats/minute, diastolic BP is greater than 100 mm Hg, or temperature is above 100°F (36.6°C). *Such findings may indicate signs of alcohol withdrawal and the need for medical intervention.*
- Minimize environmental stimuli. *Extraneous lights and noise can increase agitation and possibly cause confusion.*
- Administer prescribed sedatives. *They provide appropriate sedation as the client withdraws from the effects of alcohol.*
- Provide a safe environment for the client if he or she is extremely agitated or at risk for seizures. Place client near nurses' station if he or she requires close observation. *Anticipating safety needs prevents harm to the client. If the client is near the nurses' station, the nurses can more closely monitor his or her activities.*
- Pad side rails and keep oral suction available. *If the client has a seizure or becomes extremely agitated, padded side rails, other safety measures, and immediate availability of suction can prevent further injury.*
- If a seizure occurs, initiate seizure precautions by protecting, but not restraining, the client. Observe the client throughout the seizure. After the seizure, ensure that the airway is clear and administer oxygen briefly according to agency policy. *Restraining a client during a seizure can cause more injury. Staying with the client during and after the seizure provides protection for the client and ensures that his or her airway is patent.*

Evaluation of Expected Outcomes

The client reports relief of pain, with increased ability to sleep and rest more comfortably. He or she breathes deeply at a rate of 12 to 20 breaths/minute and maintains adequate pulmonary ventilation, as evidenced by clear lungs and 95% saturation by pulse oximetry. Fluid intake and output are balanced as evidenced by urine output of at least 50 mL/hour and normal BP and skin turgor. The client reports fewer stools and that stools have more form. Alcohol withdrawal occurs without hypertension or seizures.

• CARCINOMA OF THE PANCREAS

Carcinoma of the pancreas may occur in the gland's head, body, or tail. Some tumors are primary lesions, and others are metastases from other locations. Because tumors of the head of the pancreas tend to cause obstructive jaundice, they usually are diagnosed earlier. Most are discovered late in the disease and have a lethal prognosis.

Pathophysiology and Etiology

When sufficient malignant cells accumulate, they block the pancreatic duct, producing symptoms similar to chronic pancreatitis. Pancreatitis may be a precursor or consequence of tumor development. Tumors in the body or tail of the pancreas can press on the portal vein and lead to formation of varices and bleeding. Tumors tend to grow rapidly. When symptoms are serious enough for the client to seek medical assistance, the tumor may have spread to adjacent structures, such as the liver or spleen.

Besides pancreatitis, factors that correlate with pancreatic cancer include diabetes mellitus, a high-fat diet, and chronic exposure to carcinogenic substances (i.e., petrochemicals). A relationship may exist between cigarette smoking and high coffee consumption (especially decaffeinated coffee) and development of pancreatic carcinoma.

Assessment Findings

Symptoms may not appear until the disease is far advanced. The most common symptoms are left upper abdominal pain that may be referred to the back, jaundice, anorexia, and weight loss. The client may describe light-colored stools but dark urine, typical symptoms of obstructive jaundice. Pruritus may accompany jaundice.

A mass may be palpated in the left upper quadrant, which may be a tumor or an enlarged gallbladder that expands as a result of obstructed passage of bile. Ascites may be present in late stages of the disease.

Abdominal ultrasonography or CT scan demonstrates pancreatic enlargement. A biopsy obtained by ERCP or percutaneous needle aspiration provides evidence of malignant cells.

Elevated serum amylase, alkaline phosphatase, and bilirubin levels indicate that the pancreas is diseased but do not confirm carcinoma. The level of carcinoembryonic antigen is elevated, but this elevation is a less specific tumor marker than is CA 19–9.

Medical and Surgical Management

Prognosis is poor. Resection of a tumor at the head of the pancreas is possible by **radical pancreatoduodenectomy (Whipple procedure)** (Fig. 49.11). This surgical procedure involves removing the head of the pancreas, resecting the duodenum and stomach, and redirecting flow of secretions from the stomach, gallbladder, and pancreas into the jejunum. The tumor may be irradiated during surgery, or radioactive seeds may be implanted. Because metastasis to the spleen is so common, some surgeons also may perform a splenectomy. Rather than do an extensive resection, others are inclined to do a total pancreatectomy. This creates a malabsorption syndrome and historically brittle diabetes, which must be treated after surgery. Some complications associated with this surgery include bleeding tendencies caused by a vitamin K deficiency and liver and kidney failure.

A cholecystojejunostomy, a rerouting of pancreatic and biliary drainage, may be done to relieve obstructive jaundice. This measure is palliative only. For inoperable tumors, radiation therapy or chemotherapy with 5-fluorouracil (5-FU) or mitomycin (Mutamycin) may be tried. These treatments do not cure the disease. Despite surgery, chemotherapy, or radiation therapy, most clients die within 3 to 12 months after the onset of symptoms.

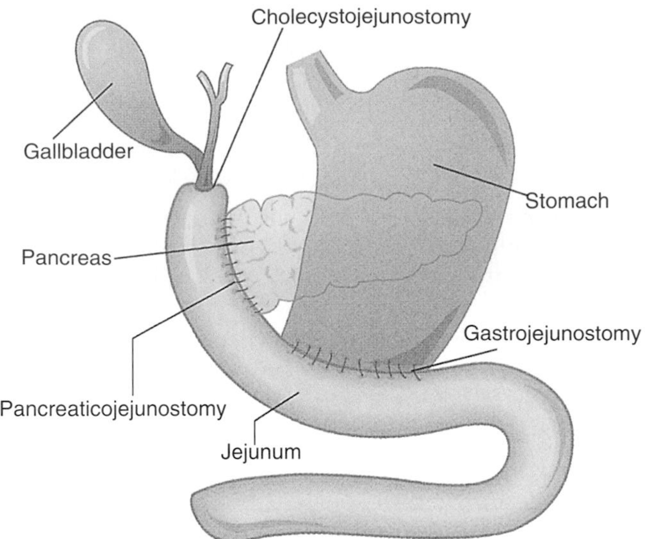

FIGURE 49.11 Radical pancreatoduodenectomy (Whipple's procedure). (From Smeltzer, S. C. & Bare, B. G. [2004]. *Brunner & Suddarth's textbook of medical-surgical nursing* [10th ed.]. Philadelphia: Lippincott Williams & Wilkins.)

Nursing Management

Nursing management for those treated medically is the same as for any client with a terminal malignant disorder (see Chap. 19). Clients undergoing palliative surgery require care similar to that of clients having general abdominal surgery. If clients have severe anorexia and weight loss, they are poor risks for immediate surgery. These clients may receive preoperative IV fluids, TPN, or a special diet to improve nutritional status and correct fluid or electrolyte imbalances. Most surgical clients have a nasogastric tube inserted. Once biliary obstruction is relieved, color of skin, stools, and urine returns to near normal. Clients undergoing the Whipple procedure or one of its variations require more intensive nursing management because of the profoundly invasive nature of the procedure.

Evaluate the client's general physical condition and obtain a history of all symptoms present before admission. Ask about the onset of symptoms, weight loss, bleeding tendencies, and the type of pain or abdominal discomfort. Physical examination includes inspection for jaundice, visual examination of stools and urine, and palpation of the abdomen for tenderness and distention. Laboratory tests include blood or urine samples for analysis and detection of glucose. Record vital signs and weight and assess nutritional status.

Observe the client after surgery for complications such as shock, pancreatic abscess formation, and hemorrhage. Immediate postoperative assessments include vital signs and a review of the chart for the type and extent of surgery. Check the surgical dressing and all drains and tubes for patency, as well as noting amount and color of drainage throughout the entire postoperative course.

Observe for signs of bleeding, such as easy bruising, blood in the urine or stool, or bleeding from the incision, drains, or tubes. Monitor for signs of infection (elevated temperature, increased pain, abdominal distention, abdominal tenderness, and purulent drainage from the incisional site).

The surgery for carcinoma of the pancreas is very serious, with potentially major complications and poor outcomes. Nursing diagnoses can include the following:

- **Acute Pain** related to surgical procedure
- **Deficient Fluid Volume** related to hemorrhage and loss of fluids
- **Ineffective Breathing Pattern** related to abdominal discomfort and drainage tubes
- **Risk for Infection** related to invasive procedure and poor physical condition
- **Risk for Imbalanced Nutrition: Less than Body Requirements** related to high metabolic requirements and decreased ability to digest food
- **Risk for Injury** related to failure to consume adequate calories or get enough insulin
- **Anticipatory Grieving** related to shortened life span and poor prognosis

Care for clients with pancreatic tumors also must include psychological and emotional support. If the client is discharged home, he or she and family members require extensive teaching and home health services. The teaching plan should address schedules and techniques for administering prescribed medications, how to check blood glucose level, recommended diet, importance of drinking fluids and eating, skin care (particularly around the incision), and future schedule for follow-up visits, radiation therapy, or chemotherapy. Review with the client and family symptoms to report to the physician: jaundice, dark urine, bleeding tendencies, vomiting, tarry stools, increased pain, swelling of the extremities, abdominal enlargement, decreased urine output, weight loss, and calf pain.

GENERAL GERONTOLOGIC CONSIDERATIONS

Although hepatitis A commonly is found in younger people, older adults may contract hepatitis through contact with younger people who have the disease, such as grandchildren, waiters, or supermarket or nursing home employees.

Older adults may recover more slowly from surgery on the gallbladder. They also are more prone to develop postoperative complications, such as pneumonia and thrombophlebitis, because of an inability to move about in bed, adequately perform deep breathing exercises, and ambulate shortly after surgery.

Disease of the gallbladder is common in older adults. Incidence of gallstones is greater in older women than in men. Approximately 33% of abdominal surgeries performed in adults older than 70 years of age are for disorders of the gallbladder and biliary tree.

With age, the liver loses weight, becomes more fibrous, and takes on a brownish color. However, function is not significantly affected unless disease is present.

Although recurrent severe pain is the predominant symptom of chronic hepatitis in young to middle-aged adults, older adults report pain with chronic hepatitis as mild or absent.

Hepatitis B vaccination is not routinely given to older adults. In general, older adults should receive the vaccine only if they are traveling to areas where they may be exposed to the disease. Immunogenicity is somewhat reduced in the older adult.

Critical Thinking Exercises

1. *A client has jaundice. What questions can you use to help determine the cause?*
2. *How would you reassure someone who is interested in becoming a nurse, yet has reservations because of potentially acquiring a blood-borne disease, such as hepatitis B?*
3. *What are the differences between a laparoscopic cholecystectomy and an open cholecystectomy?*

● NCLEX-STYLE REVIEW QUESTIONS 

1. A nursing supervisor is assessing the client population in the intensive care unit for potential transfers to the medical-surgical floor. All the following clients were admitted on the same day. Which would the nursing supervisor identify as the last to leave?
   1. A client diagnosed with Hepatitis B
   2. A client diagnosed with esophageal varices
   3. A client diagnosed with acute pancreatitis
   4. A client diagnosed with acute cholecystitis
2. Which assessment finding in a client with hepatic encephalopathy is most indicative of an increased ammonia level?
   1. Vomiting
   2. Anuria
   3. Jaundice
   4. Confusion
3. A client is being moved from the operating room stretcher to a bed following an open cholecystectomy with T-tube placement. Which instruction to the nurse's aide is most correct regarding positioning of the T-tube collector?
   1. Place the T-tube collector to the side below the incision.
   2. Secure the T-tube collector on the top of the abdomen.
   3. Dangle the T-tube collector over the bedside.
   4. Tape the T-tube collector to the thigh.

connection

Visit the Connection site at **http://connection.lww.com/go/timbyEssentials** for links to chapter-related resources on the Internet.

References and Suggested Readings

Aronson, B. S. (1999). Update on acute pancreatitis. *MEDSURG Nursing, 8,* 9–16.

Chene, B. L., & Decker, A. P. (2001). Battling hepatitis C. *RN, 64*(4), 54–58.

Elta, G. H. (1999). Approach to the patient with gross gastrointestinal bleeding: Acute upper gastrointestinal bleeding. In T. Yamada, D. H. Alpers, C. Owyang, L. Laine, & D. W. Powell (Eds.), *Textbook of gastroenterology.* Philadelphia: Lippincott Williams & Wilkins.

Farrar, J. A., & Kearney, K. (2001). Acute cholecystitis. *American Journal of Nursing, 101*(1), 35–36.

Fischbach, F. (2000). *A manual of laboratory and diagnostic tests* (6th ed.). Philadelphia: Lippincott Williams & Wilkins.

Heer, E. (March/April 2002). Hepatitis C: A public health dilemma. *Community Health Forum,* 34–37.

Holcomb, S. S. (2002). Hepatitis, part 1: Which types are trouble? *Nursing 2002, 32*(6), 32cc 1–4.

Holcomb, S. S. (2002). Hepatitis, part 2: How to support your patient. *Nursing 2002, 32*(7), 32cc 1–3.

Holcomb, S. S. (2000). Reviewing acute pancreatitis. *Nursing 2000, 30*(4), 32–35.

Klainberg, M. (1999). Clinical snapshot: Primary biliary cirrhosis. *American Journal of Nursing, 99*(12), 38–39.

Krumberger, J. (2002). When the liver fails. *RN, 65*(2), 26–29.

McConnell, E. A. (2002). Managing a T-tube. *Nursing 2002, 32*(6), 17.

Parini, S. (2003). Hepatitis C: Update your knowledge of this silent stalker. *Nursing 2003, 33*(4), 57–63.

Porth, C. M. (2002). *Pathophysiology: Concepts of altered states* (6th ed.). Philadelphia: Lippincott Williams & Wilkins.

Smeltzer, S. C., & Bare, B. G. (2004). *Brunner & Suddarth's textbook of medical–surgical nursing* (10th ed.). Philadelphia: Lippincott Williams & Wilkins.

Tasota, F. J. (2000). Eye on diagnostics: Reading liver function values. *Nursing 2000, 30*(6), 73–75.

Warren, M. L. (1999). Taking a hard look at cirrhosis. *Nursing 99, 29*(12), 32–34.

chapter 50

Introduction to the Endocrine System

Words to Know 

adrenal cortex
adrenal glands
adrenal medulla
adrenocorticotropic hormone
antidiuretic hormone
calcitonin
corticosteroids
estrogen
feedback loop
follicle-stimulating hormone
glucagon
glycogenolysis
hormones
hypophysis
hypothalamus
insulin
islets of Langerhans
luteinizing hormone
melatonin
nuclear scan
ovaries
oxytocin
pancreas
parathormone
parathyroid glands
pineal gland
pituitary gland
progesterone
prolactin
radioimmunoassay
radionuclide
somatotropin
testes
testosterone
tetraiodothyronine
thymosin
thymus gland
thyroid gland
thyroid-stimulating hormone
triiodothyronine

Learning Objectives

On completion of this chapter, the reader will:

- Identify the chief function of the endocrine glands.
- Describe the general function of hormones.
- Explain the relationship between the hypothalamus and pituitary gland.
- Discuss regulation of levels of hormones.
- List endocrine glands and the hormones they secrete.
- Outline information needed for a health history of a client with an endocrine disorder.
- Describe physical assessment findings that suggest an endocrine disorder.
- List examples of laboratory and diagnostic tests that identify endocrine disorders.
- Discuss nursing management of clients undergoing diagnostic tests to detect endocrine dysfunction.

The endocrine glands (Fig. 50.1) secrete **hormones,** chemicals that accelerate or slow physiologic processes, directly into the bloodstream. This characteristic distinguishes endocrine glands from exocrine glands, which release secretions into a duct. Hormones circulate in the blood until they reach receptors in target cells or other endocrine glands. They play a vital role in regulating homeostatic processes such as metabolism, growth, fluid and electrolyte balance, reproductive processes, and sleep and wake cycles. Table 50.1 presents an overview of the hormones involved in the endocrine system.

Stop, Think, and Respond • BOX 50-1

Give an example of hormones that affect metabolism, growth, fluid and electrolyte balance, reproductive processes, and sleep and wake cycles.

ANATOMY AND PHYSIOLOGY

Pituitary Gland

Many endocrine glands respond to stimulation from the **pituitary gland** (or **hypophysis**), connected by a stalk to the **hypothalamus** in the brain (Fig. 50.2). The pituitary gland is called the *master gland* because it regulates the function of other endocrine glands. The term is misleading, because the hypothalamus influences the pituitary gland.

Hypothalamus

The hypothalamus, a portion of the brain between the cerebrum and the brain stem, stimulates and inhibits the pituitary gland. It sends nerve impulses to the posterior

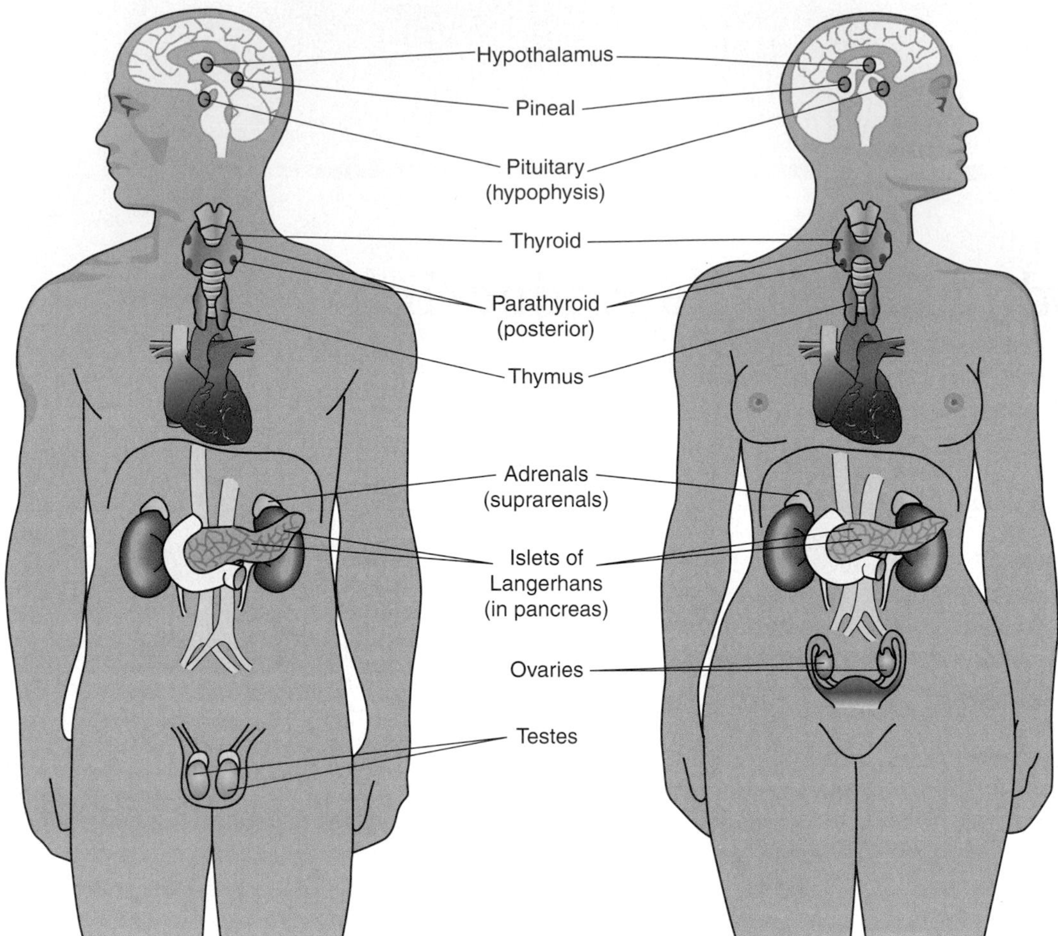

FIGURE 50.1 The glands of the endocrine system. (From Smeltzer, S. C. & Bare, B. G. [2004]. *Brunner & Suddarth's textbook of medical–surgical nursing* [10th ed.]. Philadelphia: Lippincott Williams & Wilkins.)

lobe of the pituitary gland and releasing factors to the anterior lobe. When stimulated, each lobe secretes various hormones.

Hormone Regulation

A feedback loop controls hormone levels. A **feedback loop** is a mechanism that turns hormone production off and on (Fig. 50.3). Feedback can be either negative or positive. Most hormones are secreted in response to negative feedback; a decrease in levels stimulates the releasing gland. In positive feedback the opposite occurs, keeping concentrations of hormones within a stable range at all times. Most endocrine disorders result from overproduction or underproduction of specific hormones.

Thyroid Gland

The **thyroid gland** is located in the lower neck anterior to the trachea (Fig. 50.4). It is divided into two lateral lobes joined by a band of tissue called the *isthmus.* The thyroid concentrates iodine from food and uses it to synthesize **tetraiodothyronine** (thyroxine or T_4) and **triiodothyronine** (T_3). These two hormones regulate the body's metabolic rate. Another hormone, **calcitonin,** inhibits release of calcium from bone into extracellular fluid. A rise in the serum calcium level stimulates release of calcitonin from the thyroid gland.

Parathyroid Glands

The **parathyroid glands** are four small, bean shaped bodies embedded in the lateral lobes of the thyroid (Fig. 50.5). The upper parathyroids are found posteriorly at the junction of the upper and middle thirds of the thyroid. The lower parathyroids typically lie among the branches of the inferior thyroid artery. They secrete **parathormone,** which regulates metabolism of calcium and phosphorus.

Thymus Gland

The **thymus gland** is located in the upper part of the chest above or near the heart. It secretes **thymosin,** which aids in developing T lymphocytes, a type of white blood cell involved in immunity (see Chap. 35). The thymus gland

TABLE 50.1 ENDOCRINE HORMONES

GLAND	HORMONE RELEASED	HORMONE FUNCTION	HORMONE REGULATOR
Posterior pituitary	**Antidiuretic hormone** (ADH)	Increases water absorption from kidney; raises blood pressure	Hypothalamic secretions, blood osmolarity
	Oxytocin	Stimulates contraction of pregnant uterus and release of breast milk after childbirth	Hypothalamic secretions, uterine stretch, suckling
Anterior pituitary	**Somatotropin** (growth hormone)	Stimulates bone and muscle growth; promotes protein synthesis and fat mobilization	Hypothalamic secretions
	Prolactin	Promotes production and secretion of milk after childbirth	Hypothalamic hormones
	Thyroid-stimulating hormone (TSH)	Stimulates production and secretion of thyroid hormones	Blood thyroxine levels; hypothalamic secretions
	Adrenocorticotropic hormone (ACTH)	Stimulates adrenal cortex to secrete cortisol and other steroids	Corticotropin-releasing hormone (CRH) from the hypothalamus; blood cortisol levels
	Luteinizing hormone (LH) in females and interstitial cell–stimulating hormone (ICSH) in males	Initiates ovulation and the secretion of sex hormones in both genders	Hypothalamic secretions, estrogen and testosterone levels
	Follicle-stimulating hormone (FSH)	Stimulates development of ovum in ovaries and sperm in testes	Hypothalamic secretions, progesterone
Thyroid	Tetraiodothyronine (thyroxine or T_4 and triiodothyronine or T_3)	Increases oxygen consumption and heat production; stimulates, increases, and maintains metabolic processes	TSH regulated by thyrotropin-releasing hormone (TRH) from the hypothalamus
	Calcitonin	Inhibits calcium release from bone, thus lowering blood calcium levels	Blood calcium concentrations
Parathyroids	Parathyroid hormone (PTH)	Increases blood calcium by stimulating calcium release from bone; decreases blood phosphate level	Calcium concentrations in blood
Thymus	Several thymosin and thymopoietin hormones; thymic humoral factor; thymostimulin; factor thymic serum	Stimulates T-cell development in thymus and maintenance in other lymph tissue; involved in some B cells developing into antibody-producing plasma cells	Not known
Pineal gland	Melatonin	Involved in circadian rhythms; antigonadotropic effect; exposure to light decreases release	Exposure to light–dark cycles
Adrenal medulla	Epinephrine (adrenaline)	Constricts blood vessels in skin, kidneys, and gut, which increases blood supply to heart, brain, and skeletal muscles, leads to increased heart rate and blood pressure; stimulates smooth muscle contraction; raises blood glucose levels	Sympathetic nervous system
	Norepinephrine	Constricts blood vessels; increases heart rate and contraction of cardiac muscles; increases metabolic rate	Sympathetic nervous system

(continued)

TABLE 50.1 ENDOCRINE HORMONES (Continued)

GLAND	HORMONE RELEASED	HORMONE FUNCTION	HORMONE REGULATOR
Adrenal cortex	Corticosteroids Glucocorticoids	Regulates blood glucose by affecting carbohydrate metabolism; affects growth; decreases effects of stress and anti-inflammatory agents	ACTH; stress and serum electrolyte concentrations
	Mineralocorticoids (mainly aldosterone)	Regulates sodium, water, and potassium excretion by the kidney	Renin and angiotensin
	Gonadocorticoids (mainly androgens—male sex hormones)	Contributes to secondary sex characteristics (particularly after menopause)	ACTH
Pancreas (islets of Langerhans)	Insulin	Lowers blood sugar; increases glycogen storage in liver; stimulates protein synthesis	Blood glucose concentrations
	Glucagon	Stimulates glycogen breakdown in liver; increases blood sugar (glucose) concentration	Blood glucose and amino acid concentration
Ovary follicle	Estrogens	Develops and maintains female sex organs and characteristics; initiates building of uterine lining	FSH and LH
Ovary (corpus luteum)	Progesterone and estrogens	Influences breast development and menstrual cycles; promotes growth and differentiation of uterine lining; maintains pregnancy	FSH
Testes	Androgens (mainly testosterone)	Develops and maintains male sex organs and characteristics; aid sperm production.)	FSH and ICSH

Note: Words in bold type are key terms.
(Adapted from Campbell, N. A. [1996]. *Biology* [4th ed.]. Redwood City, CA: Benjamin/Cummings.)

is large during childhood but usually shrinks by adulthood. Functional disorders of the gland are rare.

Pineal Gland

The **pineal gland** is attached to the thalamus in the brain. It secretes **melatonin,** which aids in regulating sleep cycles and mood (see Chap. 15). Melatonin is believed to play a role in hypothalamic–pituitary interaction.

Adrenal Glands

The **adrenal glands** are located above the kidneys (Fig. 50.6). The outer portion is called the *cortex,* and the

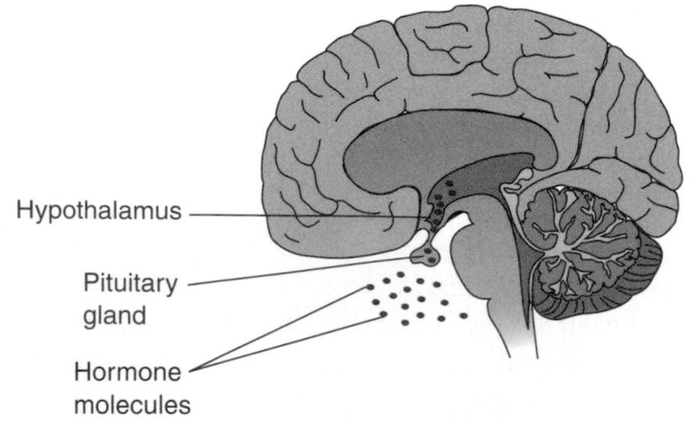

FIGURE 50.2 The hypothalamus regulates pituitary activity.

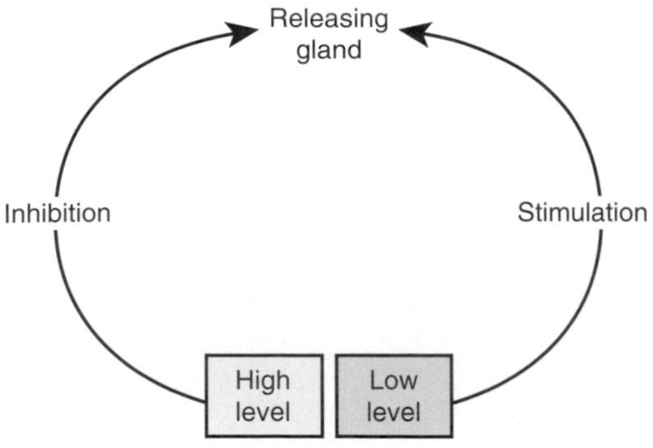

FIGURE 50.3 A feedback loop regulates hormone levels.

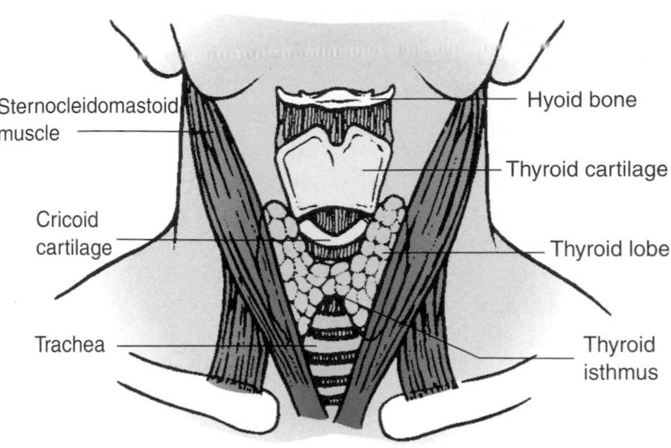

FIGURE 50.4 The thyroid gland and surrounding structures. (From Weber, J. W. & Kelley, J. [2003]. *Health assessment in nursing* [2nd ed.]. Philadelphia: Lippincott Williams & Wilkins.)

inner portion is the *medulla,* both of which secrete specific hormones.

The **adrenal cortex** manufactures and secretes glucocorticoids, mineralocorticoids, and small amounts of sex hormones, called **corticosteroids.** Glucocorticoids and mineralocorticoids are essential to life and influence many organs and structures of the body. Glucocorticoids affect body metabolism, suppress inflammation, and help the body withstand stress. Mineralocorticoids, primarily aldosterone, maintain water and electrolyte (sodium, potassium, chloride) balances.

The **adrenal medulla** secretes epinephrine and norepinephrine, which are released in response to stress or threat to life. They facilitate what has been referred to as the *fight-or-flight response.* Many organs respond to

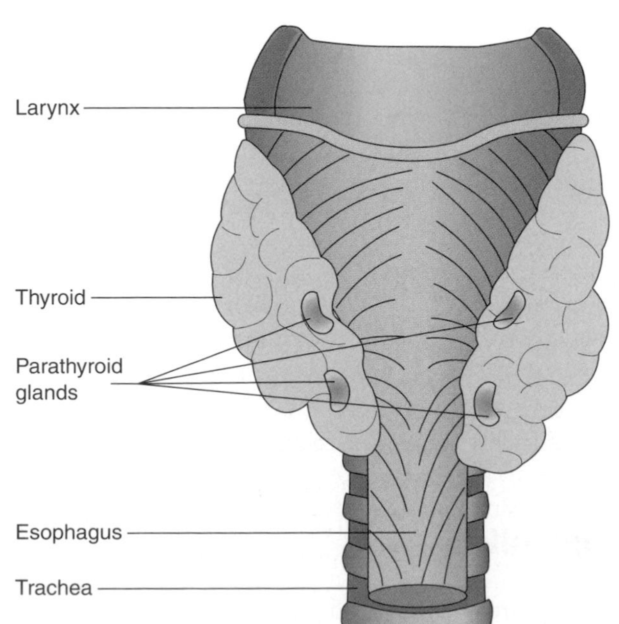

FIGURE 50.5 The parathyroid glands.

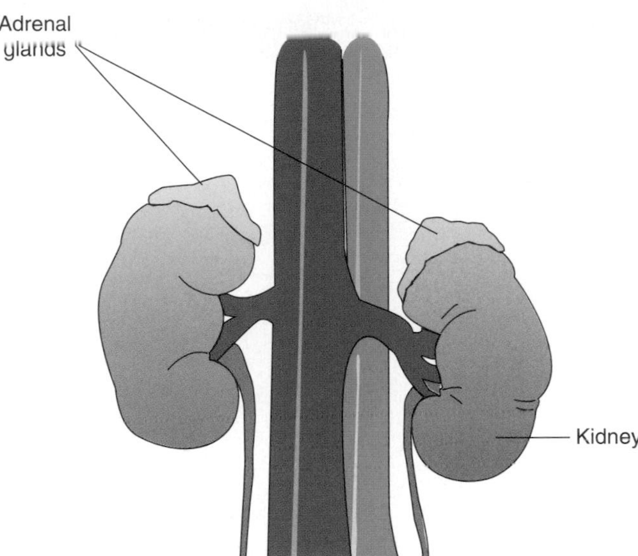

FIGURE 50.6 The adrenal glands sit on top of each kidney. (From Porth, C. M. [2002]. *Pathophysiology: Concepts of altered health states* [6th ed.]. Philadelphia: Lippincott Williams & Wilkins.)

release of epinephrine and norepinephrine. Responses include increased blood pressure and pulse rate, dilation of pupils, constriction of blood vessels, bronchodilation, and decreased peristalsis.

Pancreas

The **pancreas** lies below the stomach, with the head of the gland close to the duodenum (Fig. 50.7). It is both an exocrine and an endocrine gland. The exocrine portion secretes digestive enzymes that the common bile duct carries to the small intestine. The hormone-secreting cells of the pancreas, called the **islets of Langerhans,** release insulin and glucagon. **Insulin** is a hormone necessary for metabolism of glucose. **Glucagon** increases blood sugar levels by stimulating **glycogenolysis,** the breakdown of glycogen into glucose, in the liver. Together, glucagon and insulin maintain a relatively constant level of blood sugar.

Ovaries and Testes

The sex glands, the female **ovaries** and the male **testes,** are important in development of secondary sex characteristics, manufacture of hormones, and development of the ovum (female) and sperm (male).

Testes produce the hormone **testosterone,** which is involved with development and maintenance of male secondary sex characteristics, such as facial hair and a deep voice. Ovaries produce **estrogen** and **progesterone.** The functions and roles of these hormones are discussed in Chapters 53 and 55.

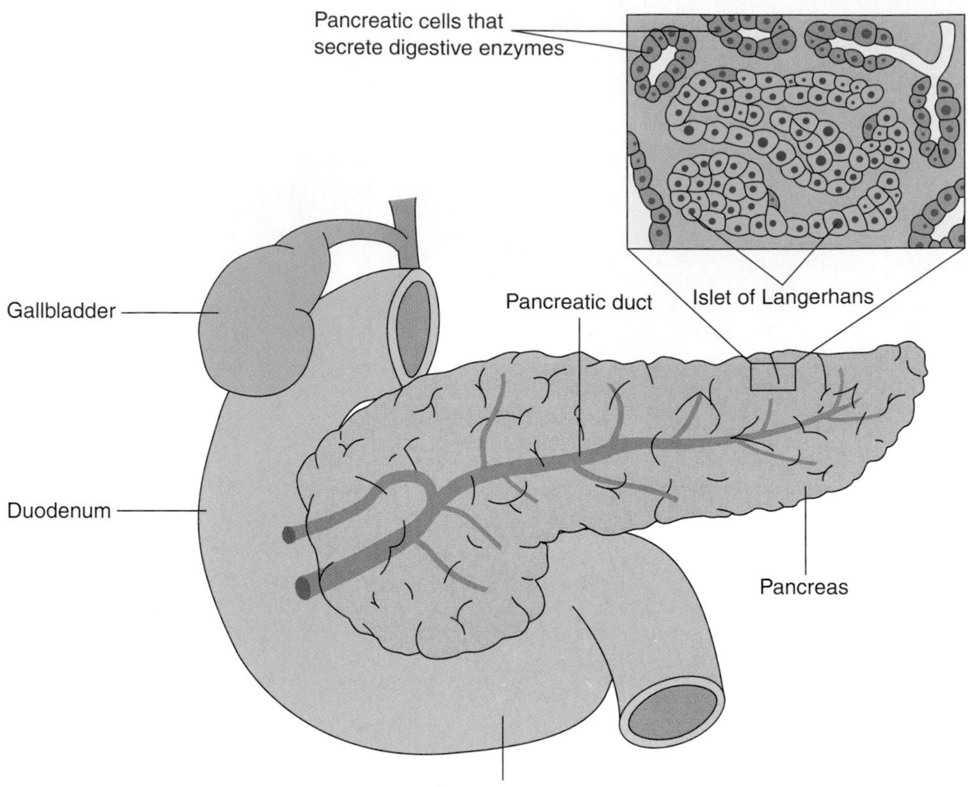

FIGURE 50.7 The pancreas secretes hormones from the isles (singular, islet) of Langerhans. Digestive enzymes are released from the common bile duct.

ASSESSMENT

History

The health history is important in diagnosing many endocrine disorders. Some are inherited or have a tendency to occur in families; therefore, a complete family history is needed. Also obtain diet and drug histories.

Document an allergy to iodine, a component of contrast dyes, or seafood, and inform the physician. Report whether the client has had a test that used iodine (e.g., intravenous pyelography, gallbladder series) within the past 3 months. This information is essential before initiating a thyroid test. Identify current symptoms, which can be vague or resemble other physical or mental disorders. Examples are fatigue, personality changes, inability to sleep, and frequent urination. At other times, symptoms are dramatic, such as a change in mental acuity or sudden weight loss.

Physical Examination

Obtain the client's height, weight, and vital signs and note his or her general physical appearance. Examine body structures to detect evidence of hypersecretion or hyposecretion of hormones (see Chaps. 51 and 52 for assessment findings unique to specific endocrine glands). Inspect the skin for excessive oiliness, dryness, excessive or absent areas of pigmentation, excessive hair growth or loss, and skin breaks that heal poorly. Examine shape and color of the nails and determine whether they are thin, thick, or brittle. Examine the eyes for *exophthalmos,* abnormal bulging or protrusion of eyes (Fig. 50.8), and periorbital swelling. Observe the client's facial expression and general features. Inspect the neck for thyroid enlargement and gently palpate the thyroid gland (Fig. 50.9). Repeated or forceful palpation of the thyroid can result in a sudden release of a large amount of thyroid hormones, which can have serious implications. Note the pulse rate and rhythm. Examine the extremities for edema and changes in pigmentation, auscultate the lungs for abnormal sounds, and examine outstretched hands for tremors. Also determine if the client has experienced any loss of motor function or decreased sensitivity to pain or touch in the extremities.

Assess the client's mental and emotional status and evaluate his or her demeanor (e.g., dull, apathetic, extremely nervous). Determine the client's ability to process information and respond to questions.

Diagnostic Tests

The type and extent of laboratory and diagnostic testing depends on the tentative medical diagnosis. Because phys-

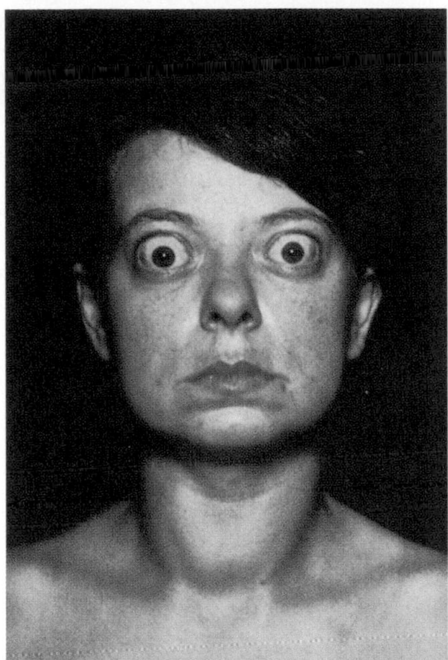

FIGURE 50.8 Exophthalmos in a person with hyperthyroidism. (From Rubin, E. & Farber, J. L. [1999]. *Pathology* [3rd ed.]. Philadelphia: Lippincott Williams & Wilkins.)

ical symptoms may be vague, multiple and varied laboratory tests may be necessary to ultimately determine the etiology of the client's symptoms. A complete blood count and chemistry profile are done to determine the client's general status and to rule out disorders.

Hormone Levels

Measuring blood hormone levels helps evaluate the functioning of some endocrine glands. These tests include cortisol levels (morning and evening) to determine adrenal hyperfunction or hypofunction, antidiuretic hormone (ADH) levels to determine presence or absence of ADH, testosterone levels to detect increased or decreased total testosterone levels, and total thyroxine to identify diseases associated with increased or decreased thyroid hormone levels.

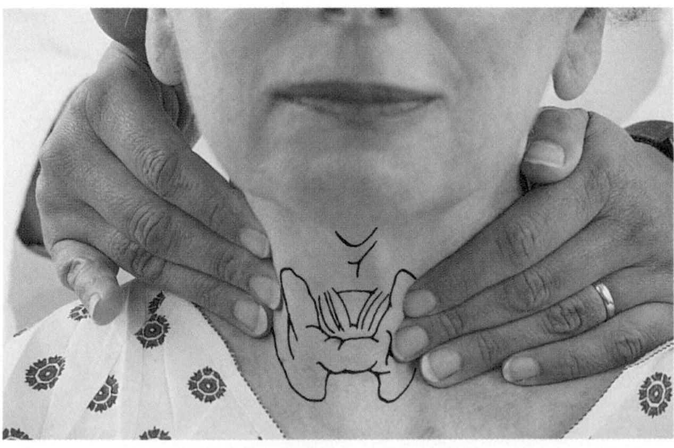

FIGURE 50.9 With the head slightly tilted to the side and the fingers laterally displacing the thyroid, the thyroid is palpated as the person swallows. The examination is repeated on the opposite side.

Radiography, Computed Tomography Scan, Magnetic Resonance Imaging

Chest or abdominal radiographs can detect tumors as well as determine organ size and placement. A computed tomography (CT) or magnetic resonance imaging scan is done to detect a suspected pituitary tumor or to identify calcifications or tumors of the parathyroid glands.

Radionuclide Studies

A **radionuclide** is an atom with an unstable nucleus that emits electromagnetic radiation as alpha, beta, or gamma particles. A radioactive iodine uptake test (RAI, ^{131}I uptake) or thyroid-stimulating hormone test are radionuclide studies done to determine thyroid function.

A **radioimmunoassay** determines concentration of a substance in plasma. Venous blood samples are required for radioimmunoassay tests. A radioactively labeled substance (e.g., hormone, protein, antibodies, antigens) is combined in the laboratory with a blood sample to determine quantity of the substance to be identified. For example, a T_3 determination by radioimmunoassay evaluates thyroid function.

A **nuclear scan** uses a radioactive substance that is taken orally or injected intravenously. The dose of the radioactive substance is larger than the dose used for radionuclide studies. Certain endocrine organs are visualized or their activity determined by means of special equipment. Examples of scans include thyroid scan, adrenergic tumor scan, and parathyroid scan.

NURSING MANAGEMENT

Prepare the client for laboratory and diagnostic testing. Explain the general purpose of the test, type of test, and how it will be done. Encourage the client and family to ask questions and discuss the results with the physician.

Nurses must consult the institution's procedure manual and physician's orders for the required preparation for each diagnostic procedure. Some tests, such as a CT scan, require no special preparation other than a general explanation. Some tests require fasting; others require temporary elimination of certain foods from the diet.

Explain to the client how to participate in the test. For example, some tests require the client to save all voided urine for some time or to return for additional testing. If a client is anxious about the use of radioactive materials for tests, offer assurance that these substances are safe and ordinarily pose no danger to the client or others.

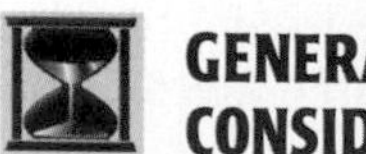

GENERAL GERONTOLOGIC CONSIDERATIONS

Older adults may forget the instructions for a diagnostic test. Nurses may give printed directions to outpatients and, when possible, review them with a family member. This is especially important if test preparation or participation in the test is complicated.

When obtaining a drug history before a diagnostic examination in an older adult, it may be necessary to consult a family member or the caregiver to confirm drugs the client is taking or those he or she has taken within the last several months.

Critical Thinking Exercises

1. *Explain why the pituitary gland is considered the master gland. Give some examples that support the terminology.*
2. *Discuss the meaning and purpose of a feedback loop.*

• NCLEX-STYLE REVIEW QUESTIONS

1. A client diagnosed with parathormone deficiency is admitted to the hospital. As the nurse initiates the care plan, which body system should be the focus of care?
   1. Skeletal
   2. Urinary
   3. Respiratory
   4. Integumentary
2. The nurse takes vital signs for a client scheduled for open heart surgery in the next few minutes and notes that the client's pulse, respirations, and blood pressure are elevated. The nurse explains to the client that the elevations are a normal response to stress and anxiety and are the result of the release of which hormone?
   1. Epinephrine
   2. Insulin
   3. Thyroxine
   4. Aldosterone
3. The nurse gently palpates the neck of a client diagnosed with a thyroid disorder. The client asks why the nurse's touch is so gentle. Which response by the nurse is most appropriate?
   1. "Forceful palpitation can result in increased thyroid hormone, causing thyroid storm."
   2. "This type of palpation is the way my instructor in nursing school taught me how to do it."
   3. "Gentle palpation prevents closing off the trachea, which would cause you to gasp for air."
   4. "Forceful palpation causes pain in an area that is already enlarged and tender to touch."

connection—

Visit the Connection site at **http://connection.lww.com/go/timbyEssentials** for links to chapter-related resources on the Internet.

References and Suggested Readings

A quick check of the endocrine system. (2000). *Nursing 2000, 30*(8), Critical Care, 32cc10–32cc11.

Bullock, B. L., & Henze, R. L. (2000). *Focus on pathophysiology.* Philadelphia: Lippincott Williams & Wilkins.

Cohen, B. J., & Wood, D. L. (2000). *Memmler's structure and function of the human body* (7th ed.). Philadelphia: Lippincott Williams & Wilkins.

Fischbach, F. T. (2004). *A manual of laboratory diagnostic tests* (7th ed.). Philadelphia: Lippincott Williams & Wilkins.

Fuller, J., & Schaller-Ayers, J. (1999). *Health assessment: A nursing approach* (3rd ed.). Philadelphia: Lippincott Williams & Wilkins.

Porth, C. M. (2002). *Pathophysiology: Concepts of altered health states* (6th ed.). Philadelphia: Lippincott Williams & Wilkins.

Watson, R. (2000). Assessing endocrine system function in older people. *Nursing Older People, 12*(9), 27–28.

chapter 51

Caring for Clients With Disorders of the Endocrine System

Words to Know

acromegaly
addisonian crisis
adrenalectomy
adrenal insufficiency
carpopedal spasm
Chvostek's sign
cushingoid syndrome
Cushing's syndrome
diabetes insipidus
goiter
hyperparathyroidism
hyperplasia
hyperthyroidism
hypoparathyroidism
hypophysectomy
hypothyroidism
myxedema
syndrome of inappropriate antidiuretic hormone secretion
tetany
thyroiditis
thyrotoxic crisis
Trousseau's sign

Learning Objectives

On completion of this chapter the reader will:

- Describe the physiologic effects of hyposecretion and hypersecretion of the pituitary, thyroid, parathyroid, and adrenal glands.
- Identify assessment findings for clients experiencing endocrine disorders.
- Discuss basic nursing management of clients experiencing endocrine disorders.
- Identify symptoms of emergency conditions resulting from endocrine disorders.
- Discuss use of the nursing process in the management of a client with hypothyroidism, hyperthyroidism, Addison's disease, and diabetes insipidus.

A disorder of any endocrine gland can profoundly affect other endocrine glands, as well as many major body systems. When caring for clients with endocrine disorders, the nurse must consider management of the endocrine disorder and the effects of the disorder on other organs and systems.

DISORDERS OF THE PITUITARY GLAND

Pituitary disorders usually result from excessive or deficient production and secretion of a specific hormone. When oversecretion of growth hormone (GH) occurs before puberty (when ends [epiphyses] of long bones are fully united), *gigantism* results. *Dwarfism* occurs when secretion of GH is insufficient during childhood. Refer to a pediatric text for further discussion of gigantism and dwarfism.

• ACROMEGALY (HYPERPITUITARISM)

Pathophysiology and Etiology

Acromegaly is a condition in which GH is oversecreted after epiphyses of long bones have sealed. It results from **hyperplasia** (increased number of cells) or a tumor of the anterior pituitary. The most common pituitary tumor is an *adenoma,* which is benign. As with other cranial tumors, it becomes a space-occupying lesion and can affect other cerebral structures (see Chap. 39).

Assessment Findings

A client with acromegaly has coarse features, a huge lower jaw, thick lips, a thickened tongue, a bulging forehead, a bulbous nose, and large hands and feet (Fig. 51.1). When the overgrowth is from a tumor, headaches caused

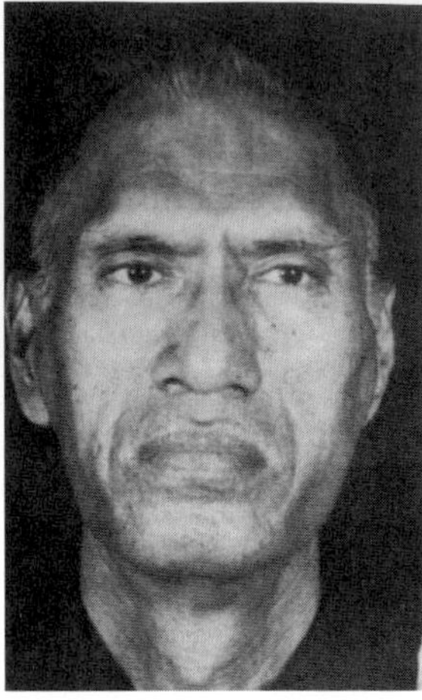
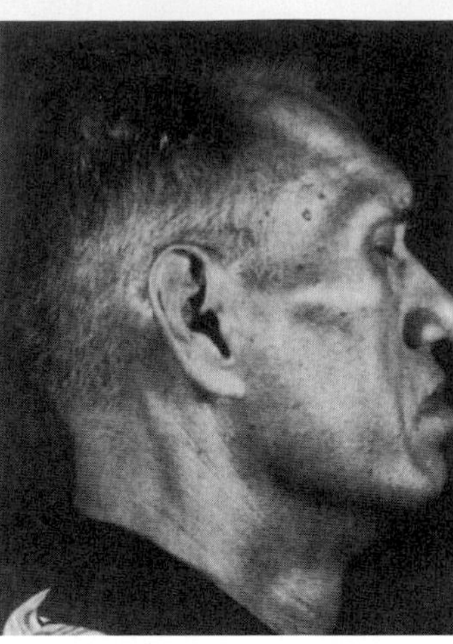

FIGURE 51.1 A 64-year-old man with acromegaly. Note the prominent, "lantern-like" jaw, the large zygomatic arches and supraorbital ridges, and the sloping "beetle brow." The bony overgrowth often results in a comparative hollowing of the temporal region. The nose and ears are enlarged, and the latter may be calcified. The skin folds are exaggerated, the skin is tough and oily, and there is enlargement of the sebaceous glands and pores.

by pressure on the sella turcica are common. Partial blindness may result from pressure on the optic nerve. The heart, liver, and spleen may be enlarged. Despite enlarged tissues, muscle weakness is common, and hypertrophied joints become painful and stiff. Osteoporosis of the spine and joint pain develop. Many men experience erectile dysfunction, and women may have amenorrhea (absence of menstruation), increased facial hair, and deepened voices.

Skull radiography, magnetic resonance imaging (MRI), and computed tomography (CT) scan reveal pituitary enlargement. Bone x-rays show thickened long bones and skull bones. Radioimmunoassay shows increased plasma levels of GH. Results of a glucose tolerance test show the same or increased levels of GH in a client with acromegaly and decreased GH levels in a person who does not have the disorder.

Medical and Surgical Management

Acromegaly is treated by surgical removal of the pituitary gland (**hypophysectomy**) or by radiation therapy with consequent destruction of the pituitary. Even if the disease is arrested successfully, physical changes are irreversible. If radiation therapy removes or destroys the tumor, replacement therapy with thyroid hormone, corticosteroids, and sex hormones is necessary.

Medical treatment includes bromocriptine mesylate (Parlodel), an antiparkinsonism drug that inhibits release of GH in clients with acromegaly. Parlodel is used alone or in conjunction with pituitary irradiation or surgery to reduce the serum GH level.

Nursing Management

Nursing priorities include correcting fluid volume excess or deficit, relieving pain, and improving nutrition. Carefully measure fluid intake and output, weigh the client daily, and observe for signs of fluid volume excess or deficit. Notify the physician of a sudden or steady weight loss or gain. Skeletal changes can cause mild to severe musculoskeletal pain. Evaluate such pain, noting type and location. Give analgesics as ordered and note whether the client reports relief from pain.

The client may experience severe psychological stress because of the prominent physical changes, erectile dysfunction, and decreased libido. Discuss such issues to help the client cope with changes. If the client expresses concern over sexual dysfunction, bring it to the physician's attention. Referral to a sex therapist could be indicated.

● DIABETES INSIPIDUS

Diabetes insipidus is an endocrine disorder that develops when antidiuretic hormone (ADH) from the posterior pituitary gland is insufficient.

Pathophysiology and Etiology

Diabetes insipidus can result from head trauma that damages the pituitary or from primary or metastatic brain tumors. Diabetes insipidus also can occur after hypophysectomy, surgical removal of the pituitary. ADH, secreted by the posterior pituitary, regulates reabsorption of water in the kidney tubules. Lack of ADH secretion causes the client to produce large volumes of dilute urine.

Assessment Findings

Urine output may be as high as 20 L/24 hours. Urine is dilute, with a specific gravity of 1.002 or less. Limiting fluid intake does not control urine excretion. Thirst is excessive and constant. The need for frequent drinking and voiding limits activities. Weakness, dehydration, and weight loss develop.

In a fluid deprivation test, fluids are withheld for 8 to 12 hours, and urine specific gravity and osmolarity are determined at the beginning and end of the test. Failure to concentrate urine during the period of fluid deprivation is characteristic of this disorder. Urinalysis reveals virtually colorless urine of low specific gravity. The 24-hour urine output is abnormally large.

Medical Management

Desmopressin (DDAVP) nasal solution and lypressin (Diapid) nasal spray are synthetic drugs with ADH activity that reduce urine output to 2 to 3 L/24 hours (Nursing Guidelines 51-1). If the client cannot take oral fluids to meet the excessive fluid volume loss, intravenous (IV) fluids are necessary.

Nursing Management

The goal is to correct fluid volume deficit. Closely monitor IV infusion rates to ensure that the prescribed amount is given. Measure fluid intake and output. If the client is acutely ill or extremely dehydrated, fails to take oral fluids, or is beginning to receive medical treatment, measure urine output every 30 minutes. Weigh the client daily to identify weight gain or loss and observe for signs of fluid excess or deficit. Notify the physician of sudden or steady weight gain or loss. Reassure the client that symptoms are controllable with treatment.

SYNDROME OF INAPPROPRIATE ANTIDIURETIC HORMONE SECRETION

The **syndrome of inappropriate antidiuretic hormone secretion** (SIADH) is characterized by renal reabsorption of water rather than its normal excretion.

Pathophysiology and Etiology

Causes of SIADH include lung tumors, central nervous system (CNS) disorders, brain tumors, cerebrovascular accident, head trauma, and drugs such as vasopressin, general anesthetic agents, oral hypoglycemics, and tricyclic antidepressants. Continued release of ADH increases fluid volume and causes *hyponatremia* (decreased serum sodium level).

NURSING GUIDELINES 51-1

Self-Administration of Lypressin Nasal Spray

1. Hold container upright.
2. Place nozzle in nostril while in sitting position.
3. Spray prescribed number of times in each nostril.
4. Avoid exceeding the number of sprays per self-administration; the excess is not absorbed and therefore wastes the volume of prescribed drug.
5. Do not inhale medication.
6. Report nasal irritation to the physician.
7. Monitor urine output and level of thirst.

Assessment Findings

Water retention, headache, muscle cramps, and anorexia develop. As the condition worsens, the client experiences nausea, vomiting, muscle twitching, and changes in level of consciousness (LOC). Diagnosis is based on symptoms and a history of a disorder associated with SIADH. Serum sodium levels and serum osmolarity are decreased. Urine sodium levels and osmolarity are high.

Medical Management

When possible, treatment aims at eliminating the underlying cause. Osmotic diuretics, such as mannitol (Osmitrol), and loop diuretics, including furosemide (Lasix), help to correct water retention. Severe hyponatremia is treated with IV administration of a 3% hypertonic sodium chloride solution.

Nursing Management

Closely monitor fluid intake and output and vital signs. Carefully assess LOC and immediately report any changes to the physician. Check closely for signs of fluid overload (confusion, dyspnea, pulmonary congestion, hypertension) and hyponatremia (weakness, muscle cramps, anorexia, nausea, diarrhea, irritability, headache, weight gain without edema).

Give client and family extensive information about the medication schedule and adverse effects of drug therapy, especially if several medications are prescribed. Stress the importance of adhering to the medication schedule and not omitting a dose.

DISORDERS OF THE THYROID GLAND

Thyroid disorders are difficult to detect because symptoms are vague until the disease advances to a severe level. Treatment often is long term, and the client requires periodic follow-up to monitor response. Thyroid disorders include hyperthyroidism, thyrotoxic crisis, hypothyroidism, thyroid tumors, and endemic and multinodular goiters.

• HYPERTHYROIDISM

Hyperthyroidism also is called *Graves' disease, Basedow's disease, thyrotoxicosis,* or *exophthalmic goiter.*

Pathophysiology and Etiology

There is no one etiologic factor for hyperthyroidism. It may be autoimmune or inherited. Hypersecretion of thyroid hormones accompanies thyroid tumors, pituitary tumors, and hypothalamic malignancies. It also may result from stress or infection. The metabolic rate increases because of oversecretion of the thyroid hormones thyroxine (T_4) and triiodothyronine (T_3). Both T_4 and T_3 increase the metabolic rate. Hyperthyroidism is more common in women than in men.

Assessment Findings

Symptoms vary from mild to severe. Clients with well-developed hyperthyroidism characteristically are restless despite feeling fatigued and weak, highly excitable, and constantly agitated. Fine tremors of the hands occur, causing unusual clumsiness (Fig. 51.2). The client cannot tolerate heat and has an increased appetite, but loses weight. Diarrhea also occurs. Visual changes, such as blurred or double vision, can develop. *Exophthalmos,* seen in clients with severe hyperthyroidism, results from enlarged muscle and fatty tissue surrounding the rear and sides of the eyeball (see Fig. 50.8). Neck swelling caused by the enlarged thyroid gland often is visible. Table 51.1 compares the signs and symptoms of hyperthyroidism and hypothyroidism.

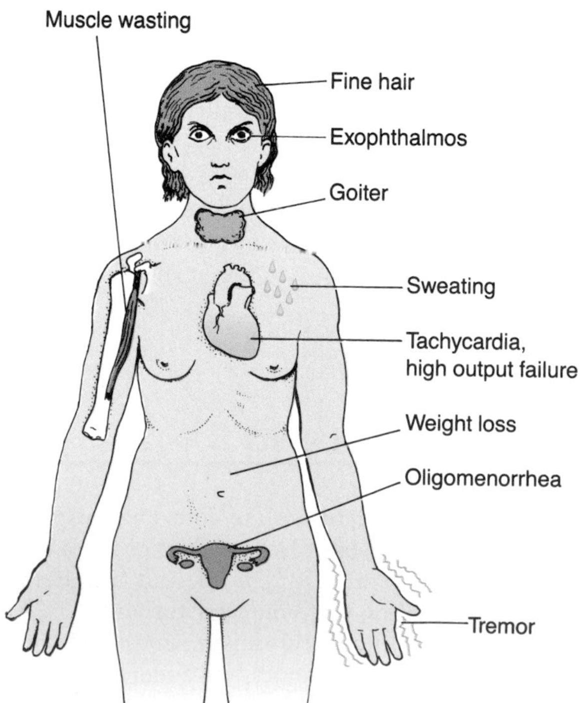

FIGURE 51.2 Clinical manifestations of hyperthyroidism.

Protein-bound iodine, free T_3, thyroglobulin, and serum T_3 and T_4 levels are elevated. The TSH level is decreased. Thyroid ultrasonography shows an enlarged thyroid gland. A thyroid scan indicates an increased uptake of radioactive iodine (RAI; ^{131}I and ^{123}I). Results of an RAI uptake study show an increased uptake of iodine.

Medical and Surgical Management

Antithyroid drugs, such as propylthiouracil (PTU, Propyl-Thyracil) and methimazole (Tapazole), are given to block production of thyroid hormone. Potassium iodide (Lugol's solution) is prescribed in combination with an antithyroid drug. Antithyroid medications are avoided during pregnancy because they can induce hypothyroidism, or cretinism, in the fetus. Drug Therapy Table 51.1 discusses these and other drugs used to treat thyroid disorders.

^{131}I is used to destroy hyperplastic thyroid tissue by radiation. The thyroid is quick to remove iodine, including RAI, from the bloodstream. Antithyroid drugs are given for 6 months or more before administration of ^{131}I. If symptoms do not improve, a second and perhaps a third dose of ^{131}I is given. About 6 to 8 weeks after the initial dose of ^{131}I, most clients notice some remission of symptoms. The extended time lag before relief of symptoms is a disadvantage of this treatment method. A more common and unfortunate result of treatment is hypothyroidism because accurately determining the precise amount of thyroid tissue that radiation will destroy is very difficult. This complication may not develop until long after administration of ^{131}I, and clients must remain under medical supervision for many years.

Subtotal thyroidectomy (partial removal of the thyroid gland) is an effective treatment for hyperthyroidism. *Total thyroidectomy* (removal of the thyroid gland) may be done if a neoplastic tumor is present. Clients commonly receive antithyroid drug therapy for several weeks before surgery to prevent a dramatic release of thyroid hormones into the bloodstream during surgery. Single thyroid nodules less than 3 cm in diameter can be removed by minimally invasive endoscopic techniques in which the surgeon makes three to four small incisions in the neck rather than the typical single incision, which is several inches long.

Complications of thyroidectomy include the following:

- Accidental removal of or alteration in the blood supply to the parathyroid glands, which are embedded in thyroid tissue, resulting in hypocalcemia
- Hemorrhage caused by vascularity of the thyroid and surrounding tissue

TABLE 51.1 SYMPTOMS OF THYROID DYSFUNCTION

BODY SYSTEM OR FUNCTION	HYPERTHYROIDISM	HYPOTHYROIDISM
Metabolism	Increased, with symptoms of increased appetite, intolerance to heat, elevated body temperature, weight loss despite increased appetite	Decreased, with symptoms of anorexia, intolerance to cold, low body temperature, weight gain despite anorexia
Cardiovascular system	Tachycardia, moderate hypertension	Bradycardia, moderate hypotension
Central nervous system	Nervousness, anxiety, insomnia, tremors	Lethargy, sleepiness
Skin and skin structures	Flushed, warm, moist	Pale, cool, dry; face appears puffy, hair coarse; nails thick and hard
Ovarian function	Irregular or scant menses	Heavy menses, may be unable to conceive, loss of fetus also possible
Testicular function		Low sperm count

DRUG THERAPY TABLE 51.1 AGENTS FOR THYROID DISORDERS

DRUG CATEGORY AND EXAMPLES	MECHANISM OF ACTION	SIDE EFFECTS	NURSING CONSIDERATIONS
Antithyroid Agents			
methimazole (Tapazole) *propylthiouracil (PTU)*	Inhibits synthesis of thyroid hormones	Paresthesias, nausea, agranulocytosis, bleeding, rash, diarrhea, vomiting	Caution clients to avoid use during pregnancy. Monitor results of blood tests for bone marrow depression. Administer in three equal doses every 8 hours. Alert client to notify the physician of fever, sore throat, unusual bleeding or bruising, or malaise.
Iodides			
strong iodine solution (Lugol's solution)	Inhibits synthesis and release of T_3 and T_4	Iodism: metallic taste, burning mouth, sore teeth and gums, nausea, abdominal pain, diarrhea, rash	Monitor for symptoms of acute iodine toxicity: vomiting, abdominal pain, diarrhea, circulatory collapse. Dilute with fruit juice or water. Advise client to drink solution with a straw to avoid staining teeth.
Radioactive Iodine			
sodium iodine ^{131}I and ^{123}I	Used in diagnostic scans; destroys thyroid tissue in hyperthyroidism and thyroid malignancies	Allergy to iodine, nausea, vomiting	Follow precautions for body fluids for 24 hours after diagnostic testing. Monitor for signs of hypothyroidism.
Beta-Adrenergic Blockers			
propranolol (Inderal)	Reduces symptoms of hyperthyroidism—tachycardia, tremors, nervousness	Nausea, vomiting, diarrhea, constipation, bradycardia, congestive heart failure, dysrhythmias, hypoglycemia	Monitor cardiac function. Administer with meals. Instruct client not to discontinue abruptly. Assess blood glucose level regularly for clients with diabetes.
Thyroid Hormone Replacement Drugs			
thyroid dessicated (Armour thyroid, S-P-T, Thyrar, Thyroid Strong) *thyroid hormones T_3 and T_4 in their natural state* *liothyronine (T_3, Cytomel, Triostat)* *liotrix (Thyrolar)*	Increases metabolic rate of body tissues	Hyperthyroidism: tachycardia, tremors, headache, nervousness, insomnia, diarrhea, weight loss, heat intolerance	Monitor response closely. Monitor thyroid function tests. Advise client that drug usually is required for lifetime. Administer drug as a single daily dose before breakfast. Thyroid preparations interact with digitalis, estrogen, beta blockers, glucagon, and anticoagulants.

- Thyrotoxicosis (or thyroid storm) as a result of excessive secretion of thyroid hormones during surgical excision
- Damage to the recurrent laryngeal nerve, which affects the function of the vocal cords. If the recurrent laryngeal nerve is damaged either temporarily or partially, breathing may be impaired because vocal cords cannot open properly during inspiration; the voice may sound weak, hoarse, or breathy; and aspiration and pneumonia may occur if the vocal cords do not close completely during swallowing.

Nursing Management

Monitor heart rate and blood pressure (BP) regularly. Record the client's sleep pattern and daily weights. Promote rest and help the client avoid excess physical stimulation. Increased caloric intake can compensate for increased metabolism. Inform the client that effects of antithyroid therapy usually are not apparent until the thyroid gland has secreted excess thyroid hormone into the bloodstream. This process may take several weeks or more. If RAI is used to destroy thyroid tissue, tell the client that it does not seriously affect other tissues. Possible transient effects after use of ^{131}I and ^{123}I are nausea, vomiting, malaise, fever, and gland tenderness. Nursing Care Plan 51-1 discusses care of the client undergoing thyroid surgery.

• THYROTOXIC CRISIS

Pathophysiology and Etiology

Thyrotoxic crisis, an abrupt and life-threatening form of hyperthyroidism, is probably triggered by extreme stress, infection, diabetic ketoacidosis, trauma, toxemia of pregnancy, or manipulation of a hyperactive thyroid gland during surgery or physical examination. Although rare, it may occur in clients with undiagnosed or inadequately treated hyperthyroidism.

Oversecretion of T_3 and T_4 is followed by a release of epinephrine. Metabolism is markedly increased. Adrenal glands produce excess corticosteroids in response to stress created by this hypermetabolic state.

Assessment Findings

The temperature may be as high as 41°C (106°F). Pulse rate is rapid, and cardiac dysrhythmias are common. The client may experience persistent vomiting, extreme restlessness with delirium, chest pain, and dyspnea.

Diagnosis is based on symptoms and a recent medical history that indicates symptoms of severe hyperthyroidism. Laboratory tests, such as serum T_3 and T_4 determinations, may be used to confirm the diagnosis. In thyrotoxic crisis, serum thyroid determinations are markedly elevated.

Medical Management

Immediate treatment is necessary. Antithyroid drugs (e.g., propylthiouracil, methimazole) block the synthesis of thyroid hormones. An IV corticosteroid may be given to replace depletion that results from overstimulation of the adrenals during the hypermetabolic state. IV sodium iodide prevents the thyroid gland from releasing thyroid hormones. Propranolol (Inderal), a beta blocker, reduces the effect of thyroid hormones on the cardiovascular system. Supportive therapy includes IV fluids, antipyretic measures, and oxygen therapy.

Nursing Management

The client with thyrotoxic crisis is acutely ill. Monitor vital signs, especially the temperature, frequently. Failure to respond to an antipyretic drug requires other measures, such as a cooling blanket or ice application. A cool room also may help reduce body temperature. Give all therapeutic treatment measures as ordered because the situation must be corrected quickly.

• HYPOTHYROIDISM

Hypothyroidism occurs when the thyroid gland fails to secrete adequate thyroid hormones.

Pathophysiology and Etiology

This condition may originate in the thyroid (primary hypothyroidism) or in the pituitary, in which case insufficient TSH is secreted. Regardless of the cause, the result of inadequate thyroid hormone secretion is a slowing of all metabolic processes (see Table 51.1). Severe hypothyroidism is called **myxedema.** Advanced, untreated myxedema can progress to myxedema coma. Signs include hypothermia, hypotension, and hypoventilation. A client with hypothyroidism experiencing infection, trauma, or excessive chills, or taking narcotics, sedatives, or tranquilizers, can lapse into a myxedema coma.

Assessment Findings

Signs and symptoms are opposite in many respects to those of hyperthyroidism. Metabolic rate and physical

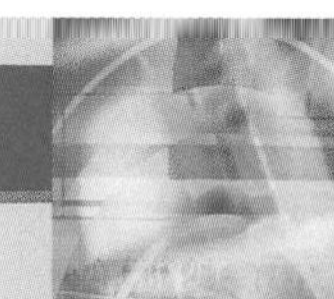

Nursing Care Plan 51-1

THE CLIENT UNDERGOING THYROID SURGERY

Assessment

- Obtain complete medical, drug, and allergy histories.
- Check and compare present weight with preillness weight.
- Measure vital signs each shift and more often if findings are abnormal.
- Perform a physical examination, but avoid palpating the thyroid gland (manipulation releases excess thyroid hormones).
- Determine client's preoperative compliance with antithyroid drug therapy.
- Explore client's knowledge of the operative procedure and perioperative care.

Nursing Diagnosis: **Risk for Ineffective Breathing Pattern** related to compression of the trachea from edema of the glottis, accumulated blood in the operative area, recurrent laryngeal nerve damage, or retained secretions

Expected Outcome: Breathing will be regular, noiseless, and effortless with SpO_2 at least 90%.

Interventions	*Rationales*
Elevate head of the bed 30° or more.	Head elevation reduces edema.
Apply ice bag to neck if prescribed.	It promotes vasoconstriction, thereby reducing edema and bleeding.
Place a tracheostomy set in client's room.	Having a means for establishing a patent airway is an emergency life-saving measure.
Assemble oral/pharyngeal suction equipment at client's bedside and suction client if he or she cannot raise respiratory secretions.	Suctioning clears the airway of substances that compromise movement of gases into and out of the lungs.
Observe for dyspnea and restlessness.	Increased breathing effort is evidence of a compromised airway.
Report signs of respiratory distress to the nurse in charge and the physician.	Sharing information aids in collaborative efforts to prevent complications.

Evaluation of Expected Outcome: Client maintains normal ventilation, with no airway obstruction.

PC: **Hemorrhage**

Expected Outcome: The nurse monitors to detect, manage, and minimize signs of hemorrhage.

Interventions	*Rationales*
Monitor vital signs every 1 to 4 hours.	Tachycardia and hypotension suggest cellular hypoxia and fluid volume deficit secondary to bleeding.
Inspect surgical dressing frequently for bleeding.	Gauze dressing material wicks blood from the surgical incision.
Check back of the neck for bloody drainage.	Gravity causes blood to drain posteriorly, which interferes with its visibility on the surface of the surgical dressing.

(continued)

Nursing Care Plan 51-1 (Continued)

THE CLIENT UNDERGOING THYROID SURGERY

Interventions	*Rationales*
Attend to client's complaints of fullness in or around the surgical incision.	Blood may accumulate beneath the sutured incision rather than drain externally.
Place suture or staple removal equipment in client's room or stock equipment in a clean utility room.	The incision may need to be opened to remove clotted blood or ligate blood vessels that continue to bleed.

Evaluation of Expected Outcome: There is no evidence of excessive bleeding in or around the operative site.

Nursing Diagnosis: **Impaired Verbal Communication** related to hoarseness secondary to recurrent laryngeal nerve damage

Expected Outcome: Client will regain normal volume and quality of speech.

Interventions	*Rationales*
Minimize unnecessary vocalizations for client.	Resting the voice reduces strain on the vocal cords.
Deliver bedside humidification.	Inhalation of moist air helps relieve hoarseness.
Provide an alternate means (pad of paper, magic slate, alphabet board) for the client to ask questions or make needs known.	Written communication provides a substitute for verbal interactions.
Ensure that client has access to a signal cord or bell with which to summon a caregiver.	A light or bell signals a need for assistance and is essential when a client cannot call for help.
Assess the quality of client's voice periodically every 2 to 4 waking hours for the first 2 postoperative days.	A weakening of the voice or loss of the ability to project sounds may indicate impaired verbal ability.

Evaluation of Expected Outcome: Speech is at the presurgical volume.

Nursing Diagnosis: **Risk for Aspiration** related to recurrent laryngeal nerve damage

Expected Outcome: Lungs will be free of food or liquids.

Interventions	*Rationales*
Prepare oral/pharyngeal suction equipment.	Suctioning provides a way to clear the airway.
Have client sit upright.	An upright position promotes the mechanics of swallowing and a more forceful cough if substances enter the airway.
Provide thickened substances initially.	Watery food and beverages are more difficult to swallow.
Encourage client to place a very small amount in his or her mouth at any one time.	Controlling ingested substances increases the potential success for swallowing the mass.

Evaluation of Expected Outcome: Client does not experience respiratory distress, and lungs are clear on auscultation.

PC: **Tetany**

Expected Outcome: The nurse will monitor to detect, manage, and minimize tetany.

(continued)

Nursing Care Plan 51-1 (Continued)

THE CLIENT UNDERGOING THYROID SURGERY

Interventions	*Rationales*
Observe for spontaneous spasm of fingers or toes, mouth twitching or jaw tightening when tapping the cheek anteriorly to the earlobe (Chvostek's sign), and spasm of the fingers toward the wrist when you inflate a BP cuff midway between systolic and diastolic pressures for 3 minutes (Trousseau's sign).	Tetany develops when the parathyroid glands, which regulate blood calcium levels, are accidentally removed during a thyroidectomy. Hypocalcemia results in neuromuscular hyperexcitability.
Note crowing respirations and dyspnea.	Manifestations of hypocalcemia include symptoms caused by laryngeal spasm.
Be prepared to implement seizure precautions.	Seizures may occur when the blood calcium level falls below normal.
Have calcium gluconate for IV administration available if prescribed by the physician.	Calcium replacement controls symptoms of tetany.

Evaluation of Expected Outcome: No complications develop.

PC: **Thyrotoxic Crisis**

Expected Outcome: The nurse will monitor to detect, manage, and minimize thyrotoxic crisis.

Interventions	*Rationales*
Assess for hyperthermia, tachycardia, chest pain, cardiac dysrhythmias, and altered level of consciousness.	Excess levels of thyroid hormones raise body temperature and accelerate cardiac activity by increasing the rate of metabolism.
Notify the physician if symptoms of thyrotoxic crisis develop.	Collaborative measures are necessary to control symptoms and their consequences.
Implement measures to reduce body temperature such as administering antipyretics or placing client on an aquathermia pad.	Measures to reduce body temperature help prevent complications such as seizures and brain damage.
Follow medical orders for measures to reduce heart rate and dysrhythmias.	Tachycardia increases myocardial demands for oxygen; unless managed, it can lead to myocardial infarction, acute heart failure, or cardiac arrest.

Evaluation of Expected Outcome: No complications develop.

and mental activity slow down. The client is lethargic, lacks energy, dozes frequently during the day, is forgetful, and has chronic headaches. The face takes on a masklike, unemotional expression, yet the client often is irritable. The tongue may be enlarged and the lips swollen, and there may be edema of the eyelids. Temperature and pulse rate are decreased; the client is intolerant to cold. Weight increases despite a low caloric intake. The skin is dry, and hair characteristically is coarse and sparse and tends to fall out. Menstrual disorders are common. Constipation may be severe. The voice is low pitched and hoarse, and speech is slow. Hearing may be impaired. The client may experience numbness or tingling in the arms or legs unrelieved by position change.

Hypothyroidism may lead to an enlarged heart caused by pericardial effusion and a tendency toward atherosclerosis and heart strain. Anemia also may be present. Early recognition of hypothyroidism is difficult because many of the symptoms are nonspecific and not sufficiently dramatic to bring the client to the physician. This condition can go untreated for years.

In primary hypothyroidism, levels of TSH are increased because of negative feedback to the pituitary gland (see Chap. 50). The RAI uptake may be decreased. T_3 and

T_4 levels show no response in primary untreated hypothyroidism but may show a response if hypothyroidism results from failure of the pituitary to secrete TSH.

Medical Management

Hypothyroidism is treated with thyroid replacement therapy (see Drug Therapy Table 51.1). Thyroid hormone in the form of desiccated thyroid extract, or with one of the synthetic products, such as levothyroxine sodium (Synthroid) or liothyronine sodium (Cytomel), are oral thyroid preparations. A low dose of thyroid hormone is given initially and then increased or decreased as needed.

Nursing Management

Obtain medical, drug, and allergy histories and a thorough description of symptoms. Check vital signs and weight. During physical examination, observe for symptoms of hypothyroidism: lethargy, fatigue, anorexia, weight gain, hair loss, brittle nails, and cold intolerance.

Once a definitive diagnosis is made, observe for adverse effects of thyroid replacement therapy. Dyspnea, rapid pulse rate, palpitations, precordial pain, hyperactivity, insomnia, dizziness, and gastrointestinal (GI) disorders—in other words, signs of hyperthyroidism—may be seen if the dose of thyroid hormone is too high. Once replacement therapy has begun, a dramatic change may be seen in a few weeks.

Assess activity tolerance. Allow adequate rest between activities. Assess bowel elimination patterns and stool characteristics. Provide high-fiber foods. Encourage adequate fluid intake and increased physical activity (e.g., short walks) within client's tolerance. Assess body temperature; report deviations from usual values. Provide extra warmth with blankets or clothing. Protect client from exposure to cold or drafts.

Teach client and family reasons for hormone replacement therapy and the therapeutic effects. Assist client to develop a schedule for taking medication each day and explain the need for continued follow-up to monitor hormone status. Recommend that the client obtain and wear a Medic Alert tag at all times.

Symptoms associated with hyperthyroidism and hypothyroidism often affect learning and retention ability. Carefully explain the treatment regimen. If a special diet is recommended, obtain a dietary consultation and review sample diets with the client. A teaching plan includes the following:

- Weigh self weekly; keep a record of symptoms and weight in case the medication dose needs adjustment.
- Avoid stressful situations.
- Maintain good nutrition.
- Notify the physician if symptoms worsen or adverse drug effects occur.

THYROID TUMORS

Tumors of the thyroid can cause hyperthyroidism. They are more commonly benign, but all nodules must be evaluated.

Pathophysiology and Etiology

A lump on the thyroid is most likely to be benign for adults with symptoms of hyperthyroidism or hypothyroidism. *Papillary carcinoma* is the most common malignant lesion, occurring in clients who have received radiation treatments to the head or neck region. It tends to spread only to nearby lymph nodes and rarely to other parts of the body. Curing thyroid cancer depends on the type of tumor present.

Assessment Findings

Symptoms are vague, and the client may be unaware of the lesion. Often a routine physical examination reveals a nodular thyroid. As the tumor enlarges, the client may notice a swelling in the neck. Benign tumors cause symptoms of hyperthyroidism in some clients. Malignant tumors can cause voice changes, hoarseness, and difficulty swallowing.

Biopsy of the lesion confirms the diagnosis. Thyroid cancer is suspected when the gland is firm and palpable and when results of RAI studies show poor concentration in the suspect area.

Medical and Surgical Management

If there are no symptoms of hyperthyroidism with a benign nodule, treatment usually is not needed. The nodule is examined yearly. If the enlargement causes such symptoms as difficulty swallowing and noticeable neck swelling, surgical removal of the lesion is considered. Although treatment of malignant lesions varies, a thyroidectomy (total or subtotal) typically is performed. A modified or radical neck dissection is indicated if there is metastasis. After a thyroidectomy, replacement therapy (consisting of thyroid hormones) is given to supply thyroid hormones and to suppress pituitary TSH so that it no longer stimulates growth of residual thyroid tissue. ^{131}I is administered to destroy remaining thyroid tissue as well as to treat lymph node metastasis, if present.

Nursing Management

If the thyroid tumor is malignant, the physician explains the planned treatment and expected outcome. Provide emotional support, especially if the tumor has metastasized and radical surgery is necessary. When RAI is used after surgery, isolate and place the client on radiation precautions (see Chap. 19). Handle body fluids carefully to prevent spread of contamination.

• ENDEMIC AND MULTINODULAR GOITERS

The word **goiter** refers to an enlarged thyroid gland.

Pathophysiology and Etiology

Endemic goiter is caused by deficiency of iodine in the diet, inability of the thyroid to use iodine, or relative iodine deficiency caused by increasing body demands for thyroid hormones. *Nontoxic goiter* (also called *simple* or *colloid goiter*) is an enlarged thyroid, usually with no symptoms of thyroid dysfunction. *Nodular goiters* contain one or more areas of hyperplasia. This type of goiter appears to develop for essentially the same reasons as an endemic goiter.

Assessment Findings

The thyroid gland enlarges. The client has a sense of fullness in the neck area. Continued gland enlargement eventually results in difficulty swallowing and breathing as the thyroid presses on the trachea and esophagus. When the gland enlarges, it is visible as a swelling in the neck. Nodular goiters also produce enlargement, but the gland has an irregular surface on palpation (Fig. 51.3).

A thyroid scan shows an enlarged gland and decreased uptake of ^{131}I. Tests of thyroid function are performed, but results are inconclusive.

Medical Management

Treatment depends on the cause. If the diet is deficient in iodine, foods high in iodine, such as seafood or iodized salt, are recommended. Potassium iodide supplements may be given. A thyroidectomy may be recommended, especially when the gland is grossly enlarged.

Nursing Management

If the client has respiratory distress because of the enlarged thyroid, closely observe respiratory status and elevate the head of the bed to relieve respiratory symptoms. Provide a diet high in iodine and iodized salt. Natural iodine content is highest in seafoods; it is also found in varying amounts in bread, milk, eggs, meat, and spinach. A soft diet may be necessary if the client has difficulty swallowing.

• THYROIDITIS

Thyroiditis, inflammation of the thyroid gland, can be acute, subacute, or chronic.

Pathophysiology and Etiology

Acute thyroiditis, most common in children, appears to result from bacterial infection of the gland. *Subacute*

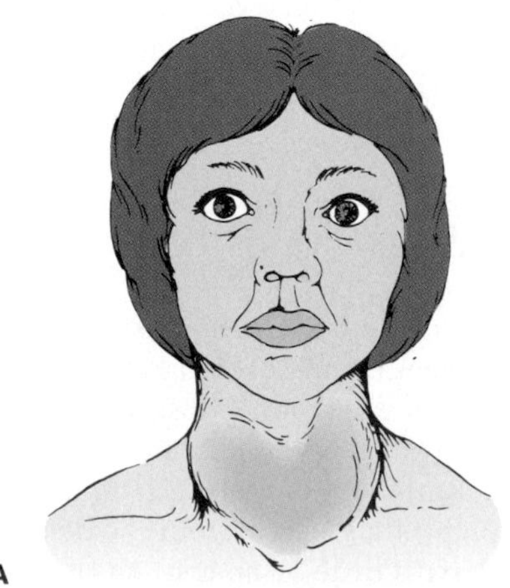

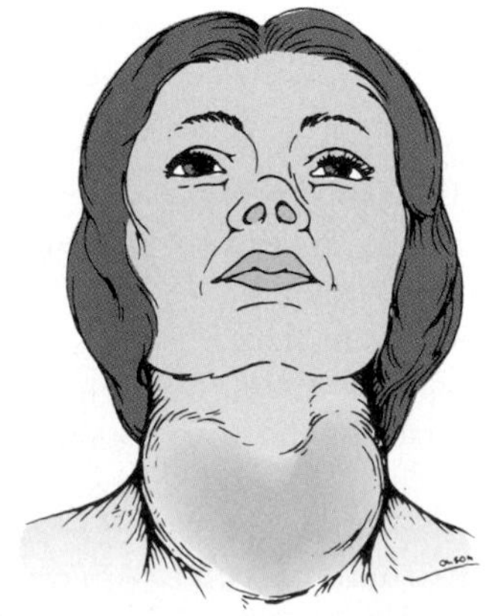

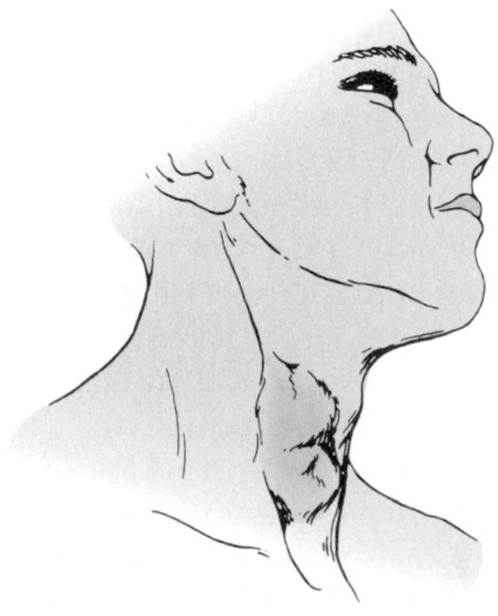

FIGURE 51.3 Thyroid abnormalities. (**A**) Diffuse toxic goiter (Graves' disease) with exophthalmos. (**B**) Diffuse nontoxic goiter. (**C**) Nodular goiter. (From Judge, R. D., Zuidema, G. D., & Fitzgerald, F. T. [Eds.]. [1982]. *Clinical diagnosis* [4th ed.]. Boston: Little, Brown.)

thyroiditis can follow an upper respiratory viral infection and is relatively rare. More common is *Hashimoto's thyroiditis,* a chronic form of thyroiditis, believed to be an autoimmune disorder.

Assessment Findings

Signs and symptoms of acute thyroiditis include high fever, malaise, and tenderness and swelling of the thyroid gland. Subacute thyroiditis produces symptoms of a swollen and painful gland, chills, fever, and malaise approximately 2 weeks after a viral infection. In Hashimoto's thyroiditis, there is an enlarged thyroid and possibly symptoms of hypothyroidism.

In acute thyroiditis, laboratory test results show an elevated white blood cell (WBC) count and normal thyroid function. In subacute thyroiditis, results of some thyroid tests, such as T_3 and T_4, are elevated. The RAI study shows a decreased iodine uptake. In Hashimoto's, there are high titers of antithyroid antibodies, and RAI studies show increased iodine uptake.

Medical and Surgical Management

Acute thyroiditis requires administration of appropriate antibiotics. Treatment of subacute thyroiditis is symptomatic and includes analgesics for pain and discomfort. Corticosteroids also may be prescribed to reduce inflammation. Treatment of Hashimoto's thyroiditis includes thyroid hormone replacement therapy. Surgery is required if the gland becomes excessively large.

Nursing Management

Management depends on the type of thyroiditis and severity of symptoms. Give antipyretics for fever. Elevate the head of the bed if the client has difficulty breathing. Offer a soft diet if the gland is markedly enlarged and the client has difficulty swallowing.

If a client has undergone surgery (see Nursing Care Plan 51-1), before discharge instruct the client in surgical wound care and to avoid excessive strain on the wound until it is healed. Because the incision is made in a neck crease, the healed scar is barely visible. If a client appears concerned about scarring, suggest that the client wear clothing that covers the neck until the scar is almost invisible.

Discuss symptoms of hypothyroidism, hyperthyroidism, and hypoparathyroidism with instructions to notify the physician immediately if they occur. If medication is prescribed, review the dosage and adverse effects of each drug. A teaching plan includes techniques for wound care, need to take thyroid replacement medication in the morning at the same time each day to avoid insomnia and CNS stimulation, and side effects that require notification of the physician (chest pain, tachycardia, and dyspnea).

Stop, Think, and Respond ● BOX 51-1

When reviewing a client's medical record, you read that the physician has detected an enlarged thyroid gland. What are some possible causes?

DISORDERS OF THE PARATHYROID GLANDS

When the parathyroid gland dysfunctions, hyperparathyroidism or hypoparathyroidism develops. Calcium and phosphorus levels are affected.

● HYPERPARATHYROIDISM

Hyperparathyroidism can be a primary or secondary condition.

Pathophysiology and Etiology

The most common cause of *primary hyperparathyroidism* is an adenoma of one of the parathyroid glands. In primary hyperparathyroidism, excessive secretion of parathyroid hormone (parathormone) results in increased urinary excretion of phosphorus and loss of calcium from bones. The bones become demineralized as calcium leaves and enters the bloodstream. Renal stones may develop as calcium becomes concentrated in the urine.

In *secondary hyperparathyroidism,* the parathyroid glands secrete excessive parathormone in response to hypocalcemia (low serum calcium level), which may result from vitamin D deficiency, chronic renal failure, large doses of thiazide diuretics, and excessive use of laxatives and calcium supplements.

Assessment Findings

Excessive serum calcium depresses responsiveness of the peripheral nerves, accounting for fatigue and muscle weakness. Muscles become hypotonic (loss of or decreased muscle tone). Cardiac dysrhythmias may develop. Because bones have lost calcium, there is skeletal tenderness and pain on bearing weight; they may become so demineralized that they break with little or no trauma (pathologic fractures). Other possible effects include nausea, vomiting, and constipation. Large amounts of calcium and phosphorus passing through the kidneys predispose the client to formation of stones in the genitourinary tract, pyelonephritis, and uremia.

Diagnosis is based on elevated serum calcium and decreased serum phosphorus levels without other causes of hypercalcemia. Results of a 24-hour urine test show increased urine calcium levels. Skeletal radiographs show calcium loss from bones. An MRI or a CT scan identifies a parathyroid adenoma if present. Parathormone levels are elevated in hyperparathyroidism.

Medical and Surgical Management

Secondary hyperparathyroidism is managed by correcting the cause (e.g., vitamin D therapy for a vitamin D deficiency, correction of renal failure, calcium-restricted diet). Sodium and phosphorus replacements often are ordered.

The only treatment for primary hyperparathyroidism is surgical removal of hypertrophied gland tissue or of an individual tumor of one of the parathyroid glands. Before surgery, the physician determines the number of glands to be removed, based on the cause of hyperparathyroidism and laboratory and diagnostic test results. One or more of the parathyroids is left in place because they are necessary for calcium and phosphorus metabolism.

Nursing Management

Closely measure the client's intake and output. Observe for signs of urinary calculi from hypercalcemia, flank pain, and decreasing urine output. Encourage a large volume of fluid to keep the urine dilute. Assess the client's ability to perform self-care, provide a safe environment to prevent falls and other injury, encourage frequent rest periods, and monitor fatigue level.

The primary nursing responsibility is teaching the client about effects of the disease, planned medical management, and importance of following prescribed treatment. If the client undergoes surgery, nursing management is similar to that for thyroid surgery. In addition, observe the client for symptoms of hypoparathyroidism.

• HYPOPARATHYROIDISM

Hypoparathyroidism is a deficiency of parathormone that results in hypocalcemia.

Pathophysiology and Etiology

Parathormone regulates calcium balance by increasing calcium absorption from the GI tract and bone resorption of calcium. Hypocalcemia affects neuromuscular functions, causing hyperexcitability resulting in spastic muscle contractions and *paresthesias* (abnormal sensations).

Common causes of hypoparathyroidism are trauma to the glands and inadvertent removal of all or nearly all these structures during thyroidectomy or parathyroidectomy. The idiopathic form of this disorder is rare but may be autoimmune in origin or caused by congenital absence of the parathyroids.

Assessment Findings

The main symptom of acute and sudden hypoparathyroidism is **tetany.** The client may report numbness and tingling in fingers or toes or around the lips. A voluntary movement may be followed by an involuntary, jerking spasm. Muscle cramping may be present. Tonic (continuous contraction) flexion of an arm or a finger may occur. When the client's facial nerve (which lies under the tissue in front of the ear) is tapped, the client's mouth twitches and the jaw tightens. The response is identified as a positive **Chvostek's sign.** Look for a positive **Trousseau's sign** by placing a BP cuff on the upper arm, inflating it between systolic and diastolic BP, and waiting 3 minutes. Observe the client for spasm of the hand (**carpopedal spasm**), evidenced by the hand flexing inward.

Laryngeal spasm can occur, causing dyspnea, with long, crowing respirations as air tries to get past the constriction. Cyanosis may be present, and the client is in danger of asphyxia and cardiac dysrhythmias. Nausea, vomiting, abdominal pain, and seizures can develop.

In chronic hypoparathyroidism, the client experiences neuromuscular irritability, constipation or diarrhea, numbness and tingling of the arms and legs, loss of tooth enamel, and muscle pain. Positive Chvostek's and Trousseau's signs may or may not be elicited, depending on the degree of hypocalcemia.

Serum calcium level is decreased, serum phosphorus level is increased, and urine levels of both are decreased. In chronic hypoparathyroidism, radiographs show increased bone density.

Medical Management

Tetany and severe hypoparathyroidism are treated immediately by administration of an IV calcium salt, such as calcium gluconate. Endotracheal intubation and mechanical ventilation may be necessary if acute respiratory distress occurs. Bronchodilators also are used.

Long-term treatment after trauma to or inadvertent removal of the parathyroids includes administration of oral calcium, vitamin D, or vitamin D_2 (calciferol), which increases the serum calcium level. The dose is related to the degree of hypocalcemia, which is determined by frequent monitoring of serum and urine calcium levels. A diet high in calcium and low in phosphorus usually is recommended.

Nursing Management

Be alert for signs of tetany and assess for Chvostek's and Trousseau's signs. Monitor the client with chronic hypoparathyroidism for increasing severity of symptoms. Prepare to administer IV calcium salt and observe the client during such administration for adverse effects, such as flushing, cardiac dysrhythmia (usually a bradycardia), tingling in the arms and legs, and a metallic taste. Local tissue necrosis may occur if IV fluid escapes into surrounding tissues. Monitor serum calcium levels to determine the effectiveness of therapy.

If the client has chronic hypoparathyroidism, obtain complete medical, drug, and allergy histories. Examine the client for symptoms of the disorder, primarily for the effect of hypocalcemia on the CNS. Assess the arms and legs for evidence of muscle spasm. Auscultate the lungs because the client may have dyspnea or other respiratory difficulty. During assessment of vital signs, attention to heart rate and rhythm is particularly important.

Keep an emergency tracheostomy tray, mechanical ventilation equipment, artificial airway, and endotracheal intubation equipment at the client's bedside if hypocalcemia is severe. Insert an IV line for the emergency administration of calcium. Observe frequently for respiratory distress and notify the physician immediately if this problem occurs.

Until hypocalcemia is corrected, assist the client with activities of daily living (ADLs). Movement, noise, and other environmental disturbances can trigger muscle contractions or convulsions. Thus, minimizing all forms of stress is essential until serum calcium levels approach normal and symptoms are relieved.

Clients who require lifetime treatment of the disorder need careful review of the prescribed treatment. Because normal calcium levels depend on drug and diet therapy, stress the importance of these two aspects of treatment. Consultation with a dietitian may be necessary to provide a list of foods to include or avoid in the prescribed diet. Give the client a list of the symptoms of hypercalcemia and hypocalcemia, either of which can occur if the dose of the prescribed drug is too high or too low or if the drug is omitted. Emphasize the need to contact the physician immediately about any symptoms. Remind the client that the physician may need to adjust the dose of the drug; therefore, recognizing the symptoms associated with hypercalcemia and hypocalcemia is essential.

DISORDERS OF THE ADRENAL GLANDS

Adrenal dysfunction includes pathology of the outer portion of the adrenal gland, the *cortex,* which synthesizes and secretes the hormones known as *steroids:* mineralocorticoids, glucocorticoids, and androgens or estrogens. Disorders of the adrenal glands also involve the *medulla,* the inner portion, which secretes the catecholamines norepinephrine (noradrenaline) and epinephrine (adrenaline). Proper secretion of these hormones is essential to life.

● ADRENAL INSUFFICIENCY (ADDISON'S DISEASE)

Adrenal insufficiency is classified as either primary or secondary.

Pathophysiology and Etiology

Primary adrenal insufficiency (Addison's disease) results from destruction of the adrenal cortex by diseases such as tuberculosis. It also may be autoimmune, in which antibodies formed by the client's immune system destroy adrenal tissue. Often, the cause is unknown.

Consequences of decreased adrenal cortical function include decreased available glucose and hypoglycemia. The glomerular filtration rate of the kidneys slows dramatically, causing decreased urea nitrogen excretion.

Secondary adrenal insufficiency is the result of surgical removal of both adrenal glands (*bilateral adrenalectomy*), hemorrhagic infarction of the glands, hypopituitarism (caused by pituitary failure or surgical removal of the pituitary), or suppression of adrenal function by the administration of corticosteroids. Clients with secondary adrenal insufficiency after bilateral adrenalectomy or surgical removal of the pituitary gland do not experience true adrenal insufficiency because corticosteroids are administered to replace hormones no longer secreted by the adrenals.

Assessment Findings

Decreased or absent adrenocortical hormones lead to symptoms of adrenal insufficiency, which are the same in primary and secondary adrenal insufficiency (Box 51-1). Clients with primary adrenal insufficiency usually experience symptoms gradually. Clients with secondary adrenal insufficiency develop symptoms suddenly or over several days to weeks.

A dose of synthetic ACTH, cosyntropin (Cortrosyn), is administered intramuscularly as a screening test for adrenal function. In primary adrenal insufficiency, an absent or a low cortisol response indicates adrenal insufficiency. In secondary insufficiency, the decrease in serum cortisol levels is less significant.

The serum cortisol level is decreased. Serum sodium and fasting blood glucose levels are low, and serum

BOX 51-1 • Signs and Symptoms of Adrenal Insufficiency

- Increased urinary excretion of sodium and retention of potassium followed by dehydration and reduced blood plasma volume
- Weakness, fatigue, dizziness, hypotension, postural hypotension, hypothermia
- Vascular collapse because of poor myocardial tone, decreased cardiac output, weak and irregular pulse
- Weight loss, anemia, anorexia, gastrointestinal symptoms
- Nervousness, periods of depression
- Hypoglycemia from a deficiency of the hormones that facilitate the conversion of protein into glucose; episodes of hypoglycemia may occur 5 to 6 hours after eating—the period before breakfast is especially dangerous
- Abnormally dark pigmentation, especially of exposed areas of the skin and mucous membranes, and decreased hair growth (primary adrenal insufficiency)

potassium, calcium, and blood urea nitrogen levels are increased. The WBC count often is elevated. A glucose tolerance test shows evidence of hypoglycemia. In Addison's disease, the glucose level in the bloodstream does not rise as high as normal and returns to its fasting level more quickly than it would under normal conditions. The fasting blood glucose level may be low. Radiographs of the adrenals show calcification. An abdominal CT scan reveals atrophy of the adrenal glands.

Medical Management

Clients with primary adrenal insufficiency require daily corticosteroid replacement therapy for the rest of their lives. Fludrocortisone (Florinef), a synthetic corticosteroid preparation that possesses glucocorticoid and mineralocorticoid properties, is often used for replacement therapy. An additional glucocorticoid can be necessary, depending on the client's response to therapy.

Treatment for secondary adrenal insufficiency caused by bilateral adrenalectomy or pituitary failure is the same as treatment for primary adrenal insufficiency. Treatment of secondary adrenal insufficiency resulting from discontinuation of corticosteroid therapy or hemorrhagic infarction of the gland varies and depends on the ability of the adrenals to return to normal function.

If the client is not given or does not take the medication, acute adrenal crisis can develop (see next section). This also applies to clients on long-term corticosteroid therapy for treatment of disorders such as allergies, rheumatoid arthritis, and collagen diseases who abruptly discontinue taking their prescribed steroid. If the drug is to be discontinued, the dose must be tapered over time. Client and Family Teaching 51-1 discusses important information to teach clients receiving corticosteroid therapy.

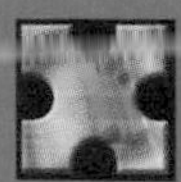

51-1 *Client and Family Teaching*
Corticosteroid Therapy for Adrenal Insufficiency

The nurse explains adrenal insufficiency and the importance of lifetime corticosteroid replacement. A teaching plan includes the following points:

- Lifetime corticosteroid replacement therapy is necessary. Never omit, increase, or decrease a dose. If the prescribed drug is not taken, adrenal insufficiency, which is life-threatening, will occur.
- The body has limited ability to handle stress of any kind. Seek medical attention for dosage readjustment whenever there is stress. Examples of stress include an infection, a motor vehicle accident (even if not noticeably hurt), a family crisis, and a heavy workload.
- Avoid exposure to infections and excessive fatigue.
- If an infection (e.g., sore throat, upper respiratory tract infection) or other type of illness occurs, contact the physician immediately. An increased medication dose may be necessary.
- Vomiting, diarrhea, or any other condition that prevents the medication from being taken orally or interferes with proper drug absorption requires immediate medical attention. Parenteral administration will be necessary.
- Wear identification, such as a MedicAlert tag or bracelet, stating that the wearer has adrenal insufficiency. If an accident or other problem occurs, medical personnel must be made aware of the need for corticosteroids.
- Follow the diet recommended by the physician.

Nursing Management

Obtain a complete health history that includes presence or absence of weight loss, salt craving, nausea and vomiting, abdominal cramps, diarrhea, muscle weakness, and decreased stress tolerance. Take vital signs frequently. Hypoglycemia may be seen in clients with primary adrenal insufficiency. These clients must never receive insulin by error because insulin would lower blood glucose to a critically low level that could result in brain damage, coma, or death.

Nursing management of the client with primary adrenal insufficiency is essentially the same as that of the client with secondary adrenal insufficiency because the major problem in both types is a lack of adrenal cortical hormones. The client with secondary adrenal insufficiency because of surgery (bilateral adrenalectomy, surgical removal of the pituitary) has a controlled deficiency that hormone replacement therapy corrects.

Keep careful records of fluid intake and urine output. Weigh client daily on the same scale, at a similar time, with similar clothing. Notify the physician if dehydration, signs of hyponatremia, or progressive weight loss occurs. Encourage client to drink fluids and eat the prescribed diet to maintain fluid and electrolyte balance. If serum sodium levels are decreased, instruct client to add salt to food. If excessive perspiration occurs, increase fluid and salt intake.

Minimize any reason for fasting, such as before a diagnostic test, because regular carbohydrate intake maintains the blood glucose level. Observe for symptoms of hypoglycemia: hunger, headache, sweating, weakness, trembling, emotional instability, visual disturbances, and, finally, disorientation, and loss of consciousness. Check client's blood glucose level with a glucometer 30 minutes before each meal, at bedtime, and whenever the client is symptomatic. Follow agency protocol for raising blood glucose level, which may include offering the client a glass of grape juice if the level is below 80 mg/dL and rechecking the level in 15 minutes. If the blood glucose level continues to be low, repeat administration of grape juice. Give client milk and graham crackers when the blood glucose level is above 80 mg/dL, because milk and graham crackers contain forms of carbohydrate that take longer to absorb and tend to maintain the blood glucose level for an extended period. Offer five or six small meals per day rather than three regular meals to control hypoglycemic episodes; if client is eating three meals per day, give between-meal snacks of milk and crackers.

• ACUTE ADRENAL CRISIS (ADDISONIAN CRISIS)

Clients with either primary or secondary adrenal insufficiency are at risk for **addisonian crisis,** a life-threatening endocrine emergency.

Pathophysiology and Etiology

Acute adrenal crisis occurs when adrenal glands suddenly fail. Because hormones of the adrenal cortex affect the body's adaptive reactions to stress, clients with Addison's disease may develop acute adrenal crisis when faced with extreme stress. Even uncomplicated surgery requires more physiologic adaptive ability than a client with Addison's disease usually possesses. Salt deprivation, infection, trauma, exposure to cold, overexertion, or any abnormal stress can cause adrenal crisis. Acute adrenal crisis can occur when corticosteroid therapy is suddenly stopped. If the condition is untreated, coma and death result.

Assessment Findings

Adrenal crisis may be sudden or gradual. It may begin with anorexia, nausea, vomiting, diarrhea, abdominal pain, profound weakness, headache, intensification of hypotension, restlessness, or fever. Unless the corticosteroid dose is increased to meet the demand, the client progresses to acute adrenal crisis. The BP markedly decreases, and shock develops.

Medical Management

Adrenal crisis is an emergency; death may occur from hypotension and vasomotor collapse. Corticosteroids are given IV in solutions of normal saline and glucose. Antibiotics are administered because of an extremely low resistance to infection.

Nursing Management

Two important nursing tasks are recognition of signs and symptoms of adrenal crisis and accurate administration of corticosteroid drugs. A client with a diagnosis of adrenal insufficiency is a candidate for acute adrenal crisis. Constantly observe such clients for this problem. Administer the correct dose of corticosteroid therapy at the correct time. Doses must never be omitted or abruptly discontinued because this can result in adrenal crisis. Once the condition is recognized, take vital signs frequently, paying special attention to heart rate and rhythm. Observe for signs of hyponatremia and hyperkalemia. Keep the client warm and as quiet as possible until treatment is instituted and the condition is stabilized.

• CUSHING'S SYNDROME (ADRENOCORTICAL HYPERFUNCTION)

Cushing's syndrome is an endocrine disorder resulting from excessive secretion of hormones by the adrenal cortex.

Pathophysiology and Etiology

Overproduction of adrenocortical hormones results from (1) overproduction of ACTH by the pituitary gland, with resultant hyperplasia of the adrenal cortex and excessive production and secretion of glucocorticoids, mineralocorticoids, and androgens; (2) benign or malignant tumors of the pituitary gland or adrenal cortex; or (3) prolonged administration of high doses of corticosteroids. Hyperadrenalism affects most body systems and causes many changes in appearance and physiology. The term **cushingoid syndrome** refers to the physical changes that accompany this disorder (Fig. 51.4), which include suppression of the inflammatory response, hyperglycemia, hypokalemia, hypernatremia with subsequent weight gain and elevated BP, peptic ulcer, demineralization of bones, and muscle weakness. Increased levels of androgenic hormone cause women to acquire male secondary sex characteristics. Both sexes experience decreased sexual drive. Many suffer from depression, and the endocrine imbalance may cause psychosis.

Assessment Findings

Physical examination reveals muscle wasting and weakness resulting from extensive protein depletion. Carbohydrate tolerance is lowered, and signs and symptoms of diabetes mellitus develop (see Chap. 52). Fat is redistributed, leading to facial fullness and the characteristic moon face and buffalo hump. The skin is thin, and the face is ruddy. The client has increased susceptibility to wounds, and healing is prolonged. The immunosuppressive effects of the disorder usually mask symptoms of infection.

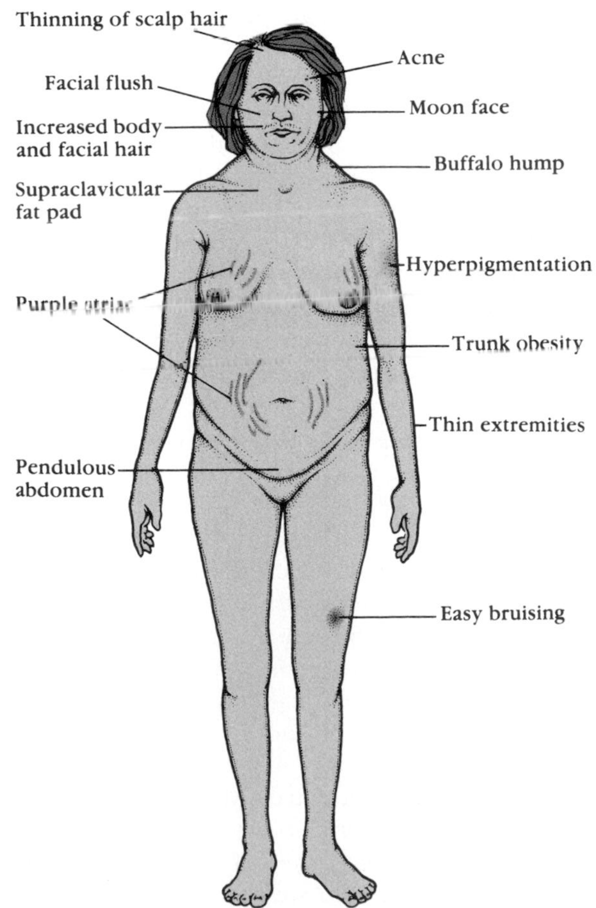

FIGURE 51.4 The symptoms of Cushing's disease. (From Beyers, M. & Dudas, S. [Eds.]. [1984]. *The clinical practice of medical surgical nursing* [p. 71]. Boston: Little, Brown.)

Because blood vessels are fragile, the client bruises easily, and striae often form over extensive skin areas. Bones become so demineralized that the client may have backache, kyphosis, and collapse of the vertebrae. He or she retains sodium and water, and peripheral edema and hypertension develop. The client reports mood changes and difficulty coping with stressors that were manageable in the past. The family may report serious mental changes. In women, Cushing's syndrome produces masculinization with hirsutism and amenorrhea. These sexual changes and alterations in appearance are reversible when adrenocortical hormone levels return to normal (Fig. 51.5).

Diagnosis is tentatively based on physical changes. Urine levels of 17-hydroxycorticosteroids (17-OHCS) and 17-ketosteroids (17-KS) almost always are increased. Plasma and urine cortisol levels are elevated. An overnight dexamethasone suppression test is used as an initial screening. The client takes 1 mg oral dexamethasone; the next morning plasma cortisol levels are obtained. If results are above normal (5 mg/dL), 0.5 mg dexamethasone is given every 6 hours, and 24-hour urine collections are tested for 2 consecutive days. Clients without the disorder will have decreased 17-OHCS and 17-KS levels; these levels remain elevated in those with Cushing's syndrome.

Laboratory blood test results also reveal increased serum sodium, decreased serum potassium, and increased blood glucose levels. Abdominal radiographs, CT scan, or MRI may show adrenal enlargement, and an IV pyelogram may show changes in the renal shadow caused by an abnormally large adrenal gland.

Medical and Surgical Management

Treatment depends on whether a tumor or adrenal hyperplasia causes the disorder. It is directed toward removing the cause and lowering plasma cortisol levels. Radiation therapy to or removal of the pituitary may be used for adrenal hyperplasia. Bilateral adrenalectomy may be preferred if both adrenals are involved.

Drug therapy includes diuretics for edema as well as an antihypertensive agent. A diet low in sodium and carbohydrates controls edema and blood glucose level. Antibiotics are used to treat infection.

If cushingoid syndrome results from exogenous administration of a corticosteroid preparation, the drug is slowly withdrawn by tapering the dose over days or weeks. In some instances, as in the treatment of a disorder such as

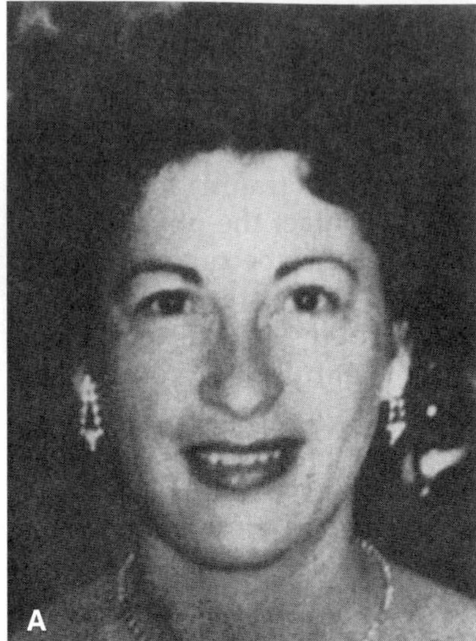
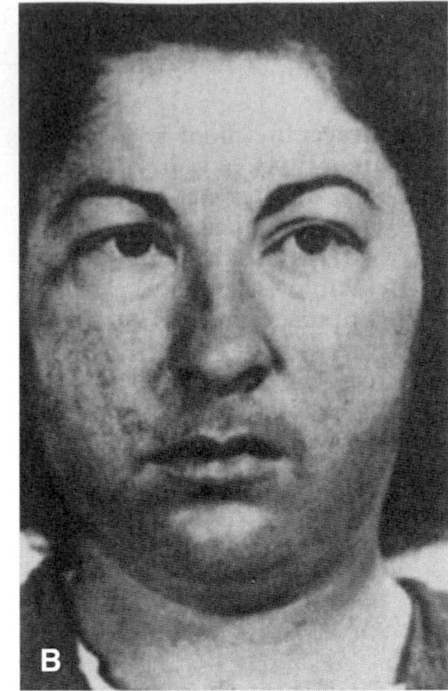
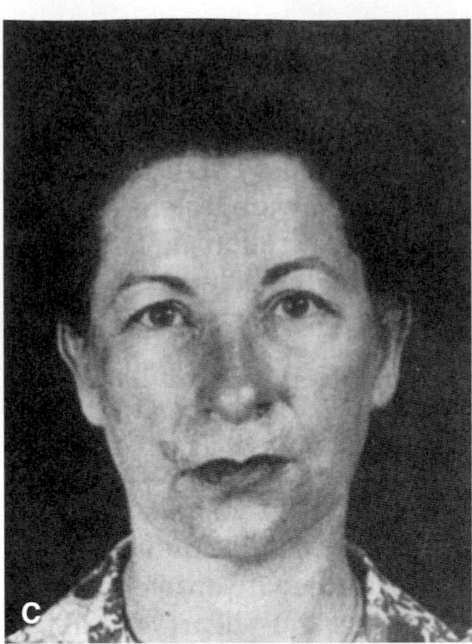

FIGURE 51.5 Progressive facial changes in a woman with Cushing's disease: (**A**) before onset of the illness, (**B**) preoperative, and (**C**) 1 year after surgery.

leukemia, or to prevent rejection of transplanted organs, the syndrome is allowed to persist.

NURSING PROCESS

The Client With Cushing's Syndrome

Assessment

Obtain thorough medical, drug, and allergy histories and observe for symptoms of an adrenal disorder: altered skin pigmentation and integrity, decreased energy level, mental changes, sexual dysfunction, and changes in mood, appetite, weight, and bowel patterns. Monitor vital signs every 4 hours and test blood, urine, or both for glucose three or four times per day. If urine tests positive for glucose or the blood glucose level is elevated, report the information to the physician.

Because the client is at risk for developing peptic ulcers, observe the color of and test each stool for occult blood. If the client reports epigastric pain or discomfort or the stool has a black appearance or tests positive for blood, make the physician aware of the findings.

Diagnosis, Planning, and Interventions

If corticosteroid therapy has caused a cushingoid appearance and the dose is to be tapered over time, give the client and family a detailed explanation of the tapering schedule. Review the directions printed on the prescription container and emphasize the importance of strictly following the tapering schedule. The client may find it helpful to use a calendar to enter the dosage for each day of the tapering schedule.

Depending on many factors, such as age and severity of the disorder, clients with Cushing's syndrome may or may not be scheduled for adrenalectomy or irradiation of the pituitary. Until such time as further treatment is scheduled, emphasize the importance of continued medical supervision. Important points to emphasize include avoiding skin trauma; contacting the physician if sores or cuts do not heal or become infected, if easy bruising occurs, or if stools are dark or black; following the recommended diet; reading food labels carefully; avoiding exposure to infection; avoiding nonprescription drugs (unless approved by the physician); weighing self weekly; and reporting marked weight gain or edema to the physician.

Excess Fluid Volume related to sodium and water retention

Expected Outcome: Fluid volume will be normal as evidenced by equivalent fluid intake and output volumes, reduced or no dependent edema, consistent daily weights, and BP measurements within normal limits.

- Examine extremities for increased or decreased edema. *Fluid retention is manifested by swelling in dependent areas, pitting when pressure is applied to the skin over a bone, tight-fitting shoes or rings, the appearance of lines in the skin from stockings, and seams in the shoes or areas where they lace. Swelling and pitting in dependent areas indicates fluid retention.*
- Measure intake and output daily, weekly, or as ordered. *Acutely ill clients require more frequent assessment. A gain of 2 pounds in 24 hours suggests 1 L of water retention.*
- Assess vital signs each shift; report systolic BP that exceeds 139 mm Hg or diastolic BP that exceeds 89 mm Hg. *Hypertension is defined as a consistently elevated BP above 139/89 mm Hg (see Chap. 29). One factor that contributes to hypertension is excess circulatory volume.*

- Administer prescribed diuretics. *They promote excretion of sodium and water.*
- Provide a sodium-restricted diet at the level prescribed by the physician. *Limiting sodium reduces the potential for fluid retention.*

Risk for Impaired Skin Integrity related to thinning of skin and edema

Expected Outcome: Skin will remain intact.

- Inspect skin daily, especially over bony prominences, for open lesions or ulcers. *The skin is thin and fragile and prone to breaking down with minimal trauma.*
- Encourage client to change positions frequently. *Relieving pressure on capillaries helps maintain a supply of oxygenated blood to cells and tissues.*
- Handle client gently; use interventions that relieve pressure on the skin. *Gentleness reduces the potential for skin abrasions and development of pressure ulcers.*
- Exercise care when performing tasks that may damage the skin, such as removing tape when discontinuing an IV infusion. *The skin's fragility increases its potential for injury.*

Disturbed Body Image related to changes in appearance

Expected Outcome: Client will express a positive self-image.

- Provide client opportunities to express feelings over physical changes. *Verbalizing feelings with a supportive person increases the client's ability to cope with stress.*
- Explain that when the cause of the disorder is eliminated, some physical changes gradually improve, but others, such as striae and kyphosis, are permanent. *Being honest and sharing accurate information promotes the client's trust and confidence.*
- Offer suggestions such as wearing loose clothing, a hat, or cap, to help disguise physical changes that the client finds difficult to tolerate. *Although the client's perception of physical changes probably is more exaggerated than others', he or she may feel more confident in social situations with techniques that minimize changes in appearance.*

Evaluation of Expected Outcomes

Fluid volume is normal, with no evidence of edema, hypertension, or weight gain. Skin is intact. The client copes effectively with physical changes.

HYPERALDOSTERONISM

Secretion of aldosterone, a mineralocorticoid, is regulated by serum levels of potassium and sodium, the renin–angiotensin mechanism, and ACTH. Hypersecretion of aldosterone creates extreme electrolyte imbalances.

Pathophysiology and Etiology

The cause of primary hyperaldosteronism may be a benign aldosterone-secreting adenoma of one of the adrenals, an adrenal malignant tumor, or unknown. Pregnancy, congestive heart failure, narrowing of the renal artery, and cirrhosis can cause secondary hyperaldosteronism.

Excessive secretion of aldosterone results in increased reabsorption of sodium and water and excretion of potassium by the kidneys. Figure 51.6 presents an overview of the renin–angiotensin–aldosterone cycle.

Assessment Findings

Headache, muscle weakness, increased urine output, fatigue, hypertension, and cardiac dysrhythmias are seen. Serum potassium levels are decreased and serum sodium levels are increased in the absence of other causes, such as diuretic therapy or diarrhea. Serum bicarbonate, serum aldosterone, and plasma renin levels are increased. CT or MRI may rule out or locate an adrenal tumor. Adrenal venography may identify small tumors that CT scanning fails to reveal.

Medical and Surgical Management

If the cause is an adrenal tumor, unilateral adrenalectomy may be performed. Medical management may include administration of spironolactone, a potassium-sparing diuretic, and an antihypertensive agent to control BP. A sodium-restricted diet may be necessary.

Nursing Management

Monitor vital signs every 4 hours or as ordered. Report marked elevations to the physician. Measure fluid intake

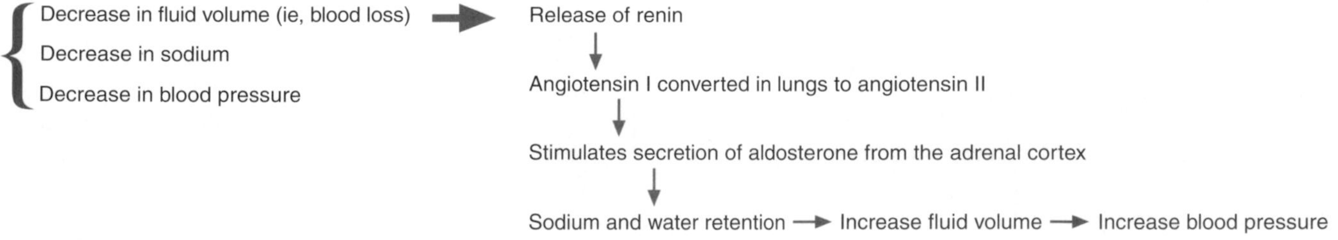

FIGURE 51.6 The renin–angiotensin–aldosterone cycle.

and output and weigh the client every 2 to 7 days. Examine the extremities for edema daily. Observe for signs of hypokalemia and hypernatremia.

● ADRENALECTOMY

Adrenalectomy is surgical removal of the adrenal gland(s), usually to remove a cancerous tumor. In some instances, removal of ovaries, testes, and both adrenal glands (which secrete male and female hormones), is considered to control cancers of the breast and prostate, which depend on hormones for growth.

The adrenals are surgically approached by means of an abdominal incision or a flank incision under and following the position of the 12th rib. The abdominal incision usually is long because adequate exposure is needed to access the adrenals, which lie posteriorly.

Nursing Management

Preoperative Period

Major goals include reduced anxiety and an understanding of preparations for surgery and possible postoperative events. Keep the client on bed rest and minimize anxiety. The client who requires surgery to halt progression of a metastatic disease may be anxious as well as depressed and needs time to discuss the surgery and anticipated results. When bilateral adrenalectomy is scheduled, the nurse may start IV administration of a solution containing a corticosteroid preparation the morning of surgery. Some surgeons prefer to initiate corticosteroid administration during removal of the adrenals. Additional preparations are the same as for the client having general surgery.

Postoperative Period

When the client returns from surgery, review the surgical record because postoperative observations and management depend on whether one or both adrenal glands were removed. In addition to complications associated with general anesthesia, observe for such problems as hemorrhage, atelectasis, and pneumothorax because adrenals are located close to the diaphragm and inferior vena cava. Monitor vital signs frequently and closely observe for signs of adrenal insufficiency (addisonian crisis, adrenal crisis), which may occur when:

- The prescribed dose of a corticosteroid preparation is inadequate to meet the client's needs (bilateral adrenalectomy).
- The remaining adrenal gland does not produce sufficient hormone to meet the client's needs (unilateral adrenalectomy).
- The prescribed dose of a corticosteroid preparation is not given.

If symptoms of adrenal insufficiency occur, notify the physician immediately. Do not omit administering a prescribed corticosteroid because corticosteroid replacement is essential to life. Acute adrenal insufficiency is managed with infusions of IV solutions, glucose, and cortisol. Client and Family Teaching 51-2 provides detailed instructions for postdischarge management of the client who has undergone bilateral adrenalectomy.

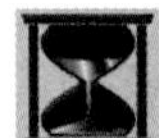

GENERAL GERONTOLOGIC CONSIDERATIONS

Changes in hormone levels may accompany aging. Although levels of T_4 tend to remain constant, levels of T_3 may decrease with age. Parathyroid hormone levels tend to increase with age. Older adults have an increased incidence of nodules and small goiters on the thyroid gland.

Symptoms of thyroid disease in older adults often are atypical or minor and easily attributed to other problems. For example, the older adult may not experience restlessness or hyperactivity and may not appear nervous. Symptoms seen most often in older adults include anorexia, weight loss, palpitations, angina, and atrial fibrillation. The most reliable thyroid function test to diagnose hyperthyroidism in an older adult is a serum T_4 level.

Hypothyroidism is difficult to identify in older adults because symptoms closely resemble normal aging—for example, anorexia, constipation, weight loss, muscular weakness and pain, joint stiffness, apathy, and depression.

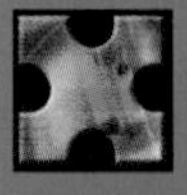

51-2 *Client and Family Teaching* Discharge Instructions After Adrenalectomy

The nurse teaches the client about the:

- Function of the adrenal glands and importance of adhering to the prescribed treatment regimen
- Care of the surgical wound until healed
- Medication schedule
- Need for obtaining adequate rest, eating a well-balanced diet, complying with ongoing medical supervision, avoiding infections and stressful situations, carrying identification indicating surgical removal of the adrenal glands, and seeking immediate medical help if unable to take the prescribed corticosteroid drug or if symptoms of adrenal insufficiency and adrenal crisis develop

Dosages of thyroid replacement drugs are lower in older adults, and drug therapy is initiated slowly and increased cautiously. The older adult receiving thyroid replacement therapy is at increased risk for adverse reactions associated with cardiac function.

Critical Thinking Exercises

1. *When caring for a client receiving fludrocortisone (Florinef) orally after bilateral adrenalectomy, nurses have a team conference to review the client's potential for acute adrenal insufficiency. What information is appropriate to discuss?*
2. *A client had a thyroidectomy this morning. It is now 8:00 PM, and she complains of difficulty swallowing clear liquids and a fullness in her throat. Her BP is normal, but her pulse rate is elevated. You see no drainage on the surface of her dressing. What actions would you take at this time?*

• NCLEX-STYLE REVIEW QUESTIONS 

1. A client diagnosed with hypothyroidism is taking a thyroid replacement. Prior to discharge from the hospital, the nurse instructs the client to report to the physician any side effects of the drug including chest pain, insomnia, and hyperactivity. What is the best explanation for the nurse's instruction?
   1. The side effects indicate that the dosage is too low and needs to be increased.
   2. The side effects determine whether the medication should be changed.
   3. The side effects of thyroid replacement often mimic those of hyperthyroidism.
   4. The side effects indicate that an adverse drug reaction is occurring.
2. A confirmation of Cushing's syndrome has been given to a hospitalized client. The client asks the nurse about the cause of the disorder. Which response by the nurse is most accurate?
   1. "Cushing's syndrome results from decreased iodine in the diet."
   2. "Cushing's syndrome results from overproduction of ACTH by the pituitary."
   3. "Cushing's syndrome is caused by a reduction of calcium from the bone."
   4. "Cushing's syndrome is caused by an elevation in blood glucose."
3. The nurse weighs a client hospitalized with cushingoid syndrome daily. What explanation can be given for the nurse's action?
   1. In clients with cushingoid syndrome, excess fluid volume relates to sodium and water retention, which causes weight gain.
   2. In clients with cushingoid syndrome, fat is frequently redistributed causing weight gain.
   3. In clients with cushingoid syndrome, sodium fluctuates, causing excess urine output and weight loss.
   4. In clients with cushingoid syndrome, excessive urine output results in fluid volume deficit and weight loss.

connection

Visit the Connection site at **http://connection.lww.com/go/timbyEssentials** for links to chapter-related resources on the Internet.

References and Suggested Readings

A quick check of the endocrine system. (2000). *Nursing 2000, 30*(8), Critical Care, 32cc10–32cc11.

Carr, S. (2001). Acromegaly management in the community. *Nursing Times, 97*(2), 32–33.

Incredibly easy! Understanding goiter. (2001). *Nursing 2001, 31* (8), 78.

Innis, J. (2002). Critical care: Recognizing lithium-induced diabetes insipidus. *Nursing 2002, 32*(6), 32cc, 12, 15.

Kaye, J., Morton, J., Bowcutt, M., et al. (2000). Stress, depression, and psychoneuroimmunology. *Journal of Neuroscience Nursing, 32*(2), 93–100.

Levin, N. A., & Greer, K. E. (2001). Cutaneous manifestations of endocrine disorders. *Dermatology Nursing, 13,* 185–186, 189–196, 201–202.

Nayback, A. M. (2000). Hyponatremia as a consequence of acute adrenal insufficiency and hypothyroidism. *Journal of Emergency Nursing, 26,* 130–133.

Sabol, V. K. (2001). Addisonian crisis: This life-threatening condition may be triggered by a variety of stressors. *American Journal of Nursing, 101*(7), Advanced Practice Extra, 24AAA, 24CCC–24DDD.

Terpstra, T. L., & Terpstra, T. L. (2000). Syndrome of inappropriate antidiuretic hormone secretion: Recognition and management. *MEDSURG Nursing, 9*(2), 61–70.

chapter 52

Caring for Clients With Diabetes Mellitus

Words to Know 

diabetes mellitus
diabetic ketoacidosis
diabetic nephropathy
diabetic retinopathy
fasting blood glucose
glycosuria
glycosylated hemoglobin
hyperglycemia
hyperosmolar hyperglycemic nonketotic syndrome
hypoglycemia
ketoacidosis
ketonemia
ketones
Kussmaul respirations
lipoatrophy
lipohypertrophy
lipolysis
metabolic syndrome
oral glucose tolerance test
polydipsia
polyphagia
polyuria
postprandial glucose
random blood glucose
renal threshold

Learning Objectives

On completion of this chapter, the reader will:

- Define and distinguish the types of diabetes mellitus.
- Identify the classic symptoms of diabetes mellitus.
- Explain the source of ketones.
- Name laboratory methods used to diagnose diabetes mellitus.
- Describe methods used to treat diabetes mellitus.
- Explain the cause of diabetic ketoacidosis.
- List goals in the treatment of diabetic ketoacidosis.
- Identify physiologic signs of hyperosmolar hyperglycemic nonketotic syndrome.
- Describe treatment of hyperosmolar hyperglycemia nonketotic syndrome.
- Explain the cause and treatment of hypoglycemia.
- List common complications of diabetes mellitus.
- Differentiate symptoms of hypoglycemia and hyperglycemia.
- Discuss the nursing management of the client with diabetes mellitus.

Diabetes mellitus, a metabolic disorder of the pancreas, affects carbohydrate, fat, and protein metabolism. It is reaching epidemic proportions in the United States. Diabetes in adults may be a consequence of **metabolic syndrome,** which includes obesity, especially in the abdominal area; high blood pressure (BP); elevated triglyceride, low-density lipoprotein, and blood glucose levels; and a low high-density lipoprotein level (see Chap. 27).

Most affected persons acquire the disease as adults. Diabetes is the seventh leading cause of death in the United States. Because of the chronic nature of diabetes, affected persons experience many debilitating and life-threatening complications before death.

DIABETES MELLITUS

There are two major forms of diabetes mellitus:

- Type 1—insulin-dependent diabetes mellitus (IDDM), also referred to as *juvenile diabetes* because it affects children and adolescents, is characterized by no insulin production by the beta cells in the islets of Langerhans of the pancreas (Fig. 52.1).
- Type 2—non–insulin-dependent diabetes mellitus (NIDDM) is characterized by insulin resistance or insufficient insulin production. Although NIDDM is more common in aging adults (half of affected clients are older than 55 years), type 2 diabetes also is being detected in obese children.

Hyperglycemia, an elevated blood glucose level, is associated with other disorders or their management, such as pancreatitis (see Chap. 49), which causes both exocrine and endocrine disturbances. When production of adrenocortical hormones is excessive, as in Cushing's syndrome (see Chap. 51), or with administration of glucocorticoid drugs for immunosuppressive purposes, secondary diabetes can develop.

Pathophysiology and Etiology

Type 1 Diabetes Mellitus

Insulin has three functions: (1) it carries glucose into body cells as the preferred source of energy, (2) it promotes storage of glucose as glycogen, and (3) it inhibits

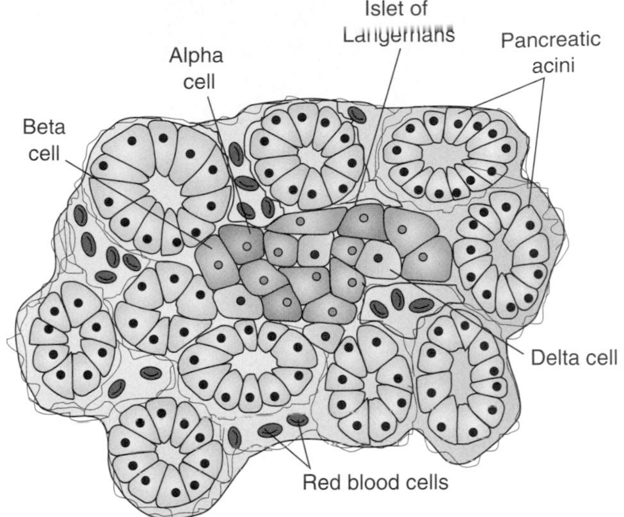

FIGURE 52.1 Islet of Langerhans in the pancreas. (Guyton, A. C. & Hall, J. E. [1996]. *Textbook of medical physiology* [9th ed.]. Philadelphia: W. B. Saunders.)

breakdown of glycogen back into glucose. In type 1 diabetes, the islet cells, or endocrine portion of the pancreas, cease to produce insulin. Without insulin, blood glucose levels rise beyond normal range, and the body breaks down fat and protein as alternative sources of cellular energy (Porth, 2002). Breakdown of fat, known as **lipolysis,** results in the accumulation of fatty acids and **ketones,** metabolic byproducts of fat metabolism. When ketones accumulate in the blood, clients with diabetes are prone to developing a form of metabolic acidosis known as **ketoacidosis.** In type 1 diabetes, ketoacidosis develops quite suddenly because of the total cessation of insulin production.

Type 1 diabetes is considered an autoimmune disorder. It has been shown that a genetic mutation causes killer (CD8) T-cell lymphocytes to attack and destroy the insulin-producing islet cells (Kolata, 2002). It is hypothesized that B-cell lymphocytes and macrophages of people with type 1 diabetes lack a protein marker that helps T cells identify natural cells as "self." T cells misidentify islet cells as unnatural and subsequently destroy them.

Type 2 Diabetes Mellitus

Diabetes mellitus, especially type 2, runs in families, although a specific diabetic gene has not been isolated. In this type of diabetes, the beta cells of the islets of Langerhans secrete insulin into the bloodstream, but blood glucose levels remain elevated because of peripheral insulin resistance and increased conversion of glycogen to glucose by the liver. Insulin resistance is linked to obesity, especially intra-abdominal obesity. The correlation of obesity and insulin resistance helps explain how dieting and weight loss control type 2 diabetes and delay, reduce, or eliminate the need for medication to treat the disease.

Lack of response to the usual amount of insulin causes beta cells to secrete even more insulin. Despite hyperinsulinemia, however, the blood glucose level remains elevated. Eventually, overstimulation exhausts beta cells, resulting in a decline in insulin production. The client with type 2 diabetes also becomes insulin deficient.

Excessive glucose levels lead to **glycosuria,** glucose in the urine, and urinary excretion. Glycosuria appears when the blood glucose level rises above 180 mg/dL. At this level, the kidneys' **renal threshold,** the ability to reabsorb glucose and return it to the bloodstream, is impaired. Hypertonicity from concentrated amounts of blood glucose pulls fluid into the vascular system, resulting in **polyuria,** excessive urine production. Increased excreted urine accompanies urinary frequency. Because so much water is lost, **polydipsia,** excessive thirst, develops.

While needed glucose is wasted, the body's requirement for fuel continues. The person with diabetes feels hungry and eats more (**polyphagia**). Despite eating more, he or she loses weight as the body uses fat and protein to substitute for glucose. Ketones, chemical intermediate products in fat metabolism, such as acetone, cause ketoacidosis when they accumulate.

The bicarbonate buffer system buffers ketones. Thus, **ketonemia** (increased ketones in the blood) causes a decreased alkali (base) reserve, leading to acidosis. **Kussmaul respirations** (fast, deep, labored breathing) are common in ketoacidosis (Fig. 52.2). Acetone can be detected on the breath by its characteristic odor. If treatment is not initiated, the outcome of ketoacidosis is circulatory collapse, renal shutdown, and death. Ketoacidosis is more common in clients with diabetes who no longer produce insulin, such as those with type 1 diabetes. Clients with type 2 diabetes are more likely to develop hyperosmolar hyperglycemic nonketotic syndrome (HHNKS; see later discussion) because with limited insulin, they can use enough glucose to prevent ketosis, but not enough to maintain normal blood glucose levels.

Stop, Think, and Respond ● BOX 52-1

Identify some differences between type 1 and type 2 diabetes mellitus.

Assessment Findings

Three classic symptoms of both types of diabetes mellitus are polyuria, polydipsia, and polyphagia. Additional symptoms include weight loss, weakness, thirst, fatigue, and dehydration. These signs and symptoms occur abruptly in clients with type 1 diabetes and more gradually in clients with type 2 diabetes. Some develop skin, urinary tract,

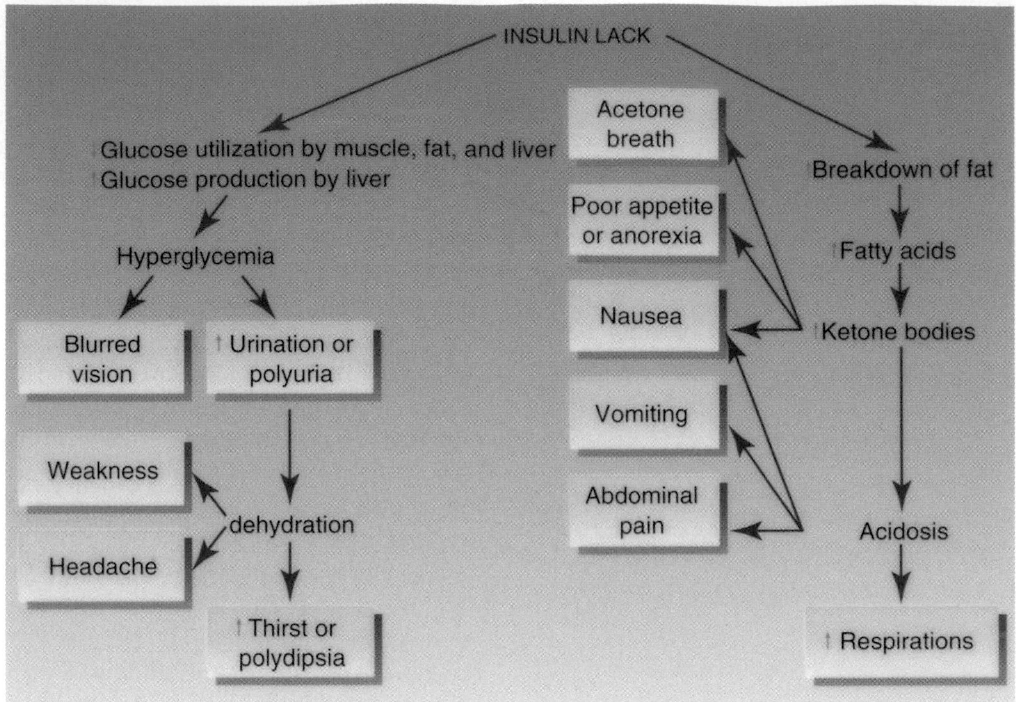

FIGURE 52.2 Abnormal metabolism that causes signs and symptoms of diabetic ketoacidosis: ↑, increased; ↓, decreased. (Pearce, M. A., Rosenberg, C. S., & Davidson, M. D. [1991]. Patient education. In M. B. Davidson [Ed.], *Diabetes mellitus: Diagnosis and treatment* [3rd ed.]. New York: Churchill Livingstone.)

and vaginal infections, possibly because elevated blood glucose levels support bacterial growth. There may be changes in visual acuity manifested by blurred vision because the hypertonicity of body fluid affects cells in the lens and retina (Porth, 2002).

Although diabetes mellitus is a highly complex disease, screening for its detection is relatively simple. Normally, urine contains no detectable glucose or ketones; in diabetes, one or both may be present. Because the body fails to use glucose adequately, it excretes glucose in the urine. If the body metabolizes fats faster than it can use the ketone bodies, ketone bodies also appear in urine. The relative ease of these urinary tests facilitates early detection of diabetes (Nursing Guidelines 52-1).

Because glycosuria and ketonuria may not become evident until glucose exceeds the renal threshold, blood tests help establish the diagnosis. They include random blood sugar, fasting blood glucose, postprandial glucose, and the oral glucose tolerance test (Table 52.1). Another method of testing for blood glucose is with a glucometer, which measures capillary blood glucose from a finger stick blood sample. Close monitoring of blood glucose levels can delay onset of complications associated with diabetes. Self-monitoring with a glucometer is helpful for those taking hypoglycemic agents to determine effects of diet, exercise, and drugs.

Once a client with diabetes receives a treatment regimen to follow, the physician can assess effectiveness of treatment and client compliance by obtaining a glycosylated hemoglobin or hemoglobin A1c test. Results reflect the amount of glucose stored in the hemoglobin molecule during its life span of 120 days. Normally, the level of glycosylated hemoglobin is less than 7%. A hemoglobin A1c of 7% is the equivalent of an average blood glucose

NURSING GUIDELINES 52-1

Performing Urine Glucose Testing

Method: Test-tape and Diastix

- Client empties the bladder to eliminate glucose and ketones that have been stored in the bladder for hours; save this specimen in case the client cannot void later.
- Encourage the client to drink water; ask the client to void in 30 minutes.
- For the client with an indwelling catheter, clamp the catheter for 30 minutes and take the specimen directly from the catheter, not the drainage bag.
- Test the second voided specimen to detect current concentration of glucose and ketones.
- Dip the testing strip into the urine and wait for the recommended time.
- Observe the color change and document the results.

TABLE 52.1 DIAGNOSTIC TESTS FOR DETECTING GLUCOSE INTOLERANCE

TEST	IMPLEMENTATION	DIAGNOSTIC RESULT
Random blood glucose	Blood specimen is drawn without preplanning.	≥200 mg/dL in the presence of symptoms is suggestive of diabetes mellitus.
Fasting blood glucose	Blood specimen is obtained after 8 hours of fasting.	In the nondiabetic client the glucose level will be between 70 and 110 mg/dL. In the diabetic client glucose is ≥ 110 mg/dL but <126 mg/dL.
Postprandial glucose	Blood sample is taken 2 hours after a high-carbohydrate meal.	In the nondiabetic client, the glucose level will be between 70 and 110 mg/dL. In the client with diabetes mellitus, the result is ≥140 mg/dL but <200 mg/dL.
Oral glucose tolerance test	Diet high in carbohydrates is eaten for 3 days. Client then fasts for 8 hours. A baseline blood sample is drawn and a urine specimen is collected. An oral glucose solution is given and time of ingestion recorded. Blood is drawn at 30 minutes and 1, 2, and 3 hours after the ingestion of glucose solution. Urine is collected simultaneously. Drinking water is encouraged to promote urine excretion.	In the nondiabetic client, the glucose returns to normal in 2 to 3 hours and urine is negative for glucose. In the diabetic client, blood glucose level returns to normal slowly; urine is positive for glucose.
Glycosylated hemoglobin or Hemoglobin A1c	Single sample of venous blood is withdrawn.	The amount of glucose stored by the hemoglobin is elevated above 7.0% in the newly diagnosed client with diabetes mellitus, in one who is noncompliant, or in one who is inadequately treated.

level of 150 mg/dL. Amounts of 8% or greater indicate that control of the client's blood glucose level has been inadequate during the previous 2 to 3 months.

Medical Management

Treatment depends on many factors, such as the type of diabetes and the ability of the pancreas to manufacture insulin. It involves combinations of diet and weight loss, exercise, insulin, oral antidiabetic agents, pancreas transplantation, and islet cell transplantation.

Diet and Weight Loss

Diet is a major component of treatment for diabetes. A diabetic diet depends on the client's sex, age, height and weight, activity level, occupation, state of health, former dietary habits, and cultural background. With prescribed dietary allowances (calories, percentages of carbohydrates, fats, and proteins), the client receives a diet prescription and list of substitutions and exchanges to vary the diet. For example, the physician determines that the client with diabetes may have 1500 calories per day. Calories are then distributed according to percentages of carbohydrates, fats, and proteins that equal the total prescribed caloric amount. A dietitian provides the client with a list of foods in six different categories—starch/bread, meat, vegetable, fruit, milk, and fat—and indicates how many items from each category the client can consume for breakfast, lunch, dinner, and snacks (Fig. 52.3). The dietitian gives the client a list of foods in each category and their equivalent amounts. The client can then exchange or substitute one food for another in the specified amount for variety (Fig. 52.4).

	1 Starch/Bread	2 Meat	3 Vegetable	4 Fruit	5 Milk	6 Fat
Breakfast	2			1	1	1
Snack time						
Lunch	2	1	1	1		1
Snack time				1		
Dinner	2	2	1	1		2
Snack time	1			1	1	

FIGURE 52.3 A diabetic meal plan for 1500 calories.

Bran cereals, concentrated	⅓ cup
Bran cereals, flaked (Bran Buds, All Bran)	½ cup
Bread	1 oz
Bulgur, cooked	½ cup
Cooked cereals	½ cup
Cornmeal, dry	1½ tsp
Grapenuts	3 tbsp
Grits, cooked	½ cup
Pasta, cooked	½ cup
Rice (white or brown), cooked	½ cup
Shredded Wheat	½ cup
Unsweetened cereals	¾ cup
Wheat germ	3 tsp
Lentils, cooked	⅓ cup
Baked beans	¼ cup
Beans and peas, cooked (kidney, split)	⅓ cup
Corn	½ cup
Corn on cob	6" 1
Lima beans	½ cup
Peas, green (canned or frozen)	½ cup
Plantain	½ cup
Potato, baked (3 oz)	1 small
Potato, mashed	½ cup
Squash, winter (acorn, butternut)	¾ cup
Yam, sweet potato, plain	⅓ cup

FIGURE 52.4 Sample of starch/bread categories.

Dietary modifications alone can control type 2 diabetes for some clients. These clients have a mild form of diabetes, with the pancreas producing some insulin. The client with diabetes who is overweight is placed on a weight reduction diet because diabetes is less easily controlled in the presence of obesity. Even moderate weight loss improves the body's use of insulin.

Exercise

Exercise helps metabolize carbohydrates, thus decreasing insulin requirements. It improves circulation, which is compromised in the client with diabetes. Exercise also lowers cholesterol and triglyceride levels and improves muscle tone. An exercise program for clients with diabetes specifies the type of exercise and the length of time to perform it and is tailored according to each client's needs and lifestyle. Clients need to exercise consistently each day. Sporadic periods of exercise are discouraged because wide fluctuations in blood glucose levels can occur. It is necessary to regulate food and insulin requirements during times of increased activities.

Insulin

All clients with type 1 diabetes must rely on insulin therapy. They require daily, multiple, or continuous injections of insulin. Clients with type 2 diabetes eventually may become dependent on insulin therapy when other antidiabetic agents are no longer effective.

TYPES OF INSULIN. Human forms of insulin generally are used. Human insulin causes fewer allergic reactions than insulin obtained from animal sources. Gastrointestinal juices inactivate insulin; therefore, insulin must be injected. Table 52.2 includes commonly used insulin preparations, which are divided into four categories: rapid acting, short acting, intermediate acting, and long acting. Some clients with type 2 diabetes maintain glycemic

TABLE 52.2 INSULIN PREPARATIONS

INSULIN	ONSET (HR)	PEAK (HR)	DURATION (HR)
Rapid acting			
insulin lispro (Humalog) aspart (Novalog)	5–15 min	1–2	3–4
Short acting			
regular insulin (Humulin R, Novolin R, Iletin II Regular)	30 min–1 hr	1–3	6–8
Intermediate acting			
isophane insulin suspension (NPH, Humulin N, Novolin N)	1–1.5	4–12	24
insulin zinc suspension (Lente)	1–2.5	7–15	24
Long acting			
extended insulin zinc suspension (Ultralente, Humulin U)	4–8	8–10	18–30
glargine (Lantus)	2–4	No peak	≥24
Insulin Mixtures			
Humulin 50/50	15 min	2–4	20–22
Humulin 70/30	30 min	7–12	16–24
Novolin 70/30	30 min		
Humalog 75/25	15 min	2	20–22

control with a once-daily injection of an intermediate-acting insulin or combination of intermediate-acting and short-acting insulin in a 70:30 or 50:50 proportion. Clients with type 1 diabetes may self-administer three to four injections or more throughout the day unless they use an insulin pump (discussed later).

Stop, Think, and Respond ● BOX 52-2

Identify which of the following insulins is rapid acting, short acting, intermediate acting, and long acting: glargine (Lantus), Lente, lispro (Humalog), Novolin R. 

ADMINISTRATION OF INSULIN. Insulin is prescribed in units. U100 means that 1 mL contains 100 units of insulin. The physician specifies both dosage and type of insulin. When combining two types of insulin in the same syringe, the short-acting regular insulin is withdrawn into the syringe *first* and the mixture is administered within 15 minutes to ensure that onset, peak, and duration of each separate insulin remains intact. Glargine (Lantus) insulin cannot be mixed with other types of insulin in the same syringe. Combination mixtures of insulin, such as Humulin 70/30, Novolin 70/30, and Humulin 50/50, eliminate the need for mixing insulins from two separate vials.

Regular insulin can be administered intravenously (IV) and subcutaneously. The IV route is used to (1) treat severe hyperglycemia or (2) prevent or control elevated blood sugar by adding it to a total parenteral nutrition solution that contains a high concentration of glucose. The subcutaneous route is used most commonly for administering insulin (Fig. 52.5). Insulin is absorbed more rapidly when injected in the abdomen than in the arms or legs. Clients with diabetes are taught to use the abdomen as the preferred site for self-administration. Subcutaneous injection sites require rotation to avoid **lipoatrophy,** breakdown of subcutaneous fat at the site of repeated injections, and **lipohypertrophy,** buildup of subcutaneous fat at the site of repeated injections, either of which eventually interferes with insulin absorption in the tissue. Other techniques for injecting insulin subcutaneously include an insulin pen, jet injector, or insulin pump.

An *insulin pen* has a cartridge containing 150 to 300 units of insulin loaded into an injecting pen with a needle attached. Once the device is loaded, the client (1) selects the number of units for injection by dialing in the dose in 1- to 2-unit increments, (2) cleans and pierces the skin, and (3) injects the programmed amount.

A *jet injector* uses high pressure and rapid speed, rather than a needle, to instill insulin through the skin. Pressure transforms the liquid into a fine mist distributed over a wide area of tissue, resulting in faster absorption (Fig. 52.6). Although a jet injector offers several advantages, such as reducing pain at the site and eliminating use of needles and their appropriate disposal, the cost tends to make this form of administration less attractive.

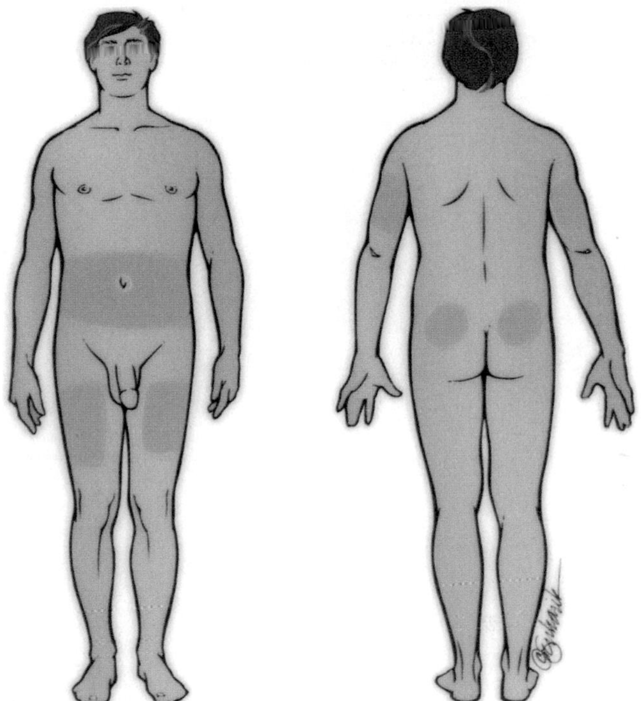

FIGURE 52.5 Suggested areas for insulin injection.

An *insulin pump* delivers insulin by continuous infusion. Its three components are pump, tubing, and needle (Fig. 52.7). The pump contains a reservoir for rapid-acting or short-acting insulin, a battery-operated infuser, and a computer chip enabling a person to regulate continuous and premeal bolus doses in 0.05- to 0.1-unit increments. The pump, worn in a pouch or belt holder, is attached to tubing with a needle. The needle is inserted in the subcutaneous tissue of the abdomen and can remain in the same site for up to 3 days. Clients interested in controlling their diabetes with an insulin pump need to consider both advantages and disadvantages (Table 52.3).

Oral Antidiabetic Agents

Oral antidiabetic drugs are prescribed for clients with type 2 diabetes who have a fasting blood glucose level less than

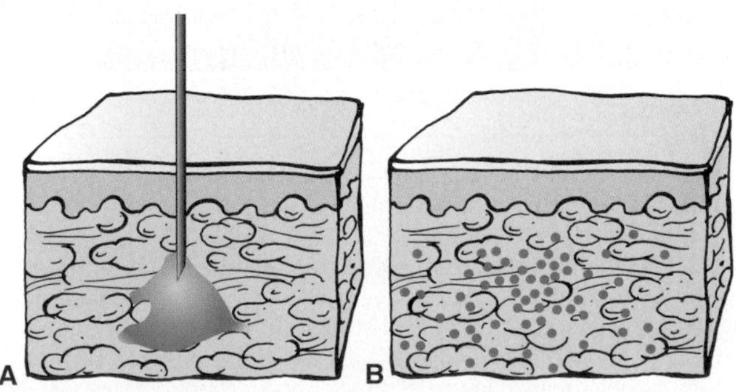

FIGURE 52.6 (**A**) Needle produces a pool of insulin beneath the skin, which is slowly absorbed. (**B**) Jet injector produces an insulin mist beneath the skin, which is absorbed more quickly.

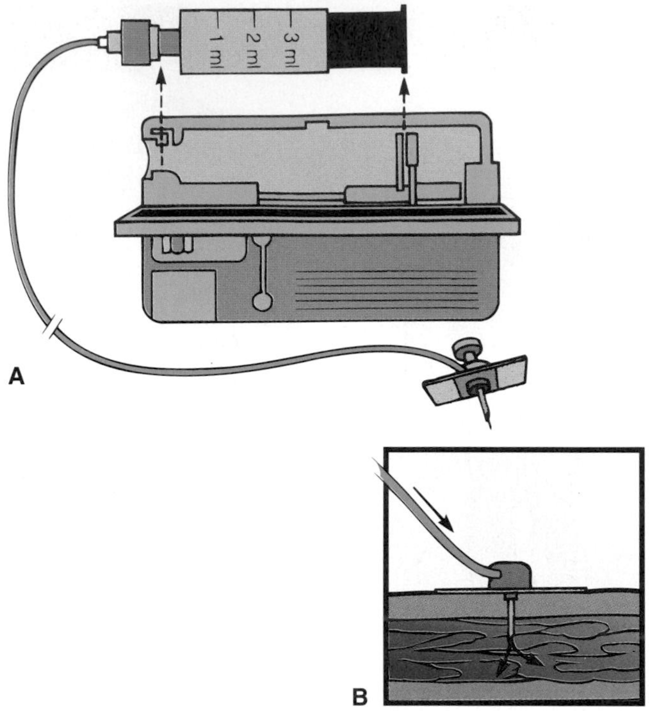

FIGURE 52.7 (**A**) Diagram of an insulin pump showing syringe in place inside pump and connection of pump through tubing to needle site. (**B**) Actual insertion site. (Smeltzer, S. C. & Bare, B. G. [2004]. *Brunner & Suddarth's textbook of medical–surgical nursing* [10th ed.]. Philadelphia: Lippincott Williams & Wilkins.)

200 mg/dL, an insulin requirement less than 40 units/day, no ketoacidosis, and no renal or hepatic disease. Traditionally, sulfonylureas were used to lower blood glucose levels. Now many new drugs help control type 2 diabetes. Recently developed drug categories include biguanides, alpha-glucosidase inhibitors, thiazolidinediones, and meglitinides. Drug Therapy Table 52.1 lists examples of oral hypoglycemic drugs.

Pancreas Transplantation

Replacing the pancreas involves a whole or partial organ transplant. The usual candidate is a client with type 1 diabetes who has renal failure and will benefit from a combined kidney and pancreas transplant. Clients with type 2 diabetes are not offered the option of a pancreas transplant because usually their problem is insulin resistance, which does not improve with a transplant.

The pancreas is both an exocrine and endocrine gland. Exocrine drainage is accomplished by establishing a duodenal or urinary bladder connection with the transplanted pancreas. Insulin is released into the portal vein, which carries blood to the liver. Although bladder connections have a lower incidence of organ rejection, they tend to cause urologic complications and are used less often.

As with any transplant, lifelong immunosuppressive drug therapy also is required, because without it, the new organ is destroyed. Because type 1 diabetes can be managed with insulin, many believe that the risks involved with immunosuppression outweigh the benefit that can be achieved with a pancreas transplant, unless a kidney transplant also is necessary.

Islet Cell Transplantation

Some clients with type 1 diabetes are recipients of islet cell transplants, rather than a transplant of the entire organ or part of the organ. Islet cells, the insulin-producing components of the pancreas, are harvested from human organ donors and from pigs.

After the pancreas is harvested, islet cells are separated from the tissue and injected through the abdominal wall into the client's peritoneal cavity, where they begin to release insulin. Islet cell transplantation surgeons use a combination of tacrolimus (Prograf), sirolimus (Rapamune), and daclizumab (Zenapax) to prevent rejection. Although only a few islet cell transplantations have been performed, most recipients require very little to no insulin and can eat whatever they want.

Nursing Management

Obtain a complete medical, drug, and allergy history, including a list of all symptoms and their duration. Deter-

TABLE 52.3 INSULIN PUMP CONSIDERATIONS

ADVANTAGES	DISADVANTAGES
Resembles the normal pancreatic release of insulin Decreases the necessity for multiple daily injections in different sites Helps maintain consistent blood sugar levels; reduces the potential for episodes of hyperglycemia and ketoacidosis Provides more flexibility for eating food at varying times during the day Facilitates the instillation of smaller doses than those of insulin syringes	Requires high motivation to control diabetes by frequently checking blood glucose levels and adjusting the infusion Creates a potential for hyperglycemia if the pump fails, the tubing becomes kinked or obstructed, or the needle is displaced Interferes or creates a nuisance factor when participating in active sports, sexual intercourse, or bathing; the pump can be temporarily disconnected without removing the needle, but doing so stops the delivery of insulin until it is reconnected

DRUG THERAPY TABLE 52.1 ORAL HYPOGLYCEMIC AGENTS

DRUG CATEGORY AND EXAMPLES	MECHANISM OF ACTION	SIDE EFFECTS	NURSING CONSIDERATIONS
First-Generation Sulfonylureas			
acetohexamide (Dymelor), chlorpropamide (Diabinese), tolazamide (Tolinase), tolbutamide (Orinase)	Stimulates insulin release in type 2 diabetes	Anorexia, nausea, vomiting, hypoglycemia	Give before breakfast and evening meal. Monitor serum and urine glucose levels. Avoid administering to pregnant women.
Second-Generation Sulfonylureas			
glimepiride (Amaryl), glipzide (Glucotrol), glyburide (DiaBeta, Glynase Pres Tab, Micronase)	Stimulates insulin release; are more potent than first-generation sulfonylureas	Increased risk of cardiovascular mortality, anorexia, nausea, vomiting, heartburn, diarrhea, hypoglycemia, allergic skin reactions, insulin "burn out"	Give before breakfast. Monitor urine and serum glucose levels. Avoid administering to pregnant women. Caution client to avoid alcohol. Teach client appropriate diet, exercise, signs and symptoms of hypoglycemia and hyperglycemia, avoidance of infection. Do not abruptly discontinue medication.
Alpha-Glucosidase Inhibitors			
acarbose (Precose), miglitol (Glyset)	Delays digestion of carbohydrates Effects are additive to sulfonylureas in type 2 diabetes	Abdominal pain, flatulence, diarrhea, hypoglycemia	Give three times a day 15 min before each meal. Monitor urine and serum glucose levels. Inform client of gastrointestinal side effects.
Biguanide Compound			
metformin (Glucophage)	Improves use of insulin in type 2 diabetes	Anorexia, nausea, heartburn, diarrhea, lactic acidosis, hypoglycemia, allergic skin reactions, flatulence	Monitor urine and serum glucose levels. Avoid administering to pregnant women. Caution client to avoid use of alcohol. Instruct client not to discontinue medication.
Insulin-Enhancing Agents			
rosiglitazone (Avandia), pioglitazone (Actos)	Increases effects of circulating insulin	Headache, pain, liver injury, hypoglycemia, hyperglycemia, infections, fatigue	Give once daily in morning.
Meglitinides			
repaglinide (Prandin)	Stimulates insulin release	Upper respiratory infections, hypoglycemia, hyperglycemia, headache	Monitor urine and serum glucose levels. Teach client appropriate diet, exercise, signs and symptoms of hypoglycemia and hyperglycemia, avoidance of infection.

mine when the client was diagnosed with diabetes and if others in the family also are diabetic. If the client is a diagnosed diabetic, ask the client to identify his or her prescribed treatment regimen and when he or she last consumed food and self-administered drugs. Weigh the client and perform a complete head-to-toe physical examination because diabetes affects many systems. Look for physical changes associated with diabetes:

- Changes in skin over insulin injection sites, impaired skin areas that appear to be healing poorly; ulcerations or evidence of skin or soft tissue infection
- Vital signs, peripheral pulses, temperature of extremities, inspection of extremities for edema or changes in color
- Decreased visual acuity and visual changes such as blurred vision
- Muscle atrophy, weakness, or loss of sensation

See Nursing Care Plan 52-1 for managing the care of a client with diabetes mellitus.

Before teaching a client with diabetes, confer with the physician regarding type of diet for the client to follow; medication regimen (insulin or oral antidiabetic agent);

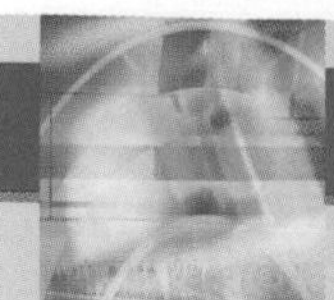

Nursing Care Plan 52-1

THE CLIENT WITH DIABETES MELLITUS

Assessment

Determine the following:

- Evidence of polyuria, polydipsia, polyphagia
- Current weight
- Vital signs, especially blood pressure in lying, sitting, and standing positions
- Blood glucose level before each meal and bedtime
- Any ketones or albumin in the urine
- Serum electrolyte, cholesterol, lipid, triglyceride, blood urea nitrogen, and creatinine levels
- Condition of the skin and feet
- Any abnormal sensations such as pain, tingling, burning, numbness
- Visual acuity and last date of ophthalmic examination
- Knowledge of therapeutic management

Nursing Diagnosis: **Imbalanced Nutrition: More than Body Requirements** related to altered satiety, decreased activity, and habituation of preillness eating habits

Expected Outcome: Client will adhere to his or her prescribed calorie-controlled diet.

Interventions	*Rationales*
Provide three meals and snacks within prescribed caloric limits.	Promotes weight loss and balances glucose with naturally produced or parenterally administered insulin
Suggest free foods such as up to 1 cup of raw vegetables like cucumbers, radishes, celery, or zucchini; unlimited sugar-free drinks; or low-sodium bouillon, if the client becomes hungry between meals or snacks.	Free foods contain *fewer* than 20 calories per serving; their consumption provides negligible calories.
Encourage client to drink 8 ounces of water before eating a meal.	Water is calorie free, distends the stomach, and provides a feeling of fullness.
Advise client to eat slowly and wait 15 seconds between chewing thoroughly, swallowing, and taking the next bite.	Prolongs the pleasure of eating and allows time for the brain to sense satiation

Evaluation of Expected Outcome: Client eats the prescribed diet and verbalizes understanding of restrictions and allowances.

PC: **Hypoglycemia**

Expected Outcome: The nurse will monitor for, manage, and minimize hypoglycemia.

Interventions	*Rationales*
Test capillary blood glucose level with a glucometer 30 minutes before each meal and at bedtime.	Hypoglycemia is more likely before the client consumes food.
Monitor for signs of hypoglycemia such as shakiness, diaphoresis, hunger, and disturbed cognition.	Low blood glucose level causes physiologic stimulation and diminishes the ability to think clearly.
Follow agency policy for administering a quick-acting source of simple carbohydrate according to lower limit of blood glucose level.	Simple carbohydrates are absorbed quickly and tend to raise blood glucose level high enough to eliminate symptoms of hypoglycemia.

(continued)

Nursing Care Plan 52-1 (Continued)

THE CLIENT WITH DIABETES MELLITUS

Interventions	Rationales
Recheck capillary blood glucose level within 15 to 30 minutes after treating a hypoglycemic episode.	Helps determine client's response to nursing intervention
Repeat administration of simple carbohydrate if client continues to be symptomatic; reassess capillary blood glucose level.	The client may need additional simple carbohydrate to successfully raise blood glucose.
Notify the physician if client's symptoms continue after two attempts to raise blood sugar with oral substances.	Parenteral interventions to raise the blood glucose level are medically prescribed.
Offer client complex carbohydrates when hypoglycemia is controlled.	Complex carbohydrates are digested and absorbed more slowly than simple carbohydrates, which reduces the potential for another hypoglycemic episode.
Withhold insulin when client must fast before laboratory or diagnostic procedures.	Eating and administration of insulin are timed according to insulin's onset, peak, and duration of action.
Ask a second nurse to double-check the vial of insulin and the number of units in the syringe before administering the injection.	Double-checking helps avoid errors in insulin administration.

Evaluation of Expected Outcome: Client eats the prescribed diet and verbalizes understanding of restrictions and allowances.

PC: **Hyperglycemia**

Expected Outcome: The nurse will monitor for, manage, and minimize hyperglycemia.

Interventions	Rationales
Monitor capillary blood glucose levels before each meal and at bedtime; check urine for ketones if glucose levels are elevated.	Elevated blood glucose level before a client eats suggests that he or she is not compliant with the diet and may require a higher dose of an oral antidiabetic agent or coverage with rapid-acting or short-acting insulin. Ketonuria increases the potential for DKA.
Assess for clinical signs and symptoms of hyperglycemia such as thirst, increased urination, and sleepiness.	Hyperglycemia has a gradual onset with symptoms similar to the undiagnosed state; hyperglycemia can progress to DKA or HHNKS.
Administer insulin or oral antidiabetic agents as prescribed.	Insufficient insulin results in elevated blood glucose level.
Implement medical orders for insulin administration according to a sliding scale established by the physician.	Insulin lowers blood glucose level.
Notify the physician if the client with hyperglycemia is noninsulin dependent.	Modifications in diet or changes in antidiabetic medications are medically prescribed.
Reinforce importance of compliance with the prescribed diet, exercise, and medication regimen.	These measures manage hyperglycemia.

Evaluation of Expected Outcome: Blood glucose levels are within 80 to 120 mg/dL in a nonfasting state.

Nursing Diagnosis: **Risk for Injury** related to orthostatic hypotension and impaired vision secondary to neuropathy and retinopathy

Expected Outcome: Client will be free from injury.

(continued)

Nursing Care Plan 52-1 (Continued)

THE CLIENT WITH DIABETES MELLITUS

Interventions	*Rationales*
Assist client when rising from a sitting or laying position.	Autonomic neuropathy causes orthostatic hypotension and the potential for fainting and falling.
Have client dangle on the side of the bed before ambulating.	Dangling allows a period during which blood flow increases in the brain.
Keep the floor dry and the environment free of clutter.	Retinopathy may interfere with the client's ability to see potential safety hazards.

Evaluation of Expected Outcome: There is no evidence of trauma.

Nursing Diagnosis: **Risk for Impaired Skin Integrity** related to loss of sensation in feet and impaired blood circulation

Expected Outcome: Skin will remain intact.

Interventions	*Rationales*
Examine skin and feet daily.	Client may be insensitive to injuries and slow to heal because of peripheral neuropathy and vascular disturbances.
Assess skin for signs of breakdown, poor healing, change in color or temperature, or infection.	Impaired blood supply compromises integrity of integument.
Dry client's skin well after bathing, especially in areas of the body that are dark and moist.	Fungal infections are common in creases and folds of skin.
Rotate insulin injection sites; give each injection ½ to 1 inch away from the previous injection.	Prevents lipoatrophy and lipohypertrophy
Inspect inside the client's shoes for foreign objects or disrepair.	Friction or pressure can impair integrity of feet.
Provide foot care with daily hygiene.	Prevents injury and skin breakdown

Evaluation of Expected Outcome: Skin is warm, dry, and intact, with no evidence of tissue breakdown in the feet.

materials for insulin administration, such as needle and syringe, insulin pen, insulin jet, or insulin pump; technique for monitoring blood glucose levels, self-testing devices (glucometer), and the suggested brand to use; materials for and frequency of urine testing; and any additional information, such as skin care, signs of diabetic ketoacidosis (DKA), hyperosmolar hyperglycemic nonketotic syndrome (HHNKS), and hypoglycemia (discussed later). Include family in a diabetic teaching program because one or more members may assume some or all responsibility for the treatment regimen. Present material in small increments. Begin teaching by explaining diabetes, why treatments are necessary, and various methods of treatment. Use audiovisual materials to enhance learning. Because treatment of diabetes is highly individualized, emphasize that treatment of one person cannot be compared with that of another.

If the client requires insulin, identify that the preferred site for injections is the abdomen and use a chart to explain how to rotate injection sites. Allow time for the client to use the glucometer and monitor his or her own blood glucose levels. Additional teaching topics include the following:

- Signs and symptoms of hyperglycemia and hypoglycemia
- The importance of weight reduction, if necessary
- Methods of terminating hypoglycemia, such as grape or orange juice, Prolycen (a commercial product containing glucose), 2 or 3 teaspoons of honey, hard candy, and glucose tablets
- Problems that require contacting the physician, such as skin infection, pain in extremities, visual problems, change in color or temperature of skin of the

extremities, frequent episodes of hypoglycemia, prolonged nausea and vomiting, and illness

- Importance of following an exercise regimen suggested by the physician. Stress that during exercise, the client needs to have some food or other physician-approved form of glucose if symptoms of hypoglycemia occur. This is especially important for clients taking insulin or those subject to episodes of hypoglycemia while taking an oral antidiabetic agent.
- How to integrate the dietary exchange list throughout the day
- Information that is printed on food labels to promote compliance with the prescribed diet
- Definitions of products labeled as "low calorie" and "dietetic" and that these terms are not synonymous with "no sugar." They may contain sugar.
- Importance of drinking adequate water, especially in warm weather, when exercising, and when perspiring
- Foot care
- Necessity for regular appointments with an ophthalmologist for comprehensive eye examinations
- Need to consult the physician regarding dosage adjustments for insulin or oral antidiabetic agent if the client becomes ill or cannot eat

ACUTE COMPLICATIONS OF DIABETES MELLITUS

Despite careful control of their disease, some clients develop serious complications. Some complications can be managed when detected early.

Diabetic ketoacidosis (DKA), a type of metabolic acidosis, occurs with acute insulin deficiency or an inability to use insulin secreted by the pancreas. **Hyperosmolar hyperglycemic nonketotic syndrome** (HHNKS) is characterized by hyperglycemia without ketosis. **Hypoglycemia,** low blood glucose level, is a potential adverse reaction for clients taking medications for diabetes.

Pathophysiology and Etiology

DKA can occur despite a client's compliance with diabetes management. Clients who develop DKA often have a severe, hard-to-control form of diabetes (brittle). Clients admitted to the hospital in DKA may have undiagnosed diabetes. Other causes of DKA include infection and noncompliance with the treatment regimen.

When the amount of glucose transported across cell membranes decreases, the liver increases glucose production, causing extreme elevation of blood glucose levels. The kidneys attempt to excrete the glucose, which is well beyond the renal threshold. Excessive amounts of water, sodium, and potassium also are excreted. The client becomes dehydrated; skin is warm, dry, and flushed. Stored fat is broken down, causing ketones to accumulate in blood and urine. As ketones mount, blood pH becomes acidotic. The client begins to breathe rapidly and deeply in an attempt to eliminate carbon dioxide and prevent formation of carbonic acid, which contributes more to the acidotic state. If DKA is severe and prolonged, the client becomes comatose, with death resulting from no or ineffective treatment.

HHNKS often results from a serious illness in which metabolic needs exceed the limits of available insulin. Because of persistent hyperglycemia (blood glucose levels well over 500 mg/dL), fluid moves from intracellular to extracellular compartments. Diuresis occurs with loss of sodium and potassium. The client still secretes some insulin, which transports glucose in the cells. Fat metabolism is minimal or unaffected and ketosis does not develop. Blood pH remains within normal range of 7.35 to 7.45. HHNKS is more common in undiagnosed or older clients with type 2 diabetes. Nondiabetic clients who receive drugs that elevate blood glucose or who are on dialysis or total parenteral nutrition also may experience HHNKS.

When too much insulin (hyperinsulinism) is in the bloodstream, hypoglycemia occurs. Blood glucose levels fall below 60 mg/dL. Because glucose is the primary source of cellular energy, especially for the brain, hypoglycemia usually presents as neurologic changes, including confusion, difficulty processing information, anxiety, irritability, and headache. The client is hungry, a homeostatic mechanism to stimulate eating. If untreated, seizures, permanent brain damage, or death can occur.

Hypoglycemia occurs when a client with diabetes is (1) not eating but taking insulin or oral antidiabetic medications, (2) not eating sufficient calories to compensate for glucose-lowering medications, or (3) exercising more than usual, which lowers available blood glucose. Alcohol consumption also interferes with the liver's ability to synthesize glucose from noncarbohydrates, placing clients with diabetes who drink at higher risk for hypoglycemia.

Assessment Findings

Symptoms for any of these conditions depend on blood glucose levels. In DKA, early symptoms are vague. Blood glucose levels are elevated to 300 to 1000 mg/dL or more. As ketones accumulate in the bloodstream, weakness, thirst, anorexia, vomiting, drowsiness, and abdominal pain develop. Cheeks are flushed, and skin and mouth are dry. The breath smells of acetone, and Kussmaul respirations often are evident. Pulse is rapid and weak and blood pressure is low. Urine contains glucose and ketones. Blood pH ranges from 6.8 to 7.3. The serum bicarbonate level is decreased. Compensatory breathing patterns lower arterial blood $PaCO_2$ levels. The client is dehydrated, as evidenced by serum sodium and potassium levels.

In HHNKS hypotension, mental changes, extreme thirst, dehydration, tachycardia, and fever develop. Neurologic signs include paralysis, lethargy, coma, and seizures. Symptoms of hypokalemia and hyponatremia usually are present. The client has dry mucous membranes and poor skin turgor. Blood glucose levels are exceedingly high and serum potassium and sodium levels are low. Serum osmolarity is increased.

The degree of hypoglycemia determines symptoms, dependent on an individual's reaction and type of insulin taken. Initial symptoms include weakness, headache, nausea, drowsiness, nervousness, hunger, tremors, malaise, and excessive perspiration. Some clients exhibit characteristic personality or behavior changes. Confusion and dizziness can occur. If not corrected, hypoglycemic symptoms can progress to difficulty with coordination, double vision, unconsciousness and seizures. Symptoms vary, with each client having a uniquely repetitious pattern of hypoglycemic symptoms that develop rapidly. Unconsciousness or seizures occur shortly after onset.

When a client with diabetes is found unconscious, DKA or hypoglycemia needs to be ruled out. These conditions are direct opposites: in ketoacidosis, blood glucose levels are high; in hypoglycemia, they are low. Clients and nurses must be familiar with symptoms of hypoglycemia and hyperglycemia to recognize and differentiate complications as they occur (Table 52.4).

Diagnosis is based on symptoms, client history, and blood glucose levels. If the client had insulin and has not eaten, most likely hypoglycemia is present. If the client has eaten and not had insulin, DKA is more likely.

Medical Management

Treatment of DKA depends on its severity. Primary goals are to (1) reduce elevated blood glucose, (2) correct fluid and electrolyte imbalances, and (3) clear the urine and blood of ketones. Insulin is given IV, which reduces production of ketones by making glucose available to tissues and restoring the liver's supply of glycogen. Regular insulin is added to an IV solution and infused continuously. The amount and rate of insulin infusion depend on blood glucose levels. Isotonic fluid is infused at a high volume for several hours. The rate is adjusted when the client is rehydrated and diuresis is less acute. As insulin lowers blood glucose levels, an IV solution with glucose is added to avoid the potential for hypoglycemia. Potassium replacements are given despite elevated serum levels to raise intracellular stores.

Treatment of HHKNS includes administration of insulin and correction of fluid and electrolyte imbalances. A central venous pressure monitor may be used to evaluate the client's response to fluid replacement. As with the other acute diabetic complications, periodic monitoring of serum electrolytes and blood glucose levels is necessary. Urine is tested for glucose and ketones.

Medical treatment of hypoglycemia is rapid administration of 15 to 20 g of simple carbohydrate. Sources include sweetened fruit juice, honey, candy, cake frosting, sugar, or glucose tablets. If the client is unconscious, glucose gel can be applied in the buccal cavity of the mouth. Glucagon, a hormone that stimulates the liver to release glycogen, or 20 to 50 mL of 50% glucose is administered IV if the client does not respond fairly quickly and blood glucose levels remain low. Once hypoglycemic symptoms are relieved, the client with diabetes is given complex carbohydrates such as graham crackers and milk to sustain and prolong adequate blood glucose levels.

TABLE 52.4 CHARACTERISTICS OF HYPERGLYCEMIA AND HYPOGLYCEMIA

CHARACTERISTIC	HYPERGLYCEMIA	HYPOGLYCEMIA
Predisposing factors	Insufficient or omitted insulin Concurrent infection Dietary indiscretion	Excessive insulin Unusual exercise Too little food
Onset	Slow; hours to days	Sudden; minutes
Mental status	Drowsy	Disoriented; eventually becomes comatose
Skin	Flushed, dry, hot	Pale, moist, cool
Blood pressure	Low	Normal
Pulse	Rapid, weak	Normal or slow, bounding
Respiration	Air hunger	Normal to rapid, shallow
Hunger	Absent	Often present
Thirst	Present	Absent
Vomiting	Present	May be absent
Urine glucose	Present in large amounts	Absent in second voided specimen
Response to treatment	Slow	Rapid

(Adapted from Lilly Research Laboratories, *Diabetes mellitus.*)

Nursing Management

Priority areas for assessment for clients with DKA and HHNKS include hydration status, intake and output, skin turgor, vital signs, and electrolyte studies. Older adults and those with cardiopulmonary or renal disorders are prone to fluid overload. Clients require close measuring of urine output and possibly an indwelling catheter to ensure adequate potassium excretion. Check serum electrolyte results, attach cardiac leads, and observe the heart's conduction pattern to detect evidence of hyperkalemia, such as peaked T waves. Measure blood glucose level frequently, and check urine for ketones. Observe client's neurologic and cognitive symptoms. Protect the client's safety if cognition is impaired and judgment is poor. Keep the physician informed of the client's response, or lack of response, to therapy. See Nursing Care Plan 52-1 for additional nursing care.

For clients with hypoglycemia who can swallow, give grape juice or sweetened orange juice, candy, warm tea or coffee with sugar, a cola beverage, honey, or an oral source of glucose. Implement medical orders for parenteral medications such as IV glucose or parenteral glucagon. In a severe reaction, provide additional carbohydrates and monitor the client's blood glucose level to evaluate effectiveness. Additional medical interventions may be necessary if symptoms do not abate. Stay with hypoglycemic clients until symptoms are corrected. Regulation of glucose metabolism can be tenuous for approximately 24 hours.

Prevent hypoglycemia as follows:

- Ensure that meals are served within 15 minutes of administering rapid-acting insulin, and within 30 minutes of short-acting insulin.
- Ensure that the client eats the prescribed diet and between-meal snacks.
- Inform the physician immediately if nausea, vomiting, or diarrhea occur, or if the client refuses to eat.
- Administer the correct type and dose of insulin at the prescribed times.
- Ask a colleague to check the label on the insulin vial and the number of units in the insulin syringe against that which is ordered before administering insulin, to avoid a medication error.

Additional nursing management of hypoglycemia depends on the symptoms presented (see Nursing Care Plan 52-1).

CHRONIC COMPLICATIONS OF DIABETES MELLITUS

Although clients with diabetes can develop many complications, extremely common ones include peripheral neuropathy, nephropathy, retinopathy, and vascular changes.

• PERIPHERAL NEUROPATHY

Neuropathy is a general term referring to pathologic changes in nerves. Neuropathies in clients with diabetes can affect motor, sensory, and autonomic nerves. Neuropathies develop 10 or more years after onset of diabetes, but incidence increases with duration. Because onset is gradual, the client usually is oblivious to development in early stages.

Pathophysiology and Etiology

Neuropathy results from poor glucose control and decreased blood circulation to nerve tissue. Manifestations of peripheral neuropathies are more common among clients with diabetes who smoke and whose blood glucose level is poorly controlled. Because nitric acid dilates blood vessels, some believe that prolonged elevated blood glucose levels lower nitric acid levels, impair circulation, and subsequently damage peripheral nerves.

When motor nerves are affected, muscles weaken and atrophy. Joint support is diminished and the feet widen. Eventually bone structure is affected, resulting in skeletal deformities, usually in feet and ankles, with subsequent changes in gait. Areas of skin and soft tissue that are subjected to friction and pressure are prone to ulcerate (Fig. 52.8). If there is infection or impaired healing, portions of the affected extremity may require amputation (see Chap. 61).

Neuropathy involving sensory nerves leads to *paresthesias,* abnormal sensations like prickling, tingling, burning, or needle-like pain in the feet, legs, and sometimes hands. In severe cases, feeling is totally lost. Lack of sensitivity increases the potential for soft tissue injury without the client's awareness.

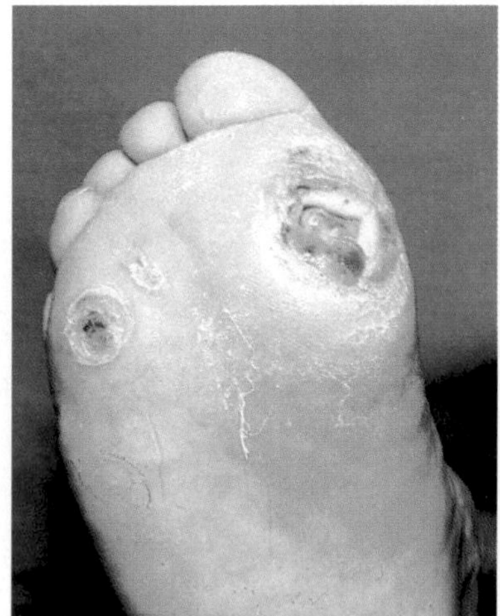

FIGURE 52.8 Neuropathic ulcers occur on pressure points in areas with diminished sensation in diabetic polyneuropathy. Pain is absent (and therefore the ulcer may go unnoticed). (Smeltzer, S. C. & Bare, B. G. [2004]. *Brunner & Suddarth's textbook of medical–surgical nursing* [10th ed.]. Philadelphia: Lippincott Williams & Wilkins.)

Assessment Findings

Pain is a major symptom that accompanies motor and sensory nerve changes. Skeletal muscles in extremities become smaller. Feet swell and become insensitive to temperature or other tactile stimuli. Disturbing sensations develop that often are intensified by maintaining a position for an extended period, such as occupational tasks that require standing in place, holding a steering wheel while driving, or performing a repetitive motion like knitting.

A neurologic examination validates that a client has decreased sensation. Loss of protective sensation, the ability to sense and differentiate hot and cold, sharp and dull, and soft and rough stimuli, occurs. Electromyography studies demonstrate a slowed conduction of electrical stimulation along nerves (see Chap. 38).

Medical Management

Diet, exercise, and medication control blood glucose levels. Several medications can reduce pain, such as non-narcotic analgesics or a tricyclic antidepressant such as imipramine (Tofranil). Anticonvulsants like gabapentin (Neurontin), carbamazepine (Tegretol), or phenytoin (Dilantin) also provide pain relief. Nonpharmacologic pain relief with transcutaneous electrical nerve stimulation may be used.

Nursing Management

Implement a teaching plan for management of diabetes and its potential complications. If possible, refer the client for classes with a diabetes educator. Emphasize compliance with prescribed medications and warn the client to avoid taking more than recommended doses of analgesics. Promote scrupulous foot care (Client and Family Teaching 52-1).

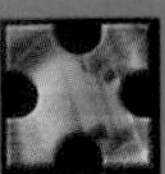

52-1 *Client and Family Teaching* Foot Care in Diabetes

The nurse instructs the client and family as follows:

- Inspect the feet daily for blisters, corns, calluses, long or ingrown nails, or reddened areas; use a mirror to visualize all of the foot.
- Wash feet daily in warm (not hot) water.
- Dry feet thoroughly, being careful to dry between toes.
- Keep toenails short and cut straight across.
- Apply moisturizer to feet daily.
- Do not use razor, abrasive, or commercial products to remove corns or calluses.
- Use lamb's wool between toes that overlap.
- Wear well-fitting shoes that fit comfortably when first worn; do not wear rubber, plastic, or vinyl shoes that cause feet to perspire. Consult physician about wearing sneakers.
- Never go barefoot.
- Visit a podiatrist regularly for foot care.
- Wash, dry, and cover injuries with sterile gauze and call healthcare provider immediately for evaluation.
- Notify the physician about a blister, abrasion, or foot injury.

• DIABETIC NEPHROPATHY

Diabetic nephropathy refers to progressive decrease in renal function that occurs with diabetes mellitus. Clients with type 1 diabetes are most likely to develop diabetic nephropathy.

Pathophysiology and Etiology

Nephropathy is a consequence of glomerular deterioration resulting in impaired filtration of blood during urine formation (see Chap 57). There are five stages of nephropathy, each characterized by successive progression of renal dysfunction (Table 52.5). Essentially, glomeruli excrete blood proteins, especially albumin, and lose their ability to excrete nitrogen waste products.

Poor glucose control contributes to onset of nephropathy. Although hypertension is an eventual consequence of diabetic nephropathy, when it occurs in the prediabetic or prenephropathic state, it accelerates the onset and progression of renal damage. Nephropathy is associated with retinopathy and systemic vascular changes (discussed later).

Assessment Findings

In early stages, the client does not manifest obvious signs and symptoms. Eventually, he or she notices swelling of feet and hands, most likely from loss of albumin, a colloid that pulls water into the vascular system. Blood pressure increases gradually. The client feels tired and weak.

A routine urinalysis or dip with a chemical strip detects albumin in urine. Blood urea nitrogen and serum creatinine become elevated. Renal creatinine clearance is decreased.

Medical Management

Controlling blood glucose levels and hypertension can prevent or delay development of diabetic nephropathy.

TABLE 52.5 STAGES OF DIABETIC NEPHROPATHY

STAGE	CHARACTERISTICS	EFFECTS	AVERAGE ONSET AFTER DIAGNOSIS OF DIABETES
Stage I	Hyperfiltration Glomerular hypertrophy	Blood flow through kidneys is increased. Kidneys are enlarged.	10 yr
Stage II	Microalbuminuria	Albumin, a blood protein, is excreted in small amounts.	
Stage III	Gross albuminuria	Large amount of albumin is excreted; urine consistently tests positive for its presence. Blood pressure becomes elevated. Excretion of nitrogen wastes is impaired.	15 yr
Stage IV	Advanced dysfunction	Severe impairment of glomerular filtration is evidenced by excessive proteinuria, hypertension, and rise in blood urea nitrogen and creatinine levels.	
Stage V	End-stage renal failure	Kidney functions are severely impaired; dialysis or renal transplantation is necessary.	20–25 yr

It is recommended that clients with diabetes maintain their BP at or below 130/85 mm Hg. Clients with diabetes and proteinuria should have a BP lower than 125/75 mm Hg. Angiotensin-converting enzyme (ACE) inhibitors like captopril (Capoten) and angiotensin II receptor antagonists such as losartan (Cozaar) slow the progressive nature of nephropathy. Moderate reduction in dietary protein is beneficial. Smoking cessation is strongly recommended.

Nursing Management

Monitor the client's blood glucose and hemoglobin A1c results. Check the urine with a test strip to detect evidence of albuminuria. Provide additional teaching if the client's blood glucose level is not controlled. Refer the client to programs that assist with smoking cessation or discuss the possibility of nicotine patches or gum to control further habituation. Explain the therapeutic regimen associated with prescribed antihypertensive drugs and dietary measures for lowering BP and complications from vascular disease (see Chap. 29). Because nephropathy is progressive, encourage the client to keep appointments for regular medical follow-up.

• DIABETIC RETINOPATHY

Diabetic retinopathy refers to pathologic changes in the retina experienced by persons with diabetes. On average, it develops 10 or more years after the onset of diabetes. The earlier retinopathy develops, the more likely it is that vision will rapidly deteriorate.

Pathophysiology and Etiology

Diabetic retinopathy is a consequence of inadequately controlled blood glucose levels, which cause vascular changes in the retina (Fig. 52.9). In nonproliferative retinopathy, a milder form, *microaneurysms* (outpouchings in retinal capillaries) develop from high vascular pressure and compromised circulation. Stasis of blood flow interferes with transferring substances between the retina and blood vessels. The deprived retinal cells swell.

In the more advanced, proliferative form of retinopathy, damaged blood vessels are replaced with new ones that grow along the surface of the retina. The newer blood vessels are more fragile and are more apt to rupture and leak blood into the vitreous, the gel-like fluid that fills the posterior portion of the eye. Inelastic scar tissue forms, altering the shape of the retina. This causes distorted vision, and pulls at the retina, increasing the potential for retinal detachment. Eventually, blindness can occur.

Assessment Findings

Clients with nonproliferative and proliferative retinopathy may not experience any visual changes for some time. When symptoms occur, clients report blurred vision, no vision in spotty areas, or seeing debris floating about the visual field.

Visual acuity is diminished. Ophthalmic examination reveals swelling near the macula of the eye, an area lateral to the optic nerve that provides acute central vision. Fluorescein angiography documents changes in retinal blood vessels photographically (see Chap. 43).

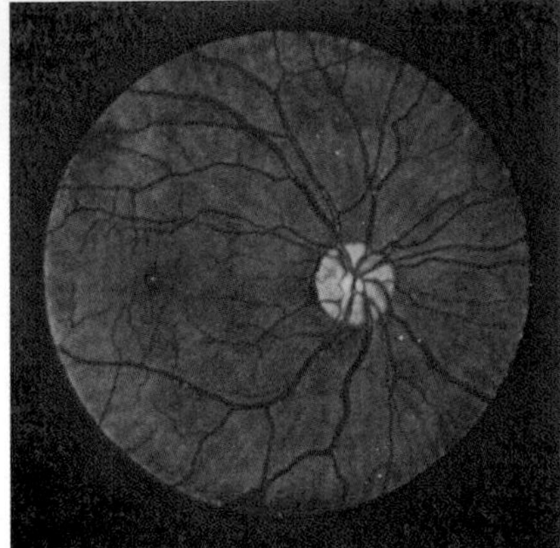

A

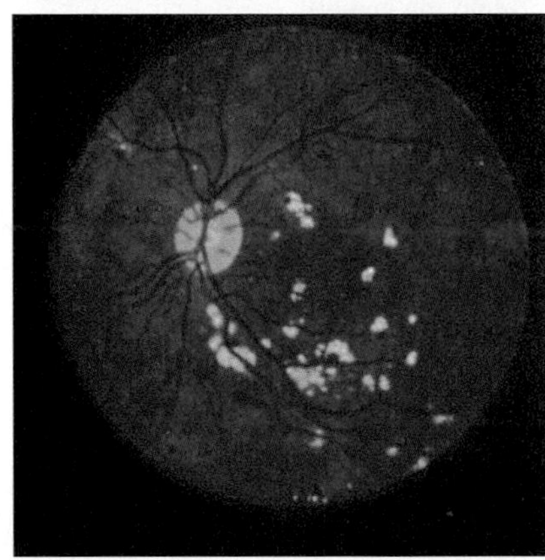

B

FIGURE 52.9 (**A**) In the normal eye, the light circular area over which several blood vessels converge is the optic disc, where the optic nerve meets the back of the eye. (**B**) In diabetic retinopathy, the fundus photograph shows characteristic waxy-looking lesions, microaneurysms, and hemorrhages.

Medical Management

Clients with diabetes are referred for an ophthalmic evaluation within 3 to 5 years after diagnosis. Some physicians suggest yearly ophthalmic examinations. If there is evidence of retinal vessel changes, an ACE inhibitor like lisinopril (Prinivil) is prescribed to dilate retinal blood vessels and improve blood flow. If vitreous hemorrhage already has occurred, some physicians prefer to let the condition resolve on its own, which may take up to 18 months. A more expeditious technique is to seal leaking or newly forming blood vessels with laser photocoagulation. A vitrectomy, removal of bloodied vitreous, also improves clarity of vision.

Nursing Management

Encourage clients with diabetes to follow the therapeutic regimen to facilitate tight glucose control. Teach clients about complications associated with diabetes and encourage regular ophthalmic examinations. When medications are prescribed, explain their purpose, techniques for self-administration, side effects, and symptoms that are important to report to the prescribing physician.

• VASCULAR DISTURBANCES

Vascular disturbances affect many tissues and organs, as described in previous discussions of peripheral neuropathy, diabetic nephropathy, and retinopathy. In clients with diabetes, all arteries and arterioles are susceptible to accelerated atherosclerotic and arteriosclerotic changes.

Pathophysiology and Etiology

A consistent finding in clients with diabetes is thickening of arterial walls. Incidence of coronary artery disease also is increased. A possible explanation for obesity among clients with diabetes is that the brain may be insensitive to leptin, a chemical that signals satiation. Lack of response to leptin promotes overeating, which contributes to hyperlipidemia.

Assessment Findings

Peripheral vascular changes are one of the most common complications associated with diabetes (see Chap. 27). Because of decreased blood supply, extremities are pale and cool. Leg cramps occur. Gangrene develops if blood supply to extremities is markedly diminished. Uncontrolled infection leads to skin ulcers. Clients with diabetes are likely to develop chest discomfort when coronary arteries are affected. Myocardial infarctions can occur at a much earlier age. Hyperlipidemia and elevated triglyceride levels correlate with a predisposition to atherosclerosis. Angiography and Doppler studies indicate peripheral vascular disease.

Medical and Surgical Management

Atherosclerosis is managed with lipid-lowering measures such as a low-fat diet, exercise, and medications. Vasodilators treat the effects of arteriosclerosis. Drugs that reduce platelet aggregation (e.g., aspirin) are prescribed prophylactically. Smoking cessation is advised. Impaired skin is managed with aggressive measures to promote healing (see Chap. 27). Uncontrolled gangrene of extremities can result in amputation. Lower extremities are involved most often. Any type of surgery or hospitalization is an enormous stressor. The diabetic client's glucose levels increase, with a concomitant increased demand for insulin. The health care team monitors the client's blood glucose levels. Either higher doses of insulin or antidiabetic drugs are prescribed, or elevated blood glucose levels are covered by administering rapid-acting or short-acting insulin before meals and at bedtime.

Nursing Management

Nursing management is geared toward the type of vascular disturbance and the signs and symptoms the client experiences.

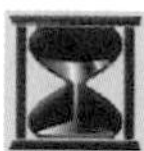

GENERAL GERONTOLOGIC CONSIDERATIONS

Diabetes mellitus is especially prevalent among older adults. Many older clients with diabetes can learn to care for themselves if they receive sufficient time, instruction, and help in overcoming disabilities.

Although it is useful for a family member to learn how to care for the older adult with diabetes, be certain to include the client unless it is evident that the client cannot safely assume responsibility for his or her own treatment.

Some older clients experience difficulty in administering their insulin because of problems such as decreased visual acuity or arthritis. Evaluate the client's ability to self-administer insulin before developing a teaching program.

A variety of aids, such as a magnifier that fits over the syringe, are available for clients who experience difficulty in preparing insulin for injection.

Eating and sleeping habits of older adults often differ from those of young or middle-aged persons. Take this into consideration when planning meals and selecting the proper type and dosage of insulin or oral hypoglycemic agent.

Good foot care is especially important in the older adult because other diseases common in this population, such as peripheral vascular disease and osteoarthritis, increase the risk of complications related to the feet. The client should consult a podiatrist at regular intervals.

Cognitive problems such as depression, dementia, or Alzheimer's disease can interfere with the management of diabetes.

Because older adults usually take several drugs, review all drugs (both prescription and nonprescription) for any that may interact with the oral antidiabetic drugs.

Critical Thinking Exercises

1. *A client with diabetes mellitus has not followed the prescribed diet. What information would you include in a teaching plan for this client? What approach would you take to reinforce the importance of diet in management of diabetes?*
2. *Explain differences between signs and symptoms of hyperglycemia and hypoglycemia.*

● NCLEX-STYLE REVIEW QUESTIONS

1. A client with type 1 diabetes mellitus inadvertently received an extra dose of insulin during shift change. Which assessment findings would indicate to the nurse that the client is developing hypoglycemia?
    1. Confusion, shakiness, and headache
    2. Thirst, chills, and nausea
    3. Increased urine output, irritability, and vomiting
    4. Fatigue, Kussmaul respirations, and fruity breath
2. A client has insulin ordered at 7:00 AM but is NPO for a test scheduled at 9:30 AM. Which action by the nurse is most appropriate regarding the administration of this medication?
    1. Give the insulin as ordered but with small sips of juice.
    2. Call the physician and request a different type of insulin.
    3. Decrease the dose by half and give the reduced dosage.
    4. Hold the drug until the client returns from the test and can eat.
3. The nurse assesses the feet of a 70-year-old client with diabetes. Which finding is most indicative of impaired circulation?
    1. Capillary refill less than 3 seconds.
    2. Client report of pain when pricked with a pin
    3. Cold, cyanotic, swollen toes
    4. Swelling of the joints of the ankle

connection—

Visit the Connection site at **http://connection.lww.com/go/timbyEssentials** for links to chapter-related resources on the Internet.

References and Suggested Readings

American Diabetes Association. (2002). One step closer to a cure. [On-line.] Available: http://ada.yellowbrix.com/pages/ada/Story.nsp?story_id=26991107&ID=ada.

Beebe, C., & O'Donnell, M. (2001). Educating patients with type 2 diabetes. *Nursing Clinics of North America, 36,* 375–386.

Braun, L. T. (2001). Lipid disorders in type 2 diabetes. *Nursing Clinics of North America, 36,* 291–302.

Cameron, B. L. (2002). Making diabetes management routine. *American Journal of Nursing, 102*(2), 26–32.

Camporeale, J. (2001). Client challenge: Teaching an insulin-dependent blind patient about self-care. *Home Healthcare Nurse, 19,* 247–250.

Chu, J. (2001). A breath of fresh insulin: Inhaled insulin may be a welcome answer for millions. *American Journal of Nursing, 101*(10), 30.

Colwell, L., & Quinn, L. (2001). Glycemic control and heart disease. *Nursing Clinics of North America, 36,* 321–331.

Conlon, P. C. (2001). A practical approach to type 2 diabetes. *Nursing Clinics of North America, 36,* 193–202.

Creviston, T., & Quinn, L. (2001). Exercise and physical activity in the treatment of type 2 diabetes. *Nursing Clinics of North America, 36,* 243–272.

Cunningham, M. A. (2001). Glucose monitoring in type 2 diabetes. *Nursing Clinics of North America, 36,* 361–374.

Cypress, M. (2001). Acute complications. *RN, 64*(4), 26–32.

Fain, J. A. (2002). Delivering insulin around the clock. *Nursing 2002, 32*(8), 54–56.

Fain, J. A. (2001). Lowering the boom on hyperglycemia. *Nursing 2001, 21*(8), 48–50.

Flood, L., & Constance, A. (2002). Diabetes and exercise safety. *American Journal of Nursing, 102*(6), 47–55.

Fritschi, C. (2001). Preventive care of the diabetic foot. *Nursing Clinics of North America, 36,* 303–320.

Hardman, L., & Young, F. T. (2001). Combating hyperosmolar hyperglycemic nonketotic syndrome. *Nursing 2001, 31*(3), Hospital Nursing: 32hn1–32hn2, 32hn4.

Insulin-Free World Foundation. (2002). [On-line.] Available: http://www.insulin-free.org.

Kanzer-Lewis, G. (October 28, 2002). Targeting Type 2 diabetes. *Advance for Nurses,* 28–29.

Kaufman, F. (October, 2002). Stop diabetes in its tracks. *A Guide to Women's Health: A Supplement to Nursing 2002,* 2–3.

Kolata, G. (2002, January 15). Doctors advance in helping body repair itself. *New York Times.* [On-line]. Available: http://www.nytimes.com.

McDonald, K. (March 18, 2002). The newest analog: Novolog. *Advance for Nurses,* 36, 42.

McDonald, K. (December 9, 2002). On the diabetes watch. *Advance for Nurses,* 33.

Merriam, M. (November 25, 2002). When diabetes is new. *Advance for Nurses,* 27–28.

Plummer, E. S. (2001). Diabetes update: Chronic complications. *RN, 64*(5), 34–36, 38–40.

Porth, C. M. (2002). *Pathophysiology: Concepts of altered health states* (6th ed.). Philadelphia: Lippincott Williams & Wilkins.

Quinn, L. (2001). Diabetes emergencies in the patient with type 2 diabetes. *Nursing Clinics of North America, 36,* 341–360.

Quinn, L. (2001). Pharmacologic management of the patient with type 2 diabetes. *Nursing Clinics of North America, 36,* 217–242.

Quinn, L. (2001). Type 2 diabetes: Epidemiology, pathophysiology, and diagnosis. *Nursing Clinics of North America, 36,* 175–192.

Rezabek, K. M. (2001). Medical nutrition therapy in type 2 diabetes. *Nursing Clinics of North America, 36,* 203–216.

Ruiz, E. K. (2001). Diabetes update: Type 2 disease in children. *RN, 64*(10), 44–48, 50, 82–83.

Sammer, C. E. (2001). How should you respond to hypoglycemia? *Nursing 2001, 31*(7), 48–50.

Treatment could end daily jabs . . . type 1 diabetes could be conquered in 10 years. (2001). *Nursing Times, 97*(5), 8.

Skelly, A. H. (2002). Elderly patients with diabetes. *American Journal of Nursing, 102*(2), 15–16.

Strowig, S., Robertson, C., & Metules, T. J. (2001). Diabetes update: Insulin therapy. *RN, 64*(9), 38–44.

Tkacs, N. C. (2002). Hypoglycemia unawareness. *American Journal of Nursing, 102*(2), 34–40.

Valentine, V. (2002). Using a laser to make a point. *Nursing 2002, 32*(10), 56–57.

Williams, J. A. (2001). Diabetes update: We make foot exams a priority. *RN, 64*(5), 40.

chapter 53

Caring for Female Clients With Disorders of Pelvic Reproductive Structures

Words to Know 

amenorrhea
carcinoma in situ
cervicitis
conization
cystocele
dilation and curettage (D and C)
dysmenorrhea
dyspareunia
endometrial ablation
endometriosis
fertilization
fibroid tumors
fistula
hormone replacement therapy
hysterectomy
implantation
Kegel exercises
menarche
menopause
menorrhagia
menstruation
metrorrhagia
oligomenorrhea
oophorectomy
ova
ovulation
Papanicolaou test
pelvic inflammatory disease
premenstrual syndrome
puberty
rectocele
salpingo-oophorectomy
sterility
toxic shock syndrome
vaginitis

Learning Objectives

On completion of this chapter, the reader will:

- Name reproductive processes associated with sexual maturation.
- Explain ovulation, fertilization, implantation, and menstruation.
- Name conditions that deviate from normal menstrual patterns.
- Discuss the nurse's role in caring for clients with menstrual disorders.
- List physiologic consequences of menopause and benefits of hormone replacement therapy.
- Describe infectious and inflammatory conditions common in women.
- Describe signs and symptoms that differentiate types of vaginal infections.
- Discuss methods that may prevent vaginal infections or their recurrence.
- Discuss nursing management of clients with pelvic inflammatory disease.
- Describe structural abnormalities of the female reproductive system and their effects on fertility or sexuality.
- Discuss treatments for endometriosis.
- List problems experienced by women who develop vaginal fistulas, and related nursing management.
- Explain the term *carcinoma in situ* and how it applies to the prognosis of women with gynecologic malignancies.
- Identify the most common reproductive cancers and methods for early diagnosis.
- Discuss nursing management for clients who undergo a hysterectomy.

Diseases or disorders of pelvic reproductive structures can profoundly affect a woman's health and sexuality. Some common problems for which adult women seek healthcare include disturbances in menstruation, infectious and inflammatory disorders, structural abnormalities, and benign and malignant tumors of the reproductive system.

ANATOMY AND PHYSIOLOGY

External and Internal Structures

The female reproductive system consists of external and internal structures. External structures include the breasts (see Chap. 54) and female genitalia (Fig. 53.1), which include the vaginal orifice (opening), labia majora, labia minora, and clitoris.

Internal structures of the female reproductive system (Fig. 53.2) consist of two ovaries, two fallopian tubes, the uterus, and the vagina. Two ovaries (female gonads) lie behind and slightly below the ends of the fallopian tubes. Each ovary contains thousands of **ova** (sing., *ovum*), all present at birth. Ovaries secrete two hormones: estrogen, responsible for secondary sexual characteristics such as breast development and the preparation of the uterus for conception, and progesterone (discussed later).

After **puberty** (the onset of sexual maturation) and up to **menopause** (the termination of female fertility), three processes occur: ovulation, pregnancy, and menstruation.

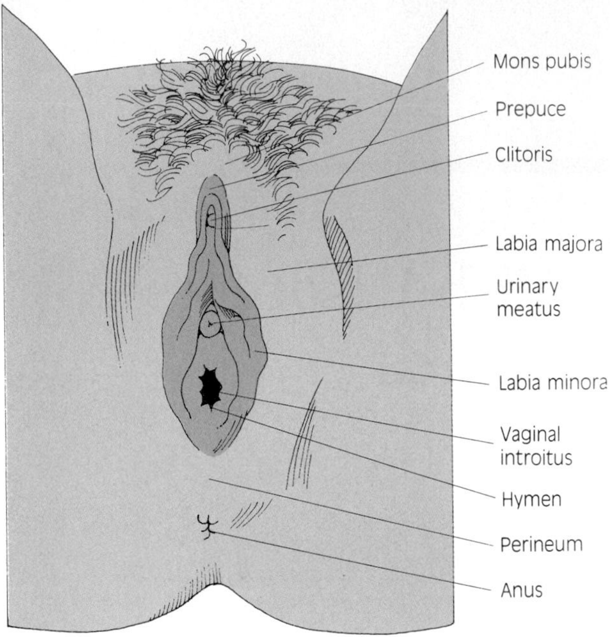

FIGURE 53.1 Female external genitalia.

Ovulation

The role of the internal reproductive structures is to release and transport ova and to support the implantation and nourishment of a fertilized ovum. Cyclical release of an ovum is known as **ovulation** and occurs under the influence of pituitary hormones.

Ovulation is initiated monthly by the anterior pituitary hormone known as follicle-stimulating hormone (FSH). It triggers maturation of a follicle in one of the ovaries and increased production of ovarian estrogen. A second pituitary hormone, luteinizing hormone (LH), causes the mature follicle to rupture, thereby releasing an ovum from the ovary. After the ovum is released, movement of the cilia at the end of the fallopian tube, combined with muscular contractions of the tube itself, draw the ovum toward the uterus.

Meanwhile, the endometrium, the inner lining of the uterus, becomes thick and vascular in response to the secretion of estrogen. The ruptured follicle is transformed into the corpus luteum, a small body filled with yellow fluid. The corpus luteum secretes progesterone, a hormone that sustains the lining of the uterus should fertilization occur.

Pregnancy

Pregnancy occurs as a result of fertilization and implantation. **Fertilization,** the union of an ovum and a spermatozoon (pl., *spermatozoa*), normally occurs in the fallopian tube. At the moment a sperm penetrates the ovum, the number of chromosomes is complete, making it possible for an embryo to develop. The fertilized ovum, or zygote, then proceeds down the uterus and attaches itself in the endometrium, a process referred to as **implantation.** Once fertilization and implantation occur, pituitary production of FSH is inhibited so that ovulation is temporarily halted. See Chapter 1 for more discussion.

Menstruation

If the ovum is not fertilized, production of progesterone by the corpus luteum begins to decrease until it changes from a yellow to a white spot on the ovary (corpus albicans). Without the high level of progesterone, the endometrium degenerates and is shed, a process referred to as **menstru-**

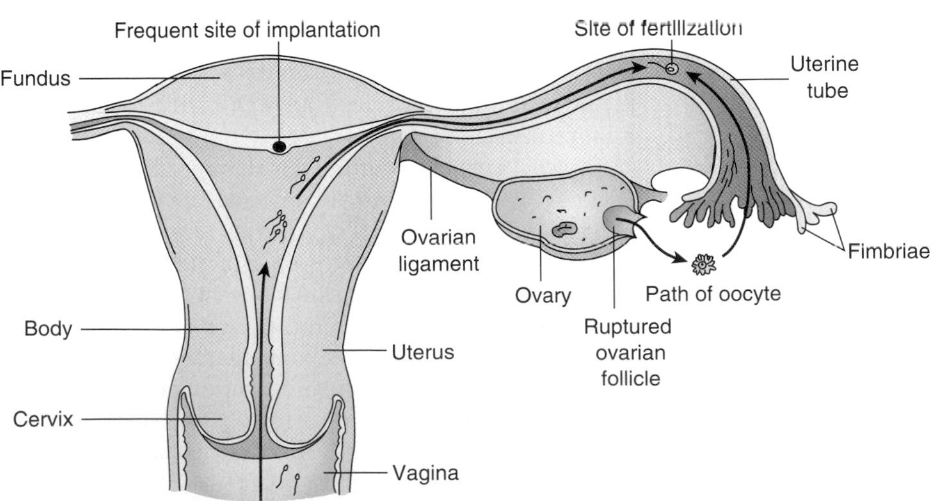

FIGURE 53.2 Schematic drawing of female reproductive organs, showing path of ovum from ovary into fallopian tube, path of spermatozoa, and the usual site of fertilization and implantation.

ation. Menstruation begins about 2 weeks after ovulation. Menstrual flow usually lasts 4 to 5 days, with a normal loss of 30 to 60 mL of blood. Women who have a heavy menses, or menstrual flow, lose more blood. After menstruation, the endometrium becomes thicker and more vascular again in preparation for a possible pregnancy. Because of these hormone-dependent changes, microscopic characteristics of the uterus are in a cyclical state of transition. Thus, it is important that each gynecologic specimen sent to the laboratory is marked with the date of the beginning of the client's last menstrual period (LMP).

ASSESSMENT

Health History

To ensure a thorough baseline history, the nurse obtains the following information:

- General health and family history
- Age of **menarche,** the first menstruation
- Date of client's LMP, description of the menstrual pattern and flow, and other symptoms associated with menstruation
- Risks for sexually transmitted infections (see Chap. 56)
- Pregnancy history: number of pregnancies, live births, stillborn births; type of fetal abnormalities
- Abortion history
- Contraceptive practices
- Age of menopause, associated symptoms, and use of hormone replacement therapy (HRT)
- Date of last gynecologic and breast examination, including mammograms and Papanicolaou tests
- Prior treatments or surgery for a gynecologic disorder
- Drug, allergy, substance abuse, and smoking history
- Symptoms of present disorder, such as painful intercourse or characteristics of vaginal discharge, and duration

Gynecologic Examination (Pelvic Examination)

A physician, clinical nurse specialist, physician's assistant, or nurse practitioner performs the gynecologic examination. Inspection of external genitalia and adjacent structures occurs first, followed by inspection of the vaginal wall and cervix using a bivalve speculum. Next, one or two fingers of a lubricated, gloved hand are placed in the vagina. By vaginal–abdominal palpation, structures beyond the vaginal orifice are examined and the position, size, and contour of the uterus, ovaries, and other pelvic structures are assessed. At the end of the examination, a gloved finger is inserted into the rectum to palpate the posterior surface of the uterus.

In preparation for the test, the nurse obtains examination gloves, lubricant, several sizes of bivalve speculums, a light source, and materials for obtaining a Papanicolaou test (discussed next). The nurse is sensitive to the fact that many women dislike having gynecologic examinations because they anticipate discomfort, are embarrassed, and have anxiety over possible diagnoses.

Diagnostic Tests

Cytologic Test for Cancer (Papanicolaou Test)

A **Papanicolaou test** (Pap test) is an important cancer screening tool. It involves obtaining a sample of exfoliated cells (dead cells that are shed). The specimens, best obtained 2 weeks after the first day of the LMP, are removed by scraping and brushing tissue during the pelvic examination. The test is used mainly to detect early cancer of the cervix and secondarily to determine estrogen activity as it relates to menopause or endocrine abnormalities. See Box 53-1 for the classification system.

The American Cancer Society recommends that all women have an initial Pap test at 18 years of age (or earlier if sexually active). Women should then have them yearly for 3 years, then every 3 years if results for the three prior tests are normal. Advise the client to avoid intercourse for 2 days and douching for 1 day before the test When assisting with the examination, obtain required materials, prepare the client, and label and preserve the specimens (Fig. 53.3). See Nursing Guidelines 53-1.

Cervical Biopsy

A cervical biopsy is performed when results from a Pap test are positive or questionable. Tissue is obtained by punching out multiple small samples or by **conization,** removing a larger cone-shaped section of cervical tissue. Conization is an invasive surgical procedure performed on an outpatient basis; it also is used to treat early-stage cervical cancer.

If the client is premenopausal, schedule the biopsy for 1 week after the end of a menstrual period, when the cervix is least vascular. Tell the client that cramps and

BOX 53-1 • Papanicolaou Classification System

Papanicolaou findings are described using the following numerical system:
Class 1—No atypical or abnormal cells
Class 2—Atypical cells but no evidence of malignancy
Class 3—Suggestive of but not conclusive for malignancy
Class 4—Strongly suggestive of malignancy
Class 5—Conclusive for malignancy

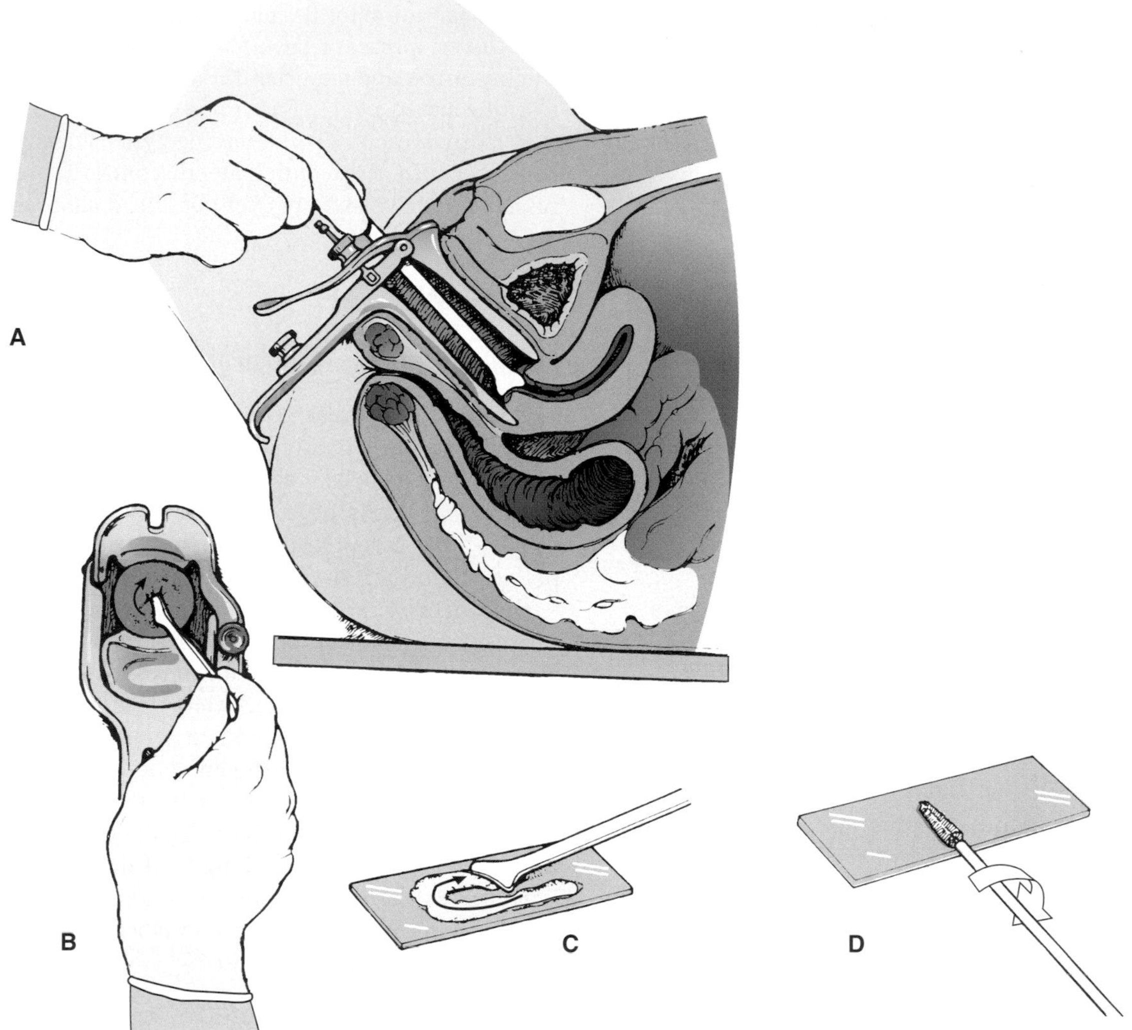

FIGURE 53.3 (**A**) With the speculum in place, the examiner uses the Ayre spatula to obtain cervical secretions. (**B**) He or she places the spatula tip in the cervical os and rotates the spatula 360°. (**C**) Examiner smears material that clings to the spatula smoothly on a glass slide and promptly places in a solution. (**D**) He or she rotates the cytobrush in the cervical os and rolls it onto a glass slide. (Smeltzer, S. C., & Bare, B. G. [2004]. *Brunner & Suddarth's textbook of medical–surgical nursing* [10th ed.]. Philadelphia: Lippincott Williams & Wilkins.)

slight spotting may occur afterward. Recommend a mild analgesic for discomfort and advise the client to report severe pain or heavy bleeding.

Endometrial Smears and Biopsy

Diagnosing cancer of the endometrium, the inner lining of the uterus, is accomplished by aspirating endometrial tissue specimens or performing an endometrial biopsy (the more accurate test). A smear is obtained by inserting a flexible cannula through the cervix and into the uterine cavity. The cannula is attached to a syringe used to aspirate secretions. This procedure usually is performed without anesthesia.

To obtain a biopsy specimen, a dilating instrument called a *uterine sound* is inserted through the cervical opening. A tissue sample is then obtained with a scraping instrument called a *curette,* or by aspiration. This procedure can be performed in the physician's office without anesthesia.

Dilation and Curettage

Dilation and curettage (D and C) is a surgical procedure in which the cervix is stretched open and the endometrium scraped (curettage). Dilation and curettage is done to diagnose or treat various gynecologic problems (e.g., abnormal uterine bleeding) and to remove fetal and placental tissue.

NURSING GUIDELINES 53-1

Assisting the Client Undergoing a Pelvic Examination

- Have the client void before the examination.
- Ask client open-ended questions to promote verbalizing anxiety.
- Provide information on what to expect during the examination and when results from tissue samples will be available.
- Answer questions and use the opportunity to educate the client on health maintenance and health promotion activities.
- Have a blanket available.
- Assist client to assume a lithotomy position immediately before the examination.
- Put pleasing posters on the walls or ceiling to help distract the client.
- Guide the client to breathe deeply during the examination.

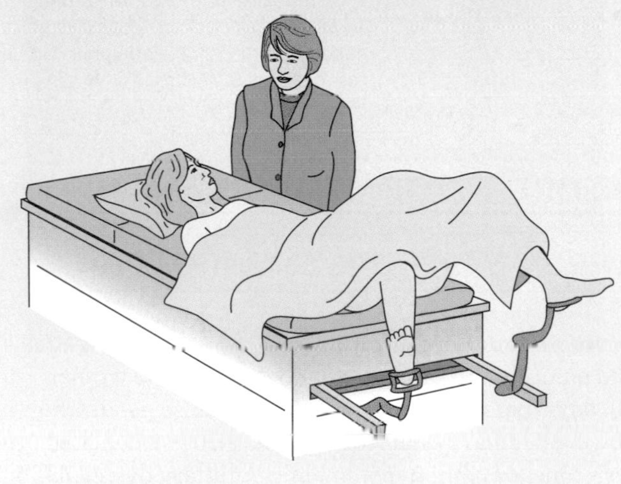

Samples of endometrial scrapings are obtained when the client is under general or light intravenous (IV) anesthesia. A vaginal and cervical pack usually is left in place and a sterile perineal pad applied before the client leaves the operating room. See Client and Family Teaching 53-1 for examples of discharge instructions.

Endoscopic Examinations

Endoscopic examinations are diagnostic procedures that use a lighted instrument inserted into the body for the purpose of visualizing structures not otherwise accessible. They are less invasive and more economical than using surgical techniques.

CULDOSCOPY. *Culdoscopy,* performed under local or general anesthesia, allows visualization of the uterus, broad ligaments, and fallopian tubes by inserting an endoscope through an incision made in the posterior vaginal wall. Ectopic pregnancy and pelvic masses can be visualized.

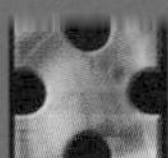

53-1 *Client and Family Teaching* Education After Dilation and Curettage

Following a D and C, the nurse instructs the client as follows:

- Expect slight cramping and a dark, bloody discharge for a few days to several weeks.
- Report bright-red bleeding, foul vaginal drainage, a fever, or pain that is intolerable despite mild analgesia.
- Change soiled perineal pads frequently and avoid tampons.
- Shower rather than take tub baths for 3 or 4 days.
- Refrain from strenuous exercises and heavy household cleaning for 4 to 5 days, after which full activity may be resumed.
- Wipe from front to back after bowel elimination to avoid introducing microorganisms into the vaginal canal or urethra.
- Delay intercourse and douching for 1 to 2 weeks or until the physician indicates that they may be resumed.

Afterward, observe client for signs of internal bleeding and symptoms of shock.

LAPAROSCOPY. Laparoscopy is an examination of the interior of the abdomen using a special endoscope called a *laparoscope* (Fig. 53.4). It is inserted through a small incision located one-half inch below the umbilicus. Two or three liters of carbon dioxide or nitrous oxide gas are introduced into the peritoneal cavity to separate the intestines from the pelvic organs and facilitate visualization. Laparoscopy is used to detect an ectopic pregnancy, perform a tubal ligation, obtain ovarian tissue for biopsy, and detect pelvic abnormalities. Tell the client undergoing laparoscopy that she will experience discomfort in the shoulder as a result of the instillation of gas. Check the incisional sites for bleeding afterward and relieve discomfort by administering a prescribed analgesic.

COLPOSCOPY. A colposcopy is a procedure used to visualize the cervix and vagina. A speculum is inserted into the vagina, and the surface areas are examined with a light and magnifying lens (colposcope). A cervical biopsy and Pap test can be taken at this time.

Hysterosalpingogram

A *hysterosalpingogram* is a radiographic examination that visualizes the uterus and fallopian tubes. It is used

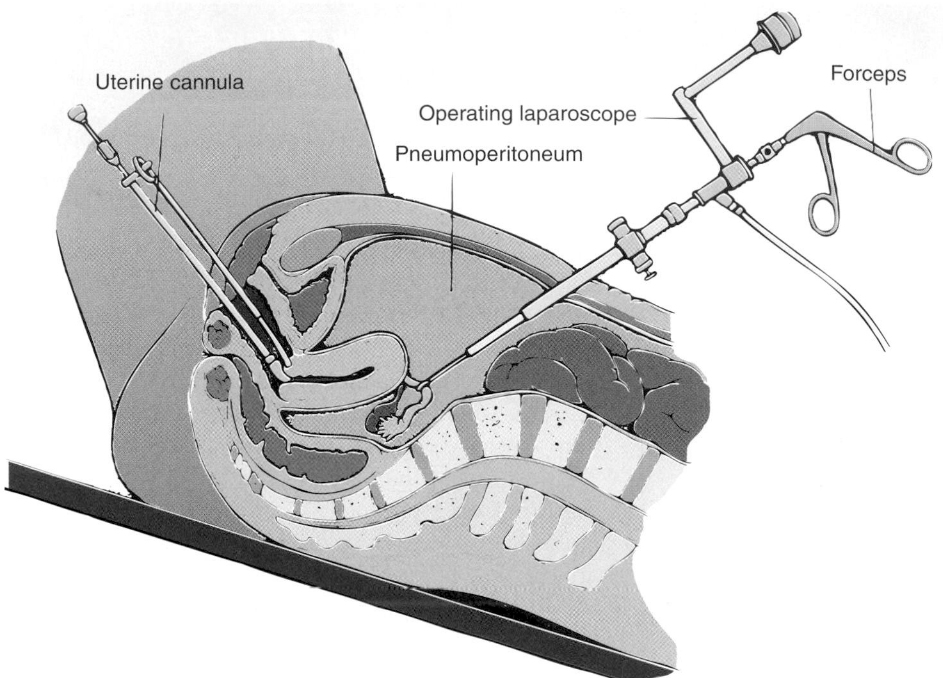

FIGURE 53.4 Laparoscopy. (Smeltzer, S. C., & Bare, B. G. [2004]. *Brunner & Suddarth's textbook of medical–surgical nursing* [10th ed.]. Philadelphia: Lippincott Williams & Wilkins.)

to detect deviations such as adhesions and to determine fallopian tube patency, other tubal abnormalities, or congenital malformations of these structures. A cannula is inserted into the cervix and contrast media injected. Fluoroscopic or radiographic films are taken. Bowel preparation usually is necessary to clear the intestine of gas and fecal material that interferes with proper visualization of the uterus and fallopian tubes.

Abdominal Ultrasonography (Sonogram)

Ultrasonography aids in visualizing soft tissue by recording the reflection of sound waves. An abdominal ultrasound detects pelvic abnormalities such as tumors and size and location of fetal and placental tissue. Instruct the client to drink at least 1 quart of water 45 minutes to 1 hour before the test and not to void until after the test is completed. A full bladder facilitates transmission of the ultrasound waves and elevates the bowel away from other pelvic organs. Solid food may be restricted for 6 to 8 hours to avoid obscuring the image with gas and intestinal contents.

Laboratory Tests

Various laboratory tests, such as a complete blood cell count, hemoglobin, and serum electrolytes, are ordered to obtain a baseline of the client's health status. Culture and sensitivity tests are ordered if an infection is suspected. Ovarian hormone activity is evaluated by tests such as total urine estrogen and urine pregnanediol.

DISORDERS OF MENSTRUATION

• PREMENSTRUAL SYNDROME

Premenstrual syndrome (PMS) is a group of physical and emotional symptoms that occur in some women 7 to 10 days before menstruation. Its cause is unknown; however, it may result from excess estrogen, deficient progesterone, or both; hypothalamic–pituitary dysregulation; or the effect of reproductive hormones on brain chemicals such as endorphins, melatonin, and serotonin. Women experience several symptoms, including weight gain; headache; nervousness; irritability; personality changes; depression; abdominal bloating; breast pain or tenderness; breast enlargement; craving for sweets; swelling of ankles, feet, and hands; anxiety; or increased physical activity. Diagnosis is based on data from a menstrual diary in which the client keeps daily recordings of her symptoms for at least 2 months. The classic finding is that the client is symptom free during the period between onset of menstruation and ovulation.

Treatment of PMS depends on severity and type of symptoms experienced. Hormonal drug therapy aims at manipulating the cyclic fluctuation in estrogen and progesterone. This is accomplished with oral contraceptives, progesterone therapy, synthetic androgens, or gonadotropin-releasing hormone (GnRH) analogs such as histrelin (Supprelin) and nafarelin (Synarel) for 6 months. Short-term therapy with tranquilizers or antidepressants may be indicated. Non-narcotic analgesics, such as mefenamic acid (Ponstel), ibuprofen (Motrin), and naproxen (Anaprox), are given for discomfort.

Encourage clients to make healthy lifestyle changes such as exercising, eating nutritiously, and managing stress more effectively to augment medical treatment. Explain how to maintain an accurate menstrual diary and help the client identify dietary sources of sodium to restrict salt consumption during the second half of her menstrual cycle. Explain drug therapy using oral contraceptives and stress the importance of taking nonsteroidal anti-inflammatory drugs (NSAIDs) with food or after meals to avoid gastric distress. Tell the client who takes a GnRH analog that, because estrogen levels are pharmacologically suppressed, she may experience vaginal dryness that can make intercourse uncomfortable and a loss of bone density similar to osteoporosis (see nursing management of menopause for additional interventions).

DYSMENORRHEA

Dysmenorrhea is painful menstruation and may be primary or secondary. Primary dysmenorrhea usually is idiopathic, and no abnormality is found. Secondary dysmenorrhea is a result of other disorders such as endometriosis, uterine displacement, or fibroid uterine tumors. Symptoms are lower abdominal pain and cramping, which may be more severe with fatigue, cold, and tension. Dysmenorrhea is treated with mild non-narcotic analgesics and by treating the underlying cause if one is identified.

For symptomatic relief of pain and discomfort, suggest local applications of heat, such as a warm shower, heating pad, or water bottle. Demonstrate how to assume a knee–chest position (Fig. 53.5) to relieve discomfort caused by retroversion (backward tilt) of the uterus. Encourage client to obtain adequate rest, nutrition, and relief from stress to facilitate coping with periodic discomfort.

AMENORRHEA AND OLIGOMENORRHEA

Amenorrhea is absence of menstrual flow. *Primary amenorrhea* is the term used when a woman of reproductive age has never menstruated. If menstruation stops after menstrual cycles have occurred, it is called *secondary amenorrhea,* which occurs normally during pregnancy, after menopause, sometimes throughout lactation, and when ovaries or uterus are surgically removed. **Oligomenorrhea** is infrequent menses. It is normal for adolescent girls to experience oligomenorrhea for 1 year or more before they establish regular menses.

Oligomenorrhea and amenorrhea usually are caused by endocrine imbalances resulting from pituitary disorders or hypothyroidism, the stress response, or severely lean body mass. Female athletes, women with anorexia nervosa, or women with debilitating diseases can have such low levels of estrogen that menstruation ceases. Treatment focuses on correction of the underlying cause. Clients with eating disorders (see Chap. 16) require referral to appropriate psychiatric specialists.

MENORRHAGIA

Menorrhagia is excessive bleeding at the time of normal menstruation. It may be quantified as menstrual flow that lasts more than 7 days, that requires the use of an additional two pads per day, or that extends 3 or more days longer than usual. It can be caused by endocrine, coagulation, or systemic disorders.

Symptomatic relief is accomplished with NSAIDs, progestins, and oral contraceptives with combinations of estrogen and progestin. NSAIDs reduce prostaglandins, biologic chemicals that exist in endometrial tissue, where they exert a stimulating effect on the uterus. Progestins, natural and synthetic forms of progesterone, transform the proliferative endometrium into a secretory endometrium

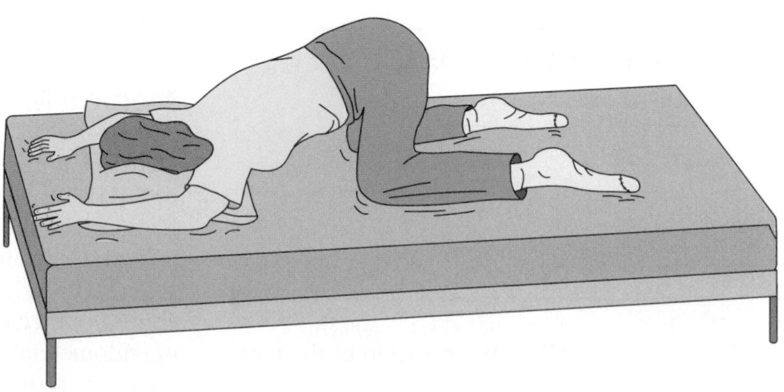

FIGURE 53.5 Knee–chest position.

that simulates a pregnant state. When combination oral contraceptives are administered, they produce a "pill period," characterized by light menstrual bleeding.

A D and C is performed for symptomatic relief; however, effectiveness sometimes lasts only 1 to 2 months. **Endometrial ablation** (detachment of the lining of the uterus) by photodynamic therapy or uterine balloon therapy is a potential nonsurgical alternative. When photodynamic therapy is used, a photosensitive substance is applied to endometrial tissue, after which a laser probe is inserted through the cervix. Absorption of laser light by tissue causes the endometrium to slough, in contrast to being removed with a surgical curette. Uterine balloon therapy produces the same effect by introducing a heated balloon into the uterus for 8 minutes. The post-treatment course is similar to that after a D and C. See Client and Family Teaching 53-1 for education guidelines.

METRORRHAGIA

Metrorrhagia is vaginal bleeding at a time other than a menstrual period. Amount of blood is not important; the fact that it occurs unexpectedly is significant. Irregular bleeding often is due to an erratic stimulation of or response to pituitary or ovarian hormones, especially in adolescent girls and perimenopausal women. Some women spot for a day or two midway between menstrual periods. This functional bleeding is attributed to ovulation and is not considered abnormal. Other causes for atypical bleeding include uterine malignancies, cervical irritation, or breakthrough bleeding that occurs with HRT or low-dose oral contraceptives. Intermenstrual or postcoital (after intercourse) bleeding needs to be evaluated promptly. Treatment depends on the underlying cause.

Advise the client with unexplained bleeding to see a physician. For metrorrhagia or any menstrual disorder, the role of the nurse is the same: gather appropriate information; assist with gynecologic examinations; offer suggestions for relieving discomfort; instruct clients about their drug therapy; prepare clients for surgical interventions; care for them during recovery; and provide specific health-teaching instructions.

Stop, Think, and Respond ● BOX 53-1

What are the differences between primary and secondary amenorrhea and menorrhagia and metrorrhagia?

MENOPAUSE

Menopause ("change of life") is the cessation of the menstrual cycle. The climacteric or perimenopausal period refers to the time during which ovarian activity gradually ceases; the postmenopausal period begins 1 year after menstruation ceases. Menopause normally occurs between the ages of 45 and 55 years. Surgical menopause, which results when ovaries are removed, occurs at any age.

Menopause is a natural physiologic process. Changes in hormone levels that accompany menopause cause a variety of reproductive and systemic effects. Symptoms may be mild and transitory or very severe. Some women seek healthcare to reduce the risk for osteoporosis and cardiovascular disease that occur when estrogen production decreases.

Physiology

Menopause occurs when ovarian function diminishes. Levels of estrogen and progesterone are reduced, ovulation gradually ceases, menstruation becomes irregular until it stops, and natural reproductive capacity ends. As levels of estrogen and progesterone drop, the hypothalamus attempts to raise them by releasing GnRH, which stimulates the anterior pituitary gland to release FSH and LH. The surge of hypothalamic–pituitary stimulation is thought to be responsible for altered temperature, sleep, and mood-regulating mechanisms. Estrogen deficiency causes thinning of vaginal walls, breast and uterine atrophy, and loss of bone density. Risks for heart disease and stroke increase with estrogen reduction. Depression, if it occurs, may be related more to an individual's perception of the social or psychological implications of menopause rather than biologic factors.

Assessment Findings

Changing menstrual patterns, including irregular periods and scanty or sometimes unusually copious menstrual flow, signal onset of menopause. Vasomotor disturbances such as hot flashes and sweats, sleep disturbance, irritability or depression, vaginal dryness, diminished libido (interest or desire for sex), or **dyspareunia** (discomfort during intercourse) are common and often are the symptoms for which women seek treatment. A cytologic examination of vaginal and cervical smears (Pap test) shows decreased estrogen production.

Medical Management

The decision to administer **hormone replacement therapy** (HRT), or estrogen combined with progestin, is made for each client on an individual basis. If HRT is indicated, it is prescribed in the lowest appropriate dose. It is believed that estrogen in small doses can help prevent osteoporosis and reduce the atherosclerotic process. The slight risk of endometrial or breast cancer is outweighed by the seriousness of future myocardial infarction, stroke, hip fracture, and kyphosis.

It may be necessary to treat some symptoms associated with menopause. Vaginal itching and drying are prevented or reduced by drugs such as an estrogen or cortisone cream or ointment. Low-dose androgens are added to the hormone replacement regimen to restore an interest in sexual activity. Antidepressants or minor tranquilizers are prescribed for women experiencing emotional problems.

Nursing Management

Collect a database that includes a menstrual, reproductive, and sexual history and prepare and support the client during physical and diagnostic examinations. Health teaching addresses topics such as normal developmental changes during middle adulthood (see Chap. 10), coping strategies, health promotion techniques, methods to achieve symptomatic relief, and treatment-related information.

Because normal and abnormal structural changes are easily confused, recommend regular gynecologic and breast examinations during and after menopause. Give the following suggestions:

- Use bland skin creams or lotions to reduce skin dryness.
- Plan an exercise program to prevent weight gain and loss of calcium from the bones.
- Increase calcium intake by eating calcium-rich foods, or take a supplement.
- Take HRT by the oral, transdermal, or vaginal route, as prescribed.
- Discuss breakthrough bleeding or menses that may occur with HRT with the physician. Changing the dose or using a different combination of hormones may eliminate this effect.
- Cultivate new interests and hobbies or resume those that have been abandoned because of other responsibilities.

INFECTIOUS AND INFLAMMATORY DISORDERS OF THE FEMALE REPRODUCTIVE SYSTEM

• VAGINITIS

Vaginitis is a condition in which the vagina is inflamed.

Pathophysiology and Etiology

Vaginal inflammation is caused by chemical or mechanical irritants such as feminine hygiene products, allergic reactions, age-related tissue changes (atrophic vaginitis with menopause), and infections. Pathogenic microorganisms frequently associated with vaginitis are the bacteria *Gardnerella vaginalis,* the protozoan *Trichomonas vaginalis,* and the yeast (fungus) *Candida albicans* (also see Chap. 56).

Although the vagina is self-protected by mucus-secreting cells and an acidic environment (pH of 3.5 to 4.5), tissue still may become disrupted. Some situations predispose to vaginitis because they alter one or the other protective mechanism. For example, antibiotics or frequent douching eliminate bacilli that promote an acidic vaginal environment. Decreased estrogen at menopause reduces the thick, moist consistency of vaginal tissue. Pregnant women, those with unregulated diabetes, and those who take oral contraceptives containing estrogen have an excess of glycogen in vaginal mucus, which supports growth of microorganisms.

Assessment Findings

Abnormal vaginal discharge is the primary symptom of vaginal infection. Characteristics of the discharge often are indicative of the infecting organism (Table 53.1). Discharge often is accompanied by itching, burning, redness, and swelling of surrounding tissues. Diagnosis is confirmed by visual and microscopic examination of secretions.

Medical Management

Infectious vaginitis is remedied by using drugs to which the microorganism is particularly sensitive. They include antifungal, antiprotozoal, and antibiotic agents (Drug Therapy Table 53-1). In some cases, the sexual partner also is infected and vaginitis recurs if both are not treated simultaneously.

Atrophic vaginitis is relieved with estrogen replacement administered as a topical cream. If the client has diabetes mellitus, regulating blood glucose is an important aspect of treatment.

Nursing Management

Inform client not to douche before the physical examination because washing away secretions removes characteristics of the vaginal discharge and interferes with obtaining an adequate diagnostic smear. After diagnosis, the nurse may insert the first dose of vaginal medication while teaching the client how to repeat the technique. Nonprescription drugs for the treatment of yeast infections are available. Inform clients that although these drugs usually are effective, the initial diagnosis of vaginitis is best made by a physician. Emphasize the importance of completing the course of therapy.

TABLE 53.1 CHARACTERISTICS OF VAGINAL INFECTIONS

MICROORGANISM	COLOR OF DISCHARGE	CONSISTENCY	ODOR	OTHER SYMPTOMS
Candida albicans	Curdy white	Thick	Strong	Burning with urination
Trichomonas vaginalis	Yellow-white	Foamy	Foul	Severe itching
Gardnerella vaginalis	Gray-white	Watery	Fishy	More discharge after intercourse

Also inform the client to avoid routine douching when asymptomatic, but to combat vaginitis, the client may douche once or twice a day for 1 week with a solution of 1 tablespoon of white vinegar to 1 pint of water. Taking *Lactobacillus acidophilus* in capsule form or eating yogurt containing active cultures of lactobacilli can replenish normal vaginal microorganisms. Sitz baths are recommended to relieve itching, burning, and swelling of the vulva and perineum. Skin protectants containing zinc oxide promote healing. Offer additional suggestions for preventing a recurrence of vaginal infections, as presented in Client and Family Teaching 53-2.

DRUG THERAPY TABLE 53.1 AGENTS TO TREAT VAGINITIS

DRUG CATEGORY AND EXAMPLES	MECHANISM OF ACTION	SIDE EFFECTS	NURSING CONSIDERATIONS
Antiprotozoal			
metronidazole (Flagyl)	Antiprotozoal–trichomonicidal Mechanism of action unknown Used to treat trichomoniasis and *Gardnerella vaginalis*	Headache, dizziness, ataxia, unpleasant metallic taste, anorexia, nausea, vomiting, diarrhea, darkening of urine	This drug is contraindicated in first trimester of pregnancy. Sexual partner may need to be treated. Instruct client to complete therapy. Administer with food if gastrointestinal upset occurs. Advise client to avoid alcoholic beverages and alcohol-containing products—a severe reaction may occur. Alert client that darkening of the urine may occur.
Antifungal			
clotrimazole (Gyne-Lotrimin), miconazole (Monistat), terconazole (Terazol), tioconazole (Vagistat)	Disrupts fungal cell membrane, causing cell death Used in the treatment of candidiasis	Cramping, nausea, vomiting, slight urinary frequency, erythema, stinging	Obtain culture before initiating therapy. Administer cream or vaginal tablets high into vaginal canal; instruct client to remain recumbent for 10–15 min or administer at bedtime. Treatment continues through menses if necessary. Instruct partner to use a condom to prevent reinfection. Partner may need treatment. Client should use a sanitary pad to prevent staining underwear.
Antibiotic			
sulfisoxazole (Gantrisin)	Prevents cell replication by competing with the enzyme involved in the synthesis of intracellular proteins Used to treat vaginitis, *Chlamydia trachomatis*	Headache, nausea, vomiting, abdominal pain, agranulocytosis, photosensitivity, hematuria	Discontinue immediately if hypersensitivity reaction occurs. Administer medication on an empty stomach with a full glass of water. Complete drug therapy as ordered. Inform client of potential side effects. Tell client to report blood in urine, rash, fever, difficulty breathing, drowsiness, nausea, vomiting, or diarrhea.

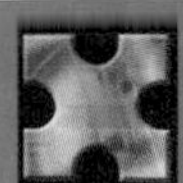

53-2 Client and Family Teaching
Preventing Vaginal Infections

The nurse teaches the client to do the following:

- Bathe daily with particular attention to perineal hygiene.
- Wipe from front to back after voiding and bowel movements.
- Avoid feminine hygiene products and douching more than once per week.
- Wear cotton undergarments and change them daily.
- Refrain from wearing layers of clothing, such as underwear plus pantyhose plus slacks, that increase warmth and interfere with air circulation about the genital area.
- Change from a wet swimsuit as soon as possible.
- Wash hands and devices that are inserted into the vagina, such as medication applicators, douche tips, and diaphragms, and store them in clean containers.
- Change sanitary pads before they become saturated; substitute a sanitary pad for a tampon at night.
- Use a condom or avoid intercourse if either client or her sex partner has genitourinary symptoms.

• CERVICITIS

Cervicitis is an inflammation of the cervix.

Pathophysiology and Etiology

Cervical inflammation is caused by infectious microorganisms, decreased estrogen levels during menopause, or trauma during gynecologic procedures, or occurs as a consequence of inserting tampons or vaginal medication applicators. Streptococcal, staphylococcal, gonorrheal, and chlamydial (see Chap. 56) infections are the most common etiologies. Potential is greater during pregnancy and after childbirth, when microorganisms can enter cervical tissue through small lacerations. Infection can travel upward through uterine and tubal structures, leading to pelvic inflammatory disease (see later discussion). Inflammation and subsequent formation of scar tissue increase potential for ectopic pregnancy or difficulty conceiving. Chronic cervicitis decreases the amount and quality of cervical mucus and alters pH, both of which are underlying causes of infertility.

Assessment Findings

Early cervicitis may fail to produce symptoms. The client eventually spots or bleeds intermenstrually or develops a vaginal discharge. Dyspareunia (painful intercourse) or slight bleeding after sexual intercourse may occur. Severe cervicitis sometimes causes a sensation of weight in the pelvis.

Diagnosis is made by visual examination of the cervix. Microscopic examination of cervical smears identifies the causative microorganism.

Medical Management

Douches and local or systemic antibiotics are the treatment of choice for acute cervicitis. Chronic cervicitis is treated with electrocautery. Frank bleeding requires cervical or vaginal packing or electric coagulation of the bleeding vessel. Healing often takes 6 to 8 weeks. Severe chronic cervicitis is treated by conization (removal of the diseased portion of the cervical mucosa). This outpatient procedure uses an instrument that simultaneously cuts tissue and coagulates the bleeding area. Dilatation is done if there is cervical stenosis. Successful treatment eliminates inflammation, relieves symptoms, and aids fertility.

Nursing Management

The client should be scheduled for treatment 5 to 8 days after the end of the menstrual period to reduce potential for bleeding. Position the client as for a gynecologic examination and explain that a momentary cramping sensation may be felt during the electrocautery procedure. After electrocautery, instruct the client to:

- Rest more than usual for 1 to 2 days.
- Avoid straining or heavy lifting.
- Rest in bed and report if slight bleeding does occur; frank bleeding requires a return visit to the physician.
- Expect a grayish-green, malodorous discharge about 3 weeks after cautery.
- Anticipate slight bleeding about the 11th day.
- Return for follow up to the physician in 2 to 4 weeks.
- Abstain from sexual relations until tissues are healed.
- Plan for healing that may take 6 to 8 weeks.

• PELVIC INFLAMMATORY DISEASE

Pelvic inflammatory disease (PID) is an infection of the pelvic organs except the uterus. These include the ovaries (oophoritis), fallopian tubes (salpingitis), pelvic vascular system, and pelvic supporting structures.

Pathophysiology and Etiology

Microorganisms enter pelvic structures through the cervix from the vagina (Fig. 53.6). The cause usually is bacterial, with gonococci and *C. trachomatis* being the most common pathogens. Infection travels up the uterus

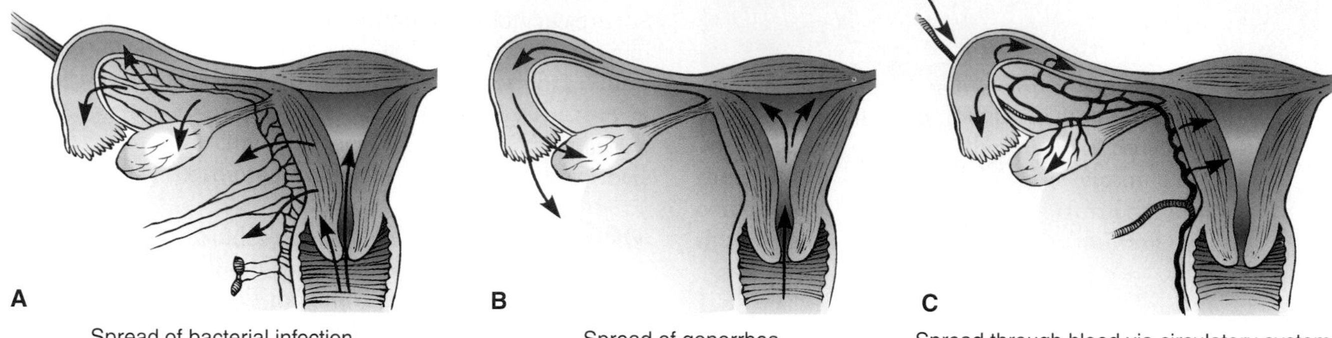

FIGURE 53.6 (**A**) Bacteria spread from the vagina and uterus through the lymphatics. (**B**) Gonorrhea spreads from the vagina and uterus through the tubes and ovaries. (**C**) Bacteria can also reach the reproductive organs through the bloodstream. (Smeltzer, S. C., & Bare, B. G. [2004]. *Brunner & Suddarth's textbook of medical–surgical nursing* [10th ed.]. Philadelphia: Lippincott Williams & Wilkins.)

to the fallopian tubes (salpingitis) and ovaries (oophoritis) and can result in pelvic abscess or peritonitis as pus from infected tubes leaks into the abdomen.

Assessment Findings

Signs and symptoms include an infectious malodorous discharge, backache, severe or aching abdominal and pelvic pain, a bearing-down feeling, fever, dyspareunia, nausea and vomiting, menorrhagia, and dysmenorrhea. Some women experience milder symptoms such as pain during a pelvic examination. Severe infection may cause urinary symptoms.

Diagnosis is based on symptoms as well as a gynecologic examination. A culture and sensitivity test of the vaginal discharge is obtained to identify the causative microorganism. Ultrasonography, magnetic resonance imaging (MRI), or computed tomography (CT) may disclose a pelvic abscess.

Medical Management

Hospitalization with complete bed rest often is necessary. Parenteral or oral antibiotics are administered as soon as culture and sensitivity tests are obtained. IV fluids are ordered if the client is dehydrated, and antipyretics are used if temperature is elevated. A ruptured pelvic abscess requires emergency surgery.

NURSING PROCESS

● The Client With Pelvic Inflammatory Disease

Assessment

Obtain a complete medical, drug, and allergy history and ask client to describe symptoms. A vaginal smear may be necessary. If the client is an outpatient, instruct the client to refrain from douching for 48 hours before being examined. If the client is admitted to the hospital and a vaginal smear is ordered, inquire if the client has douched within the last 48 hours.

Diagnosis, Planning, and Interventions

PC: Sepsis related to systemic spread of pathogenic microorganisms
Expected Outcome: The nurse will monitor to detect, manage, and minimize sepsis if it occurs.

- Monitor vital signs and results of white blood cell counts. *Increased temperature, pulse rate, and leukocytosis indicate an infectious process.*
- Maintain IV site and administer parenteral fluids and antibiotic therapy as scheduled. *Doing so treats infection and prevents further infection.*
- Keep client in a semisitting position. *This facilitates pelvic drainage and minimizes upward extension of infection.*

Risk for Infection Transmission related to direct or indirect contact with infectious microorganisms
Expected Outcome: No nosocomial infections will occur among other clients or staff that can be traced to client with primary infection.

- Follow contact isolation precautions. *Contact isolation controls spread of infectious microorganisms found in wound drainage and other body fluids.*
- Wrap and dispose soiled perineal pads in a lined biohazard container. *Confining objects reduces the potential for transmitting them to other susceptible people.*
- Bag soiled linen according to infection control policies. *This measure avoids transmitting pathogens to personnel who handle laundry.*
- Leave a disposable stethoscope, blood pressure cuff, and paper thermometers in room for assessments.

instruments used for frequent assessments are restricted to the infectious client and then destroyed.

- Wash hands after removing gloves. *Handwashing reduces pathogens on the skin.*
- Instruct housekeeping personnel to damp mop the client's room after cleaning other clients' rooms and change the mop head when finished. *A principle of medical asepsis is to always clean the most heavily soiled area last. Changing the mop head prevents spreading microorganisms to other areas.*

Risk for Impaired Skin Integrity related to excoriating potential of vaginal drainage
Expected Outcome: Vulvar and perineal tissue will be intact.

- Wash perineum well with soap and water every 4 hours. *Doing so promotes skin integrity.*
- Pat or blot the skin dry. *Touching the skin gently rather than vigorously reduces trauma to skin. Keeping skin dry reduces the potential for maceration.*
- Change perineal pads frequently. *Doing so increases the potential for absorbing and wicking drainage from skin surface.*

Evaluation of Expected Outcomes

Expected outcomes are that vital signs and white blood cell count are normal. Infection control measures are effective. The genital tissue is free of redness and excoriation.

After discharge from the hospital, tell the client to temporarily abstain from sexual intercourse to prevent extending infection and infecting the partner. In addition, explain that preventing subsequent episodes of PID can be accomplished by seeking medical attention when symptoms of infection, such as a feeling of pressure in the pelvic area, burning on urination, or vaginal drainage, first appear. Early treatment prevents infection from moving up the reproductive tract and resulting in complications such as peritonitis, abscess formation, and obstruction of the fallopian tubes. When early treatment of acute PID is delayed or inadequate, infection may become chronic.

• TOXIC SHOCK SYNDROME

Toxic shock syndrome (TSS), a type of septic shock (see Chap. 20), is a life-threatening systemic reaction to the toxin produced by several kinds of bacteria. Some causative microorganisms include *Staphylococcus aureus, Streptococcus pyogenes,* and *Clostridium sordellii.* TSS also occurs in men and in nonmenstruating women with soft tissue and postoperative infections.

Pathophysiology and Etiology

TSS is associated with use of superabsorbent tampons that are not changed frequently and internal contraceptive devices that remain in place longer than necessary. The syndrome occurs when virulent bacteria reproduce suddenly and abundantly in the body and remain unchecked by normal physiologic defense mechanisms. Bacteria produce chemicals that cause blood vessels to dilate, keeping the major portion of the blood volume in the periphery, reducing cardiac output, and causing severe hypotension (shock). The toxin also seems to inhibit the ability of affected cells to use oxygen (Porth, 2002).

Assessment Findings

A sudden onset of high fever, chills, tenderness or pain in muscles, nausea, vomiting, diarrhea, hypotension, hyperemia (increased redness and congestion) of vaginal mucous membranes, disorientation, and headache occurs. Skin is warm although the client is in shock. A rash that first appears on the palms of the hands or the body a few hours after infection later results in a shedding of the superficial layer of the skin (desquamation). Pulse is rapid and thready.

The infecting microorganism is found in cultures of specimens from the vagina, blood, urine, or other sites. Blood urea nitrogen, serum creatinine, and serum bilirubin levels are increased. The serum enzymes aspartate aminotransferase (AST) and alanine aminotransferase (ALT) are elevated. The platelet count may be decreased.

Medical Management

Circulation is supported with IV fluids while combating the infection with IV antibiotic therapy. Drugs include oxacillin (Prostaphlin), nafcillin (Nafcil), and methicillin (Staphcillin). Potent adrenergic drugs such as dopamine (Intropin) or dobutamine (Dobutrex) are given to counteract peripheral vasodilation and maintain renal perfusion. Oxygen is given to promote aerobic metabolism at the cellular level.

Nursing Management

Frequently assess vital signs. Administer the first dose of antibiotics immediately and as ordered thereafter. Apply pressure to venipuncture or injection sites to control bleeding and oozing if platelet count is low. Carefully measure intake and output and report any sudden decrease in the urinary output or a urinary output of less than 500 mL/day to the physician.

Before discharge, teach preventive measures such as using perineal pads rather than tampons or changing tampons frequently. Tell clients who use a diaphragm, vaginal sponge, or cervical cap for birth control to remove the device within 24 hours after use. Emphasize handwashing and keeping vaginal devices clean.

STRUCTURAL ABNORMALITIES

• ENDOMETRIOSIS

Endometriosis is a condition in which tissue that histologically and functionally resembles that of the endometrium is found outside the uterus. Atypical locations for endometrial tissue include the ovaries, pelvic cavity, and abdominal cavity.

Pathophysiology and Etiology

The cause of endometriosis is not clearly understood. It may result from remnants of embryonic tissue that remain in the abdominal cavity. Another possible cause is retrograde menstruation, in which the fallopian tubes expel fragments of endometrial tissue that eventually become implanted outside the uterus.

The ectopic tissue responds to stimulation by estrogen and, perhaps, to progesterone. It bleeds when the endometrium of the uterus is shed, but unfortunately there is no outlet for the extrauterine bleeding. The trapped blood causes pain and ultimately adhesions in the peritoneal cavity. If the fallopian tubes are affected, they may become occluded and result in **sterility** (inability to conceive). If endometrial tissue is enclosed in an ovary, a chocolate cyst (named because of its collection of dark blood) develops. Occasionally this cyst ruptures, spilling old blood and endometrial cells into the pelvic or abdominal cavity. The condition is naturally relieved when endometrial tissue atrophies after menopause or regresses during pregnancy.

Assessment Findings

Severe dysmenorrhea and copious menstrual bleeding are typical symptoms. The client may experience dyspareunia and pain on defecation. Rupture of a chocolate cyst results in severe abdominal pain that can mimic other abdominal pathologies such as appendicitis or bowel obstruction.

A pelvic examination reveals fixed, tender areas in the lower pelvis. Restricted mobility of the uterus from adhesions may be noted. A laparoscopy confirms the diagnosis.

Medical and Surgical Management

Endometriosis is cured by natural or surgical menopause. Many women are managed medically as long as possible to maintain the potential for having children later. Estrogen–progestin contraceptives are administered to keep the client in a nonbleeding phase of her menstrual cycle for about 9 months. The goal is to control ectopic tissue so that the client is symptom free for several years. The progestin norethindrone (Norlutin) and the synthetic androgen danazol (Danocrine) are effective in causing atrophy of endometrial tissue.

Without destroying the possibility for childbearing, surgery is performed to remove cysts, as much of the ectopic tissue as possible, and lyse adhesions caused by bleeding. Laparoscopy is used to remove small areas of endometrial tissue as well as relieve adhesions. Endometriosis that is widespread throughout the pelvic organs may necessitate a panhysterectomy: removal of the uterus, both fallopian tubes, and ovaries.

Nursing Management

Obtain a complete reproductive history, asking the client to describe all symptoms, including their duration; type and location of pain; number of days of menses; amount of menstrual flow; and regularity or irregularity of the menstrual cycle. Offer information on methods for relieving menstrual pain (see discussion of dysmenorrhea) and assist the client through the decision-making process as it applies to family planning and medical or surgical treatment of endometriosis before natural menopause. Some techniques for resolving decisional conflict include the following:

- Reinforce or clarify explanations of treatment options and consequences of each option.
- Emphasize that the condition does not require an immediate decision and avoid giving advice or influencing the client's opinions.
- Suggest that the client include her significant other in discussion of options.
- Offer the option of seeking a second medical opinion.
- Suggest listing pros and cons of each option to help determine which choice is most compatible with her values and goals.

Emphasize the importance of adhering to the prescribed medication schedule, if that is the client's choice, and the importance of regular gynecologic evaluations. Instruct the client to seek care if pain increases, menstrual flow is extremely heavy, or pregnancy occurs. Refer to information on nursing management of clients undergoing a hysterectomy (later in this chapter) for those who choose that treatment option.

• VAGINAL FISTULAS

A **fistula** is an unnatural opening between two structures. The opening may be between a ureter and the vagina (ureterovaginal fistula), between the bladder and the vagina (vesicovaginal fistula), or between the rectum and the vagina (rectovaginal fistula; Fig. 53.7).

Pathophysiology and Etiology

Vaginal fistulas are caused by cancer, radiation treatment, surgical or obstetric injury, congenital anomaly, or a complication of ulcerative colitis. They result in continuous drainage of urine or feces from the vagina. The vaginal wall and external genitalia become excoriated and often infected. The client may not void through the urethra because urine does not accumulate in the bladder.

Assessment Findings

The client reports that urine or stool leaks from the vagina. Diagnosis is made by physical examination of the vaginal wall. A sterile probe is inserted if the fistula is easily seen or a dye (usually ethylene blue) is used to detect the exact location of the fistula. When a vesicovaginal fistula is suspected, colored dye is injected into the bladder through a urethral catheter. A ureterovaginal fistula requires IV administration of the dye. An IV pyelogram (IVP) detects the flow of radiopaque dye through the lower genitourinary tract. A rectovaginal fistula is located by looking for fecal drainage on the posterior vaginal wall.

Medical and Surgical Management

Surgery is performed after inflammation and edema disappear. It may require months of treatment. Sometimes the tissues are in such poor condition that surgical repair is not possible. In the meantime, or if the fistula cannot be repaired, symptomatic treatment to reduce risk for infection and manage skin excoriation is provided.

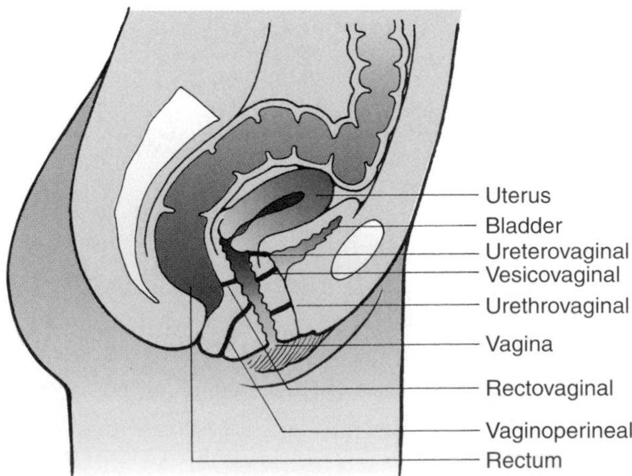

FIGURE 53.7 Types of vaginal fistulae. (Smeltzer, S. C., & Bare, B. G. [2004]. *Brunner & Suddarth's textbook of medical–surgical nursing* [10th ed.]. Philadelphia: Lippincott Williams & Wilkins.)

Nursing Management

Obtain client's history and perform a physical assessment. Ask client to describe characteristics of vaginal drainage. While wearing gloves, inspect the vaginal meatus and vault as well as the condition of the perianal skin. Help the client discuss lifestyle changes that have accompanied the vaginal fistula. Recommend that the client wear disposable, absorbent incontinence briefs or perineal pads with protective panties, and change and launder clothing or bed linens as soon as possible. Let the client know that commercial deodorizers are available for use in the home. Advise daily bathing and frequent perineal hygiene with premoistened disposable wipes. Apply a skin protectant, such as collodion, over intact skin, or a skin barrier, such as zinc oxide or karaya gum, to excoriated skin. Teach client how to take sitz baths and administer cleansing douches. Inform client that powders may cake and cause irritation or a superficial skin infection. She may use a thin dusting of plain cornstarch but must wash it off thoroughly when the area becomes soiled with feces or urine.

The nurse's focus when managing the care of a client with a vaginal fistula includes implementing and teaching measures for maintaining skin integrity, helping the client maintain self-esteem, and offering suggestions for promoting sexuality if the client experiences sexual repercussions.

Administer neomycin (Mycifradin), kanamycin (Kantrex), or another prescribed antibiotic to clean the bowel of microorganisms before repair of a rectovaginal fistula. Provide a light, low-residue diet to keep stool soft. Give an enema and cleansing vaginal irrigation the morning of surgery, and insert an indwelling catheter to keep the bladder empty.

After surgery, serosanguineous vaginal drainage on the perineal pad is normal. No urine or feces from the vagina indicates healing of the repaired fistula. Prevent pelvic pressure and stress on the suture line by monitoring catheter drainage closely. Pressure of a full bladder from an obstructed catheter may break down the surgical repair and cause the fistula to reappear. The nurse prevents and relieves pressure on perineal structures. Warm perineal irrigations and heat-lamp treatments are effective in promoting healing and lessening discomfort. Douches used during the postoperative time frame remove drainage, keep suture area clean, and lessen chances of infection. About the third or fourth postoperative day, a rectal suppository or a stool softener may be ordered to prevent straining during a bowel movement.

• PELVIC ORGAN PROLAPSE

The term *prolapse* indicates a structural protrusion. Women can experience problems of this nature in the vagina, including cystocele, rectocele, enterocele, and uterine prolapse (Fig. 53.8).

A **cystocele** is bulging of the bladder into the vagina. Herniation of the rectum into the vagina is called a **rectocele.** An enterocele is a protrusion of the intestinal wall into the vagina. A uterovaginal prolapse is a downward displacement of the cervix anywhere from low in the vagina to outside the vagina.

Pathophysiology and Etiology

Pelvic organ prolapse is a consequence of congenital or acquired weaknesses in muscles and fascia needed to support pelvic structures. Common causes include unrepaired postpartum tears; stretching during pregnancy and childbirth or with tumorous masses, ascites, and obesity; and postmenopausal atrophy. As the pelvic floor relaxes, the uterus, rectum, intestine, and bladder, alone or in combination, herniate downward. Structural displacement of the bladder and bowel leads to alterations in urinary and bowel elimination. Uterine tissue that protrudes below the vaginal orifice is subject to irritation from clothing or rubbing against the thighs while walking; ulceration and infection frequently follow. Clients with severe uterovaginal prolapse are at greater risk for cervical cancer.

Functional consequences of pelvic organ prolapse can be disruptive. The client often experiences difficulty standing for long periods, walking with ease, lifting, and other activities.

Assessment Findings

Clients with a cystocele may experience stress incontinence—a little urine seeps every time the woman coughs, sneezes, laughs, bears down, or strains. Cystitis (inflammation of the bladder), discussed in Chapter 59, results from stagnation of urine in the bladder. Constipation often is a problem for those with a rectocele. In some instances, the client has to put her finger into the vagina and apply pressure to the posterior vaginal wall to reduce herniation before being able to evacuate stool. Symptoms of a uterovaginal prolapse include backache, pelvic pain, fatigue, and a feeling that "something is dropping out," especially when lifting a heavy object, coughing, or standing for prolonged periods.

Diagnosis is confirmed during a pelvic examination and visual inspection of the vagina. Urinary tests are done to reproduce stress incontinence or to determine the volume at which a client senses an urgent need to void. A Pap test determines the client's estrogen status.

Medical and Surgical Management

A pessary is a firm, doughnut-shaped or ring device that may be inserted in the upper vagina to reposition and give support to the uterus when surgery cannot be done or the client declines surgery. **Kegel exercises,** also known as *pelvic floor strengthening exercises* (see Chap. 59), are recommended when there is stress incontinence.

Surgical repairs are done transvaginally. The surgical repair of a cystocele is called *anterior colporrhaphy.* Repair of a rectocele is called *posterior colporrhaphy.* Repair of the tears (usually old obstetric tears) of the perineal floor is called *perineorrhaphy.* A vaginal hysterectomy (see later discussion) is done to remove a completely prolapsed uterus.

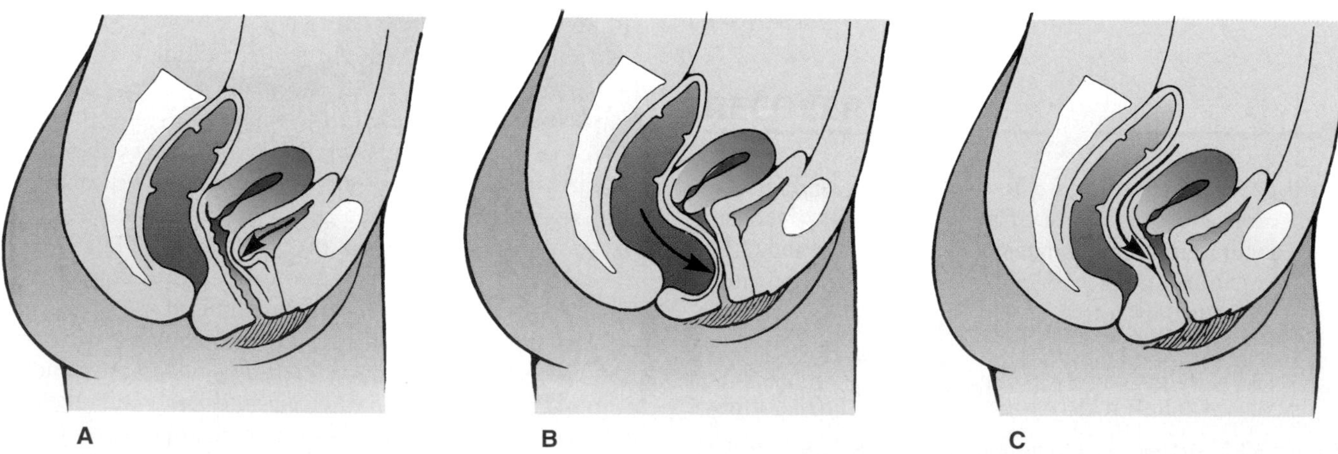

FIGURE 53.8 (**A**) Cystocele. (**B**) Rectocele. (**C**) Enterocele. (Smeltzer, S. C. & Bare, B. G. [2004]. *Brunner & Suddarth's textbook of medical–surgical nursing* [10th ed.]. Philadelphia: Lippincott Williams & Wilkins.)

Nursing Management

Obtain a comprehensive medical history, including chief complaint and symptoms; insert a catheter for diagnostic testing; assist with pelvic examination and collection of specimens; and provide appropriate health teaching based on physician's plan for treatment. Show the client how to remove, clean, and reinsert a pessary, including the following information:

- Remove pessary and then thoroughly wash it with warm, soapy water, followed by rinsing and drying.
- Inspect pessary to be sure all secretions are removed.
- Apply a sterile lubricant to pessary before it is reinserted. Discomfort may indicate it was inserted incorrectly, was moved, or is causing irritation. Contact the physician if these problems occur.
- See the physician immediately if a white or yellow vaginal discharge develops. It may indicate an infection.
- Assume the knee–chest position for a few minutes once or twice a day to keep pelvic organs and pessary in good position.
- Avoid heavy lifting and straining when having a bowel movement.

Tell clients not wishing to manage their own pessary to see their physician at least every 2 months or sooner if vaginal discharge or changes in voiding develop.

After an anterior colporrhaphy, some women have temporary difficulty voiding or emptying the bladder completely. For this reason, clients are discharged with a retention catheter in place or are taught to perform clean intermittent catheterization (see Chap. 59) for 7 to 10 days until they can void sufficiently to empty the bladder. The client learns Kegel exercises after surgical repairs.

TUMORS OF THE FEMALE REPRODUCTIVE SYSTEM

• UTERINE LEIOMYOMA

A *leiomyoma* or *myoma* is a benign uterine growth consisting of smooth muscle and fibrous connective tissue. This is the most common tumor in the female pelvis, often referred to as a **fibroid tumor.**

Pathophysiology and Etiology

Estrogen is believed to stimulate development of fibroids. Tumors may be small or large, single or multiple. Growth usually is slow except during pregnancy. They shrink during and after menopause. Fibroids can occur in various locations in the uterus: subserous (below the serous membrane), intramural (within the wall), and submucosal (below the mucous membrane; Fig. 53.9). The latter are associated most frequently with excessive menstrual bleeding.

Assessment Findings

When symptoms exist, menorrhagia is most common. There can be a feeling of pressure in the pelvic region, dysmenorrhea, anemia (from loss of blood), and malaise.

Benign uterine tumors may be detected during a pelvic examination. A Pap test is done to rule out a malignancy. A sonogram reveals uterine and fibroid size. Microscopic examination of the excised tumor confirms the diagnosis.

Medical and Surgical Management

Several factors govern treatment of benign uterine tumors. A symptomatic tumor in a woman who wishes to have children is watched closely. The client has a gynecologic examination every 3 to 6 months. A Pap test is repeated every 6 to 12 months.

When the client has abnormal bleeding, a D and C is performed to determine cause or control the bleeding. A D and C does not remove the tumor, but it may make more extensive surgery unnecessary. Surgical removal of the tumor only through an abdominal incision or with a laparoscope inserted through the cervical canal preserves the uterus. A hysterectomy is done when symptoms are

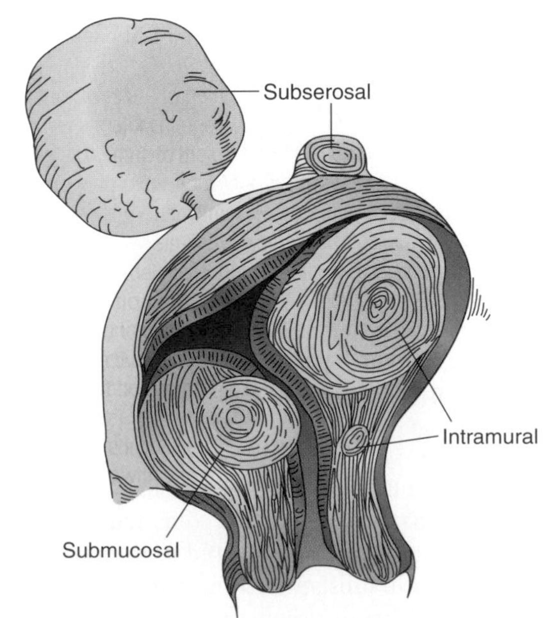

FIGURE 53.9 Submucosal, intramural, and subserosal leiomyomas.

severe and incapacitating, if the client is past childbearing years, or a future pregnancy is not wanted.

Nursing Management

Assist with the gynecologic examination, reinforce medical explanations, and provide preoperative instructions. During the postoperative time frame, assist in the safe recovery of the client who undergoes surgery similar to that discussed for cervical and endometrial cancer.

● CERVICAL AND ENDOMETRIAL CANCER

Cervical cancer, affecting the lowest portion of the uterus, is the second most frequent malignancy of the female reproductive system (breast cancer is first). Cancer of the endometrium affects the lining of the uterus, usually in the area of the fundus or corpus, and is more common in postmenopausal women.

Pathophysiology and Etiology

Cancer of the cervix has its peak incidence among women between the ages of 35 and 50 years and is associated with the following risk factors:

- Being born to mothers treated with diethylstilbestrol (DES) while pregnant
- Becoming sexually active at an early age
- Having multiple sexual partners or having intercourse with a high-risk man (one who has had multiple partners or penile condyloma [warts])
- Acquiring genital infections caused by the human papilloma virus (HPV)
- Having chronic cervicitis secondary to uterine prolapse
- Having a history of cigarette smoking
- Having had pelvic radiation

Risk of endometrial cancer increases after the age of 50 years, especially among women taking estrogens without progesterone for 5 or more years during and after menopause. Other risk factors include early menarche, late menopause, never having been pregnant (nulliparity), and obesity.

Cervical and endometrial cancers probably begin as premalignant lesions that later undergo malignant changes. The localized malignancy is referred to as **carcinoma in situ.** Untreated, it subsequently invades other areas of the uterus and adjacent tissue.

Assessment Findings

Bleeding is the earliest and most common symptom of both endometrial and cervical cancer. In early cervical cancer, spotting occurs first, especially after slight trauma such as douching or intercourse. Bleeding from endometrial cancer can be mistaken for menorrhagia in premenopausal women. Late symptoms for both include pain, symptoms of pressure on the bladder or bowel, and generalized wasting associated with advanced cancer.

All vaginal bleeding is investigated, first by a gynecologic examination, then by diagnostic tests. Cervical cancer is detected with Pap tests and biopsies of suspect tissue. Cells obtained by endocervical aspiration or endometrial biopsy during a hysteroscopy identify abnormal cells higher in the uterus. X-rays, MRI, or CT scanning determine if there is metastasis; a barium study or IVP is ordered to determine bowel or bladder metastasis. Both types of cancer are classified according to stages (Table 53.2).

Medical and Surgical Management

Treatment of cervical and endometrial cancer depends on the stage of the tumor. Prognosis depends on how early cancer is diagnosed. Methods for treating cervical and endometrial cancer include one of various **hysterectomy** (removal of uterus) procedures (Box 53-2), external or internal radiation therapy (Fig. 53.10), and chemotherapy (see Chap. 19). The uterus is removed using an abdom-

TABLE 53.2 STAGES OF UTERINE CANCERS

TYPE	STAGE	DESCRIPTION
Cervical	0	Carcinoma in situ
	I	Limited to the cervix
	II	Extends beyond the cervix to the upper two thirds of the vagina
	III	Involves the lower third of the vagina and is fixed to the pelvic wall
	IV	Involves the rectum, bladder, or extends beyond the true pelvis
Endometrial	0	Cancer in situ
	I	Confined to the corpus
	II	Involves the corpus and cervix
	III	Extends outside the uterus, but not the true pelvis
	IV	Involves the rectum, bladder, or extends outside the true pelvis

[Adapted from the Federation Internationale de Gynecologie et Obstetrique (FIGO).]

BOX 53-2 ● Types of Hysterectomies

Total hysterectomy—Removal of the entire uterus and cervix
Subtotal hysterectomy—Removal of the uterus only, with a stump of the cervix left intact
Panhysterectomy—Removal of the uterus, fallopian tubes, and ovaries
Radical hysterectomy—Removal of the uterus, cervix, ovaries, and fallopian tubes; part of the upper vagina and some pelvic lymph nodes also may be removed at this time
Pelvic exenteration—Removal of all reproductive organs, rectum, colon, bladder, distal ureters, iliac blood vessels, and pelvic lymph nodes and peritoneum

inal, vaginal, or laparoscopically assisted vaginal approach. Choice usually depends on the pathology and the client's condition.

Nursing Management

A major role of the nurse is educating women to have regular gynecologic examinations and Pap tests. Theoretically, all uterine cancers begin in situ. Regular cytologic (cell) examinations increase the potential for an early diagnosis before invasion occurs. Specific nursing management depends on selected treatment. In the interim between diagnosis and treatment, offer emotional support and information about various options for treatment. See Chapter 19 for discussion of radiation therapy or chemotherapy and nursing management.

Preoperative and Postoperative Care

Preoperative preparations vary depending on the surgeon's preference and planned surgical approach (abdominal or vaginal). A douche is given before a vaginal hysterectomy, and an enema is given before either surgery. Insert an indwelling catheter before surgery and administer an antibiotic, usually one of the cephalosporins, during or after surgery to prevent infection. See Nursing Care Plan 53-1.

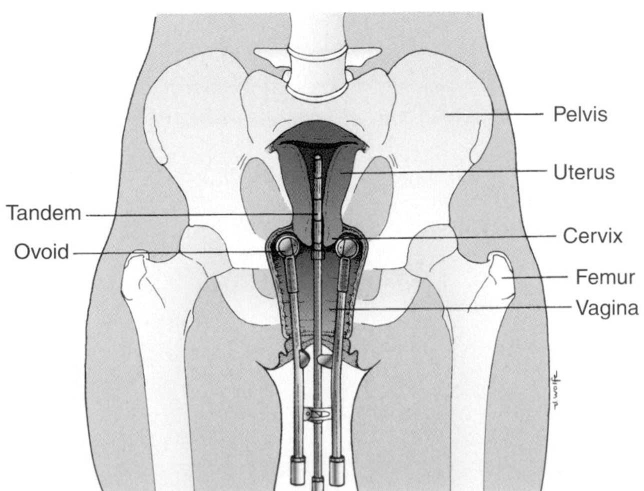

FIGURE 53.10 Placement of tandem and ovoids for internal radiation therapy. (© J. Wolfe.)

Client and Family Teaching

Depending on the client's treatment, the teaching plan includes some or all of the following:

- Take prescribed medications as ordered. Seek care if adverse drug effects occur.
- Avoid heavy lifting, sexual intercourse, vigorous physical exercise, and douching until permitted by physician.
- Ambulate at intervals and avoid sitting in one position for a prolonged period.
- Clean incision as directed.
- Seek medical care if any of the following signs and symptoms occur: fever; redness, swelling, pain, or drainage of incision; vaginal discharge that has a foul odor; vaginal bleeding; pain in chest, abdomen, or legs.
- Avoid constipation and straining to have a bowel movement. Drink plenty of fluids. If constipation occurs, contact physician.

OVARIAN CYSTS AND BENIGN OVARIAN TUMORS

A cyst is a membranous sac filled with fluid, cells, or both. Ovarian cysts, which are benign, are filled with fluid. Benign ovarian tumors are noncancerous growths of solid tissue.

Pathophysiology and Etiology

The exact cause for ovarian cysts and tumors is unknown, but endocrine dysfunction is implicated in some types. Follicular cysts may develop when a ripening ovum fails to be released. Another type forms when the corpus luteum fails to regress after ovulation and continues to produce progesterone. Chocolate cysts are secondary to endometriosis. Ovarian cysts and benign tumors tend to affect menstruation and fertility, depending on the specific type. Some benign tumors have a potential to become malignant (Porth, 2002).

Assessment Findings

The client may experience pressure in the lower abdomen, backache, menstrual irregularities, and pain, which can be

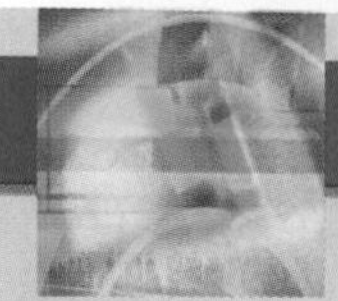

Nursing Care Plan 53-1

THE CLIENT WITH A TOTAL ABDOMINAL HYSTERECTOMY

Assessment

- Assess vital signs and level of consciousness.
- Evaluate pain intensity.
- Monitor condition of the dressing, location of drains (nasogastric, wound), and patency of urinary catheter.
- Regularly check type, volume, and rate of IV fluid, and location and appearance of IV site.
- Note presence of antiembolic stockings.

***PC:* Thrombophlebitis**

Expected Outcome: The nurse will monitor to detect, manage, and minimize thrombophlebitis.

Interventions	*Rationales*
Remove and reapply antiembolic stockings every 8 hours.	Antiembolic stockings support valves in veins and reduce venous stasis.
Encourage active leg exercises every 2 to 4 hours.	Skeletal muscle contraction propels venous blood toward the heart.
Assess for Homans' sign bilaterally every shift.	Homans' sign indicates the possibility of a thrombus in the lower extremities.
Do not place pillows beneath or raise the knees with the electric bed.	Interferes with venous circulation and promotes venous stasis and clot formation.
Ambulate as much as possible.	Walking requires skeletal muscle contraction, promoting venous circulation.

Evaluation of Expected Outcome: Homans' sign is negative bilaterally.

***PC:* Abdominal Distention, Paralytic Ileus**

Expected Outcome: The nurse will monitor to detect, manage, and minimize abdominal distention.

Interventions	*Rationales*
Palpate abdomen every 4 hours for signs of rigidity.	The abdomen loses its soft quality as it distends with gas.
Encourage ambulation.	Promotes intestinal peristalsis, which moves gas toward the rectum.
Report abdominal discomfort, nausea, abdominal distention, or diminished or faint bowel sounds to the physician.	Elimination of intestinal gas is facilitated with a rectal tube, which must be medically ordered.

Evaluation of Expected Outcome: Abdomen is soft; bowel sounds are normal; client passes flatus rectally.

***PC:* Vaginal Hemorrhage**

Expected Outcome: The nurse will monitor to detect, manage, and minimize hemorrhage.

(continued)

Nursing Care Plan 53-1 (Continued)

THE CLIENT WITH A TOTAL ABDOMINAL HYSTERECTOMY

Interventions	*Rationales*
Record number of perineal pads used.	Facilitates the assessment of blood loss.
Assess blood pressure and pulse every 15 minutes if bleeding seems severe.	Blood pressure falls and pulse rate increases in relation to loss of circulating blood volume.
Record color of bloody drainage.	Bright red bleeding correlates with arterial bleeding; dark red blood is more likely venous.
Report excessive bleeding or passage of blood clots to the physician.	A blood transfusion or increased rate of IV fluid may be necessary to maintain blood volume to prevent shock.

Evaluation of Expected Outcome: Client has normal postoperative vaginal drainage; vital signs are within normal range.

Nursing Diagnosis: **Risk for Disturbed Body Image** related to misconceptions about physical and sexual consequences of hysterectomy

Expected Outcome: Client will maintain an accurate body image after surgery.

Interventions	*Rationales*
Give client opportunity to verbalize perceptions and fears.	Clients are less apt to discuss personal problems or fears if they sense the nurse does not have time.
Clarify that a hysterectomy does not physically compromise libido or ability to achieve orgasm or cause premature aging, depression, or masculinization.	Women often accept common myths and misperceptions as fact.

Evaluation of Expected Outcome: Client has a realistic understanding of physical outcomes of surgery.

mistaken for appendicitis, ureteral stone, or other abdominal disorders. Clients with tumors associated with or influenced by hypothalamic, pituitary, or adrenal hormones can develop hirsutism (growth of facial hair), atrophy of breasts, and sterility.

Tumors and cysts may be detected during a pelvic examination. Ultrasonography and laparoscopy are used to determine tumor size. Surgery is the only means for confirming a diagnosis of a benign tumor or cyst.

Medical and Surgical Management

Some ovarian cysts and benign tumors require no treatment or are treated with oral contraceptives to provide symptomatic relief. If the cyst ruptures, surgery, which can entail complete **oophorectomy** (removal of the ovary), removal of the tissue (oophorocystectomy) only, or a **salpingo-oophorectomy** (removal of the ovary and fallopian tube), is required.

Nursing Management

Explain measures for relieving menstrual discomfort and provide referrals to support groups devoted to infertile women. Preoperative preparation and postoperative management are the same as for any client having abdominal surgery and general anesthesia. After surgery, some women develop abdominal distention, relieved by ambulating, inserting a rectal tube, or applying an abdominal binder. Inform the client who has had surgery but no hysterectomy to continue having regular gynecologic examinations and Pap tests; she is still at risk for uterine cancer.

• CANCER OF THE OVARY

Although other types of female reproductive system cancers occur with greater incidence, ovarian tumors are the leading cause of death from gynecologic malignancies.

Tumors of the ovary are so lethal largely because they present with nonspecific symptoms and frequently are far advanced and inoperable when diagnosed.

Pathophysiology and Etiology

Some ovarian tumors may have a hereditary link, whereas others arise from ovarian cysts. The more times a woman ovulates during her lifetime, the greater the risk for ovarian cancer. Certain individuals in the population tend to develop ovarian cancer more often than others. They include nulliparous women, those with a family history of ovarian cancer, and those diagnosed with other types of cancer such as endometrial, colon, or breast cancer.

Malignant tumors of the ovary are classified according to the type of cell from which they originate. Most are epithelial, followed by germ cell (an ovum) tumors. Other types are very rare.

Assessment Findings

In the beginning, clients experience vague lower abdominal discomfort. As the tumor grows larger, urinary frequency and urgency may develop because of pressure on the bladder. Later, ascites, weight loss, severe pain, and gastrointestinal symptoms occur.

A mass may be felt during a pelvic examination. Many physicians believe that ovarian enlargement found on pelvic examination requires surgical exploration. Laboratory studies measuring tumor marker antigens, such as alpha-fetoprotein, carcinoembryonic antigen, and CA 125, are done. Transvaginal and transabdominal ultrasound and Doppler imaging of ovarian vessels are used in an effort to detect early-stage ovarian cancer. An abdominal CT scan, proctoscopy, barium study, chest x-ray, and IVP are done to detect metastasis to other areas. A positive diagnosis is made by microscopic examination.

Medical and Surgical Management

Preventive measures are recommended to at-risk populations. They include having at least two full-term pregnancies followed by breastfeeding and using oral contraceptives for more than 5 years. Prophylactic bilateral oophorectomy is recommended for women at risk for hereditary ovarian cancer syndrome after 35 years of age or after childbearing is completed. The diseased ovary is removed. A total hysterectomy may be performed. If both ovaries are removed, HRT may be prescribed.

Surgical treatment, which reduces the tumor load, is followed by chemotherapy, a combination of cisplatin (Platinol) and paclitaxel (Taxol). Combinations of other drugs such as cyclophosphamide (Cytoxan) and carboplatin (Paraplatin) may be used as alternatives. Use of radiation therapy rather than chemotherapy is controversial at this time.

Nursing Management

Only a small percentage of clients with malignant tumors of the ovary survive 5 or more years, despite intensive treatment. Emotional effects of the diagnosis require support and understanding on the part of the nurse and other members of the health team. Many clients are young, treatment is difficult, and prognosis is poor. Preoperative and postoperative nursing care is similar to that of others who undergo abdominal surgery (see preoperative and postoperative care in the nursing management discussion of the client with cervical and endometrial cancer). See Nursing Care Plan 53-1 for nursing diagnoses and interventions for the client undergoing a total abdominal hysterectomy.

• CANCER OF THE VAGINA OR VULVA

Cancer of the vagina is rare and generally occurs after 40 years of age. Cancer of the vulva also is rare, occurring after 60 years of age. Women with a history of human papilloma virus (HPV) are at risk for both types of cancer. Vaginal cancer also is related to young women born of mothers who took diethylstilbestrol (DES) during early pregnancy (DES is no longer given). This type of cancer has a poor prognosis and associated complications. Vulvar cancer, if diagnosed early, is highly curable. Surgery to remove the cancer, however, can be radical.

Nursing management is directed at early treatment. Regular gynecological examinations and reporting of abnormal vaginal bleeding, dyspareunia (symptoms associated with vaginal cancer), or pruritus and genital burning (symptoms associated with vulvar cancer) are essential.

GENERAL GERONTOLOGIC CONSIDERATIONS 

Older women may develop perineal pruritus. Effort is required to discover the cause of the pruritus; it may require asking questions about diet, type of clothing worn, vaginal discharge, and so on. The client also may be tested for glucose in the blood and urine, and a pelvic examination may be performed to rule out other abnormalities, such as cervicitis, cystocele, rectocele, or cancer of the vulva, cervix, or uterus.

When an older client has a uterine prolapse, surgery may not be considered because of complicating chronic disorders. A pessary may be used to return the uterus to its normal position in the pelvis.

The female genitalia changes during aging. The vulva atrophies, causing a loss of vascularity and elasticity. This can result in irritation or excoriation of the tissue. Pubic hair thins and the labia majora and minora became smaller.

Vaginal flora changes with age, causing the environment to become more alkaline and predisposing the older woman to vaginitis.

Hot flashes, which occur in approximately 75% of all perimenopausal women, are accompanied by increased perspiration, vasodilation, and a 10% to 20% increase in pulse rate. Estrogen, progesterone, combinations of the two, or clonidine may be used to alleviate symptoms.

Critical Thinking Exercises

1. *When a client says she has "female problems," what information is important to ask?*
2. *What nursing activities are appropriate when a woman has a pelvic examination during which a Papanicolaou test will be performed?*

● NCLEX-STYLE REVIEW QUESTIONS 

1. Which nursing intervention is most effective to relieve shoulder discomfort following an ovarian tissue biopsy using laparoscopy?
    1. Reposition the client on the right side.
    2. Assist the client with ambulation.
    3. Place a pillow behind the client's back.
    4. Encourage a carbonated beverage.
2. When instructing a client with vaginitis caused by a yeast infection about prevention of recurrences, which remedy would the nurse most likely recommend?
    1. Wipe after elimination from rectum toward urethra.
    2. Wear silk underwear.
    3. Inform sexual partners of the condition.
    4. Eat cultured yogurt.

connection

Visit the Connection site at **http://connection.lww.com/go/timbyEssentials** for links to chapter-related resources on the Internet.

References and Suggested Readings

Andrist, L. C. (2001). Vaginal health and infections. *Journal of Obstetric, Gynecologic, and Neonatal Nursing, 30,* 306–315.

Choma, K. K. (2003). ASC-US: HPV testing. *American Journal of Nursing, 103*(2), 42–50.

Christman, N. J., Oakley, M. G., & Cronin, S. N. (2001). Developing and using preparatory information for women undergoing radiation therapy for cervical or uterine cancer. *Oncology Nursing Forum, 28*(1), 93–98.

Doughty, S. E. D. (November 19, 2001). The postmenopausal woman. *Advance for Nurses,* 31–33.

Duffy, M. S. (2001). Recent surgical approaches to gynecologic oncology. *Nursing Clinics of North America, 36,* 603–615.

Harris, L. L. (2002). Ovarian cancer: Screening for early detection. *American Journal of Nursing, 102*(10), 46–52.

Heer, E. (September/October 2001). Breast and cervical cancer: Taming the beast with early detection. *Community Health Forum,* 17–21.

Kim, K. H., & Lee, K. A. (2001). Symptom experience in women after hysterectomy. *Journal of Obstetric, Gynecologic, and Neonatal Nursing, 30,* 472–480.

Lee, C. O. (2000). Gynecologic cancers: Part I. Risk factors. *Clinical Journal of Oncology Nursing, 4*(2), 67–71, 89–90.

Lee, C. O. (2000). Gynecologic cancers: Part II. Risk assessment and screening. *Clinical Journal of Oncology Nursing, 4*(2), 73–77.

Maloney, C. (2002). Estrogen and recurrent UTI in postmenopausal women. *American Journal of Nursing, 102*(8), 48–51.

Munson, B. L. (2002). Myths and facts . . . about polycystic ovarian syndrome. *Nursing 2002, 32*(11), 78.

Napoli, M. (2001). A call for more research: What we don't know about hysterectomy is as significant as what we do know. *American Journal of Nursing, 101*(9), 35.

Pasacreta, J. V., Jacobs, L., & Cataldo, J. K. (2002). Genetic testing for breast and ovarian cancer risk: The psychosocial issues. *American Journal of Nursing, 102*(12), 40–47.

Porth, C. M. (2002). *Pathophysiology: Concepts of altered health states* (6th ed.). Philadelphia: Lippincott Williams & Wilkins.

Robb-Nicholson, C. (2000). By the way, doctor. . . . Differences between vaginal and abdominal hysterectomy. *Harvard Women's Health Watch, 8*(3), 7.

Rovner, E. S. (2000). Pelvic organ prolapse: A review. *Ostomy/Wound Management, 46*(12), 24–37.

Scott, L. D., & Hasik, K. J. (2001). The similarities and differences of endometritis and pelvic inflammatory disease. *Journal of Obstetric, Gynecologic, and Neonatal Nursing, 30,* 332–341.

Sharts-Hopko, N. C. (2001). Hysterectomy for nonmalignant conditions. *American Journal of Nursing, 101*(9), 32–41.

Todd, A. (2002). An alternate to hysterectomy. *RN, 65*(3), 30–34.

Wilson, A. C. (September 2, 2002). Essentials of ovarian cancer. *Advance for Nurses,* 12–14.

chapter 54

Caring for Clients With Breast Disorders

Words to Know 

breast abscess
breast cancer
breast reconstruction
breast self-examination
clinical breast examination
fibroadenoma
fibrocystic breast disease
lumpectomy
lymphedema
mammography
mammoplasty
mastalgia
mastopexy
modified radical mastectomy
partial (or segmental) mastectomy
radical mastectomy
reduction mammoplasty
sentinel lymph node mapping
simple (or total) mastectomy
subcutaneous mastectomy

Learning Objectives

On completion of this chapter, the reader will:

- List common signs and symptoms in breast disorders.
- Describe techniques for obtaining a breast biopsy.
- Describe two infectious and inflammatory breast disorders.
- Discuss health teaching related to infectious and inflammatory breast disorders.
- Contrast two benign breast disorders.
- Explain how and when to perform breast self-examination.
- Give current recommendations for mammography.
- Name groups at high risk for developing breast cancer.
- Discuss treatment methods for breast cancer.
- Describe surgical techniques used to remove a malignant breast tumor.
- Name complications of breast cancer treatment.
- Discuss nursing management of clients who undergo surgical treatment for breast cancer.
- List common sites for breast cancer metastases.
- Describe cosmetic breast procedures for clients with a mastectomy or nondiseased breasts.

The breasts are part of the female reproductive system, and they respond to the hormonal cycle associated with ovulation, menstruation, and pregnancy. Their primary function is to produce milk, referred to as *lactation.*

ANATOMY AND PHYSIOLOGY

Breasts contain mammary glands, a network of ducts that carry milk to the nipple (Fig. 54.1). Each mammary gland consists of 15 to 20 lobes divided by *adipose tissue,* which determines breast size but not the amount of milk produced. Breasts manufacture milk from elements in the blood. Prolactin, a hormone produced by the anterior pituitary gland, stimulates milk production. There is an abundant supply of blood vessels and lymphatics. Axillary lymph nodes and internal mammary lymph nodes drain the breasts.

Estrogen secreted by the ovaries causes growth and development of the mammary system. Further growth and development during pregnancy is hormone dependent. Prolactin promotes production of milk. Progesterone, secreted by the placenta, stimulates development of alveoli, which secrete the milk. Estrogen, also secreted by the placenta, stimulates increased production of tubules and ducts to transport milk to the lactiferous duct, which drains at the nipple.

ASSESSMENT

Breast Examination

Clinical breast examination is done when the client has a gynecologic examination, before a mammogram, or during a physical examination. The examiner notes breast

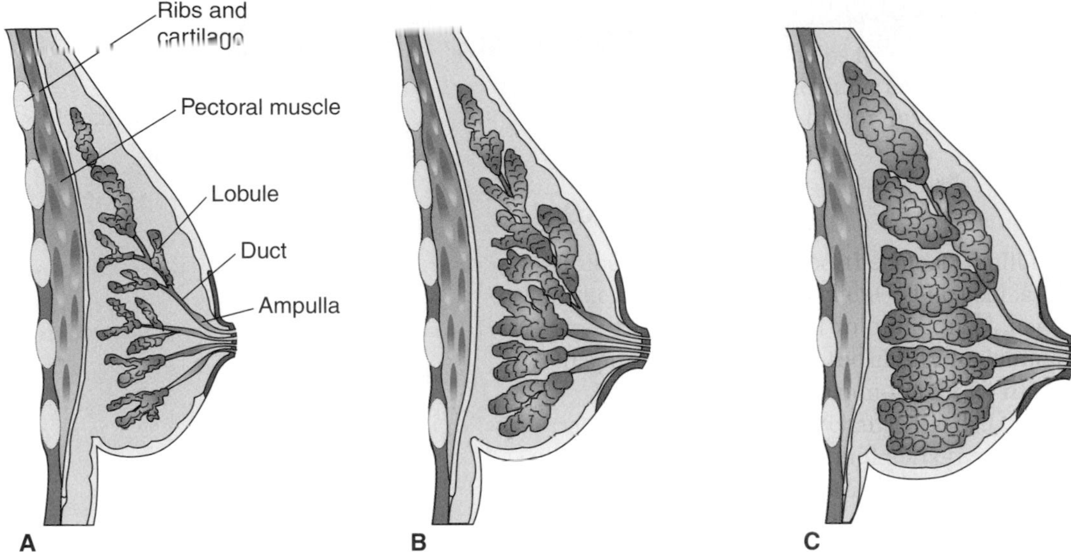

FIGURE 54.1 Breast structures. (A) Nonpregnant woman, (B) pregnant woman, and (C) lactating woman.

size and symmetry and any unusual changes in the skin of the breasts and nipples. The examiner looks for masses, dimpling, flattening, rashes, ulcerations, or nipple discharge. Using the flat part of the fingertips, the examiner palpates the breasts and axillae for masses, lymph nodes, tenderness, and other abnormalities, with the client lying down, arm raised over the head.

Breast disorders are manifested by one or more signs or symptoms in Box 54-1 among adult women. Regular **breast self-examination** (BSE), described and illustrated in Nursing Guidelines 54-1, is an important way for women to discover early breast changes, initiate early treatment, and improve outcomes of breast disorders. Breast cancer also can occur in men. Examination of the male breasts and axillae should be included in the annual physical examination.

Mammography

Mammography (mammogram) is a radiographic technique used to detect cysts or tumors of the breast, some of which are too small to palpate. Mammography is used as a screening test for breast cancer. The National Cancer Institute recommends that women begin having annual mammograms at 40 years of age (Box 54-2). The need for mammograms before age 40 years depends on factors such as a family history of breast cancer, a past history of benign breast disease, incisional or excisional breast biopsies, or other conditions that interfere with accurate BSEs.

BOX 54-1 ● Signs and Symptoms Common to Breast Disorders

- Pain, tenderness, fullness of the breast
- Breast mass(es)
- Nipple discharge
- Change in breast appearance

Ultrasonography

Ultrasonography (ultrasound) often is used with a mammogram to differentiate fluid-filled cysts from other types of breast lesions. It involves use of high-frequency sound waves to produce a visual picture. It is very useful for women with very dense breasts, such as younger women and those on hormone replacement therapy.

When a mammogram is scheduled, explain the radiographic procedure and instruct the client to omit using a deodorant with aluminum hydroxide or body talc the day of the test to avoid artifacts on the x-ray film. If the client forgets or was not provided this information, provide a premoistened wipe to cleanse axillae just before the test. Determine how often the client performs BSEs and have her demonstrate or describe the technique. For women unfamiliar with BSE, instruct and demonstrate how to perform BSE. Ensure privacy throughout the examination and advise clients to have mammograms at the same health agency or arrange for records to be transferred so that previous mammogram results can be compared.

Stop, Think, and Respond ● BOX 54-1

A 52-year-old woman tells you she has never had a mammogram and has heard they are painful. How would you respond to her?

NURSING GUIDELINES 54-1

Teaching Breast Self-Examination

- Examine your breasts 3 days after the end of menstruation or monthly on a date of your choice if you no longer menstruate.
- Begin the examination in the shower when the breasts are wet and soapy and again after the shower when lying down with a folded towel under the shoulder on the side being examined.
- Use light, medium, and firm pressure applied with the pads of three fingers when checking each breast.
- Move your fingers in circles, spokes of a wheel, or rows, but follow the same technique with each BSE.
- Feel every part of each breast, including the nipple area and the armpit to the collar bone.
- Raise your arms over your head and look at the breasts in a mirror.
- Look for changes in breast shape, size, and contour; puckering (dimpling) of the skin; or areas that appear red.
- Squeeze each nipple and look for liquid drainage.

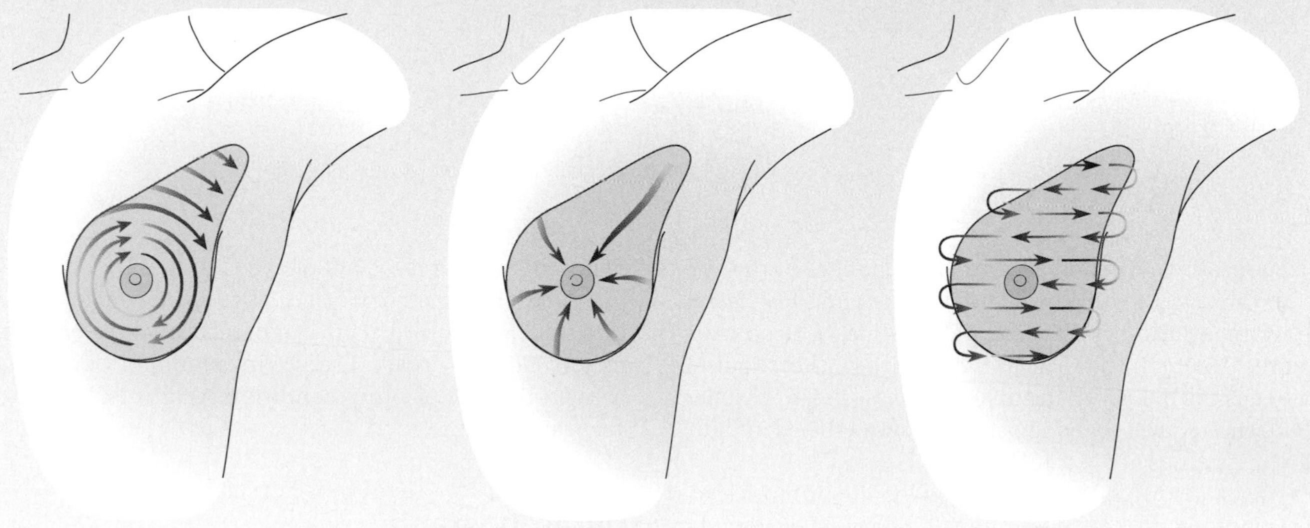

Breast Biopsy

A breast biopsy is done to determine if a breast lesion is malignant. A specimen of breast tissue may be obtained in one of three ways: incisional biopsy, excisional biopsy, or aspiration biopsy.

BOX 54-2 ● Guidelines for Mammography

The National Cancer Institute recommends that all women have a mammogram:

- Initially at age 40
- Every 1 to 2 years thereafter
- Women at higher than average risk of breast cancer should seek expert medical advice about screening before age 40 and the frequency of screening.

(Source: National Cancer Institute. [2001]. NCI Statement on Mammography Screening. [On-line.] Available: http://newscenter.cancer.gov/pressreleases/mammstatements31jan02.html.)

Types

Incisional biopsy is done in the operating room, where one or more sections of tissue are removed. The specimen is frozen quickly and examined microscopically by a pathologist while the client remains anesthetized. If tissue is negative (i.e., benign), the remainder of the benign tissue is removed (if it had not been completely removed for biopsy) If the removed specimen is found to be malignant, the surgeon may then perform the surgical procedure that offers the best chance of cure. The decision to operate immediately when there is a malignancy is thoroughly discussed with the client before surgery.

Some surgeons prefer an *excisional biopsy,* which is removal of the entire lesion. A pathologist examines the excised specimen later and more comprehensively. Clients may be discharged from the hospital before results are obtained. If the lesion is malignant, the biopsy results and proposed treatment are discussed with the client.

Aspirational biopsy, usually done on an outpatient basis, uses a needle and syringe to obtain a sample of the suspect tissue. A local anesthetic is injected around the area and a sample of tissue is removed. A pathologist examines the tissue sample. Sometimes this procedure is done in the hospital under mammographic guidance to ensure an accurate sample of suspect tissue.

Nursing Management

Allow the client time to ask questions and listen to concerns before the breast biopsy is done. The client may have concerns about not only the procedure but the results and a possible diagnosis of cancer.

An aspiration biopsy causes minimal discomfort after the procedure, but there may be redness and soreness in the area. Instruct the client to notify the physician if drainage or bleeding from the biopsy site is more than slight or if increased redness, pain, or fever occurs. Incisional and excisional biopsies require sutures, but pain usually is minimal and can be relieved with a mild analgesic.

Provide instructions regarding wound care, use of a mild analgesic, wearing a supportive brassiere, and timing of a follow-up appointment. Review signs and symptoms that suggest wound infection.

BENIGN BREAST DISORDERS

● BREAST ABSCESS

A **breast abscess** is a localized collection of pus in breast tissue.

Pathophysiology and Etiology

When an abscess occurs in the breast, it most frequently is a complication of postpartum mastitis. Purulent exudate accumulates in a confined, local area of breast tissue. *Staphylococcus aureus* is the most common cause.

Assessment Findings

The client experiences signs and symptoms of mastitis (see Chap. 3); in the case of an abscess, pus may drain from the nipple. Diagnosis is based on physical examination of the breast. A culture and sensitivity of nipple drainage identifies the infecting microorganism and appropriate antibiotic.

Medical and Surgical Management

The client may be hospitalized and placed on contact isolation precautions because soiled dressings are highly infectious. The client is started on intravenous (IV) antibiotic therapy. The abscess may be incised, drained, and packed.

Nursing Management

Remove and reapply dressings following aseptic principles. To avoid irritating skin from frequent removal of tape, use a binder to hold the dressing in place. Apply zinc oxide to surrounding skin to avoid maceration from irritating drainage or wound compresses. To reduce swelling, support the arm and shoulder with pillows. Instruct the client not to shave axillary hair on the side with the abscess until healing is complete.

The mother who is temporarily separated from her newborn needs emotional support. Help the client pump her breasts to remove milk and prevent engorgement. If the mother decides to terminate breastfeeding, apply a tight-fitting brassiere.

● FIBROCYSTIC BREAST DISEASE

Fibrocystic breast disease is a benign breast condition that affects women primarily between the ages of 30 and 50 years.

Pathophysiology and Etiology

Fibrocystic disease results from hormonal changes during the menstrual cycle. Caffeine and nicotine also may aggravate the condition.

When the disorder develops, single or multiple breast cysts appear in one or both breasts (Fig. 54.2). Cysts increase in size and become increasingly tender in proportion to secretion of estrogen. Cyst formation tends to continue throughout the reproductive years. Some disappear, although others may remain permanently. The condition resolves with menopause.

Although a correlation between fibrocystic disease and breast cancer was reported years ago, current studies do not indicate a cause-and-effect relationship between the two conditions. Women with fibrocystic disease may

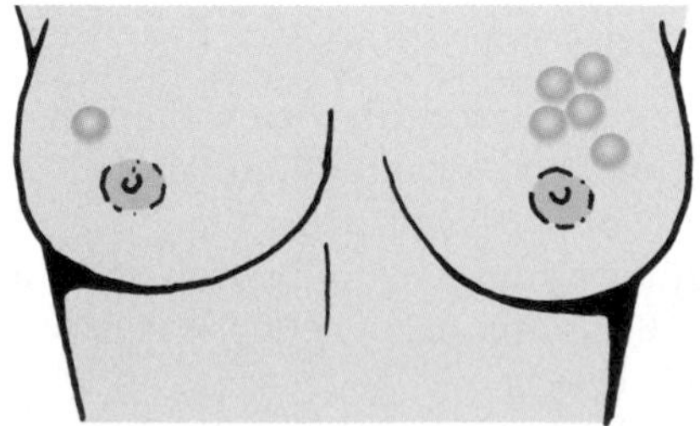

FIGURE 54.2 Depiction of single and multiple breast cysts.

mistake a cancerous mass for a fibrocystic mass and delay medical diagnosis, perform BSE less vigorously because of breast tenderness, or fail to palpate a malignant mass disguised by scar tissue from a previous incisional biopsy.

Assessment Findings

Fibrocystic disease of the breast may cause no symptoms, but many women report having tender or painful breasts and feeling one or multiple lumps within breast tissue. Symptoms are most noticeable just before menstruation and usually abate during menstruation. Size of the cyst often changes with the menstrual cycle, becoming larger before menstruation. Activities, such as weight training, can increase **mastalgia** (breast pain).

A preliminary diagnosis is made by examining the breasts. The characteristic breast mass of fibrocystic disease is soft to firm, movable, and unlikely to cause nipple retraction. Fluid from cysts is aspirated for cytologic examination, or an incisional biopsy is performed. If results are questionable, mammography and ultrasonography are done to distinguish a cystic lesion from a solid malignant tumor.

Medical and Surgical Management

Mild discomfort is relieved with an analgesic such as aspirin or ibuprofen (Advil). For severe symptoms, oral contraceptives or danazol (Danocrine), a synthetic androgen, and bromocriptine (Parlodel), a semisynthetic ergot derivative that mimics prolactin inhibitory factor, are prescribed (Drug Therapy Table 54.1). Occasionally, one or more cysts are removed surgically. Widespread disease that causes severe discomfort is treated with partial mastectomy. Care is taken to preserve the areola to provide a cosmetic appearance to the breast after surgery.

Nursing Management

Obtain a health history and ask focused questions about characteristics and timing of symptoms in relation to the menstrual cycle. During diagnostic examinations, prepare and support the client, label tissue or fluid specimens, and arrange for laboratory analysis. Teach the client with fibrocystic disease to:

- Perform BSE monthly using the same technique each time, and become familiar with the feel and location of cystic masses.
- Schedule a breast examination with a physician every 6 months or whenever a new or unusual lump develops.
- Follow the American Cancer Society's Breast Advisory Committee's Guidelines for mammography (see Box 54-2).
- Wear a well-fitting, supportive brassiere day and night.
- Take mild analgesics or prescription medications according to label directions.
- Apply cold compresses to the breasts when symptomatic.
- Avoid smoking, coffee, chocolate, and caffeinated soft drinks.
- Restrict activities that may cause breast trauma, such as playing soccer or other sports in which breasts are unprotected.
- Consult with the physician about taking vitamin E supplement or oil of evening primrose (a herbal preparation), which some clients have found helpful.

• FIBROADENOMA

A **fibroadenoma** is a solid, benign breast mass composed of connective and glandular tissue. It usually occurs during the late teens and early adulthood, but occasionally later.

Pathophysiology and Etiology

The cause of fibroadenomas is unknown. There may be a hormonal influence, because the mass grows during pregnancy and shrinks after menopause.

The benign tumor is a single nodule that grows slowly in nonpregnant women until it reaches a fixed, stable size. It usually does not enlarge and regress with each menstrual cycle, like those in fibrocystic disease, and is not considered precancerous.

Assessment Findings

A fibroadenoma presents as a painless, nontender breast lump. It usually is encapsulated, mobile, and firm when palpated. If the mass is large, the breasts may appear asymmetric.

Ultrasound can reveal physical characteristics unique to a fibroadenoma versus malignant mass with a higher degree of accuracy than mammography (Greenfield et al., 2001). In the case of very young women—an atypical age for breast cancer—an excisional biopsy is done if the mass changes or grows. If the mass is detected in a woman with a higher risk for developing breast cancer, such as one with a family history or in an older age group, a biopsy is done.

Medical and Surgical Management

Based on diagnostic findings, the client and her physician decide either to continue to observe the mass or excise it. Surgery involves removal of the benign tumor

Drug Therapy Table 54.1 AGENTS FOR SEVERE FIBROCYSTIC DISEASE

DRUG CATEGORY AND EXAMPLES	MECHANISM OF ACTION	SIDE EFFECTS	NURSING CONSIDERATIONS
Synthetic Androgen			
danazol (Danocrine)	Decreases estrogen and progesterone levels by suppressing follicle-stimulating hormone and luteinizing hormone	Acne, deepened voice, weight gain, flushing, vaginitis, enlarged clitoris, nervousness, emotional lability, fluid retention, headache, fatigue, liver dysfunction	Arrange for periodic history and physical exam; long-term use increases chances of side effects and medical supervision is required. Cancer should be ruled out before treatment is initiated. Client should begin taking the hormone during her menstrual period to ensure she is not pregnant. Instruct client to use a nonhormonal form of birth control. Inform client of possible side effects, that masculinizing can occur, and to report any unusual developments.
Progestins			
medroxyprogesterone (Provera, Amen)	Hinders estrogen's effect on breast tissue	Breakthrough bleeding, spotting, amenorrhea, rash, acne, weight gain, edema, depression, thrombophlebitis, migraine, loss of vision, photosensitivity	Arrange for periodic history and physical exam as noted above. Have client mark drug administration days on the calendar. Inform client of possible side effects, including signs and symptoms of thrombophlebitis and embolism. Instruct client to use a reliable method of birth control and sunscreen and to report any visual disturbances.
Estrogen and Progesterone Combinations			
estradiol and norethindrone (Ortho-Novum 10/11)	Oral contraceptives suppress ovarian secretion of estrogen and oppose estrogen's effect on breast tissue	Headache, dizziness, thromboembolism, nausea, breakthrough bleeding, depression, anxiety	Continued medical supervision is required; arrange for physical examination, Papanicolaou tests, and breast examinations at least yearly. Discuss side effects with client; instruct on signs and symptoms of thrombophlebitis and embolism. Instruct client not to smoke and to report any side effects.
Ergot Derivative			
bromocriptine (Parlodel)	Binds with prolactin-secreting cells of the anterior pituitary; inhibits the release of prolactin	Nausea, vomiting, diarrhea, constipation, headache, drowsiness, nasal congestion, hypotension	Administer initial dose at bedtime and with meals thereafter. Advise client to change positions slowly and to use a reliable contraceptive. Report any side effects.

but not a mastectomy. The client is discharged a few hours after recovery from anesthesia.

Nursing Management

Provide emotional support while the diagnosis is tentative because finding a mass in the breast conjures up fears that it may be malignant. Teach the client to continue monthly BSE and follow recommendations for mammography and to consult a physician if the characteristics of the mass change or if a pregnancy occurs.

If surgery is performed, include the following instructions:

- Keep the wound clean and covered until the incision heals.
- Wear a firm, supportive brassiere to reduce incisional discomfort.

- Follow label directions for taking a mild non-narcotic analgesic to relieve minor pain that may last 1 to 3 days.
- Contact the surgeon to schedule a postoperative evaluation or call immediately if there is exceptional incisional pain or if swelling, wound drainage, or a fever develops.

MALIGNANT BREAST DISORDERS

CANCER OF THE BREAST

One woman in eight develops **breast cancer,** a mass of abnormal cells. Risk for breast cancer in women increases with age. Although breast cancer does occur in men, the ratio is approximately 1:150 cases in women. In terms of cancer-related deaths in women, breast cancer is second only to lung cancer. When the disease is discovered and treated early, the 5-year survival rate for small lesions is at least 80%.

Pathology and Pathophysiology

Certain factors appear to increase risk for breast cancer. Being female, being older than 50 years of age, and having a family history of breast cancer are the most common risk factors. Relatives of women with breast cancer who carry a defective gene (BRCA1 and BRCA2) are very likely to develop breast cancer. Additional factors include exposure to ionizing radiation in childhood or adolescence, previous breast cancer, a history of colon or endometrial cancer, chronic alcohol consumption, early menarche, late menopause, obesity, and having no children or having children after 30 years of age. White women are at higher risk for breast cancer than are African Americans, but African-American women are more likely to die of it. More than 50% of women diagnosed with breast cancer demonstrate none of the identified risk factors other than age (Machia, 2001).

Each normal breast contains 15 to 20 lobes connected by ducts to smaller lobules (see Fig. 54.1). The most common malignancy is ductal carcinoma (75%), followed by infiltrating lobular carcinoma (5% to 10%), medullary carcinoma (6%), mucinous carcinoma (3%), tubular ductal carcinoma (2%), and inflammatory breast cancer (1% to 2%). Some malignant breast tumors are hormone dependent, meaning that estrogen or progesterone enhances tumor growth. Regardless of the type or its etiology, untreated cancer spreads elsewhere through the axillary lymph nodes.

Assessment Findings

The primary sign of breast cancer is a painless mass in the breast, most often in the upper outer quadrant (Fig. 54.3). The tumor may have been developing in situ for as long as 2 years before becoming palpable. Other signs of breast cancer include a bloody discharge from the nipple, a dimpling of the skin over the lesion, retraction of the nipple, peau d'orange (orange peel) appearance of the skin, and a difference in size between the breasts (Fig. 54.4). The lesion may be fixed or movable, and axillary lymph nodes may be enlarged. Many of these signs depend on several factors, such as the type, location, and duration of the tumor.

Mammography detects breast lesions earlier than they can be palpated. The radiologist often can differentiate between a benign and malignant tumor on the radiograph. Biopsy and microscopic cell examination confirm the diagnosis. Even in women who are 65 years of age or older, regular mammograms ensure an early diagnosis and decreased mortality rate from breast cancer (McCarthy et al., 2000).

Medical and Surgical Management

Treatment depends on the stage of the breast tumor (Fig. 54.5). It includes surgery, which may be combined with chemotherapy (including hormone therapy) and radiation therapy. Clinical trials using immunotherapy are in progress.

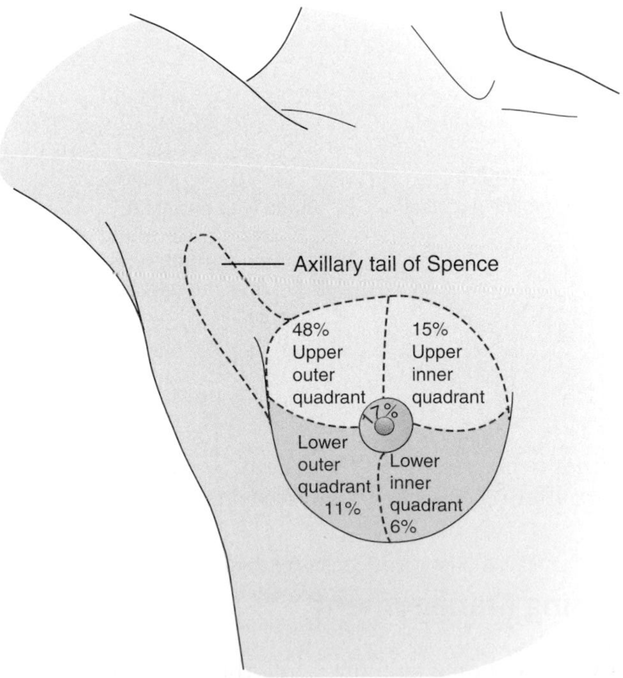

FIGURE 54.3 Locations of primary malignant breast tumors.

Dimpling

Flattening of nipple

Retraction signs

Breast cancer mass

Nipple inversion

Peau d'orange

FIGURE 54.4 Signs and symptoms of breast cancer.

Surgery

Surgery is performed immediately after obtaining results of the biopsy or shortly thereafter. The type of surgery depends on the stage of the tumor and the client's informed decision about treatment options (Table 54.1). The current trend is to perform the least mutilating procedure necessary to obtain a favorable prognosis. Compared with more extensive types of mastectomy procedures, breast-conserving surgeries such as lumpectomy, partial mastectomy, and segmental mastectomy demonstrate equivalent outcomes in terms of survival rate for treatment of early-stage breast cancer.

Removal of ovaries enhances prognosis for women whose tumors are hormone stimulated. The additional surgery inhibits growth of the primary tumor or metastatic tissue derived from the primary tumor elsewhere in the body.

A new technique, **sentinel lymph node mapping,** involves identifying the first (sentinel) lymph nodes through which breast cancer cells would spread to regional lymph nodes in the axilla. The sentinel lymph nodes are located by injecting a nuclear isotope around the breast tumor followed by instillation of blue dye. After excising the breast tumor, the surgeon passes a Geiger counter over the perimammary tissue to find the area of most intense radioactivity. A small incision is made and the

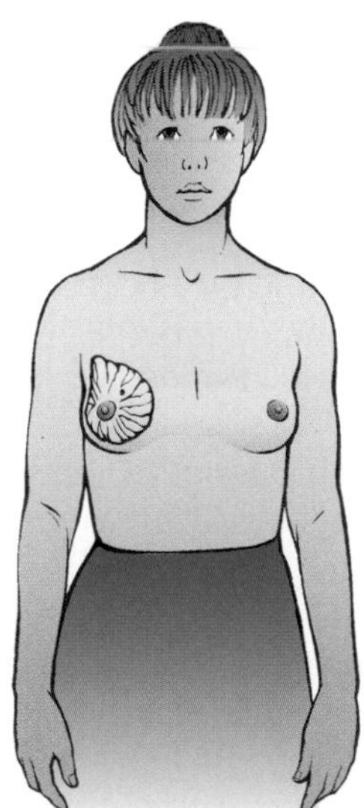

Stage I: Tumors are less than 2 cm in diameter and confined to breast.

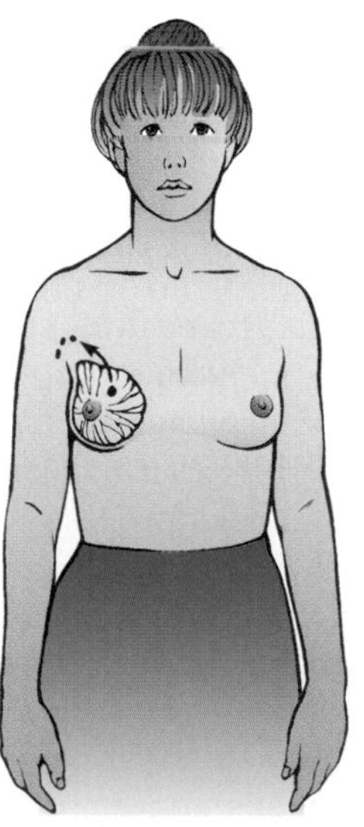

Stage II: Tumors are less than 5 cm, or tumors are smaller with mobile axillary lymph node involvement.

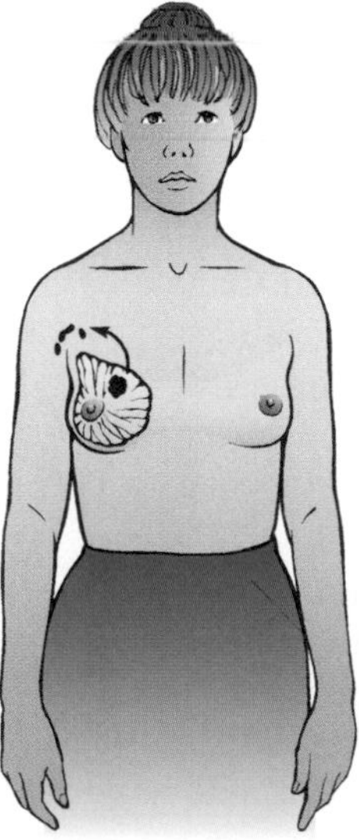

Stage IIIa: Tumors are greater than 5 cm, or tumors are accompanied by enlarged axillary lymph nodes fixed to one another or to adjacent tissue.

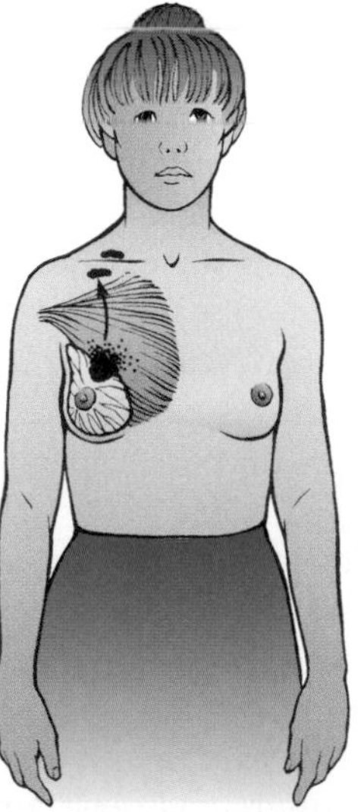

Stage IIIb: More advanced lesions with satellite nodules, fixation to the skin or chest wall, ulceration, edema, or with supraclavicular or intraclavicular nodal involvement.

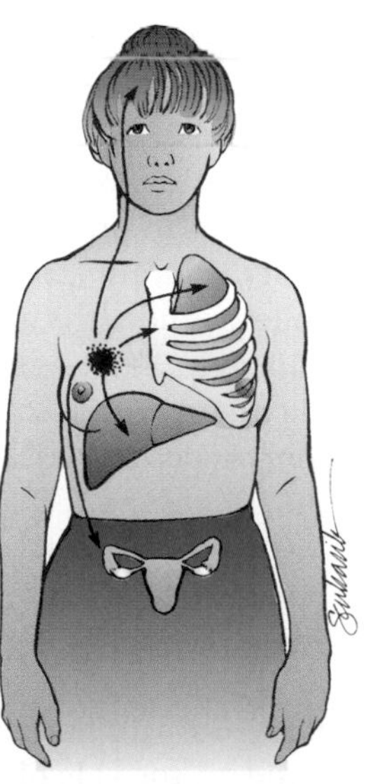

Stage IV: All tumors with distant metastases.

FIGURE 54.5 Breast cancer stages.

TABLE 54.1 SURGICAL PROCEDURES FOR BREAST CANCER

PROCEDURE	DESCRIPTION
Lumpectomy	Only the tumor is removed; some axillary lymph nodes may be excised at the same time for microscopic examination.
Partial or segmental mastectomy	The tumor and some breast tissue and some lymph nodes are removed.
Simple or total mastectomy	All breast tissue is removed. No lymph node dissection is performed.
Subcutaneous mastectomy	All breast tissue is removed, but the skin and nipple are left intact.
Modified radical mastectomy	The breast, some lymph nodes, the lining over the chest muscles, and the pectoralis minor muscle are removed.
Radical mastectomy	The breast, axillary lymph nodes, and pectoralis major and minor muscles are removed. In some instances, sternal lymph nodes also are removed.

surgeon follows the blue dye to the sentinel lymph nodes, which are removed with a minimum of surrounding tissue and investigated for cancer cells. No cancer cells in the sentinel lymph nodes suggests that all lymph nodes are free of cancer cells. Validating the lack of lymph node metastasis allows the surgeon to preserve more breast, axillary tissue, and chest muscle. Leaving many normal lymph nodes intact reduces the potential for complications, such as lymphedema (discussed later), delayed wound healing, and altered skin sensation, from the extensive disruption of lymphatic circulation.

In extensive surgical procedures such as modified radical mastectomy (radical mastectomy no longer is the standard of practice for the surgical treatment of breast cancer), drains are inserted to remove serous fluid that collects under the skin. Removing fluid promotes healing and reduces potential for infection. Also, a skin graft may be required to close the wound if a radical mastectomy is performed. Pressure dressings are applied to both the donor and recipient graft sites.

Lymphedema, soft tissue swelling from accumulated lymphatic fluid, occurs in some women after breast cancer surgery. The condition is a consequence of removing or irradiating axillary lymph nodes. It is evidenced by temporary or permanent enlargement of the arm and hand on the side of the amputated breast. Impaired lymphatic circulation predisposes to disfigurement, reduced range of motion, heaviness of the limb, skin changes, infection, and, in severe cases, tissue necrosis that may require amputation of the limb.

Depending on circumstances, chemotherapy, radiation therapy, or both are common surgical adjuncts. The choice depends on the type of cancer and stage of the tumor, any metastasis, and the client's age. Bone marrow transplantation may be used if the breast cancer resists other forms of treatment.

Stop, Think, and Respond ● BOX 54-2

A client has had a modified radical mastectomy. While trying to teach her how to care for the incision, she avoids looking at the wound. How can you help her cope with the change in body image?

Chemotherapy

The goal of chemotherapy is to destroy cancer cells that may have metastasized before or during surgery. One or more of the following drugs are given:

- An antiestrogen drug, such as tamoxifen (Nolvadex), for postmenopausal women whose tumors are hormone dependent
- An antiprogestin drug, mifepristone (RU-486), which blocks progesterone-dependent breast cancers as determined by progesterone receptor assay on excised tissue
- Androgen therapy for advanced breast cancer in postmenopausal women using testolactone (Teslac)
- Single or combined antineoplastic agents, such as cyclophosphamide (Cytoxan), doxorubicin (Adriamycin), 5-fluorouracil (5-FU), methotrexate (Rheumatrex), and prednisone (Deltasone). Antineoplastic drugs also are combined with drugs mentioned earlier that influence hormonal physiology.

Radiation Therapy

Radiation therapy can be given before or after surgery. If the surgeon finds that axillary nodes contain cancer cells, there is chest wall involvement, or the tumor is larger than 5 cm, a series of radiation treatments usually is ordered prophylactically even after a modified radical mastectomy. Side effects of radiation therapy include fatigue, skin redness similar to a bad sunburn, rash, minor discomfort, or pain (see Chap. 19).

Nursing Management

Encourage anyone who detects breast changes to see a physician immediately. Prepare the client for surgery and assist with her or his safe recovery. Men who undergo a mastectomy do not face the extreme physical changes but still require emotional support because of the diagnosis. For breast-conserving procedures, nursing care focuses on wound management and discharge instructions. Refer to Nursing Care Plan 54-1 for more specific information in managing the care of the client undergoing a modified radical mastectomy.

Prepare the client for common side effects of chemotherapy (see Chap. 19). Administering antiemetics and anxiolytic medications before chemotherapy helps lessen the potential for vomiting. Provide instructions about when and how to take medications at home to alleviate nausea and mouth sores and to boost white blood cell or red blood cell production. If alopecia is likely, offer the client a list of wig suppliers (usually provided through the American Cancer Society).

Most clients are not hospitalized long after mastectomy. Therefore, providing early discharge instructions and making arrangements for home care are important interventions. Explain wound and drain care or arrange for home health nursing. Assess availability of family assistance at home. Look for and report any signs of infection or impaired wound healing such as drainage or significant pale or dusky appearance to the skin around the incision. Stress continuation of arm exercises. Arrange for follow-up examinations by the surgeon. Instruct client on the self-administration of prescribed drug therapy. Tell client to expect some residual numbness or tingling on the chest wall and inner side of the arm from the axilla to the elbow, which may take as long as 1 year to resolve. Suggest applying cream or lotion to the arm if the skin tends to be dry.

Explain that when selecting a prosthesis, those that are filled with fluid assume natural contours like the other breast, feel like normal breast tissue, and even radiate body warmth. Advise against lifting or carrying objects that weigh more than 15 pounds and making vigorous repetitive movements with the affected arm. Discourage sleeping on the affected arm or wearing constrictive clothing that impairs circulation. Reinforce that blood pressure measurements, injections, blood donations, and IV infusions are contraindicated in the arm on the side of the mastectomy. Recommend wearing gloves while doing yard or housework to prevent injuries that may heal slowly or become infected. Advise using an electric razor for shaving axillary hair. Instruct to continue to perform monthly BSE on the intact breast and have the intact breast clinically examined each year by a physician, along with obtaining a mammogram.

• METASTATIC BREAST CANCER

Despite treatment even in early stages of breast cancer, some women develop metastatic disease (ie, affecting another part of the body). Malignant cells are spread by direct extension, through the lymphatic system, bloodstream, and cerebrospinal fluid.

Pathophysiology

Metastasis commonly involves lymph nodes. Skeletal and pulmonary involvement often occurs. The brain and liver also may become involved. Once metastasis occurs, prognosis is less favorable, but metastases progress at different rates.

Assessment Findings

Metastases often cause pain in the new site. When bone is involved, pathologic fractures are possible.

X-rays of the lungs, spine, or other areas of the body are used to detect metastases. Magnetic resonance imaging or computed tomography scanning also may be done. These studies are done before or after treating the primary tumor. Lymph node dissection is done either at the time of breast surgery or later to evaluate metastasis to lymph nodes draining the breasts.

Medical Management

Treatment aims at providing the greatest period of palliation (relieving symptoms without curing the disease) for the client. Large doses of estrogen or testosterone sometimes alleviate the pain, weight loss, and malaise of metastatic cancer. Intramuscular androgen (testosterone) therapy is used, especially when metastases are to bone. All forms of treatment carry the possibility of unpleasant effects and complications. For palliative purposes, radiation therapy may be used to treat regional or distant metastases (especially to bone) or local tumor recurrence of the chest wall. Sometimes surgery, chemotherapy, or radiation is used to slow growth of the new malignant site.

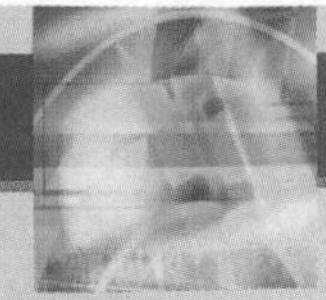

Nursing Care Plan 54-1

THE CLIENT UNDERGOING A MODIFIED RADICAL MASTECTOMY

Assessment

- Discuss client's medical, drug, allergy, and family history.
- Take vital signs and weight.
- Determine location of the breast lesion.
- Establish what diagnostic tests were done before admission.
- Discuss information the physician gave the client about the type and extent of surgery.

Nursing Diagnoses: **Anxiety** and **Fear** related to undergoing an unfamiliar experience and the potential consequences of the disease and its treatment

Expected Outcome: Client will indicate increased emotional comfort.

Interventions	*Rationales*
Provide opportunity for client to express feelings and discuss concerns.	Helps the client deal openly with feelings.
Answer all questions; consult with other team members about matters that involve their expertise.	Provides client with reality-based information and reduces exaggerated perceptions.
Collaborate with physician on arranging for a visit from a Reach to Recovery or I Can Cope volunteer sponsored by the American Cancer Society.	People who have recovered from a similar diagnosis and surgery can serve as role models and answer questions from their own personal experiences.
Do not stifle crying; stay with client when emotions are overwhelming.	Crying relieves tension when a person can find no other coping strategy.
Encourage client's significant other or whomever the client turns to for support to remain with client as much and as long as possible.	The presence of others who provide emotional support reduces anxiety.
Keep client informed of the routine that will be followed in preparation for surgery and postoperative care.	Knowledge facilitates a sense of control.

Evaluation of Expected Outcome: Anxiety is reduced.

Nursing Diagnoses: **Impaired Skin Integrity** and **Risk for Infection** secondary to surgical wound

Expected Outcome: The incision will heal; no infection will develop.

Interventions	*Rationales*
Limit movement, especially abduction, of arm on side of surgery until wound edges are intact.	Activity can disrupt approximation of the incision.
Inspect wound for swelling, unusual drainage, odor, redness, or separation of the suture line.	Wound infections are accompanied by signs of inflammation and a delay in healing.
Empty and re-establish negative pressure in closed wound drains at least once per shift.	Negative pressure (suction) pulls fluid from the incisional area, which facilitates healing.
Administer antibiotic therapy as prescribed.	Antibiotics destroy or inhibit growth of microorganisms.
Monitor trends in temperature and white blood cell counts.	Fever and leukocytosis suggest an infection is developing.
Allow client to shower after sutures and drains are removed.	Hygiene reduces number of microorganisms on the skin.

(continued)

Nursing Care Plan 54-1 (Continued)

THE CLIENT UNDERGOING A MODIFIED RADICAL MASTECTOMY

Evaluation of Expected Outcome: Incision heals without complications.

Nursing Diagnosis: **Risk for Ineffective Tissue Perfusion (lymphedema)** related to compromised flow of lymphatic fluid

Expected Outcome: Soft tissue in the arm on the side of surgery will be comparable with the opposite arm in color, size, and temperature.

Interventions	*Rationales*
Do not take blood pressures, give injections, administer IV infusions, or have blood drawn from arm on the side of the mastectomy.	Procedures that affect the circulation in the affected arm can contribute to ineffective tissue perfusion.
Support and elevate arm on the side of the mastectomy with pillows so it is higher than the heart.	Promotes gravity drainage of fluid trapped in the soft tissue.
Place arm in a sling when client ambulates initially; eventually arm can be positioned at the client's side.	A sling prevents stasis of fluid in distal areas of the arm.
Show client how to squeeze and release a soft rubber ball or a rolled pair of cotton socks several times a day.	Venous blood and lymph circulate with contraction of skeletal muscles.
Remove and reapply an elastic roller bandage from the fingers to the axilla twice a day, or insert affected arm into a pneumatic sleeve, an air-filled device that mechanically pumps the arm, for a half-hour or the prescribed time twice a day.	An elastic roller bandage or pneumatic sleeve compresses the valves in veins to promote circulation.
Assess hand for swelling, dusky color, delayed nail blanching, coldness, and tingling; report abnormal findings.	Reduces the potential for complications.

Evaluation of Expected Outcome: The circulation is maintained in the operative arm; both arms are of comparable size.

Nursing Diagnosis: **Impaired Physical Mobility** related to alteration in pectoral chest muscles

Expected Outcome: Client will achieve full range of arm motion.

Interventions	*Rationales*
Start active exercises of affected arm on first or second postoperative day, unless contraindicated.	Reduces the potential for contractures.
Begin with flexing and extending fingers, wrist, and elbow. Later, encourage client to use affected arm to perform oral hygiene, hair combing, and face washing.	Gradually restores ability to flex, extend, and abduct the arm.
Show client how to face and "finger-walk" up a wall in the room. Mark client's progress with masking tape so that the height can be exceeded with subsequent efforts.	Finger-walking increases ability to raise arm. Marking progress provides an incentive to meet or exceed heights during previous exercises.
Loop a rope or cord around a shower rod and raise and lower each arm in pulley fashion.	Facilitates rehabilitation.
Tie a string or rope to a doorknob and have client turn rope in a circular fashion.	Promotes circumduction.

(continued)

Nursing Care Plan 54-1 (Continued)

THE CLIENT UNDERGOING A MODIFIED RADICAL MASTECTOMY

Evaluation of Expected Outcome: Client improves the use of the arm and hand of operative side. The client performs postmastectomy exercises.

Nursing Diagnoses: **Risk for Disturbed Body Image, Ineffective Coping,** and **Sexual Dysfunction** related to perceived loss of physical attractiveness and sexual desirability

Expected Outcomes: Client will accept body changes, use positive coping strategies, and experience satisfactory sexual activity.

Interventions	*Rationales*
Suggest that client pad a bra with one or two cotton socks until a prosthesis is fitted in 6 to 8 weeks.	Gives outward appearance that client has both breasts. Purchasing a prosthetic bra is delayed until tissue heals completely.
Inform client that cosmetic breast reconstruction is an option to discuss with surgeon.	Provides an alternative for simulating natural breast tissue.
Advocate that client and sexual partner openly express to each other how surgery has affected them emotionally.	Facilitates mutual understanding and acceptance of body change.
Discuss methods for dealing with removed breast during sexual activities such as using no or low lighting during intercourse or wearing the upper portion of lingerie.	Modifying sexual activities reduces self-consciousness.

Evaluation of Expected Outcomes: Client adjusts to the loss of the breast.

Nursing Management

For nursing care of the client undergoing chemotherapy or radiation, see Chapter 19.

• BREAST CANCER PREVENTION

Three options are available to women with increased risk for developing breast cancer: (1) long-term follow-up, (2) bilateral prophylactic mastectomy, and (3) chemoprevention with tamoxifen (Nolvadex). Those who choose long-term follow-up receive an annual mammogram with a clinical breast examination and monthly BSE. Prophylactic bilateral mastectomy is the most invasive of the three options.

Taking the drug tamoxifen can reduce risk of breast cancer in women who are at high risk. Tamoxifen also preserves bone mineral density, thus preventing osteoporosis. It also lowers low-density lipoprotein cholesterol levels. Tamoxifen can have detrimental effects, such as increased incidences of endometrial cancer, deep vein thrombosis, pulmonary embolism, and cataracts. Other side effects are increased hot flashes, cold sweats, vaginal discharge, genital itching, and pain with intercourse.

COSMETIC BREAST PROCEDURES •

Some women undergo various cosmetic breast procedures, collectively referred to as **mammoplasty,** for several reasons, but primarily to improve their appearance.

• BREAST RECONSTRUCTION

Breast reconstruction is a surgical procedure in which the area of a mastectomy is refashioned to simulate the contour of a breast and optionally to create a nipple and an areola. It is accomplished by using either an artificial implant filled with saline or autogenous (self) tissue. Reconstruction can begin at the time of mastectomy if sufficient skin is spared, or it can be done later.

Artificial Implants

Before an implant can produce an optimum cosmetic appearance, the skin and tissue on the chest wall are expanded to provide a large enough space to fill and approximate the size of the remaining breast. Tissue expansion is achieved by stretching the chest wall over several months with an inflatable or saline-filled pocket (Fig. 54.6). Saline implants are used for breast enhancement procedures.

Autogenous Tissue

Reconstructing the breast with autogenous tissue provides a more natural look and feel to the breast. The tissue is harvested similarly to a "tummy tuck" (abdominoplasty) from the rectus abdominis muscle along with its adjoining skin and fat (Fig. 54.7). Other donor sites, such as a portion of the latissimus dorsi or gluteal muscles, may be used. Removing donor tissue tends to leave a physical deformity, parts of which may be more obvious than others.

If a woman desires a nipple, it is reconstructed from tissue from the opposite nipple, the ear, or toe. Tissue for the areola is selected from a site with a similar color, like the inner thigh or vaginal labia. It also may be created by pigmented tattoo.

• REDUCTION MAMMOPLASTY

A **reduction mammoplasty** is an overnight surgical procedure in which glandular breast tissue, fat, and skin are removed bilaterally to reduce large, pendulous breasts. Most candidates for a reduction mammoplasty wear a size D cup or larger brassiere and experience discomfort in the shoulders or back, skin irritation beneath the breasts, difficulty in finding suitable clothing, self-consciousness, or low self-esteem.

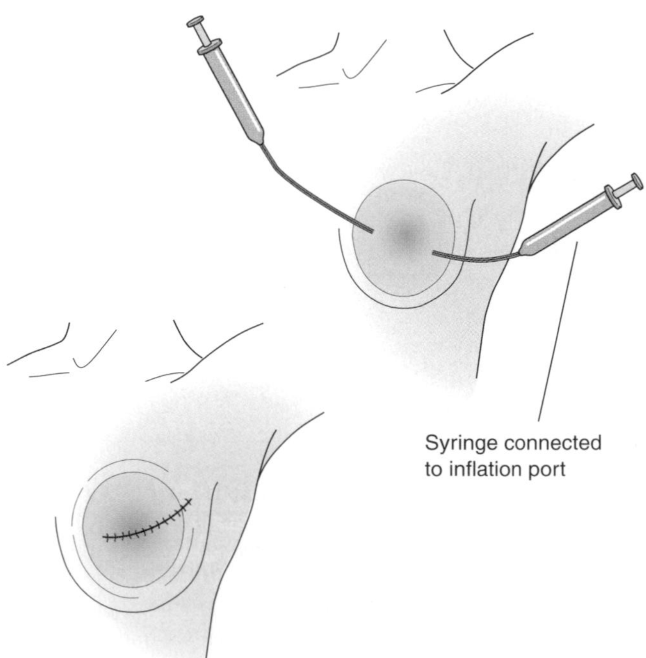

FIGURE 54.6 Tissue expander and breast implant.

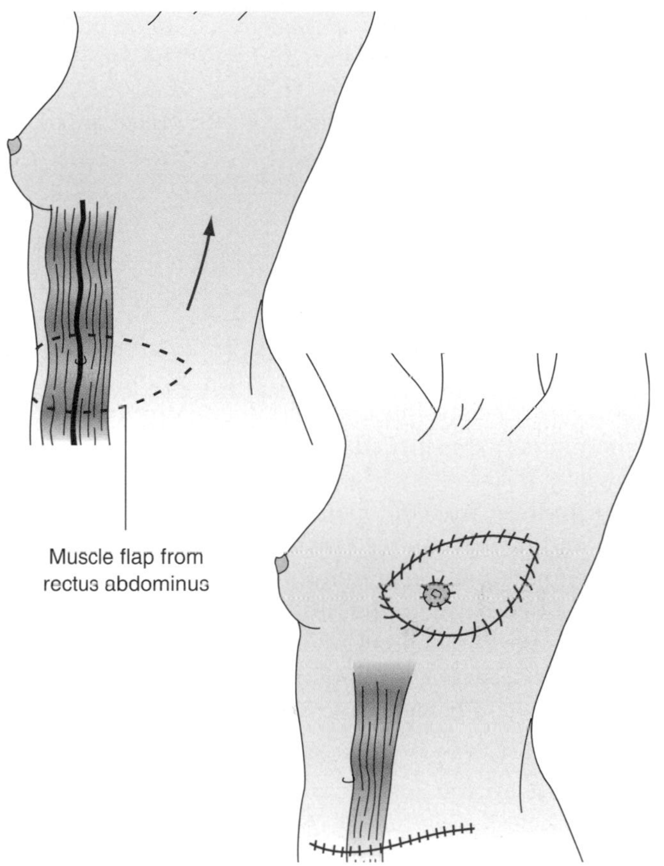

FIGURE 54.7 Autogenous breast reconstruction.

To reduce breast size, an incision is made around the nipple through which tissue is removed. Loose skin is tightened to reposition the areola and nipple. The client is discharged with a bulky chest dressing and sometimes a small wound drain.

• OPPOSITE BREAST REDUCTION

Size of a reconstructed breast is limited by the amount of tissue that remains; thus, there may be potential asymmetry. Opposite breast reduction is a surgical procedure performed to reduce a healthy breast so it more closely resembles the size of a reconstructed breast. The procedure, although done for different reasons, is the same as a reduction mammoplasty.

• BREAST LIFT

Ptosis, or drooping, of the breast(s) is corrected with a breast lift or **mastopexy.** Sagging skin and low nipple placement that accompany weight loss or aging are corrected in a procedure similar to reduction mammoplasty, although the incision and scar line are smaller and recovery time is shorter. In some cases, the size or contour of the breast is enhanced with breast augmentation techniques.

● BREAST AUGMENTATION

Women who wish to enlarge their breasts may choose breast augmentation, similar to reconstructing the breast using an artificial saline implant. When caring for women who undergo this procedure, place the client in a semi-Fowler's position after cosmetic breast surgery to promote drainage from the operative site. Give analgesics for pain and inspect the operative site for changes in color and temperature. To minimize stretching of tissues and suture line, maintain dressings and assist the client to use a support brassiere. Provide clients undergoing cosmetic breast surgery with information that applies to the type of surgery being performed. General guidelines are as follows:

- Have a mammogram to verify there are no malignancies before having cosmetic surgery.
- Continue to perform BSE and have clinical breast examinations (inspection and palpation) by the physician.
- Expect reduced sensation in the nipple, a certain amount of scarring, and temporary discomfort when moving arms and shoulders after cosmetic breast surgery.
- Wear a soft brassiere for 3 to 6 weeks after surgery except when bathing or taking a shower.
- Avoid activities, such as vigorous sports, that may result in injury to the breasts until healing is complete.

GENERAL GERONTOLOGIC CONSIDERATIONS

Many breast disorders that are hormonally influenced regress after menopause.

Risk for breast cancer increases with age. Older adult women need to continue performing monthly BSE and have yearly clinical breast examinations and mammograms.

With age, breast tissue atrophies, causing sagging and hanging of the breast. Fibrotic changes may cause some retraction of the nipple in older women.

In the older client, surgery for breast cancer may be limited to a lumpectomy or simple mastectomy.

Occasionally, breast tumors that have been present for years become more evident with age, making detection easier.

Critical Thinking Exercises

1. *How might signs and symptoms differ among women with fibrocystic breast disease, fibroadenomas, and malignant breast tumors?*
2. *What advice is appropriate for preventing breast cancer?*

● NCLEX-STYLE REVIEW QUESTIONS 

1. A client is being discharged following a mastectomy. Which discharge instruction is most essential to prevent rehospitalization?
   1. Expect numbness and tingling in the chest wall.
   2. Continue range-of-motion arm exercises at home.
   3. Perform proper wound and drain care until the next visit.
   4. Memorize date and time of the follow-up visit with the surgeon.
2. When obtaining a history from a woman diagnosed with fibrocystic breast disease, the nurse is most correct in focusing questions on:
   1. The size and shape of any lump
   2. The timing of the symptoms
   3. Any prescribed medications
   4. Any recent breast trauma
3. During a postoperative visit to the gynecologist, a 34-year-old client who has undergone a total abdominal hysterectomy is concerned about the self-breast examination schedule. Which instruction by the nurse is most helpful?
   1. "Pick a monthly date that would be easiest to remember for the examination."
   2. "Since your surgery was performed, there is no need for monthly examinations."
   3. "Examine your breasts 3 days after the end of menstruation."
   4. "Examine your breasts at mid-month on a consistent basis."

connection

Visit the Connection site at **http://connection.lww.com/go/timbyEssentials** for links to chapter-related resources on the Internet.

References and Suggested Readings

Banks, M. (November/December 2002). Richard Rountree's road to recovery from male breast cancer. *Community Health Forum*, 22–25.

Breast imaging: Mammograms still rule. (2000). *Harvard Women's Health Watch, 7*(10), 5–6.

D'Arcy, Y. (2002). What is postmastectomy pain syndrome? *Nursing 2002, 32*(11), 17.

Davis, B. S. (2001). Lymphedema after breast cancer treatment. *American Journal of Nursing, 101*(4), Continuing Care Extra: 24AAAA–24DDDD.

Greenfield, L. J., Mulholland, M. W., Oldhan, K. T., et al. (2001). *Surgery: Scientific principles and practice* (3rd ed.). Philadelphia: Lippincott Williams & Wilkins.

Harcourt, D., & Rumsey, N. (2001). Psychological aspects of breast reconstruction: A review of the literature. *Journal of Advanced Nursing, 35,* 477–487.

Harmer, V. (2000). The surgical management of breast cancer. *Nursing Times, 96*(48), 34–35.

Heer, E. (Sept./Oct. 2001). Breast and cervical cancer: Taming the beast with early detection. *Community Health Forum,* 17–21.

Jackson, L. (October 14, 2002). After breast cancer. *Advance for Nurses,* 27–28.

Judkins, A. F., & Akins, J. (2001). Breast cancer: Initial diagnosis and current treatment options. *Nursing Clinics of North America, 36,* 527–542.

Kunsman, J., & Pollard, K. (April 29, 2002). Not so radical. *Advance for Nurses,* 23–24.

Machia, J. (2001). Breast cancer: Risk, prevention, and tamoxifen. *American Journal of Nursing, 101*(4), 26–36.

McCarthy, E. P., Burns, R. B., Freund, K. M., et al. (2000). Mammography use, breast cancer stage at diagnosis, and survival among older women. *Journal of the American Geriatrics Society, 48,* 1226–1233.

Miers, M. (2001). Understanding benign breast disorders and disease. *Nursing Standard, 15*(50), 45–52.

Resnick, B., & Belcher, A. E. (2002). Breast reconstruction. *American Journal of Nursing, 102*(4), 26–33.

Sandau, K. E. (2002). Free tram flap: Breast reconstruction. *American Journal of Nursing, 102*(4), 36–43.

Thomas, S., & Greifzu, S. P. (2000). Oncology today: Breast reconstruction. *RN, 63*(4), 45–48.

U.S. Preventive Service Task Force (2003). Chemoprevention of breast cancer: Recommendations and rationale. *American Journal of Nursing, 103*(5), 107–113.

Wilmoth, M. C. (2001). The aftermath of breast cancer: An altered sexual self. *Cancer Nursing, 24,* 278–286.

Workman, L. (2002). Breast cancer: New strategies to beat an old enemy. *Nursing 2002, 32*(10), 58–63.

Zack, E. (2001a). Mammography and reduced breast cancer mortality rates. *MEDSURG Nursing, 10*(1), 17–21.

Zack, E. (2001b). Sentinel lymph node biopsy in breast cancer: Scientific rationale and patient care. *Oncology Nursing Forum, 28,* 997–1007.

Zuckerman, D. (2002). The breast cancer information gap. *RN, 65*(2), 39–41.

chapter 55

Caring for Clients With Disorders of the Male Reproductive System

Words to Know 

benign prostatic hyperplasia
cryptorchidism
digital rectal examination
ejaculation
epididymitis
impotence
orchiectomy
orchiopexy
orchitis
prostatectomy
prostate-specific antigen
retrograde ejaculation
semen
spermatogenesis
testicular self-examination
transillumination
tumor markers
vasectomy

Learning Objectives

On completion of this chapter, the reader will:

- List external and internal structures of the male reproductive system.
- Identify possible consequences of disorders affecting the male reproductive system.
- Give examples of structural disorders affecting the male reproductive system.
- Explain the technique and purpose for performing testicular self-examination.
- Describe infectious or inflammatory conditions affecting the male reproductive system.
- Discuss erectile disorders.
- Identify methods for treating impotence.
- Describe the nursing plan of care for a client who receives a penile implant.
- Explain how prostatic hyperplasia compromises urinary elimination.
- Discuss the nursing management of a client undergoing a prostatectomy.
- Contrast three male reproductive cancers in terms of age of onset, incidence, and treatment outcomes.
- List home care instructions after a vasectomy.

The physiologic functions of the male reproductive structures include generation of gender-specific sexual characteristics and the manufacture and transportation of sperm and seminal fluid. The lower urinary tract and reproductive system structures are so closely associated that disorders frequently affect both systems. Congenital or acquired structural abnormalities, infectious and inflammatory conditions, erection disorders, benign prostatic enlargement, and cancer are all threats to male reproductive health.

ANATOMY AND PHYSIOLOGY

External and Internal Structures

The external male genitalia consists of the penis and scrotum. The testes (sing., *testis*) lie within the scrotum and are responsible for **spermatogenesis,** sperm production, and secretion of testosterone. Testosterone is the male sex hormone that affects development and maintenance of secondary male sex characteristics. The structures that extend from the testes, the epididymides (sing., *epididymis*), vas deferens (or ductus deferens), seminal vesicles, prostate gland, and bulbourethral (Cowper's) glands (Fig. 55.1), form a complex secretory and ductal system. Their functions are to nurture and enhance the motility of sperm and ensure their survival once they are released from the body. The prostate gland is an accessory sex organ surrounding the urethra at the neck of the bladder. It secretes fluid that neutralizes acidic vaginal secretions.

Spermatogenesis and Ejaculation

Under the influence of follicle-stimulating hormone and testosterone, sperm are manufactured and sustained in the seminiferous tubules of the testes until they are motile—a

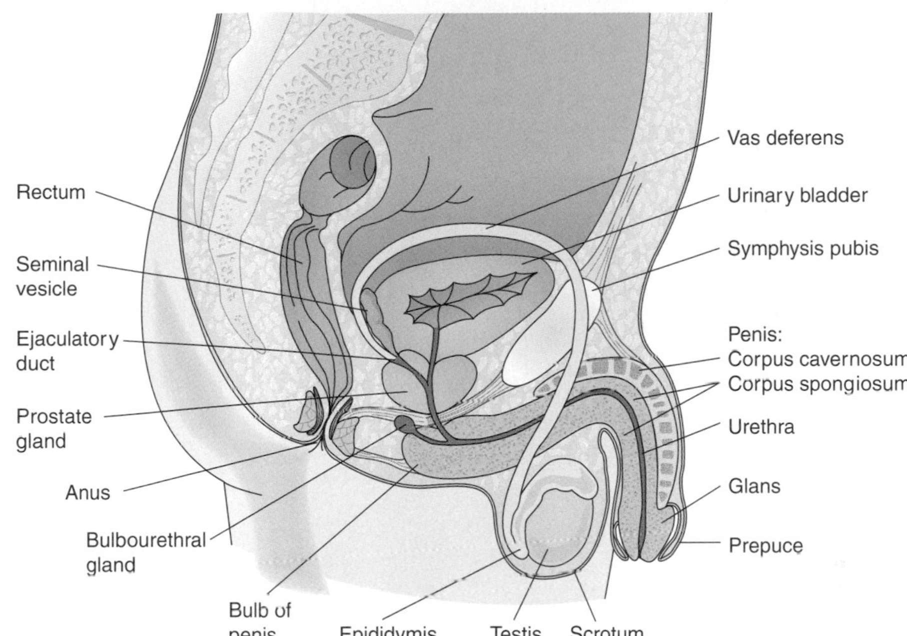

FIGURE 55.1 Anatomy of the male reproductive system.

process that takes approximately 64 days. They then pass into the epididymides and vas deferens, where they complete their maturation. The seminal vesicles that empty into the vas deferens produce seminal fluid, which adds volume to the sperm and nourishes them after ejaculation.

Ejaculation is the discharge of **semen,** the fluid that contains sperm, from the body. The process of ejaculation results from rhythmic contraction of the muscles of the vas deferens and the penis during orgasm and sexual climax. The normal volume of ejaculate is 2.5 to 6 mL, which contains an average of 400 million spermatozoa (Bullock & Henze, 2000). A count of less than 20 to 50 million spermatozoa per milliliter results in infertility.

ASSESSMENT

History

Obtain a general health and family history and a detailed sexual history. A sexual history includes questions that elicit information about risks for sexually transmitted infections (STIs), contraceptive practices, ability to achieve or sustain an erection, pain during sexual intercourse, premature ejaculation or other concerns of a sexual nature, inability of a sex partner to conceive, and prior treatments (including drug therapy, diagnostic tests, or surgery) that relate to the genitourinary system.

Physical Examination

Inspect the external genitalia, looking for abnormalities such as skin lesions and urethral discharge. Palpate the testes for tumors and examine the scrotum. **Transillumination,** shining a light through the scrotum, provides clues about the density of scrotal tissue. A **digital rectal examination** (DRE) is performed to assess the prostate for size as well as evidence of tumor (Fig. 55.2). Yearly DREs are recommended for men older than 40 to 50 years.

Diagnostic Tests

Several diagnostic tests commonly are performed to evaluate the male genitourinary tract. See Box 55-1 for appropriate nursing care.

Transrectal Ultrasonography

Transrectal ultrasonography (sonogram) is a test in which a lubricated probe is inserted into the rectum to obtain a view of the prostate gland from various angles. The test is indicated in cases in which the prostate gland is enlarged or the blood level of prostate-specific antigen (see later discussion) is elevated.

Cystoscopy

In a cystoscopy, an illuminated optical instrument called a *cystoscope* is inserted into the meatus to inspect the bladder, prostate, and urethra. This aids in evaluating the degree of encroachment by the prostate on the urethra.

Tissue Biopsy

A needle biopsy of prostatic tissue is obtained for analysis by the perineal or rectal approach. A testicular biopsy is obtained for evaluation of spermatozoa production or to diagnose a testicular malignancy.

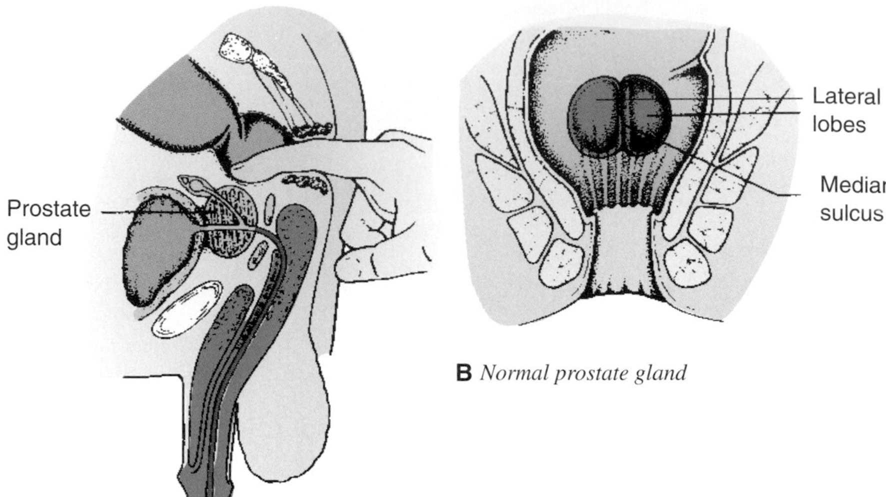

FIGURE 55.2 (**A**) Palpation of the prostate gland during digital rectal examination (DRE). (**B**) The prostate is round with a palpable median sulcus or groove that separates the two lobes.

Cultures

Cultures are obtained from urethral secretions, skin lesions, or urine. Prostatic fluid can be expressed during a DRE and also sent for culture.

Fertility Tests

Fertility studies include a semen analysis to determine sperm count, sperm motility, and any abnormal sperm. Other laboratory tests may include measuring the level of plasma luteinizing hormone (LH), which is necessary for release of testosterone from the testes. A decrease in the blood level of LH may be responsible for decreased testosterone production and infertility.

Tumor Markers

Tumor markers are substances synthesized by tumors that are released into the circulation in excessive amounts. The **prostate-specific antigen** (PSA) assay is a blood test to detect prostate cancer. Although an elevated PSA does not always indicate a malignancy, it now is possible to differentiate free PSA in total PSA. High percentages of free PSA are associated with benign disease, whereas low percentages of free PSA indicate malignancy. Regular PSA tests assist in early diagnosis and staging of prostatic cancer, and in evaluating effectiveness of cancer treatment. Other blood test findings that suggest cancer are elevated levels of alpha-fetoprotein, beta-human chori-

BOX 55-1 ● Nursing Management of the Client Undergoing Genitourinary Diagnostic Testing

Test	Preprocedure Care	Postprocedure Care
All tests	Explain procedure, answer questions in a calm and reassuring manner. Use techniques of therapeutic communication to provide an opportunity for client to express concerns. Talk with client and inform him of each step as test proceeds.	Assist client to resume a comfortable position and clean up gels or lubricants. Answer questions about when test results will be available and when normal activity can resume. Provide written post-test instructions, if applicable.
Ultrasound of the prostate	Assure client that test is not painful; administer or have client self-administer an enema; encourage client to focus on breathing slowly to reduce anxiety.	Assist client in removing excess lubricant. Explain that client may resume normal activities.
Prostatic biopsy	Inform client that a local anesthetic may be used to minimize discomfort; administer or have client self-administer an enema if a rectal approach is used.	Provide information about site care. Instruct client that sitz baths and a mild analgesic will reduce discomfort. Tell client that a prophylactic antibiotic will be given and stress that medication be taken as ordered.
Testicular biopsy	Inform client that a local anesthetic will be administered.	In the case of an incisional rather than a needle biopsy, instruct the client to refrain from tub baths until the sutures are removed.
Cystoscopy	Inform client that he will experience bladder fullness and a strong desire to void. Inform client that an anesthetic lubricant will be instilled into the urethra to minimize discomfort and facilitate passage of cystoscope.	Instruct client to monitor voiding pattern and to report any bleeding or difficulty urinating. Inform client that prophylactic antibiotics will be given and stress that medication be taken as ordered.

onic gonadotropin (hHCG), and total urine estrogens. Alkaline and acid phosphatase blood tests determine if prostatic cancer has spread to the bone.

Stop, Think, and Respond ● BOX 55-1

What health teaching is important to provide men to ensure early diagnosis and treatment of disorders that affect the male reproductive system?

STRUCTURAL ABNORMALITIES

Structural abnormalities of the male genitalia may be congenital or acquired. These various abnormalities, including torsion of the spermatic cord, disorders of the foreskin, and benign scrotal swelling, often require surgical repair. Nursing management after these surgeries is similar.

• TORSION OF THE SPERMATIC CORD

Torsion means "to twist." In this case, it is the spermatic cord that twists, kinking the artery and compromising blood flow to the testicle (Fig. 55.3). The condition occurs in prepubescent boys and in men whose spermatic cords are congenitally unsupported in the tunica vaginalis, the membrane surrounding the testes. Clients report a sudden, sharp testicular pain, with visible local swelling. The pain may be so severe that nausea, vomiting, chills, and fever occur. Torsion may follow severe exercise, but it also may occur during sleep or after a simple maneuver such as crossing the legs. Physical examination reveals an extremely tender testis. Elevation of the scrotum intensifies the pain by increasing the degree of twist.

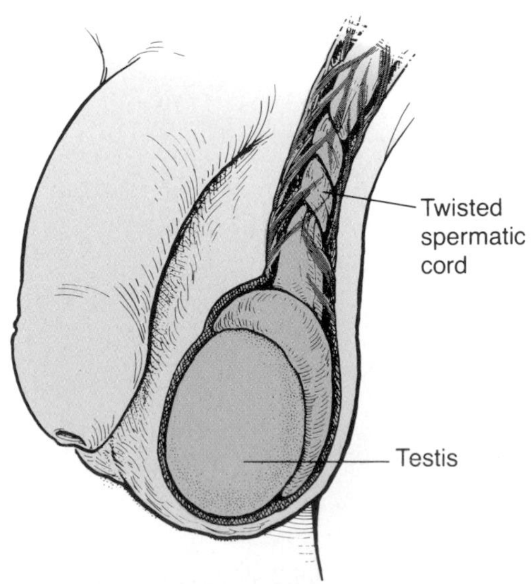

FIGURE 55.3 Torsion of the spermatic cord.

Immediate surgery is necessary to prevent atrophy of the spermatic cord and preserve fertility. Torsion is reduced, excess tunica vaginalis is excised, and the testis is anchored with sutures in the scrotum. A prophylactic procedure may be performed on the opposite side.

Preoperatively, administer prescribed analgesia to relieve pain. After surgery, apply a scrotal support, especially when the client is out of bed. Inspect the dressing for signs of drainage and give antibiotics if medically ordered. Report any sudden onset of pain to the physician.

• PHIMOSIS AND PARAPHIMOSIS

Phimosis and paraphimosis are conditions that occur among uncircumcised male clients when the opening of the foreskin is constricted. Phimosis refers to an inability to retract the foreskin (prepuce); paraphimosis is a strangulation of the glans penis from an inability to replace the retracted foreskin. These phimotic conditions often are caused by a congenitally small foreskin. Chronic inflammation at the glans penis and prepuce secondary to poor hygiene or infection also are etiologic factors. Clients with phimosis report pain with erection and intercourse and difficulty cleaning under the foreskin. Clients with paraphimosis experience painful swelling of the glans. If the condition continues, severe edema and urinary retention may occur. Circumcision is recommended to relieve these conditions permanently; if surgery is not indicated, the client is instructed to wash under the foreskin daily and seek care if he cannot retract the tissue.

• HYDROCELE, SPERMATOCELE, AND VARICOCELE

The suffix, *cele,* indicates a swelling. Hydrocele, spermatocele, and varicocele all present as a swelling of the scrotum (Fig. 55.4), but in each case, the conditions are somewhat different. Often, hydrocele and spermatocele are not clinically significant and do not require treatment; however, varicoceles are thought to be an underlying cause of male infertility and may be surgically repaired.

INFECTIOUS AND INFLAMMATORY CONDITIONS

• PROSTATITIS

Prostatitis is an inflammation of the prostate gland and is most often caused by microorganisms that reach the prostate by way of the urethra. *Escherichia coli* and microbes that cause STIs (see Chap. 56) often are responsible, but in some instances there is no evidence

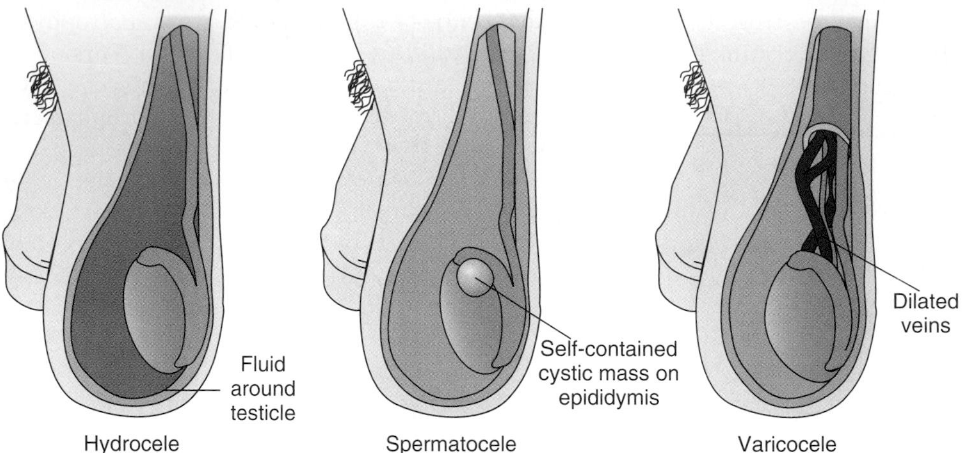

FIGURE 55.4 Causes of scrotal swelling.

of bacterial infection. A psychosexual problem may be the suspected cause of the client's symptoms. In any case, inflammation causes glandular swelling and tenderness. Because the prostate surrounds the urethra, a combination of genitourinary problems develops. Clients experience perineal pain or discomfort, an unusual sensation preceding or following ejaculation, low back pain, fever, chills, dysuria, and urethral discharge. Treatment consists of up to 30 days of antibiotic therapy, mild analgesics, and sitz baths.

Stress that sexual partners also need to be treated. Tell the client to avoid caffeine, prolonged sitting, and constipation, and regularly to drain thc prostate gland through masturbation or intercourse. Instruct the client to comply with antibiotic therapy and use a mild analgesic for pain.

• EPIDIDYMITIS AND ORCHITIS

An inflammation of the epididymis (**epididymitis;** Fig. 55.5) and testis (**orchitis;** Fig. 55.6) occurs alone or simultaneously (epididymo-orchitis). Common causes are an extension of the infectious agent causing prostatitis or an infection elsewhere in the body. Noninfectious epididymitis may result from long-term indwelling catheter use or genitourinary procedures such as cystoscopy or **prostatectomy** (excision of the prostate gland). Orchitis without epididymal involvement is associated with a viral mumps infection that occurs after puberty and may result in testicular atrophy and sterility. Bilateral epididymitis frequently leads to permanent *azoospermia* (absence of sperm), especially when infection recurs frequently or becomes chronic.

The chief complaint is pain and swelling in the inguinal area and scrotum. Fever and chills occur with bacterial infections, and the urine contains pus and bacteria. Inspection reveals a markedly swollen testis and epididymis and scrotal skin that is red and tense. It is important to differentiate epididymitis from testicular torsion because torsion is a surgical emergency. Treatment consists of bed rest, scrotal elevation, analgesics, anti-inflammatory agents, and comfort measures such as local cold applications. Antibiotic therapy is initiated to eliminate the infectious agent. An epididymectomy (excision of the epididymis) is performed on clients with recurrent, chronic, or intractable infections, but this results in sterility if performed bilaterally.

Elevate the scrotum with a folded towel, four-tail bandage, or adhesive taped across the upper thighs (Fig. 55.7) to relieve pain by lessening the weight of the testes. Place an ice bag under the tender scrotum, not on top of or leaning against it. Avoid keeping the cold bag constantly next to the skin because it may damage tissue. Use a routine such as on 60 minutes, off 30 minutes. As with any infection, encourage copious fluid intake. Home care includes instructions to continue taking prescribed antibiotics, take sitz baths, apply local heat after scrotal swelling subsides, and avoid lifting and sexual intercourse until symptoms are relieved.

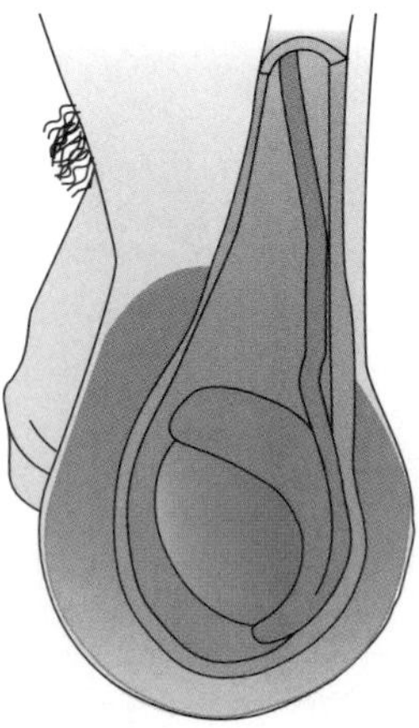

FIGURE 55.5 Acute epididymitis.

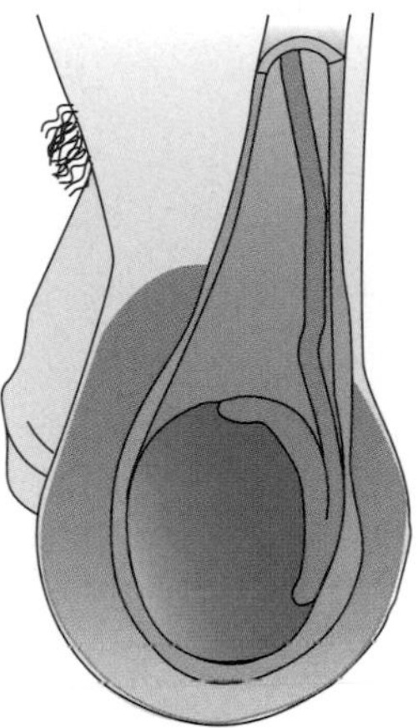

FIGURE 55.6 Acute orchitis.

ERECTION DISORDERS

• IMPOTENCE

Pathophysiology and Etiology

Impotence is the inability to achieve or maintain an erection that is sufficiently rigid for sexual activity. There must be multiple or persistent incidences of failed erection for the disorder to be considered pathologic. It often is a consequence of inadequate blood flow to the penis or rapid emptying of blood once it accumulates. Aging, testosterone insufficiency, side effects of drug therapy, atherosclerosis, hypertension, and complications of diabetes mellitus are common causes. Impotence also may be related to anxiety or depression. A nocturnal penile tumescence test determines if the client is experiencing spontaneous erections during sleep. The test involves applying paper bands about the shaft of the penis at bedtime and observing if bands are broken in the morning. Absence of nocturnal erections supports a physical rather than emotional cause for impotence.

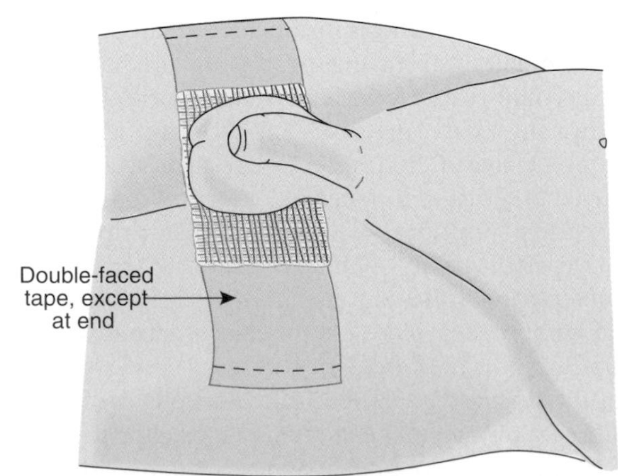

FIGURE 55.7 Technique for scrotal elevation.

Medical and Surgical Management

Several approaches exist to help restore sexual function. Substituting other drugs for those that cause impotence or treating the contributing cause may restore potency (erectile ability). Some elect to facilitate penile engorgement by attaching a vacuum device to the penis or self-injecting drugs such as papaverine (Pavatine), phentolamine (Regitine), or alprostadil (Caverject) into the corpus cavernosa to achieve an erection. Sildenafil (Viagra) facilitates penile erection by producing smooth muscle relaxation in the corpus cavernosa, facilitating inflow of blood. Sildenafil is taken orally about 1 hour before sexual activity. It has no erectile effect without sexual stimulation. Apomorphine (Uprima), a dopamine agonist, is an older drug used in the treatment of Parkinson's disease (see Chap. 39) that is an alternative to sildenafil for the treatment of erectile dysfunction. This drug, which is administered as a nasal spray, has some advantages over sildenafil: (1) it acts within 15 to 25 minutes of administration, and (2) it is safer for men with coronary artery disease. The newest drug, varadenafil HCl (Levitra), treats erectile dysfunction by increasing blood flow to the penis. It may help men to maintain an erection. Blood flow to the penis decreases after sexual activity. It has been successful in men with other health problems, such as diabetes.

Vascular surgery is an option for some clients, but many clients choose a surgically implanted penile prosthesis (Fig. 55.8). One type contains a saline reservoir that is pumped to fill the implant when sexual activity is desired and the other type maintains the penis in a semi erect state at all times. Inform the client before surgery that when a pump-type of implant is inserted, the erect penis tends to be shorter than experienced in preillness erections because cylinders do not fill the glans portion of the penis.

If the client prefers to self-inject a vasodilator, provide instruction on technique, suggested frequency of injections, and side effects. If the client undergoes a penile implant, assess for pain, swelling, bleeding, and surgical complications like infection. Reinforce information the physician identifies as possible complications after discharge, such as:

- Erosion of penile or urethral tissue from a mis-sized implant, pressure, and friction of implanted cylinders evidenced by seeing the implant through the skin
- Erosion of scrotal, bowel, or bladder tissue if an implant with a fluid reservoir is used, detected by changes in scrotal skin texture and elimination
- Migration of the cylinders, pump, or reservoir from their intended location accompanied by pain, tenderness, and dysfunction of components that are part of the device
- Malfunction of the device characterized by underinflation, bulging of the cylinders during inflation, and loss of fluid from the implant that can occur with migration, accidental trauma such as a fall, or aggressive or improper use of the device

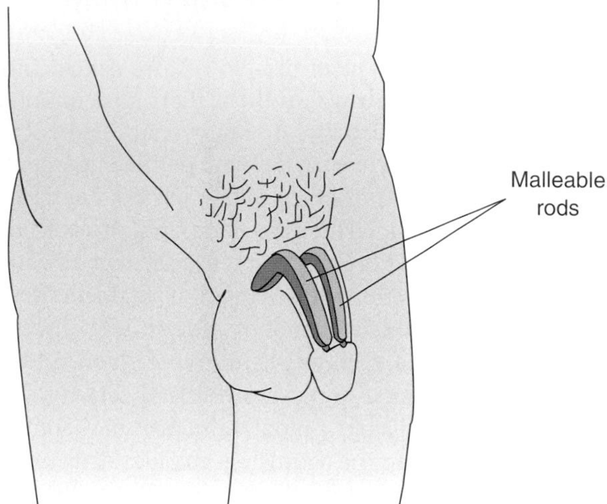

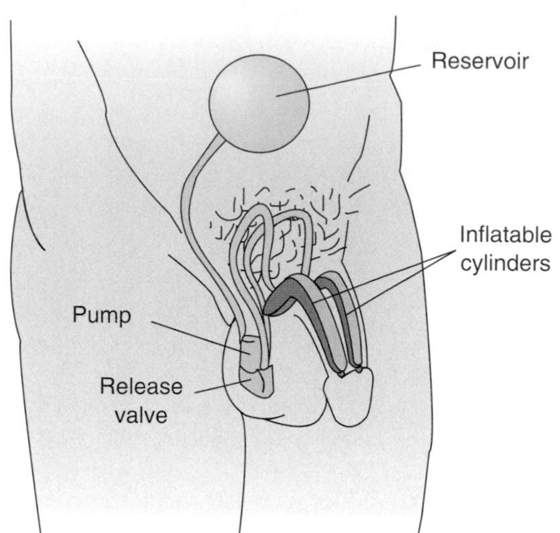

FIGURE 55.8 Examples of penile implants.

Nursing Management

Postoperative care includes assessing the client's level of consciousness and vital signs, condition of dressing and incision, level of pain, amount of penile and scrotal swelling, status of IV infusion (type of solution, drip rate, location of IV site), urinary catheter and volume of urine elimination, and client's knowledge of postoperative care and discharge instructions. The client is at risk for bleeding. Assess for frank bleeding or enlarging hematoma at operative site. Ensure that the implant is semi-rigid, which helps to provide pressure and reduce bleeding. Impaired skin integrity is another risk related to a tight prosthesis. Report signs of pale, thin skin near the glans penis, inadequate capillary perfusion, and skin erosion. Prolonged interruption of blood flow can cause tissue perfusion. Protect the client's privacy; explain the reasons for genital assessments. Provide opportunities for the client to privately share his feelings about his changed appearance. Describe techniques for concealing the semi-erect appearance of the penis, such as wearing untucked shirts and pleated trousers or pants with an elastic waist.

Postoperatively:

- Explain that the penis should be taped against the skin in a straight position for 1 week or longer, but can be untaped for voiding. Taping acts as a splint to keep the penis from moving about while healing takes place.
- Identify the period for sexual abstinence (usually 3 to 6 weeks). Sexual intercourse is safe once healing is complete.
- Instruct on how to inflate and deflate an inflatable prosthesis. An erect penis facilitates vaginal penetration; the client empties the penile implant after intercourse.
- Inform client to avoid tight-fitting underwear. Pressure and friction can cause tissue erosion and curvature of the penis.
- Advise client to avoid contact sports. The force of physical contact may alter the position or integrity of the penile implant.
- Explain that the client must avoid heavy lifting for at least 3 weeks. Straining can disrupt internal sutures and reconstructed tissue.
- Emphasize the need to report persistent pain and swelling. Pain and swelling are common signs of infection, erosion, and migration.

● PRIAPISM

Priapism is a condition in which the penis becomes engorged and remains persistently erect without sexual stimulation. The underlying etiology usually is a vascular problem, a medical condition that causes blood to thicken, or a side effect of medications, including those prescribed to treat impotence. The engorged penis produces significant discomfort and interferes with arterial blood flow and, in some cases, urinary elimination. If the erection lasts longer than 6 hours, the tissue may be sufficiently damaged to result in impotence.

Treatment options include administering vasoconstrictive medications such as terbutaline (Brethine) or phenylephrine (Neo-Synephrine) or draining trapped blood with a needle placed in the side of the penis. If these interventions fail, emergency surgery is performed to shunt blood temporarily out of the corpus cavernosum. Healthcare providers must extend respect for the client's feelings and understandable embarrassment throughout interactions.

BENIGN PROSTATIC HYPERPLASIA

Benign prostatic hyperplasia (BPH) indicates that the prostate gland contains more than the usual number of normal cells. When the gland enlarges, the condition is known as *benign prostatic hypertrophy.*

Pathophysiology and Etiology

BPH occurs as men age. Outward expansion of the gland is of no clinical importance. Inward encroachment, however, diminishes the diameter of the prostatic section of the urethra and interferes with emptying the bladder (Fig. 55.9).

Assessment Findings

Symptoms of BPH appear gradually. At first, the client notices that it takes more effort to void. Eventually, the urinary stream narrows and has decreased force. The bladder empties incompletely. As residual urine accumulates, the client has an urge to void more often and nocturia occurs. Because residual urine is a good culture medium for bacteria, symptoms of cystitis (inflammation of the bladder) may develop (see Chap. 59).

A DRE reveals an enlarged and elastic gland. Cystoscopy exposes the extent of the infringement on the urethra and effects on the bladder. Intravenous and retrograde pyelograms and blood chemistry tests give information about possible damage to the upper urinary tract from urinary retention. Measurement of a significant quantity of residual urine confirms the diagnosis. PSA test results may be slightly elevated. Transrectal ultrasonography indicates prostatic size and helps rule out the possibility that a malignancy is causing the enlargement.

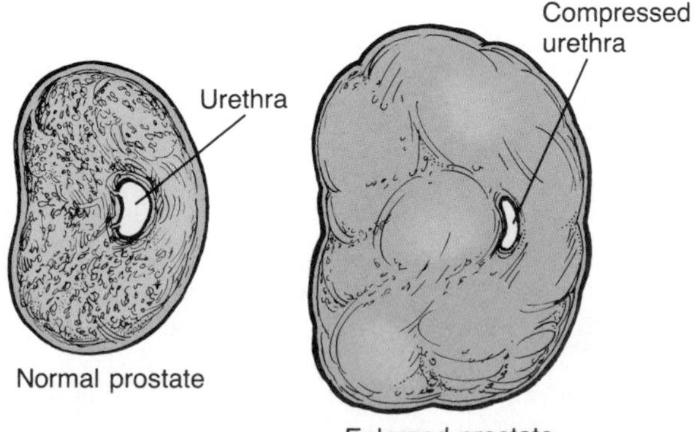

FIGURE 55.9 Comparison of normal prostate and enlarged prostate.

Medical and Surgical Management

In early stages of BPH, progression of prostatic enlargement is monitored with periodic DREs. Drug therapy is the second line of treatment (Drug Therapy Table 55.1). Terazosin (Hytrin), an alpha-adrenergic blocker, helps relax prostate muscles and relieve urinary symptoms. Finasteride (Proscar), an androgen hormone inhibitor, decreases symptoms and appears to arrest progression of prostate enlargement in some clients.

Other forms of treatment are used when glandular enlargement results in pronounced symptoms. The aim of all surgical procedures for BPH is to enlarge the bladder outlet. Table 55.1 provides a description of the various types of surgical procedures.

After a transurethral prostatectomy (TURP), clients experience **retrograde ejaculation,** a condition in which semen is deposited in the bladder rather than discharging through the urethra at the time of orgasm, rendering the client sterile. After a TURP and open prostatectomies, men may have temporary or permanent urinary incontinence. Perineal surgical approaches often result in permanent impotence, although some nerve-sparing techniques are being developed.

Nursing Management

For the client who is not yet a candidate for surgery, teach how to maintain optimal bladder emptying (Client and Family Teaching 55-1).

The surgical client requires support and information to allay anxiety and promote a postoperative period that is free of complications. Teach deep breathing and leg exercises and explain that the client will have continuous bladder irrigation for at least 24 hours after surgery. Urethral catheterization before surgery is necessary for clients with sudden or acute retention. If difficulty is encountered while inserting a urethral catheter, a coudé catheter, which has a curved tip, and instillable anesthetic lubricant are used to facilitate the procedure. If the catheter cannot be passed urethrally, a temporary suprapubic catheter is required to relieve bladder distention. For care after a prostatectomy, see Nursing Care Plan 55-1.

MALIGNANCIES OF THE MALE REPRODUCTIVE SYSTEM

• CANCER OF THE PROSTATE

Prostatic cancer is most common in men older than 50 years of age. In fact, it is the third most common cause of death from cancer in men of all ages and is the most common cause of death from cancer in men older

DRUG THERAPY TABLE 55.1 AGENTS FOR BENIGN PROSTATIC HYPERPLASIA

DRUG CATEGORY AND EXAMPLES	MECHANISM OF ACTION	SIDE EFFECTS	NURSING CONSIDERATIONS
Hormonal Agents			
finasteride (Proscar)	Inhibits the conversion of testosterone into a potent androgen (dihydrotestosterone) on which the prostate depends; causes the gland to shrink	Loss of libido, impotence, decreased ejaculate, adverse effects on fetal development	Monitor urinary output. Avoid handling the drug if pregnant. Instruct to use a condom to prevent fetal exposure. Explain that sexual changes are reversible after drug is discontinued. Inform client that it may take 6 months or longer to achieve full benefit.
Alpha-Adrenergic Blockers			
terazosin (Hytrin)	Reduces the tone of smooth muscle in the bladder neck and prostatic urethra	Hypotension, dizziness, nausea, urinary frequency, incontinence, edema, fatigue, headaches	Monitor urinary elimination patterns and postural blood pressure changes. Administer drug at bedtime to reduce orthostatic hypotension. Warn to change position slowly. Weigh regularly for evidence of fluid imbalance.

than 75 years of age. Prostatic cancer grows slowly and has a high survival rate if detected early.

Pathophysiology and Etiology

The cause of prostatic cancer is unknown, but there seems to be a relationship with increased testosterone levels and a diet high in fat. Having two or more blood relatives with prostatic cancer increases risk for developing the disease. Most prostatic carcinomas occur in the periphery of the gland. As it enlarges, it causes genitourinary symptoms similar to a variety of other conditions (e.g., BPH and cystitis). If untreated, tumor cells spread by way of the bloodstream and lymphatics to the pelvic lymph nodes and bone, particularly the lumbar vertebrae, pelvis, and hips.

TABLE 55.1 INVASIVE PROCEDURES FOR PROSTATIC ENLARGEMENT

PROCEDURE	DESCRIPTION
Transurethral Approaches (Procedures Done Through the Urethra)	
Transcystoscopic urethroplasty	The balloon tip of a catheter is inflated for 10 to 20 minutes to stretch the prostatic urethra.
Urethral stent or coils	A flexible tube is permanently placed in the urethra to dilate the lumen.
Thermotherapy	A heated instrument inserted in a urethral catheter destroys prostatic tissue but preserves the urethra.
Transurethral resection of the prostate (TURP)	Part of the prostate is removed with a cutting instrument inserted through an endoscope.
Transurethral incision of the prostate (TUIP)	No tissue is removed; the bladder outlet is enlarged by making an incision in the prostate, which relieves pressure on the urethra.
Transurethral laser incision of the prostate (TULIP)	A laser is used to incise and destroy prostate tissue.
Open Surgical Approaches (Require External Incision)	
Suprapubic prostatectomy	The prostate gland is removed by making a midline abdominal incision into the bladder. A suprapubic catheter, also known as a cystostomy tube, and a Foley catheter are inserted.
Retropubic prostatectomy	The prostate gland is removed through an abdominal incision, but the bladder is not entered.
Perineal prostatectomy	The prostate gland is removed through an incision made between the scrotum and anus.
Radical prostatectomy	The prostate gland and its capsule, seminal vesicles, and lymph nodes are removed through a retropubic or perineal incision; this procedure is reserved for clients with prostatic cancer.

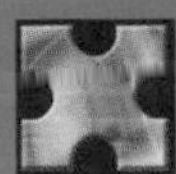

55 1 Client and Family Teaching
Optimal Bladder Function

The nurse instructs the client as follows:

- Void often and assist bladder emptying by leaning forward on toilet and "bearing down" (Valsalva maneuver), or pressing down on the bladder while seated on the toilet (Credé's maneuver).
- Drink frequent small volumes of oral fluids so that the bladder does not become extremely full at any one time.
- Note any signs and symptoms of acute urinary obstruction and urinary infection such as distended bladder, lower abdominal discomfort, inability to urinate, small and frequent urination, fever and chills, and flank pain that indicate a need for medical attention.

Assessment Findings

At first, no symptoms occur, and none may develop for years. When the tumor grows large enough, it compromises urinary flow and causes frequency, nocturia, and dysuria (difficult or painful urination). The first symptoms of metastases may be back pain or pain down the leg from nerve sheath involvement. When pain develops, the disease often is in an advanced stage.

Rectal examination detects a prostatic nodule. A PSA greater than 4 ng/mL is the basis for performing more definitive diagnostic procedures, and a PSA above 10 ng/mL indicates a prostatic malignancy. A PSA greater than 80 ng/mL indicates advanced metastatic disease. Researchers are now finding that measuring insulin-like growth factor-1 and insulin-like growth factor binding protein-3 is a more sensitive test for prostate cancer that may identify cases that PSA alone fails to detect (Kurek et al., 2000; Wolk et al., 2000).

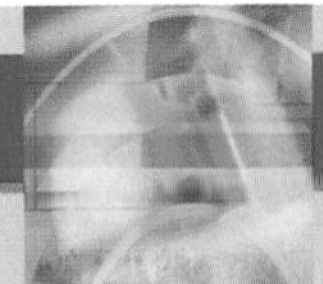

Nursing Care Plan 55-1

THE CLIENT UNDERGOING A PROSTATECTOMY

Assessment

Determine the following before surgery:

- Medical, drug, and allergy history
- Symptoms such as urgency, frequency, hesitancy, nocturia, decreased urinary stream
- Previous episodes of urinary tract infections
- Discomfort associated with an acute, sudden episode of urinary retention because this problem may require immediate preoperative attention
- Vital signs
- Weight

Determine the following after surgery:

- Level of consciousness
- Vital signs
- Level of discomfort
- Location of urinary catheter(s)
- Volume and color of urine

PC: **Risk for Hemorrhage** related to inadequate hemostasis

Expected Outcome: The nurse will monitor to detect, manage, and minimize excessive bleeding.

Interventions	*Rationales*
Monitor vital signs every 15 minutes until stable and then every 4 hours.	Hypotension and tachycardia suggest a loss of blood volume.

(continued)

Nursing Care Plan 55-1 (Continued)

THE CLIENT UNDERGOING A PROSTATECTOMY

Interventions	*Rationales*
Assess color of urine and status of dressing, if there is one, at least every 4 hours.	A change from burgundy to bright red, like catsup, suggests fresh bleeding.
Maintain traction on urinary catheter for at least 6 hours after surgery.	Traction provides pressure on blood vessels, which facilitates hemostasis.
Discourage straining to have a bowel movement, attempts to void with the catheter in place, and lifting heavy objects.	Bearing down increases blood pressure, which can trigger fresh bleeding.
Report signs of hypovolemic shock to the physician.	The physician determines the medical measures such as administering blood transfusions and medications for stabilizing the client's condition.

Evaluation of Expected Outcome: Client's urine is light pink, clear, or amber.

Nursing Diagnosis: **Risk for Urinary Retention** related to obstruction of urinary catheter with tissue debris and blood clots or urethral stricture

Expected Outcome: Catheter will remain patent.

Interventions	*Rationales*
Instill bladder irrigation solution at a rate to maintain light pink or clear urine (Fig. 55.10).	Irrigating solution dilutes blood cells and tissue debris and facilitates removal from bladder by gravity drainage.
Encourage client to drink about one glass of water every hour while awake.	A generous fluid intake keeps urine dilute and the catheter patent.
Palpate bladder and assess true urine volume every 4 hours, whenever client complains of pain, or if urine leaks around catheter.	The bladder is not palpable unless distended. True urine volume is assessed by subtracting the volume of irrigating solution from the total urinary output. Pain and leaking fluid suggest accumulated urine with no appropriate outlet.
Avoid dependent loops and kinks in urinary catheter, never clamp urinary catheter, and do not allow client to lie on the drainage tubing (Nursing Guidelines 55-1).	Interference with gravity drainage results in urine accumulation in the bladder.
Keep drainage bag below level of bladder.	Fluid (urine in this case) flows by gravity from higher to lower locations. If the urinary drainage bag is above the bladder, urine flows backward into the bladder.

Evaluation of Expected Outcome: Urine drains freely from the catheter or with spontaneous voiding.

Nursing Diagnosis: **Acute Pain** related to tissue injury or bladder spasms

Expected Outcome: Pain will be controlled within the client's level of tolerance.

Interventions	*Rationales*
Check that catheter is patent and draining before administering medication.	Obstruction in the flow of urine contributes to pain.
Administer a prescribed antispasmodic, such as a belladonna and opium suppository, or prescribed medications like oxybutynin (Ditropan) or propantheline (Pro-Banthine), or an analgesic for incisional pain.	Anticholinergics relieve bladder spasms. Analgesics interfere with the perception of pain.

(continued)

Nursing Care Plan 55-1 (Continued)

THE CLIENT UNDERGOING A PROSTATECTOMY

Explain that the large balloon holding the catheter in place, traction on the catheter, and the volume of instilling irrigant tend to produce the urge to void, but an effort to do so contributes to discomfort.	Offering the client an explanation helps to alleviate the anxiety concerning the cause of discomfort.
Use nursing measures such as placing a rolled towel beneath the scrotum, assisting with the application of an athletic support, suggesting the use of a recliner rather than sitting on a hard surface, changing position, and diversional activities.	Alternative measures enhance the response to drug therapy.

Evaluation of Expected Outcome: Pain and discomfort are tolerable.

Nursing Diagnosis: **Risk for Infection** related to impaired tissue and potential contamination of catheters and incisional drains

Expected Outcome: Client will be free of infection as evidenced by progressive wound healing, no fever, no purulent drainage, expected white blood cell count, and urine free of bacteria.

Interventions	*Rationales*
Practice conscientious handwashing before providing nursing care.	Handwashing reduces the potential for spreading microorganisms.
Keep ports used for emptying drainage clean.	A contaminated port provides a portal for microorganisms that can ascend to other structures in the urinary tract.
Reinforce or change moist dressings using surgical asepsis.	Moisture on a dressing wicks microorganisms into the wound.
Keep perineum clean after a bowel movement for clients with a perineal prostatectomy.	Stool contains many bacteria that can easily enter a perineal wound because of its close proximity to the anus.
Report tenderness, unusual drainage, foul odor, and fever.	An infection produces a cluster of common signs and symptoms.

Evaluation of Expected Outcome: There is no evidence of infection; vital signs are normal.

Nursing Diagnosis: **Urge** or **Total Urinary Incontinence** related to altered urinary sphincter or nerve damage secondary to surgical procedure if nerves have been spared

Expected Outcome: Client will disguise incontinence or regain continence.

Interventions	*Rationales*
Provide absorbent pads or underwear.	Absorbing urine reduces embarrassment associated with incontinence.
Teach pelvic floor–strengthening exercises (Nursing Guidelines 55-2).	Pelvic floor exercises strengthen the muscles that promote urinary continence.
Suggest using a penile clamp (Fig. 55.11).	A penile clamp compresses the urethra externally, preventing incontinence.

Evaluation of Expected Outcome: Continence problems are controlled.

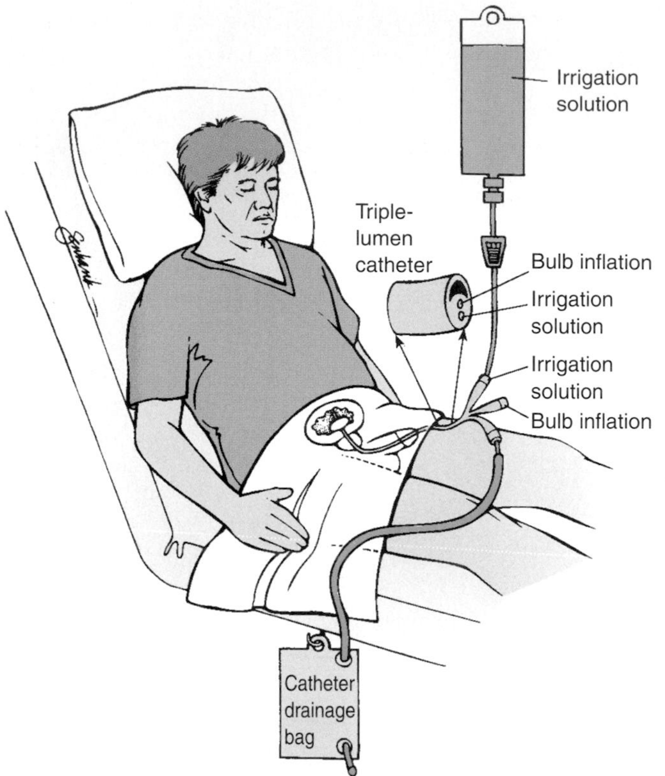

FIGURE 55.10 A three-way system for bladder irrigation.

NURSING GUIDELINES 55-2

Teaching Pelvic Floor–Strengthening Exercises

- Squeeze the pelvic floor muscles (those used to stop urination and hold back a bowel movement) for up to 10 seconds—longer is not better.
- Relax completely for 10 seconds—less is not better.
- Repeat sequence as many times as possible in 5 minutes or a cycle of 15 contractions followed by relaxation.
- Interrupt exercises when muscles can no longer be contracted tightly.
- Perform exercises in the morning and evening.
- Perform shorter pelvic floor exercises four or five times during the day:
  - Squeeze pelvic floor muscles and hold for one second.
  - Relax for 1 second.
  - Repeat five times in succession within 2 minutes.
- Continue long and short exercises for 3 to 4 months or until continent.

(Adapted from the Pelvic Floor Retraining Team, Incontinence Clinic, Beth Israel Hospital, Boston, MA, and The Prostate Cancer Infolink [1995].)

NURSING GUIDELINES 55-1

Managing Care of a Client With a Suprapubic Catheter

Purpose: To drain urine from the bladder through a catheter that is inserted through the anterior abdominal wall and anchored with external skin sutures. The client may or may not have a urethral (Foley) catheter as well.

- Stabilize the catheter by taping it to the skin of the abdomen.
- Keep the catheter connected to a sterile drainage system.
- Keep the drainage system below the level of the insertion site.
- Empty the urine from the bag periodically to reduce tension on the catheter and skin.
- Record the urine output from the suprapubic catheter separate from voided urine output or output from another catheter.
- Keep the skin clean and dry at the insertion site to avoid skin irritation and compromised skin integrity.
- For "trial voiding":
  - Clamp the catheter for 4 hours.
  - Have the client void naturally.
  - Unclamp the suprapubic catheter.
  - Measure the residual urine.
- Collaborate with the physician on removing the suprapubic catheter when the residual urine is repeatedly <100 mL.

Transrectal ultrasound confirms the presence of a mass. The definitive diagnosis is made by biopsy and microscopic examination of tissue. Sometimes the malignancy is detected after microscopic examination of tissue removed during a TURP or open prostatectomy for BPH.

Pelvic or spinal radiographs, bone scan, and magnetic resonance imaging (MRI) or computed tomography (CT)

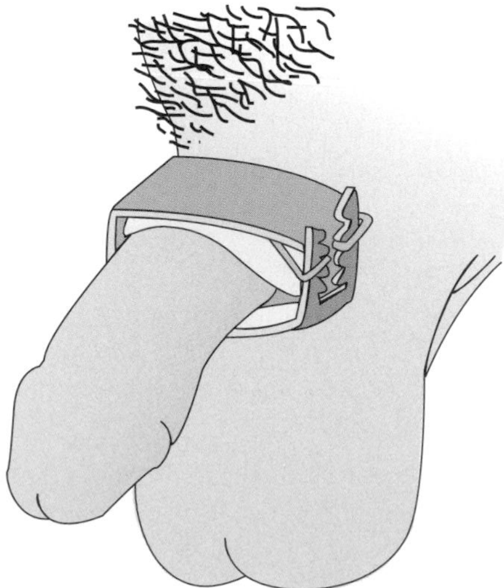

FIGURE 55.11 Penile clamp. Clamp is molded to comfortably fit penis and gently compress urethra.

scanning detect metastases to bones. An elevated serum acid phosphatase is associated with bone metastasis. An intravenous pyelogram (IVP) and other renal function studies detect kidney damage caused by long-standing urethral obstruction and urinary retention (if present).

Medical and Surgical Management

Tumor size, microscopic characteristics, and any metastases are used to establish the stage, which in turn determines treatment (Table 55.2). The client's age and general health status also are considered when planning treatment. Treatment regimens include observation, surgery, radiation, hormone therapy, or a combination of these.

If the nodule is localized, an open suprapubic prostatectomy is the treatment of choice. A radical prostatectomy, performed through a perineal or retropubic approach, is the surgical preference if the tumor is large enough to be palpated or if it has spread to adjacent tissue.

When a radical prostatectomy is performed, the entire prostate, its capsule, and the seminal vesicles are removed. The bladder neck is sutured to the membranous urethra over an indwelling urethral catheter, which is left in place for 10 to 14 days. Potential complications of this surgery include a 25% to 50% chance of impotence, difficulty with urinary control, and genital and lower extremity edema. A TURP may be done if the client has urethral obstruction and his physical status is not amenable to treatment. Occasionally, permanent suprapubic drainage may need to be established.

TABLE 55.2 STAGING AND TREATMENT OF PROSTATE CANCER

STAGE	TREATMENT	5-YEAR SURVIVAL RATE
Stage A1: Cancer is found incidentally with <5% malignant cells	Observation	98%
Stage A2: Tumor is not palpable, biopsy is positive	Observation, surgery, or radiation therapy	90%
Stage B: Tumor is palpable, confined to prostate	Surgery or radiation therapy	77%
Stage C: Local extension of tumor but no distant metastasis	Radiation therapy or combination of surgery, radiation and hormone therapy	60%
Stage D: Distant metastasis	Medical therapy	26%

A bilateral **orchiectomy** (surgical removal of the testes) may be performed to eliminate the production of testosterone in men with advanced prostatic carcinoma (stage D). Permanent side effects are impotence, loss of libido, hot flashes, and possible psychological disturbances. Many men do not accept surgical castration and low levels of testosterone are achieved with hormone therapy.

Radiation therapy (see Chap. 19) may be used alone or in conjunction with other treatment modalities, especially when there is local metastasis. Possible side effects include impotence, diarrhea, and urinary frequency and urgency.

Men with stage D carcinoma of the prostate are candidates for hormone therapy (Drug Therapy Table 55.2). With antiandrogenic (male) hormones or estrogenic hormones, progression of the malignancy may be retarded and there may be a prolonged period of palliation (comfort). Estramustine (Emcyt) is a combination of estrogen and an antineoplastic drug that also is used for palliative treatment.

Feminizing side effects occur with hormone therapy. The client's voice may become higher, hair and fat distribution may change, and breasts may become tender and enlarged. Libido and potency also are diminished. When estrogens are used in lower doses, the client may not experience these problems.

Nursing Management

Obtain a health history from the client and focus on identifying information such as changes in patterns of urinary elimination (frequency, urgency, and nocturia), hematuria, low back pain, and a family history of prostatic cancer. After extensive surgical treatment for prostatic cancer, assess the client for signs of infection, urinary incontinence, and sexual dysfunction, and reinforce health teaching that aids in detection of metastasis.

Radical prostatectomy is similar to other prostatectomy procedures and the same immediate postoperative nursing diagnoses and interventions apply. If the client is discharged with a Foley catheter in place, tell client to use soap and water to clean around the urethral meatus and several inches of the catheter at least twice a day. Demonstrate and have the client return the demonstration for keeping the connection between the catheter and leg bag clean when changing and replacing leg bags for routine cleaning. Tell the client or caregiver to clean the leg bag by using soap and water and then rinsing it with a 1:7 solution of vinegar and water.

The client may experience total urinary incontinence related to surgical compromises to internal and external urinary sphincter muscles. Teach pelvic floor retraining exercises (see Nursing Guidelines 55-2) if incontinence is not permanent. For permanent incontinence, show the client how to apply a penile clamp or an external catheter connected to a leg bag.

DRUG THERAPY TABLE 55.2 HORMONAL AGENTS FOR PROSTATIC CANCER

DRUG	MECHANISM OF ACTION	SIDE EFFECTS	NURSING CONSIDERATIONS
diethylstilbestrol (DES)	Synthetic estrogen that reduces testosterone levels	Breast enlargement, nausea, vomiting, photosensitivity, elevated blood sugar	Offer small, frequent meals to offset nausea. Monitor blood sugar, especially in clients with diabetes mellitus. Recommend using a sunscreen or wearing protective clothing.
flutamide (Eulexin)	Blocks androgens	Breast enlargement, impotence, diarrhea, anemia, leukopenia, thrombocytopenia, jaundice	Instruct clients that periodic blood tests are required. Observe if urine is dark yellow.
goserelin acetate (Zoladex)	Inhibits pituitary gonadotropin secretion, which reduces testosterone to castration levels	Hot flashes, impotence, loss of libido	Administer as a monthly injection or subcutaneous implant. Use a local anesthetic before administering injection. Repeat injection every 28 days. Drug resistance occurs after 2 to 3 years of therapy.

For the client with temporary impotence (pudendal nerve responsible for erection and orgasm is spared), explain that it may take from 3 to 12 months for sexual potency to return. See interventions for impotence for additional suggestions.

For the client with impotence related to pudendal nerve damage secondary to non–nerve-sparing radical perineal prostatectomy, recommend demonstrating sexual feelings in ways other than intercourse. Discuss the use of manual stimulation or a mechanical vibrator if it does not compromise the sex partner's moral values.

Assist the client to manage and minimize the possibility of a recurrence of the primary cancer or metastasis. Explain that the PSA level will decrease after prostatectomy; a subsequent rise indicates the cancer has reoccurred. Clarify that repeat lymph node biopsies may be part of the surgical follow-up. Inform the client that blood tests for measuring serum acid phosphatase are used to monitor evidence of bone metastasis.

As the client recovers, promote increased self-care and provide instructions for home management. The discharge plan of care includes, but is not limited to, the following:

- Maintain medical follow-up.
- Take medications as prescribed.
- Decrease dietary fat and increase fiber.
- Exercise regularly to increase lean body mass and decrease insulin levels, which is a catabolic hormone that promotes weight gain.
- Join a support group to learn more about the disease process and clinical trials of research.
- Consult with the family physician or oncologist before self-treating with herbal supplements.

• CANCER OF THE TESTES

Cancer of the testes is a rapidly metastasizing malignancy seen in men between the ages of 18 and 40 years. Although relatively rare, it is the most common type in men between 15 and 34 years of age and the leading cause of death from cancer in men between 25 and 34 years of age. Significant advancement in treatment in recent years has resulted in a high cure rate, even in clients with metastatic disease.

Pathophysiology and Etiology

Incidence is higher among men with a history of **cryptorchidism** (undescended testis) regardless of whether an **orchiopexy** (surgical procedure to anchor testes in the scrotum) was performed (see Chap. 9). Although the exact etiology is unknown, cells in the undescended testis or testes may degenerate earlier than occurs with natural aging. This leads to abnormal cellular changes. In most cases, only one testicle is affected, but the other may become cancerous if the tumor is not diagnosed early.

Nearly all testicular tumors involve sperm-forming germ cells. Those that consist of immature germ cells are called *seminomas; nonseminomas* develop among more mature, specialized germ cells. Nonseminomas grow more rapidly and tend to metastasize at a faster rate; therefore, treatment is more aggressive.

Assessment Findings

Gradual or sudden swelling of the scrotum or a lump felt on palpation always deserves prompt medical attention.

The tumor usually presents as a hard, nontender nodule of the testis with additional coexisting symptoms (Box 55-2). Unless discovered early through **testicular self-examination,** the first symptoms may be those of tumor metastasis. They may include abdominal pain, general weakness, and aching in the testes.

Tumor markers include elevated levels of alpha-fetoprotein and bHCG. An IVP may show lymph node enlargement that displaces the ureters. Lymphangiography is used to detect lymph node involvement. A CT scan or MRI can detect metastases. Because biopsy risks spreading the highly malignant tumor cells, surgery is recommended immediately.

Medical and Surgical Management

Treatment of testicular tumors depends on the stage of the disease (Table 55.3) and includes surgery, chemotherapy, and radiation. An autologous (self-donated) bone marrow transplantation may be recommended for recurrent disease or for clients resistant to drug therapy. Before medical or surgical treatment, however, the topic of sperm banking should be discussed. Locating a sperm bank and then collecting and banking sperm, which may take as long as 12 to 24 days, is omitted if the delay would jeopardize the outcome of treatment.

Surgery

A radical inguinal orchiectomy (removal of the testis) and ligation of the spermatic cord is performed. Clients with nonseminomas usually undergo radical retroperitoneal lymph node dissection as well. If only one testis is removed, sexual activity, libido, and fertility usually are unaffected. After a radical lymph node dissection, libido and erections are preserved, but surgical disruption of nerve pathways results in impaired ejaculation. New nerve-sparing techniques are being developed that preserve ejaculatory function, and therefore fertility, in most clients.

Chemotherapy

A multiple antineoplastic drug regimen usually is instituted after surgery. Types of drugs, frequency of administration, and duration of therapy depend on the type of tumor and if metastasis has occurred. Chemotherapy, which usually is aggressive initially, is modified as the tumor markers show a response. Sperm tend to be destroyed or mutated when exposed to toxic cancer drugs, but spermatogenesis eventually resumes.

BOX 55-2 ● Signs and Symptoms of Testicular Cancer

- Testicular lump that is hard or granular
- Increase in the size of one testicle
- Heavy or dragging feeling in the scrotum
- Dull ache in the groin or above the pubis
- Diminished sensitivity to testicular pressure

TABLE 55.3 STAGING AND TREATMENT OF GERM CELL TUMORS OF THE TESTIS

STAGE	TREATMENT	SURVIVAL RATE
Stage I: Tumor confined to the testis	Orchiectomy, retroperitoneal lymph node dissection	95%
Stage II: Involvement of testis plus retroperitoneal nodes	Orchiectomy, retroperitoneal lymph node dissection, possible chemotherapy	93%
Stage III: Distant metastasis	Orchiectomy, retroperitoneal lymph node dissection, four cycles of chemotherapy, surgery to resect residual masses	70%

Radiation

Seminomas are sensitive to radiation, and most clients receive radiation to the retroperitoneal lymph nodes. For clients with nonseminomas, radiation is considered an adjunct to lymphadenectomy and chemotherapy.

Nursing Management

Preoperative Period

One of nursing's chief concerns is responding to the client's emotional distress over having a life-threatening diagnosis, being unfamiliar with the surgical experience, and confronting alterations in body image and sexuality. All clients are understandably concerned over the potential change in their sexual image and fertility; however, it may be of even greater concern to men in this age group. Provide private opportunities for the client to ask questions and use therapeutic communication techniques to encourage the client to verbalize his feelings.

Postoperative Period

After an orchiectomy, apply a scrotal support. If drains have been inserted, they are connected to closed (Jackson-Pratt) or open (machine) suction. Give prophylactic antibiotics to prevent infection. Manage pain, which may be severe after a radical lymph node dissection, with narcotic analgesics. If pain is not relieved and nursing measures to augment the effect of analgesics are inadequate, collaborate with the physician to modify drug therapy.

As the client's comfort improves, discuss the effects of the diagnosis and treatment and again provide opportunities for the safe expression of anxiety, fear, and grief. Advise the client that a testicular prosthesis can be inserted at a later date if he desires and that fertility may be regained in 2 to 3 years after drug therapy is discontinued, and sooner when surgery or radiation is used. Provide the client with names of local support groups and encourage him to contact them for emotional support after discharge.

Client and Family Teaching

A teaching plan includes the following instructions:

- Drink plenty of fluids and eat a well-balanced diet to avoid constipation.
- Obtain adequate rest; avoid fatigue and heavy lifting.
- Wash incision with warm soap and water. Report redness, drainage, pain, or swelling of incision or scrotum.
- Take prescribed medication as directed.
- Perform self-examination of the remaining testicle every month and immediately report any changes.
- Seek care if any of the following occur: fever, chills, adverse drug effects, weight loss, or anorexia.

For clients concerned about future reproduction, discuss issues as appropriate for the client's particular situation. If a client has banked sperm, inform him that normal pregnancies have occurred with sperm stored up to 10 years. For clients for whom treatment has proceeded without collecting and storing sperm, identify other pregnancy options, such as donor insemination or adoption.

ELECTIVE STERILIZATION

A **vasectomy** is a minor surgical procedure done in a physician's office or clinic. It involves ligation of the vas deferens and results in permanent sterilization by interrupting the pathway that transports sperm (Fig. 55.12). On occasion, the client may complain of impotence, although the procedure has no effect on erection or ejaculation. It may take several weeks or more after surgery before ejaculatory fluid is free of sperm, and the client is informed to use a reliable method of contraception until sperm no longer are present. The client may wish to consider banking sperm before undergoing the procedure. Some men feel ambivalent about having this procedure. Provide the client with an opportunity to express these feelings.

Reinforce the following important information for home care after a vasectomy:

- Expect some bruising and incisional soreness after the local anesthetic wears off.

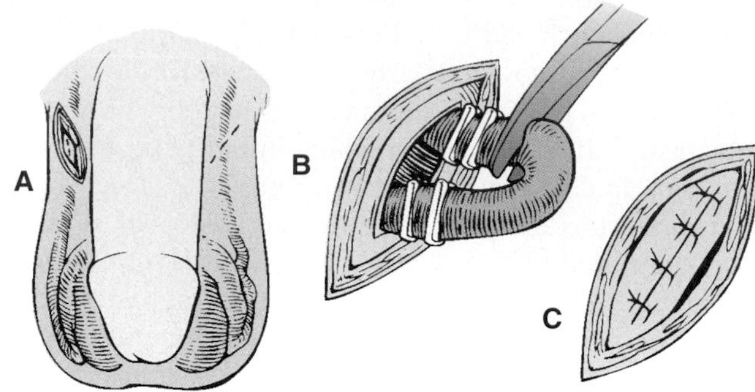

FIGURE 55.12 Vasectomy procedure. (**A**) An incision is made to expose the vas deferens. (**B**) The vas deferens is isolated and severed. (**C**) The severed ends are occluded with sutures or sealed with electrocautery.

- Apply ice packs to the scrotum to reduce swelling; remove the cold application after 20 minutes and replace again after the tissue rewarms.
- Take a mild analgesic, such as aspirin or acetaminophen, for discomfort.
- Wear an athletic support for several days for comfort.
- Resume usual activities in 2 to 3 days, but avoid strenuous exercise for up to 5 days.
- Resume sexual activity when comfort allows, usually in 1 week.
- Use a reliable method of contraception until the physician indicates that sperm no longer are present, which may be determined after 10 or more ejaculations.
- Report severe pain, fever, or swelling at the top of the testes.

A *vasovasostomy* is a surgical attempt to reverse a vasectomy by restoring patency and continuity to the vas deferens; a *vasoepididymostomy* connects the stump of the vas deferens directly to the epididymis. It may take from 3 to 6 months after reversal procedures before sperm counts and motility are normal. Lack of success usually is the result of either scar formation or sperm leakage from the surgical connection.

GENERAL GERONTOLOGIC CONSIDERATIONS 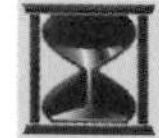

When an older man develops a varicocele when none existed before, the congestion of blood may be caused by pressure from a urologic tumor.

Impotence increases as men age; 15% to 25% of all men experience impotence by age 65 years. More than half of all men 75 years of age or older are chronically impotent.

Sperm and testosterone production gradually decreases as men age. This phenomenon possibly is the result of degenerative changes in the vascular system in the testes.

There are greater numbers of older than middle-aged men who are uncircumcised because many were born at home and the procedure was not performed. Therefore, the incidence of phimosis, paraphimosis, balanoposthitis, and penile cancer is more common in older men.

Along with a decrease in sperm production, the volume and viscosity of seminal fluid decreases with age. A loss of muscular tone causes the scrotum to become more pendulous. As the scrotum drops, there is an increased risk of trauma and injury to this area.

Impotence is not a normal part of aging. If impotence occurs, other causes should be explored such as adverse reactions to medication, atherosclerosis, or psychological problems.

Critical Thinking Exercises

1. *Assume you are attending a team conference to plan the care of a client having a suprapubic prostatectomy. What nursing interventions are appropriate?*
2. *Describe the typical client who acquires prostatic hypertrophy versus one who develops testicular cancer.*

• NCLEX-STYLE REVIEW QUESTIONS 

1. A male client presents at an infertility clinic. While completing the health history, which childhood illness should the nurse question the client about further?
   1. Rheumatic fever
   2. Mumps
   3. Epstein-Barr virus
   4. Varicella
2. A client has scrotal swelling secondary to epididymitis. Which of the following sets of nursing actions is most correct to incorporate in the client's plan of care?
   1. Administer intravenous antibiotics; give pain medication; apply heat to the scrotum.
   2. Administer a diuretic; give pain medication; maintain the client on strict bed rest.
   3. Administer intravenous antibiotics; elevate the scrotum; apply ice under the scrotum.
   4. Encourage fluids; use a scrotal support; complete regular urinary catheterization.
3. A nurse is documenting output from a client with indwelling Foley and suprapubic catheters. Which documentation procedure is most correct?
   1. Place the combined total output from both the Foley and suprapubic catheters in the urinary output section.
   2. Document the indwelling Foley catheter output in the urinary output section; ignore the suprapubic catheter output.
   3. Document the suprapubic catheter output in the urinary output section; ignore the Foley catheter output.
   4. Document the Foley and suprapubic catheter outputs separately in the urinary output section.

connection

Visit the Connection site at **http://connection.lww.com/go/timbyEssentials** for links to chapter-related resources on the Internet.

References and Suggested Readings

Allison, L. (2000). Clinical effectiveness: Testicular self-examination. *Professional Nurse, 15,* 710–713.

Bullock, B. L., & Henze, R. L. (2000). *Focus on pathophysiology.* Philadelphia: Lippincott Williams & Wilkins.

Cerrato, P. L. (2000). Complementary therapies: Diet and herbs for BPH? *RN, 63*(2), 63–64.

Chow, R. D. (2001). Benign prostatic hyperplasia: Patient evaluation and relief of obstructive symptoms. *Geriatrics, 56*(3), 33–38.

Cohen, B. J., & Wood, D. L. (2000). *Memmler's structure and function of the human body* (7th ed.). Philadelphia: Lippincott Williams & Wilkins.

Held-Warmkessel, J. (2001). Treatment of advanced prostate cancer. *Seminars in Oncology Nursing, 17,* 118–128.

Iwamoto, R. R., & Maher, K. E. (2001). Radiation therapy for prostate cancer. *Seminars in Oncology Nursing, 17,* 90–100.

Kurek, R., Tunn, W., Eckart, O., et al. (2000). The significance of serum levels of insulin-like growth factor-1 in patients with prostate cancer. *British Journal of Urology, 85,* 125–129.

Maliski, S. L., Heilemann, M. V., & McCorkle, R. (2001). Mastery of postprostatectomy incontinence and impotence: His work, her work, our work. *Oncology Nursing Forum, 28,* 985–992.

Marsche, P. S. (2001). The role of surgery in the treatment of prostate cancer. *Seminars in Oncology Nursing, 17,* 85–89.

Sneddon, D. (2000). Assessing and treating erectile dysfunction. *Journal of Community Nursing, 14*(11), 4–6, 8.

U.S. Preventive Services Task Force. (2003). Screening for prostate cancer: Recommendations and rationale. *American Journal of Nursing, 103*(3), 107–111.

Weaver, J. (2001). Combating complications of transurethral surgery. *Nursing 2001, 31*(7), Hospital Nursing: 32hn1–32hn2, 32hn4.

Weinrich, S. (2001). The debate about prostate cancer screening: What nurses need to know. *Seminars in Oncology Nursing, 17,* 78–84.

Wolk, A., Andersson, S., Mantzoros, C., et al. (2000). Can measurement of IGF-1 and IGFBP-3 improve the sensitivity of prostate screening? *Lancet, 356,* 1902.

chapter 56

Caring for Clients With Sexually Transmitted Infections

Words to Know 

autoinoculation
chancre
Charcot's joints
chlamydia
condylomas
genital herpes
gonorrhea
herpes simplex virus
human papillomavirus
neuropathic joint disease
syphilis
tabes dorsalis
venereal disease
venereal warts

Learning Objectives

On completion of this chapter, the reader will:

- Describe common sexually transmitted infections (STIs).
- Identify STIs that by law must be reported.
- Discuss contributing factors to the transmission of STIs.
- Give reasons why women acquire STIs more often than men.
- Explain ways STIs are spread.
- Discuss methods that are helpful in preventing STIs.
- Name infectious microorganisms that cause common STIs.
- Identify common complications of STIs.
- Name drugs used to treat STIs.

Sexually transmitted infections (STIs), also known as **venereal diseases,** are a diverse group of infections spread through sexual activity with an infected person, and represent a significant public health problem. Some, such as acquired immunodeficiency syndrome (AIDS; see Chap. 37), hepatitis (see Chap. 49), and skin infestations with lice and mites (see Chap. 63), are spread by additional routes as well. Pathogens that cause STIs include bacteria, fungi, parasites, protozoans, and viruses. Besides AIDS, the most common STIs are chlamydia, gonorrhea, syphilis, genital herpes, and genital warts. Chlamydia, gonorrhea, and syphilis are easily cured with early and adequate treatment. Social, sexual, and biologic factors contribute to the high incidence of venereal disease, and include the following:

- Ignorance of how STIs are transmitted or prevented
- Asymptomatic sex partner(s)
- Casual sex with partner(s) about whom little is known
- Sex with high-risk partner(s), like those who use intravenous (IV) drugs, are bisexual, or have sex with prostitutes
- Multiple concurrent or sequential sex partner(s)
- Failure to use contraceptive techniques that also reduce risk for acquiring STIs
- Sexual contact during the period between infection and manifestation of symptoms
- Failure to seek early treatment
- Noncompliance with treatment or instructions to refrain from sexual contact until treatment is complete
- Mutation and resistance of microorganisms to antimicrobial drug therapy

EPIDEMIOLOGY

Epidemiology is the study of occurrence, distribution, and causes of human diseases. The Centers for Disease Control and Prevention (CDC) collects disease statistics such as incidence of STIs. Determining exact incidence of these diseases is difficult because only a few are reportable by law (Box 56-1), and some go untreated, treated and unreported, or misdiagnosed or undiagnosed. Women acquire STIs more often than men, probably because the moist, warm vaginal environment is conducive to micro-

BOX 56-1 ● Reportable STIs

By federal law, the following STIs must be reported to the Department of Public Health:

- Gonorrhea
- Syphilis
- Chlamydia
- Chancroid
- Granuloma inguinale
- Lymphogranuloma venereum
- Acquired immunodeficiency syndrome

bial growth and because the vagina, as a receptive orifice, is more readily traumatized during sexual activity.

Obtaining a sexual history (Nursing Guidelines 56-1) is crucial when assessing clients with signs or symptoms of an STI. Asking questions nonjudgmentally also is essential. In addition to curing infection when possible (some STIs are not curable), treatment consists of education and counseling to reduce the client's risk for contracting an STI in the future (Nursing Guidelines 56-2), and screening, counseling, and treating their sexual partner(s), if needed.

NURSING GUIDELINES 56-2

Methods for Reducing the Risk for STIs

- Abstain from sexual activities.
- Have monogamous sex with an uninfected partner.
- Use latex condoms with nonoxynol-9 (a spermicide) when having oral, vaginal, or anal intercourse.
- Combine the use of male condoms with a spermicide when having vaginal intercourse, or use a female condom.
- Urinate and wash the genital and perineal areas before and immediately after having sexual intercourse.
- Wash your hands and any areas where there has been direct contact with semen or vaginal mucus.
- Refuse or terminate sexual activity that causes trauma to the genitals, internal reproductive structures, anus, and elsewhere.
- If infected, report the information to all sexual partners and encourage them to seek medical diagnosis and treatment.
- Avoid unprotected sex until you and sex partners have completed treatment.

COMMON SEXUALLY TRANSMITTED INFECTIONS

● CHLAMYDIA

Chlamydia is the most common and fastest-spreading bacterial STI in the United States. The number of new cases and reinfections amounts to as many as 3 million annually (Centers for Disease Control and Prevention, 2001).

NURSING GUIDELINES 56-1

Obtaining a Sexual History From the Client With an STI

- Are there new or multiple sexual partners in recent weeks?
- Was a condom used during sexual activity?
- Is there a past history of STI?
- Has the client engaged in vaginal, anal, or oral sex?
- Was the client a receptive partner in anal or oral sex?
- Is there a history of infection with human immunodeficiency virus?
- Is there a history of employment as a sex worker?
- Are drugs and alcohol used?
- Is there a possibility of pregnancy?

Pathophysiology and Etiology

The causative microorganism is a bacterium, *Chlamydia trachomatis*, that lives inside the cells it infects. The disease is spread by sexual intercourse or genital contact without penetration.

The microorganism invades the reproductive structures (see pelvic inflammatory disease [PID] in Chap. 53), the urethra in women, and the urethra and epididymis in men (see nongonococcal urethritis in Chap. 59). Tissue irritation, which may be permanent despite successful eradication of the bacteria, puts those with chlamydial infections at greater risk for acquiring other STIs, such as AIDS. Untreated chlamydia can cause sterility in infected women; infected pregnant women can transmit the microorganism to their infants during birth.

Chlamydial infections also can be spread to the eyes by **autoinoculation** (self-transmission to another area of the body), usually by unwashed hands. Ophthalmic infections, more common in underdeveloped countries where flies transmit the microorganism, can cause granulation of the cornea and blindness.

Assessment Findings

As many as 75% of all infected women and 25% of all infected men are asymptomatic. Symptoms, if they occur, may appear 1 to 3 weeks after infection. They include a sparse, clear urethral discharge; redness and irritation of infected tissue; burning on urination; and lower abdominal pain in women or testicular pain in men.

Diagnosis is made by microscopic examination and culture of secretions. A test kit is available that identifies the microorganism in approximately 15 minutes. It is common practice to test clients for chlamydia, gonorrhea, and syphilis because it is not unusual for clients to have concurrent infections with more than one STI.

Medical Management

Antimicrobial drugs, such as doxycycline (Vibramycin), the tetracyclines, erythromycin, clarithromycin (Biaxin), and azithromycin (Zithromax) are used for treatment.

Nursing Management

Obtain a sexual history, follow precautions for preventing infection transmission, assist in collecting a specimen for microscopic analysis, explain the course of treatment, and discuss methods for preventing transmission and reinfection (Nursing Care Plan 56-1 and Nursing Guidelines 56-3).

● GONORRHEA

Gonorrhea is a common STI with the highest incidence in the 15- to 24-year-old age group. Many women are asymptomatic—a factor that contributes to the spread of the disease.

Pathophysiology and Etiology

The infection is caused by the bacteria *Neisseria gonorrhoeae,* which can be transmitted heterosexually or homosexually. The microorganism invades the urethra, vagina, rectum, or pharynx, depending on the nature of sexual contact; it can spread throughout the body.

In untreated men, localized infection may spread to the prostate, seminal vesicles, and epididymis. Urethral strictures may develop, requiring periodic dilatation of the urethra or, possibly, reconstructive urethral surgery. In women, infection may progress upward to the cervix, endometrium, and fallopian tubes, and symptoms of PID (see Chap. 53) may develop. Gonorrhea also can be transmitted to an infant's eyes at the time of birth.

Assessment Findings

In men, symptoms usually appear 2 to 6 days after infection. The most common signs and symptoms are urethritis with a purulent discharge and pain on urination. A small proportion of men are asymptomatic. More than half of infected women experience no symptoms. When symptoms do occur, women have a white or yellow vaginal discharge, intermenstrual bleeding due to cervicitis, and painful urination. An anal infection is accompanied by painful bowel elimination and a purulent rectal discharge; the throat is sore when the pharynx is infected. If the microorganism disseminates (scatters) throughout the body, the client may manifest a skin rash, fever, and painful joints.

Specimens of drainage from infected tissue are examined microscopically immediately after they are collected or are inoculated on a culture medium and incubated to reveal the causative organism.

Medical Management

Because of the increasing resistance of *N. gonorrhoeae* to penicillin, gonorrhea is now treated with a single intramuscular dose of ceftriaxone (Rocephin) or a single oral dose of ciprofloxacin (Cipro). Coinfection with chlamydia is common, and clients also are given oral doxycycline (Vibramycin) for 7 to 10 days. Clients with complicated gonococcal infections, as in PID or disseminated infection, are hospitalized and treated with IV multiple-drug therapy. Repeat therapy with different antibiotics may be required.

Nursing Management

The nursing management and client teaching are similar to those provided clients with chlamydia. However, when a culture is collected from a woman, the vaginal speculum is moistened with water rather than lubricated, which may destroy the gonococci and cause inaccurate test results (see Nursing Care Plan 56-1).

● SYPHILIS

Syphilis is a curable STI that also can be transmitted from the blood of an infected person, directly from the lesion, or across the placenta to an unborn infant. Incidence of syphilis in the United States has risen in certain groups, particularly young African American men and women. The disease has been declining in the United States since 1995, however.

Pathophysiology and Etiology

The spirochete *Treponema pallidum* is the causative microorganism of syphilis. The time between infection and first occurrence of symptoms is about 21 days. If untreated, syphilis progresses through three distinct

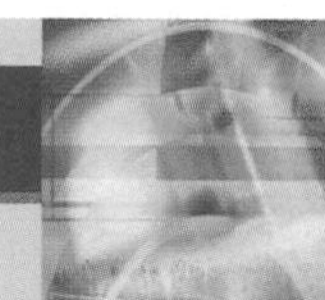

Nursing Care Plan 56-1

THE CLIENT WITH AN STI

Assessment

Determine the following:

- Vital signs
- Health history with a focus on the onset and course of current symptoms
- Similar symptoms in sexual partner(s)
- Presence of oral, vaginal, rectal, or genitourinary lesions
- Characteristics of discharge (vaginal, urethral, rectal), if any is evident
- Evidence of skin rash or abnormal appearance of integument
- Accompanying symptoms such as joint or abdominal pain or pain during intercourse
- Failure to become pregnant if pregnancy is desired
- Drug and allergy history

Nursing Diagnoses: **Impaired Skin Integrity** and **Impaired Mucous Membranes** related to inflammation of local tissues and scratching secondary to infectious process

Expected Outcomes: (1) Skin lesions will heal. (2) Integrity of mucous membranes will be restored.

Interventions	*Rationales*
Provide information on appropriate topical skin applications.	Various over-the-counter and prescription medications can be applied to the skin to relieve inflammation, reduce itching, lubricate the skin, and dry lesions.
Advise client to pat rather than rub skin dry.	Patting reduces friction and the itch–scratch–itch cycle.
Reinforce compliance with medical treatment.	Taking prescribed medications according to directions ensures eradication or control of the infecting microorganism.

Evaluation of Expected Outcomes: Skin and mucous membranes are intact; no lesions are evident.

Nursing Diagnosis: **Risk for Infection Transmission** related to infectious drainage and viral shedding

Expected Outcome: The infection will remain confined and not be transmitted to any other susceptible host.

Interventions	*Rationales*
Follow standard precautions before diagnosis and contact precautions after diagnosis is confirmed.	Standard precautions reduce the risk of transmission of a blood-borne infection before a diagnosis is made. Transmission-based precautions interfere with the routes by which specific pathogens are spread.
Advise client to have all sexual partners tested and treated.	STIs often are transmitted between both sexual partners; to eradicate the infection, sexual partners must be treated as well.

(continued)

Nursing Care Plan 56-1 (Continued)

THE CLIENT WITH AN STI

Interventions	Rationales
Identify methods for preventing STIs such as abstinence, barrier and chemical types of contraceptives, and voiding and washing after sexual intercourse.	STIs are spread by direct contact; methods that prevent direct contact reduce the potential for disease transmission.
Recommend early prenatal care to pregnant women.	Some STIs can be transmitted during childbirth.
Explain how to manage articles used for personal hygiene and items to avoid sharing with noninfected people.	Keeping personal hygiene items separate from others and preventing indirect contact with contaminated items can reduce the potential for disease transmission.
Direct client to take medications as prescribed and return for medical follow-up.	Compliance and medical follow-up help ensure that the infection responds to treatment.

Evaluation of Expected Outcome: No other person acquires the STI from the infected person.

Nursing Diagnosis: **Ineffective Sexuality Patterns** related to shame about revealing the risk for an STI to sexual partner(s)

Expected Outcome: Client will resume sexual relationships with modifications that help to avoid STI transmission.

Interventions	Rationales
Role-play situations in which client communicates his or her STI status to a significant other.	Role-playing with an uninvolved person helps a person rehearse and prepare for a situation that evokes anxiety.
Suggest that the client and sexual partner(s) discuss and select methods that will facilitate sexual activity without transmitting the STI.	Open communication facilitates a mutual plan for reducing the potential for disease transmission.

Evaluation of Expected Outcome: Client discusses and implements modifications for sexual expression.

Nursing Diagnoses: **Risk for Ineffective Therapeutic Regimen Management** and **Risk for Noncompliance** related to lack of knowledge or abandoning recommendations

Expected Outcomes: (1) Client will understand the regimen for curing or controlling the STI. (2) Client will comply with the plan of care.

Interventions	Rationales
Provide specific client teaching that is appropriate for the particular STI.	STIs result from various pathogens; treatment varies.
Stress completing the full course of drug therapy.	Drug therapy may cure or slow the progression of the STI and relieve symptoms.
Provide client with a telephone number for obtaining objective and authoritative information.	Clients may be more inclined to ask questions about an STI and its treatment if their identity can remain anonymous.
Schedule an appointment for follow-up care.	Medical follow-up promotes compliance with therapeutic regimen.

Evaluation of Expected Outcomes: Client paraphrases the plan for treatment and carries out prescribed interventions.

NURSING GUIDELINES 56-3

Educating the Client With an STI

- Take prescribed medication according to label directions for the full length of time that it is prescribed.
- Stop having sex until retesting indicates that the infection is gone.
- Urge any and all sex partners to be examined and follow-through with concurrent treatment.
- Use a condom, a contraceptive barrier device, consistently and correctly (Nursing Guidelines 56-4) before any and all sexual contact after completing medical treatment.
- Do not assume that successful treatment means there is any permanent immunity; reinfection can and does occur if preventive sexual practices are not implemented.
- Seek treatment as soon as possible if the symptoms continue or if they recur after successful treatment.

stages: primary, secondary, and tertiary. It is infectious only during the primary and secondary stages. In the third stage, the client becomes demented and dies from complications involving other organ systems.

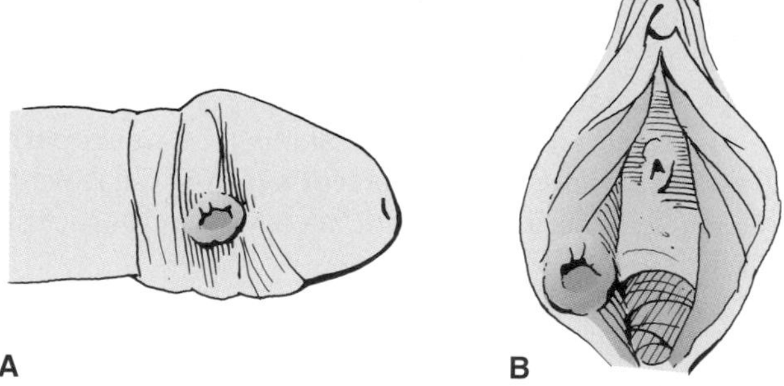

FIGURE 56.1 Syphilitic chancres. (**A**) Penile chancre. (**B**) Vulvar chancre.

Assessment Findings

In the primary (early) stage, a **chancre** (painless ulcer) appears on the genitals, anus, cervix, or other parts of the body (Fig. 56.1). At first, it resembles a small papule, which later ulcerates. The chancre heals in several weeks. Without treatment, the client progresses to the secondary stage of syphilis.

Symptoms of secondary syphilis include fever, malaise, rash, headache, sore throat, and lymph node enlargement. Late, or tertiary, syphilis is noninfectious because the

NURSING GUIDELINES 56-4

Teaching Clients How to Use a Condom

- Purchase condoms that are made in the United States because they are of high quality and have been tested for reliability.
- Select condoms that are lubricated with a spermicide or silicone.
- Natural-membrane condoms are porous and although they act as a barrier to sperm, viruses may pass through.
- Keep condoms in a cool, dry place.
- Discard condoms beyond their expiration date or if they are more than 5 years old.
- Never unroll or examine a condom before its use or use one that appears to have deteriorated.
- Unroll the condom over the erect penis while pinching the space at the condom tip.
- Use additional water-based lubricant to reduce friction and prevent tearing the condom; avoid oil-based lubricants, which can weaken latex.
- Remove the condom from the vagina before the penis becomes limp.
- Dispose of the condom in a lined container.
- Apply a new condom for each sex act.
- Breakage and slipping rates may be higher during anal sex.
- Condom breakage rate can be reduced by using a silicone-based lubricant; silicone does not deteriorate latex.

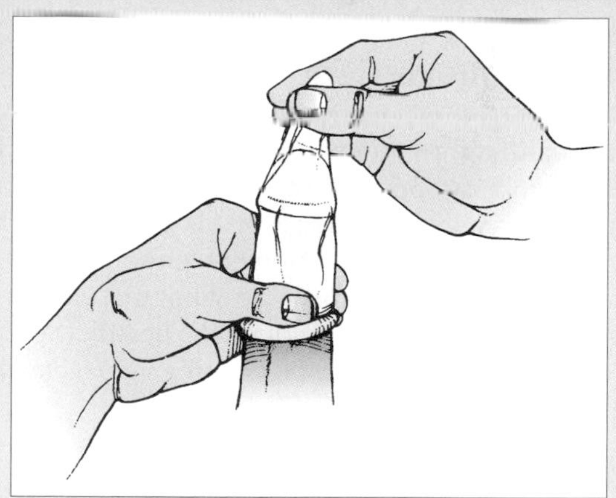

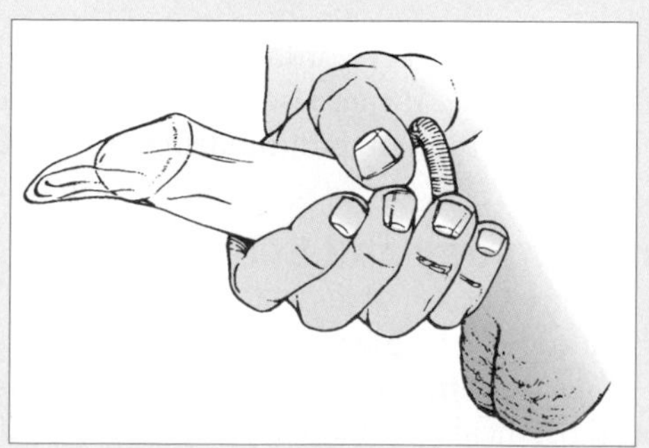

(Adapted from American Social Health Association. [2001]. Condoms—do's and don'ts. [On-line.] Available: http://www.ashastd.org/stdfaqs/condom_dd.html.)

microorganism invades the central nervous system (CNS) as well as other organs of the body. Symptoms of tertiary syphilis include **tabes dorsalis** (a degenerative condition of the CNS that results in loss of peripheral reflexes and of vibratory and position senses), ataxia, and **neuropathic joint disease,** also called **Charcot's joints.** Cardiovascular complications include aortic aneurysm and aortic valve insufficiency.

Diagnosis is made by detecting the spirochete in microscopic examination of scrapings from the chancre, by a positive Venereal Disease Research Laboratory (VDRL) test or rapid plasma reagin (RPR) on blood serum, and a positive fluorescent treponemal antibody absorption test (FTA-ABS). Occasionally, the FTA-ABS test is falsely positive in clients with systemic lupus erythematosus, a connective tissue disease, and rheumatoid arthritis. When a person develops CNS symptoms, the cerebrospinal fluid is examined.

Medical Management

Penicillin is used to treat primary and secondary syphilis. Clients who are allergic to the penicillins are given tetracycline or doxycycline. Follow-up examinations and laboratory tests are recommended 3, 6, and 12 months after initial treatment. Those with tertiary syphilis require larger doses of penicillin. Response is poor in those with cardiovascular syphilis.

Nursing Management

Gather health information and a sexual history, ask about the client's allergy history in anticipation of antibiotic treatment, prepare the client for diagnostic laboratory tests, support the client emotionally at the time the diagnosis is confirmed, and inform the client that case-finding is reported to the department of public health. (See Nursing Care Plan 56-1 for more on nursing management.)

• HERPES INFECTION

Herpes infection is a very contagious STI that is controllable but not curable. It increases risk for cervical cancer and infection with human immunodeficiency virus (HIV).

Pathophysiology and Etiology

Although **herpes simplex virus** type 2 (HSV-2), also known as **genital herpes,** is primarily responsible for genital and perineal lesions, herpes simplex virus type 1 (HSV-1), associated with cold sores around the nose and lips, also can cause anogenital lesions. One in five people older than 12 years of age are infected with the virus that causes genital herpes (Sexually Transmitted Disease Information Center, 2000). Transmission of these viruses is by direct contact with oral or genital secretions from a person during an active stage of the disease, sexual contact during periods of asymptomatic viral shedding, or autoinoculation. Either virus may be introduced into the eye, the mouth, the genital area, or a skin site.

Genital herpes increases risk for cervical cancer and HIV infection. Transmission also can occur from mother to infant during a vaginal birth and carries a neonatal mortality rate of 50%.

Herpes recurs because after initial infection, the virus remains dormant in the ganglia of nerves that supply the area. Symptoms usually are more severe with the initial outbreak. Subsequent episodes usually are shorter and less intense. When the virus is active, shedding viral particles are infectious.

Most victims have at least 1 outbreak per year, and many clients report 5 to 10 outbreaks per year. Some clients note that stress, emotional situations, exposure to sunlight, menstruation, and fever reactivate the disease.

Assessment Findings

After a short incubation period, HSV-2 causes single or multiple vesicles on the penis, prepuce, buttocks, thighs, introitus, or cervix (Fig. 56.2). The HSV-2 lesions burn and itch before becoming fluid-filled blisters. Vesicles rupture in 1 to 3 days and are followed by painful, reddened ulcers that scab over and eventually disappear. The outbreak may be accompanied by swelling of inguinal lymph nodes, flulike symptoms, and headache. The initial attack lasts 3 to 4 weeks; subsequent attacks usually last 10 days.

Diagnosis of HSV-1 and HSV-2 infection is tentatively made by inspecting lesions. Smears and scrapings from lesions are examined microscopically using special stains to confirm the clinical impression.

Medical Management

Because an outbreak of HSV-1 infection often is self-limiting, treatment may be unnecessary. If treated, either

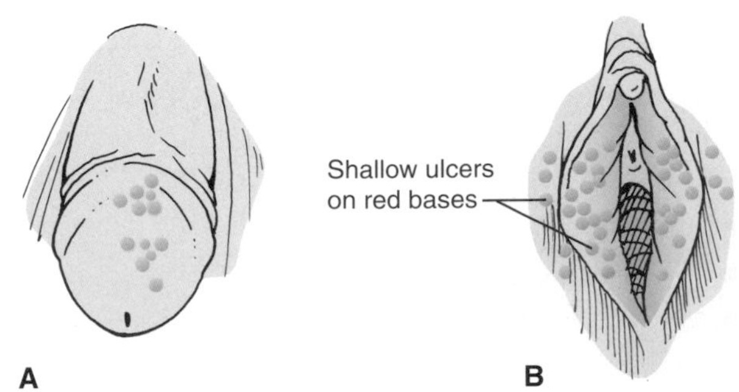

FIGURE 56.2 Herpes genitalis lesions. (**A**) Penile lesions. (**B**) Vulvar lesions.

type of herpes responds to the antiviral drugs acyclovir (Zovirax) and valacyclovir (Valtrex) (Drug Therapy Table 56.1). IV acyclovir is used if there is a severe episode of HSV-2 or if the client is immunocompromised. Acyclovir and valacyclovir shorten subsequent active episodes and tend to reduce frequency of outbreaks. Cesarean delivery is performed on pregnant women with active lesions.

DRUG THERAPY TABLE 56.1 AGENTS TO TREAT STIs

DRUG CATEGORY AND EXAMPLES/USE	SIDE EFFECTS	NURSING CONSIDERATIONS
Antibiotics		
	Allergy, anaphylaxis (applies to all antibiotics listed below)	Inquire about allergies and past reactions to medications. Be aware that clients allergic to cephalosporins also may be allergic to penicillin antibiotics. Inform client to seek treatment if rash, hives, fever, or difficulty breathing occur.
penicillin G: syphilis, gonorrhea	Allergy, stomatitis, nausea, vomiting, diarrhea, rash, fever, wheezing, pain at injection site	Give intramuscularly into gluteus maximus only. Massage site. Have client wait for 30 min after injection in case allergic reaction occurs.
erythromycin: syphilis, gonorrhea, chlamydia, chancroid, lymphogranuloma venereum, prophylactically to prevent eye infection in newborns	Allergy, abdominal cramps, diarrhea, vomiting, rash, emotional lability, altered thinking, ototoxicity, hepatitis	Reassure client that emotional and cognitive side effects, should they occur, are temporary. Report tinnitus and jaundice.
doxycycline: syphilis, gonorrhea, granuloma inguinale, lymphogranuloma venereum	Allergy, anorexia, nausea, vomiting, diarrhea, sensitivity to light, liver failure, discoloration of developing teeth, liver damage	Suggest taking with meals if gastrointestinal upset occurs. Inform client to report dark-colored urine or light-colored stools. Use a sunscreen. Strongly encourage client to return for all follow-up visits to ensure that organism has been eradicated.
ceftriaxone: gonorrhea	Allergy, anorexia, nausea, vomiting, diarrhea, rash, fever, decreased hematocrit, disulfiram-like reaction with alcohol	Avoid alcohol during and for 3 days after drug therapy. Inform client of possible side effects and to report unusual fatigue.
tetracycline: syphilis, gonorrhea, chlamydia	Allergy, nausea, vomiting, diarrhea, discoloration of developing teeth, phototoxicity, superinfections	Take on an empty stomach. Avoid antacids, dairy products, and iron supplements. Do not use outdated drugs because they are nephrotoxic. Use a sunscreen. Report appearance of oral or vaginal yeast infections.
ciprofloxacin: gonorrhea	Headache, dizziness, nausea, diarrhea, vomiting	Take on an empty stomach and avoid antacids within 2 hr of antibiotic dose. Drink plenty of water. Report any side effects.
Antivirals		
acyclovir: decreases severity and frequency of herpes outbreaks	Transient burning at application site	Apply with a rubber glove or finger cot. Inform client that drug does not cure the disease. Clients should avoid sexual activity during outbreaks and wear a condom at other times.
Caustics		
podophyllum resin: venereal warts	Peripheral neuropathy, thrombocytopenia and leukopenia when absorbed systemically, irritation of normal tissue	Highly toxic and should be applied only by the physician. Surrounding skin may be protected with petroleum jelly. Use minimal amount possible. Warn client that local irritation may occur in 12–48 hr.

Strongly encourage all clients to return for all follow-up visits to ensure that organism has been eradicated.

Nursing Management

Collect appropriate health and sexual data, use standard precautions when inspecting lesions, obtain specimens, and provide related health teaching. More on nursing management appears in Nursing Care Plan 56-1.

Instruct clients with HSV-2 infections to:

- Inform all potential sexual partners of HSV infection, even if inactive.
- Use a condom during sexual activity even if disease is dormant.
- Avoid sexual contact if there is any question that infection is active; condoms do not protect skin and mucous membrane that are left exposed.
- Keep lesions dry using alcohol, peroxide, witch hazel, and warm air from a hair dryer.
- Check with the physician about taking warm baths with Epsom salts or baking soda to relieve discomfort.
- Wear loose clothing that promotes air circulation about the genitals.
- Perform thorough handwashing after direct contact with lesions, and keep personal hygiene articles separate to avoid inadvertent use by others.
- Use one towel to pat lesions dry and another when drying other body parts to avoid autoinoculation.
- Have annual Pap smears to detect cervical cancer.
- Investigate stress management strategies because reducing stress tends to decrease frequency of outbreaks.

● VENEREAL WARTS

Venereal (genital) **warts,** also called **condylomas,** are an STI that tends to recur even after treatment. Anyone can become infected with venereal warts, but people with AIDS and others with an immunodeficiency are particularly susceptible. One fourth of people in the United States carry the virus and are infectious, but do not manifest symptoms.

Pathophysiology and Etiology

The **human papillomavirus** (HPV) causes venereal warts. HPV is transmitted by genital-genital, genital-anal, or genital-oral contact with an infected person and is contagious as long as warts are present. Sexual penetration is not necessary to transmit HPV, and warts also can be spread to other body areas by autoinoculation. Warts can grow in the mouth and throat of infants infected at birth. There is an increased risk of cancer of the vulva and vagina in women with genital warts. Cervical infection with HPV is associated with cervical cancer.

Assessment Findings

Genital warts usually are painless and appear as a single lesion or cluster of soft, fleshy growths on the genitalia (Fig. 56.3) or cervix, in the vagina, or on the perineum, anus, throat, or mouth. Sometimes warts are so small that they are inconspicuous. They can become large and raised—resembling a cauliflower. Large warts may narrow or obstruct the urethra, vagina, anus, or throat.

Venereal warts turn white when vinegar is applied to the lesion. The highlighted tissue is then examined with a magnifying glass.

Medical and Surgical Management

Warts are removed in various ways: laser therapy, electrocautery (heat), cryosurgery (freezing), or treating them with chemicals. Three major drugs are used to eradicate the warts: trichloroacetic acid, podophyllum solution in tincture of benzoin, and 5-fluorouracil (5-FU). Eradication does not mean the condition is cured; the person is temporarily noncontagious once warts are destroyed.

Nursing Management

Provide information about STI transmission to sexually active people and prepare affected individuals for medical examination, diagnosis, and treatment. Nursing management is discussed further in Nursing Care Plan 56-1.

Tell clients with venereal warts to:

- Avoid intimate contact until warts are removed.
- Advise all sexual contacts to be examined and treated.

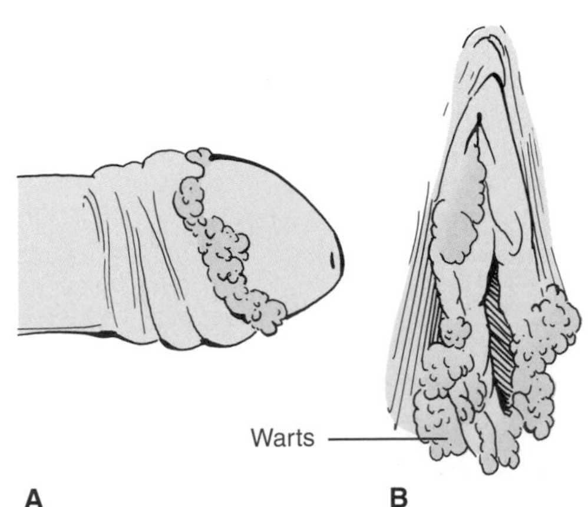

FIGURE 56.3 Venereal warts. (**A**) Penile warts. (**B**) Vulvar warts.

- Seek treatment at an STI clinic or with a private physician when, and if, warts return.
- Use a condom even when lesions are absent, and suggest that the sex partner wash his or her genitals or other skin areas immediately after intimate contact.
- Provide information about diagnosis and treatment in future health histories, especially if a pregnancy occurs.
- Avoid stress and genital trauma, which appear to be factors in reactivating the virus (Porth, 2002).
- Obtain yearly examinations for possibility of reproductive cancers.

Stop, Think, and Respond ● BOX 56-1

Which STI is associated with the following signs?

1. *Painless ulceration on the genitals or other areas of sexual contact*
2. *Discharge from the vagina, urethra, or both; burning on urination; and abdominal pain in women*
3. *Cluster of soft, fleshy growths about the genitals or other places of sexual contact*
4. *Burning and itching about the genitals before an outbreak of multiple vesicles that become painful after rupture*

GENERAL GERONTOLOGIC CONSIDERATIONS

Nurses must abandon biases that older adults are sexually inactive. Therefore, when taking a health history, nurses must include questions about sexuality and behaviors that put them at risk for STIs.

Older clients who are sexually active have the same risks of acquiring an STI as other age groups.

Some older clients have limited knowledge about STIs and therefore may not recognize the symptoms or seek treatment.

Older adults who are not in monogamous relationships may not understand that barrier and chemical contraceptives are appropriate for preventing STIs.

Syphilis causes approximately 10% of cases of heart disease in those older than 50 years of age. The most frequently seen valvular disorder as the result of syphilis is aortic insufficiency. Damaged valves may need to be replaced with a ball-valve prosthesis.

Some older adults with an STI are embarrassed and may not seek medical attention. Careful assessment is necessary to help the older adult obtain medical treatment as quickly as possible.

Critical Thinking Exercises

1. *Discuss STI information that is appropriate to provide for a person who confides that he or she is having unprotected sexual intercourse with more than one person.*
2. *Explain information a person who has never used a condom should know.*

● NCLEX-STYLE REVIEW QUESTIONS 

1. When preparing to obtain a vaginal culture from a woman with a suspected sexually transmitted infection, which nursing action may cause inaccurate results?
   1. Using a nonsterile vaginal speculum to obtain the culture.
   2. Using latex gloves for the examination and culture.
   3. Moistening the vaginal speculum with lubricant.
   4. Moistening the vaginal speculum with water.
2. Which of the following statements by a client with active herpes simplex virus type 2 indicates a need for further teaching?
   1. "Alcohol will help keep the lesions dry."
   2. "Condoms protect against all disease transmission."
   3. "Warm baths will help relieve discomfort."
   4. "I will continue to wear boxer type underwear."
3. A client must inform a significant other of a newly diagnosed sexually transmitted infection. Which instructional strategy encouraged by the nurse would be most helpful in preparing the client?
   1. Obtain Web site addresses for information on disease transmission.
   2. Offer the client printed information to share with the significant other.
   3. Role-play situations in which the client discusses the problem.
   4. Provide phone numbers for counseling and support groups.

connection—

Visit the Connection site at **http://connection.lww.com/go/timbyEssentials** for links to chapter-related resources on the Internet.

References and Suggested Readings

American Social Health Association. (2001). Facts & answers about STIs. [On-line.] Available: http://www.ashaSTI.org/STIfaqs/syphilis.html.

Bielan, B. (2001). Clinical snapshot: Herpes simplex. *Dermatology Nursing, 13,* 372.

Centers for Disease Control and Prevention. (1999). Syphilis continues to retreat: Nation sets sights on elimination. [On-line.] Available: www.cdc.gov/nchstp/od/nchstp/html.

Centers for Disease Control and Prevention. (2001). Tracking the hidden epidemics: Trends in STIs in the United States 2000. [On-line.] Available: http://www.cdc.gov/STI.

Coombes, R. (2000). Return of the dirty dozen . . . sexually transmitted infections. *Nursing Times, 96*(36), 12–13.

Gleave, T. (2000). Keeping an eye on chlamydia. *Nursing Times, 96*(27), 51.

Hinds, P. (2000). Improving screening practices in the fight against chlamydia. *Community Nurse, 6*(8), 31–32.

Kobayashi, A., Miaskowski, C., Wallhagen, M., et al. (2000). Recent developments in understanding the immune response to human papilloma virus infection and cervical neoplasia. *Oncology Nursing Forum, 27,* 643–653.

Martin, Y. (September 10, 2001). Recognizing and treating the silent STI. *Advance for Nurses,* 28–30.

Natinsky, P. (November/December 2002). The return of syphilis. *Community Health Forum,* 2–3.

Patient Handout. (August 19, 2002). Protecting yourself from STIs. *Advance for Nurses,* 39.

Porth, C. M. (2002). *Pathophysiology: Concepts of altered health states* (6th ed.). Philadelphia: Lippincott Williams & Wilkins.

Rogers, D. (2003). New meaning for safe sex. *RN, 66*(1), 38–41.

Sheff, B. (2001). Microbe of the month: *Chlamydia trachomatis. Nursing 2001, 31*(1), 71.

Sheff, B. (2000). Microbe of the month: *Neisseria gonorrhoeae. Nursing 2000, 30*(7), 76.

Thomas, D. J. (2001). Sexually transmitted viral infections: Epidemiology and treatment. *Journal of Obstetric, Gynecologic, and Neonatal Nursing, 30,* 316–323.

U.S. Preventive Services Task Force. (2002). Screening for chlamydial infection: Recommendations and rationale. *American Journal of Nursing, 102*(10), 87–92.

chapter 57

Introduction to the Urinary Tract

Words to Know 

blood urea nitrogen
costovertebral angle
creatinine
creatinine clearance test
cystogram
cystometrogram
cystoscope
cystoscopy
intravenous pyelogram
postvoid residual
renal arteriogram
retrograde pyelogram
ultrasonography
urinalysis
urine protein test
urine specific gravity
urodynamic studies
uroflowmetry
voiding cystourethrogram

Learning Objectives

On completion of this chapter, the reader will:

- Name parts of the urinary system.
- Define primary functions of the kidney and other structures in the urinary system.
- List tests performed for diagnosis of urologic and renal system diseases.
- Identify laboratory tests performed to diagnose urologic and renal system diseases.
- Discuss nursing management for a client undergoing diagnostic evaluation of the urinary tract.

The urinary system consists of the kidneys, renal pelves (sing. *pelvis*), ureters, urinary bladder, and urethra. The kidneys have many functions, including urine formation, excretion of excess water and nitrogenous waste products of protein metabolism; a role in maintenance of acid-base and electrolyte balance; production of the enzyme *renin,* which helps regulate blood pressure; and production of the hormone *erythropoietin,* which stimulates red blood cell production. The remainder of the urinary system is involved in transport (ureters and pelves), storage (bladder), and excretion (urethra) of urine.

Urologic nursing assessment focuses on changes in urine production, transport, storage, and elimination. Other responsibilities of urologic nurses involve caring for clients with conditions that affect the reproductive systems, discussed in Chapters 53 and 55.

ANATOMY AND PHYSIOLOGY

The upper urinary tract is composed of the kidneys, renal pelves, and ureters. The lower urinary tract consists of the bladder, urethra, and pelvic floor muscles (Fig. 57.1). The two kidneys are paired, bean-shaped organs located in the upper abdomen on either side of the vertebral column. They span from the level of the 12th thoracic vertebra to the 3rd lumbar vertebra. A thin, fibrous capsule encloses each kidney; the peritoneum separates the kidneys from the abdominal cavity anteriorly. Blood supply to each kidney consists of a renal artery, which arises from the aorta, and a renal vein, which empties into the vena cava. Kidneys receive 25% of the total cardiac output.

A cross-section of the kidney (Fig. 57.2) helps to illustrate the inner structures. There are two main areas: renal pelves and the *parenchyma,* which is made up of a cortex (outer layer) and a medulla (inner core). Within each cortex are microscopic nephrons that carry out kidney functions. Each kidney contains about 1 million *nephrons,* the smallest functioning units of the kidney. Each nephron has a *glomerulus, afferent arteriole, efferent arteriole, Bowman's capsule, distal* and *proximal convoluted tubules,* the *loop of Henle,* and the *collecting tubule* (Fig. 57.3). The medulla contains calyces (pyramids), cone-shaped structures that open to the pelvis, a large funnel-like structure in the center of the kidney. The renal pelvis then empties into the ureter, which carries urine to the bladder for storage.

The bladder, urethra, and pelvic floor muscles form the urethrovesical unit. The urinary bladder, located just behind the pubis, is a hollow, muscular organ. Its shape

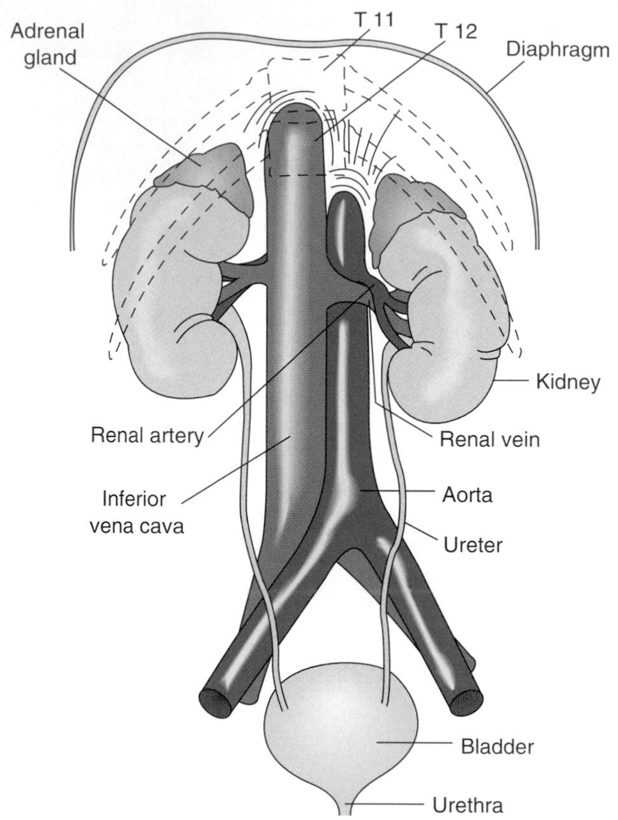

FIGURE 57.1 Kidneys, ureters, and bladder. The right kidney is usually lower than the left.

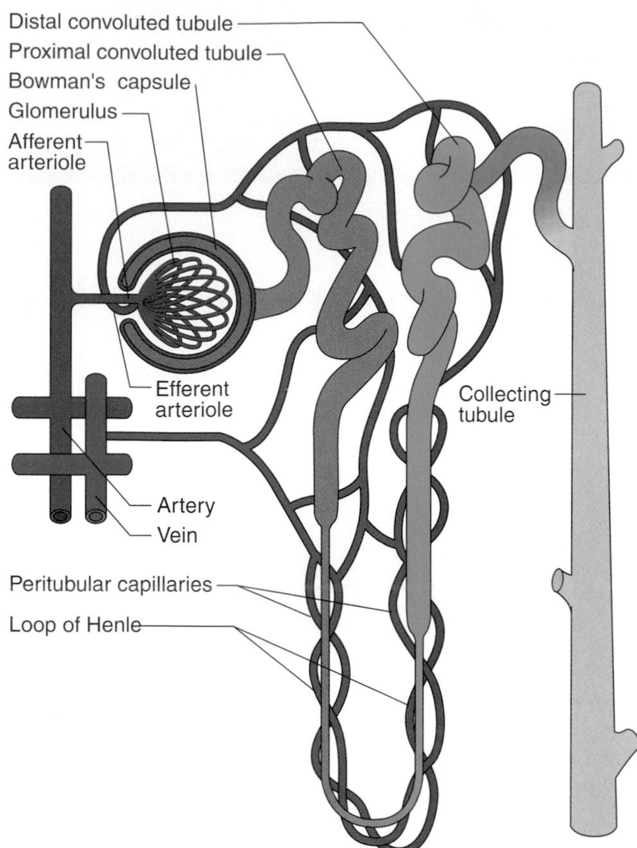

FIGURE 57.3 Representation of a nephron.

and size vary with the amount of urine it contains as well as the person's age. Adult bladders hold approximately 300 to 500 mL of urine. The urethra is a hollow tube that begins at the bladder neck and ends at the external meatus. It serves as a conduit during urination and has a sphincter mechanism to prevent urine leakage. The male urethra extends approximately 24 cm (10 inches) from the bladder neck through the prostate and the penile shaft to the glans penis. The female urethra extends about 4 cm (1.5 to 2 inches) from the bladder neck to the external meatus, anterior to the vagina. The pelvic floor muscles constitute the final part of the urethrovesical unit. These muscles form a sling that supports the bladder and urethra, rectum, and some reproductive organs.

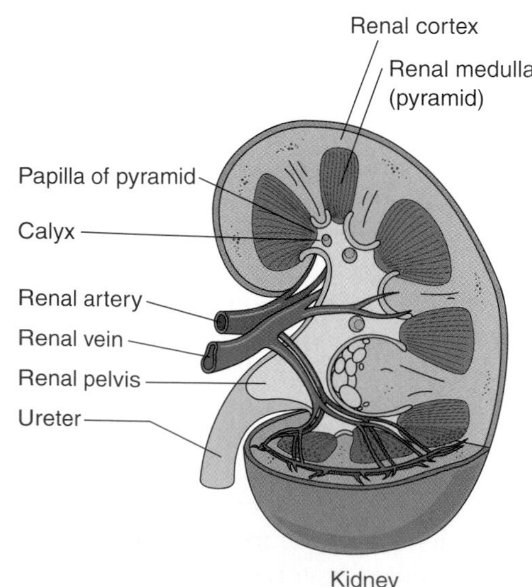

FIGURE 57.2 Internal structure of the kidney. (Adapted from Willis, M. C. [1996]. *Medical terminology: The language of healthcare.* Baltimore: Williams & Wilkins.)

There are three steps in the complex process of urine formation:

- *Glomerular filtration*—involves the filtration of plasma by the glomerulus (see Fig. 57.3). Filtered substances include water, sodium, chloride, bicarbonate, potassium, glucose, urea, creatinine, and uric acid.
- *Tubular reabsorption*—the filtrate enters Bowman's capsule and then moves through the tubular system of the nephron and is either reabsorbed (placed back into the systemic circulation) or excreted as urine.
- *Tubular secretion*—formed urine drains from the collecting tubules, into the renal pelves, and down each ureter to the bladder.

The filtrate secreted as urine usually contains water, sodium, chloride, bicarbonate, potassium, urea, creatinine, and uric acid. Amino acids and glucose typically are reabsorbed and not excreted in the urine. Protein molecules, except for periodic small amounts of globulins and albumin, also are reabsorbed. Transient proteinuria in small amounts (< 150 mg/dL) is not considered a problem. Persistent and elevated proteinuria may indicate glomerular damage. Glycosuria (glucose in the urine) occurs when glucose concentration in the blood and glomerular filtrate exceeds the ability of tubules to reabsorb the glucose (Porth, 2002).

Urine flows from the renal pelvis through the ureter into the bladder. Peristaltic waves help move urine to the bladder. Normally, urine flows in one direction because of this peristaltic action and because ureters enter the bladder at an oblique angle (Bullock & Henze, 2000). Reflux of urine (urine that flows backward) can occur secondary to an overdistended bladder or other problems, and may cause infections (see Chapter 59).

The desire to urinate comes from feeling bladder fullness. A nerve reflex is triggered when approximately 150 mL of urine accumulates. During urination, the bladder muscle contracts and sphincter muscles relax, forcing urine out of the bladder and urethra through the urethral meatus. If there is any interference or abnormality of these muscles, the bladder may not empty completely or empty uncontrollably (incontinence).

Stop, Think, and Respond ● BOX 57-1

What factors influence the amount of urine produced?

ASSESSMENT

History

Obtain information about general health, childhood and family illnesses, past medical history, allergies, sexual and reproductive health, exposure to toxic chemicals or gas, and history of present complaint, such as voiding changes, pain with voiding, or other abnormal symptoms. In addition to the client's chief complaint and medical history, a medication history is important. Older clients in particular may be taking multiple medications, which may affect renal function. Obtain information about voiding patterns, which may indicate renal or urologic problems (Table 57.1).

Physical Examination

Before beginning the physical examination, ask the client to void. Inspection includes observing the abdomen for scars, symmetry, abdominal movements, and pulsations. Examine the back and note any bulging, bruising, or scars. The experienced examiner auscultates the abdomen for bruits (abnormal vascular sounds heard over a blood vessel). In addition, he or she percusses the area over the bladder beginning 2 inches above the symphysis pubis and moving toward the base of the bladder. Percussion usually produces a tympanic sound; it produces a dull sound if the bladder is filled. The examiner can palpate the suprapubic area but can palpate the bladder only if it is moderately distended. Assessing the kidneys for tenderness or pain is done by lightly striking the fist at the **costovertebral angle** (CVA), which is where the lower ribs meet the vertebrae (Fig. 57.4). Normally, the client experiences a dull thud. Pain or tenderness may indicate a renal disorder. Also assess for signs of electrolyte and water imbalance.

In addition to evaluating the client's general health, evaluate the client for signs or symptoms of periorbital edema (swelling around the eyes), edema of the extremities, cardiac failure, and mental changes. All these signs or symptoms may indicate urinary tract disorders. Also obtain vital signs and weight.

Diagnostic Tests

In the male client, diseases and disorders of the reproductive system also affect the urinary system. In addition to diagnostic tests discussed in the following sections, tests that may be performed on the male client are discussed in Chapters 55 and 56.

Radiography

An x-ray study of the abdomen includes x-rays of the kidneys, ureters, and bladder (KUB). It shows the size and position of the kidneys, ureters, and bony pelvis as well as any radiopaque urinary calculi (stones), abnormal gas patterns (indicative of renal mass), and anatomic defects of the bony spinal column (indicative of neuropathic bladder dysfunction). An x-ray of the pelvis, chest, or other area may reveal metastatic bone lesions that could be a result of renal or bladder tumors.

Ultrasonography

Renal **ultrasonography** identifies the kidney's shape, size, location, collecting systems, and adjacent tissues. Other uses include identification of renal cysts or obstruction sites, assistance in needle placement for renal biopsy or nephrostomy tube placement, and drainage of a renal abscess. There are no contraindications to this procedure. It is not invasive and does not require the injection of a radiopaque dye or require fasting or bowel preparation for a renal or bladder sonogram.

Computed Tomography Scan and Magnetic Resonance Imaging

A computed tomography (CT) scan or magnetic resonance imaging (MRI) of the abdomen and pelvis may be

TABLE 57.1 PROBLEMS ASSOCIATED WITH CHANGES IN VOIDING

PROBLEM	DEFINITION	POSSIBLE ETIOLOGY
Frequency	Frequent voiding—more than every 3 hours	Infection, obstruction of lower urinary tract leading to residual urine and overflow, anxiety, diuretics, benign prostatic hyperplasia, urethral stricture, diabetic neuropathy
Urgency	Strong desire to void	Infection, chronic prostatitis, urethritis, obstruction of lower urinary tract leading to residual urine and overflow, anxiety, diuretics, benign prostatic hyperplasia, urethral stricture, diabetic neuropathy
Dysuria	Painful or difficult voiding	Lower urinary tract infection, inflammation of bladder or urethra, acute prostatitis, stones, foreign bodies, tumors in bladder
Hesitancy	Delay, difficulty in initiating voiding	Benign prostatic hyperplasia, compression of urethra, outlet obstruction, neurogenic bladder
Nocturia	Excessive urination at night	Decreased renal concentrating ability, heart failure, diabetes mellitus, incomplete bladder emptying, excessive fluid intake at bedtime, nephrotic syndrome, cirrhosis with ascites
Incontinence	Involuntary loss of urine	External urinary sphincter injury, obstetric injury, lesions of bladder neck, detrusor dysfunction, infection, neurogenic bladder, medications, neurologic abnormalities
Enuresis	Involuntary voiding during sleep	Delay in functional maturation of central nervous system (bladder control usually achieved by 5 years of age), obstructive disease of lower urinary tract, genetic factors, failure to concentrate urine, urinary tract infection, psychological stress
Polyuria	Increased volume of urine voided	Diabetes mellitus, diabetes insipidus, diuretics, excess fluid intake, lithium toxicity, certain types of kidney disease (hypercalcemic and hypokalemic nephropathy)
Oliguria	Urine output less than 400 mL/day	Acute or chronic renal failure (see Chap. 58), inadequate fluid intake
Anuria	Urine output less than 50 mL/day	Acute or chronic renal failure (see Chap. 58), complete obstruction
Hematuria	Red blood cells in the urine	Cancer of genitourinary tract, acute glomerulonephritis, renal stones, renal tuberculosis, blood dyscrasia, trauma, extreme exercise, rheumatic fever, hemophilia, leukemia, sickle cell trait or disease
Proteinuria	Abnormal amounts of protein in the urine	Acute and chronic renal disease, nephrotic syndrome, vigorous exercise, heat stroke, severe heart failure, diabetic nephropathy, multiple myeloma

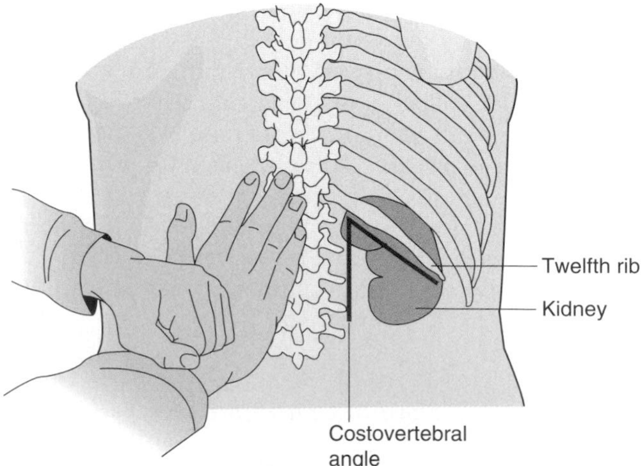

FIGURE 57.4 Assessing for CVA tenderness.

done to diagnose renal pathology, determine kidney size, and evaluate tissue densities with or without contrast material. An iodine-based contrast medium may be injected intravenously (IV) after the initial scan to enhance the images, especially when vascular tumors are suspected. The CT scan also is useful in identifying calculi, congenital abnormalities, obstruction, infections, and polycystic disease. An MRI produces sharp images of the kidneys and can delineate the renal cortex from the medulla. It also is useful in identifying bladder tumors, staging renal cell carcinoma, and imaging the vascular system.

Angiography

A renal angiogram (**renal arteriogram**) provides details of arterial supply to the kidneys, specifically the location and number of renal arteries (multiple vessels to the kidney are not unusual) and patency of each renal artery. A catheter is passed up the femoral artery into the aorta to the level of the renal vessels. Contrast medium is then injected into the catheter and serial x-rays are taken. Radiopaque dye first outlines the aorta in the area of the renal artery, then enters the renal artery and the kidney. A series of x-rays is taken. The catheter tip also may be passed into each renal artery for additional images. The procedure lasts 30 to 90 minutes. This procedure is contraindicated if a client is allergic to iodine contrast material.

Ask the client about allergy to iodine or seafood and any previous dye reactions. Review pertinent laboratory tests (blood urea nitrogen [BUN], creatinine) to assess renal function, record vital signs, and assess peripheral pulses. Instruct the client to void before the procedure. If ordered, administer a sedative to promote relaxation before the procedure. After the procedure, the physician applies a pressure dressing to the femoral area, which remains in place for several hours. Palpate the pulses in the legs and feet at least every 1 to 2 hours for signs of arterial occlusion. Monitor the pressure dressing to note frank bleeding or hematoma formation. If either condition occurs, immediately notify the physician. Another important assessment is for hypersensitivity responses to contrast material. Clients remain on bed rest for 4 to 8 hours. Also monitor and document intake and output. See Client and Family Teaching 57-1.

Cystoscopy

Cystoscopy is the visual examination of the inside of the bladder using an instrument called a *cystoscope*. When the urethra is examined, the procedure is called *cystourethroscopy*. The **cystoscope** consists of a lighted tube with a telescopic lens (Fig. 57.5). It identifies the cause of painless hematuria, urinary incontinence, or urinary retention. It helps to evaluate structural and functional changes of the bladder. The cystoscope is inserted through the urethra into the bladder. Local anesthesia is usual; however, spinal or general anesthesia also may be used. The procedure lasts 30 to 45 minutes. Biopsy samples (tissue examination), cell washings (cytologic analysis), and urine samples may be obtained.

Preoperative sedatives or antispasmodics may be ordered. Cystoscopy can aggravate any abnormality of the urinary tract. A urine culture should be done before testing. If a urinary infection was present before the cystoscopy, chills, fever, and possibly septicemia may occur. Observe the client for these and other symptoms and report findings to the physician. Clients receive antibiotics after a cystoscopy. Record vital signs before and after the procedure. If general anesthesia is used, monitor vital signs every 15 to 30 minutes until the client is stable. Significant prostatic obstruction may result in pain and complete urinary retention after a cystoscopy. Administer medications for pain or bladder spasms postprocedure as ordered.

Stop, Think, and Respond ● BOX 57-2

A client having a cystoscopy has the potential for complications. What are these?

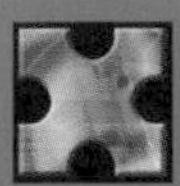

57-1 *Client and Family Teaching*
The Client Undergoing Renal Angiography

The nurse reviews the following points:

- Drink extra fluids on the day before the test; do not eat any food or fluids (per protocol) before testing; IV fluids will be given before, during, and after the test; medication will be given to promote relaxation; local anesthesia is administered.
- Expect a burning sensation or feeling of heat, pain, or nausea while contrast material is injected. These reactions are normal and transient.
- Remain on strict bed rest for 4 to 8 hours or more as per protocol. A urinal or bedpan must be used in the meantime.
- Drink extra fluids (2000 to 3000 mL over the 24-hour postprocedure period).

Intravenous Pyelogram and Retrograde Pyelogram

An **intravenous pyelogram** (IVP) is a radiologic study to evaluate structure and function of the kidneys, ureters, and bladder. It locates urinary tract obstructions and

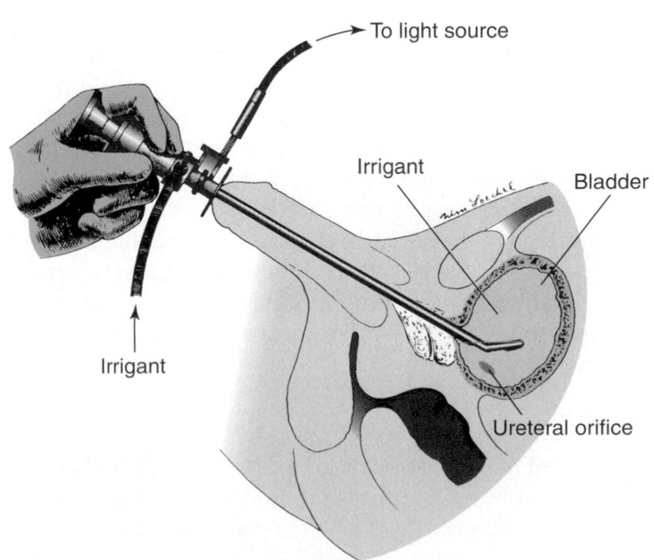

FIGURE 57.5 Cystoscopic examination.

investigates the causes of flank pain, hematuria, or renal colic. It is based on the ability of the kidneys to excrete a radiopaque dye (also called a *contrast medium*) in urine. The IV radiopaque dye outlines kidney pelves, ureters, and bladder as blood containing the dye passes through the urinary tract. After IV injection of contrast material, x-rays of the urinary tract are taken after 1 minute (kidney visualization), at 3 to 5 minutes (renal collecting system visualization), at 10 minutes (ureters visualization), and at 20 to 30 minutes (bladder filling visualization). A postvoiding film shows the emptying of the bladder.

Because radiopaque dye usually contains iodine, the physician may inject a minute amount of radiopaque dye IV and observe the client for 5 to 10 minutes to determine any allergy to iodine. Radiopaque dyes that do not contain iodine, called *nonionic contrast agents,* are available and produce fewer allergic reactions.

A **retrograde pyelogram** may be done for better visualization of the complete ureter and renal pelvis. A flexible radiopaque ureteral catheter is inserted in each of the ureteral orifices (opening at the terminal end of the ureter), which lie on the lower posterior wall of the bladder. This is done during a cystoscopy. Visualization of ureters and renal pelves is possible after sterile contrast medium is instilled into the renal collecting system. This procedure also evaluates ureteral stent or catheter placement. Retrograde pyelography carries a risk of sepsis and severe urinary tract infection.

Nursing Guidelines 57-1 provide information on the care of the client undergoing a pyelogram. After the IVP or retrograde pyelogram, instruct the client to consume an adequate fluid intake. In addition, the client continues to receive IV fluid replacement. Monitor and document the intake and output, making sure that urine output is at least 30 mL/hour. Clients who are dehydrated are at high risk for renal failure from the toxic effect of the contrast medium on the kidney tissues. Also monitor vital signs. If additional radiographic films are to be taken in the next 24 hours (if the excretory function of the kidney is abnormal), the physician or radiology department provides instructions regarding the food and fluid intake.

The client undergoing a retrograde pyelogram may experience a dull ache caused by distention of the renal pelves with radiopaque dye. Observe the client for signs and symptoms of pyelonephritis (see Chap. 58) 24 to 48 hours postprocedure because of the instrumentation and injection of material. If there are symptoms, report them to the physician and obtain a urine specimen for culture and analysis. Antibiotic agents are administered as directed.

Biopsy

Biopsies of urinary tract tissue are taken to diagnose cancer, assess prostatic enlargement, diagnose and monitor progression of renal disease, and assess and evaluate treatment of renal transplant rejection. Bladder biopsies are obtained during cystoscopy. Information about prostate biopsy can be found in Chapter 55. Table 57.2 describes renal biopsy techniques. There is risk of postprocedure bleeding because the kidneys receive up to 25% of the cardiac output each minute.

Reassure the client undergoing a renal biopsy and explain the procedure and its purpose. In addition, record vital signs and review pretest coagulation studies, urinalysis, IVP, and renal scan. After the procedure, the client remains on bed rest. Observe the urine for signs of hematuria. It is important to assess the dressing frequently for signs of bleeding, monitor vital signs, and evaluate the type and severity of pain. Severe pain in the back, shoulder, or abdomen can indicate bleeding. Notify the physician of these signs and symptoms immediately. Also assess the client for difficulty voiding. Encourage the client to

NURSING GUIDELINES 57-1

Care of Client Undergoing Intravenous or Retrograde Pyelogram

- Check client's allergy history, especially to intravenous contrast dye (iodine) or seafood. Inquire about previous reactions to x-ray studies that used contrast media. Report allergies to the physician or radiography department personnel.
- Instruct client to fast from food for 8 to 12 hours before the pyelogram. Fluid is permitted.
- Cleanse the bowel so there is no interference with visualization of the kidneys on the radiographic film. It is important that the bowel preparation is effective because poor cleansing of the intestinal tract may require that the test be repeated. Clients with a peptic ulcer or ulcerative colitis usually require modification of the bowel-cleansing preparation.
- Document baseline vital signs.
- Explain the procedure and its purpose. Tell clients that a series of x-rays will be taken after injection or instillation of IV contrast material and that the entire test requires 1 to 1½ hours to complete.
- Caution clients that they may experience burning, hot flushing sensations, unpleasant (metallic) taste in the mouth, or nausea or vomiting as the contrast is given. Half the clients experience nausea or vomiting. Reassure clients that these reactions are transient.
- Encourage adequate fluid intake postprocedure and voiding within 8 hours postprocedure. A burning sensation on voiding and small amounts of blood-tinged urine are normal and should disappear after the third voiding.
- Advise the use of warm tub baths to decrease urethral discomfort or spasms after a retrograde pyelogram. These reactions should disappear within 24 hours.
- Instruct client to abstain from alcohol 48 hours postprocedure to avoid irritating the bladder.
- Discuss taking antibiotics for 1 to 3 days postprocedure. Teach client to report flank pain, chills, fever, dysuria, or bleeding. Advise client to notify physician should symptoms present.

TABLE 57.2 TECHNIQUES FOR RENAL BIOPSY	
TYPE OF BIOPSY	**DESCRIPTION**
Needle biopsy	• Minimally invasive • Renal tissue is removed through a needle • Useful when CT or MRI findings are inconclusive
Fine-needle aspiration biopsy	• Minimally invasive • Performed under local anesthesia in the operating room • Needle placement guided by fluoroscopy
Open biopsy	• Small incision made into flank • Usually performed if needle biopsy tissue samples are not satisfactory

have adequate fluid intake after the biopsy. If the client is to be discharged the following day, instruct him or her to:

- Maintain limited activity for several days to avoid bleeding.
- Complete prophylactic antibiotic therapy as indicated.
- Report signs of systemic infection (fever, malaise), urinary tract infection (dysuria, frequency, discolored urine, malodorous urine), or bleeding (hematuria, lightheadedness, flank pain, or rapid pulse). Advise the client to notify the physician immediately should symptoms occur.

Cystogram and Voiding Cystourethrogram

A **cystogram** evaluates abnormalities in bladder structure and filling through instillation of contrast dye and radiography. A **voiding cystourethrogram** (VCUG) is similar to a cystogram except the client is instructed to void (the urine contains the radiopaque dye), and a rapid series of x-rays are taken. Urinary tract infection is a contraindication to a cystogram or VCUG.

Urodynamic Studies

Urodynamic studies evaluate bladder and urethral function and are done to assess causes of reduced urine flow, urinary retention, and urinary incontinence. Two of the main tests are uroflowmetry and cystometrogram.

Uroflowmetry (determination of the urinary flow rate) is done to evaluate bladder and sphincter function. This noninvasive procedure measures the time and rate of voiding, volume of urine voided, and pattern of urination. Results are compared with normal flow rates and urinary patterns and vary by age and sex. See Table 57.3 for normal uroflowmetry values. The client usually is catheterized afterward for **postvoid residual,** which is the amount of urine left in the bladder after voiding and provides information about bladder function. Normal postvoid residual is 0 to 30 mL, but retention of up to 100 mL may be acceptable in the older adult.

A **cystometrogram** (CMG) evaluates bladder tone and capacity. A retention catheter is inserted into the bladder after the client voids. The bladder is slowly filled with sterile saline and the client indicates at what point the first urge to void is felt and when the bladder feels full. These measurements indicate whether the client's bladder capacity is normal. Most clients feel a mild urge to void at approximately 120 mL and a strong urge to void at about 250 mL. By comparison, clients with a neurogenic bladder (see Chap. 59) may not feel an urge to void until 500 mL or more is instilled. In many instances, the client with a neurogenic bladder never feels an urge to void and instillation is terminated at this point. The client is assessed for bladder contractions that he or she cannot control, leakage around the catheter, or leakage of urine when asked to cough. Pressures within the bladder are also assessed. The client may be given antibiotics for a day or two after a CMG.

Laboratory Tests

URINALYSIS. Much information about systemic diseases and the condition of the kidneys and lower urinary tract can be learned by **urinalysis,** a study of the components and characteristics of urine. It also is useful in monitoring effects of treatment of known urinary or renal conditions. Characteristics of normal urine and possible causes contributing to abnormal results are listed in Table 57.4. A clean-catch midstream specimen from the first voiding of the morning is preferred. See Nursing Guidelines 57-2 for instructing the client how to collect a clean-catch specimen.

URINE CULTURE AND SENSITIVITY. When infection is suspected, a urine specimen may be taken for culture by collecting a clean-catch midstream specimen or by urinary

TABLE 57.3 NORMAL URINE FLOW RATES			
GENDER	**YOUNG ADULT**	**MIDDLE-AGED ADULT**	**OLDER ADULT**
Male	21 mL/second	12 mL/second	9 mL/second
Female	18 mL/second	15 mL/second	10 mL/second

TABLE 57.4 URINALYSIS CHARACTERISTICS

CHARACTERISTIC AND NORMAL VALUE	ABNORMAL FINDINGS	POSSIBLE CAUSES
Color: yellow	Colorless	Overhydration, diabetes insipidus, chronic renal disease, diuretic therapy, diabetes mellitus
	Red, pink	Hematuria, foods (beets, rhubarb, blackberries), drugs (phenothiazines, rifampin)
	Dark yellow or orange	Bilirubin, dehydration, drugs (multiple vitamins, Pyridium, azogantrisin)
	Green	*pseudomonas* infection, bilirubin, drugs (methylene blue, amitriptyline, vitamin B complex)
	Brown	Dehydration, urobilinogen, drugs (cascara, Flagyl)
	Dark brown to black	Melanin, drugs (Macrodantin, quinine, methyldopa)
Clarity: clear	Cloudy	Phosphaturia
	Turbid	Pyuria, bacteriuria, parasitic disease
	Hazy	Mucus
	Smoky, milky	Prostatic fluid, sperm, lipids
	Pinkish precipitates	Hyperuricemia
Specific gravity: 1.003–1.029	Dilute (1.00–1.010) or concentrated (1.029–1.030)	Low: diabetes insipidus, kidney disorders High: false reading due to pus, albumin, protein, glucose, or dextran in urine
pH: 4.5–7.5	>7.5	Urinary tract infection, metabolic acidosis, Cushing's syndrome, low-protein diet with large vegetable intake, diet high in dairy and citrus fruit, drugs (sodium bicarbonate, thiazides)
Ketones: none	Ketonuria	Starvation, fasting, abnormal carbohydrate metabolism, diabetes mellitus, pregnancy, pernicious anemia, vomiting, high-protein diet
Protein: none	Proteinuria	Cancer, severe heart failure, renal disease, glomerulonephritis, nephrotic syndrome, trauma, fever, heavy exercise
Glucose: none	Glycosuria	Diabetes mellitus, gestational diabetes
Red blood cells: 0–3 RBCs/high-power field	>3 RBCs/high-power field	Renal disorders (glomerulonephritis, calculus, cancer, trauma, cysts), systemic disease (lupus, sickle cell, hypertension)
White blood cells: 0–4/high-power field	>4/high-power field	Urinary tract infection (acute pyelonephritis, cystitis, urethritis), renal disease, urinary stones
Bilirubin: none	Bilirubinuria	Hepatitis, biliary obstruction
Urobilinogen: <1 mg/dL	>1 mg/dL	Hepatitis, cirrhosis, congestive heart failure, hemolytic anemia
Casts: 0–2 hyaline casts/low-power field	>2/low-power field	Granular casts (glomerulonephritis, renal disease); fatty casts (nephrotic syndrome); cellular casts (glomeruli or tubule infection); hyaline casts (fever, strenuous exercise, congestive heart failure)
Crystals: none to few	Many	Urolithiasis, chronic renal failure, gout, urinary tract infection
Bacteria: negative per high-power field	Positive	Urinary tract infection, pyelonephritis, cystitis

catheterization. It is important that the urine specimen not be contaminated by skin bacteria. The container is labeled with the client's name and the time and date of the voiding. To prevent the growth of bacteria in the urine and decomposition, ensure delivery of the urine specimen immediately to the laboratory or refrigerate it promptly until it can be taken to the laboratory.

24-HOUR URINE COLLECTION. Sometimes the entire 24-hour volume of urine is collected, such as a 24-hour urine for 17-ketosteroids. The client is initially instructed to void and discard urine. The collection bottle is marked with the time the client voided. Thereafter, all urine is collected for 24 hours. The last urine is voided at the same time the test originally began. The entire specimen is refrigerated to prevent bacterial growth. To prevent any part of the specimen from being lost or contaminated, tell the client to use separate receptacles for voiding and defecation. If any urine is discarded by mistake or lost while defecating, stop the test. The loss of even a small amount of urine can invalidate the test.

URINE SPECIFIC GRAVITY. **Urine specific gravity** is a measurement of the kidney's ability to concentrate and excrete urine. Specific gravity measures urine concentration by measuring density of urine and comparing it with the density of distilled water, which is 1 (1 mL of distilled water weighs 1 g). The number, weight, and size of urine solutes

NURSING GUIDELINES 57-2

Instructing Client on Obtaining a Clean-Catch Midstream Specimen

Tell the client to:

- Wash hands and remove the lid from the specimen container without touching the inside of the lid.
- Open antiseptic towelette package and cleanse the urethral area. Tell the female client to hold labia apart with one hand and wipe down one side of the urethra with the first towelette and discard, wipe down the other side with the second towelette and discard, and wipe down the center with the third towelette and discard. Emphasize wiping one time only, from front to back. Tell the male client to retract foreskin if uncircumcised and to clean the urethral meatus in a circular motion using each towelette one time.
- Instruct the client to begin voiding into the toilet, urinal, or bedpan; tell the female client to continue to hold labia apart while voiding.
- Tell the client to void 30 to 50 mL of the midstream urine into the collection container and then finish urinating into the toilet, bedpan, or urinal. Emphasize not to contaminate the container.
- Tell the client to carefully replace the lid, dry the container if necessary, and wash his or her hands.

(particles) determine its specific gravity (density). Normally, specific gravity is inversely proportional to urine volume. On a hot day, a person who is perspiring profusely and taking little fluid has low urine output with a high specific gravity. Conversely, a person who has a high fluid intake and who is not losing excessive water from perspiration, diarrhea, or vomiting has copious urine output with a low specific gravity. When kidneys are diseased, the ability to concentrate urine may be impaired and the specific gravity remains relatively constant, no matter what the water needs of the body are or how much the client drinks.

URINE PROTEIN. The **urine protein test** is used to identify renal disease. Normally, protein is minimally present in urine. Increased urine protein levels may be seen with salt depletion, strenuous exercise, fever, or dehydration. Proteinuria in an individual urine specimen may be detected by dipping a test reagent stick (dipstick method) in the urine and comparing color changes with the provided color chart.

CREATININE CLEARANCE TEST. A **creatinine clearance test** is used to determine kidney function and creatinine excretion. **Creatinine** is a substance that results from breakdown of phosphocreatine (an amino acid waste product), present in muscle tissue. It is filtered by glomeruli and excreted at a fairly constant rate by kidneys. The total amount of excreted creatinine is called *creatinine clearance*. Renal tubules increase creatinine secretion with any decrease in glomerular filtration (renal failure). Muscle necrosis and atrophy greatly increase urinary creatinine owing to accompanying protein catabolism. For this test a 4-, 12-, or 24-hour urine specimen and a sample of blood (serum creatinine) are collected. The blood sample is obtained either at the midpoint or at the beginning and end of urine collection (varies per protocol). Both urine and blood samples are sent to the laboratory.

BLOOD CHEMISTRIES. When nephrons fail to remove waste products efficiently from the body, blood chemistry is altered. Deterioration in renal function is manifested by rises in the **blood urea nitrogen** (BUN) and creatinine values, both of which are protein breakdown products. Table 57.5 shows normal values of common blood studies performed on clients with signs and symptoms of a urinary system disorder, as well as renal implications regarding abnormal results. A moderate decrease in renal function occurs, however, before these values rise.

Nursing Management for Diagnostic Testing for Renal or Urologic Disorders

Interview the client to determine past experience with the test or other urologic procedures. Ask the client to discuss the nature of past experiences and expectations for the current tests. If the client had preparations before the test, check to see that preparations are complete. Also review the client's history and determine if there is any allergy history to contrast agents, if applicable.

Take the client's vital signs and weigh the client if required. Depending on the test, ask the client to void. If informed consent is required (necessary for invasive procedures), check for the signed consent form. Client and family members need teaching and reassurance about the purpose of the test and what the procedure involves. They also need to know the care required after the procedure.

Clients undergoing diagnostic testing often are anxious and worried. Clients having urologic testing may feel embarrassed and afraid that testing will be painful. It is important to provide privacy, reassurance, and information and to maintain a professional and empathic attitude. Administer sedative medications as ordered; they reduce anxiety. In addition, provide understandable explanations, repeating instructions as needed.

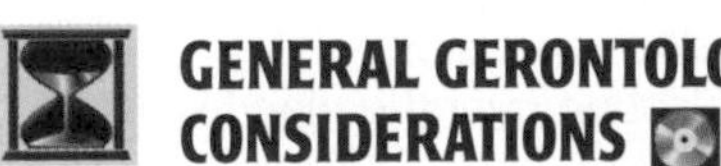

The older client may have difficulty following directions when collecting a 24-hour urine specimen. The directions may need to be repeated and the client supervised at frequent intervals.

Age-related changes in kidney function, such as decreased glomerular filtration rate and thickening of the renal tubules, can alter the excretion of drugs in older adults, increasing the risk of drug toxicity.

TABLE 57.5 NORMAL SERUM VALUES AND RENAL DISEASE

PARAMETER	NORMAL VALUE	CHANGE SEEN IN RENAL DISEASE
Calcium	8.8–10 mg/dL	Decreased in renal failure
Carbon dioxide combining power	23–30 mmol/L	Decreased in acute renal failure
Magnesium	1.3–2.1 mEq/L	Decreased in chronic renal disease
Phosphate, inorganic phosphorus	2.7–4.5 mg/dL	Increased in renal failure
Potassium	3.5–5.0 mEq/L	Increased in renal failure
Total protein	6.0–8.0 g/dL	Increased in poor renal function; decreased in nephrotic syndrome
Sodium	135–148 mmol/L	Decreased in severe nephritis; increased in renal disease
Blood urea nitrogen	7–18 mg/dL	Increased in renal disease and urinary obstruction
Creatinine	Male: 0.7–1.3 mg/dL Female: 0.6–1.1 mg/dL	Increased in renal disease or insufficiency
Albumin	>60 yr: 3.4–4.8 g/dL <60 yr: 3.5–5 g/dL	Decreased in renal failure
Chloride	98–107 mEq/L	Decreased in renal failure (onset)
Uric acid	Male: 4.5–8 ng/dL Female: 2.5–6.2 ng/dL	Increased in renal failure

Nephrotoxicity is more likely to occur in older adults than in younger adults receiving prolonged or high doses of nephrotoxic drugs. It is important for the nurse to identify and report signs of nephrotoxicity (increased BUN or serum creatinine levels, oliguria, or proteinuria).

Critical Thinking Exercises

1. *A client is scheduled for a cystoscopy and retrograde pyelogram. He is very nervous and asks many questions about the procedure. What could you do to try to decrease his anxiety?*
2. *A client has possible renal disease and is scheduled for many tests on her upper and lower urinary tract and gastrointestinal tract. What would you do to be sure one test does not interfere with another test?*

• NCLEX-STYLE REVIEW QUESTIONS 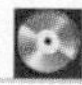

1. The nurse assesses the abdomen of a 70-year-old female client. Which assessment finding requires further evaluation?
    1. A gently rounded abdomen
    2. A pulsation just above the umbilicus
    3. Stretch marks on the abdomen
    4. A dull percussion sound over the bladder
2. The nurse is preparing a client scheduled for a renal angiogram. Which information is the most important for the nurse to document prior to the test?
    1. Client allergies to iodine or shellfish
    2. The client's tolerance to pain
    3. When the client last ate or drank
    4. The client's height and weight
3. Following an intravenous pyelogram (IVP), the nurse is providing a client with post-procedure instructions. Which instruction is the most important?
    1. Drink as much water as possible.
    2. Request medication if pain is intolerable.
    3. Avoid eating or drinking for the next 24 hours.
    4. Remain flat on the back for 12 hours.

connection

Visit the Connection site at **http://connection.lww.com/go/timbyEssentials** for links to chapter-related resources on the Internet.

References and Suggested Readings

Albaugh, J. (1999). Unlocking the mystery of urodynamics. *Urologic Nursing, 19,* 202, 206–208.

Bullock, B. A., & Henze, R. L. (2000). *Focus on pathophysiology.* Philadelphia: Lippincott Williams & Wilkins.

Fischbach, F. (2002). *Nurses' quick reference to common laboratory and diagnostic tests* (3rd ed.). Philadelphia: Lippincott Williams & Wilkins.

Porth, C. M. (2002). *Pathophysiology: Concepts of altered health states* (6th ed.). Philadelphia: Lippincott Williams & Wilkins.

Smeltzer, S. C., & Bare, B. G. (2004). *Brunner & Suddarth's textbook of medical–surgical nursing* (10th ed.). Philadelphia: Lippincott Williams & Wilkins.

Weber, J. R. (2001). *Nurses' handbook of health assessment* (4th ed.). Philadelphia: Lippincott Williams & Wilkins.

chapter 58

Caring for Clients With Disorders of the Kidneys and Ureters

Words to Know 

acute renal failure
acute tubular necrosis
anasarca
anuria
arteriovenous fistula
arteriovenous graft
azotemia
bruit
calciuria
calculus
casts
chronic renal failure
colic
dialysate
dialysis
dialyzer
disequilibrium syndrome
end-stage renal disease
extracorporeal shock-wave lithotripsy
glomerulonephritis
hematuria
hemodialysis
hydronephrosis
nephrectomy
nephrolithiasis
nephrostomy tube
nocturia
oliguria
osteodystrophy
periorbital edema
peritoneal dialysis
pyelonephritis
pyeloplasty
pyuria
thrill
uremia
uremic frost
ureteral stent
ureterolithiasis
ureteroplasty
urolithiasis

Learning Objectives

On completion of this chapter, the reader will:

- Differentiate pyelonephritis and glomerulonephritis.
- Name problems the nurse manages when caring for clients with glomerulonephritis.
- Explain the pathophysiology and associated renal complications of polycystic disease.
- Give examples of conditions that predispose to renal calculi.
- Identify methods for eliminating small renal calculi and larger stones.
- Discuss the nursing management of a client with a nephrostomy tube.
- Describe conditions that cause a ureteral stricture.
- Explain the classic triad of symptoms associated with renal cancer.
- Discuss problems the nurse manages when caring for a client with a nephrectomy.
- Differentiate acute and chronic renal failure.
- Explain pathophysiologic problems associated with chronic renal failure.
- Describe sources of organs for kidney transplantation.
- Identify nursing methods for managing pruritus.
- Explain purposes and methods of dialysis.
- Discuss nursing assessments performed when caring for clients undergoing dialysis.

The most common urologic disorders are infectious and inflammatory conditions. Those that affect the kidneys are extremely dangerous because damage to the nephrons can result in permanent renal dysfunction. The same is true of other upper urinary tract disorders such as kidney and ureteral stones and tumors. Consequences can lead to acute or chronic renal failure.

INFECTIOUS AND INFLAMMATORY DISORDERS OF THE KIDNEY

Infectious and inflammatory disorders of the kidney affect structures such as the renal pelvis, the nephrons, or both.

• PYELONEPHRITIS

Pyelonephritis is an acute or chronic bacterial infection of the kidney and lining of the collecting system (kidney pelvis). *Acute pyelonephritis* presents with moderate to severe symptoms that usually last 1 to 2 weeks. If treatment of acute pyelonephritis is unsuccessful and infection recurs, it is termed *chronic pyelonephritis.*

Pathophysiology and Etiology

Bacteria ascend to the kidney and kidney pelves by way of the bladder and urethra. Normal fecal flora such as

Escherichia coli, Klebsiella pneumoniae, Proteus mirabilis, Streptococcus fecalis, Pseudomonas aeruginosa, and *Staphylococcus aureus* are the most common bacteria that cause acute pyelonephritis. *E. coli* accounts for about 85% of infections. Additional risk factors for chronic pyelonephritis, such as urinary obstruction and reflux, are listed in Box 58-1.

In acute pyelonephritis, inflammation causes the kidneys to grossly enlarge. The cortex and medulla develop multiple abscesses. The renal calyces and pelves also can become involved. Resolution of inflammation results in fibrosis and scarring. Chronic pyelonephritis develops after recurrent episodes of acute pyelonephritis. Kidneys manifest irreversible degenerative changes and become small and atrophic. If destruction of nephrons is extensive, renal failure develops. Renal dysfunction may not occur for 20 or more years after onset of the disease. About 10% to 15% of clients with chronic pyelonephritis require dialysis.

Stop, Think, and Respond ● BOX 58-1

Explain why a client with an indwelling catheter is at risk for acute pyelonephritis.

Assessment Findings

Flank pain or tenderness, chills, fever, and malaise occur in clients with acute pyelonephritis. Frequency and burning on urination are present if there is accompanying cystitis (bladder infection). Some clients with chronic pyelonephritis are asymptomatic; others have a low-grade fever and vague gastrointestinal complaints. Polyuria and nocturia develop when the tubules of the nephrons fail to reabsorb water efficiently.

BOX 58-1 ● Risk Factors for Pyelonephritis

ACUTE PYELONEPHRITIS

- Instrumentation of the urethra and bladder (catheterization, cystoscopy, urologic surgery)
- Inability to empty the bladder
- Pregnancy
- Urinary stasis
- Urinary obstruction (tumors, strictures, calculi, prostatic hypertrophy)
- Diabetes mellitus
- Other renal disease (polycystic kidney disease)
- Neurogenic bladder (stroke, multiple sclerosis, spinal cord injury)
- Women with increased sexual activity, diaphragm, spermicide use, failure to void after intercourse, history of recent urinary infection
- Men who perform anal intercourse, infection with HIV

CHRONIC PYELONEPHRITIS

- Recurrent episodes of acute pyelonephritis
- Chronic obstruction (e.g., strictures and stones)
- Reflux disorders that allow urine to flow backward up the ureters

A urinalysis demonstrates multiple abnormalities. The chief abnormality is **pyuria,** or pus (a combination of bacteria and leukocytes) in the urine. A urine culture identifies the causative microorganism. A cystoscopy, or intravenous pyelogram (IVP) or retrograde pyelogram, demonstrates obstruction or damage to structures of the urinary tract. An x-ray of the kidneys, ureters, and bladder may reveal calculi, cysts, or tumors in the kidney or other urinary structures. Diagnosis of chronic pyelonephritis is based on a history of repeated acute pyelonephritis. Serum creatinine and blood urea nitrogen (BUN) levels, if elevated, indicate impaired renal function.

Medical and Surgical Management

Treatment of acute pyelonephritis includes relieving fever and pain and prescribing antimicrobial drugs such as trimethoprim-sulfamethoxazole (Septra) or ciprofloxacin (Cipro) for 14 days. Antispasmodics and anticholinergics, such as oxybutynin (Ditropan) and propantheline (Pro-Banthine), are additional pharmacologic interventions that relax smooth muscles of the ureters and bladder, promote comfort, and increase bladder capacity. Symptoms usually disappear within a few days of antibiotic therapy. Four weeks of drug therapy is prescribed for clients with a history of frequent relapsing infections with the same microorganism.

The goal of treatment for chronic pyelonephritis is to prevent progressive kidney damage. When possible, any urinary tract obstruction is relieved. An effort is made to improve the client's overall health. A **nephrectomy,** surgical removal of a kidney, is performed if severe hypertension develops and if the other kidney has adequate function.

Nursing Management

Obtain complete medical, drug, and allergy histories and assess vital signs, reporting abnormal findings such as elevated temperature or blood pressure. Continued and regular monitoring of vital signs is important to detect any evidence of changes. Determine the location of discomfort and any signs of fluid retention such as peripheral edema or shortness of breath. Observe and document the characteristics of the client's urine. A clean-catch urine specimen is collected for urinalysis and urine culture. Measure intake and output. Encouraging a liberal daily fluid intake of approximately 2000 to 3000 mL helps flush infectious microorganisms from the urinary tract. Administer prescribed medications. Evaluate laboratory test results such as BUN, creatinine, serum electrolytes, and urine culture to determine the client's response to therapy. If chronic pyelonephritis develops, the treatment often is lengthy. Poor health and prolonged medical therapy are discouraging. Urge the client to follow recommendations of the physician and adhere to the prescribed medication regimen.

Client and family teaching includes the following information:

- Explanation of the disease, its cause, related risk factors, treatment, and preventive measures
- Discussion of purpose, dosage, side effects, and toxic effects of prescribed medications
- Instructions to complete the entire regimen of antimicrobial therapy as indicated, even if symptoms abate
- Reinforcement of the importance of consuming a large volume of oral fluids daily
- Suggestions to consume acid-forming foods such as meat, fish, poultry, eggs, grains, corn, lentils, cranberries, prunes, plums, and their juices to prevent calcium and magnesium phosphate stone formation
- Recommendation to avoid alcohol and caffeine products if bladder spasms are present or until a clinical response to therapy is verified
- Explanation of the purpose and protocols for diagnostic procedures
- Teaching how to collect a clean-catch urine specimen for subsequent medical follow-up at 2 weeks and 3 months after treatment
- Referring client to resources where blood pressure can be monitored intermittently
- Identification of the signs of recurring or worsening pyelonephritis or lower urinary tract infection (frequency, urgency, burning, cloudy urine, and fever) and emphasis on the need to consult the primary care provider
- Discussion of methods to prevent reinfection—women should wipe from front to back after defecation and wear cotton undergarments. The nurse tells all clients to void every 2 to 3 hours when awake and before and after intercourse.

• ACUTE GLOMERULONEPHRITIS

The term *nephritis* describes a group of inflammatory but noninfectious diseases characterized by widespread kidney damage. **Glomerulonephritis** is a type of nephritis that occurs most frequently in children and young adults. It can affect people of any age. The exact incidence of the disease is unknown, but it occurs twice as often in men as in women. Most clients recover spontaneously or with minimal therapy without sequelae. Some develop chronic glomerulonephritis.

Pathophysiology and Etiology

Symptoms of acute glomerulonephritis appear about 2 to 3 weeks after an upper respiratory infection with group A beta hemolytic streptococci. Impetigo (skin infection) and viral infections such as mumps, hepatitis B, or human immunodeficiency virus also may precede acute glomerulonephritis (Smeltzer & Bare, 2004). The relationship between infection and acute glomerulonephritis is not clear. Microorganisms are not present in the kidney when symptoms appear, but glomeruli are acutely inflamed. Most believe that the inflammatory response is from antigen–antibody stimulation in the glomerular capillary membrane. Disruption of membrane permeability causes red blood cells (RBCs) and protein molecules to filter from glomeruli into Bowman's capsule and eventually become lost in the urine.

Assessment Findings

Approximately 50% of clients with glomerulonephritis have no symptoms. Early symptoms may be so slight that the client does not seek medical attention. Occasionally, onset is sudden with pronounced symptoms such as fever, nausea, malaise, headache, generalized edema, or **periorbital edema,** puffiness around the eyes. Some clients experience pain or tenderness over the kidney area and mild to moderate hypertension. A routine physical examination may reveal the disorder. More often, the client or family notices that the person's face is pale and puffy and that slight ankle edema occurs in the evening. Appetite is poor, and **nocturia** (urination during the night) may be present. Irritability and shortness of breath also develop. As the condition progresses, the client develops **hematuria** (blood in the urine), anemia (from the hematuria), convulsions associated with hypertension, congestive heart failure, **oliguria** (low urine output of 100 to 500 mL/day), and perhaps **anuria** (<100 mL of urine over 24 hours). Fluid retention and hypertension contribute to visual disturbances, often as a result of papilledema or hemorrhage in the eye, and epistaxis (nosebleeds).

Gross or microscopic hematuria gives urine a dark, smoky, or frankly bloody appearance. Laboratory findings include proteinuria (primarily as albumin in the urine) and an elevated anti-streptolysin O titer from the recent streptococcal infection. There is decreased hemoglobin, slightly elevated BUN and serum creatinine levels, and an elevated erythrocyte sedimentation rate. If renal insufficiency develops, serum electrolyte levels indicate hyperkalemia, hypermagnesemia, hypocalcemia, and dilutional hyponatremia. Percutaneous renal biopsy reveals cellular changes characteristic of an antigen–antibody response and the extent of damage.

Medical Management

No specific treatment exists for acute glomerulonephritis. Treatment is guided by symptoms and underlying abnormality. Treatment may consist of bed rest, a sodium-restricted diet (if edema or hypertension is present), and antimicrobial drugs to prevent a superimposed infection in the already inflamed kidney and abolish any remaining streptococci from the recent infection. Diuretics to reduce edema and antihypertensive agents for severe hypertension may be necessary. Vitamins are added to the diet to improve general resistance, and oral iron supplements may be needed to counteract anemia. Corticosteroids and immunosuppressive agents may be given to treat a rapidly progressive inflammatory process. Any increase in hematuria, proteinuria, or blood pressure indicates a need for aggressive treatment. The client is not considered cured until urine is free of protein and RBCs for 6 months. Return to full activity usually is not permitted until urine is free of protein for 1 month.

Nursing Management

The client must maintain bed rest when blood pressure is elevated and edema is present. Collect daily urine specimens to assist with evaluating the client's response to treatment. Assess blood pressure every 4 hours or as ordered. Encouraging adequate fluid intake and measuring intake and output are important. Although the diet may be restricted in sodium and protein, the client needs adequate carbohydrate intake to prevent the catabolism of body protein stores.

Provide teaching based on the following guidelines:

- Identify the specific amount of sodium allowed and sources of sodium to avoid.
- Explain the purpose of diuretic therapy or other prescribed medications, the dosing regimen, and side effects.
- Recommend regular blood pressure monitoring.
- Caution client to avoid contact with persons who have infections.
- Emphasize compliance with medical appointments and necessity for repeated urinalyses.
- Advise client to contact the physician if urinary volumes diminish, there is unexplained weight gain, or headaches or nosebleeds occur.

• CHRONIC GLOMERULONEPHRITIS

Chronic glomerulonephritis is a slowly progressive disease characterized by inflammation of the glomeruli, causing irreversible damage to nephrons. The course of the disease is highly variable. Some clients live for years with no or occasional symptomatic episodes, while for others, the disease is rapidly fatal unless they receive dialysis for the renal failure.

Pathophysiology and Etiology

A small number of those with chronic glomerulonephritis have had repeated acute glomerulonephritis, but many do not have that history. Complications of autoimmune connective tissue disorders, such as lupus erythematosus (see Chap. 61), also may cause chronic glomerulonephritis.

Chronic inflammation leads to ever-increasing bands of scar tissue that replace nephrons, the vital functioning units of the kidney. Decreased glomerular filtration eventually can lead to renal failure. Chronic glomerulonephritis accounts for approximately 40% of people on dialysis.

Assessment Findings

Some clients do not experience symptoms until renal damage is severe. Generalized edema, known as **anasarca,** is common, caused by the shift of fluid from the intravascular space to interstitial and intracellular locations. The fluid shift results from depletion of serum proteins, particularly albumin, which is lost in urine. Clients remain markedly edematous for months or years. They may feel relatively well, but the kidney continues to excrete albumin. The fluid burden and subsequent renal failure contribute to fatigue, headache, hypertension, dyspnea, and visual disturbances.

Low RBC volume is detected through complete blood counts, caused by excretion of erythrocytes in urine and reduced production of erythropoietin. **Azotemia,** accumulation of nitrogen waste products in blood, is evidenced by elevated BUN, serum creatinine, and uric acid levels. Urine contains protein (albumin), sediment, **casts** (deposits of minerals that break loose from the walls of the tubules), and red and white blood cells. Urinary creatinine clearance is reduced. Serum electrolyte changes indicate nephron dysfunction.

Chest x-ray and echocardiography evaluate cardiac size because cardiac enlargement is common. A percutaneous kidney biopsy may be done to confirm the diagnosis and to determine severity. In late stages, kidneys are too small to safely perform a biopsy.

Medical Management

Treatment is nonspecific and symptomatic. Management goals include controlling hypertension with medications and sodium restriction, correcting fluid and electrolyte imbalance, reducing edema with diuretic therapy, preventing congestive heart failure, and eliminating urinary tract infections with antimicrobials. Renal failure eventually may necessitate dialysis or kidney transplantation, discussed later in this chapter.

Nursing Management

Monitor fluid and electrolyte balance by checking blood values, intake and output, and skin turgor, and looking for any edema. Assess the client's neurologic, cardiac, and mental status.

Caring for the client with chronic glomerulonephritis involves close observation for changes in fluid and electrolyte status and kidney function. Clients may experience anxiety or depression and require emotional support.

Weigh client daily at the same time on the same scale with client wearing similar clothing each time. Plan with client to proportionately distribute restricted fluid volumes over 24 hours. Request that the dietitian instruct the client on sodium restriction and adequate caloric intake. Suggest herbs or spices that increase palatability of food. Administer prescribed diuretics.

Clients also experience fatigue related to anemia, retention of waste products, and edema. Provide periods of rest and promote uninterrupted sleep at night. Facilitate an adequate nutritional intake that includes some complete protein and iron-rich foods. Eliminate any unnecessary activities of daily living (ADLs). Assist client with ADLs when he or she shows evidence of tachycardia or dyspnea.

Evaluate the client's ability to manage home care and the availability of a support system before developing discharge plans. If the client lacks a support system from the family or extended family members, consult with the physician for a referral to a social agency or home health care agency. Develop a teaching plan with the following instructions:

- Follow diet and fluid regimen recommended by the physician and as outlined by the dietitian.
- Take medications exactly as directed on the container label. Do not omit or discontinue any medication unless ordered to do so by the physician. Do not take nonprescription drugs unless a physician approves their use.
- Monitor and record temperature and weight daily. (In some instances, clients may be asked to monitor their blood pressure.)
- Follow the physician's recommendations as to physical activity and exercise. Take frequent rest periods if fatigue occurs.
- Contact the physician with any question about the medication, if symptoms become worse, or if fever, chills, blood in the urine, weight gain, swelling of the arms or legs or periorbital edema, difficulty in breathing, difficulty in thinking, severe fatigue, excessive sleepiness, constipation, loss of appetite, or an upper respiratory infection occurs.
- Emphasize that frequent follow-up visits and laboratory tests are necessary to monitor response to treatment.

CONGENITAL KIDNEY DISORDERS: POLYCYSTIC DISEASE

Individuals may be born with various malformations of renal structures. Most of these are unpredictable because they are the result of errors in fetal development. Polycystic disease is the result of a hereditary trait.

The adult form has its onset between 30 to 50 years of age and progresses to renal insufficiency. Once renal failure develops, polycystic disease usually is fatal within 4 years, unless the client receives dialysis or an organ transplant. Women and men are affected equally. Death usually results from renal failure or complications of hypertensive cardiovascular disease.

Pathophysiology and Etiology

Adult polycystic kidney disease is inherited as an autosomal dominant trait, which means that an affected parent passes the gene for the disease to his or her children. Each child has a 50:50 chance of acquiring the defective gene.

This disorder is characterized by the formation of multiple bilateral kidney cysts (Fig. 58.1). Cysts interfere with kidney function and lead to renal failure. Fluid-filled cysts cause great enlargement of the kidneys, from their normal size of a fist to that of a football. As cysts enlarge, they compress renal blood vessels and cause chronic hypertension. Bleeding into cysts causes flank pain. People with polycystic disease are susceptible to kidney infections and kidney stones. In addition to renal

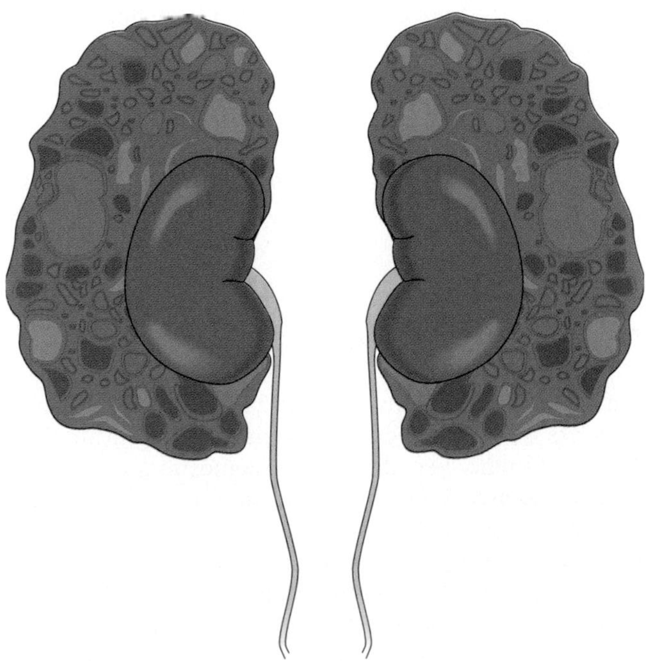

FIGURE 58.1 Normal kidneys in comparison with polycystic kidneys.

failure, complications include cysts on the pancreas and liver, enlarged heart, mitral valve prolapse, and brain aneurysm.

Assessment Findings

Hypertension is present in approximately 75% of affected clients. Pain from retroperitoneal bleeding, lumbar discomfort, and abdominal tenderness are caused by the size and effects of cysts. Clients may experience **colic** (acute spasmodic pain) when there is ureteral passage of clots or calculi.

A family history is a diagnostic indicator. Urinalysis shows mild proteinuria, hematuria, and pyuria. A complete blood count may show decreased or increased RBCs and hematocrit. An increase is seen because erythropoietin production sometimes is accelerated. Abdominal ultrasound, computed tomography (CT) scan, magnetic resonance imaging (MRI), and IVP reveal enlarged kidneys with indentations caused by cysts. Laboratory tests such as BUN and serum creatinine indicate the degree of current kidney dysfunction.

Medical and Surgical Management

Polycystic disease has no cure, but some interventions reduce rate of progression. Hypertension is treated with antihypertensive drugs, diuretic medications, and sodium restriction, but is difficult to control. When and if urinary infections develop, they are treated promptly with antibiotics. Low RBC counts are treated with iron supplements, injections of erythropoietin (Epogen), or blood transfusions. Nephrotoxic medications, such as nonsteroidal anti-inflammatory drugs (NSAIDs) and cephalosporin antibiotics, are avoided at all costs.

Dialysis substitutes for kidney function when renal failure occurs and while the client awaits an organ transplant. Surgical removal of one or both kidneys may be required.

Nursing Management

Many clients with polycystic disease are treated as outpatients by primary care physicians or nephrologists, physicians who specialize in the diagnosis and treatment of renal diseases. When hospitalization is necessary, assess vital signs, especially blood pressure, and report any significant elevations. Monitor laboratory test results for indicators of renal function. Inspect the urine for signs of bleeding or infection. Measure and document intake and output at least every 8 hours. Report any decrease in or absence of urine output. For further information about complications or advanced stages, refer to Nursing Process: The Client With Renal Calculi, and the Nursing Management sections in the discussions of the client with renal failure and dialysis.

OBSTRUCTIVE DISORDERS

Urinary obstruction at any point in the urinary tract can occur in clients of all ages for various reasons. Obstructing conditions include urinary tract stones, strictures, and tumors. Table 58.1 lists causes of urinary tract obstruction.

• KIDNEY AND URETERAL STONES

Urolithiasis refers to a condition of stones (**calculus;** pl. *calculi*) in the urinary tract. A calculus is a precipitate of mineral salts ordinarily dissolved in urine. About 70% to 80% of renal calculi in the United States are composed of calcium oxalate, calcium phosphate, or both (Porth, 2002). Others are composed of calcium phosphate, uric acid, cystine, and magnesium ammonium phosphate, or struvite. Stones may be smooth, jagged, or staghorn shaped.

Calculi occur anywhere in the urinary tract from the kidney pelvis and beyond. When a stone forms, the condition is called *urolithiasis.* **Nephrolithiasis** refers to a kidney stone, the size of which may range from microscopic to several centimeters. **Ureterolithiasis** is a stone

TABLE 58.1 CAUSES OF URINARY TRACT OBSTRUCTION

LEVEL OF OBSTRUCTION	CAUSE
Renal pelvis	Renal calculi Papillary necrosis
Ureter	Renal calculi Pregnancy Tumors that compress the ureter Ureteral stricture Congenital disorders of the ureterovesical junction, and ureteropelvic junction strictures
Bladder and urethra	Bladder cancer Neurogenic bladder Bladder stones Prostatic hyperplasia or cancer Urethral strictures Congenital urethral defects

(From Porth, C. M. [2002]. *Pathophysiology: Concepts of altered health states* [6th ed]. Philadelphia: Lippincott Williams & Wilkins.)

in the ureter. Ureteral stones usually are small; some may be no larger than a grain of sand.

Pathophysiology and Etiology

The reason urinary calculi form is not fully understood. Predisposing factors include the following:

- **Calciuria,** excessive calcium in the urine, as may accompany hyperparathyroid disease, administration of calcium-based antacids, and excessive intake of vitamin D
- Dehydration
- Urinary tract infection with urea-splitting organisms such as *P. mirabilis,* which makes urine alkaline, a condition that promotes precipitation of calcium
- Obstructive disorders, such as an enlarged prostate gland, which foster urinary stasis
- Metabolic disorders, such as gout, in which uric acid crystallizes
- Osteoporosis, in which bone is demineralized
- Prolonged immobility from paralysis secondary to spinal injuries or other incapacitating conditions that result in sluggish emptying of urine from the urinary tract

Calculi traumatize the walls of the urinary tract and irritate the cellular lining, causing pain as violent contractions of the ureter develop to pass the stone along. But ureteral spasms may just as easily hold a stone in place. If a stone totally or partially obstructs passage of urine beyond its location, pressure increases in the area above the stone. Pressure contributes to pain, and urinary stasis promotes secondary infection. Retained urine distends the renal pelvis, a condition called **hydronephrosis.** Eventually, there may be compression of the glomeruli and tiny arterioles that supply blood to the kidney, which can result in permanent kidney damage.

Assessment Findings

Symptoms of a kidney or ureteral stone vary with size, location, and cause. Small stones may pass unnoticed. Sudden, sharp, severe flank pain that travels to the suprapubic region and external genitalia is the classic symptom of urinary calculi. Pain is accompanied by renal or ureteral colic, painful spasms that attempt to move the stone. It comes in waves radiating to the inguinal ring, the inner aspect of the thigh, and to the testicle or tip of the penis in men, or the urinary meatus or labia in women. Severity of the pain usually is inversely proportional to the size of the stone. Smaller stones travel more rapidly down the ureter, causing more forceful ureteral spasm and, therefore, greater pain. Nausea, vomiting, and shock can all occur.

If an infection develops, the client may experience chills, fever, and serious hypotension. Urinary retention or dysuria may accompany obstruction. The kidney pelvis and ureter may become markedly enlarged as a consequence of urinary obstruction, and a mass may be palpated. The client also may experience renal tenderness.

Urinalysis shows evidence of gross or microscopic hematuria from trauma as the calculus tears at tissue as it moves downward. It also may show a pH conducive to stone formation, increased specific gravity, mineral crystals, and casts. Leukocytes in urine and an elevated white blood cell count indicate an infectious process. A urine culture identifies specific infectious microorganisms.

Radiography identifies most translucent kidney stones. If visualization is inconclusive, an IVP shows dye-filling defects caused by a stone. The dye stops at a certain point in the ureter and demonstrates enlargement above the obstruction. Kidney ultrasonography also detects obstructive changes. Depending on how long the stone has been present, some blood chemistry values, such as serum creatinine, BUN, and serum uric acid, may be elevated. Analysis of stone content is useful in preventing recurrence.

Medical Management

Small calculi are passed naturally with no specific interventions. If the stone is 5 mm or less in diameter and moving, pain is tolerable, and there is no obstruction, the client is managed medically with vigorous hydration, analgesics (including opioids and NSAIDs), antimicrobial therapy, and drugs that dissolve calculi or eventually alter conditions that promote their formation (Drug Therapy Table 58.1).

For larger stones, **extracorporeal shock wave lithotripsy** (ESWL), a procedure that uses 800 to 2400 shock waves aimed from outside the body toward soft tissue to dense stones, may be used. Stones are shattered into smaller particles that are passed from the urinary tract. ESWL is administered with the client in a water bath or surrounded by a soft cushion while under light anesthesia or sedation. Stones also can be pulverized with laser lithotripsy. To do so, a fine wire, through which the laser beam passes, is inserted into the ureter by means of a cystoscope. Repeated bursts of the laser reduce the stone to a fine powder, which is then passed in the urine.

Other stone removal procedures are performed with ureteroscopic approaches in which the endoscope is inserted from the urethra into the upper urinary tract under anesthesia to grasp, crush, and remove stones from the kidney pelvis or ureter. Afterward, a catheter or **ureteral stent,** a slender supportive device, is left in place for 3 days to splint the ureter or divert the urine past any possible tear in the ureteral wall (Fig. 58.2). If the stone cannot be removed, a ureteral catheter is left in place for 24 hours to dilate the ureter in the hope that the

DRUG THERAPY TABLE 58.1 AGENTS TO TREAT PYELONEPHRITIS

DRUG CATEGORY AND EXAMPLES	MECHANISM OF ACTION	SIDE EFFECTS	NURSING CONSIDERATIONS
Antispasmodics			
oxybutinin chloride (Ditropan) flavoxate (Urispas), belladonna and opium suppositories	Inhibits the action of acetylcholine and relaxes smooth muscle of the ureters and bladder	Dizziness, drowsiness, blurred vision, dry mouth, constipation, increased heart rate, delirium	Do not administer to clients with closed-angle glaucoma or hypotension.
Anticholinergics			
propantheline (Pro-Banthine), hyoscyamine (Levsinex), tincture of belladonna	Reduces spasms and smooth muscle contractions by inhibiting the effects of acetylcholine, thereby increasing bladder capacity	Same as above	Same as above
Oral Antibiotics			
trimethoprim-sulfamethoxazole (Bactrim, Septra), ciprofloxacin (Cipro)	Inhibits bacterial growth and destroys microorganisms	Same as above	Drugs can be used for up to 14 days. Clients do not require hospitalization unless nausea, vomiting, or signs of septicemia develop.

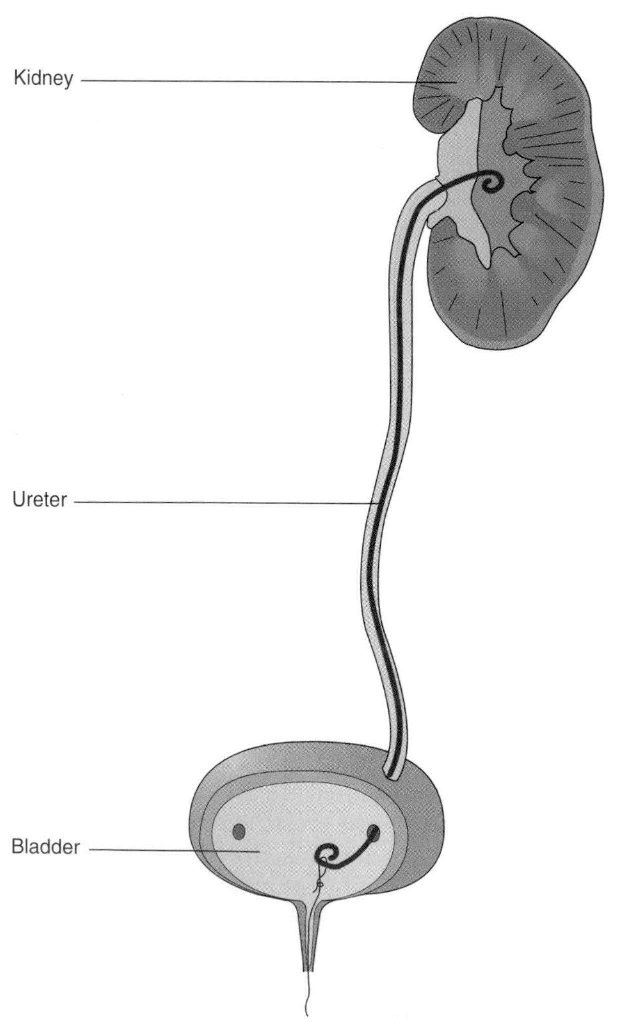

FIGURE 58.2 Example of a ureteral stent; in this case, a double J stent.

stone will pass through it or that it will be pulled into the bladder when the catheter is removed.

Surgical Management

Calculi that are large or complicated by obstruction, ongoing urinary tract infection, kidney damage, or constant bleeding require surgical removal. Drainage of urine from the affected kidney is accomplished with a nephrostomy tube during the postsurgical healing process. A **nephrostomy tube** is a catheter inserted through the skin into the renal pelvis. A nephrostomy tube is used to manage obstruction to urine flow above the bladder. The tube is kept in place with a suture through the skin. Unlike the bladder, the kidney pelvis can hold only 5 to 8 mL of urine. If a blood clot or kinking or compression of the tubing impairs urinary drainage for even a short time, hydronephrosis and damage to surgically repaired tissue can result. The client complains of pain if the renal pelvis becomes distended with urine.

Surgical options include percutaneous nephrolithotomy, an endoscopic procedure. A nephroscope is tunneled into the kidney through a tiny skin incision while the client is under general anesthesia (Fig 58.3). Ultrasound is used to crush the stone. The fragments are removed through the endoscope.

Other options include a ureterolithotomy, pyelolithotomy, or nephrolithotomy. With the client anesthetized, a suprapubic abdominal or flank incision is made and the stone is removed under direct visualization. A **pyeloplasty,** surgical repair of the ureteropelvic junction or

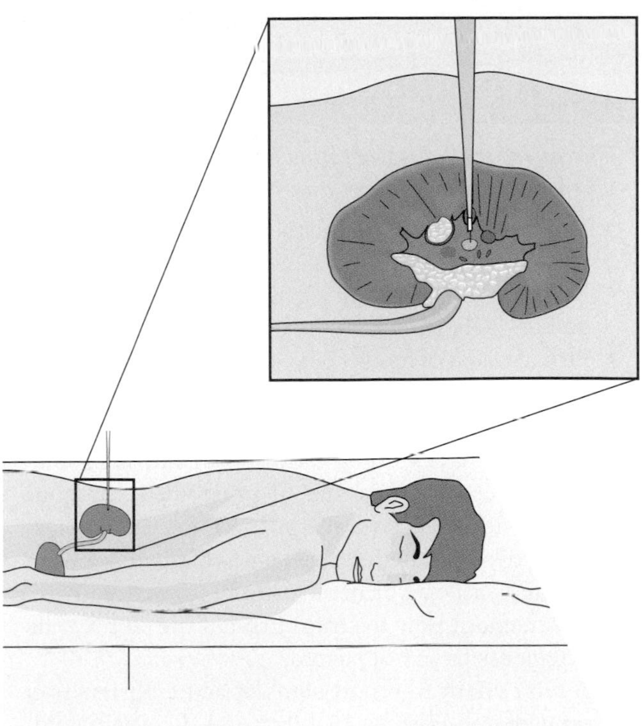

FIGURE 58.3 A nephroscope is inserted through a surgically created tunnel when a percutaneous nephrolithotomy is performed.

other anatomic anomalies, may be done at the same time. The additional surgery is done to correct conditions that contribute to the development of stones and prevent their recurrence. A nephrectomy is indicated if a stone has permanently and severely damaged a kidney beyond adequate function. The other kidney must be fully functional.

NURSING PROCESS

● The Client With Renal Calculi

Assessment

Obtain a complete history, including a drug and allergy history, family history, history of immobility, episodes of dehydration, urinary tract infections, and diet. Assess pain intensity and location and associated symptoms such as nausea and vomiting. Monitor vital signs and assess all urine for stones by straining it through a gauze or wire mesh and closely inspecting it. Save solid material for laboratory analysis. Urine may show evidence of hematuria. In some instances, the client may experience anuria related to bilateral obstruction and have abdominal distention.

Diagnosis, Planning, and Interventions

Three goals when caring for a client with urinary calculi include improving urinary output, relieving pain, and preventing or treating infection. Clients often are frightened because of excruciating pain, and require emotional support as well as pain management. Typical diagnoses, expected outcomes, and interventions include, but are not limited to, the following:

Pain related to increased pressure in the renal pelvis or renal colic

Expected Outcome: Pain will decrease within 30 minutes of a nursing measure.

- Administer prescribed narcotic analgesic. *It assists in decreasing pain related to ureteral colic during an acute episode and promotes muscle relaxation.*
- Provide supplemental nonpharmacologic interventions such as a comfortable position, guided imagery, and distraction. *These measures promote relaxation, redirect attention, and enhance coping ability.*
- Encourage ambulation and liberal fluid intake when the client is comfortable. *The supine position can increase colic; ambulation relieves it. Increased fluid intake promotes the passage of a stone and prevents urinary stasis or the formation of new stones.*

PC: Hydronephrosis related to ureteral obstruction

Expected Outcome: The nurse will manage and minimize hydronephrosis.

- Monitor intake and output. *This record provides information about kidney function and indicates any complications such as hydronephrosis.*
- Administer antibiotics as ordered. *Antimicrobials treat the cause of urinary tract infection associated with urolithiasis and urinary stasis.*
- Manage a nephrostomy tube by following Nursing Guidelines 58-1. *Proper management ensures that the*

NURSING GUIDELINES 58-1

Managing a Nephrostomy Tube

- Connect nephrostomy tube to a closed drainage system.
- Have a second nephrostomy tube available at the bedside for the physician's use in case the present one is displaced.
- Secure the tube to the client's flank with tape to ensure that it does not become dislodged.
- Keep the urine collection bag below the level of insertion.
- Never clamp the nephrostomy tubing.
- Check that the nephrostomy and drainage tubing are not kinked or that the client is not compressing the tubing.
- Use no more than 5 to 8 mL of sterile normal saline to maintain patency if an irrigation is medically ordered.
- Record the urine output from the nephrostomy tube separately from other urinary volumes.
- Assess the tube insertion site for bleeding and drainage.
- Change the dressing around the nephrostomy tube if and when it becomes damp. Apply a skin barrier ointment around the incision to prevent excoriation.
- Notify the physician immediately if the nephrostomy tube becomes dislodged or if there is an absence of urinary drainage.

nephrostomy tube remains in place, urine drains properly, and infection is prevented.

Risk for Infection related to urinary stasis

Expected Outcome: Urinary tract infection will not develop as evidenced by urine free of pus and microorganisms and normal temperature and white blood cell count.

- Administer antimicrobial therapy as prescribed. *Urinary tract infections potentiate stone formation. Antibiotics treat the infection.*
- Encourage fluid intake to 3000 mL/day unless contraindicated. *Increased hydration flushes bacteria, blood, and other debris, and may expedite stone passage.*
- Maintain patency of all catheters or encourage client to void every 2 to 3 hours. *Adequate urinary flow or frequent voiding prevents urinary stasis and eliminates bacteria, blood, and other particles.*
- Follow aseptic principles when changing dressings or urinary drainage equipment. *Strict asepsis prevents introduction of microbes into the urinary tract.*

Risk for Altered (Renal) Tissue Perfusion related to increased fluid pressure in ureter and kidney pelvis

Expected Outcome: Kidney will remain adequately perfused with blood as evidenced by normal serum creatinine, BUN, and distribution of radiopaque dye after IVP.

- Monitor laboratory and diagnostic test results. *Elevated BUN, creatinine, and electrolyte levels indicate kidney dysfunction and assist in evaluating hydration status and effectiveness of other interventions.*
- Prepare client safely but quickly for treatment measures that promote urinary drainage if it becomes apparent that kidney function is compromised. *Prompt intervention may prevent serious complications.*

Evaluation of Expected Outcomes

Pain is reduced. Urine output is balanced with intake. Urine is clear. The client is afebrile. Findings from urine and blood tests indicate adequate renal function.

For clients undergoing surgical procedures, explain the procedure and follow standards for perioperative care. After lithotripsy, endoscopy, or surgery, assess vital signs, measure fluid intake and output, and inspect the color of urine, which may be grossly bloody for a time. After ESWL, inspect the flank for ecchymosis, which is expected. Document the location of discoloration. Clients require analgesics for postprocedural discomfort.

If a ureteroscopy is performed and a urethral catheter is in place, attach the catheter to a closed drainage system. Pink-tinged urine may be seen, but if frank blood appears in the urine or the client complains of severe abdominal pain, notify the physician immediately. If a ureteral stent is present, check for the suture, which extends from the urinary meatus and is used for stent removal. It is important that the client maintain a total daily fluid volume of approximately 3000 mL. For more information, see Client and Family Teaching 58-1.

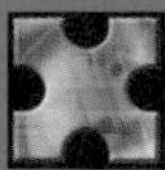

58-1 *Client and Family Teaching* Renal Calculi

The nurse includes the following recommendations when teaching the client and family:

- Explain the causes of and methods to prevent renal calculi.
- Recommend drinking plenty of liquids; water is one of the best.
- Provide a list of foods (Box 58-2) restricted to small amounts if the stones are composed of calcium oxalate.
- Review the self-administration of antimicrobial and analgesic drugs and, if prescribed, antigout medications. Discuss the purpose for the medications, dosing schedule, and side effects to report.
- Discuss catheter or nephrostomy tube care.
- Teach client how to strain urine if the stone or its fragments have not passed.
- Advise client to report signs of acute obstruction immediately, such as inability or difficulty in voiding, or pain.
- Identify signs of infection such as fever, chills, dysuria, frequency, urgency, and cloudy urine. Review the relationship between urinary calculi and infection.
- Provide discharge teaching after a treatment procedure that includes activity level, hygiene measures, dietary modifications, goals for oral fluid intake, and wound care.
- Emphasize consulting with the physician before self-administering any over-the-counter medications.

BOX 58-2 ● Sources of Calcium and Oxalate

Apples	Grapes
Asparagus	Ice cream
Beer	Milk
Beets	Oranges
Berries	Parsley
Black pepper	Peanut butter
Broccoli	Pineapples
Cheese	Rhubarb
Chocolate	Spinach
Cocoa	Swiss chard
Coffee	Tea
Cola	Turnips
Collards	Vitamin C
Figs	Yogurt

• URETERAL STRICTURE

A stricture is a narrowing of a lumen. A ureteral stricture is the narrowing of a ureter.

Pathophysiology and Etiology

A ureteral stricture is relatively rare, but incidence is higher among those with chronic ureteral stone formation. Recurrent inflammation and infection cause scar tissue to accumulate in the ureter. Other conditions that can interfere with urine passing through the ureter are congenital anomalies or conditions that mechanically compress the ureter, such as pregnancy or tumors in the abdomen or upper urinary tract.

In many instances the ureter is only partially narrowed. Symptoms develop over time as the area of the ureter above the stricture dilates with urine (*hydroureter*) and the kidney pelvis slowly enlarges. Stasis of urine promotes an upper urinary tract infection.

Assessment Findings

Flank pain or discomfort and tenderness at the costovertebral angle from enlargement of the renal pelvis often develops. The client experiences back or abdominal discomfort, which tends to increase during periods of elevated fluid intake. A voiding cystourethrogram and ultrasonography identify structural changes consistent with impaired passage of urine.

Medical and Surgical Management

Various measures are used to treat strictures. Management depends on location, density, and length of the stricture. The ureter can be stretched by inserting a dilator called a *filiform* or *urethral sound,* a curved metal rod, followed by others that are sequentially larger.

If obstruction persists, the physician performs a **ureteroplasty,** removal of the narrowed section of ureter and reconnection of the patent portions. This is the preferred procedure for a mid-ureteral stricture. A ureteral stent is placed in the ureter to provide support to the walls of the ureter, relieve obstruction, and maintain flow of urine through the ureter and into the bladder. Lower ureteral strictures are treated by removing the narrowed portion of the ureter and reimplanting the remaining section into the bladder wall.

Besides correcting strictures, ureteral surgery is done to remove tumors, repair accidental ligation of the ureter during abdominal surgery (the highest incidence is seen in hysterectomies), and to extricate a ureteral stone that cannot be removed by other means.

Nursing Management

Follow the standards of care for the perioperative client if the client undergoes surgery. If a ureteral catheter is inserted before surgery, measure the urine output from the catheter hourly. Immediately report lack of urine output from the ureteral catheter.

On return from surgery, all urinary drainage tubes and catheters are connected to a closed drainage system or to the type of drainage system ordered by the physician. The main complication associated with ureteral surgery is failure of the ureter to transport urine from the kidney to the bladder. Contact the physician if:

- Signs of shock appear.
- Urinary output from the ureteral catheter is decreased or absent.
- The client complains of significant abdominal pain, which may indicate leakage of urine into the peritoneal cavity.
- Signs of a urinary tract infection develop, such as fever and chills, or the urine is cloudy or has a foul odor.

Depending on the surgical procedure, instruct the client in the care of the ureteral or urethral catheter(s), the management of the drainage collection system, incision care, and a review of the prescribed diet and medication schedule.

TUMORS OF THE KIDNEY •

A *hypernephroma* (renal adenocarcinoma) is the most common malignant tumor of the kidney in adults. Squamous cell tumors are second. Men are affected more than women.

Pathophysiology and Etiology

The cause of kidney tumors is unknown. Incidence is higher in older adults, which suggests chronic exposure to a carcinogen whose metabolites involve renal excretion. Bladder cancer (see Chap. 59) is associated with carcinogenic effects of long-term cigarette smoking. It is possible that renal tumors are similarly initiated through this mechanism or exposure to some other environmental toxin (e.g., asbestos) or volatile solvent (e.g., gasoline). Box 58-3 lists risk factors for renal cancer.

Because kidneys are deeply protected in the body, tumors can become quite large before causing symptoms.

BOX 58-3 ● Risk Factors for Renal Cancer

- Gender: Affects men more than women
- Tobacco use
- Occupational exposure to industrial chemicals, such as petroleum products, heavy metals, and asbestos
- Obesity
- Unopposed estrogen therapy
- Polycystic kidney disease

As tumors enlarge, they occupy space, extending into adjacent renal structures and interfering with urine flow. Tumor cells tend to metastasize via the renal vein and vena cava to the lungs, bone, lymph nodes, liver, and brain. Lung metastases predominate. The first symptom may occur when the hypernephroma has metastasized to other organs.

Assessment Findings

The classic triad of renal cancer is painless hematuria, flank pain, and a palpable mass. Additional symptoms include weight loss, malaise, and unexplained fever. Later, there is colic-like discomfort during the passage of blood clots.

An abdominal mass found on a routine physical examination or on radiographic examination for other purposes suggests a kidney tumor. An IVP, cystoscopy with retrograde pyelograms, ultrasonography, MRI, renal angiography, and CT scan are used to locate the tumor. Sequential urine samples contain RBCs as well as malignant cells.

Medical and Surgical Management

Nephrectomy, including removal of the tumor, adrenal gland, surrounding perinephric fat, and fascia, is the treatment for a malignant renal tumor. When a tumor arises in the collecting system or the ureter, a complete nephroureterectomy (removal of the kidney and ureter) is done. A cuff of bladder tissue is removed as well because the recurrence rate in any stump of ureter left behind is high. Surgery may be followed by radiation therapy, chemotherapy, or both. If extensive metastases are found, only palliative treatment is given. When medical management is limited to palliative treatment because of metastases, the physician explains that the treatment measures are not curative.

Nursing Management

In addition to the standard preoperative preparations, implement other prescribed procedures that facilitate the postoperative assessment and recovery of the client, such as inserting a urethral catheter and nasogastric tube. On the client's return from surgery, assess vital signs frequently. Inspect and identify the type and location of drains or catheters. The indwelling (Foley) catheter drainage system is placed below the level of the bed. Drains in or around the incision may drain by closed negative pressure (i.e., Jackson-Pratt) or low mechanical suction.

Clients are at risk for internal hemorrhage related to bleeding from the ligated renal artery or vein. Decreased intravascular volume results in hypotension and tachycardia. Frequent monitoring assists in detecting changes in intravascular volume. Report decreased blood pressure, increased pulse, restlessness, or sudden onset of flank pain. Administer IV fluids and blood transfusions as ordered. Note and record the color of drainage from each tube and catheter. Contact the surgeon about any frank bleeding or a sudden decrease in urine output. Although pink-tinged drainage is normal for several days after surgery, frank bleeding, sudden decreased urine, or both indicate complications.

Administer prescribed analgesia and supplement drug therapy with nursing measures that promote comfort. Splint the incision when repositioning the client or during efforts to cough and deep breathe. This reduces tension on the surgical site and prevents or reduces pain-related movement.

Clients who have had a nephrectomy usually have the drains (if any) removed before discharge. A dressing over the incision may or may not be required. If the physician orders a dressing applied and changed at home, the nurse shows the client and family how to change the dressing and provides a list of the necessary materials for dressing changes (Client and Family Teaching 58-2).

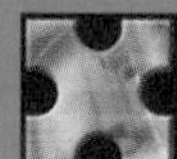

58-2 *Client and Family Teaching*
Home Care After Nephrectomy

The teaching plan should include the following:

- Change the dressing as ordered by the physician.
- Wash hands thoroughly before and after each dressing change.
- Drink plenty of fluids and follow the diet recommended by the physician.
- Avoid exposure to others who have possible infections.
- Take prescribed medication as directed on the container. Do not omit a dose.
- Contact the physician immediately if pain, fever, or chills occurs or if the urine becomes bloody, cloudy, or foul smelling.

RENAL FAILURE

Renal failure is inability of nephrons in the kidneys to maintain fluid, electrolyte, and acid-base balance; excrete nitrogen waste products; and perform regulatory functions such as maintaining calcification of bones and producing erythropoietin. There are two types of renal failure: acute and chronic. **Acute renal failure** (ARF) is characterized by sudden and rapid decrease in renal function. ARF potentially is reversible with early, aggressive treatment of its contributing etiology. **Chronic renal failure** (CRF) is characterized by progressive and irreversible damage to nephrons. It may take months to years for CRF to develop.

Pathophysiology and Etiology

Acute Renal Failure

Renal failure can develop as a consequence of prerenal, intrarenal, and postrenal disorders (Table 58.2). Prerenal disorders are nonurologic conditions that disrupt renal blood flow to the nephrons, affecting their filtering ability. Intrarenal conditions are conditions in the kidney itself that destroy nephrons. Postrenal disorders usually are obstructive problems in structures below the kidney(s) that have damaging repercussions for the nephrons above.

Acute renal failure progresses through four phases.

INITIATION PHASE. The initiation phase begins with onset of the contributing event. It is accompanied by reduced blood flow to nephrons to the point of acute tubular necrosis. **Acute tubular necrosis** refers to death of cells in collecting tubules of nephrons where reabsorption of water and electrolytes and excretion of protein wastes and excess metabolic substances occur.

OLIGURIC PHASE. The oliguric phase is associated with excretion of less than adequate urinary volumes. This phase begins within 48 hours after the initial cellular insult and may last for 10 to 14 days or longer (Porth, 2002). Fluid volume excess develops, leading to edema, hypertension, and cardiopulmonary complications. Azotemia, marked accumulation of urea and other nitrogenous wastes such as creatinine and uric acid in blood, creates potential for neurologic changes such as seizures, coma, and death.

Currently there is better treatment of many prerenal causes of ARF, so clients excrete urinary volumes greater than 500 mL/day. Urine has a very low specific gravity, because it lacks normal amounts of excreted substances such as excess potassium and hydrogen ions to maintain homeostasis. Hyperkalemia, metabolic acidosis, and **uremia,** a toxic state caused by accumulation of nitrogen wastes, develop regardless of excreted water volume.

DIURETIC PHASE. Diuresis begins as nephrons recover. Despite increased water content of urine, excretion of wastes and electrolytes continues to be impaired. The BUN, creatinine, potassium, and phosphate levels remain elevated in the blood.

RECOVERY PHASE. It may take 1 or more years of recovery while normal glomerular filtration and tubular function are restored. Some clients recover completely, whereas others develop varying degrees of permanent renal dysfunction.

Chronic Renal Failure

CRF is associated more often with intrarenal conditions or is a complication of systemic diseases such as diabetes mellitus and disseminated lupus erythematosus. In CRF, kidneys are so extensively damaged that they do not adequately remove protein byproducts and electrolytes from the blood and do not maintain acid-base balance. There are three stages of CRF:

- Reduced renal reserve—40% to 75% of nephron function is lost; client usually exhibits no symptoms.
- Renal insufficiency—75% to 90% of nephron function is lost; serum creatinine and BUN rise, with the

TABLE 58.2 CAUSES OF RENAL FAILURE

PRERENAL	INTRARENAL	POSTRENAL
Hypovolemic shock	Ischemia	Ureteral calculi
Cardiogenic shock secondary to congestive heart failure	Nephrotoxicity secondary to drugs such as aminoglycosides	Prostatic hypertrophy
Septic shock	Acute and chronic glomerulonephritis	Ureteral stricture
Anaphylaxis	Polycystic disease	Ureteral or bladder tumor
Dehydration	Untreated prerenal and postrenal disorders	
Renal artery thrombosis or stenosis	Myoglobinuria secondary to burns	
Cardiac arrest	Hemoglobinuria secondary to transfusion reaction	
Lethal dysrhythmias		

kidney losing its ability to concentrate urine and anemia developing. The client may report polyuria and nocturia.

- **End-stage renal disease**—less than 10% of nephron function remains. This is when a regular course of dialysis or kidney transplantation is necessary to maintain life, because kidney functions are severely impaired.

Because damage to nephrons is slow, declining renal function is less apparent until the end stage. The BUN and serum creatinine levels gradually rise. Hyponatremia is a reflection of diluted sodium ions in an excess volume of water in blood. Actual electrolyte imbalances include hyperkalemia, hyperphosphatemia, hypermagnesemia, and hypocalcemia. Skin becomes the excretory organ for substances the kidney usually clears from the body. A precipitate, referred to as **uremic frost,** may form on the skin.

Metabolic acidosis develops because tubules cannot convert carbonic acid in blood to water and bicarbonate ions. Erythropoietin production is inadequate, causing anemia. Susceptibility to infection increases as a result of a deficient immune system, particularly cellular immunity (see Chap. 35), as well as a decreased white blood cell count. Edema and hypertension are consequences of impaired urinary elimination. **Osteodystrophy,** a condition in which bones become demineralized, occurs from hypocalcemia and hyperphosphatemia. The parathyroid glands secrete more parathormone to raise blood calcium levels.

TABLE 58.3 SYSTEMIC COMPLICATIONS OF CHRONIC RENAL FAILURE

BODY SYSTEM	COMPLICATION
Cardiovascular	Congestive heart failure, hypertension, cardiac dysrhythmias, edema
Metabolic	Electrolyte imbalance, metabolic acidosis
Respiratory	Shortness of breath, pulmonary edema
Gastrointestinal	Malnutrition, vitamin deficiencies, anorexia, nausea, bleeding
Integumentary	Dry skin, pruritus
Neurologic	Lethargy, confusion, depression, seizures, coma
Sensory	Peripheral neuropathies
Musculoskeletal	Bone demineralization, muscle cramps, joint pain
Immunologic	Impaired immune function, decreased antibody production, increased incidence of hepatitis B and other infections

Assessment Findings

In both ARF and CRF, clients have elevated blood pressure and weight gain. Urine output usually is decreased. Those with CRF develop other symptoms as the disease worsens. Facial features appear puffy from fluid retention. Skin is pale. Ulceration and bleeding of the gastrointestinal tract may occur. Oral mucous membranes bleed, and blood may be found in feces. Clients report vague symptoms such as lethargy, headache, anorexia, and dry mouth. Later, other problems develop such as pruritus and dry, scaly skin. The breath and body may have an odor characteristic of urine. Muscle cramps, bone pain or tenderness, and spontaneous fractures can develop. Mental processes progressively slow as electrolyte imbalances become marked and nitrogenous wastes accumulate. The client may experience seizures. Table 58.3 lists the systemic manifestations of CRF.

Laboratory blood tests reveal elevations in BUN, creatinine, potassium, magnesium, and phosphorus. Calcium levels are low. RBC count, hematocrit, and hemoglobin are decreased. The pH of blood is on the acidotic side. Urinalysis reveals a decreased specific gravity. An IVP provides evidence of renal dysfunction. In clients with severe renal failure, dye excretion usually is delayed. A percutaneous renal biopsy shows destruction of nephrons. Radiography and ultrasonography demonstrate structural defects in kidneys, ureters, and bladder. Renal angiography identifies obstructions in blood vessels.

Medical Management

Prevention of ARF is an important function of physicians. Clients at risk for dehydration are adequately hydrated. Risks for dehydration include surgery, diagnostic studies that require fluid restriction and contrast agents, and treatment for cancer or metabolic disorders. Shock and hypotension are treated as quickly as possible with replacement fluids and blood. Treating infections promptly and thoroughly also is important, and greatly assists in preventing sepsis. Continuous monitoring of renal function is very important for clients at risk for ARF. Nurses are crucial in monitoring renal function, as well as preventing toxic drug effects (Smeltzer & Bare, 2004).

In ARF, treatment begins quickly to remedy the primary cause of renal failure. Renal damage can be limited by aggressive administration of parenteral fluids to increase plasma volume, vasodilating and diuretic drugs, and dopamine (Intropin) to improve cardiac output and perfuse the renal arteries.

To reduce complications and keep the client alive during the 2 or 3 weeks that the tubules are regenerating, hemodialysis (discussed later), a technique in which the blood is filtered externally with a machine, is done. When hemodialysis is a temporary measure, blood is removed and returned through a double-lumen catheter or twin central venous catheters (Fig. 58.4). Another option is

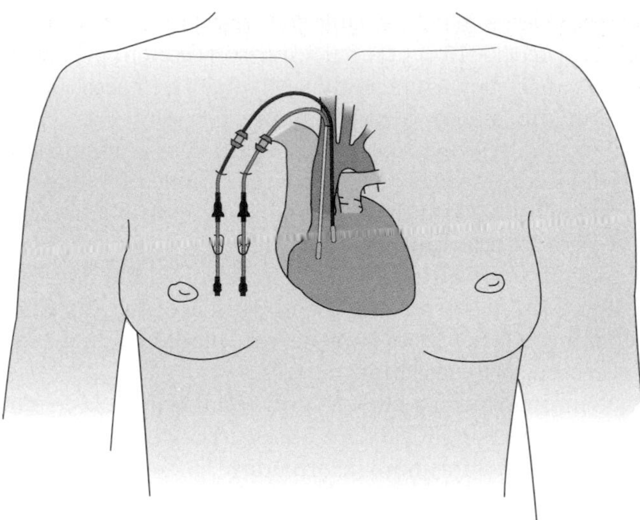

FIGURE 58.4 Twin catheters used for emergency hemodialysis.

peritoneal dialysis, a much slower process (discussed later) in which fluids and electrolytes are removed by osmosis and diffusion across the peritoneum, which acts as a semipermeable membrane.

Fluid and dietary restrictions that include low protein, high calories, low sodium, and low potassium are required as the client is stabilized. Sodium polystyrene sulfonate (Kayexalate), an ion-exchange resin, is prescribed for oral or rectal administration to remove excess potassium when hyperkalemia occurs. IV glucose and insulin also facilitate movement of potassium within the cell. Acid-base balance is restored by administering IV sodium bicarbonate if renal function is insufficient to do so.

Medical management of CRF is similar to that for ARF, except the period of treatment is lifelong (unless a kidney transplantation is performed). Rather than administer blood transfusions to correct chronic anemia, epoetin alfa (Epogen) is administered to stimulate bone marrow production of RBCs.

Surgical Management

Some clients in the end stage of CRF are candidates for kidney transplantation. One healthy kidney can perform the work of two. Donors for a transplant are selected from compatible living donors who may or may not be relatives or from organ donors who are brain dead and whose next of kin give permission for harvesting organs. Any potential donor with a history of hypertension, malignant disease, or diabetes is excluded from donation. To facilitate matching a recipient with a donor, a client is placed on a national computerized transplant waiting list. Whenever an organ becomes available, the computer searches for the recipient who is the best match.

When a transplantation is done, the donor kidney is inserted through an abdominal incision and the nonfunctioning kidneys are left in place unless the client is extremely hypertensive. The blood vessels from the donor kidney are sutured to the iliac artery and vein and the ureter is implanted in the bladder (Fig. 58.5).

A perfect match does not guarantee that a transplanted organ will not be rejected. Some less than perfectly matched transplanted organs are successful because of immunosuppressive drugs such as:

- azathioprine (Imuran)
- corticosteroids (prednisone)
- cyclosporine—available as a microemulsion (Neoral), which provides a more sustained concentration
- tacrolimus (Prograf; formerly FK-506)—similar to cyclosporine but more potent

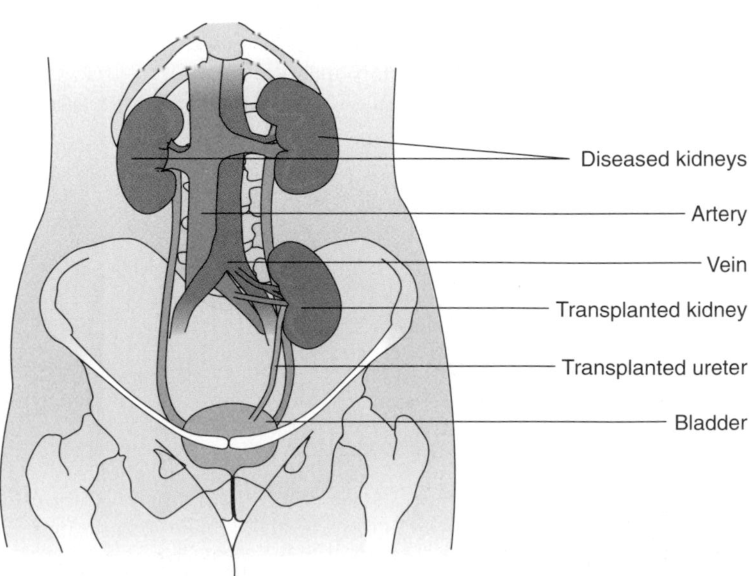

FIGURE 58.5 Transplanted kidney and ureter.

- mycophenolate mofetil (CellCept; formerly RS-61433)—specifically for preventing kidney transplant rejection (Smeltzer & Bare, 2004)
- muromonab-CD-3 (Orthoclone OKT3)—a monoclonal antibody

If rejection occurs, the client resumes hemodialysis and waits for another transplant.

Nursing Management

Before conducting an initial interview and physical assessment, attempt to learn the cause (if known), type (acute versus chronic), and prognosis of the renal disorder. Clients may be unable to give an accurate history because of the effect of renal failure on thought processes or because they are acutely ill. It may be necessary to obtain information from the family. Nursing care for the client undergoing renal transplantation is complex and specialized. Standard postoperative nursing interventions are applicable, with the added consideration of assessing for signs of rejection and prevention of infection. Signs and symptoms of transplant rejection include oliguria, edema, fever, increasing blood pressure, weight gain, swelling or tenderness over the transplanted kidney, and increased serum creatinine levels.

Nursing care for clients with renal failure is extensive. See Nursing Care Plan 58-1 and Client and Family Teaching 58-3 for more information.

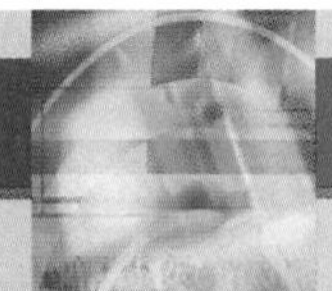

Nursing Care Plan 58-1

THE CLIENT WITH CHRONIC RENAL FAILURE

Assessment

- Assess fluid status, including problems related to imbalanced intake and output.
- Monitor nutritional status, making sure the client follows the appropriate restrictions.
- Assess emotional status to provide relevant support.

Nursing Diagnosis: **Excess Fluid Volume** related to impaired renal function

Expected Outcome: Client will maintain appropriate body weight without excess fluid.

Interventions	*Rationales*
Weigh client daily under the same conditions: time, clothing, scale.	Information provides a baseline and database for monitoring changes. A gain of 1 kg (2.2 lb) equals 1 L of fluid.
Record output accurately.	Output determines intake. Usually, client is allowed 500 mL intake (equals insensible fluid losses) plus the volume of excreted urine per day.
Assess lung sounds, respiratory rate and effort, and heart sounds. Inspect for jugular vein distention.	Findings provide a baseline and database to determine fluid volume excess, needed interventions, and effects of treatments. Fluid overload may cause pulmonary edema.
Monitor laboratory studies.	Results assist in identifying fluid excess and promote earlier interventions.
Administer prescribed diuretics and antihypertensives.	These drugs reduce fluid excess and decrease cardiac workload.
Prepare client for dialysis.	Dialysis reduces uremic toxins, corrects electrolyte imbalances, and decreases fluid overload.

Evaluation of Expected Outcome: Client demonstrates appropriate urine output/fluid balance as evidenced by stable weight, vital signs within normal range for the client, no edema, and only slightly elevated electrolyte levels.

Nursing Diagnosis: **Imbalanced Nutrition: Risk for Less than Body Requirements** related to anorexia, increased metabolic needs, and dietary restrictions

Expected Outcome: Client will maintain adequate nutritional intake.

(continued)

Nursing Care Plan 58-1 (Continued)

THE CLIENT WITH CHRONIC RENAL FAILURE

Interventions	Rationales
Monitor and record client's dietary intake.	Findings provide a database for nutritional changes and effects of interventions.
Provide frequent small feedings.	They minimize nausea and anorexia and promote the intake of high-calorie, nutritious foods.
Encourage client to be involved with food choices and times for meals.	Involving the client promotes interest and control and considers dietary habits and preferences.
Explain restrictions and provide a list of nutritional needs and acceptable food choices.	Doing so promotes client's understanding of the relationship of food intake to kidney disease and provides a positive approach to dietary restrictions.

Evaluation of Expected Outcome: Client maintains weight, unrelated to fluid volume, following dietary needs and restrictions.

PCs: **Hypertension, Azotemia, Electrolyte Imbalances, Anemia**

Expected Outcome: Nurse will minimize and manage potential complications.

Interventions	Rationales
Administer prescribed antihypertensive and diuretic medications as ordered.	They lower blood pressure and increase urine output from partially functional kidneys.
Restrict protein intake to foods that are complete proteins (contain all essential amino acids) within prescribed limits.	Complete proteins provide positive nitrogen balance needed for healing and growth.
Provide sufficient calories from carbohydrates and fats.	Doing so prevents catabolism of muscle and body stores of protein.
Monitor cardiac rhythm.	Hyperkalemia and other electrolyte imbalances can cause dangerous dysrhythmias.
Restrict sources of potassium usually found in fresh fruits and vegetables.	Hyperkalemia can cause life-threatening changes.
Be prepared to administer glucose and regular insulin.	They promote transfer of potassium from extracellular to intracellular locations.
Restrict sodium intake as ordered.	Doing so prevents excess sodium and fluid accumulation.
Administer calcium supplements, vitamin D supplements, and phosphate binders (Amphogel); at same time, limit phosphorus-containing foods such as dairy products, dried beans, and soft drinks.	CRF causes numerous physiologic changes that affect calcium, phosphorus, and vitamin D metabolism, requiring supplementation and dietary restrictions.
Administer prescribed iron and folic acid supplements or Epogen.	Iron and folic acid supplements are needed for RBC production. Epogen stimulates bone marrow to produce RBCs.

Evaluation of Expected Outcome: Blood pressure is 140/90 mm Hg. BUN and creatinine levels are slightly elevated. Serum electrolyte levels are minimally elevated. RBC and hemoglobin levels are within normal levels.

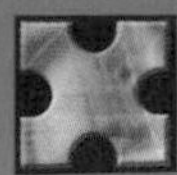

58-3 *Client and Family Teaching* The Client With Chronic Renal Failure

Develop a teaching plan based on the following:

- Follow the diet and fluid intake recommended by the physician. Do not use salt substitutes (which often contain potassium) unless allowed by the physician.
- Take medications exactly as prescribed by the physician.
- Do not use any nonprescription drug unless use is approved by the physician.
- Measure and record fluid intake and urine output. Limit fluids as recommended.
- Avoid exposure to those with any type of infection (e.g., colds, sore throats, flu).
- Monitor blood pressure as recommended by the physician.
- Keep skin clean and dry. Take brief showers with tepid water, pat skin to dry, use moisturizing lotions or creams like Eucerin, Nivea, Alpha Keri, or Lubriderm. Avoid scratching.
- When doing laundry, use a mild laundry detergent. Use an extra rinse cycle to remove all detergent or add 1 tsp of vinegar per quart of water to the rinse cycle to remove detergent residue.
- Keep a record of daily weight, and report any rapid weight gain to the physician.
- Take frequent rest periods; avoid heavy exercise.
- If any of the following occurs, contact the physician immediately: inability to urinate, slow decrease in daily urine output, weight gain (more than 5 lb or amount recommended by physician), chills, fever, sore throat, cough, blood in the urine or stool, easy bleeding or bruising, lethargy, extreme fatigue, persistent headache, nausea, vomiting, or diarrhea.

Stop, Think, and Respond ● BOX 58-2

Clients who have a kidney transplant are at risk for infection. What nursing measures help to prevent infection?

DIALYSIS

Dialysis is a procedure for cleaning and filtering blood. It substitutes for kidney function when kidneys cannot remove nitrogenous waste products and maintain adequate fluid, electrolyte, and acid-base balances.

During dialysis, the client's blood is filtered by diffusion and osmosis. Substances such as water, urea, creatinine, and dangerously high levels of potassium move from blood through the semipermeable membrane to the **dialysate,** the solution used during dialysis that has a composition similar to normal human plasma. Dialysis is performed by hemodialysis and peritoneal dialysis. Either technique can be done at home or in a dialysis center. Each type has advantages and disadvantages (Table 58.4).

● HEMODIALYSIS

Hemodialysis requires transporting blood from the client through a **dialyzer,** a semipermeable membrane filter in a machine (Fig. 58.6). The dialyzer contains many tiny hollow fibers. Blood moves through hollow fibers. Water and wastes from the blood move into the dialysate fluid that flows around the fibers, but protein and RBCs do not (see Fig. 58.6). Filtered blood is returned to the client. The entire cycle takes 4 to 6 hours and is done three times a week.

There are several methods for facilitating removal and return of the client's dialyzed blood. One technique uses tunneled central venous catheter access. Two others more commonly used for clients with CRF are (1) arteriovenous (AV) fistula and (2) AV graft.

An **arteriovenous fistula** is a surgical anastomosis (connection) of an artery and vein lying in close proximity (Fig. 58.7). Fistulas are preferred over grafts because there are fewer complications.

An **arteriovenous graft** is a type of vascular access method that uses a tube of synthetic material (e.g., Gore-Tex or polytetrafluoroethylene) to connect a vein and artery in the upper or lower arm (see Fig. 58.7). The graft pulsates with blood flow. AV grafts can be used 14 days after their insertion. Although the graft reseals after each needle puncture, the expected life of the graft is 3 to 5 years with repeated use.

Nursing Management

Assess and record vital signs before and after hemodialysis as well as weighing the client and obtaining blood for laboratory testing. To prepare for vascular access:

TABLE 58.4 COMPARISON OF HEMODIALYSIS AND PERITONEAL DIALYSIS

TYPE OF DIALYSIS	ADVANTAGES	DISADVANTAGES
Hemodialysis	Rapid removal of solutes and water Takes less time No risk for peritonitis Personnel perform procedure in a dialysis center	Bulge from fistula or graft is obvious Risk for vascular complications, infection, distal ischemia, carpal tunnel syndrome, hypotension, and disequilibrium Strict fluid and dietary restrictions Lifestyle cycles around dialysis appointments Home hemodialysis requires space for the machine and training to use it
Peritoneal	Simple to perform Facilitates independence Easier access No anticoagulation Fewer problems with hypotension or disequilibrium Less rigid dietary and fluid restrictions More flexibility in lifestyle and activities	More time-consuming Weight gain from glucose in the dialysate Peritonitis is a potential complication Requires training and motivation

- Inspect the skin over the fistula or graft for signs of infection.
- Palpate for a **thrill** (vibration) over the vascular access or listens for a **bruit,** a loud sound caused by turbulent blood flow. If absent, postpone further use and report findings.
- Note color of skin and nailbeds and mobility of fingers.
- Wash the skin over the fistula or graft with soap and water or antiseptic.
- Avoid puncturing the same site that was used previously.
- After dialysis is done, do not administer injections for 2 to 4 hours. This allows time for metabolism and excretion of heparin, which is administered during dialysis, to reach safe levels.
- Before discharging the client, observe for disequilibrium syndrome.

Disequilibrium syndrome is a neurologic condition believed to be caused by cerebral edema. Shift in cerebral fluid volume occurs when concentrations of solutes in blood are lowered rapidly during dialysis. Decreasing solute concentration lowers plasma osmolality. Water then floods brain tissue. The syndrome is characterized by headache, disorientation, restlessness, blurred vision, confusion, and seizures. Symptoms are self-limiting and disappear within several hours after dialysis as fluid

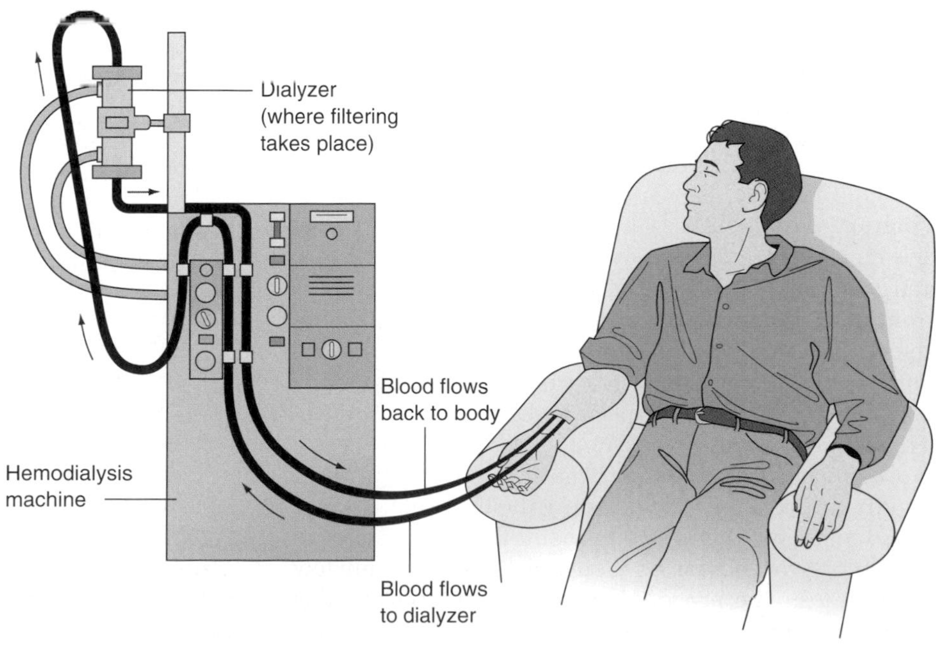

FIGURE 58.6 Hemodialysis machine and dialyzer.

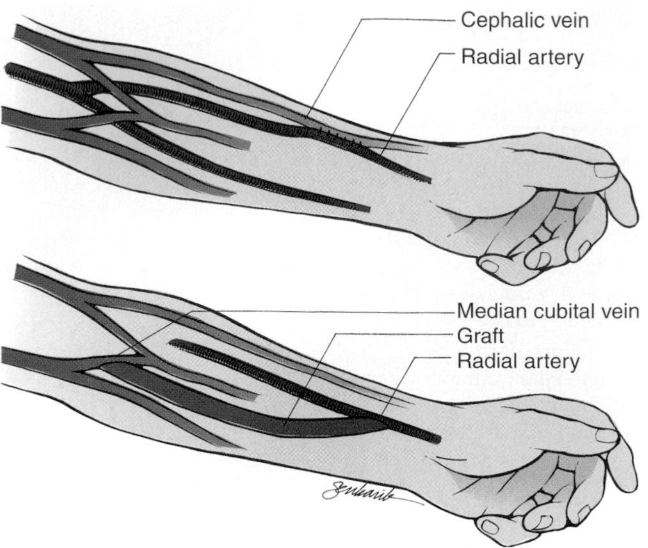

FIGURE 58.7 An internal arteriovenous fistula (*top*) is created by a side-to-side anastomosis of the artery and vein. A graft (*bottom*) can also be established between the artery and vein.

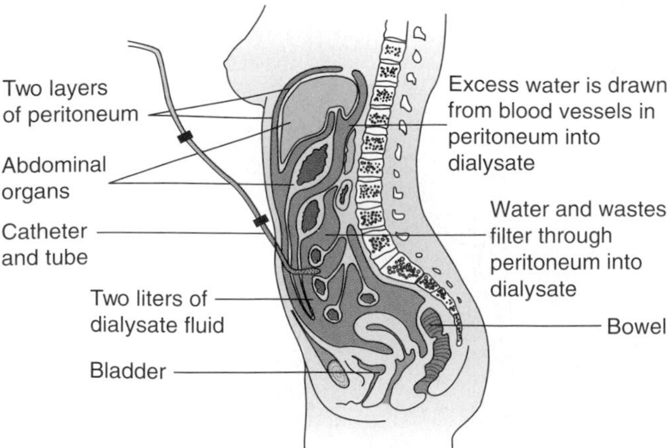

FIGURE 58.8 Peritoneal dialysis.

and solute concentrations equalize. The syndrome can be prevented by slowing the dialysis process to allow time for gradual equilibration of water.

Teach the client undergoing hemodialysis the following:

- Avoid carrying heavy items in the arm with the fistula or graft.
- Wear clothing with loose sleeves or made of fabrics that will not obstruct blood flow.
- Do not sleep on the vascular access arm.
- Do not permit venipunctures, injections, or blood pressures in the arm with the vascular access.
- Wash the skin over the vascular access daily.
- Assess for a thrill or bruit daily.
- Report signs of an infection or signs of impaired blood flow to dialysis personnel or physician immediately.

• PERITONEAL DIALYSIS

Peritoneal dialysis uses the peritoneum, the semipermeable membrane lining the abdomen, to filter fluid, wastes, and chemicals (Fig. 58.8). Dialysate is instilled and drained from the abdominal cavity by means of a catheter. Substances pass from tiny blood vessels in the peritoneal membrane into the dialysate. The catheter, which has many perforations, is sutured in place and a dressing is applied. There are three types of peritoneal dialysis.

Continuous ambulatory peritoneal dialysis (CAPD) uses gravity for instilling and draining the dialysate. It takes approximately 40 minutes to instill fluid. The solution dwells for 4 to 6 hours and then drains for approximately 40 minutes. The process is repeated four times a day continuously.

With *continuous cyclic peritoneal dialysis (CCPD)*, a machine is connected to the dialysis catheter. It automatically fills and drains dialysate from the abdomen when the person sleeps.

Intermittent peritoneal dialysis (IPD) is done with the same type of machine as used for CCPD, but the process occurs periodically, with perhaps several days between dialysis treatments. Sessions may last 24 hours. Total time spent on IPD is between 36 and 42 hours per week.

Nursing Management

Obtain and review laboratory test findings before dialysis and record vital signs and weight. If the client is acutely ill, it may be necessary to use a bed scale. It also may be necessary to weigh the client as often as every 8 hours while the procedure is in progress. Peritonitis is a major complication of peritoneal dialysis. Monitor and report fever, nausea, vomiting, and severe abdominal pain, rigidity, or tenderness before, during, or after dialysis.

Stop, Think, and Respond ● BOX 58-3

Consider why a client may not be a good candidate for CAPD.

When a client performs peritoneal dialysis at home, provide the following information:

- Keep dialysis supplies in a clean area away from children and pets.
- Avoid using dialysate solutions that are expired or look cloudy, discolored, or contain sediment.
- Wash hands before handling the catheter.
- Prevent infection by using sterile gloves during cleaning and exchanges of dialysate.
- Wear a mask when performing exchanges if you have an upper respiratory infection.
- Clean the catheter insertion site daily with an antiseptic.

- Inspect the catheter insertion site for signs of infection.
- Keep the catheter stabilized to the abdomen above the belt line to avoid constant rubbing.
- Avoid using scissors during dressing changes to prevent puncturing or cutting the catheter.
- Call the physician if:
  - A fever develops
  - There is redness, pain, or pus draining around the catheter
  - The external length of the catheter increases
  - Nausea, vomiting, or abdominal pain develop

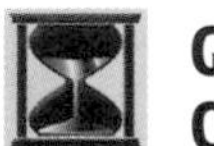

GENERAL GERONTOLOGIC CONSIDERATIONS

Acute glomerulonephritis in the older adult usually occurs in those with pre-existing chronic glomerulonephritis. Symptoms in the older adult are subtle and may go undetected.

Urinary obstruction is the most common cause of pyelonephritis in the older adult. When present, the older adult may not experience the fever and difficulty voiding common in younger adults.

The older adult is at high risk for acute renal failure because of a decline in the glomerular filtration rate, loss of nephrons, and reduced glomeruli. Although the aging kidney can recover from acute renal failure, survival rates are only approximately 50%.

Elderly clients often have slightly abnormal renal function test results. Mild abnormalities are caused by the aging process and usually are of no clinical significance.

Elderly clients usually are not considered candidates for kidney transplants, but may be able to use CAPD. Supervision of the procedure by a family member may be necessary. More frequent monitoring of the client's progress is required when this technique is used.

Critical Thinking Exercises

1. *A client with a ureteral stone is experiencing severe pain. Another nurse believes the client has a low pain tolerance. What action is appropriate at this time? Why?*
2. *A client who had a left nephrectomy is having discomfort when coughing, deep breathing, and changing positions. What nursing measures could relieve her discomfort?*
3. *If you had CRF and must decide to have either hemodialysis or peritoneal dialysis when end-stage disease develops, explain which choice you would make and the reasons for that choice.*

● NCLEX-STYLE REVIEW QUESTIONS 

1. A woman brings her 10-year-old son to the clinic. She reports that the boy has smoky-colored urine, a fever, and a puffy face; he also has not urinated for 12 hours. Which follow-up question from the nurse is most appropriate?
   1. "Has your son had a recent injury to the abdomen?"
   2. "Has your son had strep throat in the past 3 weeks?"
   3. "Has your son been taking aspirin?"
   4. "Has your son had any tick or mosquito bites?"
2. A client is being admitted to the hospital for treatment and management of renal calculi. The nurse orients the client to his room and surroundings. Which instructions should the nurse include?
   1. "Save and strain all of your urine."
   2. "Request medication if pain is unbearable."
   3. "Don't drink anything until the physician visits you."
   4. "Be sure to lie on your left side."
3. A client with chronic renal failure receives hemodialysis treatment every 2 days. The morning of a scheduled treatment, the nurse assesses the arteriovenous graft for patency. Which assessment finding requires further evaluation?
   1. Absence of a thrill or bruit
   2. Capillary refill less than 3 seconds
   3. Bruising at the puncture site
   4. A bulge in the forearm

connection

Visit the Connection site at **http://connection.lww.com/go/timbyEssentials** for links to chapter-related resources on the Internet.

References and Suggested Readings

Astle, S. M. (2001). A new direction for dialysis. *RN, 64*(7), 56–60.

Bullock, B. L., & Henze, R. L. (2000). *Focus on pathophysiology.* Philadelphia: Lippincott Williams & Wilkins.

Campbell, D. (2003). How acute renal failure puts the brakes on kidney function. *Nursing 2003, 33*(1), 59–63.

Hayes, D. D. (2003). Performing peritoneal dialysis. *Nursing 2003, 33*(3), 17.

Innes, C. P. (2001). An overlooked option for renal patients. *RN, 64*(9), 29–32.

Kaplow, R., & Barry, R. (2002). Continuous renal replacement therapies. *American Journal of Nursing, 102*(11), 26–29.

Kear, T. M. (April 15, 2002). *Advance for Nurses,* 31–32.

King, B. (2000). Meds and the dialysis patient. *RN, 63*(7), 54–60.

Lehman, S., & Dietz, C. A. (2002). Double-J stents: They're not trouble free. *RN, 65*(1), 54–59.

McConnell, E. A. (2002). Protecting a hemodialysis fistula. *Nursing 2002, 32*(11), 18.

McConnell, E. A. (2001). Clinical do's and don'ts: Preventing nosocomial urinary tract infections. *Nursing 2001, 31*(5), 17.

McConnell, E. A. (2001). Myths & facts . . . about kidney stones. *Nursing 2001, 31*(1), 73.

Porth, C. M. (2002). *Pathophysiology: Concepts of altered health states* (6th ed.). Philadelphia: Lippincott Williams & Wilkins.

Smeltzer, S. C., & Bare, B. G. (2004). *Brunner & Suddarth's textbook of medical–surgical nursing* (10th ed.). Philadelphia: Lippincott Williams & Wilkins.

Weil, C. M. (2000). Exploring hope in patients with end stage renal disease on chronic hemodialysis. *Nephrology Nursing Journal, 27,* 219–224.

Young, J. (2000). Actionstat: Kidney stone. *Nursing 2000, 30*(7), 33.

chapter 59

Caring for Clients With Disorders of the Bladder and Urethra

Words to Know 

cystectomy
cystitis
cystostomy
diverticulum
fulguration
incontinence
litholapaxy
neurogenic bladder
residual urine
retention
stricture
urethritis
urethroplasty
urinary diversion
urosepsis

Learning Objectives

On completion of this chapter, the reader will:

- Differentiate urinary retention and urinary incontinence.
- Discuss nursing management of a client with urinary retention and incontinence.
- Describe pathophysiologic changes seen in cystitis, interstitial cystitis, and urethritis.
- Discuss the cause and treatment of urethral strictures.
- Identify the most common early symptom of a malignant tumor of the bladder.
- Describe various types of urinary diversion procedures.
- Identify components of a teaching plan for a client having a urinary diversion procedure.

Disorders of the bladder and urethra are common and can be the source of severe problems that become chronic, altering a client's lifestyle. Many disorders affecting the bladder and urethra are treated on an outpatient basis; more serious disorders require hospitalization.

VOIDING DYSFUNCTION

Urinary **retention** is inability to urinate or effectively empty the bladder. Urinary **incontinence** is inability to control voiding of urine. Clients experiencing either retention or incontinence face temporary or permanent alterations in their ability to urinate normally.

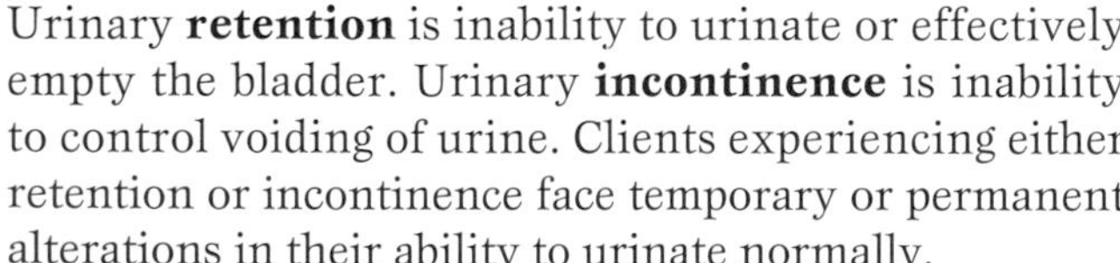

• URINARY RETENTION

Pathophysiology and Etiology

Urinary retention may be either acute or chronic. Acute urinary retention is seen in complete urethral obstruction, after general anesthesia, or with administration of certain drugs such as atropine or a phenothiazine. Chronic urinary retention often is seen in clients with disorders such as prostatic enlargement or neurologic disorders resulting in a **neurogenic bladder** (a bladder that does not receive adequate nerve stimulation).

The client with acute urinary retention usually cannot void at all. The client with chronic urinary retention may be able to void but does not completely empty the bladder (retention with overflow). **Residual urine** is urine retained in the bladder after the client voids. Amounts may vary from 30 mL to several hundred milliliters.

Assessment Findings

Symptoms of acute urinary retention are sudden inability to void, distended bladder, and severe lower abdominal pain and discomfort. Chronic urinary retention may produce no symptoms because the bladder has stretched over time and accommodates large volumes without producing discomfort. The overstretched bladder does not contract effectively, and the client is unaware that the bladder is not emptying completely. If the amount of residual urine is large, the client may void frequently in small amounts. Signs of a bladder infection (e.g., fever, chills, pain on urination) and dribbling of urine also may be present.

Urinalysis may show an increased number of white blood cells, indicating an acute or chronic bladder infection. Catheterization or ultrasound can determine post-void residual volume.

Medical and Surgical Management

Acute urinary retention requires immediate catheterization. If a catheter cannot be inserted through the urethra, special urologic instruments that dilate the urethra may be used.

Chronic retention is managed by permanent drainage with a urethral catheter, suprapubic **cystostomy** tube (a catheter inserted through the abdominal wall directly into the bladder), or clean intermittent catheterization (CIC). Permanent catheterization of the bladder carries risk of bladder stones, renal disease, bladder infection, and **urosepsis,** a serious systemic infection from microorganisms in the urinary tract invading the bloodstream. Because incidence of complications is lower, CIC is the preferred treatment. Other methods, particularly for clients who lack nervous system control secondary to disease or injury, are to use Credé voiding or abdominal strain (Valsalva voiding). Box 59-1 describes these methods. CIC may not be possible for clients who lack the mobility or cognitive functioning to perform the procedure. Some male clients who cannot perform CIC can avoid complications of permanent indwelling catheters by undergoing surgery to release the urethral sphincters. Urine then drains freely out the urethra and the client wears a condom catheter. If it is possible to remove the cause, such as excising excess prostatic tissue, surgery is done, although it does not always result in restoration of normal voiding.

External collection systems for women are available but proper fit is a problem. Women who cannot accomplish CIC usually are treated with a permanent indwelling catheter.

BOX 59-1 ● Credé or Valsalva Voiding

CREDÉ

Apply gentle downward pressure to the bladder during voiding. This maneuver may be done by the client or family member. The client also may do this by sitting on the toilet and rocking back and forth gently.

VALSALVA

Instruct the client to bear down as with defecation. Do not teach this method to a client with cardiac problems or who may be adversely affected by a vagal response (heart rate slows).

Nursing Management

The conscious client is able to verbalize pain and discomfort associated with urinary retention. Clients with Alzheimer's disease or psychiatric disorders, or comatose, anesthetized, or spinal cord-injured clients, may be unable to communicate or feel pain and discomfort. Important nursing responsibilities are measuring intake and output, palpating the abdomen for a distended bladder, promoting complete urination, and monitoring the voiding pattern of clients.

Stop, Think, and Respond ● BOX 59-1

If the priority nursing diagnosis for a client with urinary retention is ***Urinary Retention*** *related to high urethral pressure secondary to prostate enlargement, which of the following is a priority nursing intervention?*

1. *Obtain a history from client about duration of this problem.*
2. *Ask client if he has any problems with bowel elimination.*
3. *Initiate a bladder log, which includes information about urine output and fluid intake.*
4. *Catheterize client to relieve a full bladder and to measure urine output*

Acute Urinary Retention

Acute retention that is likely to resolve quickly (e.g., after anesthesia) probably will be treated by intermittent catheterization. Clients with acute retention unlikely to resolve without surgical intervention (e.g., retention caused by an enlarged prostate) probably will have an indwelling catheter.

Collaborate with the physician to determine (1) if the catheter is to be left in place or removed after the bladder is emptied, and (2) the size and type of catheter to be used. Catheters are sized according to the French system (e.g., 14 F to 24 F); the higher the number, the larger the diameter of the catheter. Examples of the various types of catheter tips are shown in Figure 59.1.

Clients with an obstruction may be more easily catheterized with a coudé catheter. The curved tip slides over obstructing tissue more readily than a straight-tipped catheter. Select the appropriate catheter and insert it under sterile conditions, noting characteristics and volume of urine returned. If the volume is large (> 700 mL), it may be necessary to clamp the catheter before the bladder has emptied completely to prevent bladder spasms or loss of bladder tone. This practice varies, so it is important to check agency policy.

If the client is going to be managed by CIC, the client and nurse establish the schedule. Clients are catheterized every 4 to 6 hours depending on the amount of urine

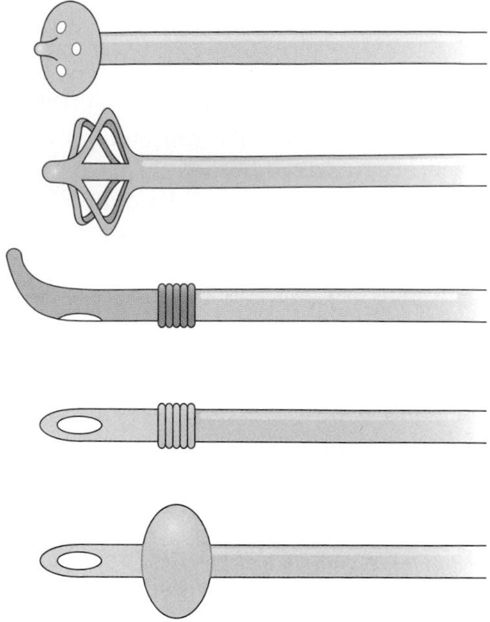

FIGURE 59.1 Catheter tips (top to bottom): de Pezzer catheter, Malecot catheter, coudé catheter, Foley catheter, Foley catheter with balloon inflated. The de Pezzer and the Malecot catheters are inserted by the physician with a stylet that temporarily straightens the tip. The Foley and coudé catheters are retained by inflating the balloon.

obtained and fluid intake. The bladder should not be allowed to get distended beyond 350 mL because bladder overdistention results in loss of bladder tone, decreased blood flow to the bladder, and reduction in the layer of mucin that protects the bladder mucosa. CIC continues until the postvoid residual volume is less than 30 mL. To obtain accurate residual volumes, it is important that clients have the opportunity to void first and that catheterization occur immediately after the attempt. Record both the volume voided (even if it is zero) and the volume obtained by catheterization. Postoperative urinary retention usually resolves within 24 to 48 hours.

Chronic Urinary Retention

Chronic urinary retention may go unrecognized. During an initial health assessment, ask clients about voiding frequency, amount (e.g., small, moderate, large) of urine passed each time, presence of pain or discomfort in the lower abdomen, pain or discomfort on voiding, and difficulty in starting the urinary stream. Gently palpate or percuss the lower abdomen to determine if the bladder is distended. In addition, obtain a complete medical, drug, and allergy history and report suspected chronic urinary retention to the physician.

Intermittent Catheterization

Intermittent catheterization performed in the hospital setting is a sterile procedure. When performed by clients or family members in the home, clean rather than aseptic technique is used. A commercially prepared straight catheterization kit is available in hospitals that includes a straight-tipped catheter, sterile gloves, lubricant and a sterile collection container. At home, the client uses a red rubber catheter that can be washed and reused for 2 to 3 months before replacing. Gloves are not required, but clients must wash their hands thoroughly before and after the procedure. The client can drain urine into a clean container or directly into the toilet bowl.

The schedule is usually three to four times per day, although frequency can be increased depending on residual volume. If more than 400 mL is returned, the client should be catheterized more often. Client education in technique, catheter care, and follow-up care is an important function of the nurse both in acute and home care settings.

Indwelling Catheters

A urethral indwelling catheter is one route for permanent bladder catheterization. A cystostomy tube, also called a *suprapubic catheter,* is inserted through an abdominal incision into the bladder. Clients require catheter care, including careful cleansing of the urethral meatus or cystostomy site and proximal catheter, maintenance of the integrity of the closed drainage system, proper anchoring of the tube to avoid tension and promote drainage, and scheduled changes of the catheter and drainage system according to facility policy.

Stop, Think, and Respond ● BOX 59-2

What methods should nurses use to prevent nosocomial infections in catheterized clients? 

● URINARY INCONTINENCE

Urinary incontinence affects many clients and is a major healthcare concern. It is estimated that at least one third of older adults living in the community and one half of older clients in institutions suffer from incontinence. Not only is incontinence a psychosocial problem, it is a physical problem in that skin breakdown and urinary tract infection may result from incontinence.

Pathophysiology and Etiology

Urinary incontinence may result from either bladder or urethral dysfunction (or both). The bladder can contract without warning, fail to accommodate adequate volumes of urine, or fail to empty completely and become overstretched, resulting in overflow incontinence. These conditions result from neurologic disease, bladder outlet obstruction, or trauma in all clients; bladder prolapse or low estrogen levels in women; and prostatic enlargement in men.

Another cause of incontinence is failure of the urethral sphincters to hold urine in the bladder. This may result from trauma, prostate surgery, or relaxed pelvic muscles. Impingement of the spinal nerves, such as in spinal cord tumors or injuries or herniated disks, can interfere with the impulse conduction to the brain, resulting in a neurogenic bladder and incontinence. A neurogenic bladder may be spastic, causing incontinence, or it may be flaccid, causing retention.

Assessment Findings

Clients complain of urgency, frequency, leaking small amounts when coughing or sneezing, or complete inability to control urine, depending on the underlying cause. Tests such as a urine culture and sensitivity, cystoscopy, or urodynamics determine the type of incontinence.

Medical and Surgical Management

Treatment aims at correcting the disorder causing incontinence (when possible), providing medication to control incontinence, correcting situational problems that contribute to functional incontinence, or instituting a bladder retraining program. Pharmacologic agents that can improve bladder retention, emptying, and control include drugs such as oxybutynin chloride (Ditropan), which reduces bladder spasticity and involuntary bladder contractions, and phenoxybenzamine hydrochloride (Dibenzaline), which may be useful in treating problems with sphincter control. Bethanechol (Urecholine) helps to increase contraction of the detrusor muscle, which assists with emptying of the bladder. Sometimes medication to control incontinence results in retention and must be discontinued. Occasionally clients who can easily perform CIC may opt for medication-induced retention and CIC because it allows them to stay dry.

Surgeries to improve urinary control include:

- Bladder augmentation—a procedure that increases the storage capacity of the bladder
- Implantation of an artificial sphincter that can be inflated to prevent urine loss and deflated to allow urination (Fig. 59.2)
- Surgeries to provide better support for urinary structures
- Urethroplasty—surgery to repair structures damaged by trauma

Nursing Management

Goals when caring for a client with urinary incontinence include maintaining continence as much as possible, preventing skin breakdown, reducing anxiety, and initiating a bladder-training program. Determine if the client is truly incontinent or if situations prevent the client from getting to the bathroom. Such situations include impaired mobility, physical restraints, and use of sedatives. In addition to assessing for functional causes of incontinence, obtain details regarding the pattern of incontinence and use of medications that may play a role in the problem. Assess for skin breakdown and determine methods the client has used to manage incontinence.

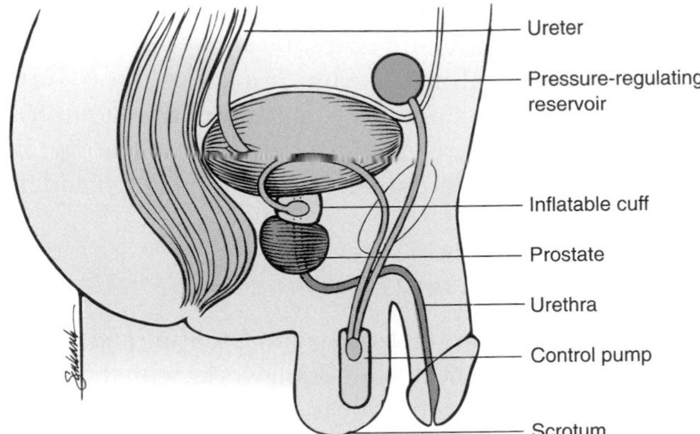

FIGURE 59.2 Artificial urinary sphincter. An inflatable cuff is inserted surgically around the urethra or bladder neck. To empty the bladder, the cuff is deflated by squeezing the control pump located in the scrotum.

Instruction centers on exercises to increase muscle tone and voluntary control (Kegel exercises), techniques to assist bladder emptying, and bladder training. Success of a bladder-training program depends not only on the cause of incontinence, but on the motivation of the client and the amount of skillful help and encouragement received from the healthcare team.

Bladder Training

One method of bladder training for the client with an indwelling urethral catheter is to alternately clamp and unclamp the catheter, which begins to re-establish normal bladder function and capacity. In the beginning, the catheter may be unclamped for 5 minutes every 1 or 2 hours. The length of time is gradually increased to every 3 or 4 hours, giving the bladder a chance to fill more completely. When possible, teach the client to release the clamp at scheduled times. The catheter eventually is removed.

At this point, or when training clients who have not had an indwelling catheter, instruct the client to try to void every hour. Usually the client cannot retain urine longer than 1 hour, and frequent voiding is necessary to prevent incontinence. Gradually the client lengthens the interval between voidings to 2, 3, or 4 hours. At first, many clients do not empty the bladder and they must be catheterized after voiding to remove residual urine. Record the amount removed.

When they cannot control storage and passage of urine or when a bladder-training program fails, clients may be anxious and depressed. Offer constant encouragement throughout the bladder-training program. Anxiety may be reduced once the client notes the effort, concern, and interest of the healthcare team. If an accident occurs, change the bed linen promptly and assure the client that accidents are to be expected. Reducing anxiety may, in some instances, contribute to the success of a bladder-training program.

Barrier Garments and External Collection Devices

If it is not possible to establish a voiding routine and incontinence persists, the healthcare team works with the client to devise a system of collecting the urine. Male clients can use a condom catheter over the penis and connect the tubing to a closed drainage system or disposable urinary drainage bag. External drainage systems are available for women, but it is difficult to get the devices to fit securely. Male and female clients may choose to wear protective pants with a plastic outside layer and absorbent material inside. These pants can be pinned or snapped in place. Liners also are available and are worn next to the skin. They are nonabsorbent, and thus the urine passes through them to the absorbent layer. Liners dry quickly and leave skin dry and free of urine, even though the absorbent material is soaked.

Clients who are incontinent may have problems with odor and maintaining skin integrity. Urea-splitting microorganisms, such as *Micrococcus ureae,* cause urea in urine to react with water, creating ammonia and causing urine odor, skin breakdown, and ammonia dermatitis. One way to protect the skin is to avoid any contact with urine. When contact is unavoidable, instruct the client to use soap and water after each episode to clean the skin thoroughly. It also is important to dry the skin completely and apply a skin barrier or moisture sealant to protect the skin. When possible, encourage the client to expose the affected area to air.

Client and Family Teaching

Encourage clients to actively participate in whatever methods are used to empty the bladder. Demonstrate procedures as needed for the client and family to understand. A teaching plan is based on the client's individual needs to include one or more of the following:

- Control odors by frequent cleansing of the perineum, changing clothes and incontinence briefs (e.g., Attends, Depends) when they become wet, and using an electric room deodorizer.
- Avoid using perfume or scented powders, lotions, or sprays. Mixing a perfumed scent with a urine odor may intensify odor, irritate skin, or cause a skin infection.
- Wash garments as soon as possible in warm, soapy water.
- Use plastic to cover objects, such as a mattress and chairs, to prevent staining and lingering odors. The plastic must be washed with mild soapy water daily or more often if needed. Instruct the client to place a sheet or blanket between the skin and the plastic.
- Follow physician's recommendations about clamping and unclamping the catheter (when this method is prescribed) or changing the catheter or cystostomy tube.
- Keep a record of fluid intake. Drink plenty of fluids during waking hours. Drink most of the required fluids in the morning and early afternoon hours and decrease the intake toward evening.
- Follow the recommended bladder-training program. Time is required to achieve success.
- Contact the physician if any of the following occurs: increased discomfort, rash around the perineal area, pain in the lower abdomen, fever, chills, or cloudy urine.

INFECTIOUS AND INFLAMMATORY DISORDERS

Infections and inflammations of the bladder and urethra are common. Although usually able to be treated on an outpatient basis, they can require more invasive treatment.

• CYSTITIS

Pathophysiology and Etiology

Cystitis is an inflammation of the urinary bladder, usually caused by a bacterial infection. Bacteria invade the bladder from an infection in the kidneys, lymphatics, and urethra. Because the urethra is short in women, ascending infections or microorganisms from the vagina or rectum are more common. Causes of cystitis include urologic instrumentation (e.g., cystoscopy, catheterization), fecal contamination, prostatitis or benign prostatic hyperplasia, indwelling catheters, pregnancy, and sexual intercourse.

The bladder lining provides a natural resistance to most bacterial invasions by preventing an inflammatory reaction from occurring. If bacteria do survive in the bladder, they adhere to the mucosal lining of the bladder and multiply. The bladder surface becomes edematous and reddened, and ulcerations may develop. When urine contacts these irritated areas, the client experiences pain and urgency, magnified in the presence of even slight bladder distention.

Assessment Findings

Symptoms of cystitis include urgency (feeling a pressing need to void although the bladder is not full), frequency, low back pain, dysuria, perineal and suprapubic pain, and hematuria. If bacteremia is present, the client also may have chills and fever. Chronic cystitis causes similar, but usually less severe, symptoms.

Microscopic examination of the urine reveals increased red and white blood cells. Culture and sensitivity studies are used to identify the causative microorganism and appropriate antimicrobial therapy. If repeated episodes occur, intravenous pyelogram (IVP) or cystoscopy with or without retrograde pyelograms may be done to identify the possible cause, such as chronic prostatitis or a bladder **diverticulum** (weakening and outpouching of the bladder wall), which encourages urinary stasis and infection.

Medical Management

Medical management includes antimicrobial therapy and correction of contributing factors. Examples of drugs that may be used include trimethoprim-sulfamethoxazole (Septra, Bactrim) and nitrofurantoin (Macrodantin). Cranberry juice or vitamin C may be recommended to keep bacteria from adhering to the bladder wall, promoting their excretion and enhancing the effectiveness of drug therapy. When there is a partial urethral obstruction, no treatment of cystitis is fully effective until adequate drainage of urine is restored. In some instances, treatment may be prolonged and may need to be repeated.

Nursing Management

Advise the client to drink extra fluids. Cranberry juice provides a less favorable climate for bacterial growth. Emphasize the importance of finishing the prescribed course of therapy. Instruct the client in the prevention of repeated cystitis (Nursing Guidelines 59-1).

NURSING GUIDELINES 59-1

Preventing Cystitis

Tell clients with recurrent cystitis to:

- Increase fluid intake to 2 to 3 L a day.
- Avoid coffee, teas, colas, and alcohol.
- Shower rather than bathe in a tub.
- Cleanse perineum after each bowel movement with front-to-back motion.
- Avoid irritating substances such as bubble bath, bath salts, perineal lotions, vaginal sprays, nylon underwear, scented toilet paper.
- Wear cotton underwear.
- Void every 2 to 3 hours while awake.
- Empty bladder completely with each voiding.
- Void after sexual intercourse.
- Notify physician of the following: urgency, frequency, burning with urination, difficulty urinating, or blood in the urine.
- Take medication exactly as prescribed.

Stop, Think, and Respond ● BOX 59-3

Your 30-year-old client tells you that she has had four urinary tract infections (UTIs) in the past 6 months. What information should you get before providing the client with instructions about preventing future UTIs?

● URETHRITIS

Pathophysiology and Etiology

Urethritis (inflammation of the urethra) is seen more commonly in men than in women. Urethritis caused by microorganisms other than gonococci is called *nongonococcal urethritis.* Gonorrhea, an STI, is a specific form of infection that can attack the mucous membrane of a normal urethra (see Chap. 57).

In women, urethritis may accompany cystitis but also may be secondary to vaginal infections. Soaps, bubble baths, sanitary napkins, or scented toilet paper also may cause urethritis. In men, a common cause of urethritis is infection with *Chlamydia trachomatis* or *Ureaplasma urealyticum,* which causes a sexually transmitted infection (STI). The distal portion of the normal male urethra is not totally sterile. Bacteria that normally are present cause no difficulty unless these tissues are traumatized, usually after instrumentation such as catheterization or cystoscopic examination. Under such conditions, bacteria may cause a nonspecific urethritis. Other causes of nonspecific urethritis in men include irritation during vigorous intercourse, rectal intercourse, or intercourse with a woman who has a vaginal infection.

Assessment Findings

Infection of the urethra results in discomfort on urination varying from a slight tickling sensation to burning or severe discomfort and urinary frequency. Fever is not common, but fever in the male client may be due to further extension of the infection to areas such as the prostate, testes, and epididymis.

The client's history and symptoms often provide a tentative diagnosis. In men, a urethral smear is obtained for culture and sensitivity to identify the causative microorganism. In women, a urinalysis (clean-catch specimen) may identify the causative microorganism.

Medical Management

Treatment includes appropriate antibiotic therapy, liberal fluid intake, analgesics, warm sitz baths, and improvement of the client's resistance to infection by a good diet and plenty of rest. If urethritis is due to an STI, it is treated with appropriate antibiotic therapy (see Chap. 56). Failure to seek treatment for gonococcal urethritis may result in a urethral stricture in men.

Nursing Management

Reinforce the need to complete antibiotic therapy, drink plenty of fluids, and take warm sitz baths and analgesics for pain. Urethritis may be seen in clients with indwelling urethral catheters. To prevent or decrease urethritis, be vigilant with sterile technique, as well as exercise gentleness when changing catheters. Provide frequent perineal care, especially if the client is incontinent of feces. In addition to washing around the anus and buttocks, also clean the meatus and labia of the female client. When cleaning the anal area, wiping away from the urethra ensures that there is no contamination. See Client and Family Teaching 59-1.

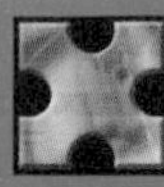

59-1 *Client and Family Teaching* Caring for Bladder and Urethreal Infections

The nurse teaches the client and family as follows:

- Take the medication as directed. Do not stop taking the medication even though symptoms have disappeared. It is important to complete the entire course of therapy.
- Take warm tub baths if discomfort is severe.
- Drink at least eight large glasses of fluids per day. Include one or more glasses of cranberry juice in the daily fluid intake. Avoid fluids that are urinary tract irritants, such as coffee, tea, alcohol, and colas. Fluids include water, cranberry juice, clear carbonated beverages, or any food (e.g., flavored gelatin, ice cream) that is liquid at room temperature. If on a special diet (e.g., low-sodium or diabetic diets), check with the physician about drinking juices or beverages or eating foods that are liquid at room temperature. Some of these liquids either must be considered part of the daily dietary allowances or may not be allowed because they contain substances that must be eliminated from the diet. In some diets, a limited amount of certain liquids may be allowed.
- Notify the physician if symptoms persist after the course of drug therapy is completed, if the symptoms become worse, or if fever or chills occur.
- Follow recommendations preventing future episodes of infection or inflammation.

NURSING PROCESS

● The Client With an Infection of the Bladder or Urethra

Assessment

Ask about present symptoms, specifically seeking information related to pain and changes in urination, including frequency, urgency, and burning. Assess the client's sexual practices, including methods of contraception and personal hygiene. Ask the client to void—measure the volume and check the urine for color, cloudiness, concentration, odor, and presence of blood.

Diagnosis, Planning, and Interventions

Pain related to infection and inflammation of the bladder and or/urethra

Expected Outcome: The client will express relief of pain and discomfort.

- Assure the client that pain and discomfort will decrease with treatment. *Antibacterial and antispasmodic medications are quickly effective in relieving the pain and discomfort associated with urinary tract infections.*
- Administer analgesics and antispasmodics as indicated. *Prompt administration of prescribed medications ensures that effective blood levels are maintained for treatment of infection. Antispasmodics relieve bladder irritability.*
- Encourage the client to use warm sitz baths two or three times a day to relieve discomfort. *Promotes relief of pain and reduces spasm.*
- Encourage the client to increase daily fluid intake to 2 to 3 L/day, excluding coffee, tea, alcohol, and colas. *Promotes renal blood flow and flushes bacteria from the urinary tract. Coffee, tea, alcohol, and colas are urinary tract irritants.*
- Instruct the client to void at regular intervals, even if uncomfortable. *Frequent voiding promotes emptying the bladder, which contributes to lower bacterial counts, reduction of urinary stasis, and prevention of reinfection.*

Deficient Knowledge regarding inflammation and infection of the bladder and urethra related to disease process and treatment

Expected Outcomes: (1) Client will verbalize understanding of condition, prognosis, and treatment. (2) Client will participate in the treatment regimen.

- Review the treatment plan. *Doing so provides a time for the client to ask questions.*
- Instruct client about medications, dosage, frequency, expected effects, and possible side effects. *Providing clients with accurate information promotes adherence to drug regimen.*
- Emphasize the need to complete the entire course of medications, even after symptoms have subsided. *Complete antibiotic therapy eradicates infection and prevents recurrence.*
- Teach client the importance of increased fluid intake. *Increased fluid intake flushes the urinary tract and removes bacteria.*
- Review client's hygiene practices. *Poor hygiene practices, such as back-to-front perineal cleansing, especially after a bowel movement, or soaking in dirty bath water can contribute to the introduction of bacterial contaminants to the urinary tract.*
- Teach client methods to prevent future infections. *Appropriate personal hygiene, increased fluid intake (promotes voiding and dilution of urine), and frequent voiding prevent urinary tract infection.*

Evaluation of Expected Outcomes

The client reports relief of pain and discomfort and states that he or she is adhering to the medication regimen. He or she demonstrates understanding of the treatment plan as evidenced by intake of at least 2 L of water, frequent voiding, and appropriate personal hygiene practices.

OBSTRUCTIVE DISORDERS

Obstruction of the lower urinary tract is a blockage in the bladder or urethra. Many obstructions are related to congenital anomalies, but in adults, obstructions occur from stones that block passage of urine, or from a narrowing that occurs as a result of a trauma, inflammation, or infection. General signs of an outflow obstruction are straining to empty the bladder, a feeling that one has not completely emptied the bladder, hesitancy, weak stream, frequency, overflow incontinence, and bladder distention.

• BLADDER STONES

Pathophysiology and Etiology

Stones may form in the bladder or originate in the upper urinary tract and travel to and remain in the bladder. Large bladder stones develop in those with chronic urinary retention and urinary stasis. Clients who are immobile (e.g., the unconscious client or those with paraplegia or quadriplegia) also may have a tendency to form bladder stones.

Assessment Findings

Symptoms of bladder stone formation include hematuria, suprapubic pain, difficulty starting the urinary stream, symptoms of a bladder infection, and a feeling that the bladder is not completely empty. Some clients may have few or no symptoms.

Cystoscopy, a kidney–ureter–bladder (KUB) study, IVP, or ultrasound studies detect the presence of bladder stones. Blood chemistries and 24-hour urine collection for serum calcium and uric acid may identify the possible cause of stone formation.

Medical and Surgical Management

Bladder stones may be removed through the transurethral route, using a stone-crushing instrument (lithotrite). This procedure, called a **litholapaxy,** is suitable for small and soft stones and is performed under general anesthesia. Larger, noncrushable stones must be removed through a surgical (suprapubic) incision into the bladder.

When it is possible to determine the chemical composition of stones that have passed or been removed, dietary treatment may be attempted to adjust the urine's pH to keep the urinary salts in solution and prevent formation of stones. These diets are not fully effective. Usually, clients are told to increase fluid intake significantly and to restrict sodium and protein. Despite dietary changes and urine pH regulation, some clients continue to form stones in the urinary tract.

Nursing Management

Obtain a complete medical, drug, and allergy history, asking the client to describe the symptoms, including type and location of pain. Determine if the client is allergic to iodine or seafood, because iodine-containing radiopaque substances may be used during diagnostic tests to locate the obstruction. Monitor vital signs every 4 hours or as ordered, and notify the physician if the client's temperature is higher than 101°F (38.3°C) orally. Document intake and output and the color of the urine.

If there is evidence of gross hematuria, report it immediately. Encourage the client to drink fluids (unless contraindicated by heart failure or renal disease), because extra fluids help pass stones and reduce the chance of infection or inflammation. Filter the urine for stones by straining all urine through gauze or wire mesh. If solid material is found, send it in a labeled container to the laboratory for analysis. If the client has moderate to severe pain, administer a narcotic analgesic as ordered. If the analgesic fails to relieve at least some of the pain or if the pain becomes worse, notify the physician, and provide details regarding the effects of medical or surgical procedures.

If a litholapaxy successfully removes the stone, a urethral catheter may be left in place to keep the bladder continuously empty for 1 to 2 days after the procedure. Administer antibiotics as ordered. Once oral fluids are tolerated, encourage the client to drink extra fluids to reduce inflammation of the bladder mucosa. Monitor the urine output and voiding pattern.

If open removal is required, the bladder is incised and the stone removed. A urethral catheter may be left in place for a week or more to keep the bladder empty and prevent tension on the bladder sutures. In addition to standard postoperative care, nursing management involves providing the same care as for the client having a suprapubic prostatectomy (see Chap. 55). Closely monitor the client's voiding once the catheter is removed to prevent urinary retention.

Teach the client to:

- Strain urine and send any stone found to the laboratory for examination.
- Follow the dietary recommendations.
- Take the prescribed medications as directed.
- Contact the physician if symptoms return.
- Drink plenty of fluids (at least 10 large glasses each day) and exercise regularly.
- Contact the physician if hematuria, burning, chills, fever, or pain occurs.

• URETHRAL STRICTURES

Pathophysiology and Etiology

Strictures of the urethra are caused by infections such as untreated gonorrhea or chronic nongonococcal urethritis. Other causes include trauma to the lower urinary tract or pelvis, such as accidents, childbirth, intercourse, or surgical procedures. Urethral strictures may be congenital.

A **stricture** (narrowing) in the urethra obstructs the flow of urine and can cause complications in the bladder or upper urinary tract. The kidney pelves can become distended with the backflow of urine. The bladder distends when the urethra is obstructed and a diverticulum (outpouching) of the muscular bladder wall may form (Fig. 59.3). In some instances more than one diverticulum may be seen. Urine becomes trapped in the diverticulum, stagnates, and becomes a culture medium for bacteria. For this reason, infection occurs often and is difficult to control until the obstruction is corrected.

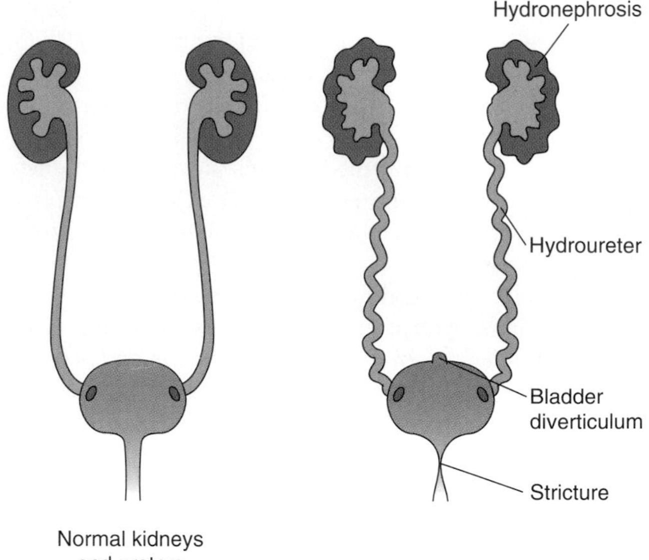

FIGURE 59.3 Urethral stricture can result in hydroureters, hydronephrosis (dilation of the ureters and kidneys), and bladder diverticulum.

Men experience urethral stricture more frequently than women, secondary to the anatomic differences and the length of the urethra. A urethral stricture may result in acute or chronic urinary retention.

Assessment Findings

Symptoms include slow or decreased force of stream of urine, hesitancy, burning, frequency, nocturia, and retention of residual urine in the bladder. Urinary retention may lead to bladder distention and infection. The client may be able to pass more urine after voiding and waiting a few minutes. The final quantity of urine comes from the diverticulum and may be malodorous.

The stricture may be seen on cystoscopy, retrograde pyelogram, and IVP. A voiding cystourethrogram also may show the stricture as well as the presence of a bladder diverticulum.

Medical and Surgical Management

Urethral strictures are treated by dilation, which is the use of specially designed instruments called *bougies, sounds, filiforms,* and *followers* (Fig. 59.4) passed gently into the urethra, although this procedure usually is painful. Because forceful stretching of the urethra may cause bleeding and further stricture formation, dilation begins with a 6-F or 8-F urethral dilator. During subsequent treatments, the physician increases the size of the dilator until 24 F or 26 F is tolerated. Depending on the cause of the stricture and the response to the therapy, the condition may sub-

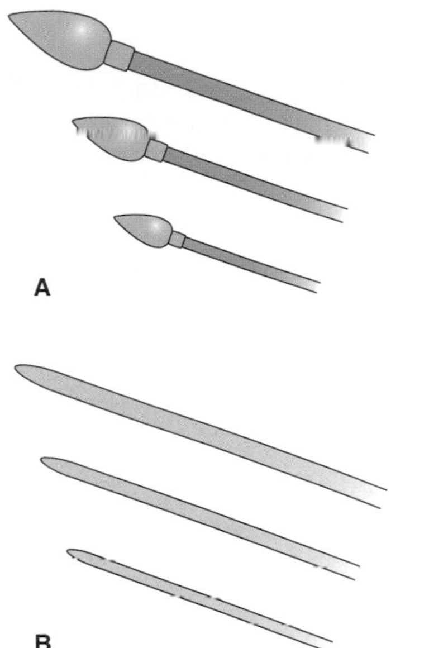

FIGURE 59.4 Bougies (**A**) and filiforms (**B**) are used to dilate the urethra.

side after one or two treatments. Periodic dilations usually are required indefinitely or until the condition is corrected surgically.

If dilation is unsuccessful, a **urethroplasty** (surgical repair of the urethra) may be attempted. Urine is diverted from the urethra by a cystostomy tube until the urethra is repaired. In one method of reconstructing the urethra, the constricted area is resected, and a mucosal graft (which may be taken from the bladder) is inserted to restore continuity of the urethra. After surgery, the client has a splinting catheter in the urethra that remains until healing occurs. This operation may be performed in two stages: urinary diversion at the first operation and plastic repair at the second.

Nursing Management

Advise the client that the urine may be blood tinged after urethral dilation and that it may burn when voiding. Sitz baths and non-narcotic analgesics may relieve discomfort. Encourage the client to drink extra fluids for several days after the procedure. Remind the client to keep appointments for follow-up dilations and not to wait until there is a marked reduction in the urinary stream or other symptoms of obstruction. Instruct the client to take all of the antibiotics and to contact the physician if difficulty voiding or frank bleeding occurs.

If a urethroplasty is done, it is most important that the urethral catheter remains in place and securely anchored. After surgery, turning and repositioning requires special attention to prevent excessive tension on the urethral catheter.

MALIGNANT TUMORS OF THE BLADDER

Malignant tumors of the bladder are frightening for clients. Bloody urine often is the first sign of a problem and the reason clients seek medical attention.

Pathophysiology and Etiology

Malignant tumors of the bladder are the most common tumors in the urinary system. They occur more frequently in men than in women and usually affect clients 50 years of age or older. Environmental and occupational health hazards thought to be associated with bladder tumors include cigarette smoking and second-hand smoke; exposure to industrial dyes, paint, ink, leather, or rubber; occupational exposure to sewage; coal gas; bladder stones; high urinary pH; high cholesterol intake; pelvic radiation therapy; and cancers arising from the prostate, colon, and rectum in men (Smeltzer & Bare, 2004).

The most common type of bladder tumor is a transitional cell carcinoma, which develops in the bladder's epithelial lining. Tumors are classified as papillary or nonpapillary. Papillary lesions are superficial and extend outward from the mucosal layer. Nonpapillary tumors are solid growths that grow inward, deep into the bladder wall. This type is more likely to metastasize, usually to lymph nodes, liver, lungs, and bone. Other types include squamous cell carcinoma and adenocarcinoma.

Assessment Findings

The most common first symptom of a malignant tumor of the bladder is painless hematuria. Additional early symptoms include UTI with symptoms such as fever, dysuria, urgency, and frequency. Later symptoms are related to metastases and include pelvic pain, urinary retention (if the tumor blocks the bladder outlet), and urinary frequency from the tumor occupying bladder space. If bleeding has been present for some time, the client also may have symptoms of anemia (fatigue, shortness of breath) caused by blood loss.

> **Stop, Think, and Respond ● BOX 59-4**
>
> *A 55-year-old man is admitted with blood in the urine. The medical diagnosis is "Rule out bladder cancer." When the nurse admits this client, what is an important question to ask?*

The tumor usually is seen by cystoscopic examination and confirmed by microscopic biopsy. A retrograde pyelogram may be obtained to detect kidney damage if the tumor is obstructing one of the ureteral orifices. A computed tomography scan and radiographs of the pelvis may show a tumor shadow or bony metastases. Ultrasonography also may show tumor size and location. Routine laboratory tests may be done to evaluate kidney function and determine the degree of anemia due to persistent hematuria.

Medical Management

Treatment varies according to grade and stage of the tumor. Metastases usually have not occurred if the tumor has not penetrated the muscle wall of the bladder. Small, superficial tumors may be removed by cutting (resection) or coagulation (**fulguration**) with a transurethral resectoscope (the same instrument used in transurethral resection of the prostate). Bladder tumors removed in this manner have a high incidence of recurrence; consequently, a cystoscopic examination is performed every 2 to 3 months. Clients having no recurrence of the tumor for at least 1 year require cystoscopic examinations every 6 months for the rest of their lives so that recurrence of the tumor or a new malignant growth can be detected early.

Topical application of an antineoplastic drug may be used after resection and fulguration of a tumor. The drug, in liquid form, is instilled into the bladder by means of a catheter (intravesicular injection). Fluid intake usually is limited before and during this procedure so that the drug remains concentrated and in contact with the bladder mucosa for about 2 hours. The client then voids and is given extra oral fluids to flush the drug from the bladder.

Intravesicular injection of BCG (bacille Calmette-Guérin) Live, a weakened strain of *Mycobacterium bovis,* also may be used. It appears that BCG causes an inflammatory reaction in the bladder wall that in turn destroys malignant cells. Another form of therapy includes administration of interferon alfa-2a (Roferon-A) injected intravenously (IV) or directly into the bladder. Interferon appears to stimulate production of lymphocytes and macrophages that may destroy malignant cells.

Photodynamic therapy also may be used in the treatment of bladder cancer. This involves IV injection of a photosensitizing agent that is absorbed in concentration by malignant cells. A laser, inserted through a cystoscope, is used to destroy those cells that have a high concentration of the photosensitizing agent.

Radiation therapy may be done if surgery is planned for the client. This reduces the size and extent of the tumor and decreases the risk of metastasis.

Surgical Management

A **cystectomy** (surgical removal of the bladder) and a urinary diversion procedure often are necessary when the tumor has penetrated the muscle wall. When a cystectomy is performed, the bladder and lower third of both ureters are removed. If the tumor extends through the bladder wall, the surgeon may perform a radical cystectomy.

In women, a radical cystectomy usually includes removal of the bladder, lower third of both ureters, uterus, fallopian tubes, ovaries, anterior vaginal wall, and urethra. In men, a radical cystectomy usually includes removal of the bladder, lower third of both ureters, prostate, and seminal vesicles.

Once a cystectomy is done, urine must be diverted to another collecting system. This is called a **urinary diversion.** Although urinary diversion procedures are used to treat bladder tumors, they also are used for extensive pelvic malignancies and severe traumatic injury to the bladder. Some urinary diversions require external ostomy bags to collect the urine (referred to as *cutaneous urinary diversions*) (Fig. 59.5). Others create a reservoir within the body that is catheterized to drain the urine—these are called *continent urinary diversions.* In some instances the urine is diverted to the colon and the client voids rectally—this also is referred to as a continent urinary diversion. Each procedure has advantages and disadvantages. The type of procedure used depends on many factors, such as age and physical condition of the client, procedure that can produce the best results for the client, and extent of metastases.

Nursing Management

Preoperative Period

Obtain a complete medical, drug, and allergy history on admission and ask the client or family member to describe symptoms. Assess general physical and emotional status, vital signs, and weight.

Caring for a client during the preoperative period includes reducing anxiety and increasing understanding of preparations for surgery and postoperative care. The client may display various emotional responses before surgery. The client faces drastic changes in the manner of excreting urine from the body, diagnosis of cancer, and changes in body image. Encourage the client to talk about the surgery and changes that will occur. Suggest a visit from a member of a local ostomy group to provide emotional support as well as information. The enterostomal therapist should meet with the client to discuss placement of the stoma and collection devices. Photographs or drawings are useful in showing placement of the stoma and urostomy pouch.

Determine the client's ability to manage stoma care or self-catheterization by assessing manual dexterity, level of understanding, and vision. Explain all preoperative preparations to the client and family and give them time to ask additional questions about the surgery, preparations for surgery, and management after surgery.

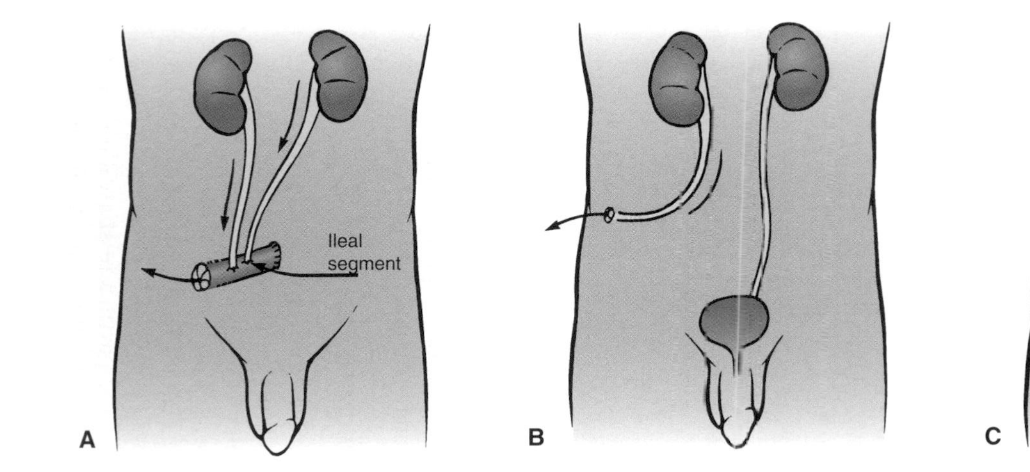

Conventional ileal conduit. Ureters are transplanted to an isolated section of the terminal ileum (ileal conduit), bringing one end to the abdominal wall.

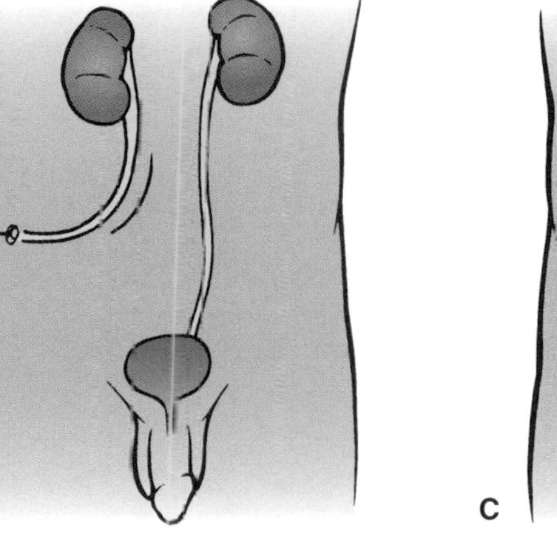

Cutaneous ureterostomy. The detached ureter is brought through the abdominal wall and attached to an opening in the skin.

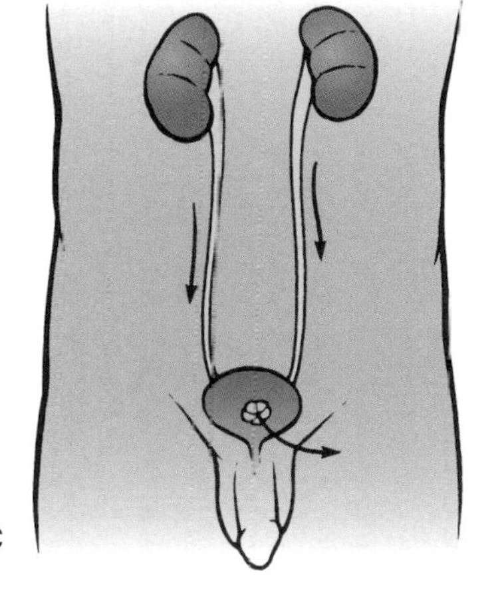

Vesicostomy. The bladder is sutured to the abdominal wall and an opening (stoma) is created through the abdominal and bladder walls for urinary drainage.

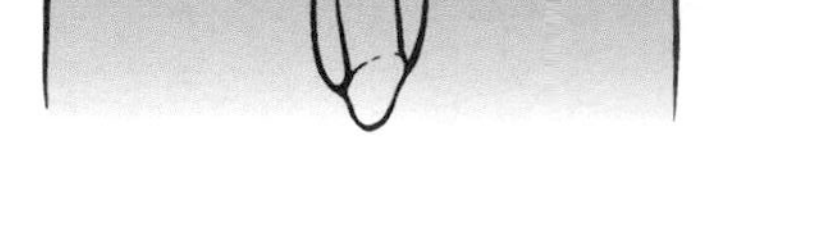

Nephrostomy. A catheter is inserted into the renal pelvis via an incision into the flank or, by percutaneous catheter placement, into the kidney.

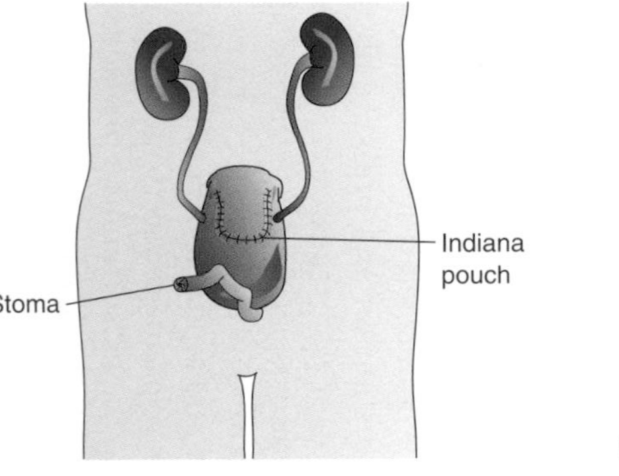

Indiana pouch. The ureters are introduced into a segment of ileum and cecum. Urine is drained periodically by inserting a catheter into the stoma.

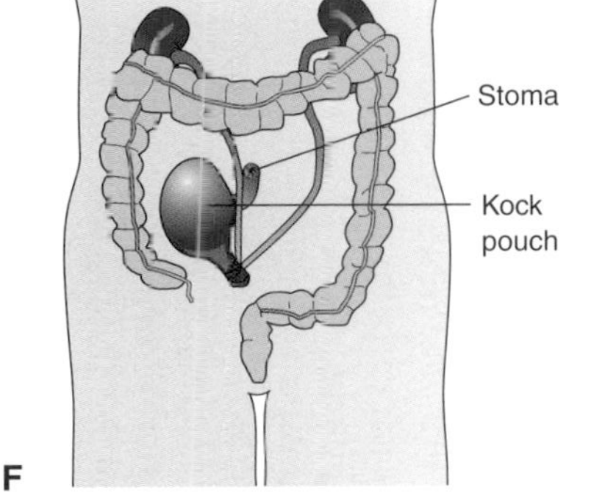

Continent ileal urinary diversions (Kock pouch). The ureters are transplanted to an isolated segment of small bowel, and an effective continence mechanism or valve is created. Urine is drained by inserting a catheter into the stoma.

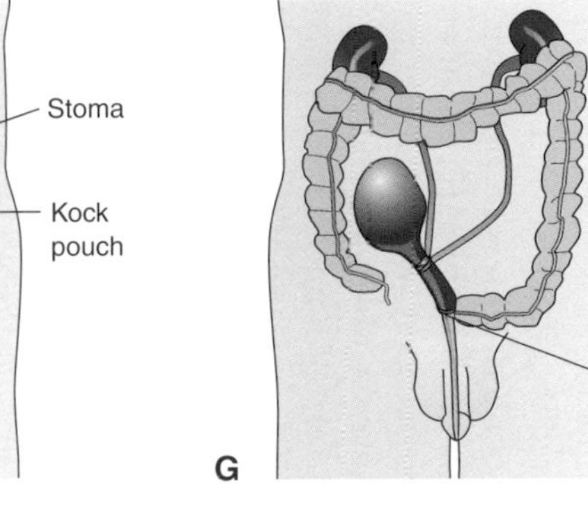
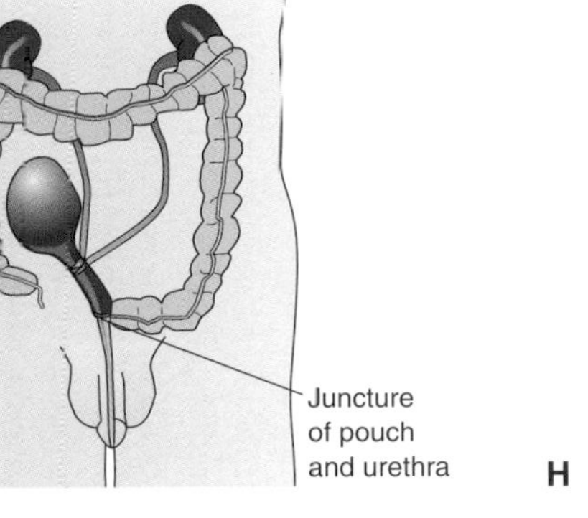

In male patients, the *Kock pouch* can be modified by attaching one end of the pouch to the urethra, allowing more normal voiding. The female urethra is too short for this modification.

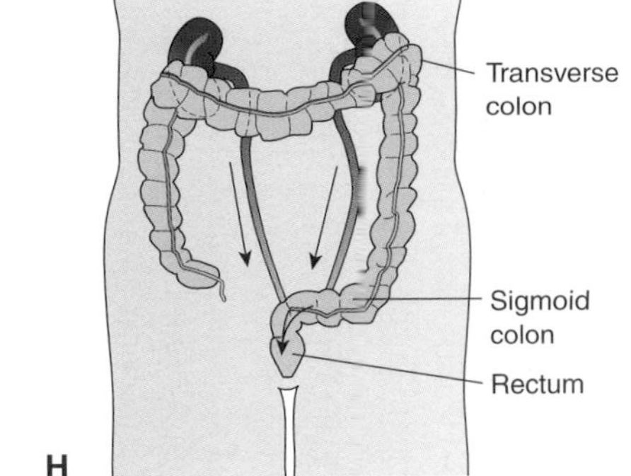

Ureterosigmoidostomy. The ureters are introduced into the sigmoid, thereby allowing urine to flow through the colon and out of the rectum.

FIGURE 59.5 Types of cutaneous diversions include (**A**) the conventional ileal conduit, (**B**) cutaneous ureterostomy, (**C**) vesicostomy, and (**D**) nephrostomy. Types of continent urinary diversions include (**E**) the Indiana pouch, (**F** and **G**) the Kock pouch, also called a continent ileal diversion, and (**H**) a ureterosigmoidostomy.

Depending on the extent and type of surgery, preoperative preparations may include insertion of a nasogastric tube, placement of IV and central venous pressure lines, administration of cleansing enemas, and adherence to a low-residue diet several days before surgery. Laxatives and enemas and a drug such as kanamycin (Kantrex) or neomycin (Mycifradin) may be given if a ureterosigmoidostomy (see Fig. 59.5) is to be performed. These agents decrease the number of microorganisms in the bowel and lessen the possibility of infection as a complication of connecting the ureters to the bowel. Clients scheduled for an ileal conduit (see Fig. 59.5) or continent urinary diversion procedure also may have the bowel prepared in this manner.

Postoperative Period

Clients undergoing urinary diversion are subject to the same conditions and complications as any surgical client. Management issues related specifically to urinary diversion procedures include observing for leakage of urine or stool from the anastomosis, maintaining renal function, assessing for signs and symptoms of peritonitis, maintaining integrity of the urinary diversion and urine collection devices, maintaining skin and stomal integrity, promoting a positive body image, and teaching the client how to manage the diversion.

Check the client's chart for information regarding the type and extent of surgery and orders for connection of catheters or drains, IV fluids, and analgesics. Clients will have multiple drainage tubes, ureteral stents, and a nasogastric tube. All urinary drainage tubes must be labeled, and urine output from each catheter or stoma must be measured and recorded hourly.

Maintain accurate intake and output measurements during the postoperative period, because this indicates both renal function and the integrity of the urinary diversion structures. Obstruction of urine flow can severely damage the kidneys. If urinary drainage stops or decreases to less than 30 mL/hour, or if the client complains of back pain, notify the physician immediately. Inspect the urine for color, clarity, and any blood. Immediately report concentrated, cloudy, or bloody urine to the physician. Ureteral stents remain in place for several days after surgery.

The nasogastric tube is connected to low intermittent suction. This prevents distention and pressure on the suture line from collection of gas in the bowel. The nasogastric tube is removed once peristalsis has returned and the diet can be advanced. Review all laboratory reports as soon as they are received and report abnormalities to the physician promptly. The following sections address management issues specific to the most common procedures.

For clients with an *ileal conduit,* a transparent ostomy bag is applied over the stoma to make stomal assessment easier. Contact the physician immediately if there is excessive bleeding, changes in the color of the stoma (e.g., from a normal to a cyanotic color), or separation of the stoma edges from the surrounding skin. Use gauze pads to clean mucus away from the stoma. Because the intestinal anastomosis can leak fecal material or the ileal conduit may leak urine into the peritoneal cavity, observe for and promptly report symptoms of peritonitis (e.g., abdominal tenderness or distention, fever, severe pain). Management of the urinary stoma is similar to management of a fecal stoma (see Chap. 48). The skin needs protection, surgical dressings must be changed promptly when they become wet, and appliances need care and cleansing.

Clients with a *continent urinary diversion (Kock pouch, Indiana pouch)* require irrigation of the pouch, if ordered, to prevent mucus plugs or blood clots. Teach the client how to perform intermittent self-catheterization. Initially, this is done every 1 to 2 hours but eventually will be performed every 4 to 6 hours.

Clients with a *ureterosigmoidostomy* have a catheter inserted in the rectum to drain urine continuously. Check the amount and color of drainage from the rectal catheter every 1 or 2 hours and inspect the anal and gluteal areas for signs of early skin breakdown. The catheter is removed when peristalsis returns. Because the sigmoid colon reabsorbs urinary constituents, clients are prone to fluid and electrolyte imbalances throughout the postoperative period (as well as for the rest of their lives). Observe for signs of electrolyte losses. Teach the client exercises to improve sphincter control. Once good control is achieved, instruct the client to void (rectally) every 2 hours to prevent reabsorption of fluid and electrolytes. Clients must never have enemas, suppositories, or laxatives. See Client and Family Teaching 59-2.

NURSING PROCESS

● Psychosocial Care of the Client Undergoing Urinary Diversion

Assessment

Assess the client's knowledge about the effects of surgery on sexual function. Up to 85% of men experience erectile dysfunction after urinary diversion. Women may have painful intercourse and lack lubrication. Ask the client about current level of social activity and what changes he or she thinks will occur after surgery. Assess the client's understanding of long-term postoperative care.

Diagnosis, Planning, and Interventions

Risk for Ineffective Sexuality Patterns related to erectile dysfunction (male) or dyspareunia (female)
Expected Outcome: Client will regain erectile function or ease painful intercourse.

- Tactfully ask the client if he or she has any questions. *Asking provides an opportunity to discuss sexuality issues.*
- Encourage client and partner to share their feelings about alteration in sexual function. *Acknowledging the*

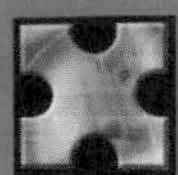

59-2 *Client and Family Teaching* Urinary Diversions

The material included in a client teaching plan varies according to the type of surgery or the physician's specific discharge orders. In addition to the points discussed previously, the nurse considers the following when preparing a teaching plan:

- Clients with a ureterosigmoidostomy must know the signs of fluid and electrolyte imbalances. To ensure understanding, give the client a written or printed list of the symptoms.
- Closed collection containers always should be below the level of the stoma. The tubing that connects the catheter or collection appliance to the closed drainage system must be kept straight so that urine does not collect in a curve of the tube. Avoid kinks that prevent the drainage of urine.
- Adequate fluids are necessary. Note the color of the urine. If the urine appears darker than usual, more fluids may be needed. Dark urine, despite an adequate fluid intake, is brought to the attention of the physician.
- Medications are taken as prescribed by the physician. Do not omit or stop taking the drugs. Do not take or use any nonprescription drug without first checking with the physician. Those with a ureterosigmoidostomy must not use laxatives or enemas.
- Odors can be controlled with cranberry juice, yogurt, or buttermilk. Avoid foods that may impart an odor to the urine, such as asparagus, cheese, or eggs.
- The enterostomal therapist recommends skin care techniques. The skin must be kept clean. When the adhesive wafer (to which the urostomy collection bag is attached) is changed, all remaining adhesive is removed before application of a new wafer.
- The continent urostomy should be drained four times a day or as directed by the physician.
- The urinary collection pouch needs to be washed thoroughly after changing. Rinse the pouch with or soak in a solution of vinegar and water if crystals form in the pouch.

The physician is contacted if any of the following occur:

- Fever
- Chills
- Blood in the urine
- Failure of a stoma or catheter to drain urine
- Skin problems around the stoma
- Weight loss (> 5 lbs)
- Loss of appetite (more than a few days)
- Inability to insert the catheter in the continent urostomy
- Pain in the flank (kidney area or lower abdomen)
- Signs of fluid or electrolyte imbalance
- Any unusual symptom or problem

importance of sexual function and expression may assist the client and partner to seek sexual counseling and to explore alternative methods of expressing sexuality.

- Discuss alternatives to sexual intercourse such as closeness and giving pleasure to a partner. Provide information about penile prostheses for men and water-soluble lubricants for women. Inform women that Kegel exercises may ease painful intercourse. Discuss masturbation, either individual or mutual, as an option. *Alternatives to sexual intercourse enable and enhance sexual satisfaction that physical limitations may otherwise impede.*

Disturbed Body Image related to change in appearance and function

Expected Outcome: Client will accept altered appearance and perform self-care.

- Assess client's willingness to look at the stoma. Accept client's response and reinforce that anxiety is normal. Reassure client that nursing staff will provide care until he or she is ready. *Gradual exposure is part of rehabilitation.*
- Discuss change in function and let client know what to expect when recovery from surgery is complete. Suggest a visit from an ostomate who can provide valuable personal information, support, and resources. *Providing information and group support assists the client to know that he or she is not alone and will be prepared to care for himself or herself.*
- Help client gain independence by reinforcing that self-care is quite manageable and providing time for practice. *Encouragement and support promote confidence and move the client from a dependent to an independent role.*

Risk for Social Isolation related to fear of accidents or urine odor

Expected Outcome: Client will maintain social relationships.

- Explain that odor-proof pouches or pouches with carbon filters or other odor barriers are available. A few drops of liquid deodorizer or diluted white vinegar also may assist in controlling odors. Suggest avoiding odor-producing foods, such as asparagus, eggs, or cheese. *A client may become socially isolated from the odors produced by the urinary diversion. Information about how to control odors will assist the client to implement measures and then to feel that friends, coworkers, and acquaintances will accept him or her.*

- Oral ascorbic acid may help to control odors. *Ascorbic acid helps to acidify urine and suppress urine odors.*
- Teach client to care for the pouch and to change it every 3 days if it is a one-piece pouch or every 4 to 7 days if it is a two-piece pouch. *Appropriate care assists in reducing odors and contributes to the client's level of confidence.*
- Tell client to empty the bag before it gets half full to prevent tension on the adhesive wafer and to eliminate source of odors. Inform the client to carry a spare pouch in case adhesive loosens while out. *These measures prevent accidents or embarrassment and provide the client with a sense of control and positive well-being.*
- Suggest drinking cranberry juice or using an appliance deodorant. *These measures reduce odors and assist the client to feel in control.*
- Suggest that the client contact the urostomy association for suggestions and additional support in alleviating anxiety. Instruct client with a ureterosigmoidostomy to avoid gas-forming foods. *Receiving support and accurate information contributes positively to a client's sense of well-being.*

Evaluation of Expected Outcomes

The client discusses methods for resuming sexual activity and alternatives to sexual intercourse. He or she states methods to avoid accidents and control urine odor. The client verbalizes a willingness to maintain social activity.

TRAUMA

Trauma to the bladder or urethra is potentially harmful and frequently requires surgical intervention.

Pathophysiology and Etiology

Various types of injury can affect the urinary tract. Gunshot and stab wounds, crushing injuries, and forceful blows can result in tears, hemorrhage, or penetration of one or more parts. Some penetrating bladder injuries are small, whereas others are large with a rapid collection of urine in the peritoneal cavity. Injuries to the kidney area may result in bruising or tearing of the kidney and its capsule. Depending on the severity of injury, blood and urine may leak into the peritoneal cavity.

Assessment Findings

Symptoms vary according to the area affected and the type of injury. Anuria, hematuria, abdominal pain (which may indicate bleeding or leakage of urine into the abdominal cavity), bladder or kidney pain, and symptoms of shock may be indicators of urinary tract injury. During treatment of a client with extensive injury, an indwelling catheter may be inserted, and hematuria or lack of urine output may be the first sign of a traumatic injury to the urinary tract. Certain other types of injuries, such as stab or gunshot wounds, may be immediately identified because of outward signs of injury (e.g., entry wounds on skin surface).

Injury to the urinary tract initially may be overlooked when the client has incurred widespread, massive injuries. Abdominal x-rays, cystoscopy, IVP, and exploratory surgery may be used to identify the type and location of the injury.

Surgical Management

Treatment depends on the type, location, and extent of injury as well as on the condition of the client. For example, a stab wound in the kidney area may require emergency exploratory surgery. Once the kidney is exposed, the physician needs to determine if the trauma to the kidney can be repaired or if the kidney must be removed immediately. Examples of surgeries that may be performed for urinary tract trauma include cystostomy (temporary or permanent), nephrectomy, insertion of a nephrostomy tube, repair (reanastomosis) of the ureter, and cystectomy.

Nursing Management

The most important nursing task is recognition of abnormal findings. Lack of urinary output, diffuse and severe abdominal pain, and hematuria are examples of signs and symptoms that may indicate an injury to the urinary tract. In some instances, the injury may be such that symptoms do not appear for several hours or days after the initial trauma.

Other nursing management depends on the surgical interventions performed and the symptoms the client experiences. Focus on the client's physical and emotional needs related to the trauma.

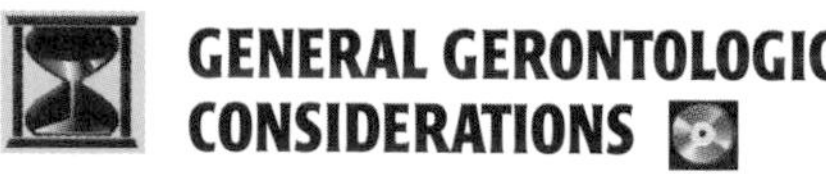

GENERAL GERONTOLOGIC CONSIDERATIONS

The older adult may have some form of incontinence. In some, involuntary leakage of urine may occur when the client coughs or sneezes, whereas others may be completely incontinent.

Some older adults may be unable to follow the instructions of a bladder rehabilitation program; others may have involuntary relaxation of the bladder sphincter, making rehabilitation extremely difficult.

Older clients with continence problems must not be treated like infants or scolded for their behavior (e.g., bed-wetting, soiling clothes). Make every effort to help rehabilitate the client. If bladder rehabilitation is not successful, try other methods to keep the client clean, dry, and odor free.

Carefully assess the cause of incontinence in the older adult. Older adults may be incontinent simply because environmental or physical conditions prevent them from maneuvering quickly enough to get to the bathroom before urination occurs. In these situations, a change in the environment or an assistive device may alleviate the incontinence.

If the elderly client is incontinent, the perineal area is particularly susceptible to skin breakdown.

Clients must not be made to feel isolated when they have a problem with urinary continence. Planned exercise and social activities should be a part of a bladder rehabilitation program.

Critical Thinking Exercises

1. *A client has recurrent cystitis. Her physician wants to perform a cystoscopy and retrograde pyelograms. She asks you why she needs these tests because medication she took in the past cured her problem. What explanation would you give?*
2. *A client has a ureterosigmoidostomy. What teaching will you do regarding long-term follow-up and care?*

• NCLEX-STYLE REVIEW QUESTIONS 

1. A nurse educator instructs a group of staff nurses on a medical-surgical unit to inform clients with frequent urinary tract infections to minimize intake of coffee, tea, cola, and alcohol. One staff nurse asks why limiting such beverages is important. Which explanation by the educator is most accurate?
   1. "They increase urine output, which can cause dehydration."
   2. "They lack vitamin C, needed for normal urinary flora."
   3. "They cause urinary retention, which can lead to infection."
   4. "They are known to cause urinary tract irritation."
2. The nurse prepares a teaching plan for a client with urinary incontinence. Which information regarding fluid intake should the nurse include in the teaching plan?
   1. Avoid fluids as much as possible.
   2. Drink most fluids in the early part of the day.
   3. Limit fluids to sips when taking medications.
   4. Drink fluids liberally and as desired.
3. The nurse assesses a client who recently had placement of an ileal conduit. Which assessment finding requires further investigation?
   1. Urinary drainage is pink tinged.
   2. Mucus is present in the stoma.
   3. The stoma is blue in color.
   4. The stoma is approximated to the surrounding skin.

connection—

Visit the Connection site at **http://connection.lww.com/go/timbyEssentials** for links to chapter-related resources on the Internet.

References and Suggested Readings

Bullock, B. A., & Henze, R. L. (2000). *Focus on pathophysiology.* Philadelphia: Lippincott Williams & Wilkins.

Castine, S., Boyington, A., & Dougherty, M. (2002). Urinary incontinence: If we don't ask, patients won't tell. *American Journal of Nursing, 102*(8), 85–87.

Executive Summary. (2003). The state of the science of urinary incontinence. *American Journal of Nursing, 103*(3), 45–49.

Gilchrist, K. J. (November 5, 2001). Skin integrity and incontinence. *Advance for Nurses,* 33.

Gray, M., Ratliff, C., & Donovan, A. (2002). Tender mercies: Providing skin care for an incontinent patient. *Nursing 2002, 32*(7), 51–54.

Gray, M. (2000a). Urinary retention: Management in the acute care setting. Part 1. *American Journal of Nursing, 100*(7), 40–47.

Gray, M. (2000b). Urinary retention: Management in the acute care setting. Part 2. *American Journal of Nursing, 100*(8), 36–44.

Hanchett, M. (2002). Techniques for stabilizing urinary catheters. *American Journal of Nursing, 102*(3), 44–48.

Kuiest, K. R., & McGovern, P. (2002). Using the umbilicus for catheterization. *RN, 55*(8), 26–30.

Mayo Clinic. (2001). Overactive bladder: How to keep it from controlling your life. *Women's HealthSource, 5*(11), 1–2.

McConnell, E. A. (2001). Clinical do's and don'ts: Preventing nosocomial urinary tract infections. *Nursing 2001, 31*(5), 17.

McConnell, E. A. (2000). Tech update: New catheters decrease nosocomial infections. *Nursing Management, 31*(6), 52.

Newman, D. K., & Giovannini, D. (2002). The overactive bladder: A nursing perspective. *American Journal of Nursing, 10*(6), 36–45.

Patient Handout. (November 5, 2001). Kegel exercises for urinary incontinence. *Advance for Nurses,* 28.

Patouillet, M. (August 5, 2002). Nursing perspective on diagnostic imaging. *Advance for Nurses,* 17–19.

Porth, C. M. (2002). *Pathophysiology: Concepts of altered health states* (6th ed.). Philadelphia: Lippincott Williams & Wilkins.

Schofield, C. (2002). My patient may have a UTI—what next? *Nursing 2002, 32*(10), 17.

Shultz, J. M. (2002). Urinary incontinence: Solving a secret problem. *Nursing 2002, 32*(11), 53–55.

Smeltzer, S. C., & Bare, B. G. (2004). *Brunner & Suddarth's textbook of medical–surgical nursing* (10th ed.). Philadelphia: Lippincott Williams & Wilkins.

Wooldridge, L. (2000). Ultrasound technology and bladder dysfunction. *American Journal of Nursing, 100*(6), 3–14.

chapter 60

Introduction to the Musculoskeletal System

Words to Know 

arthrocentesis
arthrogram
arthroscopy
bone scan
bursa
calcification
cancellous bone
cartilage
cortical bone
diaphyses
epiphyses
joint
ligament
ossification
osteoblasts
osteoclasts
osteocytes
periosteum
red bone marrow
resorption
skeletal muscles
tendon
yellow bone marrow

Learning Objectives

On completion of this chapter, the reader will:

- Describe major structures and functions of the musculoskeletal system.
- Discuss elements of the nursing assessment of the musculoskeletal system.
- Identify common diagnostic and laboratory tests used in the evaluation of musculoskeletal disorders.
- Discuss the nursing management of clients undergoing tests for musculoskeletal disorders.

The musculoskeletal system consists of bones, muscles, joints, tendons, ligaments, cartilage, and bursae. It supports the body and facilitates movement. Other functions include storage of calcium, phosphorus, magnesium, and fluoride; production of blood cells in the bone marrow; and protection and support to body organs, such as the lungs, heart, and brain. Injury to or disease in any part of the musculoskeletal system can cause pain, immobility, or disability and potentially affect quality of life.

ANATOMY AND PHYSIOLOGY

Bones

The human body has 206 bones. Bones of the skeleton are classified as:

- *Short bones,* such as those in fingers and toes
- *Long bones,* such as the femur and ulna
- *Flat bones,* such as the sternum
- *Irregular bones,* such as vertebrae

There are two types of bony tissue. The first is **cancellous bone,** or spongy bone, which is light and contains many spaces. The second is **cortical bone,** or compact bone, which is dense and hard. Both types are found in varying amounts in all bones. Cancellous bone is found at the rounded, irregular ends, or **epiphyses,** of long bones. Cortical bony tissue covers bones and is found chiefly in the long shafts, or **diaphyses,** of bones in arms and legs. The combination of the two types of bony tissue provides strength and support, yet keeps the skeleton light to promote endurance during activity.

Bone is composed of cells, protein matrix, and mineral deposits. Cells that build bones are called **osteoblasts.** They secrete bone matrix (mostly collagen), in which inorganic minerals, such as calcium salts, are deposited. This process of **ossification** and **calcification** transforms blast cells into mature bone cells, called **osteocytes,** which are involved in maintaining bone tissue. During rapid bone growth or bone injury, osteocytes function as osteoblasts to form new bone. **Osteoclasts** are the cells involved in destruction, resorption, and remodeling of bone.

During growth, bones primarily lengthen. Diameter also increases when osteoclasts break down previously formed bone, however, making the central canal wider. When skeletal growth is complete, the osteoclasts, part of the mononuclear phagocyte system (blood cells involved in ingesting particulate matter—or recycling old cells), continue with remodeling of bones by balancing bone **resorption** with new bone cell replacement. Bone formation and resorption continue throughout life. The greatest activity occurs from birth through puberty. Table 60.1 reviews factors that affect bone formation.

A layer of tissue called **periosteum** covers bones (but not the joints). The inner layer of periosteum contains osteoblasts necessary for bone formation. The periosteum is rich in blood and lymph vessels and supplies the bone with nourishment.

Inside bones are two types of bone marrow: red and yellow. **Red bone marrow,** primarily in the sternum, ileum, vertebrae, and ribs, manufactures blood cells and hemoglobin. Long bones have **yellow bone marrow,** consisting primarily of fat cells and connective tissue. If blood cell supply is compromised, yellow marrow may take on characteristics of red marrow and begin producing blood cells.

TABLE 60.1 FACTORS THAT AFFECT BONE FORMATION

BONE FORMATION FACILITATORS	BONE FORMATION RETARDANTS
Calcium	Estrogen/androgen deficiency
Phosphorus	Vitamin deficiency
Estrogen	Starvation
Testosterone	Diabetes
Calcitonin	Steroids
Vitamins D, A, C	Inactivity/immobility
Growth hormone	Heparin
Exercise	Excess parathyroid hormone
Insulin	

Muscles

There are three kinds of muscles. **Skeletal muscles** are voluntary muscles; impulses that travel from efferent nerves of the brain and spinal cord control their function. Skeletal muscles promote movement of bones of the skeleton. Examples of skeletal muscles are the biceps in the arms and the gastrocnemius in the calves.

Skeletal muscle is composed of muscle fibers that contain several myofibers. Sliding filaments called *sarcomeres* make up myofibers. They are the contractile units of skeletal muscle. Impulses from the central nervous system cause release of acetylcholine at the motor end plate of the motor neuron that innervates muscle. As a result, calcium ions are released, which stimulates actin and myosin in the sarcomeres to slide closer together, resulting in muscle contraction. When calcium is depleted, the actin and myosin fibers move apart, causing relaxation of the sarcomeres, and thus the muscle.

Smooth and *cardiac muscles* are involuntary muscles; their activity is controlled by mechanisms in their tissue of origin and by neurotransmitters released from the autonomic nervous system. Smooth muscles are found mainly in the walls of certain organs or cavities of the body, such as the stomach, intestine, blood vessels, and ureters. Cardiac muscle is found only in the heart.

Joints

A **joint** is the junction between two or more bones (Table 60.2). Free moving joints, or diarthrodial joints, make up most skeletal joints. They allow certain movements. Terms related to diarthrodial joint movement are presented in Box 60-1. Surfaces of diarthrodial joints are covered with hyaline cartilage, which reduces friction during joint movement. The space between is the joint cavity, enclosed by a fibrous capsule lined with synovial membrane. This membrane produces synovial fluid, which acts as a lubricant.

TABLE 60.2 TYPES OF JOINTS

TYPE	CHARACTERISTIC	EXAMPLE
Synarthrodial joints	Immovable	At the suture line of skull between the temporal and occipital bones
Amphiarthrodial joints	Slightly movable	Between the vertebrae
Diarthrodial joints (also called *synovial joints*)	Freely movable	Gliding joint: fingers Hinge joint: elbow Pivot joint: ends of radius and ulna Condyloid joint: between the wrist and forearm Saddle joint: between the wrist and metacarpal bone of the thumb Ball and socket joint: hip

BOX 60-1 ● Glossary of Diarthrodial Movement

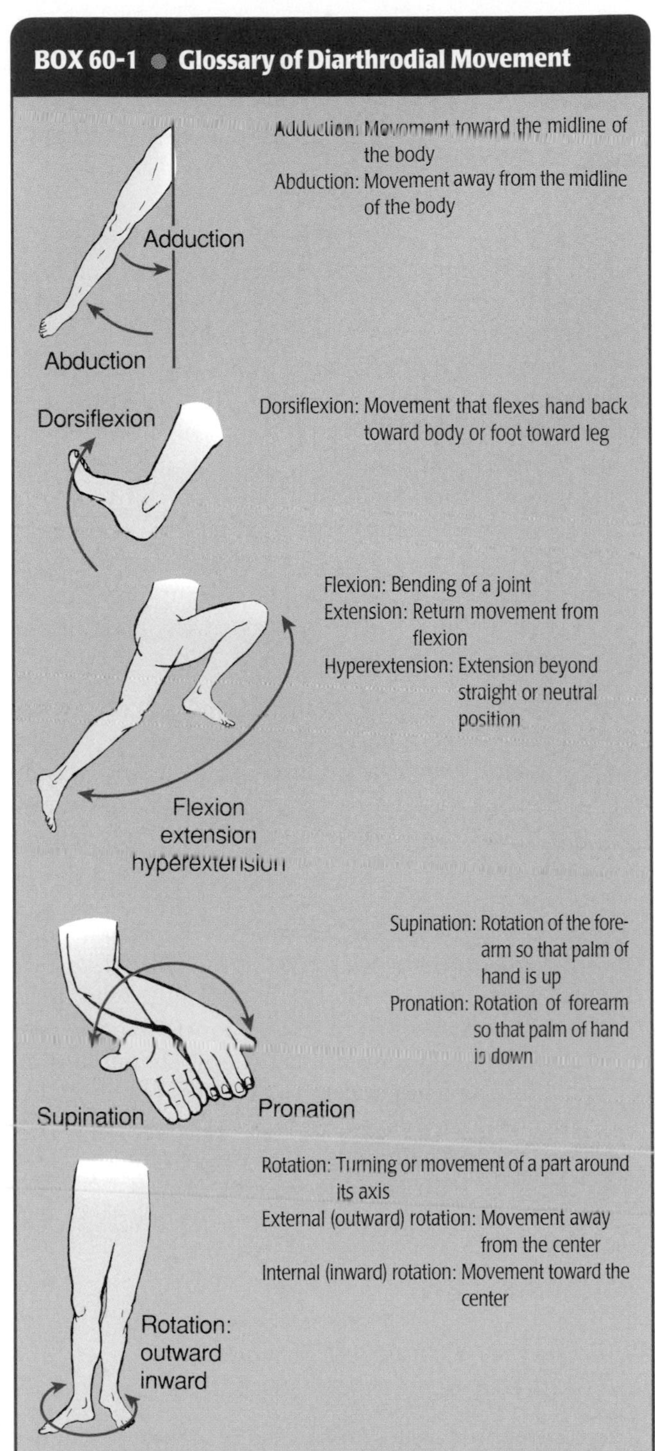

Tendons

Tendons are cordlike structures that attach muscles to periosteum of the bone. A muscle has two or more attachments. One is called the *origin* and is more fixed. The other is called the *insertion* and is more movable. When a muscle contracts, both attachments are pulled, and the insertion is drawn closer to the origin.

Ligaments

Ligaments consisting of fibrous tissue connect two adjacent, freely movable bones. They help protect joints by stabilizing their surfaces and keeping them in proper alignment. In some instances, ligaments completely enclose a joint.

Cartilage

Cartilage is a firm, dense type of connective tissue consisting of cells embedded in a substance called the *matrix*. The matrix is firm and compact, enabling it to withstand pressure and torsion. Primary functions of cartilage are to reduce friction between articular surfaces, absorb shocks, and reduce stress on joint surfaces.

Hyaline or articular cartilage covers the surface of movable joints, such as the elbow, and protects the surface of these joints. Other types of cartilage include costal cartilage, which connects the ribs and sternum; semilunar cartilage, one of the cartilages of the knee joint; fibrous cartilage, found between vertebrae (intervertebral discs); and elastic cartilage, found in the larynx, epiglottis, and outer ear.

Bursae

A **bursa** is a small sac filled with synovial fluid. Bursae reduce friction between areas, such as tendon and bone and tendon and ligament. Inflammation of these sacs is called *bursitis*.

ASSESSMENT

History

The focus of the initial history depends on whether the client has a chronic disorder or a recent injury. If the disorder is long-standing, obtain a thorough medical, drug, and allergy history. If the client is injured, find out when and how the trauma occurred. Compile a list of symptoms that includes information about onset, duration, and location of discomfort or pain. Determining whether activity makes symptoms better or worse is important. Identify associated symptoms, such as muscle cramping or skin lesions, and ask the client if the problem interferes with activities of daily living. If the client has an open wound, ascertain when the client last received a tetanus immunization.

Obtain a history of past disorders and medical or surgical treatments as soon as possible. Attention to chronic or concurrent disorders, such as diabetes mellitus, is essential. Obtain a family history, especially when relatives have had similar symptoms, and an occupational history.

Stop, Think, and Respond ● BOX 60-1

A neighbor calls you and states that he tripped and fell, spraining his ankle. When you arrive to help him, what questions should you ask? What should you observe?

Physical Examination

For a general musculoskeletal assessment, observe the client's ability to ambulate, sit, stand, and perform activities requiring fine motor skills, such as grasping objects. Examine the client for symmetry, size, and contour of extremities and random movements. A spinal inspection includes identifying spinal curvatures (Fig. 60.1):

- *Kyphosis*—exaggerated convex curvature of the thoracic spine (humpback)
- *Lordosis*—excessive concave curvature of the lumbar spine (swayback)
- *Scoliosis*—lateral curvature of the spine

Palpate the muscles and joints to identify swelling, degree of firmness, local warm areas, and any involuntary movements. To test the client's muscle strength, apply force to the client's extremity as the client pushes against that force. Perform a neurovascular assessment, which includes assessing range of motion for the joints, taking care not to force movement. Note any abnormal muscle movements such as spasms or tremors. In addition:

- Look for abnormal size or alignment and symmetry, comparing one side with the other.
- Inspect and palpate for pain, tenderness, swelling, and redness.
- Observe the degree of movement and range of motion, but never persist beyond the point of pain.
- Test for muscle strength.
- Inspect for muscle wasting.

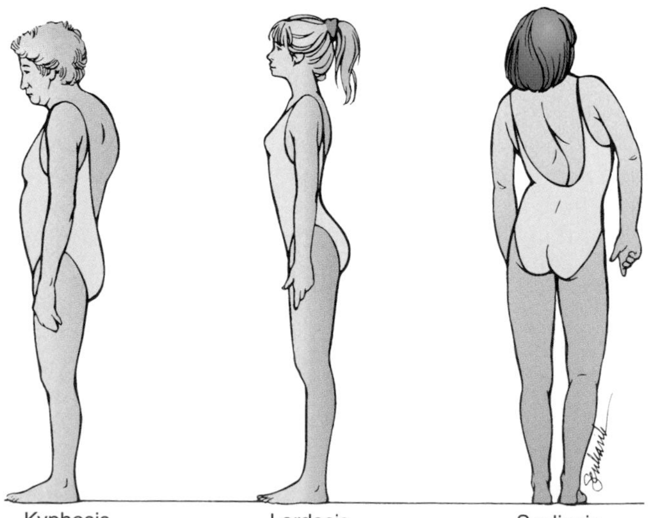

FIGURE 60.1 Common spinal curvatures.

Depending on symptoms and findings, additional assessments may include looking for changes in gait and body posture, favoring one side over the other, and ability to bend and twist the trunk, head, and extremities.

If the client has a traumatic injury, physical assessment begins with taking vital signs. Further assessment depends on the type and area of injury. During the assessment, maintain standard precautions. Cut the clothing from around an injured area if there is no other way to examine the client. Comparing structures and assessment findings on one side of the body with those on the opposite side helps determine the degree of injury. It is important to be gentle, recognizing that assessment techniques may increase pain. In addition:

- Observe for swelling, external bleeding, or bruising.
- Palpate the peripheral pulses.
- Evaluate peripheral circulation; assessing peripheral pulse (rate and character), skin coloration (pink, gray, pale, ashen), temperature, and capillary refill time.
- Check the sensation of the injured part.
- Look for broken skin, open wounds, superficial or embedded debris in or around the wound, or protrusion of bone or other tissue from the wound.
- Examine for injury beyond the original area; for example, auscultate the chest and abdomen if an abdominal or thoracic injury occurred or check the pupils and mental status if a head injury occurred.
- Look for malalignment of the injured limb.
- Assess for pain, noting type and location.

Diagnostic Tests

Radiography, Computed Tomography, and Magnetic Resonance Imaging

X-rays, computed tomography, and magnetic resonance imaging help identify traumatic disorders, such as fractures and dislocations, and other bone disorders, such as malignant bone lesions, joint deformities, calcification, degenerative changes, osteoporosis, and joint disease.

Arthroscopy

Arthroscopy is internal inspection of a joint using an instrument called an *arthroscope.* Its most common use is to visualize the knee joint, a common site of injury. After administering a local or general anesthetic, the physician inserts a large-bore needle into the joint and injects sterile normal saline solution to distend the joint. After inserting the arthroscope, the examiner inspects the joint for signs of injury or deterioration. Joint fluid may be removed and sent to the laboratory for examination. Depending on findings, the physician sometimes can use the arthroscope to perform therapeutic procedures, such as removing bits of torn or floating cartilage.

Afterward, the client's entire leg is elevated without flexing the knee. A cold pack is placed over the bulky dressing covering the site where the arthroscope was inserted. A prescribed analgesic is administered as necessary. See Nursing Guidelines 60-1.

Arthrocentesis

Arthrocentesis is aspiration of synovial fluid. The client receives local anesthesia just before this procedure. The physician inserts a large needle into the joint and removes fluid. Synovial fluid may be aspirated to relieve discomfort caused by an excessive accumulation in the joint space or to inject a drug, such as a corticosteroid preparation. Removed synovial fluid may be sent to the laboratory for microscopic examination or for culture and sensitivity studies. Arthrocentesis also may be performed during an arthrogram or arthroscopy.

Arthrogram

An **arthrogram** is a radiographic examination of a joint, usually the knee or shoulder. The physician injects a local anesthetic and then inserts a needle into the joint space. Fluoroscopy may be used to verify correct placement of the needle. Synovial fluid in the joint is aspirated and sent to the laboratory for analysis. A contrast medium is then injected, and x-ray films are taken. After arthrography, the client is informed that he or she may hear crackling or clicking noises in the joint for up to 2 days. Noises beyond this time are abnormal and should be reported.

> **NURSING GUIDELINES 60-1**
>
> ***Assisting the Client Through Arthroscopy***
>
> *Before the Procedure*
>
> 1. Explain the procedure.
> 2. Ensure that the client has signed the informed consent form.
> 3. Verify that the client has been NPO for at least 6 hours.
> 4. Administer preoperative medications, if ordered.
>
> *After the Procedure*
>
> 1. Instruct client to report unusual pain, bleeding, drainage, or swelling at the arthroscopic site.
> 2. Advise client to resume usual diet as tolerated.
> 3. Review discharge instructions with the client and explain medication regimen.
> 4. Inspect dressing before discharge.

Synovial Fluid Analysis

Synovial fluid is aspirated and examined to diagnose disorders such as traumatic arthritis, septic arthritis (caused by a microorganism), gout, rheumatic fever, and systemic lupus erythematosus. Normally, synovial fluid is clear and nearly colorless. Laboratory examination of synovial fluid may include microscopic examination for blood cells, crystals, and formed debris present in the joint space after an injury. If an infection is suspected, culture and sensitivity studies are ordered. A chemical analysis for substances such as protein and glucose also may be done.

Bone Densitometry

Bone densitometry estimates bone density. Radiography of the wrist, hip, or spine helps to determine bone mineral density. Bone sonometry or ultrasound measures the quantity and quality of heel bone and provides an estimate of bone density.

Bone Scan

A **bone scan** uses the intravenous injection of a radionuclide to detect the uptake of radioactive substance by bone. A bone scan may be ordered to detect metastatic bone lesions, fractures, and certain types of inflammatory disorders. The radionuclide is taken up in areas of increased metabolism, which occur in bone cancer, metastatic bone disease, and osteomyelitis (bone infection).

Electromyography

Electromyography tests electric potential of muscles and nerves leading to muscles. It evaluates muscle weakness or deterioration, pain, and disability and differentiates muscle and nerve problems. The physician inserts needle electrodes into selected muscles and uses electrical current to stimulate muscles. An oscilloscope records responses to electrical stimuli. If the client experiences discomfort after the study, warm compresses to the area help relieve discomfort.

Biopsy

A biopsy is done to identify composition of bone, muscle, or synovium. The specimen may be removed with a needle or excised surgically while the client is under general anesthesia. Afterward, observe the site for signs of bleeding or swelling, assess for pain, apply ice to the site, and administer analgesics as indicated.

Blood Tests

A complete blood count (includes a red blood cell count, hemoglobin level, white blood cell count, and differential) may be ordered to detect infection, inflammation, or anemia. Other diagnostic blood tests and findings of various musculoskeletal disorders include:

- Elevated alkaline phosphatase level—may indicate bone tumors and healing fractures
- Elevated acid phosphatase level—may indicate Paget's disease (a disorder characterized by excessive bone destruction and disorganized repair) and metastatic cancer
- Decreased serum calcium level—may indicate osteomalacia, osteoporosis, and bone tumors
- Increased serum phosphorus level—may indicate bone tumors and healing fractures
- Elevated serum uric acid level—may indicate gout (treated or untreated)
- Elevated antinuclear antibody level—may indicate lupus erythematosus, a connective tissue disorder

Urine Tests

When ordered, collect 24-hour urine samples for analysis to determine levels of uric acid and calcium excretion. In gout, the 24-hour excretion of uric acid is elevated. Elevated calcium levels are found in metastatic bone lesions and in clients with prolonged immobility.

NURSING MANAGEMENT

Some diagnostic tests are done while the client is assessed in the emergency department, on an outpatient basis, or after admission for treatment of the disorder. Implement protocols necessary to prepare the client for the diagnostic examination, identify and send collected specimens to the laboratory, and manage the client's safe recovery after invasive procedures.

If the client has a chronic disorder, obtain a general medical history and a description of the current symptoms. Compile drug and allergy histories. An allergy to iodine and seafood may be a contraindication to performing an arthrogram or other test in which a contrast medium is instilled.

No special care is required after most laboratory tests, general x-rays, or a bone scan. If the client has had an invasive joint examination, inspect the area for swelling, bleeding, or serous drainage. Change or reinforce dressings as needed. If the client has severe pain in the area, notify the physician, who may order the application of ice and an analgesic for pain or discomfort.

In the case of a traumatic injury, obtain information regarding the injury from the client, the person accompanying the client, or paramedics and ambulance personnel. Take vital signs during the initial examination and at frequent intervals until the client's condition stabilizes. Check the neurovascular status of the affected limb, including circulation, motion, and sensation. Keeping the client calm and promoting comfort are essential measures. For example, if the client has an arm injury, prepare a sling to ease pain until treatment can be initiated.

NURSING PROCESS

The Client With a Musculoskeletal Injury

Assessment

Assess the injury in terms of its location, nature, and effects on mobility. Determine circulatory status to the injured area by checking circulation, sensation, and mobility, if indicated. Assess the client's level of pain. Monitor vital signs and closely observe for signs of shock.

Diagnosis, Planning, and Interventions

Describe diagnostic tests or treatments briefly, because the client will find it difficult to comprehend details while anxious. Provide information about how long the test or examination will take, where it will be done, and what preparations (if any) are necessary. Allow the client an opportunity to ask questions or make comments.

Invasive procedures, such as arthroscopy, and treatment procedures require the client to sign a consent form. The physician is responsible for explaining the purpose of the procedure, its risks and benefits, and available alternatives. Repeat or clarify the physician's explanations. After an outpatient procedure, the physician often gives the client special instructions for self-care. Because recalling information from memory can lead to confusion or injury, provide written discharge instructions. See Client and Family Teaching 60-1.

Pain related to tissue injury

Expected Outcome: Client will have relief from pain.

- Minimize or avoid moving the painful body part. *Doing so prevents increased pain and helps the client to relax.*
- If the client must be moved from a stretcher, wheelchair, or an examination table, request sufficient help and support the joints above and below the area of discomfort during transfer. *Sufficient support prevents pain and avoids increasing discomfort.*
- Support an acutely or chronically inflamed joint in a comfortable position. *Maintaining a neutral position reduces pain.*
- Elevate a swollen extremity as long as doing so does not potentiate the trauma from an injury. Alternatively, cradle a painful arm in a sling when the client

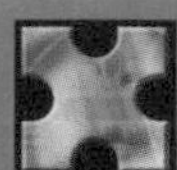

60-1 *Client and Family Teaching* Musculoskeletal Care

The nurse includes the following information:

- Signs or symptoms that clients must report, such as excessive pain or throbbing, prolonged or fresh bleeding, swelling, skin color changes, decrease in sensation, or purulent drainage
- Any special body position that the client must maintain
- When to resume bathing and activity
- How soon the client may return to work
- Purpose of prescribed drugs, how to take them, and possible side effects
- Approximate date for a follow-up appointment with the physician, if one is required
- How to remove and reapply dressings, and how to apply an immobilizer or sling, if needed
- Demonstrations of safe crutch-walking gait, if needed

is up and about. *These measures reduce swelling and, subsequently, pain.*

- Observe for signs of respiratory depression if administering a prescribed narcotic analgesic for pain relief. *Opioids may cause respiratory depression and lead to sedation in a client susceptible to shock after a traumatic injury.*
- Notify physician if pain increases or is unrelieved. *Persistent pain may indicate further injury or sequelae to trauma.*

Risk for Impaired Tissue Perfusion related to swelling, inflammation, or inactivity imposed by injury

Expected Outcome: Client will maintain tissue perfusion in the injured area as evidenced by normal neurovascular assessment findings.

- Keep a swollen body part above the level of the heart. *This position promotes venous circulation and relieves edema.*
- Consult with the physician about applying a cold pack if an injury is recent. *Cold reduces circulation to the affected area and may impair neurovascular health.*
- In cases of head injury, elevate the client's head slightly while keeping the neck neutral. *Such positioning reduces the risk of further injury.*
- Report the absence of a peripheral pulse and severe pain immediately. *These findings may indicate ischemia.*

Anxiety related to pain and injury, its treatment, and the potential for altered mobility

Expected Outcome: Client's anxiety will be reduced as evidenced by vital signs within normal range and no signs of being overly alert or easily startled.

- Relieve discomfort as much as possible. *Doing so eliminates at least one aspect of the client's concerns.*
- Call the client by name; be empathic and attentive. *Attention to the client's needs promotes relaxation and comfort.*
- Instill confidence by demonstrating technical skill and competence in explanations or preparations for tests or treatments. *A confident nurse can help reduce a client's anxiety.*
- Speak quietly in simple sentences that the client can understand. *Understanding reduces anxiety.*
- Allow a supportive family member to stay with the client if possible. *This measure can comfort the client.*

Evaluation of Expected Outcomes

The client states that medication and positioning relieved pain. Neurovascular status remains intact, as evidenced by good perfusion, strong pulses, ability to tense muscles, and appropriate sensation. The client has a calm demeanor and states that he or she is less anxious.

GENERAL GERONTOLOGIC CONSIDERATIONS

Women older than 45 years of age have a 9% to 10% decrease in cortical bone per decade.

Older adults are more prone to skeletal fractures because bone resorption is more rapid than bone formation.

Maintaining an active lifestyle delays the decline in muscle strength and bone mass among older adults.

With age, the fibrocartilage of intervertebral disks becomes thinner and drier, causing compression of the disks of the spinal column, and the water content of joint cartilage decreases, leading to a height loss of as much as 1.5 inches to 3 inches (3.75 cm to 7.5 cm).

Estrogen deficiency, which occurs at menopause, is considered the leading factor in osteoporosis among aging women.

Critical Thinking Exercises

1. *A client for whom you are caring in a nursing home falls. What assessments would you make?*
2. *What signs and symptoms would indicate that the tissue in an injured extremity is not being adequately perfused?*

● NCLEX-STYLE REVIEW QUESTIONS

1. A nurse is called to the scene of a bike accident. Upon arrival, the nurse notes that the victim's leg is deformed with the tibia protruding through the skin. Which of the following actions is the initial priority?
    1. Apply gentle traction to align the fracture for correct healing.
    2. Cover the broken skin and splint in the position of the deformity.

   3. Wrap with a tight, clean cloth to apply gentle traction to the deformity.
   4. Support the leg upon moving, with no further nursing action needed.

2. Which of the following nursing actions is most important in maintaining tissue perfusion following an arm injury?
   1. Apply an ice pack to the injured arm area.
   2. Position the arm above the level of the heart.
   3. Dangle the arm to the side of the body.
   4. Maintain alignment of the arm on the side of the body.

3. When responding to a traumatic injury, which of the following is the initial action in assessment?
   1. Obtaining a history
   2. Elevating the client's head
   3. Obtaining vital signs
   4. Assessing for pain

connection—

Visit the Connection site at **http://connection.lww.com/go/timbyEssentials** for links to chapter-related resources on the Internet.

References and Suggested Readings

Bullock, B. L., & Henze, R. L. (2000). *Focus on pathophysiology.* Philadelphia: Lippincott Williams & Wilkins.

Fischbach, F. (2002). *Common laboratory and diagnostic tests* (3rd ed.). Philadelphia: Lippincott Williams & Wilkins.

Lawrence, B. L., & Tasota, F. J. (2003). Detecting neuromuscular problems with electromyography. *Nursing 2003, 33*(4), 82.

Smeltzer, S. C., & Bare, B. G. (2004). *Brunner & Suddarth's textbook of medical-surgical nursing* (10th ed.). Philadelphia: Lippincott Williams & Wilkins.

chapter 61

Caring for Clients With Orthopedic and Connective Tissue Disorders

Words to Know 

ankylosis
arthritis
arthroplasty
avascular necrosis
avulsion fracture
Bouchard's nodes
bursitis
callus
carpal tunnel syndrome
cast
closed reduction
compartment syndrome
contusion
degenerative joint disease
dislocation
ecchymosis
epicondylitis
external fixation
fasciotomy
fracture
gout
hallux valgus
hammertoe
Heberden's nodes
hyperuricemia
internal fixation
involucrum
lupus erythematosus
Lyme disease
open reduction
osseous ankylosis
osteomalacia
osteomyelitis
osteoporosis
palsy
pannus
rheumatoid arthritis
rheumatic disorders
sequestrum
sprain
strain
subluxation
synovitis
tophi
traction
Volkmann's contracture

Learning Objectives

On completion of this chapter, the reader will:

- Differentiate strains, contusions, and sprains.
- Describe signs and symptoms and common treatments of a fracture.
- Identify principles for maintaining traction.
- Discuss complications associated with a fractured hip.
- Contrast rheumatoid arthritis and degenerative joint disease.
- Describe positioning precautions after a total hip replacement.
- State the pathophysiology of gout and bursitis.
- Explain the inflammatory process associated with Lyme disease.
- Identify causes of osteomyelitis.
- Discuss the multisystem involvement associated with systemic lupus erythematosus.
- State who is at risk for development of osteoporosis.
- Differentiate bunions and hammertoe.
- Explain the cause of carpal tunnel syndrome.
- Discuss characteristics of malignant bone tumors.
- Identify reasons for performing orthopedic surgery.
- Describe principles to follow when wrapping a stump.
- Discuss nursing management for a client with a sprain, dislocation, or cast; who is in traction or undergoing orthopedic surgery; or with an amputation.

The musculoskeletal system consists of structures the body uses for support and movement. It also protects body organs. Disorders affecting the musculoskeletal system affect a person's ability to perform activities of daily living (ADLs) and to remain active, mobile, and physically fit.

TRAUMATIC INJURIES

• STRAINS, CONTUSIONS, AND SPRAINS

A **strain** is an injury to a muscle when stretched or pulled beyond capacity. A **contusion** is a soft tissue injury resulting from a blow or blunt trauma. **Sprains** are injuries to the ligaments surrounding a joint.

Pathophysiology and Etiology

A strain results from excessive stress, overuse, or overstretching. Small blood vessels in the muscle rupture, and muscle fibers sustain tiny tears. The client experiences inflammation, local tenderness, and muscle spasms.

In contusions, injury is confined to soft tissues and does not affect the musculoskeletal structure. Many small blood vessels rupture, causing bruises (**ecchymosis**) or a hematoma (collection of blood). Applying cold packs alleviates local pain, swelling, and bruising. A contusion usually resolves within 2 weeks.

Areas most subject to sprains are the wrist, elbow, knee, and ankle. A sprain of the cervical spine is called a *whiplash injury*. Sprains result from sudden, unusual movement or stretching about a joint, common with falls or other accidental injuries. The force twists the joint in a direction it was not designed for or displaces it beyond its normal range of motion (ROM) by partially tearing or rupturing the attachment of ligaments. Damage usually is confined to ligaments and adjacent soft tissue. In severe traumatic sprains, a chip of bone to which the ligament is attached may become detached. This injury is called an **avulsion fracture.** A hematoma that may develop subsequently contributes to pain because it exerts additional pressure on nerve endings in the area.

Assessment Findings

The injured area becomes painful immediately, and swelling usually follows. The person typically avoids full weight bearing or using the injured joint or limb. Later, ecchymoses may appear. In cases of extensive ligamental tearing, the joint may be unstable until it heals.

In most cases, diagnosis is made by examination of the affected part and symptoms. X-rays may show a larger-than-usual joint space and rule out or confirm fracture. Arthrography demonstrates asymmetry in the joint as a result of damaged ligaments, or arthroscopy may disclose trauma in the joint capsule.

Medical and Surgical Management

Treatment consists of applying ice or a chemical cold pack to the area to reduce swelling and relieve pain for the first 24 to 48 hours. Elevation of the part and compression with an elastic bandage also may be recommended. The acronym RICE refers to *r*est, *i*ce, *c*ompression, and *e*levation—a method for remembering treatment for strains, contusions, and sprains. After 2 days, when swelling no longer is likely to increase, applying heat reduces pain and relieves local edema by improving circulation. Full use of the injured joint is discouraged temporarily. Nonsteroidal anti-inflammatory drugs (NSAIDs) ease discomfort.

Continued trauma during healing may result in a permanently unstable joint or formation of fibrous adhesions that may limit full ROM. Occasionally, a removable splint or light cast is applied for several weeks. A soft cervical collar limits motion if the client has a neck sprain. When sufficient healing occurs, progressively active exercises are prescribed.

Stop, Think, and Respond ● BOX 61-1

You are at a playground when you notice a man, who has been playing basketball with his son, fall and grab his ankle. He says his ankle hurts very badly, and he does not think that he can walk. What action should you take?

● DISLOCATIONS

Dislocations occur when the articular surfaces of a joint are no longer in contact. The shoulder, hip, and knee commonly are affected. A partial dislocation is referred to as a **subluxation.**

Pathophysiology and Etiology

In adults, trauma usually causes dislocations. Diseases of the joint may result in dislocations when ligaments supporting a joint are torn, stretched, or relaxed. Separation of adjacent bones from their articulating joint interferes with normal use and produces a distorted appearance. The injury may disrupt local blood supply to structures such as the joint cartilage, causing degeneration, chronic pain, and restricted movement. **Compartment syndrome** (a condition in which a structure such as a tendon or nerve is constricted in a confined space) also may develop. The syndrome affects nerve innervation, leading to subsequent **palsy** (decreased sensation and movement). If compartment syndrome occurs in an upper extremity, it may lead to **Volkmann's contracture,** a clawlike deformity of the hand resulting from obstructed arterial blood flow to the forearm and hand. The client is unable to extend his or her fingers and complains of unrelenting pain, particularly if attempting to stretch the hand. There also are signs of compromised circulation to the hand.

Another possible complication of dislocations during the healing process involves insufficient deposit of collagen during the repair stage. The ligaments may have reduced tensile strength and future instability, leading to recurrent dislocations of the same joint.

Assessment Findings

The client often reports hearing a "popping" sound when dislocation occurs, or the joint suddenly "gives out" (becomes unstable or nonsupportive). If the dislocation is related to trauma, the client usually experiences considerable pain from injury or resultant muscle spasm.

On inspection, the structural shape is altered. A depression may be noted about the joint's circumference, indicating that bones above and below are no longer aligned.

If the dislocation affects an extremity, the arm or leg may be shorter than its unaffected counterpart as a result of displacement of one of the articulating bones. ROM is limited. Evidence of soft tissue injury includes swelling, coolness, numbness, tingling, and pale or dusky color of the distal tissue.

X-rays show intact yet malpositioned bones. Arthrography or arthroscopy may reveal damage to other structures in the joint capsule.

Medical and Surgical Management

The physician manipulates the joint or reduces the displaced parts until they return to normal position, then immobilizes the joint with an elastic bandage, cast, or splint for several weeks. This allows the joint capsule and surrounding ligaments to heal. The client may receive a local or general anesthetic before manipulation is done. Some dislocations may require surgery to correct the dislocation or repair damage caused by injury.

Nursing Management

Relieve client's discomfort by administering prescribed analgesics, elevating and immobilizing the affected limb, and applying cold packs to the injury. Perform neurovascular assessments every 30 minutes for several hours and then at least every 2 to 4 hours for the next 1 or 2 days to detect complications such as compartment syndrome. See Chapter 60 for more information about neurovascular assessments.

• FRACTURES

A **fracture** is a break in the continuity of a bone. Fractures may affect tissues or organs near the bones as well. Fractures are classified according to type and extent (Box 61-1).

BOX 61-1 ● Types of Fractures

Avulsion—a pulling away of a fragment of bone by a ligament or tendon and its attachment
Comminuted—a fracture in which bone has splintered into several fragments
Compound—a fracture in which damage also involves the skin or mucous membranes
Compression—a fracture in which bone has been compressed (seen in vertebral fractures)
Depressed—a fracture in which fragments are driven inward (seen frequently in fractures of skull and facial bones)
Epiphyseal—a fracture through the epiphysis
Greenstick—a fracture in which one side of a bone is broken and the other side is bent
Impacted—a fracture in which a bone fragment is driven into another bone fragment
Oblique—a fracture occurring at an angle across the bone (less stable than transverse)
Pathologic—a fracture that occurs through an area of diseased bone (bone cyst, Paget's disease, bony metastasis, tumor); can occur without trauma or a fall
Simple—a fracture that remains contained; does not break the skin
Spiral—a fracture twisting around the shaft of the bone
Transverse—a fracture that is straight across the bone

Pathophysiology and Etiology

When force applied to a bone exceeds maximum resistance, the bone breaks. Sudden direct force from a blow or fall causes most fractures; however, some result from indirect force—for example, from a strong muscle contraction, such as during a seizure. A few fractures result from underlying weakness created by bone infections, bone tumors, or more bone resorption than production (as occurs in clients who are inactive or aging).

For 10 to 40 minutes after a bone breaks, muscles surrounding the bone are flaccid. Then they go into spasm, often increasing deformity and interfering with vascular and lymphatic circulations. Tissue surrounding the fracture swells from hemorrhage and edema. Healing begins (Fig. 61.1) when blood in the area clots and a fibrin network forms between the broken bone ends. The fibrin network changes into granulation tissue. Osteoblasts, which proliferate in the clot, increase secretion of an enzyme that restores the alkaline pH. As a result, calcium is deposited and true bone forms. The healing mass is called a **callus.** It holds the ends of the bone together but cannot endure strain. Bone repair is a local process. About 1 year of healing must pass before bone regains its former structural strength, becomes well consolidated and remodeled (reformed), and possesses fat and marrow cells.

Although fractures are common, they are associated with various complications, particularly when they are very complex. Table 61.1 briefly describes the types of possible complications, which include compartment syndrome, thromboembolism, fat embolism, delayed healing, nonunion, malunion, infection, and **avascular necrosis** (death of bone from an insufficient blood supply). Clients who are inactive during convalescence are prone to pneumonia, thrombophlebitis, pressure sores, urinary tract infection, renal calculi, constipation, muscle atrophy, weight gain, and depression.

Assessment Findings

Signs and symptoms of a fracture vary, depending on the type and location. They include the following:

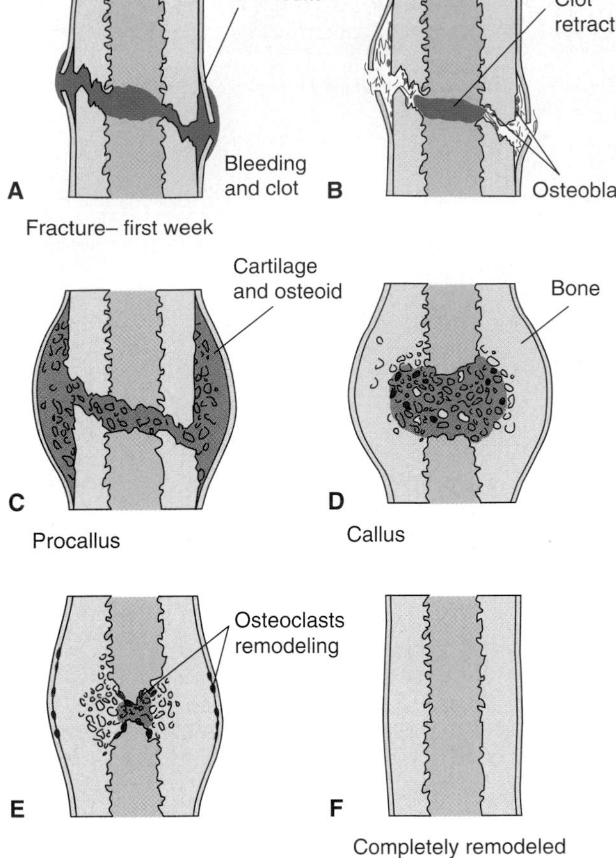

FIGURE 61.1 Process of bone healing. (**A**) Immediately after a bone fractures, blood seeps into the area, and a hematoma (blood clot) forms. (**B**) After 1 week, osteoblasts form as the clot retracts. (**C**) After about 3 weeks, a procallus forms and stabilizes the fracture. (**D**) A callus with bone cells forms in 6 to 12 weeks. (**E**) In 3 to 4 months, osteoblasts begin to remodel the fracture site. (**F**) If the fractured bone has been accurately aligned during healing, remodeling will be complete in about 12 months.

- Pain—The most consistent symptom of a fracture is pain, which may be severe. Attempts to move the part and pressure over the fracture increase pain.
- Loss of function—Skeletal muscular function depends on intact bone.
- Deformity—A break may cause an extremity to bend backward or to assume another unusual position.
- False motion—Unnatural motion occurs at the site of the fracture.
- Crepitus—The grating sound of bone ends moving over one another may be audible (this term also refers to a popping sound caused by air trapped in soft tissue).
- Edema—Swelling usually is greatest directly over the fracture.
- Spasm—Muscles near fractures involuntarily contract. Spasm, which accounts for some of the pain, may cause a limb to shorten when the fracture involves a long bone.

If sharp bone fragments tear through sufficient surrounding soft tissue, there is bleeding and black and blue discoloration of the area. If a nerve is damaged, paralysis may result.

Stop, Think, and Respond ● BOX 61-2

You are cross-country skiing with a friend and notice that a person ahead of you has fallen. When you get closer, this person tells you that she has hurt her arm. What signs would indicate that this woman probably has a fractured humerus?

One or more x-rays of the area almost always demonstrate altered bone structure. Stress fractures may not be apparent radiographically for a few weeks. A bone scan usually identifies a nondisplaced or stress fracture before radiographic changes are evident. A computed tomography (CT) scan or magnetic resonance imaging (MRI) may be necessary.

Medical and Surgical Management

The goal is to re-establish functional continuity of the bone. Treatment includes one or more methods: traction, closed or open reduction, internal or external fixation, or cast application. The treatment method depends on many factors, including first aid given, location and severity of the break, and age and overall physical condition of the client.

Traction

Traction is a method of pulling structures of the musculoskeletal system, which requires *countertraction,* a force opposite to the mechanical pull. Countertraction usually is supplied by the client's own weight. Traction relieves muscle spasm, aligns bones, and maintains immobilization.

Skin traction applies devices to the skin that indirectly affect the muscles or bones. An example is Buck's traction; another example is Russell traction. *Skeletal traction* is applied directly to a bone by using a wire (Kirschner), pin (Steinmann), or cranial tongs (Crutchfield). General or local anesthesia may be used when inserting these devices. The pull is achieved by connecting the attachment from the client to a system of ropes, pulleys, and weights on an orthopedic bed frame. A Thomas splint with a Pearson attachment often is used to suspend a leg in traction. This is referred to as *balanced suspension traction.* Nursing care measures for a client in traction are presented in Nursing Guidelines 61-1.

Closed Reduction

In a **closed reduction,** bone is restored to normal position by external manipulation. A bandage, cast, or traction then immobilizes the area. X-rays are taken to ensure correct alignment of the bone. Depending on the site and

TABLE 61.1 COMPLICATIONS OF FRACTURES

COMPLICATION	DESCRIPTION	NURSING IMPLICATIONS
Shock	Hypovolemic shock related to blood loss and loss of extracellular fluid from damaged tissue. If untreated, the client's condition will deteriorate.	Administer blood and fluid volume replacements as prescribed to prevent further losses.
Fat embolism	Fat globules released after fractures of pelvis or long bones, or after multiple injuries or crushing injuries. Globules combine with platelets to form emboli. Onset is rapid, with client experiencing respiratory distress and cerebral disturbances.	Monitor client for symptoms, which usually occur within 48–72 hours. To prevent fatty emboli, provide early respiratory support, ensure rapid immobilization of fracture, and observe client closely for signs of respiratory and nervous system problems.
Pulmonary embolism	Thromboembolism may occur after fracture or surgery to repair fractures. These lead to pulmonary emboli in some clients and can be fatal.	Promote circulation and prevent venous stasis to avoid pulmonary embolism. Administer low-dose heparin subcutaneously as prescribed to prevent clot formation.
Compartment syndrome	Tissue perfusion in the muscle compartment (muscle covered by inelastic fascia) is compromised secondary to tissue swelling, hemorrhage, or a cast that is too tight. If circulation is not restored, ischemia and tissue anoxia lead to permanent nerve damage, muscle atrophy, and contracture.	Monitor client for signs and symptoms of compartment syndrome such as unrelenting pain, unrelieved by analgesics. Elevate the extremity, apply ice, and perform neurovascular checks to help prevent this complication. As indicated, relieve pressure by loosening cast or preparing the client for a **fasciotomy** (surgical incision of fascia and separation of muscles).
Delayed bone healing	Bone fails to heal at the expected rate. Delayed healing may result from nonunion, characterized by the ends of the fractured bone failing to unite and heal, or it may result from malunion, characterized by the ends of the fractured bone healing in a deformed position.	Delayed union may require surgical intervention to promote bone growth, and correct the incorrect union. If necessary, prepare the client for use of electrical stimulation measures that promote bone growth, or for a bone graft.
Infection	The potential for infection increases with compound fractures, application of skeletal traction, or surgical procedures.	Perform careful assessments and maintain aseptic technique to prevent infections. Monitor for early signs of infection because early detection promotes early correction of the problem.
Avascular necrosis	This condition occurs from interruption of the blood supply to the fracture fragments, after which the bone tissue dies; most common in the femoral head.	Be alert for client reports of pain and decreased function of the affected limb. If necessary, prepare the client for surgery, such as bone graft, bone prosthesis, joint replacement, joint fusion, or amputation.

type of fracture, the client receives a local (nerve block) or general anesthetic for this procedure.

Open Reduction

In an **open reduction,** done in the operating room, bone is surgically exposed and realigned. Usually the client receives a general or spinal anesthetic. Radiographic studies, taken while the client is still anesthetized, show whether realignments are needed.

Internal Fixation

If **internal fixation** is needed to stabilize the reduced fracture, the surgeon secures the bone with metal screws, plates, rods, nails, or pins. A cast or other method of immobilization is then applied. Open reduction is required when:

- Soft tissue, such as nerves or blood vessels, is caught between the ends of the broken pieces of bone.
- The bone has a wide separation.
- Comminuted fractures are present.
- Patella and other joints are fractured.
- Open fractures are evident.
- Wound debridement is necessary.
- Internal fixation is needed.

External Fixation

In **external fixation,** the surgeon inserts metal pins into bone or bones from outside the skin surface and

NURSING GUIDELINES 61-1

Managing the Care of the Client in Traction

- Assess neurovascular status frequently. Compare assessment findings in the affected limb with those in the unaffected limb.
- Check traction equipment for:
  - Proper alignment (position client so that the body is in an opposite straight line to the pull of traction)
  - Correct attachment
  - Prescribed amount of weight
  - Freely hanging weights and freely moving ropes over unobstructed pulleys
  - Maintenance of countertraction and continuous traction
- Monitor client for signs of pressure areas.
- Encourage client to be as mobile as possible and to perform exercises as indicated.
- If traction is applied to the lower extremity, observe foot position and prevent footdrop.
- If skeletal traction is applied, follow procedure for pin care.
- Cover tips of any protruding metal pins or rods with corks or other protective material.

then attaches a compression device to the pins. Some complex or comminuted fractures may require an external fixation device to stabilize and position the bone. Because pin sites are an entry for infection, monitor for redness, drainage, and tenderness. Nursing Guidelines 61-2 describe pin care.

NURSING GUIDELINES 61-2

Providing Pin Care

Scrupulous pin care assists in preventing localized infection at the pin sites and systemic infection and osteomyelitis:

- Assess pin sites for redness, swelling, increased tenderness, and drainage.
- Examine pins for signs of breakage, bending, or shifting.
- Wearing gloves, use cotton-tipped applicators and saline to cleanse pin sites.
- Use at least one applicator per pin—do not use applicator more than once.
- Clean pin site from pin outward.
- Gently remove crusted areas.
- Avoid applying ointment to pin sites unless specifically ordered.
- Obtain culture if purulent drainage is present.
- Teach client not to touch pin sites.
- Instruct family member in pin care if client is discharged.

Casts

A **cast** is a rigid mold that immobilizes an injured structure while it heals. Casts usually are made of fiberglass, polyester, or thermoplastic material. Plaster of Paris may be used, but these cases require several hours for drying, whereas other materials dry rapidly.

There are basically three types of casts. A *cylinder cast* encircles an arm or leg, leaving fingers or toes exposed. A *body cast* is a larger form of a cylinder cast that encircles the trunk from about the nipple line to the iliac crests. A *spica hip cast* surrounds one or both legs and the trunk. It may be strengthened by a bar that spans a casted area between the legs. It is trimmed open in the anal and genital areas to facilitate elimination.

To keep aligned bone fragments from becoming displaced, the cast is applied from the joint above the break to the one below it. The joint is slightly flexed to decrease stiffness. Some fractures (e.g., a stress fracture) do not require surgical reduction or manual manipulation because the fractured bone is already aligned. If a closed or open reduction is required, the client receives an analgesic or a general or local anesthetic to relieve pain.

When applying the cast, the client is positioned to ensure proper alignment of the part to be immobilized. The client's buttocks may be supported on a casting frame when a body cast or spica cast is applied so the casting material can be wrapped around the client's trunk. A nurse or an assistant holds the arm or leg in place during application of a cylinder cast (Box 61-2). If the client is awake, healthcare providers explain that the cast material will feel warm during application as a result of being mixed with water.

A wet cast must be kept uncovered so that water can evaporate. Most physicians prefer natural evaporation but may order a cast dryer to speed evaporation. Intense heat never is used. There is a danger not only of burning the client, but of cracking the outside of the cast while leaving the inside damp and hospitable to mold. The drying cast should be supported on pillows. If necessary, healthcare personnel can reposition the casted arm or leg with the palms of the hands. Using fingertips or compressing the cast on a hard surface can lead to a pressure sore later.

BOX 61-2 ● Applying a Cast

In general, the physician or nurse practitioner applies a cast as follows:

- Clean and dry the skin surface.
- Cover the skin with stockinette, a tubular knitted material.
- Wrap padding around the limb, especially over bony prominences.
- Apply rolls or strips of cast material over the stockinette and padding.
- Smooth the layers and edges of the cast.
- Fasten the stockinette in cufflike fashion to the outside of the cast.
- Arrange for an x-ray study after casting to check bone alignment.

After the cast dries, a cast window, or opening, may be cut. This usually is done when the client reports discomfort under the cast or has a wound that requires a dressing change. The window permits direct inspection of the skin, a means to check the pulse in a casted arm or leg, or a way to change a dressing. Once a window is cut, the solid piece of cast is replaced in its original site and secured with adhesive tape or a roller bandage. Leaving the window open may allow the skin and soft tissue to bulge through the opening.

Once a cast is applied, it may be bivalved, or cut in two. This is done if the arm or leg swells, causing the rigid cast to compress tissue and interfere with its blood supply. A bivalved cast also may be used for a client being weaned from a cast, when a sharp x-ray is needed, or as a splint for immobilizing painful joints when a client has arthritis.

Casts are removed with a mechanical cast cutter. Cast cutters are noisy and frightening, and the client needs reassurance that the machine will not cut into skin. Once the cast is off, the skin appears mottled and may be covered with a yellowish crust composed of accumulated body oil and dead skin. The client usually sheds this residue in a few days. Lotions and warm baths or soaks may help to soften the skin and remove debris.

The now uncasted limb feels surprisingly light, and the client may report weakness and stiffness. For some time, the limb will need support. An elastic bandage may be wrapped on a leg, the client may use a cane, and an arm may be kept in a sling until progressive active exercise and physical therapy help the client regain normal strength and motion.

Nursing Management

When caring for the client with a fracture, assess the client for neurovascular and systemic complications. General nursing measures include administering analgesics, providing comfort measures, assisting with ADLs, preventing constipation, promoting physical mobility, preventing infection, maintaining skin integrity, and preparing the client for self-care. Because the client may be discharged shortly after application of an immobilization device or a cast, review care with the client and family. In addition, reinforce instructions regarding exercise and ambulatory activities.

If a client is in traction, provide simple and direct explanations about the traction and its purpose. Provide pin care as indicated. Inform client of activities that are allowed or contraindicated and identify the approximate duration of restrictions. When the traction is discontinued, prepare the client for further treatment, such as casting, and the appearance of the affected area—skin and muscles. Reassure the client that, with gradual exercise and use, muscles will regain strength and tone, and joints will be flexible. For more information about managing problems related to casting, refer to Nursing Guidelines 61-3.

When indicated, elevate the extremity, which reduces swelling and pain. Apply ice pack to site of injury. Change client's position within prescribed limits to relieve pressure on bony prominences and promote comfort. Perform neurovascular assessments frequently, reporting any compromise immediately. Capillary refill should be brisk (within 3 seconds), skin should be warm and normally colored, and the client should be able to move the extremity. Diminished or absent peripheral pulses, pale or mottled skin, cool to cold skin, or increased pain (especially with movement) can indicate arterial obstruction. Changes in sensation such as numbness, tingling, or prickling may indicate nerve compression and damage, compartment syndrome, or both. Encourage client to actively move toes, fingers, and unaffected extremities, which promotes circulation and indicates neurologic and motor function. Apply elastic stockings if indicated.

Instruct client in active and passive ROM exercises for affected and unaffected extremities, within physical and medical restrictions. See Nursing Care Plan 61-1 for more interventions related to orthopedic surgery.

• FRACTURED FEMUR

A fracture of the femur commonly occurs in automobile accidents but may occur in falls from ladders or other high places, or in gunshot wounds. Multiple injuries often accompany fractures of the femur, because they usually occur with severe trauma.

Assessment Findings

Severe pain, swelling, and ecchymosis may be seen. The client usually cannot move the hip or knee. If a compound fracture is present, there is an open wound or a protrusion of bone. X-rays show the type and location of the fracture.

Medical and Surgical Management

Fractures of the femur usually are treated initially with some form of traction to prevent deformities and soft tissue injury. Skeletal traction or an external fixator aligns the fracture in preparation for future reduction if the fracture occurred in the lower two thirds of the femur. Once the femur is aligned, a spica cast may be used to maintain the corrected position.

Nursing Management

Because the client is confined to bed, implement measures to prevent complications of immobility and inactivity.

NURSING GUIDELINES 61-3

Caring for the Client With a Cast

Before Cast Application

- Inspect the condition of the skin that will be covered with a cast.
- Assess circulation, sensation, and mobility to establish a baseline.
- Evaluate the client's pain level.
- Remove clothing that will be difficult to remove after the cast is applied.
- Explain the procedure to the client. Remember to tell the client that the cast will feel warm—even hot—as it is applied, but that it will not burn the skin.

After Cast Application

- Leave the cast uncovered.
- Assess circulation, sensation, and mobility in exposed fingers and toes every 1 to 2 hours.
- Monitor for signs of complications related to cast application. Report abnormal findings immediately.
- Handle wet cast with the palms of the hands, not the fingers.
- Elevate casted extremity so that it is higher than the heart.
- Reposition the client frequently while cast is drying so that the cast dries as evenly as possible.
- Apply ice packs to the cast where surgery was performed.
- Circle areas where blood seeped through and write the time on the circle.
- Petal cast edges with strips of adhesive tape to prevent chipping and to cover any remaining rough areas.
- Replace windows in the hole from which they were cut to prevent tissue from bulging through the opening.
- Ambulate client as soon as indicated.

Discharge Teaching

- Elevate casted extremity for 24 to 48 hours after cast application, and as indicated.
- If the client has a leg cast, show him or her how to ambulate safely.
- Exercise joints proximal and distal to the cast as indicated to prevent muscle atrophy, weakness, and loss of joint mobility.
- Keep the cast clean and dry. A damp cloth may be used.
- Explain that the skin under the cast may feel itchy, and caution client not to insert objects like straws, combs, eating utensils, knitting needles, and the like.
- Report the following to the physician or nurse: unusual and sudden pain, painful or decreased movement, or persistent pain; fever, foul odors, or increased warmth of extremity; drainage from under the cast; changes in circulation, mobility, or sensation (burning, numbness, tingling, or cold).

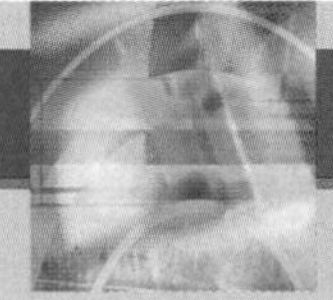

Nursing Care Plan 61-1

THE CLIENT UNDERGOING ORTHOPEDIC SURGERY

Assessment

- When client returns from surgery, review orders regarding immobilization, movement or turning, and positioning of the extremity. Inspect the dressing over the incision. If a wound drain is present, assess patency of the drain and type and amount of drainage in the collection receptacle. Assess neurovascular status of the affected extremity. Monitor vital signs frequently until they stabilize, and routinely thereafter. Maintain infusing IV fluids as ordered. Assess respiratory status. Encourage client to identify pain levels and the effectiveness of analgesics.
- Within the first 24 to 72 hours after orthopedic surgery, complications, such as a fat embolus, may occur (see Table 61.1). Symptoms are similar to those of a pulmonary embolus. In addition, petechial hemorrhages may appear on the skin of the chest. Report severe chest pain or unrelieved incisional pain to the physician immediately.

Nursing Diagnosis: **Risk for Ineffective Breathing Pattern** related to mucus and inability to mobilize secretions from the airway

Expected Outcome: Client will demonstrate effective respiratory rate and depth with clear breath sounds.

(continued)

Nursing Care Plan 61-1 (Continued)

THE CLIENT UNDERGOING ORTHOPEDIC SURGERY

Interventions	Rationales
Instruct client to deep breathe and cough every 2 hours until he or she can ambulate.	These measures expand the lungs and mobilize mucus, preventing pooling of secretions.
Encourage client to use an incentive spirometer to increase deep breathing. Evaluate client's efforts.	Increasing respiratory effort improves client's respiratory status.
Turn client at least every 2 hours and encourage activity within the prescribed limits.	Movement facilitates lung expansion and prevents pooling of secretions.
Auscultate lung sounds every 4 hours.	Immobility can cause hypoventilation, predisposing a client to atelectasis, pooling of respiratory secretions, and pneumonia.

Evaluation of Expected Outcome: Client effectively deep breathes and coughs. Lung sounds are clear.

Nursing Diagnosis: **Pain** related to surgery

Expected Outcome: Client will report relief of pain.

Interventions	Rationales
Gently move client or adjust position.	Gentle handling minimizes discomfort.
Administer analgesics as prescribed. Instruct client in the use of patient-controlled analgesia if ordered.	Regular administration of analgesics controls and prevents escalation of pain.
Elevate affected extremity and use cold applications.	These measures reduce swelling.
Report client's complaints of severe or sudden and unrelenting pain.	These findings may indicate a complication of surgery (see Table 61.1).

Evaluation of Expected Outcome: Client reports pain relief with analgesics and positioning.

Nursing Diagnosis: **Risk for Disuse Syndrome** related to immobility imposed by casting, traction, and non–weight-bearing status

Expected Outcomes: Client will maintain full ROM of unaffected joints, intact skin, good peripheral blood flow, and normal bowel and bladder function.

Interventions	Rationales
Encourage client to do ROM exercises as indicated.	They help maintain muscle strength and tone and prevent contractures.
Position client so that joints are in normal anatomic alignment.	Proper positioning prevents joint deformities and damage to peripheral nerves and blood vessels.
Get client up as soon as indicated, either in chair, ambulating, or on a tilt table.	Early mobilization prevents complications related to prolonged bed rest.
When getting client up after bed rest, do so slowly, monitoring for signs of postural hypotension, tachycardia, nausea, diaphoresis, or syncope.	When sitting or standing after even 3 to 4 days of bed rest, a client can experience postural hypotension.
Turn client every 2 hours; inspect skin for signs of pressure.	Frequent turning relieves pressure and identifies problems, allowing for early intervention.

(continued)

Nursing Care Plan 61-1 (Continued)

THE CLIENT UNDERGOING ORTHOPEDIC SURGERY

Interventions	*Rationales*
Protect bony prominences from pressure. Massage them and skin surfaces subjected to pressure.	These measures promote circulation and prevent injury.
Apply antiembolism stockings as indicated.	They help prevent deep vein thrombosis (DVT).
Encourage client to actively move fingers and unaffected extremities.	Doing so promotes circulation and indicates neurologic and motor function.
Monitor peripheral circulation, particularly noting skin color, pulses, or any swelling.	Prolonged bed rest, orthopedic surgery, and venous stasis can cause DVT and pulmonary embolism.
Monitor bowel function daily. Provide increased fluids and fiber.	Immobilization causes constipation secondary to inactivity and food intake.
Encourage client to increase fluid intake to 2000 mL/day unless contraindicated.	This intake promotes normal bladder function and prevents constipation, kidney stones, and other related complications of prolonged bed rest.

Evaluation of Expected Outcomes:

- Client can maintain full ROM of unaffected joints.
- Skin remains intact without signs of pressure or breakdown.
- Peripheral circulation is adequate to sustain tissue perfusion.
- Client has adequate urine output and regular bowel movements.

Nursing Diagnosis: **Risk for Infection** related to compromised skin integrity

Expected Outcome: Client will remain free of infection.

Interventions	*Rationales*
Inspect pins or wire sites used in traction or external fixation devices and the surgical incision, or beneath a cast window for signs of infection.	Regular inspection promotes early detection of and prompt intervention for infection.
Practice standard precautions and conscientious handwashing.	They prevent infection.
Use aseptic principles when changing dressings and performing pin care.	Asepsis prevents introduction of microorganisms into wounds and incisions.
Keep wound drainage system below the level of the incision.	Doing so prevents backflow of drainage into the incision.
Administer prescribed antibiotics.	They reduce microorganisms and control infection.
Report purulent wound drainage, elevated temperature, chills, and increased white blood count.	These are signs of infection that require intervention.

Evaluation of Expected Outcome: Client is free of infection, as evidenced by normal temperature, clean incisions and pin sites, and no purulent drainage.

Nursing Diagnosis: **Self-Care Deficit: Bathing and Hygiene, Feeding, Dressing, and Toileting** related to musculoskeletal impairment

Expected Outcome: Client will gradually perform ADLs as independently as possible.

(continued)

Nursing Care Plan 61-1 (Continued)

THE CLIENT UNDERGOING ORTHOPEDIC SURGERY

Interventions	*Rationales*
Collaborate with client to determine tasks that he or she may perform independently.	Doing so promotes independence and provides client with a sense of control.
Plan activities and rest.	Doing so conserves energy and prevents fatigue.
Consult with physical therapist (PT) and occupational therapist (OT) about client's needs related to ADLs.	PT and OT will determine adaptive equipment needed, as well as client's strengths and abilities to master self-care tasks.
Provide pain medication 45 minutes before activity.	Pain relief promotes participation in self-care.

Evaluation of Expected Outcome: Client can partially bathe and feed himself or herself, dress upper body, and use the bedside commode.

Position the client in line with the pull exerted by the traction. Clean pin sites with a prescribed agent to prevent infection (see Nursing Guidelines 61-2).

• FRACTURED HIP

Usually a hip fracture affects the proximal end of the femur (Fig. 61.2). It commonly results from a fall and occurs more frequently in older adults with osteoporosis. Usually falls are not traumatic, but the client's condition contributes to the resulting fracture. Fractures may occur in the femoral neck (intracapsular or inside the hip joint capsule), between the trochanters (intertrochanteric-extracapsular or outside the hip joint capsule), or below the trochanters (subtrochanteric-extracapsular). Older adults are prone to complications after a hip fracture; some die from associated complications.

Assessment Findings

The client reports severe pain that increases with leg movement. Pain frequently radiates to the knee, and the client may sense pressure in the outer aspect of the hip. Discontinuity of bone and muscle spasm cause shortening and external rotation of the leg. A large blood loss

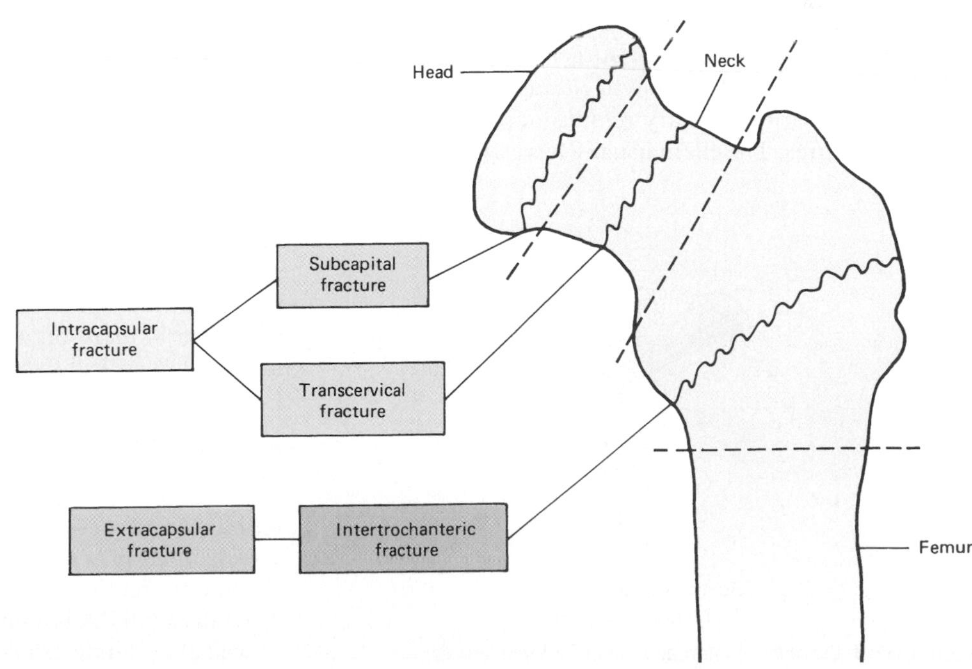

FIGURE 61.2 Types of hip fractures.

may accompany subtrochanteric and intertrochanteric fractures, leading to hypovolemic shock. There also may be extensive bruising and swelling in the hip, groin, and thigh. Femoral neck fractures are intracapsular, so bleeding is more likely to be contained within the joint capsule. X-rays reveal the exact location of the fracture, which may be within or outside the joint capsule.

Medical and Surgical Management

Buck's extension or other skin traction may be applied to relieve muscle spasm and pain until surgery is done. Open reduction-internal fixation, accomplished with a nail or an intramedullary rod (a rod inserted in the center of the bone with wires around the bone for stabilization), is done most commonly for fractures of the hip, particularly extracapsular fractures. See Figure 61.3 for an example. Intracapsular hip fractures are prone to nonunion and avascular necrosis from disrupted blood supply. Therefore, the fractured head and neck may be removed and replaced with a metal device such as an Austin-Moore or Thompson prosthesis. This procedure is referred to as *hemiarthroplasty*. A total hip arthroplasty is discussed later in the chapter.

Bone heals around the metallic device, which holds the bone together. The bone is united immediately, and clients ambulate much earlier. Plates, bands, screws, and pins may be removed after bone heals. More often, they are left in place permanently. Precautions with hemiarthroplasty are greater because the surgeon must dislocate the hip to replace the femoral head.

Nursing Management

Most clients with a fractured hip are older adults and prone to complications. After surgery, implement measures to prevent skin breakdown, wound infection, pneumonia, constipation, urinary retention, muscle atrophy, and contractures. The client usually has a wound drain in place for 1 to 2 days after surgery. Monitor the drainage and administer antibiotics as prescribed.

Show the client how to use the overhead trapeze bar safely for independent movement and activity. When client is recumbent, place a trochanter roll beside the hip to maintain a neutral position so that the repaired hip stays in place. Put abductor pillows between the client's legs when turning the client from side to side.

If a hip prosthesis is inserted, instruct the client to avoid adduction of the affected leg until it heals. The client must use abductor pillows at all times. Soon after surgery, the nurse or physical therapist assists the client to transfer from the bed to a chair, which must have an elevated seat so that the client does not flex the hips beyond 90°. The client usually requires much encouragement and assistance. Eventually the client progresses to ambulating with a walker. Before discharge, explore ways to ensure safety in the client's home to avoid future injuries and falls. Refer to Nursing Care Plan 61-1 for more information related to management of a client who requires orthopedic surgery.

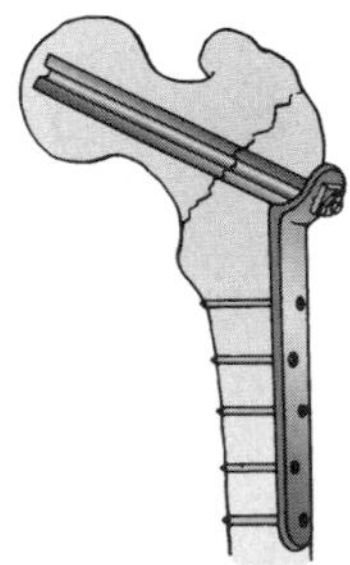

Smith-Petersen nail
with McLaughlin plate

FIGURE 61.3 Example of internal fixation for hip fractures.

INFLAMMATORY AND INFECTIOUS DISORDERS

Arthritis is a general condition characterized by inflammation and degeneration of a joint. **Rheumatic disorders** include more than 100 different types of recognized inflammatory disorders, making this collective group the most common orthopedic problem. These disorders involve inflammation and degeneration of connective tissue structures, especially joints. Infectious disorders also may affect the musculoskeletal system, causing temporary or chronic problems with musculoskeletal function. Inflammatory and infectious disorders have potential to interfere with mobility and ADLs. Clients with inflammatory and infectious disorders may need assistance with tasks most people take for granted. These disorders affect a client's physical, psychological, and social functions.

The discussion in this chapter is limited to rheumatoid arthritis, osteoarthritis, gout, bursitis, Lyme disease, osteomyelitis, and lupus erythematosus. Many clients with inflammatory and infectious disorders affecting the musculoskeletal system are treated as outpatients. A few may require hospitalization in the acute phase of the disorder, for surgery on a degenerative joint, or for other medical or surgical therapies.

● RHEUMATOID ARTHRITIS

Rheumatoid arthritis (RA) is a systemic inflammatory disorder of connective tissue/joints characterized by chronicity, remissions, and exacerbations. Potential for disability with RA is great and related to effects on joints, as well as systemic problems.

Pathophysiology and Etiology

The nature of RA, a crippling disease, is not fully understood. Its cause is unknown, although it is believed to be an autoimmune disease. Genetic predisposition and other factors may be involved. RA strikes in the most productive years of adulthood, usually between 20 and 40 years. The disorder also can be found in young children and older adults. Young adult women appear to be affected more than men, but incidence equalizes as adults age. Typically, RA affects small joints early and involves large joints later (Bullock & Henze, 2000).

The autoimmune reaction from RA occurs primarily in the synovial tissue. Approximately 70% to 80% of people with RA have a substance called *rheumatoid factor* (RF), an antibody that reacts with a fragment of immunoglobulin G (IgG). This self-produced (autologous) antibody forms immune complexes (IgG/RF). It is uncertain why. Theories include viral infections that alter the IgG so that it is seen as foreign, or genetic predisposition. Sixty percent of individuals with RA have other factors known as major histocompatibility complex (MHC) antigen and human leukocyte antigen (HLA) (Porth, 2002).

The autoimmune reaction involves lymphocytes in the inflammatory infiltrate of the synovial tissue that produce RF. Polymorphonuclear leukocytes, monocytes, and lymphocytes are attracted to the area and cause phagocytosis of the immune complexes. During this process, lysosomal enzymes are released, causing destructive changes in the joint cartilage (Fig. 61.4). The changes produce more inflammation, perpetuating the entire process of RA:

1. The inflammatory process (**synovitis**) advances as congestion and edema develop in the synovial membrane and joint capsule.
2. Synovial tissue experiences reactive hyperplasia.
3. Vasodilation and increased blood flow cause warmth and redness.
4. Increased capillary permeability causes swelling.
5. Rheumatoid synovitis advances, leading to **pannus** formation (destructive vascular granulation tissue, characteristic of RA).
6. Pannus destroys adjacent cartilage, joint capsule, and bone.
7. Pannus eventually forms between joint margins, reducing joint mobility and leading to potential **ankylosis** (joint immobility).
8. Disease progression causes further inflammation and structural changes (Bullock & Henze, 2000; Porth, 2002).

Most clients with RA experience exacerbations and remissions. For some clients, progression is steady, relentless, and not necessarily responsive to therapy. Box 61-3 lists articular and extra-articular manifestations of RA.

Assessment Findings

Signs and Symptoms

In most clients, onset of symptoms is acute. Joint involvement usually is bilateral and symmetric. Localized symptoms include joint pain, swelling, and warmth; erythema; mobility limitation/stiffness; spongy tissue on joint palpation; and fluid on joints. Over several weeks, more joints become involved. Swelling and pain come and go. Fatigue, malaise, anorexia, and weight loss are common. Fever may develop. Tolerance for any kind of stress decreases, as does tolerance for environmental temperature changes. Although dietary iron intake is adequate, clients characteristically have persistent anemia resulting from the effects of RA on the blood-forming organs. Other systemic features include vasculitis, neuropathy, scleritis, pericarditis, splenomegaly, and Sjögren's syndrome (dry eyes and mucous membranes).

In some clients, subcutaneous nodules, known as *rheumatoid nodules,* develop. Appearing in more advanced

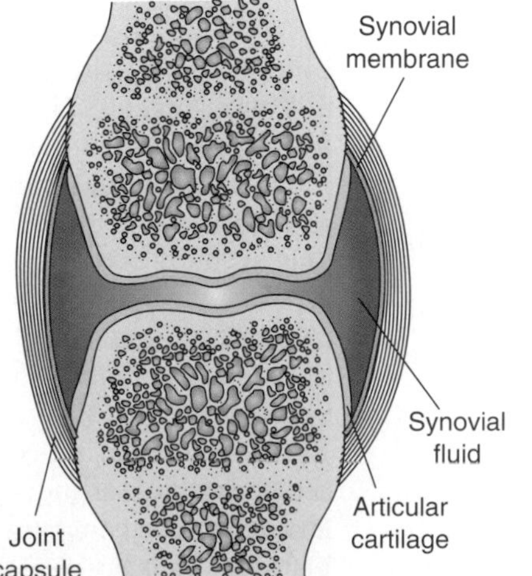

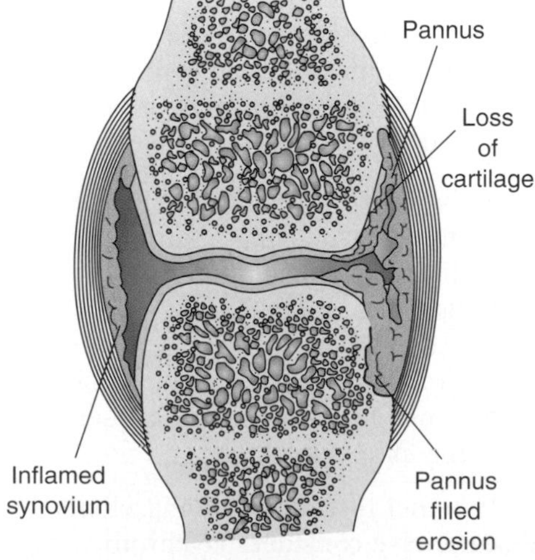

FIGURE 61.4 Joint changes in rheumatoid arthritis.

BOX 61-3 ● Articular and Extra-articular Manifestations of Rheumatoid Arthritis

- **Subcutaneous nodules:** Firm, freely movable, rubbery or granular nodules caused by deposition of extra-articular granulation tissue. Usually found at joint points such as knuckles and elbows.
- **Synovial cysts:** Called *Baker's cysts* in popliteal fossa; filled with synovial fluid that may be found in periarticular areas in elbow, shoulder, or small joints.
- **Arthritis:** Bilateral involvement of the small joints and later the large joints; hand joints usually are swollen and may be red. Inflammation leads to disability from destruction of cartilage, bone, and tendons. Flexion contractures are common. Osteoporosis, vertebral compression fractures, and avascular necrosis of the femoral head are common and may relate to treatment with corticosteroids. Usually at least three joint areas are involved.
- **Systemic rheumatoid vasculitis:** Immune complex–mediated inflammation in small and medium-sized arteries. It may be life-threatening if in a critical area. Causes pericardial, cardiac, pulmonary, and other types of lesions. Digital necrosis is common.
- **Compression neuropathy:** Mainly causes peripheral nerve entrapment with carpal tunnel syndrome. Paresthesias, pain, burning, muscle wasting, and weakness are common symptoms.
- **Cardiac disease:** Pericardial lesions and effusions are common and may or may not be symptomatic. Conduction system abnormalities from blockages due to rheumatic nodules around the atrioventricular node may cause heart block.
- **Pleuropulmonary disease:** Pleural effusions or pleuritic chest pain are relatively common. Pulmonary fibrosis or progressive interstitial lung disease may be seen with or without rheumatoid nodules in the lung parenchyma.
- **Episcleritis and scleritis:** Episcleritis is an inflammatory condition of the connective tissue between the sclera and conjunctiva. Scleritis is an inflammatory condition of the sclera and can cause scleral perforation.
- **Sicca syndrome:** A condition of dry eyes and dry mouth that can result from infiltration of the lacrimal and salivary glands with lymphocytes.

stages of RA, they usually are nontender and movable and evident over bony prominences, such as the elbow or the base of the spine.

Muscles weaken and atrophy (shrink), partially from disuse. Connective tissue and neurovascular changes lend a smooth, glossy appearance to the extremities, which may be cold and clammy. Flexion contractures are common.

As the disease progresses, muscle wasting around affected joints accentuates the appearance of swelling. Proximal finger joints swell the most, showing classic deformities:

- Swan neck deformity—Hyperextension of the proximal interphalangeal joint with fixed flexion of the distal interphalangeal joint
- Boutonniere deformity—Persistent flexion of the proximal interphalangeal joint with hyperextension of the distal interphalangeal joint
- Ulnar deviation—Fingers deviating laterally toward the ulna

Whether resting or moving, clients in this stage of the disease have considerable chronic pain, typically worse in the morning after a night's rest. Symptoms may subside suddenly for no apparent reason. Inflammation leaves joints that were sore and red; the client is not stiff, has no fever, and pain is gone. Yet symptoms almost invariably return after the client has had a symptom-free period. Inflammation causes more joint damage, followed by another remission. The pattern of remissions and exacerbations can continue for years.

Without treatment (and sometimes with it), joint destruction may be total. As bony growth replaces the synovial space, the joint loses motion. Once the joint becomes immobile, the pain of the inflammation decreases, but discomfort continues because of contractures and immobility.

Diagnostic Findings

Radiographic films show characteristic joint changes and the extent of damage. Narrowed joint spaces and bony erosions are characteristic of later disease. An arthrocentesis may be done, which is aspiration of synovial fluid (the client receives a local anesthetic) for microscopic examination. In RA, synovial fluid usually appears cloudy, milky, or dark yellow, and contains many inflammatory cells, including leukocytes and complement (a group of proteins in blood that affect the inflammatory process and influence antigen-antibody reactions). Arthroscopic examination also may be carried out to visualize the extent of joint damage as well as to obtain a sample of synovial fluid.

A positive C-reactive protein (CRP) test, low red blood cell count and hemoglobin levels in later stages, and positive RF are laboratory findings that support the diagnosis. The erythrocyte sedimentation rate (ESR) may be elevated, particularly as the disease progresses. C4 complement component is decreased. Antinuclear antibody (ANA) test results also may be positive. Serum protein electrophoresis may disclose increased levels of gamma and alpha globulin but decreased albumin.

Medical and Surgical Management

Although RA cannot be cured, much can be done to minimize damage. Treatment goals include decreasing joint inflammation before bony ankylosis occurs, relieving discomfort, preventing or correcting deformities, and maintaining or restoring function of affected structures. Early treatment leads to the best results.

Optimal health conditions must be maintained because supporting resistance of the body to inflammation is one of the few truly therapeutic steps medicine has to offer. Rest, systemic and local, is balanced carefully with exercise. Unless the client has other medical complications, such as diabetes or hypertension, the diet need not be modified.

Local applications of heat and cold are used concurrently with drug therapy to relieve swelling and pain. Drug therapy is not curative but relieves pain and, in some instances, suppresses the inflammatory process (Drug Therapy Table 61.1). In early stages, therapeutic

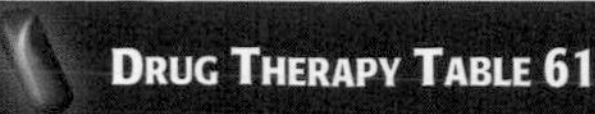

AGENTS FOR RHEUMATOID ARTHRITIS

DRUG CATEGORY AND EXAMPLES	MECHANISM OF ACTION	NURSING CONSIDERATIONS
Nonsteroidal Anti-inflammatory Drugs (NSAIDs)		
diclofenac sodium (Voltaren), fenoprofen (Nalfon), ibuprofen (Motrin), indomethacin (Indocin), naproxen (Naprosyn), piroxicam (Feldene), sulinidac (Clinoril)	Blocks undesirable effects of prostaglandins, which contribute to the inflammatory response Reduces pain and inflammation	Give with food or milk. Monitor client for decreased RBC and blood in urine. Assess client for abdominal pain, unusual bleeding or bruising, and tinnitus. Advise client not to take other NSAIDs or salicylates.
Salicylates		
aspirin	Relieves mild to moderate pain Interferes with the inflammatory response	Give with food or milk. Monitor for tinnitus, GI distress, unusual bleeding or bruising, dark-colored stools.
Cyclooxygenase-2 (COX-2) Inhibitors		
celecoxib (Celebrex), rofecoxib (Vioxx)	Blocks the enzyme involved in inflammation, thus relieving pain and inflammation	Do not administer with other NSAIDs. These drugs are less likely to cause gastric symptoms or unusual bleeding or bruising.
Disease-Modifying Antirheumatic Drugs (DMARDs)		
Gold Salts		
auranofin (Ridaura)	Anti-inflammatory, antiarthritic, and immunomodulating	Take with milk or food. May cause abdominal cramps, nausea, vomiting, loose stools, or sun sensitivity.
Immunosuppressant Agents		
azathioprine (Imuran)	Suppresses lymphocyte proliferation, interfering with the inflammatory response	These drugs decrease ability to fight off infection; report fever, chills, or cough.
Antineoplastic Agents		
methotrexate (Rheumatrex)	Interferes with purine metabolism, which then releases adenosine, which is an anti-inflammatory	These drugs may cause nausea and vomiting, loss of appetite, diarrhea, hair loss, unusual bleeding and bruising.
Antirheumatic		
penicillamine (Cuprimine, Depen)	Suppresses immune response by lowering immunoglobulin M associated with rheumatoid factor	Give on empty stomach; withhold food and drugs for 1 hr after administering. Assess for fever after 2–3 wk of therapy. These drugs diminish taste. Use with caution in clients who are allergic to penicillin. Monitor for rash or other skin changes.
Antimalarials		
hydroxychloroquine (Plaquenil)	Reduces inflammation	Give with food or milk. Monitor blood counts. Do not give with other anti-inflammatories or gold compounds. Consult with physician before giving to clients with ophthalmic, neurologic, hepatic, or GI disorders. Inform client that urine will appear brown. Monitor for muscle weakness, visual changes, skin lesions, hypotension, and electrocardiographic changes.
Glucocorticoids		
prednisone (Meticorten), hydrocortisone (Cortef)	Anti-inflammatory and immunosuppressant	Give with food or milk. Decrease dose and frequency gradually. With long-term therapy monitor for GI distress, hyperglycemia, edema, poor wound healing, personality changes, or pathologic fractures.
Biologic-Response Modifiers		
entanercept (Enbrel), infliximab (Remicade)	Reduces inflammatory responses	Do not give live vaccines if client is receiving these medications. Discontinue if client gets a serious infection. Give with caution to clients with multiple sclerosis or other demyelinating disorders.

doses of NSAIDs or salicylates (aspirin) are given. A new class of NSAIDs, referred to as cyclooxygenase type 2 (COX-2) inhibitors, now are being used as treatment for RA. COX is an enzyme involved in the inflammatory process; COX-2 inhibitors block this enzyme, but do not interfere with the enzyme that protects the stomach lining (Smeltzer & Bare, 2004).

Physicians initiate aggressive pharmacologic treatment after initial diagnosis. NSAIDs relieve inflammation and pain by inhibiting production of prostaglandins, which can damage joints. Salicylates also relieve pain and inflammation. Disease-modifying antirheumatic drugs (DMARDs) such as antimalarials (hydroxychloroquine), gold salts (auranofin, aurothioglucose), penicillamine, or sulfasalazine are initiated early. If there are bony erosions, methotrexate (Rheumatrex), an antineoplastic agent, is started. It is faster acting than DMARDs and often used first in long-term treatment of RA. Cyclosporine, an immunomodulator, may be added to enhance effects of methotrexate. Azathioprine (Imuran), an immunosuppressant, may be used in clients with severe classic RA that does not respond to more conventional therapies. Glucocorticoids such as prednisone are used at low doses for short-term relief of pain and inflammation.

For many clients, combination therapy is initiated. Although still considered experimental, early studies show effectiveness (Porth, 2002). A typical drug combination is hydroxychloroquine, azathioprine, and methotrexate or gold plus methotrexate, in addition to an NSAID. As symptoms abate and remission occurs, drug doses are tapered. Biologic response modifiers are now being used to treat RA when other treatments have failed. Etanercept (Enbrel) and infliximab (Remicade) appear to inhibit progression of structural damage by blocking tumor necrosis factor, which plays a role in inflammation and destruction of joints in RA. These biologic agents also target specific components of the immune system, while leaving other components intact, which in turn produces fewer side effects (Arthritis Foundation, 2002).

A nondrug therapy approved for clients with RA is Prosorba therapy. This method uses a protein A immunoadsorption column called Prosorba. Blood is taken from one arm and run through an apheresis machine to separate plasma from red blood cells and other blood components. The plasma then passes through the Prosorba column, where some of the antibodies associated with RA are removed. The plasma, red blood cells, and other components are rejoined and returned to the client in the other arm. The procedure is done in 12 weekly sessions for 2 to $2\frac{1}{2}$ hours each session. About 30% of the clients who receive these treatments experience limited relief (Arthritis Foundation, 2002; Smeltzer & Bare, 2004).

Another new treatment is injection of viscosupplements (Hyalgan, Synvisc, and Supartz). These products act as a lubricant, substituting for hyaluronic acid, the substance that provides joint fluid viscosity. Pain relief appears to last 6 to 13 months. Side effects include swelling, redness, or heat at the injection site. Clients allergic to eggs should not receive these injections (Arthritis Foundation, 2002).

Several surgical techniques may be performed to minimize or correct joint deformities of RA (Box 61-4). Many individuals with various types of arthritis undergo an **arthroplasty,** or reconstruction of the joint, using an artificial joint that restores previously lost function and relieves pain. Reconstructive joint surgery is discussed more fully with the surgical management of degenerative joint disease.

Nursing Management

Nursing management involves teaching clients about the disease and providing information about maintaining general health, relieving pain, reducing stress, decreasing the inflammatory process, and preserving joint mobility. Instruct clients about the medication regimen, particularly therapeutic and adverse effects. Other nursing activities center on how to apply heat and cold packs locally or how to use a transcutaneous electrical nerve stimulation (TENS) unit to relieve pain in a particular joint. A TENS unit has electrodes that are applied to the skin from a portable stimulation unit that the client learns to operate.

Collaborate with occupational therapists to provide equipment, utensils, and instruction regarding energy conservation and maintenance of joint alignment. Physical therapists (PTs) plan an appropriate exercise regimen. Home care planning involves providing nursing assistance for ADLs and ensuring the home environment is safe. Out of consideration for typical pain and morning stiffness, teach the nursing assistant to allow extra time for completing hygiene or other procedures.

When joints are severely inflamed, the use of a splint may reduce but not totally eliminate active motion. Even during an acute episode, encourage the client to move affected parts gently to help lessen the possibility of ankylosis, muscle wasting, osteoporosis, and the debilitating

BOX 61-4 ● Surgical Procedures for Rheumatoid Arthritis

Arthrodesis: Fusion of a joint (most often the wrist or knee) for stabilization and pain relief
Arthroplasty: Total reconstruction or replacement of a joint (most often the knee and hip) with an artificial joint to restore function and relieve pain
Osteotomy: Cutting and removal of a wedge of bone (most often the tibia or femur) to change the bone's alignment, thereby improving function and relieving pain
Synovectomy: Removal of enlarged and hypertrophied synovium to prevent the formation of pannus and delay destruction in the joint (most often the fingers, wrist, elbow, and knee)

effects of prolonged rest. Clients must avoid positions of flexion.

Continue to urge the client to eat nutritious, well-balanced meals despite anorexia. As joints become deformed and destroyed, techniques and equipment used to perform ADLs may require modification. Clients need assistance to deal with chronic pain, changes in function, changes in appearance, and related depression and feelings of helplessness. Education about the disease is essential because many people spend large sums of money on unscientific treatments in hopes of a cure.

Stop, Think, and Respond ● BOX 61-3 

A 35-year-old woman recently diagnosed with RA asks you if her disease happened because she experimented with marijuana and drank a lot of alcohol in her adolescence. How would you respond?

● DEGENERATIVE JOINT DISEASE

Degenerative joint disease (DJD), also referred to as osteoarthritis (OA), is the most common form of arthritis. It also is known as the "wear and tear" disease and typically affects weight-bearing joints. It is characterized by slow and steady destructive changes in weight-bearing joints and those repeatedly used for work. Unlike RA, DJD has no remissions and no systemic symptoms, such as malaise and fever. Table 61.2 compares OA and RA.

Pathophysiology and Etiology

A lifetime of repeated trauma leads to degenerative joint changes. Hips, knees, spine, and distal interphalangeal joints in hands commonly are affected. Risk factors include increasing age, previous joint injury, obesity, congenital and developmental disorders, hereditary factors, and decreased bone disease. OA may be classified as *primary*, disease without a known etiology, or *secondary*, when OA has an underlying cause such as injury or a congenital disorder (Bullock & Henze, 2000).

The degenerative process begins when cartilage that covers bone ends becomes thin, rough, and ragged. Malacia or soft spots develop. The cartilage no longer springs back into shape after normal use. As cartilage wears away, the joint space decreases, so that bone surfaces are closer and rub together. In an attempt to repair the damaged surface, new bone develops in the form of bone spurs, bone cysts, or osteophytes, which are extended margins of the joints. The joint becomes deformed, and the client experiences pain and limited joint movement. Ankylosis does not occur, but the resulting deformity may partially dislocate the joint. Degenerative changes may be seen in

TABLE 61.2 COMPARISON OF RHEUMATOID ARTHRITIS AND OSTEOARTHRITIS

	RHEUMATOID ARTHRITIS	OSTEOARTHRITIS
Age	Usually between ages 20 and 50	Usually after age 40
Sex	More common in women than men	Before age 45, more common in men; after age 45, more common in women, especially in the hands
Onset	May develop suddenly (weeks or months)	Develops slowly over many years
Symptoms		
Pain	General achiness; nocturnal pain; pain at rest	Deep, aching pain with motion early in the disease; later, pain at rest
Stiffness	Morning stiffness that lasts at least 1 hr	Stiffness localized to involved joints, which rarely exceeds 20 min; often related to weather
Joint motion	Decreased	Limited
Other	Depression, fatigue, low-grade fever, anorexia, malaise, weakness, weight loss	Instability of weight-bearing joints; crepitus; crackling
Physical signs	If multiple joints involved, usually symmetric Joints typically involved are hands (small joints), feet (small joints), wrists, elbows, knees, ankles, shoulders. Hand deformities include ulnar deviation and subluxation of metacarpophalangeal joints Joints may be tender, swollen, and red. Synovial fluid is thin and cloudy with elevated protein and polymorphonuclear cell levels.	One or many joints involved; asymmetric Joints typically involved are hands (first carpometacarpal joint), feet (first metatarsophalangeal joint), hips, knees, cervical and lumbar spine Joints—bony proliferation or occasional synovitis; local tenderness; crepitus; muscle atrophy; effusions Synovial fluid—high viscosity with mild leukocytosis (<2000 WBC:mm³)
Laboratory values	Rheumatoid factor (RF) elevated in 80% of clients with RA Elevated ESR Decreased RBC and C4 complement	No specific test ESR and hematologic survey results are normal No systemic manifestations

joint capsule, synovial membrane, ligaments, and muscles and tendons surrounding the affected joints. Figure 61.5 depicts the joint changes seen in osteoarthritis.

Assessment Findings

Early symptoms are brief joint stiffness and pain after a period of inactivity. Pain usually increases with heavy use and is relieved by rest. Later, even rest may not adequately relieve the pain. Eventually the joint undergoes enlargement and increased limitation of movement. When DJD afflicts the hands, fingers frequently develop painless bony nodules on the dorsolateral surface of the interphalangeal joints: **Heberden's nodes** (bony enlargement of the distal interphalangeal joints) and **Bouchard's nodes** (bony enlargement of the proximal interphalangeal joints). Crepitus may be heard and felt when the joint is moved. The ROM of the affected joint becomes progressively limited, and stiffness and pain increase.

Radiographic films demonstrate disruption of the joint cartilage and bony changes. Some clients may have a slightly elevated ESR.

Medical and Surgical Management

Nonpharmacologic treatment includes local rest of affected joints. Heat applied to the painful part may afford some relief. Weight loss is recommended for obese clients. Splints, braces, canes, or crutches may reduce discomfort, relieve pain, and prevent further joint destruction of the affected joints. An exercise program helps to preserve joint ROM and strength. Clients should not engage in activity that places excessive stress on affected joints. A TENS unit may help reduce joint pain.

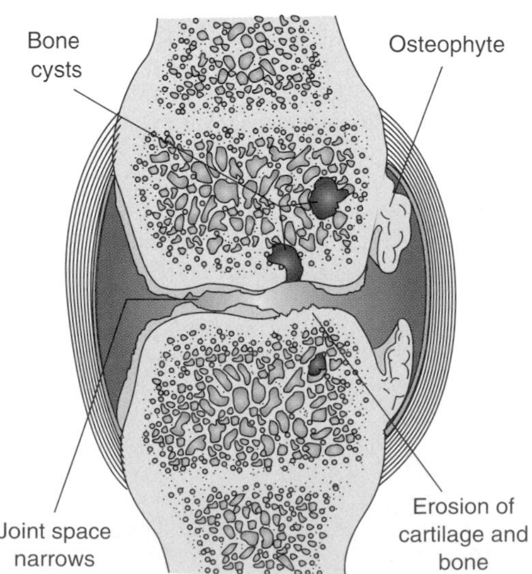

FIGURE 61.5 Joint changes in osteoarthritis.

Large doses of acetaminophen may be used initially, along with nonpharmacologic treatments. If acetaminophen is ineffective, systemic anti-inflammatory drugs, such as aspirin and NSAIDs, are prescribed. Although they do not prevent or cure DJD, they may decrease its severity. Corticosteroids may be injected into acutely inflamed joints with limited success. When possible, long-term use of these agents is avoided. Use of narcotics is deferred because of the disorder's chronic nature.

Reconstructive joint surgery is performed when mobility and quality of life are compromised. The two joints most frequently replaced are the knee and hip. Other joints that may be replaced are the shoulder, ankle, wrist, and finger joints. Total joint replacement is not strictly for clients with DJD. This type of procedure also may be done for individuals with RA, trauma, hip fracture, or a congenital deformity.

Materials used in an artificial joint are metal and high-density polyethylene (Fig. 61.6). Special bone cement or a specialized coating on the prosthesis pieces, which pro-

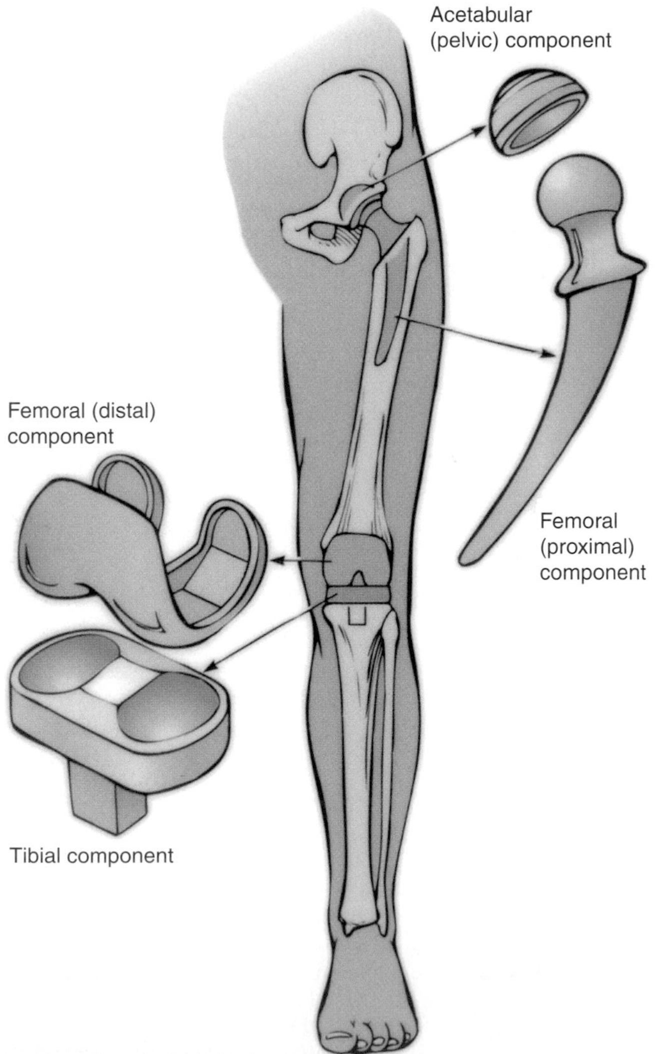

FIGURE 61.6 Hip and knee replacement.

motes bone growth on the implant, holds the prosthesis parts in place. Postoperative complications include hemorrhage, subluxation or dislocation of the artificial hip, infection, thromboembolism, and avascular necrosis. A cemented prosthesis may loosen many years later.

Some clients may want to pre-donate their own blood for use if a transfusion is needed. Anticoagulant therapy and early ambulation are implemented to prevent clot formation. Clients with a knee or hip replacement may use a continuous passive motion (CPM) machine after surgery, which promotes healing and flexibility in the joint and increases circulation to the operative area. The physician orders the amount of extension and flexion produced by the machine as well as the frequency of use. The amount of flexion and frequency of movement are increased daily for clients with knee replacements. By discharge, the client's goal is the ability to bend the knee 90°. The amount of flexion for clients with hip replacements should never exceed 30° in a CPM machine.

Nursing Management

Teach the client about the purpose of drug therapy, administration times, and therapeutic and side effects. Because aspirin and NSAIDs can cause gastric bleeding, advise clients to take the medication with food. Instruct client to maintain moderate activity, including the type, vigor, and frequency according to the symptoms experienced. If the client is overweight, provide explanations about dietary changes to promote weight loss. Remind the client to assume good posture to avoid unusual stress on a joint. If the client needs ambulatory aids such as crutches, a cane, or a walker, refer him or her to a PT for fitting and practice.

If a client is scheduled for joint replacement or other surgery, withhold aspirin before surgery to reduce risk for excessive bleeding. Monitor the complete blood count, prothrombin time, and bleeding and clotting times to ensure that the client's ability to control bleeding is not compromised. If the client will use a CPM machine after surgery, it is useful for the client to be fitted for this before surgery.

When the client returns from surgery, review the physician orders concerning movement, turning, or positioning of extremities. Usually, the head of the bed remains at 45° or less. The client with a total hip replacement needs to have legs abducted and extended because the opposite positions of adduction and flexion beyond 90° can dislocate the prosthetic femoral head from the acetabulum. Clients with a total hip replacement need to sit in an elevated chair or on a seat raised by pillows, so that the flexion remains less than 90°. Ice packs help reduce pain and inflammation to the incisional site (particularly after knee surgery). Box 61-5 provides information about avoiding hip dislocation after total hip replacement.

BOX 61-5 ● Avoiding Hip Dislocation After Replacement Surgery

Until the hip prosthesis stabilizes after hip replacement surgery, the client needs to learn about proper positioning so that the prosthesis remains in place. Dislocation of the hip is a serious complication of surgery that causes pain and necessitates reoperation to correct the dislocation. Desirable positions include abduction, neutral rotation, and flexion of less than 90°. When the client is seated, the knees should be lower than the hip.

Guidelines for avoiding displacement are as follows:

- Keep the knees apart at all times.
- Put a pillow between the legs when sleeping.
- Never cross the legs when seated.
- Avoid bending forward when seated in a chair.
- Avoid bending forward to pick up an object on the floor.
- Use a raised toilet seat.
- Do not flex the hip to put on clothing such as pants, stockings, socks, or shoes.

If CPM devices are prescribed to promote gentle flexion and extension of the knee after knee replacement, the nurse or PT increases flexion as indicated up to the goal of 90°. If CPM devices are used after hip surgery, the flexion should not exceed 30°.

Preventing postoperative complications after joint replacement is an important role of the nurse. Table 61.3 presents strategies to prevent postoperative complications after joint replacement surgery. Nursing Care Plan 61-1 provides more information related to clients having orthopedic surgery.

● GOUT

Gout, a painful metabolic disorder involving an inflammatory reaction in the joints, usually affects the feet (especially the great toe), hands, elbows, ankles, and knees.

Pathophysiology and Etiology

The disorder tends to be inherited and affects more men than women. Gout may occur secondary to other diseases marked by decreased renal excretion of uric acid. It also occurs among clients who have received organ transplants and the antirejection drug cyclosporine.

Gout is characterized by **hyperuricemia** (accumulation of uric acid in blood), caused by alterations in uric acid production, excretion, or both. Hyperuricemia occurs from one or a combination of the following pathologies:

- Primary hyperuricemia
  - Severe dieting or starvation
  - Excessive ingestion of purines (organ meats, shellfish, sardines)
  - Heredity

TABLE 61.3 PREVENTING POSTOPERATIVE COMPLICATIONS AFTER JOINT REPLACEMENT SURGERY

POTENTIAL COMPLICATION	POTENTIAL RISK FACTORS	PREVENTION STRATEGIES
Dislocation of prosthesis	Positioning beyond recommended flexion or extension Malfunction of prosthesis	Position client as prescribed. Instruct client to maintain appropriate position. Use pillows, splints, immobilizers, or slings to maintain prescribed position. Report increased pain, swelling, or change in mobility.
Infection	Elderly, debilitated clients Malnourishment Other infections such as urinary tract infections or dental abscesses Incision, wound drains, catheters, or IVs Hematoma	Monitor vital signs. Assess wound appearance and drainage. Practice aseptic technique when changing dressings and emptying drainage devices. Administer prophylactic antibiotics as prescribed. Teach client that for at least 3 months after surgery there is a potential for infection; he or she may require prophylactic antibiotics for dental cleaning or other invasive procedures. Report increased pain, elevated temperature, redness, swelling, or change in drainage from the incision.
Neurovascular compromise	Trauma Edema Immobilization devices	Assess neurovascular status frequently, including color, temperature, capillary refill, pulses, edema, pain, mobility, and sensation. Report client complaints of deep, unrelenting pain; feelings of tightness; numbness; and decreased mobility. Elevate extremity. Release constricting dressings, wraps, casts, or immobilizers.
Deep vein thrombosis	Surgical procedure Immobility	Apply elastic stockings/wraps as prescribed. Assess peripheral pulses. Change position frequently as allowed. Increase activity as indicated. Encourage client to perform passive ROM exercises. Assess for Homans' sign. Prevent pressure on popliteal vessels.

- Secondary hyperuricemia
  - Abnormal purine metabolism
  - Increased rate of protein synthesis with overproduction or underexcretion of uric acid
  - Increased cellular turnover, as in leukemia, multiple myeloma, and other cancers; some anemias; and psoriasis
  - Altered renal tubular function related to use of diuretics and salicylates and excessive alcohol intake, leading to underexcretion of uric acid (Smeltzer & Bare, 2004)

Urate (a salt of uric acid) crystallizes in body tissues and is deposited in soft and bony tissues, causing local inflammation and irritation. Collections of urate crystals, called **tophi,** are found in cartilage of the outer ear (pinna), the great toe, hands, and other joints, ligaments, bursae, and tendons. As deposits accumulate, they destroy the joint, producing a chronically swollen, deformed appearance. Uric acid also may precipitate in urine, causing renal stones.

Assessment Findings

A gout attack is characterized by sudden onset of acute pain and tenderness in one joint. The skin turns red and the joint swells so that it is warm and hypersensitive to touch. Fever may be present. Tophi may be palpated around fingers, great toes, or earlobes, particularly if the client has chronic and severe hyperuricemia. The attack may last for 1 or 2 weeks, but moderate swelling and tenderness may persist. A symptom-free period usually is followed by another attack, which may occur any time. Repeated episodes in the same joint may deform the joint.

Diagnosis usually is based on obvious clinical signs and hyperuricemia. Synovial fluid aspirated from the joint during arthrocentesis contains urate crystals. The urate deposits also may be identifiable with a radiographic examination. Elevated uric acid levels in serum and urine (24-hour urine collection) correlate with gout, but these findings are common to other disorders as well.

Medical and Surgical Management

Although gout cannot be cured in terms of removing the basic metabolic difficulty of constant or recurrent hyperuricemia, attacks usually can be controlled. The aim of treatment is to decrease sodium urate in extracellular fluid so that deposits do not form.

Two main treatment approaches involve (1) using uricosuric drugs that promote renal excretion of urates by inhibiting the reabsorption of uric acid in the renal tubules, and (2) decreasing ingestion of purine. The regimen is individualized and may be changed in response to the changes in the course of the disease.

Pain during a severe acute attack may require NSAIDs, such as ibuprofen and indomethacin. Acute attacks of gout also may be treated with colchicine or phenylbutazone (Butazolidine). Colchicine is administered every 1 or 2 hours until pain subsides or nausea, vomiting, intestinal cramping, and diarrhea develop. When one or more of these symptoms occurs, the drug should be stopped temporarily. Drugs used for long-term gout management include colchicine, allopurinol (Zyloprim), probenecid (Benemid), indomethacin (Indocin), and sulfinpyrazone (Anturane). To prevent future attacks, drug therapy continues after the acute attack subsides (Drug Therapy Table 61.2). Salicylates inactivate uricosurics, and clients with a history of gout should not use them.

Because the body can synthesize purines, emphasis on strict diet restriction has decreased, with more focus on use of uricosuric drugs. The prescribed diet includes adequate protein with limitation of purine-rich foods. The diet should be relatively high in carbohydrates and low in fats because carbohydrates increase urate excretion and fats retard it. Overweight clients are encouraged to lose weight. A high fluid intake helps increase excretion of uric acid. Alcohol is restricted because it can trigger an attack.

Surgery may be done to remove large tophi of advanced gout. Surgery also may be used to correct crippling deformities that may result from treatment delays or to fuse unstable joints and increase their function.

Nursing Management

Place a bed cradle over the affected joint to protect it from the pressure of the bed linen. If colchicine is prescribed, explain about hourly administration until side effects occur or acute pain subsides. Instruct the client to report gastrointestinal (GI) symptoms. Measure intake and output, especially when diarrhea accompanies colchicine therapy for acute gout. Provide clear explanations of long-term drug and diet therapy before discharge.

• BURSITIS

Bursitis is an inflammation of the bursa, a fluid-filled sac that cushions bone ends to enhance a gliding movement. The elbow, shoulder, and knee are common sites of bursitis.

Pathophysiology and Etiology

Trauma is the most common cause of acute bursitis. Other causes include infection and secondary effects of gout and RA. Typical of any inflammation, pain and swelling occur with compromised function.

DRUG THERAPY TABLE 61.2 SELECTED ANTIGOUT MEDICATIONS

DRUG	MECHANISM OF ACTION	NURSING CONSIDERATIONS
colchicine	Lowers the deposition of uric acid and interferes with leukocytes and kinin formation, thus reducing inflammation Does not alter serum or urine levels of uric acid Used in acute and chronic management	*Acute management:* Administer when attack first begins. Dosage is increased until pain is relieved or diarrhea develops. *Chronic management:* Prolonged use may decrease vitamin B_{12} absorption. Drug causes GI upset in most clients.
probenecid (Benemid)	Uricosuric agent; inhibits renal reabsorption of urates and increases the urinary excretion of uric acid Prevents tophi formation	Be alert for nausea, rash, and constipation.
allopurinol (Zyloprim)	Xanthine oxidase inhibitor; interrupts the breakdown of purines before uric acid forms Inhibits xanthine oxidase because it blocks uric acid formation	Be alert for side effects, including bone marrow depression, vomiting, and abdominal pain.

Assessment Findings

Painful movement of a joint, such as the elbow or shoulder, is common. A distinct lump may be felt. If the bursa ruptures, tissue in the area may become edematous, warm, and tender. An x-ray study may reveal a calcified bursa, and aspiration of fluid may demonstrate a few leukocytes in transparent fluid if the etiology is trauma, a large collection of leukocytes if the cause is sepsis, colonies of staphylococcal or streptococcal microorganisms, or urate crystals in bursitis secondary to gout. Cholesterol crystals, common in clients with bursitis and RA, may cause the fluid from the bursa to appear cloudy.

Medical and Surgical Management

Joint rest usually is recommended. Salicylates or NSAIDs may be prescribed. If the problem persists, a corticosteroid preparation may be injected into the joint to reduce inflammation. After pain and inflammation are reduced, ongoing therapy involves mild ROM exercises.

Nursing Management

Review the prescribed medication and exercise regimens with the client and allow time for questions and answers. Advise the client not to traumatize or overuse the recovering joint but to use it normally. Failure to use the joint after pain and inflammation are controlled may result in partial limitation of joint motion.

• LYME DISEASE

Lyme disease (Lyme borreliosis) gained wide recognition in the 1970s when residents of Lyme, Connecticut experienced an epidemic of progressive symptoms, beginning with a characteristic rash and eventually involving the cardiac, neurologic, and musculoskeletal systems.

Pathophysiology and Etiology

Typically, Lyme disease is prevalent during warmer months, when ticks are abundant, but it may occur at any time. It is most common in the northeast and mid-Atlantic states, and in other northern areas of the United States, where deer ticks (*Ixodes dammini*) are more prevalent. The ticks feed on white-tailed deer or white-footed mice, and then become carriers of the spirochetal bacterium *Borrelia burgdorferi.* When ticks bite humans, they transmit the bacteria, which results in a chronic inflammatory process and multisystem disease.

Assessment Findings

If untreated, the disease moves through three stages. Early stage 1 symptoms for about one third of clients include a red macule or papule at the site of the tick bite, a characteristic bull's-eye rash with round rings surrounding the center, headache, neck stiffness, and pain. Secondary pruritic lesions may accompany fever, chills, and malaise. The initial papule may not develop until 20 to 30 days after the bite. Some clients experience nausea, vomiting, and sore throat.

Midstage symptoms occur as the organism proliferates throughout the body and cardiac and neurologic involvement becomes evident. Cardiac problems include dysrhythmias and heart block. Neurologic symptoms such as facial palsy, meningitis, and encephalitis are possible. Some clients have problems with weakness, pain, and paresthesia (abnormal sensations).

Later symptoms (at least 4 weeks after the bite) include arthritis and other musculoskeletal problems. Joints, particularly knees, become warm, swollen, and painful. Joint erosion may result from the inflammatory process.

Diagnosis is based on presenting signs and symptoms. Diagnosis of Lyme disease is assisted by serologic studies for IgG antibodies for *Borrelia,* which can be detected 6 weeks after the tick bite.

Medical and Surgical Management

Treatment includes administering antibiotics and supportive measures. If the disease is treated early, prognosis is favorable. Permanent multisystem problems may occur if treatment is delayed.

Nursing Management

Nursing management involves teaching the client and family about the disease and its treatment. It is extremely important to educate clients about avoiding Lyme disease (Box 61-6).

• OSTEOMYELITIS

Osteomyelitis is an infection of the bone. Limited blood supply, inflammation of and pressure on the tissue, and formation of new bone around devitalized bone tissue make osteomyelitis a difficult and challenging condition

BOX 61-6 ● Tips for Avoiding Lyme Disease

PERSONAL PROTECTION
- Wear light-colored clothing to increase tick visibility.
- Wear long-sleeved shirts and long pants (tuck pants into socks or boots).
- Treat clothing with tick repellant.
- Wear a hat; pull long hair back so that it does not brush against shrubs or other vegetation.
- Walk in the center of a path surrounded by grass, brush, or woods.
- Do a tick check after being outside—ticks are particularly attracted to hairy areas such as the scalp, groin, and armpits, as well as the back of knees and neck.

ENVIRONMENTAL PROTECTION
- Remove leaf, grass, and brush litter.
- Clear brush and tall grass from around house and other structures, as well as gardens and flower beds.
- Keep grass mowed.
- Place a 3-foot wood chip barrier along lawn edges that border woods.
- Erect fences to keep deer away from houses and gardens.
- Prune low-lying shrubs to let in more sunlight.
- Keep woodpiles neat, dry, and off the ground.
- Keep ground bare under bird feeders, place them away from house, and suspend feeding when ticks are most active.

(Adapted from Wade, C. F. [2000]. Keeping Lyme disease at bay. *American Journal of Nursing, 100*[7], 26–31.)

to treat. In adults, osteomyelitis may become chronic, greatly affecting quality of life.

Pathophysiology and Etiology

Staphylococcus aureus causes 70% to 80% of bone infections. Other organisms include *Proteus vulgaris* and *Pseudomonas aeruginosa,* as well as *Escherichia coli.* There is increased incidence of penicillin-resistant, nosocomial, gram-negative, and anaerobic infections. Acute osteomyelitis results from bacteria reaching the bone through the bloodstream. Acute localized osteomyelitis occurs when bone is contaminated directly by trauma, such as penetrating wounds or compound fractures. Occasionally, surgical contamination or direct extension of bacteria from an infected area adjacent to the bone, such as pin sites of skeletal traction, can cause osteomyelitis.

Microorganisms appear to migrate to the area just below the epiphysis of a long bone where blood supply is more generous, but circulation through the area is limited. As microorganisms multiply, they spread down to the bone shaft. Pressure from the collecting exudate elevates the periosteum. New bone cells (**involucrum**) are deposited on the periosteum while underlying bone becomes necrotic. The pocket of necrotic bone (**sequestrum**) may remain sequestered for years or eventually drain by forming a sinus tract through to the skin. Infection tends to linger in a chronic state because it is difficult to penetrate the infected tissue by administering systemic antibiotic drugs.

In its weakened condition, infected bone is prone to pathologic fracture. Diseased bone may lengthen as bone growth is stimulated, or it may shorten because of destruction of the epiphyseal plate. Other complications of osteomyelitis include septicemia, thrombophlebitis, muscle contractures, pathologic fractures, and nonunion of fractures.

Assessment Findings

Evidence of an acute infection appears suddenly: high fever, chills, rapid pulse, tenderness or pain over the affected area, redness, and swelling. Chronic infection may be characterized by a persistent draining sinus.

With acute osteomyelitis, laboratory tests usually show an elevated leukocyte count and ESR, and possibly a blood culture positive for infective organisms. Identification of the causative organism may require aspiration of subperiosteal pus for culture and sensitivity. Radiographic findings may be inconclusive in the early stages of infection, but later studies demonstrate irregular bone decalcification, bone necrosis, elevation of the periosteum, and new bone formation. Bone scans and MRI are useful in definitive diagnoses.

Radiographic studies for chronic osteomyelitis show large cavities, sequestra or dense bone formations, and raised periosteum. Areas of infection are delineated by bone scan. Blood studies reveal a normal leukocyte count and ESR and possible anemia.

Medical and Surgical Management

Management of osteomyelitis includes the following:

- Immobilization with a cast or immobilizer to decrease pain and prevent fracture. The cast may be windowed to provide access for wound care.
- Application of warm saline soaks to affected area for 20 minutes several times a day to increase circulation to affected area
- Identification of causative organism to initiate appropriate and ongoing antibiotic therapy for infection control. Intravenous (IV) antibiotic therapy is administered for 3 to 6 weeks. Oral antibiotics then follow for as long as 3 months.
- Surgical debridement of necrotic tissue and sequestrum to remove infected areas
- Closed irrigation with saline or an antibiotic solution and low suction to affected area to flush away necrotic tissue
- Antibiotic-impregnated beads may be directly applied in wound for 2 to 4 weeks

- Bone grafts for the debrided cavity to stimulate bone growth
- Muscle flaps grafted to affected area to enhance blood supply

Nursing Management

Clients with osteomyelitis experience pain, inflammation, swelling, and impaired mobility because of pain and inability to bear weight. Handle the arm or leg or related area gently to prevent additional pain or fracture. Protect the infected area from injury. Instruct the client to elevate the area and to bear weight only as indicated. Protect the skin from breakdown, administer prescribed antibiotics and pain medications, and inform the client about the expected therapeutic effects and possible side effects. Clients with chronic osteomyelitis require extensive emotional support, related to the long-term nature of this illness. See Nursing Care Plan 61-1.

Stop, Think, and Respond • BOX 61-4

Which of the following clients is at greatest risk for osteomyelitis?

- *A 65-year-old client recently diagnosed with osteoarthritis*
- *A 70-year-old client who recently sustained an open compound fracture of the tibia after a motor vehicle accident*
- *A 40-year-old client diagnosed with Lyme disease*

• LUPUS ERYTHEMATOSUS

Lupus erythematosus is a diffuse connective tissue disease. The major type is systemic lupus erythematosus (SLE), which, as the name implies, affects multiple body systems such as the skin, joints, kidney, serous membranes of the heart and lungs, lymph nodes, and GI tract.

Pathophysiology and Etiology

Lupus erythematosus is more common in women than in men. Most clients have this disorder in the third or fourth decade of life, but it may be seen in young children and in middle-aged and older adults. It is believed to be autoimmune, but the triggering mechanism is still unknown. There is a strong familial tendency, suggesting that certain inherited cellular antigenic markers confuse the ability of T cells to distinguish self from nonself. By mistake, helper T cells alert B cells to produce antibodies against normal cells, or suppressor T cells may be ineffective in controlling a B-cell response once it has been initiated. The disease may have periods during which it is in a subacute form or even in remission. Exposure to ultraviolet light is a factor in reactivating the disease.

Antibodies destroy connective tissues of the body. Affected structures undergo inflammation, fibrosis, scarring, and dysfunction. Polymorphonuclear leukocytes (neutrophils) engulf the nuclei of attacked cells. Laboratory studies confirm this finding, which is considered diagnostic.

Assessment Findings

Signs and Symptoms

According to Porth (2002), SLE is known as the *great imitator* because clinical signs resemble many other conditions. Early signs and symptoms of SLE may include fever, weight loss, pain in joints (arthralgia), malaise, muscle pain, and extreme fatigue. These symptoms are vague and may persist for several months to 2 years before more prominent symptoms develop and the client seeks medical advice.

A prominent sign for about half of the clients with SLE is a red, butterfly-shaped rash on the face over the bridge of the nose and the cheeks (Fig. 61.7). Another skin manifestation is discoid lupus erythematosus (DLE), which involves a chronic rash on the face and scalp with erythematous papules or plaques and scaling. DLE can lead to scarring and pigmentation changes. Scalp involvement usually results in patchy loss of hair (alopecia). These symptoms also may be seen in people with SLE. Subacute cutaneous lupus erythematosus, presenting as papulosquamous lesions, also may occur.

Clients also may exhibit behavioral disturbances (confusion, hallucinations, irritability), chest pain (as a result of involvement of pleura or pericarditis), fluid retention,

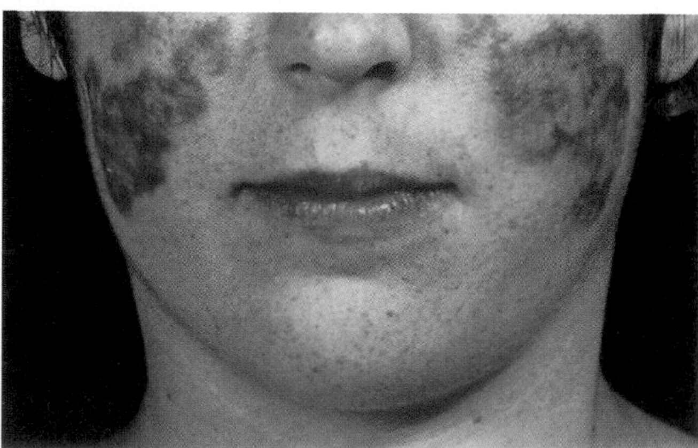

FIGURE 61.7 Characteristic butterfly rash.

proteinuria, and hematuria (as a result of renal involvement), progressive weight loss, nausea and vomiting, and, in women, irregular or heavy menses. Other signs include the following:

- Nonspecific electrocardiographic changes
- A pericardial friction rub
- Pulmonary changes seen on radiographic studies
- Enlargement of spleen and lymph nodes
- Raynaud's phenomenon (vasospasm of the smaller vessels of hands and feet resulting in blanching of skin and, at times, pain and cyanosis of extremities)
- Musculoskeletal problems, such as arthralgias and arthritis, including joint swelling, tenderness, pain on movement, and morning stiffness

Diagnostic Findings

Diagnosis of SLE is based on presenting symptoms and blood tests. Blood studies show anemia, thrombocytopenia, leukocytosis or leukopenia, and positive ANA. Other laboratory studies may indicate multisystem involvement, such as an elevated creatinine level with kidney involvement. Additional tests, such as a renal biopsy and urinalysis, may be done to determine the effect of the disorder on other body systems.

Medical Management

There is no specific treatment for this disorder. Medical management aims at producing a remission and preventing or treating acute exacerbations of the disorder. High doses of corticosteroids are used initially. Those with severe disease or for whom steroid-related side effects are problematic may be treated with cytotoxic drugs such as azathioprine (Imuran) and cyclophosphamide (Cytoxan). Simple analgesics such as aspirin or an NSAID may be prescribed for fever and joint discomfort. Topical corticosteroids may be used for skin manifestations. Renal impairment may be treated with dialysis or kidney transplantation. Cardiac, GI, and central nervous system complications are treated symptomatically.

Nursing Management

Review the medical record and diagnostic findings to evaluate the stage of disease and appropriate interventions. Assess the client's understanding of the nature of the disorder, its treatment, and the limitations imposed by the disease process. Inspect the skin for rashes, purpuric lesions, and other skin changes and ask about the client's degree of sensitivity to sunlight. Inspect for ulcerations in the mouth and throat (signs of GI involvement). In addition, listen to the heart for pericardial friction rub and to the lungs for abnormal sounds, which might suggest pleural involvement.

Nursing management focuses on measures to minimize exacerbations and to alleviate symptoms. Administer prescribed medications and monitor for side effects. Before discharge, client education efforts involve reminding the client of the need for close medical follow-up and thorough medication instruction (i.e., never abruptly discontinue taking a prescribed corticosteroid without consulting the physician, and follow the dosage regimen exactly, particularly if the drug dose is being decreased gradually).

Assist client to maintain appropriate body alignment and neutral positioning during periods of inactivity to prevent contractures and increase mobility. Encourage moderate and progressive exercise as indicated. Advise client to use moist heat before performing ROM exercises to relax muscles and reduce resistance to ROM exercises. Urge client to wear supportive shoes and use assistive devices for ambulation as needed.

Because the disease and drugs alter body image, assist the client to verbalize feelings and implement effective coping mechanisms. If the client desires, arrange a referral to the Lupus Foundation of America, which is dedicated to providing information about the disease, or to a local support or self help group.

Because SLE is a chronic disease, treated mainly on an outpatient basis, much nursing management revolves around teaching. Clients and their families need accurate and complete information about the disease, its treatment and prognosis, and self-care measures to increase comfort and promote health. Specific measures are discussed in Client and Family Teaching 61-1.

STRUCTURAL DISORDERS

Structural disorders of the musculoskeletal system involve metabolic conditions that alter bone structure. These alterations result in pain, bone deformity, and fracture.

• OSTEOPOROSIS

Osteoporosis, loss of bone density, occurs principally in older adults and affects more women than men.

Pathophysiology and Etiology

Normally, processes of bone formation and bone reabsorption occur evenly. In osteoporosis, loss of bone

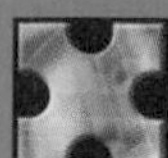

61-1 *Client and Family Teaching* Systemic Lupus Erythematosus

The nurse typically addresses the following with the client:

- Lifestyle modifications are necessary as related to musculoskeletal restrictions and systemic involvement. For example, because sunlight tends to exacerbate the disease, avoid sunlight and ultraviolet radiation. When outdoors, apply effective sunscreens with a sun protection factor (SPF) of 15 or higher and wear clothing that covers arms and legs and a wide-brimmed hat to shade the face. Sunlamps and tanning booths are taboo.
- Pace activities. Because fatigue is a major issue, allow for adequate rest along with regular activity to promote mobility and prevent joint stiffness. Avoid activities that cause severe pain or discomfort.
- Maintain a well-balanced diet and increase fluid intake to raise energy levels and promote tissue healing.
- Avoid crowds when possible and people with known infections, such as colds.
- Periodically review medication regimen with healthcare providers, particularly effects and adverse effects of medications and related signs and symptoms that require attention and need to be reported to the physician (increased severity of symptoms, involvement in other joints or areas of the body, weight loss, prolonged anorexia, nausea, vomiting, fever, cough, shortness of breath, difficult urination, infection, or any other unusual occurrence).
- Take medications exactly as directed and do not stop medication if symptoms are relieved unless advised to do so by the physician.
- If symptoms become worse, do not increase dosage unless advised to do so by the physician. Do not use over-the-counter drugs unless a physician approves their use.
- Use nonpharmacologic comfort measures. For instance, a moist form of heat may relieve joint stiffness. Use warm, not hot, soaks, wraps, or towels hot from the clothes dryer and take care not to burn the skin.
- Inform physicians and dentists of current therapy before any treatment, surgery, or drugs are prescribed.

substance exceeds bone formation. Total bone mass is reduced, resulting in bones that become progressively porous, brittle, and fragile. Compression fractures of vertebrae are common. Aging contributes to osteoporosis in the following ways:

- Levels of calcitonin, which inhibits bone reabsorption and promotes bone formation, decrease with aging.
- Levels of estrogen, which inhibits bone breakdown, decrease in postmenopausal women.
- Levels of parathyroid hormone, which increases bone reabsorption, increase with aging.

Small-framed, thin white women are at greatest risk for osteoporosis. African American women have a greater bone density and thus are less susceptible to osteoporosis. Men have an increased bone mass and do not have hormonal changes, and thus do not acquire osteoporosis as frequently and get it at a later age.

Other causes of osteoporosis, occurring in all ages and both sexes, include Cushing's syndrome, hyperparathyroidism, prolonged use of high doses of corticosteroids, prolonged immobility, hyperthyroidism, malabsorption syndromes, renal or liver failure, alcoholism, lactose intolerance, and dietary deficiency of vitamin D and calcium. Some medications that interfere with the body's ability to use and metabolize calcium include thyroid supplements, anticonvulsants, isoniazid, aluminum-containing antacids, tetracycline, and heparin.

Assessment Findings

Clients with osteoporosis frequently complain of lumbosacral pain, thoracic back pain, or both. Bone pain or tenderness results from tiny compression fractures in the vertebrae. Radiographic examination of bones shows bone loss once it is 25% or more. Bone deformities (especially in the spine), such as kyphosis and lordosis, and pathologic fractures in long bones also may be seen. Dual-energy x-ray absorptiometry is a test that measures bone mass at the spine and hip. Ultrasonic heel density (bone sonometer) provides baseline information for diagnosing osteoporosis and predicting fractures. Results of laboratory studies usually are normal, but studies may be done to rule out other disorders such as multiple myeloma, hyperparathyroidism, or metastatic bone lesions.

Medical Management

A diet rich in calcium and vitamin D throughout life can prevent osteoporosis. It cannot be treated directly, but medical management can slow rate of bone reabsorption. Bone pain or tenderness may respond to mild analgesics such as aspirin. Oral calcium preparations (calcium gluconate, calcium lactate, calcium carbonate, or dibasic calcium phosphate) may be recommended. Some preparations also contain vitamin D, needed for absorption of calcium in the intestine. New medications, such as the bisphosphonate alendronate sodium (Fosamax), inhibit bone resorption. Administration of calcitonin also inhibits bone reabsorption. Adequate rest and exercise, especially weight-bearing exercise such as walking, are part of the treatment regimen. Hormone replacement therapy may also be part of the treatment plan.

Nursing Management

In providing care for clients with osteoporosis, emphasize the need for a nutritious, well-balanced diet high in calcium, vitamin D, and protein—all recommended to delay or prevent osteoporosis. Advise women to drink three glasses of milk daily or eat other dairy products to acquire approximately 1000 to 1500 mg of calcium; those who smoke cigarettes may require more. Orange juice fortified with calcium is a nutritious alternative. If the client takes antacids, suggest those containing calcium. Recommend activity that promotes bone formation, such as regular, aerobic exercise (e.g., walking).

Stop, Think, and Respond ● BOX 61-5

A 45-year-old female client tells you that she has never liked milk and usually avoids dairy products because she thinks they are too fattening. What do you need to assess to ascertain if she is at risk for osteoporosis? What teaching does she need?

● OSTEOMALACIA

Osteomalacia, a metabolic bone disease, is characterized by inadequate mineralization of bone resulting from a calcium or phosphate deficiency.

Pathophysiology and Etiology

The defect in osteomalacia results from insufficient calcium absorption caused by insufficient calcium intake or resistance to the action of vitamin D. Alternatively, it may occur from phosphate deficiency related to increased renal losses or decreased intestinal absorption. Large amounts of new bone fail to calcify. Bone mass is structurally weaker and bone deformities occur. Other risk factors include chronic renal failure, gastrectomy, anticonvulsant therapy, and poor nutrition.

Assessment Findings

Clients with osteomalacia experience bone pain and weakness. They also complain of tenderness if bones are palpated. Bone deformities, such as kyphosis and bowing of the legs, occur as disease advances. Clients exhibit a waddling type of gait, putting them at risk for falls and fractures.

Radiographic studies demonstrate demineralization of the bone. Serum levels of calcium and phosphorus are low. Alkaline phosphatase levels typically are elevated.

Medical and Surgical Treatment

Treatment aims at correcting the underlying cause. This includes supplements of calcium, phosphorus, and vitamin D; adequate nutrition; exposure to sunlight; and progressive exercise and ambulation. Bone deformities may require braces or surgery for correction.

Nursing Management

The nurse is in a primary role of educating the client about the disease and its treatment and therefore includes teaching in the care plan. Teach the client about methods and medications used to relieve pain and discomfort. Allow the client to verbalize self-concept issues related to deformities and activity restrictions.

DISORDERS OF THE FEET

Many foot disorders are treated on an outpatient basis or encountered by nurses when caring for clients with other disorders. Common foot disorders are bunions and hammertoes.

Hallux valgus (*bunion*) is a deformity of the great (large) toe at its metatarsophalangeal joint (Fig. 61.8A). **Hammertoe** is a flexion deformity of the interphalangeal joint and may involve several toes (see Fig. 61.8B).

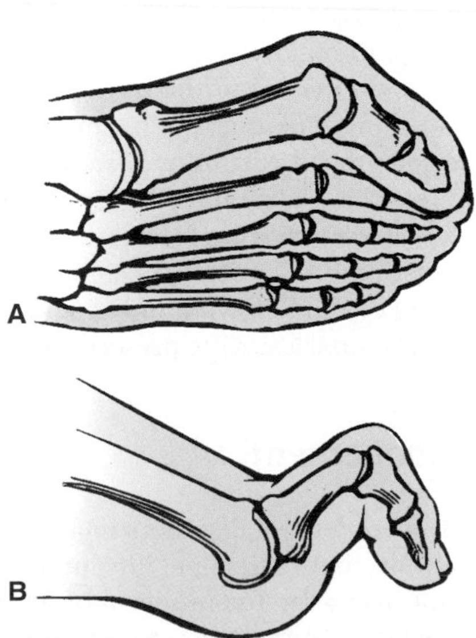

FIGURE 61.8 Common foot problems: (**A**) Bunion; (**B**) hammertoe.

Pathophysiology and Etiology

Bunions are associated with heredity, arthritis, or improperly fitting shoes. Women tend to be affected more than men. The first metatarsal bone enlarges on the medial side. The metatarsal bone protrudes at an acute angle toward the midline of the body while the great toe points laterally. There is an overgrowth of soft tissue (bursa), which actually is the bunion. The foot widens and the arch flattens. The malalignment results in pain from stress on the joint, improper support and distribution of body weight, and inflammation of bursa.

Like bunions, hammertoe also results from wearing poorly fitting shoes. Toes are pulled upward by the shoe, as the ball of the foot is pulled down. Corns (small, round, elevated overgrowths of epidermis) usually develop on top of the toes. Calluses (wide, thickened layers of skin) form under the metatarsal area.

Assessment Findings

Malalignment typical of bunions results in pain from the stress on the joint, improper support and distribution of body weight, and inflammation of bursa. The client complains of pain on walking or flexing the foot, tenderness, and redness of joint. The typical appearance of the foot deformity is obvious. In hammertoe, the foot deformity is evident. Corns and calluses are easily seen. The client complains of discomfort with ambulation. Radiographic films of the foot reveal the degree of joint deformity.

Medical and Surgical Management

No treatment is necessary for bunions if pain is not severe and the client has little or no difficulty. Low-heeled, properly fitted shoes are recommended. A bunionectomy, the surgical procedure to remove the bunion and correct the deformity, may be done when the individual has pain and difficulty walking. Treatment of hammertoe includes exercises, wearing properly fitting or open-toed shoes, use of pads to protect the joints, and surgery to correct the malalignment. Both surgeries are done on an outpatient or short-term admission basis, with the client discharged in the late afternoon or the following morning. Rest, elevation of the foot, and analgesics are prescribed.

Nursing Management

Nursing management of foot disorders includes relieving pain and discomfort, improving mobility, and instructing clients about the necessity for proper foot attire. Many clients are treated in an outpatient setting. Nurses in these settings usually are charged with teaching the client about the foot condition, treatment, medications, and postoperative care if the client had surgery. Instruct the client to apply ice postoperatively as with other orthopedic surgeries. If the client experiences a change in sensation or inability to move toes, or if toes are cool to touch and pale or blue, tell him or her to call the physician immediately. Teach client about wound care, cast care (if applicable), and mobility restrictions. See Nursing Care Plan 61-1.

DISORDERS OF THE UPPER EXTREMITY

Frequent sites of injury and pain in the upper extremity include the shoulder, elbow, and wrist. Among disorders frequently encountered are painful shoulder syndrome, epicondylitis, ganglion, and carpal tunnel syndrome.

The shoulder frequently is a site of injury and pain. Common conditions include tendinitis, tears and rupture of the rotator cuff, and bursitis. These result in painful shoulder syndrome.

Epicondylitis (tennis elbow) is a painful inflammation of the elbow. A ganglion is a cystic mass that develops near tendon sheaths and joints of the wrist. **Carpal tunnel syndrome** is a term for a group of symptoms located in the wrist where the carpal bones, carpal tendons, and median nerve pass through a narrow, inelastic canal.

Pathophysiology and Etiology

Primary causes of shoulder injuries are trauma and repeated stress. Injury also is responsible for epicondylitis, which occurs when tendons of the medial or lateral radial and ulnar epicondyles sustain damage. Injury typically follows excessive pronation and supination of the forearm, such as when playing tennis, pitching a ball, or rowing. Ganglion cysts form through defects in the tendon sheath or joint capsule and occur most commonly in women younger than 50 years of age.

Carpal tunnel syndrome results from repetitive wrist motion that traumatizes the tendon sheath or ligaments in the carpal canal. Trauma produces swelling that compresses the median nerve against the transverse carpal ligament. Those affected tend to be in occupations that perform repetitive hand movements such as cashiers, typists, musicians, and assemblers.

Assessment Findings

Shoulder injuries are marked by pain and inflammation, which can spread to surrounding tissues. In epicondylitis, clients report pain radiating down the dorsal surface of the forearm and a weak grasp. Clients with ganglion cysts experience pain and tenderness in the affected area. Clients with carpal tunnel syndrome describe pain or burning in one or both hands, which may radiate to the forearm and shoulder in severe cases. Pain tends to be more prominent at night and early in the morning. Shaking the hands may reduce the pain by promoting movement of edematous fluid from the carpal canal. Sensation may be lost or reduced in the thumb, index, middle, and a portion of the ring finger. The client may be unable to flex the index and middle fingers to make a fist. Flexion of the wrist usually causes immediate pain and numbness.

In general, x-ray studies identify abnormalities and rule out fracture and other problems. In carpal tunnel syndrome, results of electromyography, which relies on a mild electrical current to stimulate the nerve, show a delay in motor response in muscles innervated by the median nerve. Other tests are Tinel's sign, which is a test that elicits tingling, numbness, and pain for clients with carpal tunnel syndrome, and Phalen's sign, which involves having the client flex the wrist for 30 seconds to determine if pain or numbness occurs (a positive sign for carpal tunnel syndrome). The examiner percusses the median nerve, located on the inner aspect of the wrist, to elicit this response.

Medical and Surgical Management

Shoulder treatment includes applications of cold (ice) and heat, exercise, anti-inflammatory medications, local injection of corticosteroids, analgesics, NSAIDs, and rest. Surgery may be necessary to repair tears and ruptures. Clients with injuries of the shoulder or other portions of the upper extremity are referred for physical therapy. Treatment for epicondylitis is similar to that for shoulder injuries, and splinting is added to rest and support the joint structures. Corticosteroids may be injected locally. Treatment of the ganglion cyst includes aspiration of the ganglion, corticosteroid injection, and surgical excision.

Carpal tunnel treatment involves resting hands when possible and splinting the hand and wrist. NSAIDs and periodic injections of a corticosteroid preparation may relieve inflammation and discomfort. If conservative treatment fails, surgery to release pressure of the ligament on the median nerve may be done.

Nursing Management

Provide information about medications. If the client is taking NSAIDs, stress taking these medications with food. If corticosteroid injections are ordered, explain what the client can expect and mention that the injection itself may cause some discomfort.

Show clients how to use and care for prescribed splints and braces and perform related ROM exercises. Some clients find that hand exercises are less painful if performed with the hand under warm water. Additional management activities involve exploring ways to perform ADLs or alter job responsibilities to relieve stress and reduce injury to joints.

Key teaching points include the following:

- Rest the joint in a position that reduces stress.
- Support the affected arm joint on pillows while sleeping.
- Apply cold for the first 24 to 48 hours to reduce swelling and pain.
- Gradually increase joint movement.
- Avoid working or lifting above shoulder level. Do not push objects with the arm joint, particularly the shoulder.
- Perform ROM and strengthening exercises as prescribed by the physician or physical therapist

BONE TUMORS

Bone tumors may be malignant or benign. Malignant tumors are primary, originating in the bone, or secondary, originating from elsewhere in the body (i.e., breast, lung, prostate, or kidney) and traveling to the bone (metastasis). Secondary or metastatic bone tumors are more common than primary bone tumors. Benign tumors of the bone also are more common than malignant bone tumors.

• BENIGN BONE TUMORS

Benign bone tumors have the potential to cause fractures of bones. They are not life-threatening and usually cause few symptoms.

Pathophysiology and Etiology

Benign tumors usually result from misplaced or overgrown clusters of normal bone or cartilage cells that cause the structure to enlarge and impair local function. They grow slowly and do not metastasize. Their growth can weaken the bone structure by compressing or displacing normal tissue.

Assessment Findings

Clients with benign bone tumors may experience pain or discomfort that worsens when bearing weight. Bone appears deformed and swelling may appear over the involved area. If the tumor is in a bone of the extremities, movement may be decreased and pathologic fractures may occur easily. Radiography, bone scans, and tumor biopsy determine the diagnosis.

Medical and Surgical Management

Medical management includes treating pain and preventing fractures. Surgery is done if the tumor does not stop growing, bone deformity is present, or pain is interfering with ADLs and mobility.

Curettage (scraping) or local excision is the usual procedure. Bone grafts may need to be done to promote bone growth and healing. Splints or casts are applied until bone heals. Clients require close monitoring after surgery because benign bone tumors can recur.

Nursing Management

Provide adequate explanations to the client and alleviate anxiety. Emphasize the nature of the tumor, prognosis, and treatment. Allow time for questions and expressions of fear and anxiety. Administer pain medications as indicated. Teach the client methods to reduce pain and swelling and encourage the client to elevate the affected extremity. See Nursing Care Plan 61-1.

• MALIGNANT BONE TUMORS

Malignant bone tumors are abnormal osteoblasts or myeloblasts (marrow cells) that exhibit rapid and uncontrollable growth.

Pathophysiology and Etiology

Prior exposure to radiation and toxic chemicals is associated with growth of some malignant bone tumors. A hereditary link in which a tumor suppressor gene may be absent or impaired also is suspected because the same type of tumor may appear among siblings in the same family. Primary tumors include osteosarcoma, Ewing's sarcoma, chondrosarcoma, and fibrosarcoma.

Malignant bone tumors usually are located around the knee in the distal femur or proximal fibula; a few are found in the proximal humerus. As the tumor expands, it lifts the periosteum in much the same way as osteomyelitis. Metastasis occurs through the circulatory or lymphatic system. Metastasis to the lungs is common.

Assessment Findings

A pathologic fracture may be the event that leads the client to seek treatment. Clients with malignant bone tumors complain of persistent pain, swelling, and difficulty in moving the involved extremity. A limp or abnormal gait may be present. By the time the client experiences symptoms, the tumor usually has spread beyond its primary site.

Bone appears abnormal on radiographic examination, MRI, or bone scan. Biopsy identifies abnormal cells. A malignancy of the skeletal system is associated with an elevated serum alkaline phosphatase level.

Medical and Surgical Management

Treatment of primary malignant bone tumors involves surgical removal of the tumor by amputating the extremity or by wide local resection. Radiation therapy and chemotherapy may be used as well. Chemotherapy after surgery aims to destroy tumor cells that escape from the original tumor site.

Nursing Management

Clients with malignant bone tumors require extensive emotional support and information about the disease, treatment, and prognosis. Implement preoperative and postoperative measures for clients having surgery. Refer to the section on amputations for specific nursing care for amputees. As in other orthopedic surgeries, general nursing responsibilities include keeping the affected extremity elevated to reduce swelling, assessing neurovascular status frequently (see Chap. 60), and monitoring closely for complications if the affected limb is immobilized after surgery. See Nursing Care Plan 61-1.

AMPUTATION •

Amputation is removal of a limb. It may occur as a result of trauma (traumatic amputation) or in an effort to control disease or disability (therapeutic amputation).

Etiology

Conditions for which an amputation may be done include malignant tumors, long-standing infections of bone and tissue that prohibit restoration of function, extensive trauma to an extremity, death of tissues from peripheral vascular insufficiency or peripheral vasospastic diseases such as Raynaud's disease, thermal injuries, deformity of a limb rendering it a useless hindrance, and life-threatening disorders, such as arterial thrombosis and gas bacillus infections.

Medical and Surgical Management

Unless emergency surgery is done, the client is treated for any disorder that may influence healing (e.g., uncontrolled diabetes mellitus, dehydration, infection, electrolyte imbalances, poor nutrition, chronic respiratory disorders). When it is decided that amputation must be done as a life-saving measure, the following factors help the surgical team decide at which level to amputate the arm or leg (e.g., above or below the knee, above or below the elbow):

- Amount of tissue that must be removed to eliminate the disorder
- Level at which blood supply is adequate to preserve circulation to tissue that will remain
- Number of joints that can be preserved
- Length of residual limb that will promote fitting a prosthesis, an artificial limb, for rehabilitation

Levels of some commonly planned amputations include below the knee (BK), above the knee (AK), below the elbow (BE), and above the elbow (AE). The objective is to create a gently tapering stump with muscular padding over the end. Occasionally, knee disarticulations (amputation through a joint), ankle disarticulations, and partial foot amputations are done.

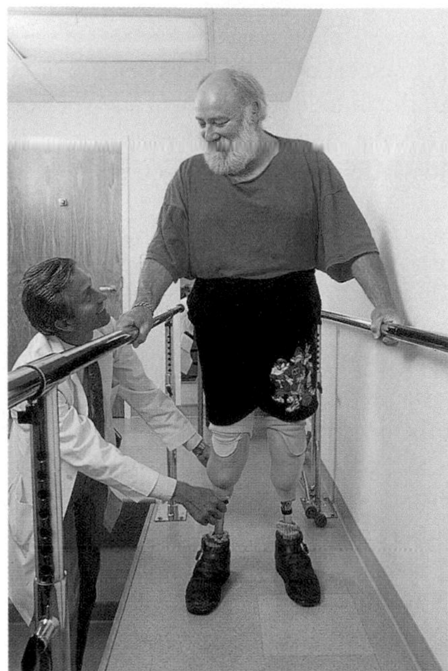

FIGURE 61.9 Many amputees receive prostheses soon after surgery and begin learning how to use them with the help and support of the rehabilitation team, which includes nurses, physicians, physical therapists, and others.

Amputation Methods

An amputation may involve using an open or closed method. In an open amputation (guillotine amputation), the end of the residual limb (or stump) is temporarily open with no skin covering it. Open amputations usually are done in cases of infection. Skin traction is applied, and the infected area is allowed to drain. Traction must be continuous. The surgeon may arrange traction so that the client can turn over in bed.

In the more common closed amputation (flap amputation), skin flaps cover the severed bone end. Clients with a closed amputation return from surgery with either a soft compression dressing or rigid plaster shell covering the residual limb. The compression dressing consists of gauze over which elastic roller bandages are wrapped to create pressure to control bleeding. There may be a walking pylon, a type of temporary prosthesis composed of a metal post and molded foot, attached to the rigid plaster shell (Fig. 61.9). It may be weeks before the postoperative client is referred to a prosthetist, a professional who creates and fits artificial limbs.

Arm Amputation

The amputation of an arm, particularly the arm with the dominant hand, requires great physical and emotional adjustment during the preoperative as well as postoperative periods. Fortunately, most clients with arm amputations can be measured for a prosthesis shortly after the surgical scar heals.

Three types of prostheses are available for arm amputees. A shoulder harness with cables that attach to a mechanical terminal device, referred to as a *hook,* performs the functions of the hand and fingers when the amputee moves the scapula and expands the chest, activating the cables attached from a shoulder harness to the mechanical device. The *cosmetic hand,* which can be attached to the same cables as the hook, has the appearance of a natural hand, but lacks the capacity for performing fine motor skills. The *myoelectric arm* has a realistic-looking hand that is activated by electrical impulses from muscles in the upper arm. It has three advantages: it eliminates the need to wear a harness, the terminal device looks natural, and it has somewhat better function than the cosmetic hand. It is not rugged enough to do the work of the mechanical terminal device.

Leg Amputation

Leg amputation is more common. The AK amputation is more disabling than a BK amputation; therefore, every attempt is made to amputate below the knee.

The trend is to have a temporary prosthesis attached to the plaster shell covering the residual lower limb immediately after surgery. It reduces psychological trauma for the client because it promotes a more intact sense of body image after surgery. Also, the walking pylon facilitates early ambulation. Almost immediately, the client is allowed to stand and place a limited amount of weight on the residual limb. As the stump heals and edema disappears, a second cast may be reapplied or a temporary socket made of lightweight polypropylene may be constructed. Ultimately, a conventional prosthesis is custom-made to conform to the stump as well as to the client's needs. Leg prostheses may be held in place by means of a pelvic belt or suction.

Complications

Hematoma, hemorrhage, and infection are potential complications in the immediate postoperative period. A potential complication late in the postoperative course is chronic osteomyelitis (after persistent infection).

Phantom Limb and Phantom Pain

The surgeon informs the client of the potential phenomenon of phantom limb sensation, a feeling that the amputated portion of the limb still remains. It is a normal, frequently occurring physiologic response after amputation. Phantom sensations can persist for months or decades, or can come and go. Although clients are aware of phantom sensations, they usually learn to ignore them.

Phantom pain is pain or other discomfort, such as burning, tingling, throbbing, or itching, in the missing limb. Pain felt from the phantom limb can be an extremely serious problem in relation to the client's emotional status and ability to use a prosthesis. Severe, prolonged phantom limb pain may require surgical removal of nerve endings at the end of the stump.

Rehabilitation

The amputee's rehabilitation depends on variables such as age, type of amputation, condition of stump, physical status, condition of remaining limb, concurrent debilitating illness, visual motor coordination, motivation, acceptance, and cooperation. Clients vary greatly in their learning capacity and ability to master use of a prosthesis. The period allotted for training also varies with each client. It is vital that all involved maintain realistic expectations throughout the rehabilitation period.

Nursing Management

Presurgical nursing management involves considerations for any surgery, specifically taking a complete medical, drug, and allergy history and evaluating the client for mental and emotional acceptance of the surgical procedure. Assessing motor strength and flexibility of other joints is important to determine potential problems involving rehabilitation. If the client is acutely ill, such as with a gangrenous limb and related fever, disorientation, and electrolyte imbalances, monitor circulation in the limb for changes, such as severe pain, color changes, and lack of peripheral pulses. Inform the physician of problems as they occur because surgery may become an emergency.

Relieve pain and anxiety and support the client as he or she begins to grieve loss of the limb and adapt to potential changes. Administer narcotic analgesics before surgery to clients with severe pain. Other comfort measures include handling the painful limb gently, elevating a swollen limb, encouraging family presence and support, being available especially at times when the client is alone, helping the client to express concerns, and clarifying misperceptions.

Before surgery, explain all the routine preoperative preparations and reinforce what the physician has discussed with the client and family regarding the extent of physical disability; the psychological, aesthetic, social, and vocational implications; and the realistic possibilities for prosthetic restoration. Review postoperative management, such as deep breathing, coughing, positioning, and routine exercises, and encourage the client to practice the exercises, if time and the client's condition permit.

Clients vary in their reactions to the impending loss of a limb. The amount of grief is thought to be proportional to the symbolic significance of the part and the resultant degree of disability and deformity. Anger and depression are common emotions. Acknowledge the client's feelings and remain objective and nonjudgmental as the client expresses negative emotional responses. Reassuring the client that his or her reaction is normal may provide comfort.

Monitor vital signs to determine any changes, particularly elevations in temperature (indicating possible infection), pulse, and BP. Review the client's medical record for information about the reason for and type and level of the amputation. Inspect the dressing or plaster shell and, when changing the dressing, assess the wound for signs of infection, excessive drainage, or separation of wound edges. Evaluate the client's general condition as well as level of pain and discomfort, and implement measures to relieve it. Implement measures to prevent infection, promote healing, and avoid skin breakdown. See Nursing Care Plan 61-1 for additional resources.

A client who has a leg amputation needs to be placed in the prone position several times a day. This position promotes stump extension and prevents contractures. Position the client so that he or she is in normal anatomic alignment. Improper positioning may injure peripheral nerves and blood vessels and cause joint deformities. On the first or second postoperative day, assist client to stand to regain a sense of balance. Stepping on the floor with the temporary prosthesis and weight bearing of about 10% of body weight usually is permitted at this time. Expect the client with a temporary prosthesis to progress to walking with crutches or a walker or in parallel bars 2 to 4 days after amputation (full weight bearing on the unaffected leg). This activity will promote the client's independence.

Client and Family Teaching

Client and family education begins before amputation surgery and extends beyond hospitalization. After surgery, discharge teaching depends on many factors, including length of hospitalization, type and location of amputation, age and physical condition of the client, and type of dressing or prosthesis the client wears. Explore factors related to the home environment and determine a plan for continued rehabilitation before discharge. Some clients need to modify their living arrangements, use a wheelchair, or make other accommodations or changes.

If the client has to bandage the stump at home, teach both client and family how to apply the bandage and care for the stump (Nursing Guidelines 61-4), as well as how to wash bandages, rinse them well, and lay them flat to dry because hanging tends to decrease the elasticity. When bandages are dry, they must be rolled without stretching. Include the following general points in the discharge instructions:

- Follow the physician's recommendations regarding caring for the stump, applying a stump dressing, washing the stump, and elevating the stump when sitting.
- Do not apply nonprescription drugs (ointments, creams, topical pain relievers) to the stump unless the physician has approved the use of a specific product.
- Adhere to the plan of scheduled exercises and complete each group of exercises as outlined by the physical therapist.
- Do not exceed the physician's recommendations regarding weight bearing and joint flexion.
- Eat well-balanced and nutritious meals or follow the diet recommended by the physician. Avoid gaining excess weight during the recovery period because weight gain may interfere with use of a leg prosthesis.
- Expect that phantom limb sensation, if present, may persist for some time, which is normal.
- Avoid injury to the stump, even though it appears to be healed. Report any skin impairment immediately.
- Continue deep breathing exercises until fully mobile.
- Contact the physician if fever, chills, productive cough, bleeding or oozing from the stump, purulent drainage from the incision, new or different pain in the stump, or any change in the appearance of the stump occurs.

NURSING GUIDELINES 61-4

Stump Care and Bandaging

Stump Care

- Assess the covering over the stump frequently to determine the type and amount of drainage from the incision. Expect some oozing of blood, but if a gauze dressing is used, it may need to be reinforced.
- Keep a tourniquet in plain view at bedside and if hemorrhage occurs, apply it and notify the physician.
- In most cases, elevate the stump for the first 24 to 48 hours to prevent edema. In some cases, such as an AK amputation, a slight Trendelenburg position is preferred to elevating the stump on pillows because bending the hip promotes a flexion contracture. A bed board or a firm mattress provides skeletal support.
- If the client has a rigid plaster cast with walking pylon, loosen the harness, which suspends the cast from the waist, when the client is in bed. Slightly tighten the harness when the client is ambulatory.

Bandaging

Before a permanent prosthesis can be made, the stump must shrink and be shaped. This is done with elastic bandages that are wrapped about the stump. Unlike leg stumps, arm stumps do not need as massive a shrinkage over as long a period. Various bandaging techniques are appropriate, but several principles are observed:

- Remove and rewrap the bandage at least twice during the day and before the client retires for the night.
- Bandage joints in a way that promotes a neutral or extended position.
- Avoid circular turns, which act like a tourniquet and interfere with blood flow.

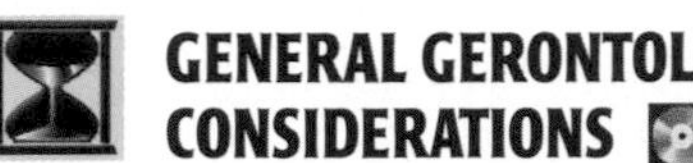

GENERAL GERONTOLOGIC CONSIDERATIONS

Women older than 45 years of age have a 9% to 10% decrease in cortical bone per decade.

Older adults are more prone to skeletal fractures because bone resorption takes place more rapidly than bone formation.

Maintaining an active lifestyle delays the decline of muscle strength and bone mass among older adults.

With age, the fibrocartilage of intervertebral disks becomes thinner and drier, causing compression of the disks of the spinal column and leading to a loss of height amounting to as much as 1.5 to 3 inches (3.75 to 7.5 cm).

Estrogen deficiency, which occurs at menopause, is considered the leading factor in osteoporosis among aging women.

Critical Thinking Exercises

1. *A male client had a total hip replacement 3 days ago and wants to use the toilet for a bowel movement. Explain how to assist this client.*
2. *A female client has just returned from the recovery unit after an AK amputation. Fresh blood has saturated the stump dressing. What actions should you take at this time?*
3. *A young man, admitted with a fractured radius, complains of increasing pain in his hand after a cast was applied, despite having received a narcotic analgesic 30 minutes ago. What assessments are important to make at this time?*

● NCLEX-STYLE REVIEW QUESTIONS 

1. A 14-year-old fractured his left femur during a school football game in October. Before football camp the following August, what instruction would the nurse give to the football player?
   1. "Your fracture is well healed after 6 months; you may resume regular training."
   2. "Your fracture will not heal fully until October; you will not have your former strength."

3. "Your femur will never have the same strength; restricted activity is required."
4. "Your femur is not completely healed; you will need to sit out this football season."

2. When managing the care of a client with a lower extremity in traction, which nursing assessment would require traction adjustment?
   1. Weights dangling freely over the bed frame
   2. Client alignment straight in an opposite line to the pull of the traction
   3. Foot position dropped with the toes pointing to the end of the bed
   4. Pulleys unobstructed with freely moving ropes

3. When assisting the physician during plaster cast application, which procedure is most correct until the cast dries?
   1. Handle the wet cast with the tips of the fingers.
   2. Place the cast on a pillow until the cast dries.
   3. Cover the cast with plastic wrap to prevent damage.
   4. Handle the wet cast with the palms of the hand.

connection

Visit the Connection site at **http://connection.lww.com/go/timbyEssentials** for links to chapter-related resources on the Internet.

References and Suggested Readings

Arthritis Foundation. (2002). Arthritis today: Drug guide. [Online.] Available: www.arthritis.org.

Bryant, G. (2001). Stump care. *American Journal of Nursing, 101*(2), 67–71.

Bullock, B. A., & Henze, R. L. (2000). *Focus on pathophysiology.* Philadelphia: Lippincott Williams & Wilkins.

Curry, L. C., & Hogstel, M. O. (2002). Osteoporosis. *American Journal of Nursing, 102*(1), 26–32.

D'Arcy, Y. (2002). How to treat arthritis pain. *Nursing 2002, 32*(7), 30–31.

Ferrari, R. (2001). The strain of cervical sprains. *American Journal of Nursing, 101*(1), 11.

Fort, C. W. (2002). Getting a fix on a long-bone fracture. *Nursing 2002, 32*(6), 32hn1–32hn6.

Hayes, D. D. (2003). How to wrap an above-the-knee amputation stump. *Nursing 2003, 33*(1), 70.

Kozuh, J. L. (2000). NSAIDs and antihypertensives: An unhappy union. *American Journal of Nursing, 100*(6), 40–42.

McConnell, E. A. (2002). Assessing neurovascular status in a casted limb. *Nursing 2002, 32*(9), 20.

Mewshaw, E. (October 14, 2002). The many faces of rheumatoid arthritis. *Advance for Nurses,* 17–19.

Munz, P. M. (November 5, 2002). Bisphosphanates. *Advance for Nurses,* 35, 38.

Overdorf, J. (2001). Osteoporosis: There's so much we can do. *RN, 64*(12), 30–35.

Pasero, C., & McCaffery, M. (2001). Pain control: Selective COX-2 inhibitors. *American Journal of Nursing, 101*(4), 55–56.

Patient Handout. (March 3, 2003). Osteoporosis. *Advance for Nurses,* 27.

Pauldine, E. F. (2003). Taking a bite out of Lyme disease. *Nursing 2003, 33*(4), 49–52.

Peloso, P. M. (2000). NSAIDs: A Faustian bargain. *American Journal of Nursing, 100*(6), 34–39.

Plummer, E. (August 19, 2002). Hip fractures. *Advance for Nurses,* 37–38.

Porth, C. M. (2002). *Pathophysiology: Concepts of altered health states* (6th ed.). Philadelphia: Lippincott Williams & Wilkins.

Ramsburg, K. L. (2000). Rheumatoid arthritis. *American Journal of Nursing, 100*(11), 40–43.

Schafer, M. C. (February 3, 2003). Hip fracture prevention. *Advance for Nurses,* 34–35.

Sharkey, N. A., Williams, N. I., & Guerin, J. B. (2000). The role of exercise in the prevention and treatment of osteoporosis and osteoarthritis. *Nursing Clinics of North America, 35,* 209–221.

Smeltzer, S. C., & Bare, B. G. (2004). *Brunner & Suddarth's textbook of medical–surgical nursing* (10th ed.). Philadelphia: Lippincott Williams & Wilkins.

Urquhart, B. S. (2001). Emergency: Anterior shoulder dislocation. *American Journal of Nursing, 101*(2), 33–35.

U.S. Preventive Services Task Force. (2003). Screening for osteoporosis in postmenopausal women. Recommendations and rationale. *American Journal of Nursing, 103*(1), 73–81.

Wade, C. F. (2000). Keeping Lyme disease at bay. *American Journal of Nursing, 100*(7), 26–31.

Walls, M. (2002). Orthopedic trauma. *RN, 65*(7), 52–56.

chapter 62

Introduction to the Integumentary System

Words to Know 

apocrine glands
debridement
dermis
eccrine glands
epidermis
integument
keratin
melanin
pressure sores
sebaceous glands
sebum
shearing
skin tear
stratum corneum
subcutaneous tissue
sweat glands

Learning Objectives

On completion of this chapter, the reader will:

- Describe structures and functions of the integumentary system.
- Identify the purpose of sebum and melanin.
- Differentiate eccrine and apocrine glands.
- Discuss assessments pertinent to the integumentary system.
- Give characteristics of normal skin.
- Discuss criteria for staging pressure sores.
- Explain diagnostic tests performed to determine the etiology of skin disorders.
- Identify medical and surgical techniques for treating skin disorders.

The **integument** includes structures that cover the body's exterior surface. The primary structure is the skin, which contains sebaceous and sweat glands and sensory nerve endings (Fig. 62.1). The integument also includes accessory structures such as hair and nails. Structures that make up the integument protect the body from environmental injuries, help regulate body temperature, serve as sensory organs, and facilitate synthesis of vitamin D.

ANATOMY AND PHYSIOLOGY

Skin

Skin is composed of two layers. The **epidermis,** the outermost layer, contains an outer layer of dead skin cells, the **stratum corneum,** that forms a tough protective protein called **keratin.** The epidermis is constantly shed and replaced with epithelial cells from the dermis. The **dermis,** or true skin, lies below the epidermis. It consists of connective tissue and contains elastic fibers, blood vessels, sensory and motor nerve fibers, sweat and sebaceous (oil) glands, and hair follicles (roots). The **subcutaneous tissue** is the layer of skin attached to muscle and bone and composed primarily of connective tissue and fat cells. Skin has a tremendous capacity to stretch with little subsequent damage, as is evident after soft tissue injury and pregnancy.

Skin color is determined by a pigment called **melanin,** manufactured by melanocytes located in the epidermis. Production of melanin is under the control of the middle lobe of the pituitary gland, which secretes melanocyte-stimulating hormone. The more melanin found in the epidermis, the darker the skin color. Exposure to ultraviolet light temporarily stimulates production of melanin to absorb harmful radiation.

Functions of the skin include protection, temperature regulation, sensory processing, and chemical synthesis. The skin forms a protective barrier between the outside world and underlying organs and structures of the body. The barrier it provides blocks microorganisms and other foreign substances from contact with structures below the epidermis. It also prevents a loss of water from structures below the skin surface.

To maintain an even body temperature, skin heats or cools structures below. The body continuously produces internal heat during cellular metabolism. To generate heat and prevent heat loss at the body's surface, erector muscles around shafts of hair contract. Elevation of skin hairs interferes with local air circulation and maintains warmth of skin.

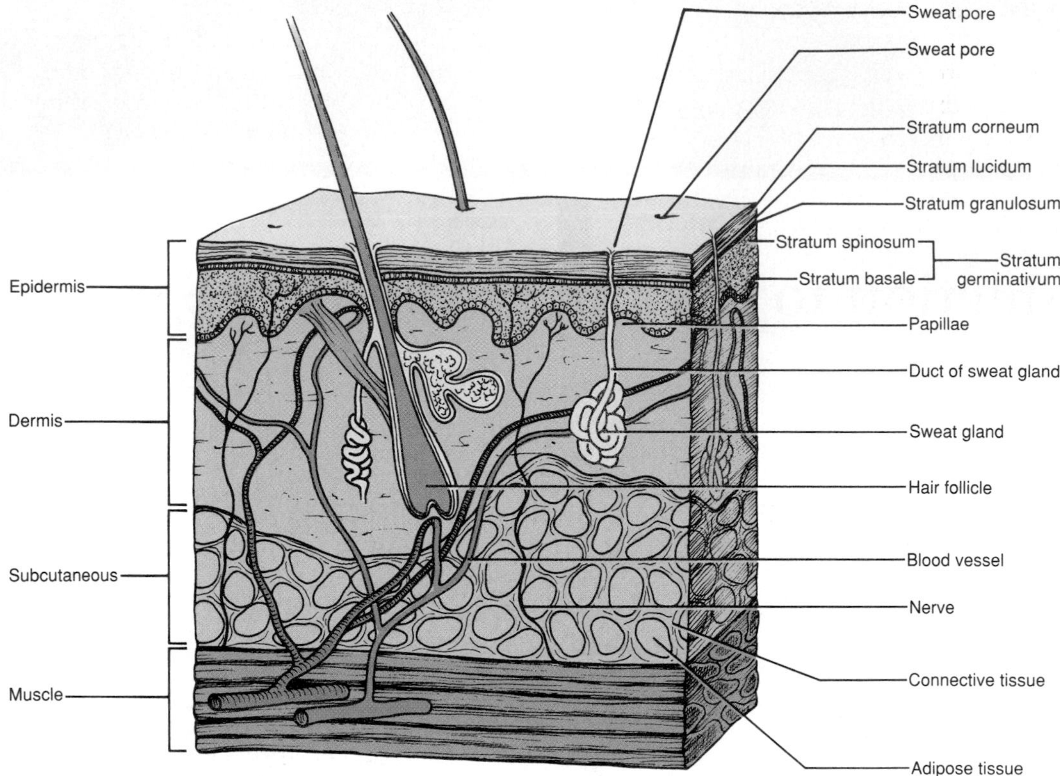

FIGURE 62.1 A cross-section of the skin.

Heat dissipates through skin and respiration. It is lost by four methods:

- *Radiation*—the transfer of surface heat in the environment, such as escape of heat from the surface of warm skin into cooler air.
- *Conduction*—the transfer of heat through contact, such as placing a cool cloth on warm skin.
- *Evaporation*—the loss of moisture or water. Water on the body surface is warmed. As moisture vaporizes, the body is cooled. Evaporation occurs unnoticed (insensible loss) and when there is obvious perspiration.
- *Convection*—the transfer of heat by means of currents of liquids or gasses in which warm air molecules move away from the body, such as a cool breeze that blows across the body surface.

When temperature and humidity outside the body rise, radiation, evaporation, and convection are ineffective. The only way heat is transferred under these conditions is by conduction. This is why exposure to warm temperatures and densely saturated moist air can raise the body temperature and result in heat stroke.

Skin serves as a means of monitoring the outside environment, as well as warning of danger. Specialized nerve endings in skin respond to pressure, pain, heat, and cold.

Skin forms a chemical substance called 7-dehydrocholesterol, which facilitates synthesis of vitamin D when the skin is exposed to ultraviolet light (sunlight). Vitamin D is necessary for healthy formation of bones and teeth. Dark-skinned people do not synthesize vitamin D as readily as light-skinned people. Cloudy environments and air pollutants that block sunlight also interfere with vitamin D synthesis. Therefore, vitamin D is added to some food sources, such as milk.

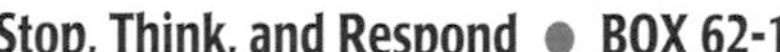

Stop, Think, and Respond ● BOX 62-1

Discuss the importance of keeping the skin intact. 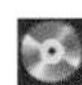

Hair

Hair originates in hair follicles in the dermis. It is formed from hundreds of strands of keratin linked together with amino acids. Melanin, produced by melanocytes in the hair root, influence hair color. The three types of melanin are brown, black, and yellow. Types of melanin are genetically inherited, as are hair texture, shape, and rate of growth. Scalp hair grows more rapidly than any other. Illness, hormone levels, nutrition, aging, and other factors can affect hair growth and loss.

Hair covers all parts of the body except the palms, soles, dorsum of fingers, lips, penis, labia, and nipples. In some areas, such as the pubis, axilla, and chest, hair is more coarse. Men of some ethnic groups (e.g., Native Americans) have less facial and body hair than their Euro-American counterparts.

Sebaceous and Sweat Glands

Sebaceous glands are connected to each hair follicle and secrete an oily substance called **sebum,** a lubricant that prevents drying and crackling of the skin and hair. As sebum fills the glandular duct, it enters the hair follicle, from which it eventually is released. During puberty, sebaceous glands in the forehead, nose, chest, and back become more active.

The two types of **sweat glands** are eccrine and apocrine. **Eccrine glands** release water and electrolytes, such as sodium and chloride, in the form of perspiration. Rate of perspiration is related to body temperature. Adults can produce as much as 3 L under extremely hot conditions. The pH of perspiration is slightly acidic, which helps in providing a hostile environment for microbial colonization. Frequent washing with alkaline soaps removes sebum and reduces the acid mantle of protection.

Apocrine glands are found around the nipples, in the anogenital region, in the eyelids (Moll's glands), in the mammary glands of the breast, and in the external ear canals—where the secretion is referred to as *cerumen.* The function of apocrine secretions in humans is unknown, although the onset of secretions coincides with puberty.

In general, perspiration, which includes secretions from both eccrine and apocrine glands, is odorless. An odor develops when perspiration mixes with bacteria on the skin.

Nails

Fingernails and toenails are layers of hard keratin that have a protective function. In primates and humans, nails may be a biologic diversification of claws. Animal species that have claws use them to catch and tear prey, whereas primates and humans developed nails on fingers and toes because of a greater biologic need for grasping limbs and manipulating primitive tools or utensils.

The nail root lies buried beneath the nail's exposed surface in a fold of skin. The nails have an abundant blood supply. Their semitransparent appearance facilitates circulatory assessment.

ASSESSMENT

History

Initial assessment of the client begins with a thorough history based on symptoms. Include the following questions:

- When did the disorder first begin and where did it first appear?
- Where are lesions located?
- Have there been any changes in the disorder since it first appeared (an increase or decrease in symptoms; in appearance or color; in location)?
- Has the problem spread?
- What physical sensations pertain to the disorder (pain, itching, burning, and intensity)?
- Do other physical or emotional problems appear to be associated with the disorder?
- Was a specific event associated with onset of the disorder?
- What factors appear to make the condition better or worse?
- Do you or anyone in your family have known or suspected allergies?
- What prescription and nonprescription medications have you taken recently?
- Have you made changes in personal products, such as soaps, deodorants, and cosmetics?
- Have there been recent changes in your work or living environment, such as pets, plants, sprays, dust, and pollutants, that might have precipitated this problem?

Physical Examination

During a physical examination, inspect and palpate the structures of the integument.

Skin Assessment

Examine the skin on all areas of the body during the head-to-toe assessment or as a focused assessment. Good lighting is essential. Skin should be smooth, unbroken, of uniform color according to the person's ethnic or racial origin, warm, and resilient. It should feel neither wet nor unusually dry.

Color deviations have several possible causes (Table 62.1). While examining the skin, the nurse may detect

TABLE 62.1 COMMON SKIN COLOR VARIATIONS

COLOR	TERM	POSSIBLE CAUSES
Pale, regardless of race	Pallor	Anemia, blood loss
Red	Erythema	Superficial burns, local inflammation, carbon monoxide poisoning
Pink	Flushed	Fever, hypertension
Purple	Ecchymosis	Trauma to soft tissue
Blue	Cyanosis	Low tissue oxygenation
Yellow	Jaundice	Liver or kidney disease, destruction of red blood cells
Brown	Tan	Racial variation, sun exposure, pregnancy, Addison's disease

changes in its structure or integrity such as those listed in Table 62.2. Document the sites of any abnormalities.

Assess temperature by placing the dorsum of the hand on the skin surface. Detect moisture with the palmar surface. Determine the quality of skin turgor by grasping the skin, such as that over the chest, between the thumb and forefinger. Normally the skin returns to its original position immediately after being released. Tight, shiny skin

TABLE 62.2 TERMS FOR VARIOUS SKIN LESIONS

TYPE OF LESION	DESCRIPTION	EXAMPLES	DEPICTION
Macule	Flat, round, colored	Freckles, rash	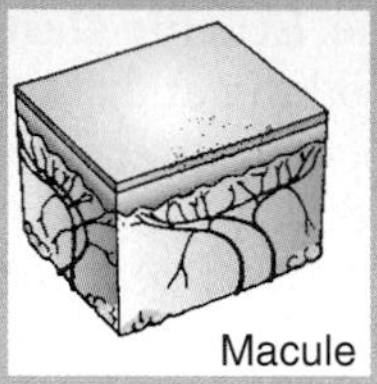 Macule
Papule	Elevated, obvious raised border, solid	Wart	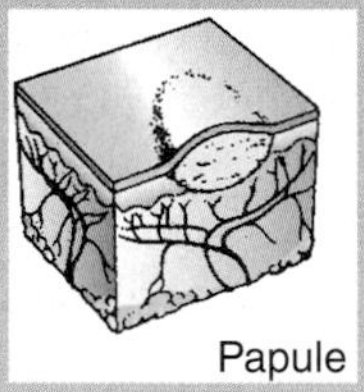 Papule
Vesicle	Elevated, round, filled with serum	Blister	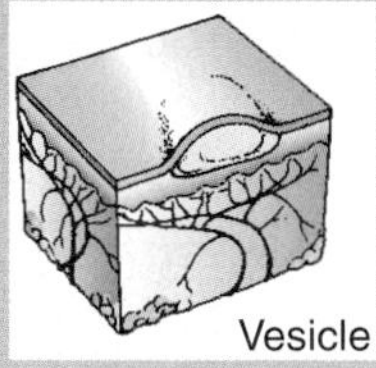 Vesicle
Wheal	Elevated, irregular border, no free fluid	Hives	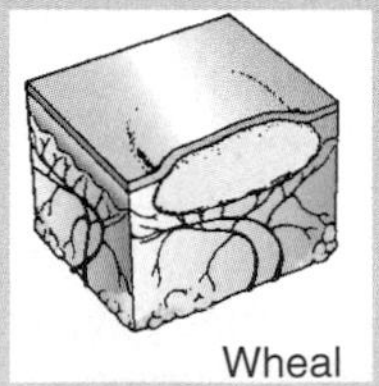 Wheal
Pustule	Elevated, raised border, filled with pus	Boil	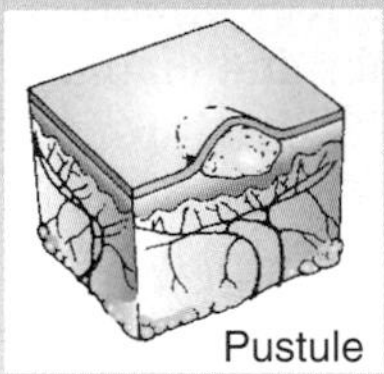 Pustule
Nodule	Elevated solid mass, extends into deeper tissue	Enlarged lymph node	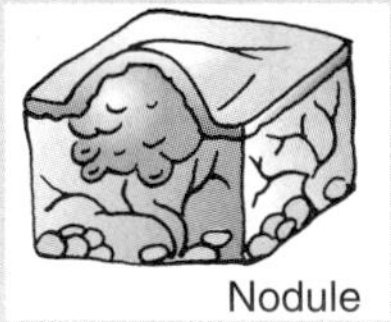 Nodule
Cyst	Encapsulated, round, fluid-filled or solid mass beneath the skin	Tissue growth	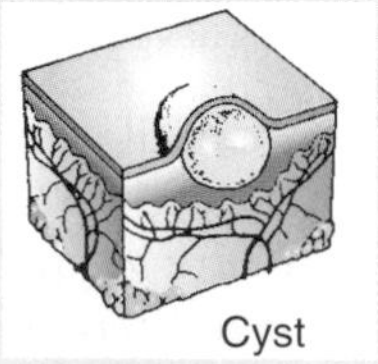 Cyst

suggests fluid retention; loose, dry skin may indicate dehydration.

Stop, Think, and Respond ● BOX 62-2

What type of skin lesion does a client have if it is described as follows:

A. Elevated, round, and filled with serum?
B. Flat, round, and red?
C. Elevated, solid, with a raised border?
D. Elevated, raised border, filled with pus? 

Pressure Sore Staging

Pressure sores, also known as *decubitus ulcers,* occur when capillary blood flow to the area is reduced. This may happen when skin over a bony prominence is compressed between the weight of the body and a hard surface for a prolonged period. Common locations include skin over the coccyx and sacrum in the lower spine, hips, heels, elbows, shoulder blades, ears, and back of head. Prevention of pressure sores first involves identifying persons who are at greatest risk, such as those with dehydration, diaphoresis, emaciation, immobility, inactivity, incontinence, localized edema, malnutrition, sedation, or vascular disease. Inactive, immobile, or sedated clients are also at risk. Pressure sores are categorized into one of four stages depending on the extent of tissue injury.

Stage I pressure sores are characterized by redness of the skin. The reddened skin of a beginning pressure sore fails to resume its normal color, or blanch, when pressure is relieved.

A *stage II* pressure sore is red and accompanied by blistering or a shallow break in the skin, sometimes described as a **skin tear.** This impairment leads to microbial colonization and infection of the wound.

Pressure sores classified as *stage III* are those in which superficial skin impairment progresses to a shallow crater extending to subcutaneous tissue. They may be accompanied by serous drainage from leaking plasma or purulent drainage (white or yellow-tinged fluid) caused by a wound infection. Although a stage III pressure sore is a significant wound, the area is relatively painless.

Stage IV pressure sores are the most traumatic and life-threatening. Tissue is deeply ulcerated, exposing muscle and bone. Dead tissue produces a rank odor. Local infection easily spreads throughout the body, causing a potentially fatal condition referred to as *sepsis.*

Once at-risk clients are identified, implement measures that reduce conditions under which pressure sores are likely to form:

- Turn and reposition the client frequently.
- Keep client's skin clean and dry.
- Massage bony prominences if the client's skin blanches with pressure relief.
- Use a moisturizing skin cleanser rather than soap.
- Apply pressure-relieving devices to the bed and chairs.
- Pad body areas subject to pressure and friction.
- Avoid **shearing,** a physical force that separates layers of tissue in opposite directions, such as when a seated client slides downward.

Scalp and Hair Assessment

Assess the scalp by separating the hair at random areas and inspecting the skin. The scalp normally is smooth, intact, and free of lesions.

Hair assessment not only applies to that which covers the head, but to other locations such as eyebrows, eyelashes, chest, arms, pubis, and legs. Note color, texture, and distribution, keeping sex- and age-related variations in mind. Nits, eggs from a louse infestation, scales, and flaking skin are abnormal findings.

Nail Assessment

Normal nails appear slightly convex with a 160° angle between the nail base and the skin (Fig. 62.2). Concave-shaped nails, referred to as *spooning,* are a sign of iron deficiency anemia. Clubbing of the nails, evidenced by an angle greater than 160°, suggests long-standing cardiopulmonary disease. Although nail thickness varies from 0.3 mm to 0.65 mm, nails thicken when there is a fungal infection and poor circulation. There may be evidence of other nail abnormalities (Fig. 62.3).

Observe the color of the nailbeds. Pink nailbeds suggest adequate oxygenation, but nails may be darker in other than Anglo-American clients. To assess tissue perfusion, compress the nailbeds, causing them to blanch, and then release them. Color returns normally in 3 seconds or less. This is called *capillary refill time.*

Diagnostic Tests

Diagnosis of a skin disorder is made chiefly by visual inspection. Some disorders may require additional testing, including the following types:

- Biopsy—performed to identify malignant or premalignant lesions. It also is of value in helping to identify some skin disorders.

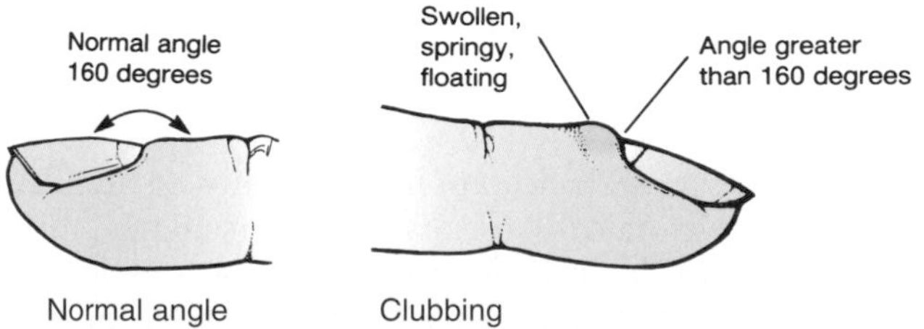

FIGURE 62.2 Normal nail angle and clubbed nail.

Onychorrhexis
- Brittle, fragile, uneven nail edge
- Associated with malnutrition, overhydration, thyrotoxicosis, chemical damage, radiation, aging

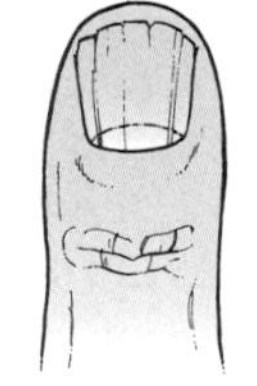
Onychorrhexis

Splinter Hemorrhage
- Blood streaks
- Associated with heart disease, hypertension, rheumatoid arthritis, neoplasms, trauma

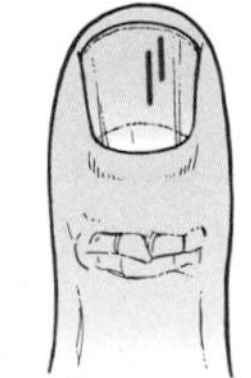
Splinter hemorrhage

Onychauxis
- Nail hypertrophy
- Associated with trauma, aging, fungal infections

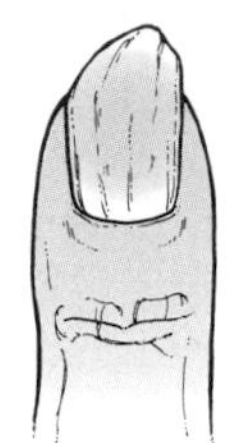
Onychauxis

Subungual Hematoma
- Blood clot
- Associated with trauma

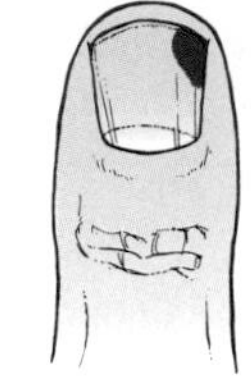
Subungual hematoma

Beau's Lines
- Tranverse furrows in nail plate
- Associated with malnutrition, severe illness

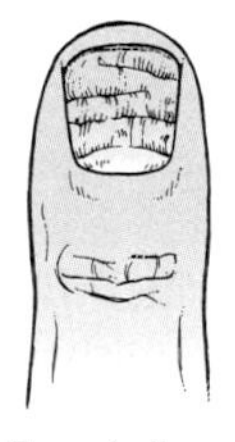
Beau's lines

FIGURE 62.3 Nail abnormalities.

- Culture and sensitivity tests—performed on lesions suspected or known to contain microorganisms.
- Allergy tests—intradermal injection, scratch test, and patch test are used to confirm an allergy to one or more substances (see Chap. 35).

MEDICAL AND SURGICAL TREATMENT OF SKIN DISORDERS

Various types of therapies are used to treat or manage skin disorders. They include drug therapy, wet dressings, therapeutic baths, surgical excision, radiation therapy, photochemotherapy, hyperbaric oxygenation, and lifestyle changes.

Drug Therapy

Topical and systemic medications are used to treat skin disorders:

- Corticosteroids are applied topically or administered systemically (orally, intramuscularly, intravenously) to relieve inflammatory and allergic symptoms. When used systemically, they can have serious toxic effects and thus are used primarily to relieve acute problems. Continued long-term use brings greater risk and is justified only when the disease itself is serious and other treatments cannot relieve it. Used as directed, topical application of a corticosteroid does not result in pronounced adverse effects seen with systemic administration, and can be used for longer periods.
- Antihistamines frequently are prescribed when allergy is a factor. They relieve itching and shorten the duration of the allergic reaction.
- Antibiotic, antifungal, and antiviral agents are used to treat infectious disorders. They are applied topically or administered systemically.
- Scabicides and pediculicides are used in the treatment of infestations with the scabies mite and lice.
- Local (topical) anesthetics are applied to relieve minor skin pain and itching.
- Emollients, ointments, powders, and lotions, which may be combined with other agents, soothe, protect, and soften the skin.
- Antiseborrheic agents are applied directly to the scalp or incorporated into shampooing products to control dandruff.
- Antiseptics are used to reduce bacteria on the skin.
- Keratolytics dissolve thickened, cornified skin such as warts, corns, and calluses, which causes the treated area to soften and swell, facilitating removal.

Use Standard Precautions when applying any topical medication to impaired skin or changing dressings that cover an open lesion. Infected, draining, or weeping lesions may require contact precautions as well. Apply topical medication as prescribed, such as a thin layer evenly spread over the area, or a thick layer dabbed on the area. Take care when applying medication so that lesions are not broken or skin surfaces abraded.

Wet Dressings

Wet dressings are used to apply a solution to a skin lesion. They have a cooling and soothing effect. The nature of the skin lesion (open or intact) determines whether sterile technique is required. First, a dry dressing consisting of gauze or other porous material is applied to the area. The dressing is then saturated with prescribed liquid. Dressings can be temporarily anchored with nonallergenic tape or roller gauze.

Some wet dressings are left in place until dry as a method of **debridement,** a technique for removing damaged tissue from a wound. When dried gauze is removed it usually contains bits of trapped debris in the gauze mesh. Removing dead and dying tissue provides an environment that fosters and promotes regeneration of healthy tissue and closure of the wound.

Therapeutic Baths

A therapeutic bath is one in which various solutions, powders, and oils, but no soap, are added to water into which the client's entire body or only a part is submerged. They relieve inflammation and itching and aid in the removal of crusts and scales. Examples of products used include cornstarch, sodium bicarbonate (baking soda), oatmeal colloid bath preparations, and mineral oil.

The tub or container is filled with lukewarm water. The drug or product is then added and the water stirred so that the preparation mixes thoroughly. A washcloth or a compress is used to apply the solution gently without rubbing the face and any other parts not covered by the solution.

Surgical Excision

When necessary to remove a skin lesion, such as a benign or malignant growth, tissue may be excised conventionally or with a laser, cryosurgery, or electrodesiccation. Surgical excisions are done under local or general anesthesia.

Laser stands for *l*ight *a*mplification by *s*timulated *e*mission of *r*adiation. Lasers convert a solid, gas, or liquid substance into light. The energy of laser light vaporizes tissue and coagulates bleeding vessels. Lasers also are used to remove tattoos and pigmented skin lesions such as hemangiomas and nevi. When a laser procedure is done, the eyes must be protected, precautions taken for preventing fires and burns from heated instruments, and vaporized fumes removed.

Cryosurgery is the application of extreme cold to destroy tissue. Liquid nitrogen circulates through a probe that is touched to skin or inserted to the center of the lesion. After application of extreme cold, the area thaws and becomes gelatin-like in appearance. A scab forms at the site. Healing takes approximately 4 to 6 weeks.

Electrodesiccation (or electrosurgery) uses electrical energy converted to heat, which destroys tissue. Plantar warts and skin tumors are examples of disorders treated by this method.

Radiation Therapy

Radiation therapy is used to treat malignant skin lesions. For more information on radiation therapy, see Chapter 19.

Photochemotherapy

Photochemotherapy involves a combination of psoralen methoxsalen and type A ultraviolet light. It is one method used to treat psoriasis, a chronic skin condition (see Chap. 63). Psoralen methoxsalen is taken 1 to 2 hours before exposure to ultraviolet A.

Lifestyle Changes

Some skin disorders grow worse when the person is tired or under emotional stress. Therefore, rest and sleep are an important part of treatment. Diet also is important, because certain foods contribute to or aggravate skin disorders in some individuals and must be eliminated from the diet.

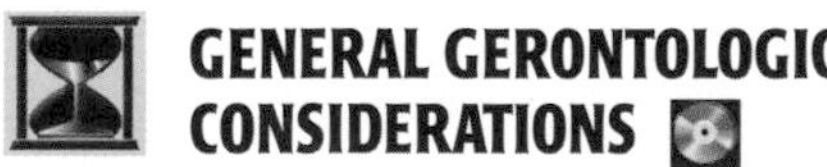

GENERAL GERONTOLOGIC CONSIDERATIONS

Melanin production decreases with aging; older adults develop gray hair.

Facial hair, and sometimes chest hair, appears in postmenopausal women as a result of decreased production of estrogen.

Loss of skin elasticity and subcutaneous tissue causes wrinkles to form among older adults. Skin in the upper arms becomes fleshy and loose. The eyelids, cheeks, chin, and breasts tend to sag.

The skin becomes dry and flaked as sebum production is reduced.

Small, brown, pigmented, benign lesions, known as *liver spots* or *senile lentigines,* form on the hands and forearms.

Small, yellow or brown, raised lesions called *senile keratoses* appear on the face and trunk. Senile keratoses are precancerous and require close observation by the nurse for any change in size, color, or form.

These lesions may be removed by freezing, chemical peel, cauterization, or topical creams.

Critical Thinking Exercise

1. *A client has developed a rash over her arms and thorax. What additional data are important to obtain before contacting the physician?*

● NCLEX-STYLE REVIEW QUESTIONS 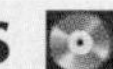

1. An older adult comes to the clinic for a routine appointment. The nurse notes that the client's skin is loose, dry, and flaky. Which follow-up question would be the most important?
    1. "How much fluid do you drink per day?"
    2. "When did your skin first become like this?"
    3. "Does anyone in your family have this condition?"
    4. "Are you also having any itching or redness?"
2. A nursing home resident confined to bed has a stage III pressure ulcer over the coccyx. The nurse instructs the patient care technician (PCT) about the resident's care. Which instruction given to the PCT is the most accurate?
    1. Check for incontinence at the end of the shift.
    2. Assist the resident to turn every 2 hours.
    3. Apply lotion to the coccyx once per shift.
    4. Pull the resident up when her feet touch the footboard.
3. When assessing a hospitalized client, the nurse notices that the client's face and body are flushed. Based on this finding, which nursing action is the most appropriate?
    1. Call the physician and request oxygen therapy.
    2. Ask if the client has been coughing or crying.
    3. Check the client's respiratory rate.
    4. Take the client's temperature.

connection

Visit the Connection site at **http://connection.lww.com/go/timbyEssentials** for links to chapter-related resources on the Internet.

References and Suggested Readings

Baranoski, S. (2000). Skin tears: Staying on guard against the enemy of frail skin. *Nursing 2000, 30*(9), 41–47.

Kohr, R. (2001). Clinical focus: Wound care. Moist healing versus wet-to-dry. *Canadian Nurse, 97*(1), 17–19.

Lawton, S. (2000). Assessing pigmented skin. *Nursing Times, 96*(27), NT plus: 14.

LeLievre, S. (2000). Skin care for older people with incontinence. *Elderly Care, 11*(10), 36–38.

Penzer, R., & Finch, M. (2001). Promoting healthy skin in older people. *Nursing Standard, 15*(34), 46–52.

Rader, J., Jones, D., & Miller, L. (2000). The importance of individualized wheelchair seating for frail older adults. *Journal of Gerontological Nursing, 26*(11), 24–32.

chapter 63

Caring for Clients With Skin, Hair, and Nail Disorders

Words to Know

acne vulgaris
alopecia
carbuncle
comedone
dermabrasion
dermatitis
dermatome
dermatophytes
dermatophytoses
erythema
furuncle
furunculosis
herpes zoster
onychocryptosis
onychomycosis
photochemotherapy
podiatrist
pruritus
psoriasis
shingles

Learning Objectives

On completion of this chapter, the reader will:

- Describe types of dermatitis.
- Explain factors that lead to acne vulgaris.
- Differentiate a furuncle, furunculosis, and carbuncle.
- Describe the appearance and cause of psoriasis.
- Identify skin disorders caused by a mite, a fungus, and a virus.
- Discuss factors that promote skin cancer.
- Describe conditions and their etiology characterized by hair loss.
- Discuss factors that promote fungal infections of the nails.
- Identify techniques for preventing onychocryptosis (ingrown toenails).

Disorders of skin, hair, and nails are common. Because self-image is inextricably related to how a person looks, disorders that affect appearance have personal and social consequences. In addition to requiring medical or surgical treatment, clients with skin disorders need empathic support while coping with chronic or acute conditions.

SKIN DISORDERS

• DERMATITIS

Dermatitis is a general term referring to an inflammation of the skin (Fig. 63.1). It is a common sign of many skin disorders accompanied by a red rash. An associated symptom is **pruritus,** or itching. Dermatitis and pruritus may be localized or generalized. Because both are nonspecific symptoms, it is essential that the cause be diagnosed and treated. Two common types are allergic and irritant dermatitis.

Pathophysiology and Etiology

Allergic contact dermatitis develops in people sensitive to one or more substances, such as drugs, fibers in clothing, cosmetics, plants (e.g., poison ivy), and dyes. Primary irritant dermatitis is a localized reaction that occurs when skin comes into contact with a strong chemical such as a solvent or detergent.

In clients with allergies, sensitized mast cells in the skin release histamine, causing a red rash, itching, and localized swelling (see Chap. 36). An allergy does not cause irritant dermatitis. Rather, the caustic quality of the substance damages the protein structure of the skin or eliminates secretions that protect it.

Assessment Findings

The skin response is characterized by dilation of blood vessels, causing redness and swelling, and sometimes by *vesiculation* (blister formation) and oozing. Itching is a

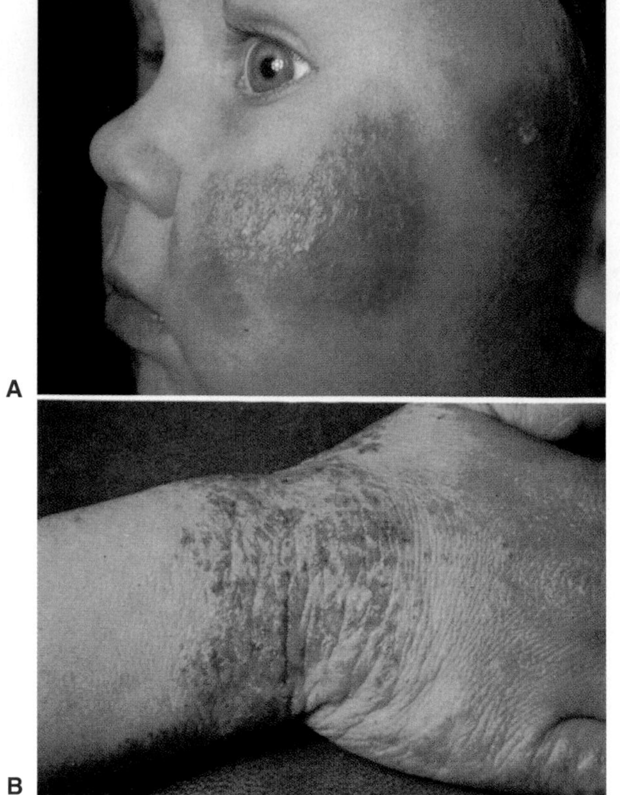

FIGURE 63.1 Contact dermatitis of the (**A**) face and (**B**) wrist.

prominent symptom. Primary irritant dermatitis may cause soreness or discomfort from irritation, itching, redness, swelling, and vesiculation.

Diagnosis is made by visual examination. A detailed and thorough history helps identify offending substances as well as the type of dermatitis. In difficult cases, a skin patch test may identify an allergic substance.

Medical Management

Treatment of both types of dermatitis is to remove substances causing the reaction. This is done by flushing the skin with cool water. Topical lotions, such as calamine, or systemic drugs, such as diphenhydramine (Benadryl) or cyproheptadine (Periactin), are prescribed to relieve itching. Moisturizing creams with lanolin restore lubrication. In more severe cases, wet dressings with astringent solutions, such as Burow's solution (aluminum acetate), are prescribed. Corticosteroids taken orally or applied topically also provide relief.

Nursing Management

Advise clients to wear rubber gloves when coming in contact with any substance such as soap or solvents, put all clothes through a second rinse cycle when laundering to remove soap residue, and avoid use of cosmetics or any topical drug or substance until the etiology of the dermatitis is identified. To reduce itching or preserve skin integrity, tell clients to:

- Keep nails short and clean.
- Use light cotton bedding and clothes that allow normal evaporation of moisture from the skin (avoid wool, synthetics, and other dense fibers).
- Wear white cotton gloves if prone to scratching during sleep.
- Avoid regular soap for bathing; hypoallergenic or glycerin soaps can be used without causing skin irritation or itching.
- Use tepid bath water; pat rather than rub the skin dry.
- Inform the physician if the drug therapy fails to restore skin integrity or relieve itching.

● ACNE VULGARIS

Acne vulgaris, which tends to coincide with puberty, is an inflammatory disorder affecting sebaceous glands and hair follicles. Its severity varies from minimal to severe.

Pathophysiology and Etiology

It is believed that acne is related to hormonal changes that occur when secondary sex characteristics are developing. It is aggravated by cosmetics as well as picking and squeezing blemishes that form. Correlation with specific food items (e.g., chocolate) is more myth than fact.

Sebum, keratin, and bacteria accumulate and dilate the follicle. The collective secretions form a **comedone,** or a *blackhead.* The dark appearance results from oxidation of the core material. The follicle becomes further distended and irritated, causing a raised papule in the skin. If the follicular wall ruptures, the inflammatory response extends into marginal areas of dermis. In serious cases, inflamed nodules and cysts develop. Severe acne, if neglected, leads to deep, pitted scars that leave skin permanently pockmarked. Acne vulgaris improves after adolescence.

Assessment Findings

Comedones and pustules appear on the face, chest, and back, where skin is excessively oily (Fig. 63.2). Oiliness of the scalp often accompanies acne. Diagnosis is made by visual examination of the affected areas.

Medical Management

Mild cases of acne improve with gentle facial cleansing and nonprescription drying agents containing benzoyl

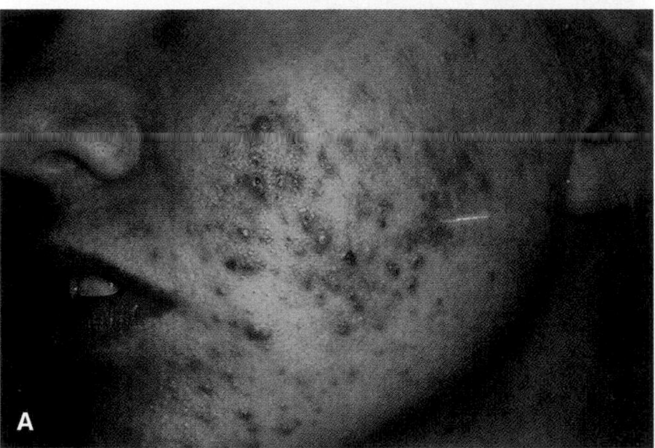

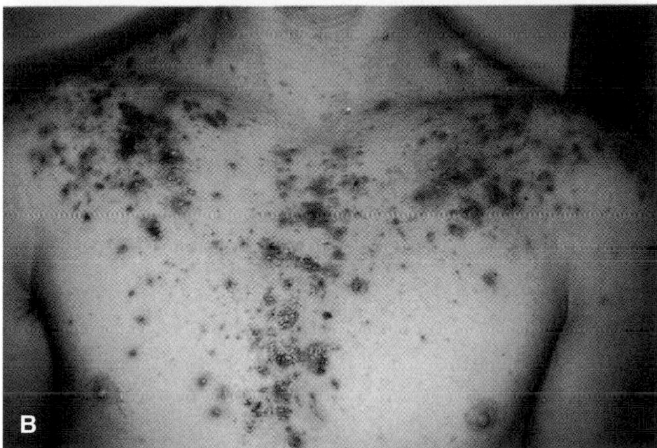

FIGURE 63.2 Acne of (A) the face and (B) the chest.

peroxide. Drug therapy includes topical application of tretinoin (Retin-A) or oral administration of isotretinoin (Accutane). Topical and systemic antibiotics such as tetracycline and erythromycin, in low doses, also are used for severe acne and have produced good results. Comedones can be removed and the pustules drained with special instruments.

Surgical Management

Dermabrasion is a method of removing surface layers of scarred skin. It is useful in lessening scars such as pitting from severe acne. The outermost layers of skin are removed by sandpaper, a rotating wire brush, chemicals (chemical face peeling), or a diamond wheel. A local anesthetic, such as an ethyl chloride and Freon mixture, is used during the procedure. Afterward, the skin looks and feels raw and sore, and some crusting from serous exudate occurs. Clients frequently say that the discomfort is similar to that from a burn. The client is instructed not to wash the area until it heals sufficiently. The client must avoid picking and touching the area because this contact might cause infection or produce marking of tissues.

Nursing Management

Advise the client to keep the face and hair clean and avoid cosmetics that contribute to oily skin. Explain that manipulating the lesions worsens the condition. Warn female clients about the risk of birth defects associated with oral isotretinoin. Explain that women for whom this drug is prescribed must (1) have a negative pregnancy test 2 weeks before beginning therapy, (2) comply with contraceptive measures while taking the drug, and (3) continue reliable contraception for 1 month after discontinuing therapy. Teaching measures include the following:

- Keep hair short, clean, and away from the face and forehead.
- Wash hair frequently; daily shampooing does not damage hair.
- Avoid makeup, lotions, hair sprays, and skin products unless a physician approves their use.

FURUNCLES, FURUNCULOSIS, AND CARBUNCLES

A **furuncle** is a boil. **Furunculosis** refers to having multiple furuncles. A **carbuncle** is a furuncle from which pus drains.

Physiology and Etiology

The cause of furuncles and carbuncles is skin infections with organisms that usually exist harmlessly on the skin surface. When an injury such as that caused by squeezing a lesion impairs skin integrity, microorganisms can enter and colonize the skin. Furunculosis also is associated with diabetes mellitus because an elevated blood glucose level promotes microbial growth. Other predisposing factors include poor diet and general health and any disorder that lowers resistance.

Assessment Findings

The lesion, which may appear anywhere on the body, but especially around the neck, axillary, and groin regions, appears as a raised, painful pustule surrounded by erythema. The area feels hard to touch. After a few days, the lesion exudes pus and later a core. The client also may experience a fever, anorexia, weakness, and malaise. A culture of the exudate identifies the infectious organism.

Medical and Surgical Management

Hot wet soaks are used to localize infection and provide symptomatic relief. It may be the only treatment necessary.

Antibiotics are used in some instances, especially when a fever is present or if the lesion is a carbuncle. Surgical incision and drainage may be necessary.

Nursing Management

Follow strict aseptic technique when applying or changing a dressing to prevent spread of the infection to other body parts or to others. Teach the client also to do so. Inform the client to:

- Never pick or squeeze a furuncle—drainage is infectious, and this practice can spread infection to surrounding tissues or even to the bloodstream.
- Wash hands thoroughly before and after applying topical medications.
- Keep hands away from infected areas.
- Use separate face cloths and towels from those used by others.
- Wash clothing, towels, and face cloths separately from family laundry in hot water and bleach.

• PSORIASIS

Psoriasis is a chronic, noninfectious inflammatory skin disorder affecting young and middle adult men and women. Although there are many types of psoriasis, the most common is plaque psoriasis (Fig. 63.3). Periods of emotional stress, hormonal cycles, infection, and seasonal changes appear to aggravate the condition.

Pathophysiology and Etiology

The cause of psoriasis is unknown, but a genetic predisposition is likely because many report a family history of the disorder. The disorder seems to require a triggering mechanism such as systemic infection, injury to skin, vaccination, or injection. This also suggests a link with the immune system. Psoriasis has periods of exacerbation and remission.

In psoriasis, skin cells called *keratinocytes* react as if there is a need to repair a wound. Cells of the epidermis proliferate much faster than normal, so that the upper layer of cells cannot be shed fast enough to make room for newly produced cells. The excessive cells accumulate and form elevated, scaly lesions called *plaque.* The area around the lesion becomes red from increased blood supply needed to nourish the rapidly developing skin cells.

Assessment Findings

Psoriasis is characterized by patches of **erythema** (redness) covered with silvery scales, usually on extensor surfaces of the elbows, knees, trunk, and scalp. Itching usually is absent or slight, but occasionally it is severe. Lesions are obvious and unsightly, and scales tend to shed.

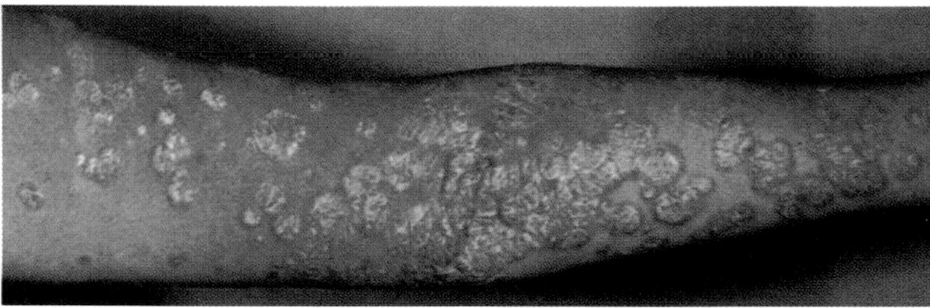

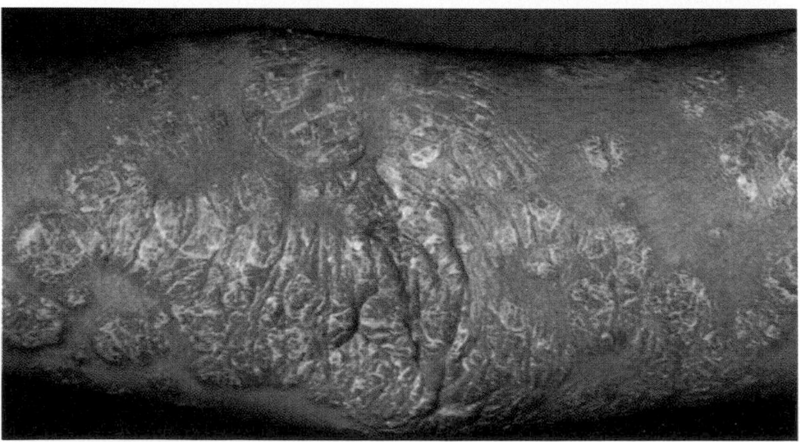

FIGURE 63.3 Psoriasis on the elbows. (Roche Laboratories)

Diagnosis is made by visual examination of lesions. A skin biopsy reveals increased proliferation of epidermal cells.

Medical Management

Psoriasis has no cure. Symptomatic treatment to control scaling and itching includes use of topical agents such as coal tar extract, corticosteroids, or anthralin. Anthralin, a distillate of crude coal tar, is applied to thick plaques; it tends to irritate unaffected skin areas. Topical corticosteroids are beneficial. Methotrexate, an antimetabolite used in the treatment of cancer, is prescribed for clients with severe disease that does not respond to other forms of therapy. It inhibits production of cells that divide rapidly (cancer cells, cells composing the skin and mucous membranes) and is capable of reducing plaque formation. Dosage is carefully individualized because the drug causes serious adverse effects.

Etretinate (Tegison) is related to retinoic acid and retinol (vitamin A) and is used to treat psoriasis that does not respond to other therapies. It is recommended only for those who can reliably understand and carry out the treatment regimen, are capable of complying with mandatory contraceptive measures, and do not intend to become pregnant. Another treatment is injection of triamcinolone acetonide (Kenacort), a corticosteroid, into isolated psoriatic plaques.

Photochemotherapy, a combination of ultraviolet light therapy and a photosensitizing psoralen drug such as methoxsalen (Oxsoralen-Ultra), also is used for severe, disabling psoriasis that does not respond to other methods of treatment. The extent of exposure is based on the client's skin tolerance. Treatments are given once every other day or less because phototoxic reactions may appear 48 hours or more after light exposure. Once psoriasis clears, the client is placed on a maintenance treatment program.

Some clients respond well to treatment; others receive only minor relief. The condition tends to recur.

NURSING PROCESS

● The Client With Psoriasis

Assessment

Inspect and evaluate skin integrity in a well-lit environment. Compare the pathologic appearance of affected skin with characteristics of normal skin. Ask the client whether there is a family history of psoriasis and determine onset, duration, and possible triggering factors.

Diagnosis, Planning, and Interventions

Show acceptance of clients with skin lesions, who need understanding and emotional support. Explain that treatment usually is for life, and that the client must follow the plan of therapy. Reassure clients for whom more than one form of treatment has failed that other, untried modalities may offer improved control of symptoms. Instruct the client receiving photochemotherapy to avoid exposure to sunlight for 8 hours after treatment because it takes that long for the body to excrete methoxsalen.

Impaired Skin Integrity related to decreased protective function of epidermal tissue

Expected Outcome: Client will achieve smoother skin with control of lesions and increased protective skin function.

- Instruct client that repeated trauma to the skin (cuts, abrasions, sunburn) may exacerbate psoriasis. *Facts can help the client manage the disorder.*
- Advise client not to pick or scratch lesions. *Disruption of lesions causes secondary trauma.*
- Inspect skin regularly for signs of infection. *Impaired skin integrity provides a portal through which pathogens can enter.*
- Wash affected area with warm water and pat dry. Apply moisturizing or medicated topical ointments as ordered. *Clean, moisturized skin not irritated by friction during drying helps maintain skin integrity.*

Disturbed Body Image related to embarrassment of appearance of skin and self-perception of uncleanliness

Expected Outcome: Client will acquire self-acceptance regarding skin changes.

- Inform client that psoriasis has no permanent cure, but the condition usually can be controlled or cleared. *The reality of the prognosis facilitates the development of mechanisms for coping with the skin disorder.*
- Assist client to carry out cosmetic efforts to decrease visibility of lesions. *Camouflaging the skin lesions reduces self-consciousness.*
- Encourage client to join a psoriasis support group. *A support group helps the client understand that many others have the same disorder and similar problems. Group work better facilitates coping than does working alone.*

Evaluation of Expected Outcomes

Expected outcomes are improved integrity and appearance of the skin. Itching is reduced or eliminated. The client understands clearly what the diagnosis of psoriasis means in terms of duration and length of treatment. He or she copes effectively with the altered appearance.

● DERMATOPHYTOSES

Dermatophytoses are superficial fungal infections; they have been given many unscientific names. For example, a common term for one dermatophytosis is *ringworm,* which is a misnomer because a worm does not cause the infection. Other examples are *athlete's foot* for a foot infection and *jock itch* for an infection in the groin.

Pathophysiology and Etiology

Dermatophytes (also called *tinea*) are parasitic fungi that invade the skin, scalp, and nails (discussed later). The terms *tinea pedis, tinea capitis, tinea corporis,* and *tinea cruris* identify the skin areas of infection, namely, feet, head, body, and groin, respectively.

Assessment Findings

Tinea corporis appears as rings of papules or vesicles with a clear center in nonhairy areas of the skin (Fig. 63.4). Several clusters of rings may be found in the same general location. The affected skin often itches and becomes red, scaly, cracked, and sore. In tinea pedis, the infection begins in skin between toes and spreads to the soles of the feet. Tinea capitis, which is more common in children, invades the hair shaft below the scalp, followed by breaking of the hair, usually close to the scalp.

Diagnosis is made by visual examination of affected areas. Lesions are scraped and examined microscopically. When a Wood's light is used, affected areas fluoresce green-yellow.

Medical Management

Treatment of tinea pedis includes topical use of antifungal agents, such as benzoic and salicylic acid ointment, Burow's solution, undecylenic acid, and tolnaftate (Tinactin). Oral griseofulvin (Grisactin), a systemic antifungal agent, also is useful in treatment. The drug may be required for many weeks to eradicate infection. Tinea capitis may be treated with oral griseofulvin, which is taken with meals. A topical antifungal agent also may be prescribed to destroy fungi present on hair shafts above the surface of the scalp. Treatment of tinea corporis includes the use of topical antifungal agents for less severe infections. Oral griseofulvin is prescribed for more severe infections. Tinea cruris often responds to topical application of tolnaftate or miconazole (Micatin). Tinea onychomycosis (discussed later) may respond to oral griseofulvin, but long-term therapy usually is necessary.

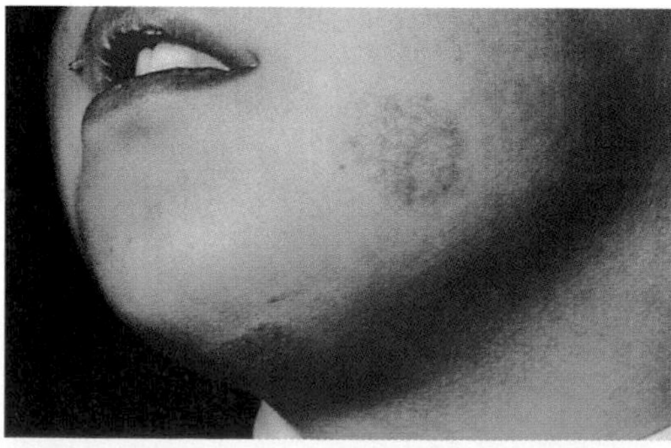

FIGURE 63.4 Tinea corporis of the face, which is commonly referred to as ringworm because of its circular appearance.

Nursing Management

If an oral or topical antifungal agent is prescribed, review directions for use. Explain that the infected person must use separate towels, washcloths, grooming articles, and clothing because the disorder is contagious. Stress that keeping the affected areas dry reduces the spread of the infection. After a bath or shower, recommend thoroughly drying all areas of the body, including skin folds. To prevent infection and reinfection of tinea cruris, suggest avoiding excessive heat and humidity, not wearing tight-fitting clothing or nylon next to the skin (in hot, humid weather), and keeping the skin as dry as possible.

To avoid acquiring or spreading a fungal infection of the feet, advise against sharing towels and slippers or going barefoot in locker rooms or community bathrooms. Recommend keeping the feet (particularly the area between the toes) dry, which increases resistance to the infection. Advise clients whose feet perspire freely to apply powder between the toes, keep the area dry, wash and thoroughly dry the feet daily, and put on clean, dry socks and a different pair of shoes after coming home from work or school.

• SHINGLES

Shingles, also known as **herpes zoster,** is a skin disorder that develops years after an infection with varicella (chickenpox). It is more frequent in middle-aged to older adults, as well as in those who are immunocompromised.

Pathophysiology and Etiology

Herpes zoster is an acute reactivation of the varicella-zoster virus, which lies dormant in nerve roots. When aging, cancer, drugs, or AIDS suppresses a client's immune system, the virus migrates along one or more cranial or spinal nerve routes. Viral reactivation produces inflammatory symptoms in the **dermatome,** a skin area supplied by the nerve (Fig. 63.5). Raised, fluid-filled, and painful skin eruptions accompany inflammation.

If herpes zoster affects the ophthalmic branch of the trigeminal nerve (third cranial nerve), corneal (eye) ulcerations may occur. Involvement of the vestibulocochlear nerve (eighth cranial nerve) can lead to vertigo

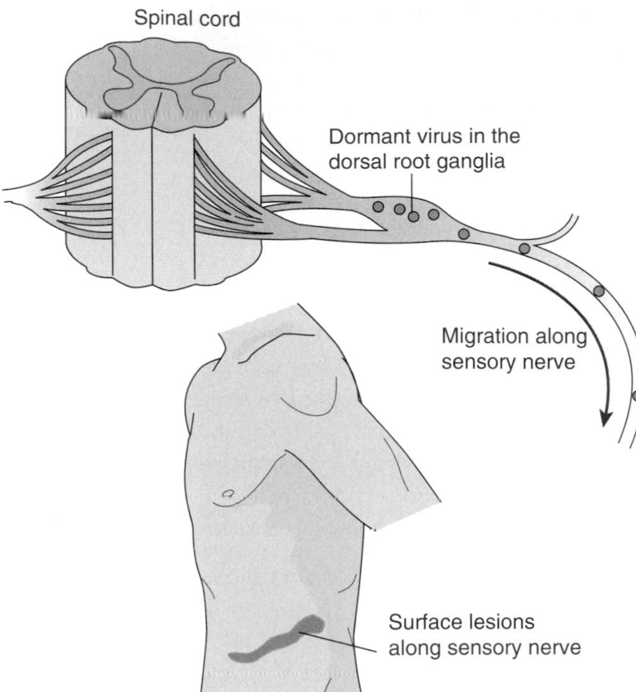

FIGURE 63.5 Reactivation of the varicella-zoster virus causing eruptions typical of shingles.

and permanent hearing loss. Cerebral vasculitis (inflammation of cerebral vessels) is the most serious complication because involvement of the internal carotid arteries can result in a stroke. The virus rarely spreads to the brain, resulting in encephalitis.

Susceptible individuals exposed to someone in the early stages of herpes zoster infection can acquire varicella. The virus is contagious until crusts from ruptured lesions are dry and fall off the skin. Herpes zoster infection also can recur.

Assessment Findings

Initial symptoms include a low-grade fever, headache, and malaise. An area of skin along a dermatome develops a red, blotchy appearance that begins to itch or feel numb. In about 24 to 48 hours, vesicles appear on the skin along the nerve's pathway. Usually eruptions are unilateral (one side) on the trunk, neck, or head. They become severely painful. Severe itching soon follows. Like chickenpox lesions, vesicles rupture in a few days and crusts form. Scarring or permanent skin discoloration is possible. Pain (postherpetic neuralgia) and itching may persist for months or as long as 2 years or more. Secondary skin infections may occur from scratching the area. Diagnosis is made primarily by examination of the lesions and symptoms.

Medical Management

Oral acyclovir (Zovirax) taken within 48 hours of the appearance of symptoms reduces their severity and prevents development of additional lesions. Topical acyclovir also may be applied to lesions. A brief course of corticosteroid therapy reduces pain. Lesions of the ophthalmic division of the trigeminal nerve require immediate examination and treatment by an ophthalmologist.

Additional treatment is symptomatic. Analgesics and liquid preparations with a drying or antipruritic effect are applied to the affected area once crusts fall off. Skin may be so sensitive that any clothing or application of topical drugs intensifies pain or itching. A narcotic analgesic such as codeine often is necessary during the first few days to weeks.

Nursing Management

Nursing personnel who have not had chickenpox must avoid contact with a client with herpes zoster. Instruct clients with crusted lesions to avoid contact with immunocompromised people and those who have not had chickenpox. Advise the client that application of cool or warm compresses or warm showers may relieve pain and itching; it may be necessary to experiment with both to determine which provides the most relief. Tell the client to wear loose clothing and avoid scratching the area. If oral acyclovir is prescribed, review the dose regimen, as printed on the prescription label.

• SKIN CANCER

Skin cancer is the most common cancer in the United States. It can involve any of three types of cells in the epidermis: squamous cells (flat and scaly); basal cells (round); and melanocytes (contain color pigment).

Pathophysiology and Etiology

Increased exposure to ultraviolet (UV) radiation, especially UVB and UVC, harmful components in the spectrum of sunlight, predisposes to malignant skin changes and other health risks, including cataracts and premature aging of the skin. Fair-skinned people are more susceptible to skin cancer than are dark-skinned people.

Several factors predispose to malignant changes in the skin:

- Thinning layer of ozone, a naturally occurring gas in the earth's atmosphere. Ozone absorbs UVB and UVC radiation. Ozone depletion occurs primarily from release of chlorofluorocarbons (CFCs) in refrigerants, aerosol propellants, and other industrial pollutants.

- Residence in high-altitude areas where the atmosphere is thinner than at sea level or in areas with a regular cloud cover
- Decreased melanin in skin, especially individuals who sunburn easily and tan minimally; black- or brown-skinned people rarely are affected.
- Prolonged, repeated exposure to UV rays such as those who do farming, fishing, road construction, and so on, or those who frequent tanning salons and use sunlamps
- Prior radiation therapy for an unrelated form of cancer
- Ulcerations of long duration and scar tissue (both prone to malignant changes)

Malignant skin growths (Table 63.1) usually are primary lesions, that is, they originate in the skin. Prompt removal of the malignant tissue prevents its spread to other parts of the body or tissues.

Assessment Findings

Symptoms vary, but usually the new appearance of a growth or a change in skin color is the first symptom the client notices. The lesion can be smooth or rough, flat or elevated, and itchy or tender. It may bleed. Diagnosis is made by visual inspection and confirmed by biopsy.

Medical and Surgical Management

Depending on size and location of the lesion, treatment of squamous cell and basal cell carcinomas may involve electrodesiccation, surgical excision, cryosurgery, or radiation therapy. The client is followed regularly for at least 3 to 5 years to be sure regrowth does not occur.

Treatment of melanoma involves radical excision of the tumor and adjacent tissues, followed by chemotherapy. Administration of melphalan (Alkeran) and prednisone is an example of an initial antineoplastic therapy regimen. Interferon alfa-n3 (Alferon N) has controlled metastases in some persons. Clinical trials of other types of therapies are being conducted. In some instances, skin grafting may be necessary to replace large areas of defect when a wide excision of the tumor is necessary.

Nursing Management

Examine and measure abnormal-appearing skin lesions, especially those in sun-exposed areas such as the face, nose, lips, and hands. Determine facts about the lesion, including when the lesion first was noticed, whether it has undergone any recent changes, and, if so, what kind.

Surgery for a malignant melanoma may involve structures of the head and neck, trunk, or extremities. Specific nursing management of those having radical surgery for this malignancy depends on original site of tumor and extent of surgery. Give emotional support to those having disfiguring surgery.

Encourage all those with any type of skin change to seek medical attention. Advise those in high-risk groups for malignant skin lesions to examine all areas of their body and scalp for new lesions or changes in moles, other growths, or pigmented lesions. If a client notes any change, he or she should make an appointment for a medical examination as soon as possible.

Educate clients about measures to prevent skin cancer:

- Always use a sunscreen with a sun protection factor (SPF) of at least 15; higher SPFs are beneficial for clients who sunburn easily.
- Reapply sunscreen at least every 2 hours or more often if swimming or perspiring.
- Use a lip balm with sunscreen.
- Wear a hat with a wide brim and cover the back of the neck.
- Stay in the shade when outdoors.
- Wear tightly woven, but loose-fitting clothing.
- Avoid prolonged sun exposure between 10:00 AM and 4:00 PM.
- Avoid artificial tanning.

Recommend that at-risk clients consult the UV forecast, a daily report that rates the UV conditions from 0 to 10+ in 30 metropolitan areas. Depending on the numerical rating, called the UV index, sun-sensitive people are advised to take protective measures (Fig. 63.6). A sensometer, a credit card–sized device, also is available for a person to determine the UV level in his or her immediate locale.

SCALP AND HAIR DISORDERS

Some conditions are unique to the scalp and hair. They include inflammatory and noninflammatory scalp conditions and disorders that cause hair loss.

• SEBORRHEA, SEBORRHEIC DERMATITIS, AND DANDRUFF

Seborrhea and dandruff are noninflammatory conditions that usually precede or accompany seborrheic dermatitis. Seborrheic dermatitis has an inflammatory component.

TABLE 63.1 TYPES OF SKIN CANCER

TYPE	INCIDENCE	LOCATION	APPEARANCE	CHARACTERISTICS
Basal cell carcinoma	Most common, especially in light-skinned individuals Increases with age	Sun-exposed areas	Small, shiny, gray or yellowish plaque that undergoes central ulceration 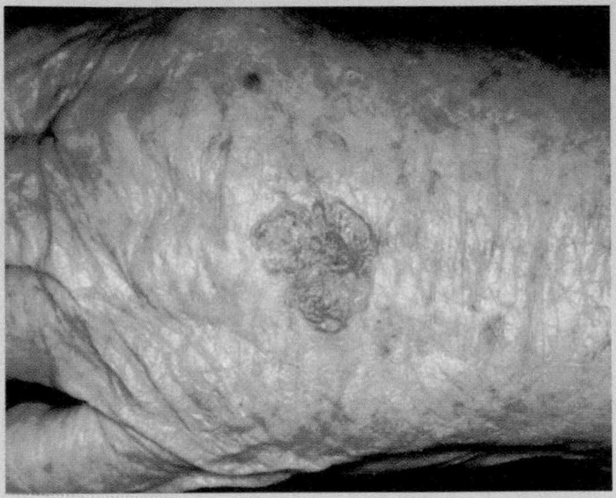	Slow growing, rarely metastasizes; commonly recurs
Squamous cell carcinoma	Second after basal cell in those with fair skin	Sun-exposed areas such as ears, nose, hands, scalp of bald persons	Scaly, elevated lesion with an irregular border; shallow, large ulcerations form in untreated advanced lesions 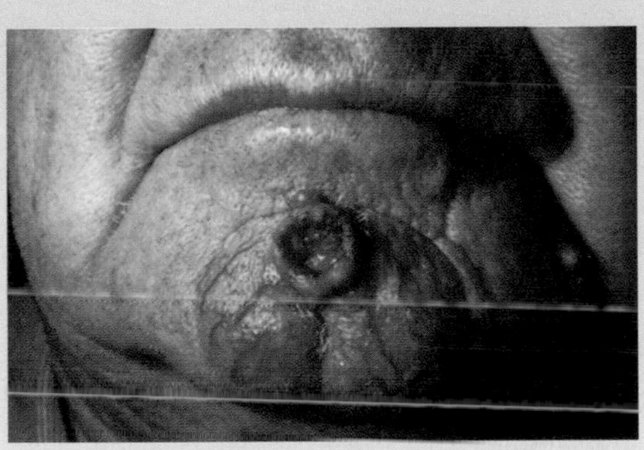	Can metastasize through blood and lymph
Malignant melanoma	Increasing in incidence	Arises from pre-existing moles anywhere on the body	Raised brown or black lesion In some cases, satellite lesions occur adjacent to the primary cancer 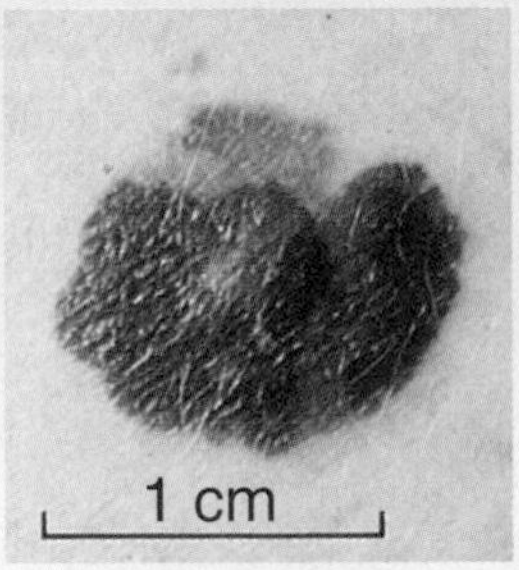 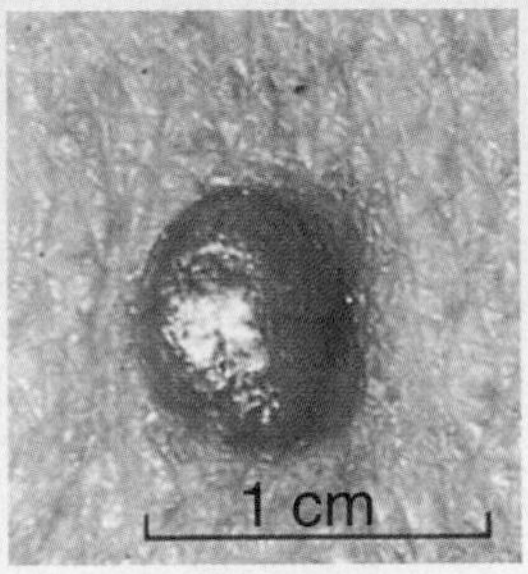 1 cm 1 cm	Poor prognosis because of distant metastases

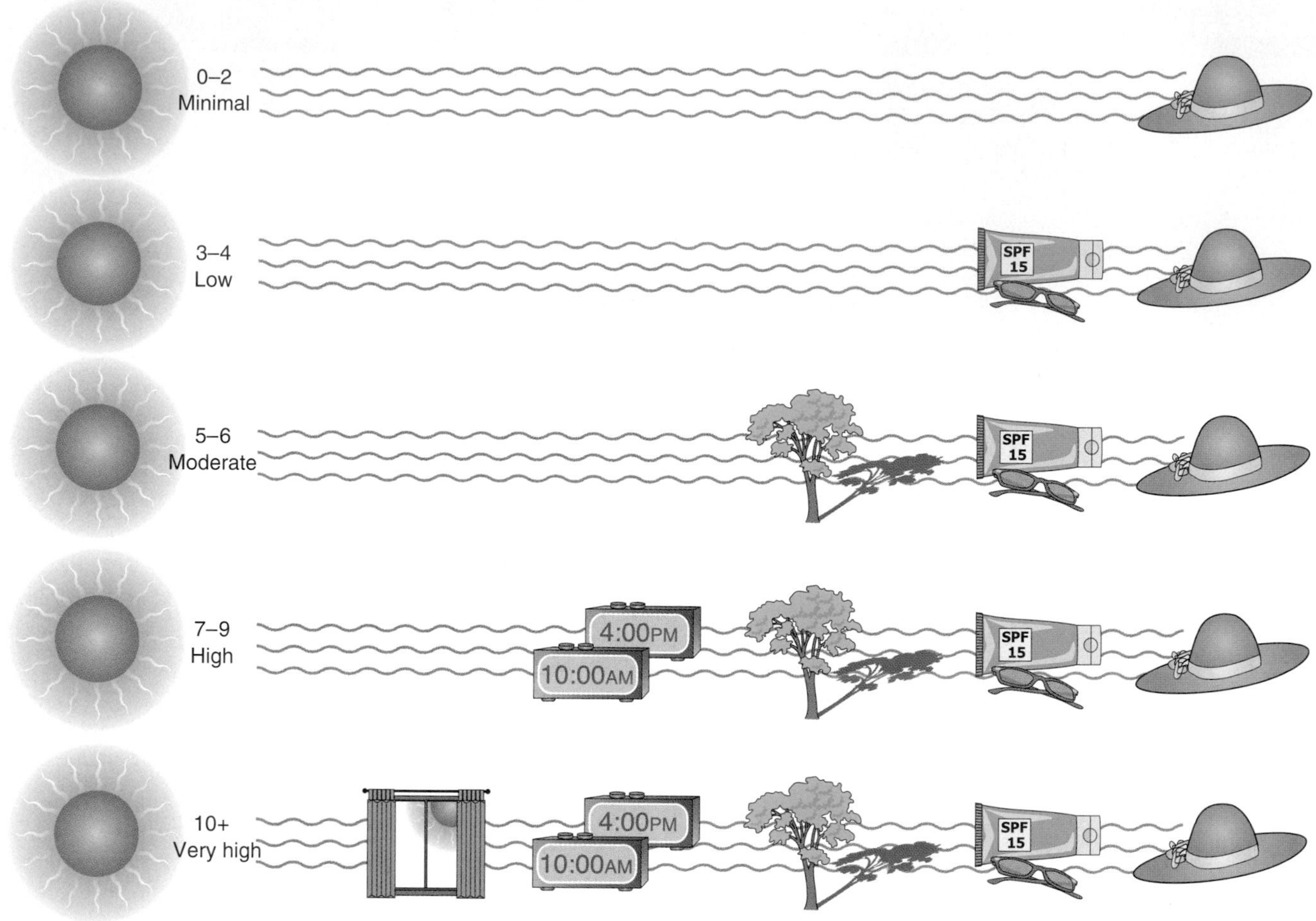

FIGURE 63.6 Sun protection measures based upon the UV index.

Pathophysiology and Etiology

Seborrhea is a dermatologic condition associated with excessive production of secretions from sebaceous glands. Although not always confined to the scalp, it is one of the primary sites. *Seborrheic dermatitis* presents as red areas covered by yellowish, greasy-appearing scales. *Dandruff* is loose, scaly material of dead, keratinized epithelium shed from the scalp in clients who may or may not have seborrheic dermatitis. Dermatologists believe that a tiny fungus known as *Pityrosporum ovale* causes dandruff. Most people harbor this fungus, yet only some people develop dandruff. Some possible factors for this phenomenon include excessive perspiration, inadequate diet, stress, and hormone activity.

Scalp conditions cause more of a cosmetic rather than a health problem. They usually necessitate retreatment. They do not progress or transform into other serious skin disorders.

Assessment Findings

Clients note that hair is unusually oily. There may be red or scaly patches on the scalp. White flakes fall from hair and become more obvious when they collect on the shoulders of dark clothing. Inflamed areas may itch.

No diagnostic testing is necessary unless the condition does not respond to treatment. In that case, a skin biopsy or laboratory blood work is performed to eliminate the possibility that the condition was misdiagnosed.

Medical Management

Frequent shampooing with or without a medicated product helps reduce oil in scalp and hair. Effective medicated shampoos contain tar, zinc pyrithione, selenium sulfide, sulfur, or salicylic acid. Some clients require topical applications of corticosteroids.

Nursing Management

Explain the underlying cause. Review directions and frequency for using medications. Inform clients that the disorder may recur and persistent treatment is necessary for control.

● ALOPECIA

Alopecia means "baldness." The condition affects hair follicles and results in partial or total hair loss. It is normal to shed 50 to 100 hairs a day, replaced by new ones from the same hair follicles. In some cases, hair loss is excessive, which may be temporary or permanent.

Alopecia is not life-threatening, but whenever men or women lose their hair, most experience self-consciousness and lose self-confidence. Many spend great sums of money on unscientific methods for restoring hair growth. Although not everyone can be helped, several options are available to clients with hair loss.

Pathophysiology and Etiology

Hair loss can develop for several reasons. In cases of temporary hair loss, possible causes include medications such as antineoplastic drugs, inadequate diet, thyroid disease, tinea infection, improper application of hair care products, and hair styles that pull hair tightly.

Alopecia areata and androgenetic alopecia are two chronic conditions that are difficult to reverse. Alopecia areata is believed to be an autoimmune disorder characterized by patchy areas of hair loss about the size of a coin. It can progress to total hair loss and even loss of hair from the entire body. Antibodies attack and destroy the hair follicle.

Androgenetic alopecia is a genetically acquired condition, referred to as *male pattern baldness.* The term is somewhat inaccurate because it also affects women, although to a milder degree. A person inherits androgenetic alopecia from his or her mother or father. When testosterone, an androgenic hormone, combines with an enzyme, 5-alpha-reductase, in the hair follicle, hair production stops. This condition begins in adolescence or early adulthood and progresses with age.

Assessment Findings

Clients note that their hair is thinning or falling out in patches in several areas of the scalp. Those with a family history of baldness tend to lose hair in the lateral frontal areas or over the vertex of the head. Women report thinning in the frontal, parietal, and crown regions. Primary hair loss is not associated with any other physical health problems.

Diagnostic tests are done to determine any physical disorder contributing to the hair loss. When results are negative, the family history and pattern of hair loss suggest hereditary baldness or an autoimmune disorder.

Medical Management

If a medical disorder causes hair loss, relieving the cause usually restores hair growth. Some drugs can retard hair loss and promote hair growth. One drug is minoxidil (Rogaine); however, hair growth that is stimulated has a downy texture. If a client discontinues minoxidil, hair growth stops and baldness recurs. Young clients who begin drug therapy when hair loss is minimal obtain the best results. A hair addition is a technique for giving the appearance of more hair by attaching extra hair to the client's natural hair.

Surgical Management

Some balding clients prefer a more permanent solution with hair replacement surgery or other surgical techniques. Hair grafting is a technique for transplanting hair-bearing scalp from the back and sides of the head into bald areas. Each graft contains from one to eight hairs. A bald area that is approximately 3 inches square requires approximately 500 to 600 hair grafts. Unfortunately, because of the progressive nature of androgenetic alopecia, transplanted hairs may not survive permanently.

A procedure that disguises hair loss is a scalp reduction that surgically removes a bald area. A scalp reduction usually is done along with hair grafts. Another surgical technique is to transfer a skin flap. The flap transfers the greatest amount of hair in a short amount of time. However, the scalp may have to be expanded before surgery to stretch the flap area because the flap remains attached in its original location at one end.

Nursing Management

Support clients who may not have the financial means for medical or surgical treatment. Reassure them they can cope with hair loss. Suggest consulting a cosmetologist who can provide a haircut and style that minimizes the appearance of hair loss. Tell women to opt for loose styling rather than ponytails or braids. Recommend using a conditioner or detangler after shampooing to avoid pulling hair from the head and a wide-toothed comb or brush with smooth tips.

NAIL DISORDERS ●

Nails, especially toenails, are subject to disorders. Two common conditions include fungal infections, known as *onychomycosis,* and ingrown toenails, technically called *onychocryptosis.*

● ONYCHOMYCOSIS

Onychomycosis is a fungal infection of fingernails or toenails. A fungus is a tiny, plantlike parasite that thrives in warm, dark, moist environments. Fungi can spread unchecked from one nail to another. They more commonly affect toenails because conditions inside shoes are perfect for breeding fungi.

Pathophysiology and Etiology

Onychomycosis and tinea pedis (athlete's foot) often occur together. Older adults and immunocompromised clients are at greater risk for fungal infections. Incidence of fungal fingernail infections has increased among women who have artificial nails. Unsanitary cleansing of nail application utensils between customers in salons seems to be the mode of transmission.

Fungi relocate themselves from surrounding skin to beneath the nail plate. The fleshy portion underneath the nail becomes inflamed. The nail becomes elevated, thickens, loosens, and changes color. Eventually the nail plate is destroyed. The longer the infection is present, the more difficult it is to cure.

Assessment Findings

One or more nails appears grossly different from normal. They are much thicker, causing them to be elevated and distorted. They are yellowed and friable. Because they are difficult to trim, the infected nail(s) may be long and jagged. Pressure and friction from thickened toenails can lead to pain because shoes do not fit comfortably and socks may wear through.

Diagnosis usually is made on the basis of appearance. Microscopic examination of nail scrapings can confirm the diagnosis.

Medical and Surgical Management

Treatment involves prolonged systemic drug therapy with either of two antifungal agents: itraconazole (Sporanox) and terbinafine (Lamisil). Both drugs inhibit fungal enzymes that regulate cell membrane permeability and result in fungal death. Clients take medications daily for 2 weeks for fingernail infections and 3 weeks for toenail infections. Terbinafine also can be administered in a pulse-dosing regimen consisting of 1 week of medication followed by a 3-week rest period. Repeated pulse dosing is necessary to eradicate infection. Drug therapy is more than 50% effective. Because nails grow slowly, it may take as long as 12 months before the nail appears normal.

A more radical solution involves removal of the infected nail. This usually is a last resort because it causes permanent cosmetic changes. Surgery is considered when the condition results in chronic pain or causes difficulty in wearing shoes.

Nursing Management

Reinforce that the condition is chronic and to remain compliant with drug therapy for the duration of treatment. Explain the dosing regimen, side effects that may develop, and drug interactions. To prevent reinfection, remind clients to:

- Alternate pairs of shoes daily.
- Purchase leather shoes that promote evaporation of foot moisture.
- Never go barefoot.
- Wear footwear at communal pools or when showering in gyms or fitness centers.
- Avoid damage to the skin around the nail, which makes it easier for fungi to colonize.

● ONYCHOCRYPTOSIS

Onychocryptosis is the medical term for an ingrown toenail. This common condition can affect all people, although some are more predisposed than others. It usually affects the inside edge of the great toe. Recurrence tends to be a significant problem.

Pathophysiology and Etiology

Some people have an inherited trait that causes a curvature in the growing nail plate. These clients have a higher incidence of ingrown toenails despite the fit of their shoes or methods for keeping nails trimmed. The latter two factors, along with fungal nail infections, explain why most others acquire ingrown toenails. Athletes or those who are physically active seem to have repeated episodes as a result of recurring trauma.

When the nail curves during growth, a corner of the nail becomes trapped under skin. As the nail grows, it cuts into the flesh at the lateral border of the nail. The trauma causes local inflammation. The impaired skin provides an opportunity for bacteria secondarily to invade traumatized tissue.

Assessment Findings

The client feels local pressure from abnormal nail growth. Redness, swelling, and pain occur where the nail pierces

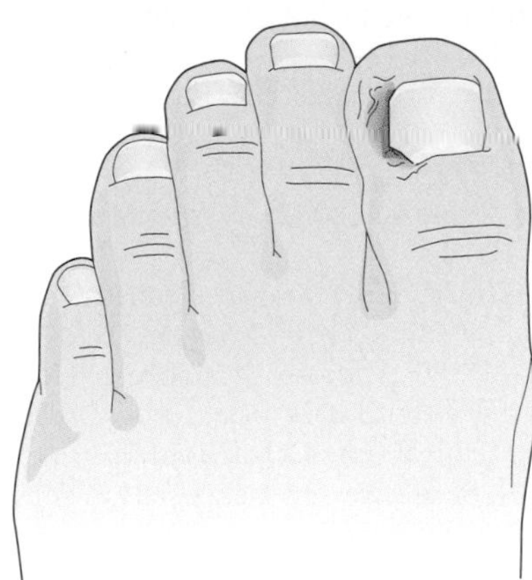

FIGURE 63.7 Infected ingrown toenail.

the adjacent tissue (Fig. 63.7). The corner of the upper nail is embedded in tissue. Purulent drainage and an odor are evident if the tissue is infected. Some people develop compensatory gait and postural changes in an effort to relieve pain. Physical examination is sufficient for diagnosis.

Medical and Surgical Management

Treating the infection, if present, is as important as correcting the nail disorder. Local or systemic antibiotic therapy sometimes is prescribed. Applications of hydrogen peroxide are used to loosen and remove exudate. To promote healing, the foot is soaked in warm water and Epsom salts, followed by thorough drying. A wedge of cotton may be inserted to lift the corner of the nail. Clients with diabetes or peripheral vascular disease are referred to a **podiatrist,** a person trained to care for feet. Older clients and those with chronic diseases are especially susceptible to traumatic complications that can impair circulation and necessitate amputation.

For persistent or recurrent ingrown toenails, surgery is indicated. Various techniques are used to remove the nail border, not the entire nail, and its root. Surgical procedures are done in the physician's office using local anesthesia or a laser to vaporize the abnormal tissue. Chemical cauterization controls bleeding, and no sutures are required. The client temporarily may need to wear a slipper or shoe from which the toe has been cut out until the swelling and discomfort subsides, but he or she can resume most activities immediately.

Nursing Management

Explain how to perform foot-soaking regimens and techniques to relieve pressure around the ingrown nail. If surgery is done, instruct the client how to change the dressing, frequency of dressing changes, and signs of infection or compromised circulation to report immediately to the surgeon. Provide the following information to affected clients:

- Wear wide shoes and loose socks with sufficient room for the toes.
- Use nail clippers rather than scissors to trim toenails.
- Trim toenails so that they are slightly longer than the end of the toes; do not round off the corners.
- Keep feet clean and dry.
- Avoid physical activities that involve sudden stops, such as playing basketball, which jams toes into the front of the shoe.
- Obtain regular foot and nail care from a podiatrist if there is a history of diabetes, diminished vision, or vascular problems.

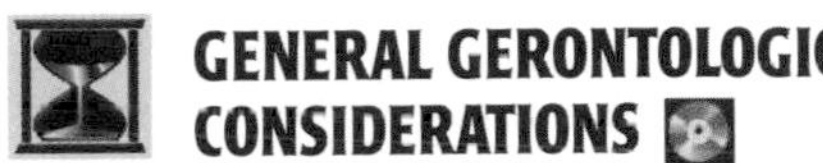

GENERAL GERONTOLOGIC CONSIDERATIONS

Advise older adults with any type of skin lesion to seek medical attention; caution against self-treatment. Early treatment of skin lesions helps prevent infection and complications.

Explain that excessive drying of skin may result in pruritus and infection. Encourage older clients to apply creams and lotions to the skin, especially during winter or when living in a hot, dry climate. A daily bath is not necessary.

Carefully assess older debilitated clients or clients with dementia for scabies and head lice (see Chap. 9). These clients may be unable to inform the nurse of these problems or manifest the typical symptoms. Instead, they may become increasingly confused or agitated.

Critical Thinking Exercises

1. *What health teaching is appropriate for keeping the skin, hair, and nails in healthy condition?*
2. *Name a skin disorder that is more common in younger adults and one that is more common in older adults. Discuss the factors that make these age groups particularly susceptible to the disorder.*

● NCLEX-STYLE REVIEW QUESTIONS 

1. A client comes to the clinic complaining of a rash on the side and back. Assessment findings reveal red areas and vesicles. The physician suspects herpes zoster. Which question by the nurse will help confirm the diagnosis?
   1. "Have you come in contact with poison ivy?"
   2. "Did you change soap or detergent recently?"
   3. "Have you had a recent fungal infection?"
   4. "Did you have chickenpox as a child?"

2. A nurse teaches a class about skin cancer to a group of construction workers. The nurse explains that a common cause of skin cancer is:
   1. Prolonged exposure to sun
   2. A history of smoking
   3. Working with asbestos
   4. Tattoos and body piercings

connection—

Visit the Connection site at **http://connection.lww.com/go/timbyEssentials** for links to chapter-related resources on the Internet.

References and Suggested Readings

Aly, R., Forney, R., & Bayles, C. (2001). Treatments for common superficial fungal infections. *Dermatology Nursing, 13,* 91–94, 98–101.

Ayello, E. A., Cuddigan, J., & Kerstein, M. O. (2002). Skip the knife. *Nursing 2002, 32*(9), 58–63.

Barry, M. (2003). Using human skin equivalents to heal chronic wounds. *Nursing 2003, 33*(3), 68–69.

Bielan, B. (2001). Clinical snapshot: Scabies. *Dermatology Nursing, 13,* 300.

Bielan, B. (2000). What's your assessment? . . . Tinea corporis. *Dermatology Nursing, 12,* 350–351.

Faherty, K. (September 30, 2002). Under pressure. *Advance for Nurses,* 31–33.

Fishman, T. D. (2000). Wound assessment and evaluation . . . Contact dermatitis. *Dermatology Nursing, 12,* 194–195.

Gradewell, C. (2000). Teaching patients to cope with psoriasis. *Practice Nurse, 20,* 543–544, 546, 548.

Graves, P. B. (April 1, 2002). Itching for more information? *Advance for Nurses,* 27–29.

Hayes, J. L. (2003). Are you assessing for melanoma. *RN, 66*(2), 36–40.

Hess, C. T. (2002a). Assessing a fistula. Part 1. *Nursing 2002, 32*(8), 22.

Hess, C. T. (2002b). Managing an external fistula. Part 2. *Nursing 2002, 32*(9), 22–24

Hewitt, H., Wint, Y., Talabere, L., et al. (2002). The use of papaya on pressure ulcers. *American Journal of Nursing, 102*(12), 73–77.

Jackson, R. A. (June 10, 2002). Neat and clean. *Advance for Nurses,* 31–32.

Kloth, L. C. (2002). How to use electrical stimulation for wound healing. *Nursing 2002, 32*(12), 17.

Letuzua, M. (2001). Addressing alopecia: Helping patients with cancer deal with hair loss. *American Journal of Nursing, 101*(4), Critical Care Extra: 24LL.

Lowe, J. (2000). Skin care: Over exposed . . . dermatitis. *Nursing Times, 96*(3), 55–56.

Madison, L. K. (2001). Shingles update: Common questions in caring for a patient with shingles. *Dermatology Nursing, 13,* 51, 54–55.

Mulinari-Brenner, F., & Bergfeld W. F. (2001). Hair loss: An overview. *Dermatology Nursing, 13,* 269–272, 277–278.

Porth, C. M. (2002). *Pathophysiology: Concepts of altered health states* (6th ed.). Philadelphia: Lippincott Williams & Wilkins.

Raftery, K. (September 16, 2002). Life's an itch. *Advance for Nurses,* 22–23, 34.

Schweon, S. J., & Novatnack, E. (2002). What's causing that itch? *RN, 65*(8), 43–46.

Scott, F. (2000). Shingles: Diagnosis and treatment. *Nursing Times, 96*(50), 36–37.

Squires, A. (2003). Documenting surgical incision site care. *Nursing 2003, 33*(1), 74.

Stewart, K. B. (2000). Combating infection: Stopping the itch of scabies and lice. *Nursing, 30*(7), 30–31.

Thompson, J. (April 2003). Maximizing your pressure ulcer care. *RN's TNT,* 16–24.

U.S. Preventive Services Task Force. (2002). Screening for skin cancer: Recommendations and rationale. *American Journal of Nursing, 102*(5), 97–101.

Venna, S., Fleisher, A. B., Jr., & Feldman, S. R. (2001). *Dermatology Nursing, 13,* 257–262, 265–266.

Winslow, E. H., & Jacobson, A. F. (2000). Research for practice: Can a fashion statement harm the patient? *American Journal of Nursing, 100*(9), 63, 65.

Zulkowski, K. (2003). Protecting your patient's aging skin. *Nursing 2003, 33*(1), 84.

chapter 64

Caring for Clients With Burns

Words to Know 

allograft
autograft
closed method
debridement
epithelialization
eschar
escharotomy
full-thickness graft
heterograft
open method
slit graft
split-thickness graft

Learning Objectives

On completion of this chapter, the reader will:

- Explain how the depth and percentage of burns are determined.
- Identify life-threatening complications of serious burns.
- Differentiate open and closed methods of wound care for burns.
- Describe three sources for skin grafts.
- Discuss priority nursing diagnoses for the care of a client with burns.

According to the American Burn Association (2000), there were more than 1 million burn injuries in the United States in 2000. Approximately 4500 people die from burns each year. Risk is highest among children and adults older than 60 years. The most common causes of burns in older adults are smoking materials, scaldings, and lighting trash fires or furnaces.

BURN INJURIES

A burn is a traumatic injury to skin and underlying tissues. Causes are heat, chemicals, or electricity. Burns from electricity are characteristically the most severe because they are deep. Electricity moving through the body follows an undetermined course from entrance to exit, causing major damage in its path.

Pathophysiology and Etiology

The immediate initial cause of cell damage is heat. Severity of the burn is related to temperature of the heat source, its duration of contact, and thickness of tissue exposed to the heat source. Location of the burn also is significant. Perineal burns are at increased risk for infection from organisms in stool. Burns of the face, neck, or chest can impair ventilation. Burns involving hands or major joints can affect dexterity and mobility.

Thermal injuries cause protein in cells to coagulate. Chemicals such as strong acids, bases, and organic compounds yield heat during a reaction with substances in cells and tissue. This liquefies tissue and loosens the attachment to nutritive sublayers in skin. Electrical burns and lightning also produce heat, which is greatest at the points of entry to and exit from the body. Because deep tissues cool more slowly than those at the surface, the extent of internal damage is difficult to assess. Cardiac dysrhythmias and central nervous system complications are common among victims of electrical burns.

The initial burn injury is complicated by inflammatory processes affecting tissue below the initial surface injury. Protease enzymes and chemical oxidants are proteolytic, compounding injury to healing tissue and deactivation of tissue growth factors. Neutrophils phagocytize debris and consume available oxygen at the wound site, contributing to tissue hypoxia. Injured capillaries thrombose, causing localized ischemia and tissue necrosis. Bacterial colonization, mechanical trauma, and topically applied antimicrobial agents further damage viable tissue.

Serious burns cause various neuroendocrine changes within the first 24 hours. Adrenocorticotropic hormone and antidiuretic hormone are released in response to stress and hypovolemia. Stimulation of the adrenal cortex releases glucocorticoids, causing hyperglycemia, and aldosterone, causing sodium retention. Sodium retention leads to peripheral edema as a result of fluid shifts and oliguria. The client eventually enters a hypermetabolic state that requires increased oxygen and nutrition to compensate for accelerated tissue catabolism.

After a burn, fluid from the body moves toward the burned area, accounting for edema at the burn site. Some fluid is trapped in this area and rendered unavailable for use by the body, leading to fluid loss. Fluid also is lost from the burned area, often in extremely large amounts, in the forms of water vapor and seepage. Decreased blood pressure follows. If physiologic changes are not immediately recognized and corrected, irreversible shock is likely. These changes usually happen rapidly and the client's status may change hourly. Clients with burns need intensive care by skilled personnel.

Fluid shifts, electrolyte deficits, and loss of extracellular proteins like albumin from the burn wound affect fluid and electrolyte status. Anemia develops because heat literally destroys erythrocytes. The client with a burn experiences hemoconcentration when the plasma component of blood is lost or trapped. Sluggish flow of blood cells through blood vessels results in inadequate nutrition to healthy body cells and organs.

Myoglobin and hemoglobin are transported to the kidneys, where they may cause tubular necrosis and acute renal failure. Release of histamine as a consequence of the stress response increases gastric acidity. A client with a burn is prone to developing gastric ulcers. Inhalation of hot air, smoke, or toxic chemicals, accompanying injuries such as fractures, concurrent medical problems, and the client's age increase the mortality rate from burn injuries.

Depth of Burn Injury

The extent of burn injuries is measured by assessing its depth. Classification includes superficial (first degree), partial thickness (superficial and deep second degree), and full thickness (third and fourth degree; Fig. 64.1). Burn depth is determined by assessing color, skin characteristics, and sensation in the area of the burn injury (Table 64.1).

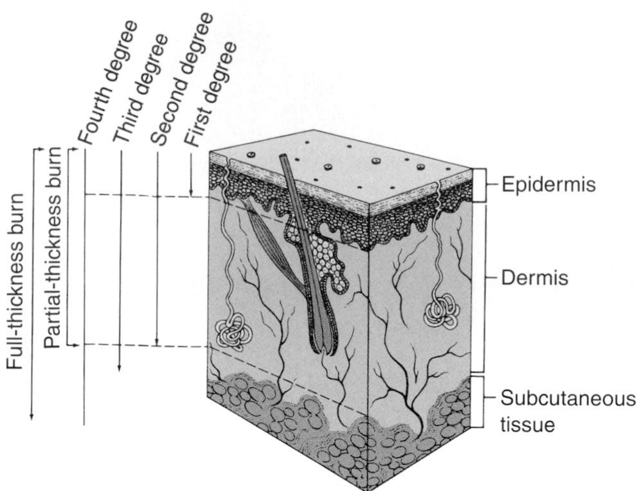

FIGURE 64.1 Depths of burn injury.

Zones of Burn Injury

Determining depth of a burn is difficult initially because there are combinations of injury zones in the same location (Fig. 64.4). The *zone of coagulation* at the center of the injury is where injury is most severe and usually deepest. The area of intermediate burn injury is referred to as the *zone of stasis.* Blood vessels are damaged, but tissue has potential to survive. If circulation is secondarily impaired, however, injured tissue in the zone of stasis can convert to a zone of coagulation. The *zone of hyperemia* is the area of least injury, where the epidermis and dermis are only minimally damaged. Because early appearance of the burn injury can change, the estimate of burn depth may be revised in the first 24 to 72 hours.

TABLE 64.1 DEPTH OF BURN INJURIES

TYPE	DEPTH	CHARACTERISTICS
Superficial (first degree)	Epidermis and part of dermis	Painful with pink or red edema, but subsides quickly; no scarring
Superficial partial thickness (second degree)	Epidermis and dermis, hair follicles intact	Mottled pink to red; painful; blistered or exuding fluid; blanches with pressure; heals within 2 weeks; pigment changes are possible (Fig. 64.2A)
Deep partial thickness (second degree)		Variable color from patchy red to white, wet or waxy dry; does not blanch with pressure, sensitive to pressure only; takes more than 3 weeks to heal; may need debridement and require skin grafts (Fig 64.2B)
Full thickness (third degree)	Epidermis, dermis, subcutaneous tissue	Red, white, tan, brown, or black; leathery covering (eschar); painless
Full thickness (fourth degree)	Epidermis, dermis, subcutaneous tissue; may include fat, fascia, muscle, and bone	Black; depressed; painless; scarring; requires debridement and skin grafts; injury may cause sepsis and contractures (Fig. 64.3)

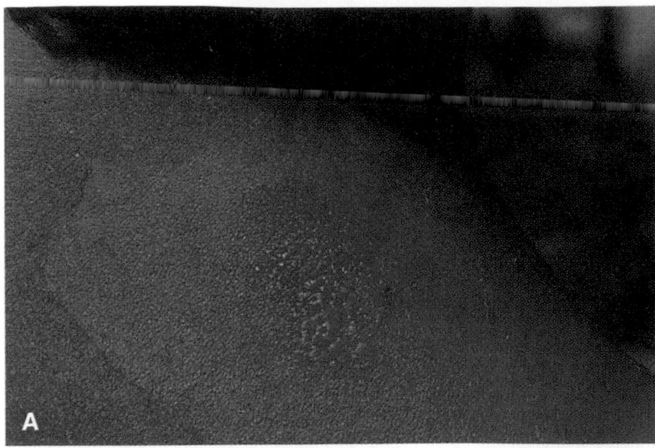

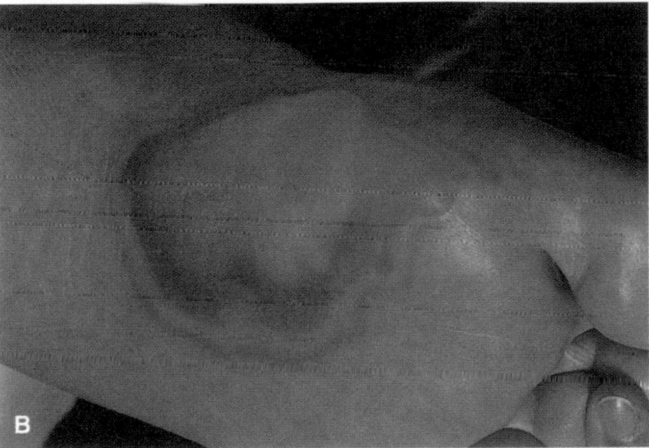

FIGURE 64.2 (**A**) Superficial second-degree burn. (**B**) Full-thickness second-degree burn.

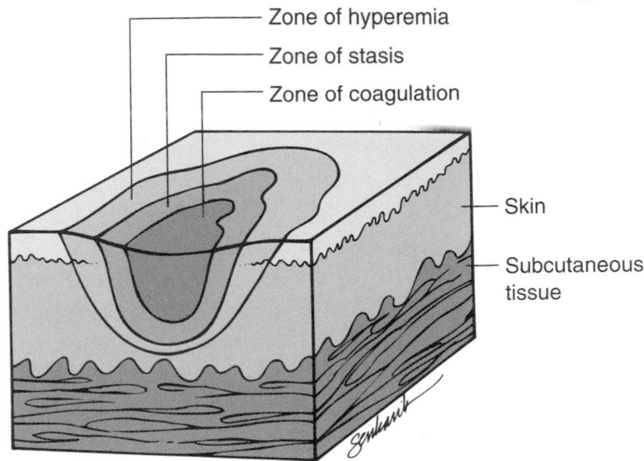

FIGURE 64.4 Zones of burn injury.

Extent of Burn Injury

In addition to determining burn depth and zones, burn severity also is determined by assessing the percentage of burn injury. The "rule of nines" (Fig. 64.5) is a quick initial method of estimating how much skin surface is involved. Special charts and graphs provide more precise estimates for determining the percentage of the total body surface area (TBSA) that is burned. A quick assessment technique is to compare the client's palm with the size of the burn wound. The palm is approximately 1% of a person's TBSA.

Stop, Think, and Respond ● BOX 64-1

Using the rule of nines, calculate the TBSA burned if the burn includes one arm and the anterior chest.

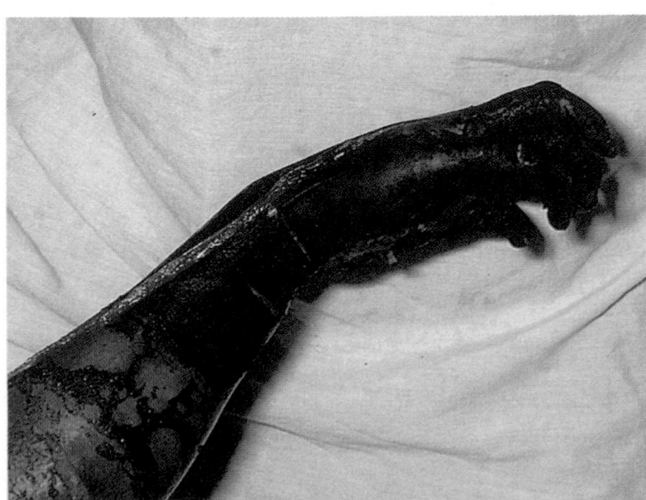

FIGURE 64.3 Third-degree burn.

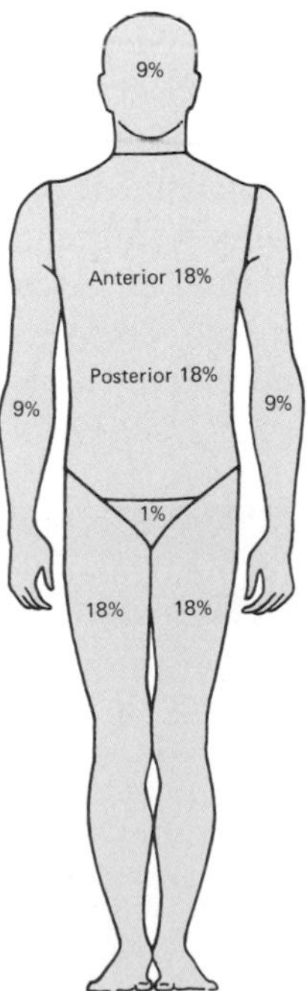

FIGURE 64.5 Rule of nines.

Assessment Findings

Skin color ranges from light pink to black depending on burn depth. There may be edema or blistering. Pain occurs in all areas except those of full-thickness burns. Clients with extensive burns may exhibit symptoms of hypovolemic shock, such as hypotension, tachycardia, oliguria, or anuria. Breathing may be compromised. The client experiences sore throat; singed nasal hairs, eyebrows, and eyelashes; hoarseness; carbon in sputum; soot around mouth or nose; shortness of breath; and stridor. Electrical burns usually show entrance and exit wounds.

Diagnosis is made by physical inspection. X-rays identify secondary injuries such as fractures or compromised lung function in inhalation injuries.

Medical Management

Outcome of a burn injury depends on initial first aid provided and subsequent treatment in the hospital or burn center. Any one of three complications—inhalation injury, hypovolemic shock, and infection—can be life-threatening. Clients with major burns are transported to a regional burn center (Box 64-1).

Initial First Aid

At the scene of a fire, the first priority is to prevent further injury to the affected person. If clothing is on fire, the client is placed in a horizontal position and rolled in a blanket to smother the fire. This prevents fire, hot air, and smoke from rising toward the head and entering respiratory passages. The client is taken to a hospital immediately for examination. During transport, those burned around the face or neck or who may have inhaled smoke, chemicals, steam, or flames are observed closely for respiratory difficulty. Inhalation of such substances can damage or severely irritate the mucous membrane lining the respiratory passages, resulting in edema of the respiratory passages. Secretion of mucus may be excessive, making breathing difficult. Oxygen is administered, and intravenous (IV) fluid therapy is begun en route.

BOX 64-1 ● Criteria for Major Burns

- Full-thickness burn greater than 10%
- Partial-thickness burn greater than 25%
- Burn in a critical location (face, eyes, ears, hands, perineum/genitalia, feet)
- Burn complicated by inhalation or electrical injury, fractures, or other major trauma
- Preexisting medical disorder (e.g., diabetes, heart disease)
- Age younger than 2 years or older than 60 years
- Circumstances of burn suggest abuse (child abuse, spouse abuse)

Acute Care

When the client with a burn arrives, the medical team works quickly to assess the extent of burn injury and additional trauma such as fractures, head injury, and lacerations. Team members ensure adequate ventilation and fluid resuscitation. For clients with difficulty breathing or edema of the face and neck, the team inserts an endotracheal tube.

Blood samples are drawn. Fluid resuscitation begins according to the severity of the burn injury. IV analgesics are administered for pain, which often is severe. An indwelling urethral catheter is inserted and attached to a closed drainage system. Tetanus immunization and antibiotics are administered.

Wound Management

Staphylococcus aureus, Pseudomonas aeruginosa, and *Candida albicans* are common microorganisms causing infection in burned tissue. As soon as possible, all clothing is removed. Body hair around the perimeter of the burns is shaved because hair is a source of bacterial wound contamination. When the head, neck, and upper chest are burned, singed eyebrows and eyelashes are clipped, scalp hair is shaved, lips and mouth are cleansed, and lips are lubricated. Eye ointments or irrigations are used to remove dirt and to lubricate lid margins.

Burned areas are cleansed to remove debris. There are two methods of wound management of burns (Table 64.2).

OPEN METHOD. The **open method** (exposure method) exposes burned areas to air. With the advent of effective topical antimicrobials, it is used only on a small scale for areas such as the face and perineum to which applying dressing materials is difficult. If the open method is used, the client is placed in isolation in a bed with sterile linen. Health team members and visitors wear sterile gowns and masks. The client is sensitive to drafts and temperature changes, so a bed cradle or sheets are placed over the client. The room is kept warm and humidified.

A hard crust forms over a partial-thickness burn in 2 or 3 days, and **epithelialization** (regrowth of skin) is completed in about 2 or 3 weeks. At this time, the crust falls off, is debrided, or is loosened by whirlpool baths. **Eschar,** a hard, leathery crust of dehydrated skin, forms in areas of full-thickness burns. If the eschar constricts the area and impairs circulation, an **escharotomy** (an incision into the eschar) is done to relieve pressure on the affected area. A dressing may be used to cover the exposed areas as the eschar is removed. New skin cannot grow beneath eschar.

CLOSED METHOD. The **closed method** is the current preferred method of wound management. The burn area is covered with nonadherent and absorbent dressings, consisting of gauze impregnated with petroleum jelly or ointment-based antimicrobials and fluffed gauze pads.

TABLE 64.2 OPEN AND CLOSED METHODS OF BURN CARE

TYPE	ADVANTAGES	DISADVANTAGES
Open method	Reduces labor-intensive care Causes less pain during wound care Facilitates inspection Decreases expense	Contributes to wound dessication (dryness) Promotes loss of water and body heat Exposes wound to pathogens Contributes to pain during repositioning Compromises modesty
Closed method	Maintains moist wound Promotes maintenance of body temperature Decreases cross-contamination of wound Provides wound debridement during dressing removal Keeps skin folds separated Reduces pain during position changes	Requires more time Adds to expense Enhances growth of pathogens beneath dressings Interferes with wound assessment Causes more blood loss with removal Can interfere with circulation if tightly applied

The final covering is an occlusive or semiocclusive dressing made of polyvinyl, polyethylene, polyurethane, and hydrocolloid materials. Occlusive dressings prevent bacteria from contact with the wound but are minimally permeable to water and oxygen. Various topical antimicrobials are applied to the burn wound to discourage growth of pathogens or control or eliminate any infection that develops.

Stop, Think, and Respond ● BOX 64-2

If a person is seriously burned, which method of wound management would you expect the burn unit to use? Give at least three reasons for your answer.

ANTIMICROBIAL THERAPY. Three major antimicrobials are used to treat burns: silver sulfadiazine (Silvadene) 1% ointment, mafenide (Sulfamylon), and silver nitrate ($AgNO_3$) 0.5% solution. Other commonly used drugs are povidone-iodine (Betadine), gentamicin (Garamycin) 0.1% cream, nitrofurazone (Furacin), mupirocin (Bactroban), clotrimazole (Lotrimin), and ciclopirox (Loprox). Povidone-iodine is contraindicated with some skin substitutes discussed later because it can damage new tissue growth in the wound bed.

Topical antimicrobials have various advantages and disadvantages, and no one preparation appears superior to another. All drugs are applied using sterile technique. Because infection is the rule rather than the exception, the client may require systemic antibiotics and antifungals. Some examples include amphotericin B (Fungizone) and penicillin G (Pfizerpen).

Surgical Management

Additional treatment modalities to promote healing include debridement, skin grafting, application of a skin substitute, and application of cultured skin.

Debridement

Wound **debridement** is removal of necrotic tissue and accomplished in one of four ways:

1. Naturally, as the nonliving tissue sloughs away from uninjured tissue
2. Mechanically, when dead tissue adheres to dressings or is detached during cleansing
3. Enzymatically, through the application of topical enzymes to the burn wound
4. Surgically, with the use of forceps and scissors during dressing changes or wound cleansing

After dead tissue is removed, it is imperative that healthy tissue be covered with a skin graft, a temporary skin substitute, or cultured skin.

Skin Grafting

Superficial burns heal when keratinocytes from the periphery and beneath the dermis proliferate to regenerate the epidermis (Schulz et al., 2000). Skin grafting is necessary for deep partial-thickness and full-thickness burns because skin layers responsible for regeneration are destroyed. Unassisted healing (healing without use of skin grafts or substitutes) results in proliferation of granulation tissue. Granulation tissue contains fibroblasts, which create hypertrophic scars that contract and pull the edges of the wound together, causing contractures. Wounds greater than 2 cm may not be able to granulate fully, resulting in a chronic open wound (Schulz et al., 2000). Purposes of a skin graft are to lessen the potential for infection, minimize fluid loss by evaporation, hasten recovery, reduce scarring, and prevent loss of function.

SOURCES FOR SKIN GRAFTS. Several sources are available for skin grafting. An **autograft** uses the client's own skin transplanted from one part of the body to another. Only autograft or skin transplanted from one identical twin to another can become a permanent part of the client's own skin.

An **allograft** or homograft is human skin obtained from a cadaver. Allografts temporarily cover large areas of tissue. Although allografts slough away after approximately 1 week, they last for the critical period until the client's own skin can be used for skin grafting. Cadaver skin usually is in short supply; although tissue is screened for human immunodeficiency virus and hepatitis, concerns remain that it could be a source of other pathogens.

A **heterograft** or xenograft is obtained from animals, principally pigs. Like allografts, heterografts are temporary and serve the same purposes. Allografts and heterografts are rejected in days to weeks and must be removed and replaced at that time.

TYPES OF AUTOGRAFTS. Human skin from the client with a burn is harvested under general anesthesia. Either a split-thickness or full-thickness graft is removed. In a **split-thickness graft,** the epidermis and a thin layer of dermis are harvested from the client's skin. Split-thickness autografts vary in thickness (0.008 to 0.024 inch), size, and shape and usually are obtained from the buttocks or thighs. Split-thickness autografts have more successful outcomes than other types, but their cosmetic appearance is less than desirable. They are less elastic, and hair does not grow from their surface.

A **full-thickness graft,** which may be 0.035 inch thick, includes epidermis, dermis, and some subcutaneous tissue. This type of graft is used when the burned area is fairly small or involves hands, face, or neck. Full-thickness grafts are more comparable in appearance to normal skin and can tolerate more stress once they become permanently attached to the burn wound.

A **slit graft** (also called a *lace* or an *expansile graft*) is used when the area available as a donor site is limited, as in clients with extensive burns. Skin is removed from the donor site and passed through an instrument that slits it; thus, a smaller piece of skin is stretched to cover a larger area (Fig. 64.6).

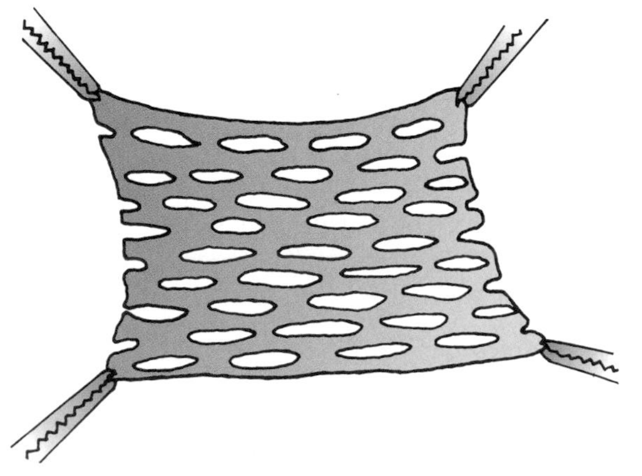

FIGURE 64.6 A slit graft. The slits allow for stretching to cover a larger area of tissue.

Harvesting the client's own tissue has several disadvantages: (1) it compounds the client's pain because it creates a new wound, (2) the donor site has potential for scarring and atypical pigment changes, (3) there is a potential for donor site infection, (4) there is a delay in wound closure while waiting for the donor site to heal and be reharvested, and (5) delays caused by waiting for harvest sites to heal increase costs and challenge the client's ability to cope with a prolonged hospitalization. It may be virtually impossible to harvest sufficient skin to totally close a full-thickness burn wound that is greater than 60% TBSA (Schulz et al., 2000).

Once the skin graft heals, pressure garments made of elasticized cloth or plastic are applied over the grafted area. They smooth the grafted skin, reducing scarring and the potential for wound contractures. The client may need to wear a pressure garment for up to 2 years.

Skin Substitutes

Scientists are creating alternative materials referred to as *skin substitutes* that cover the wound and promote healing. These bioengineered coverings promote wound healing by interacting directly with body tissues. Skin substitutes can be applied all over the burn wound as soon as the skin is cleaned and debrided instead of having to wait until enough skin is available for grafting purposes.

One example of a skin substitute is Biobrane, a nylon–silicone membrane coated with a protein derived from pig tissue. Another is Integra, a two-layer membrane: one is a synthetic epidermal layer; the other contains cross-linked collagen fibers that mimic the dermal layer of skin. The pseudodermal layer becomes a permanent cover; the outer layer, which provides a barrier against pathogens, is removed in 2 to 3 weeks and replaced with a thin autograft. The thin autograft heals in only a few days and provides a better cosmetic appearance.

Cultured Skin

Another alternative to wound closure is to culture the client's skin in a laboratory. Cultured skin is a wound closure product that is developed by growing the client's own skin cells in a laboratory culture medium. From a piece of postage stamp-sized skin, it is possible to grow sufficient skin to cover nearly the entire body in 3 weeks. A skin substitute is used to cover the burn wound while the skin culture is growing.

Once sufficient cultured cells are available, they are combined with a fabric material made from collagen that dissolves after it is applied to the wound. The burn wound heals in 2 to 3 weeks without traditional skin grafting. The only current disadvantage to cultured skin is that pigmentation does not perfectly match original skin color.

Nursing Management

Assess the wound and how the burn injury affects the client's status. Calculate fluid replacement requirements and infuse the prescribed volume according to the agency's protocol. Quickly recognize and efficiently treat signs of shock (see Chap. 20). Administer prescribed analgesics to relieve or reduce pain. Clean the wound, apply an antimicrobial agent, and cover the wound with the prescribed dressing. Monitor the wound to determine any infection. Help the client and family cope with the change in body image; encourage the client to perform exercises that minimize contractures. Before discharge, teach the client about use of a pressure garment and methods for skin care. See Nursing Care Plan 64-1.

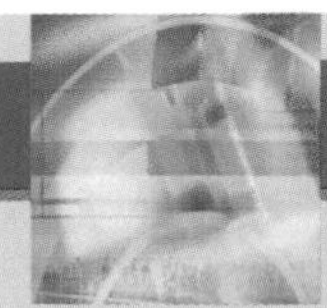

Nursing Care Plan 64-1

THE CLIENT WITH BURNS

Assessment

- Determine type of burn (thermal, chemical, electrical) and when it occurred.
- Assess vital signs.
- Look for evidence of inhalation injury.
- Determine oxygen saturation and respiratory effort.
- Evaluate pain intensity.
- Determine volume and characteristics of urine.
- Note percentage and depth of burn.
- Auscultate bowel sounds.
- Assess for concurrent medical problems, and review results of laboratory tests.

Depending on the extent and degree of burns, some or all of the following nursing diagnoses may apply. Diagnoses change as the client progresses through treatment and the stages of healing.*

Nursing Diagnosis: **Acute Pain** related to tissue injury

Expected Outcome: Pain will be within client's level of tolerance.

Interventions	*Rationales*
Assess pain intensity as needed and whenever you measure vital signs.	Assessing pain is the fifth vital sign.
Administer prescribed IV analgesia.	The IV route facilitates drug distribution when absorption is impaired at other parenteral routes.
Give analgesics prophylactically 30 minutes before dressing changes or debridements.	Preventing severe pain is easier than relieving it.
Implement nonpharmacologic methods of pain relief: imagery, self-hypnosis, and distraction.	Alternative methods for relieving pain supplement pharmacologic methods.
Place client on a CircOlectric bed or other type of turning frame to facilitate turning and repositioning.	Pain is reduced when the bed turns the client mechanically and passively.
Exercise caution and gentleness when removing and reapplying dressings.	Pain is intensified when movement stimulates intact sensory nerves.

Evaluation of Expected Outcome: Client responds to pain-relieving techniques.

Nursing Diagnosis: **Hypothermia** related to impaired ability to regulate body temperature

Expected Outcome: Temperature will be in normal range.

(continued)

Nursing Care Plan 64-1 (Continued)

THE CLIENT WITH BURNS

Interventions	*Rationales*
Reduce evaporation from burn wound by humidifying the environment, preventing drafts, and covering the burn wound with ointment, creams, and dressings.	Impaired skin cannot regulate body temperature; reducing the potential for heat loss helps maintain body temperature.

Evaluation of Expected Outcome: Temperature is normal.

PC: **Infection** related to impaired skin integrity

Expected Outcome: Nurse will monitor to detect, manage, and minimize infection.

Interventions	*Rationales*
Assess temperature every 4 hours; monitor results of blood counts and cultures.	Fever, leukocytosis, and bacterial growth from a wound culture indicate infection.
Use sterile or clean linen.	Surgical and medical asepsis reduce the potential for infection.
Wear sterile or clean caps, gowns, and masks.	Using outer garments reduces the transmission of pathogens from contaminated clothing to the client.
Restrict infectious people from visiting or caring for client.	Limiting contact with sources of infection protects a susceptible host.
Apply and administer prescribed antimicrobial and antibiotic therapy.	Antimicrobials and antibiotics suppress the growth of pathogens.
Inspect burn areas for healing, drainage, formation of eschar, infection, and stability of the skin graft or wound covering.	Direct observation of the wound and comparing normal and abnormal findings help determine the client's response to treatment.
Accurately record all findings.	

Evaluation of Expected Outcome: Wound infections are eliminated, and the wound heals.

PC: **Skin Graft Disruption**

Expected Outcome: Nurse will monitor to detect, manage, and minimize skin graft disruption.

Interventions	*Rationales*
Avoid excessive pressure on grafted area; minimize movement.	Relief of pressure and restricting movement promote vascularization.
Assist physician with dressing changes.	Graft disruption is minimized when the nurse assists the physician and client.
Monitor color and odor in the area of grafted tissue.	A pale color suggests ischemia. A dark appearance suggests poor venous outflow. A foul odor suggests colonization with bacteria.

Evaluation of Expected Outcome: The burn wound is covered; skin grafts are viable.

(continued)

Nursing Care Plan 64-1 (Continued)

THE CLIENT WITH BURNS

PC: **Gastric and Intestinal Paresis (Hypomotility)** and **Peptic Ulcer**

Expected Outcome: Nurse will monitor to detect, manage, and minimize gastrointestinal hypomotility and peptic ulcer.

Interventions	*Rationales*
Assess for abdominal distention and status of bowel sounds.	Abdominal distension and diminished or no bowel sounds suggest impaired peristalsis.
Insert a prescribed nasogastric tube; connect it to low intermittent suction.	Negative pressure removes gas and secretions from the upper gastrointestinal tract.
Administer IV histamine antagonists and drugs such as metoclopramide (Reglan).	Histamine antagonists raise the pH of gastric secretions and reduce the potential for gastric mucosal irritation.
Instill antacid through nasogastric tube; clamp for 30 minutes before reconnecting to suction.	Metoclopramide promotes stomach emptying.
Assess pH of gastric secretions every shift; report if pH is less than 3.	Antacids neutralize stomach acid.

Evaluation of Expected Outcome: Bowel sounds are active in all abdominal quadrants; client experiences no epigastric distress.

Nursing Diagnosis: **Impaired Physical Mobility** related to pain, bulky dressings, and contracted skin secondary to scar formation

Expected Outcome: Range of motion and muscle strength will be preserved or restored.

Interventions	*Rationales*
Keep joints in burned areas neutral: extended rather than flexed.	A neutral position facilitates functional use.
Exercise uninvolved joints actively; exercise involved joints during hydrotherapy.	Exercise promotes muscle tone and strength. Exercising in water reduces resistance to work.
Encourage performance of activities of daily living (ADLs), such as brushing teeth and eating.	Performing ADLs is a form of active exercise that maintains the flexibility of joints and muscle tone.

Evaluation of Expected Outcome: Client regains functional use of joints in burn areas.

Nursing Diagnosis: **Risk for Disturbed Thought Processes** related to reduced mental stimulation, sleep deprivation, social isolation, fluid and electrolyte imbalance, narcotic administration, and sepsis

Expected Outcome: Client will remain oriented and have realistic perceptions.

Interventions	*Rationales*
Assess mental status every shift.	Focused assessments facilitate the early detection of problems.
Reorient the confused client.	Providing facts helps the client reorder thinking.
Have a calendar and clock within client's view.	Environmental cues help prevent disorientation.

(continued)

Nursing Care Plan 64-1 (Continued)

THE CLIENT WITH BURNS

Interventions	*Rationales*
Discuss current events; encourage visits from family.	Interacting with others and staying aware of current events help stimulate the mind.
Cluster nursing activities to facilitate continuous sleep.	Sleep deprivation contributes to confusion and disorientation.

Evaluation of Expected Outcome: Client logically processes verbal and environmental cues.

Nursing Diagnoses: **Risk for Ineffective Coping** and **Risk for Ineffective Family Coping** related to inadequate emotional resources for managing multiple stressors

Expected Outcome: Client and family will adapt and use strategies for effective coping.

Interventions	*Rationales*
Explain methods and reasons for treatment.	Information helps clarify the plan and assists the client to strive to meet goals.
Acknowledge signs of progress.	Objective evidence of progress sustains motivation.
Involve client and family in long-range planning, physical therapy, and vocational rehabilitation.	A client and family who feel they are part of a team willingly participate in achieving goals.
Refer family to counseling for assistance in managing conflicts.	Health professionals with specialized expertise can help clients and family members solve problems.

Evaluation of Expected Outcome: Client and family cope effectively and use resources wisely to manage client's care.

*Other potential nursing diagnoses include **Risk for Ineffective Airway Clearance, Risk for Impaired Gas Exchange, PC: Hypovolemic Shock, Risk for Constipation, PC: Anemia,** and **Risk for Imbalanced Nutrition: Less than Body Requirements.**

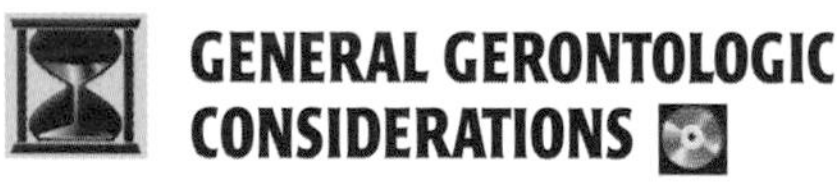

GENERAL GERONTOLOGIC CONSIDERATIONS

Burns can result in serious complications in the elderly because of diminished renal, cardiac, and respiratory functions associated with the aging process.

Critical Thinking Exercise

1. *Discuss methods used to reduce the potential for infection in a burn wound.*

• NCLEX-STYLE REVIEW QUESTIONS 

1. The family of a client who experienced burns 5 days ago asks the nurse why she is taking the client's temperature so frequently. Which explanation is most appropriate?
   1. "Fever is a sign of infection, which is common."
   2. "I need to carry out the physician's orders."
   3. "A fluid shift causes the temperature to rise."
   4. "Clients with burns are usually warm to touch."
2. Which nursing action is most appropriate prior to changing a dressing of a client with a partial thickness burn?
   1. Administer analgesics 30 minutes prior to the procedure.
   2. Turn up environmental temperature in the client's room.
   3. Don clean gloves and hair and shoe covers.
   4. Change the dressing just before mealtime.
3. A client is hospitalized with a partial thickness burn over 50% of the body. During the healing process, which of the following foods would the nurse be most likely to advise the client to increase consumption of?
   1. Butter
   2. Cereal
   3. Orange juice
   4. Meat

connection

Visit the Connection site at **http://connection.lww.com/go/timbyEssentials** for links to chapter-related resources on the Internet.

References and Suggested Readings

American Burn Association. (2000). Burn incidence and treatment in the US: 2000 fact sheet. [On-line.] Available: http://www.ameriburn.org/pub/factsheet.htm.

Badger, J. M. (2001). Understanding secondary traumatic stress. *American Journal of Nursing, 101*(7), 26–33.

Cole, M. R. (2000). Burn trauma: More than just skin deep. *Nursing Spectrum (Greater Chicago/NE Illinois, NW Indiana Edition), 13*(17), 32–33.

DuKamp, A. (2000). Managing burn blisters. *Nursing Times, 96*(4), NT plus: 19–20.

Jones, M. L. (2001). Burns. *Practice Nurse, 22*(6), 41–42, 44.

Jordan, K. S. (2000). Fluid resuscitation in acutely injured patients. *Journal of Intravenous Nursing, 23*(2), 81–87.

Kagan, R. J., & Smith, S. C. (2000). Evaluation and treatment of thermal injuries. *Dermatology Nursing, 12,* 334–335, 338–344, 347–350.

McKirdy, L. (2001). Burn wound cleansing. *Journal of Community Nursing, 15*(5), 24, 26–27, 29.

Regojo, P. S. (2003). Burn care basics. *Nursing 2003, 33*(3), 50–53.

Schulz, J. T., III, Tompkins, R. G., & Burke, J. F. (2000). Artificial skin. *Annual Reviews, 51*(1), 231–244. [On-line.] Available: http://www.AnnualReviews.org.

Sheridan, R. L. (2000). Evaluating and managing burn wounds. *Dermatology Nursing, 12,* 17–18, 21–28, 30–31.

Weinberg, K., Birdsall, C., Vail, D., et al. (2000). Pain and anxiety with burn dressing changes: Patient self-report. *Journal of Burn Care and Rehabilitation, 21,* 155–161.

Wiebelhaus, P., Hansen, S., & Hill, H. (2001). Helping patients survive inhalation injuries. *RN, 64*(10), 28–32.

Wiebelhaus, P., & Hansen, S. L. (2001). What you should know about managing burn emergencies. *Nursing, 31*(1), 36–42.

chapter 65

Leadership Roles and Management Functions

Words to Know 

accountability
advocacy
autocratic leadership
collaboration
delegation
democratic leadership
laissez-faire leadership
leadership
management
multicratic leadership
power
resource management
responsibility
supervision
time management

Learning Objectives

On completion of this chapter, the reader will:

- Differentiate between leadership and management.
- Define three styles of leadership.
- Outline the purpose of power in the leadership role.
- Describe the role of the licensed practical/vocational nurse (LPN/LVN) in managing client care.
- Distinguish delegation and supervision.
- Compare responsibility and accountability.
- Discuss potential problems with delegation and supervision.
- Describe the role of the LPN/LVN in collaboration and advocacy.
- Explain the role of the LPN/LVN in resource management.
- Discuss methods to manage time effectively.

Licensed practical/vocational nurses (LPN/LVNs), in their role of providing care to clients, must organize client care, supervise care provided by unlicensed personnel, collaborate with other healthcare personnel, manage time and resources, and be accountable for assigned client care. Although primarily educated to provide direct client care, LPN/LVNs need a basic understanding of management and supervisory principles to function in leadership roles in various healthcare settings. This chapter provides an overview of theory related to leadership and management, with a focus on the role of the LPN/LVN in delegation and supervision.

LEADERSHIP AND MANAGEMENT

In many ways, leadership and management are interrelated concepts; discussing one is impossible without reference to the other. **Leadership** involves qualities related to a person's character and behaviors, as well as roles within a group or organization. It is the ability to guide and influence another person, group, or both to think in a certain way, achieve common goals, or provide inspiration for change. Marquis and Huston (1998) state that leaders:

1. May or may not have delegated authority, but can obtain power through other means
2. Have a wider variety of roles than managers
3. Frequently are not part of a formal organization
4. Focus on group process, information gathering, feedback, and empowering others

Any healthcare provider can be a leader in terms of influencing a group or exercising power in a particular situation. LPN/LVNs may be leaders, informally or formally. For example, an LPN working on a medical–surgical unit may assume responsibility for organizing social events for fellow employees. A more formal leadership role is acting as co-chairperson of the unit's staffing policy committee.

Management entails assigned functions such as planning, organizing, directing, and controlling to meet specific objectives within an organization (Ellis & Hartley, 2000). The overall goal is to coordinate and direct resources, including work space, supplies, equipment, budgetary concerns, and services (Harrington & Terry, 2003). Managers direct and coordinate the work of assigned employees. They (1) are assigned a position in an organization,

(2) have a legitimate source of power, (3) are expected to carry out specific functions, and (4) emphasize control, decision-making, decision analysis, and results (Marquis & Huston, 1998). A key feature is the individual manager's responsibility and accountability for accomplishing tasks (Ellis & Hartley, 2000).

The Relationship of Leadership and Management

To be effective, leaders and managers must possess certain qualities:

- An ability to gain respect of others through competence and shared goals
- Expertise in communication skills, both oral and written
- A capacity to motivate others to achieve a particular purpose or accomplish goals

Ideally, a good manager is also a good leader, and a good leader is a good manager. In reality, some managers do not possess good leadership skills, and some leaders are ineffective managers. People can learn leadership and management skills. Improving and developing skills through education and experience enhances a person's ability to lead and manage.

Integrated leaders/managers (Marquis & Huston, 2002) have traits that distinguish them from just leaders or managers. They include thinking in the long term; seeing the big picture; influencing others outside their own group; emphasizing vision, values, and motivation; being politically astute; and embracing change and modification (Gardner, 1990). In addition, integrated leaders/managers set reasonable goals, think positively, and are willing to take risks.

Leadership Styles

Lewin (1951) identified three prevalent leadership styles that managers use, consciously or unconsciously, to accomplish goals and tasks. The styles vary in the amount of control the manager exerts and the degree of input subordinates have in the decision-making process.

The first leadership style is the authoritarian or **autocratic leadership** style. Strong control by the manager over the work group characterizes this style. The manager gives and asks for little input from staff for decisions. Communication flows from top to bottom. The focus is on accomplishing tasks; as such, decisions are made quickly and lines of authority and policies are clear. The work is very controlled and dictated, and leaders may create hostility and dependency. Autocratic leadership works best in bureaucracies and with employees with limited education and training.

The second leadership style, **democratic leadership,** involves more participation in decision-making by the work group. Leaders with this style view themselves as coworkers or colleagues, as opposed to superiors. They emphasize communication, consensus, and teamwork (Ellis & Hartley, 2000). Communication is mutual, and employees are motivated and involved in goals of the organization. Decisions may take longer, and the manager's role may not be acknowledged. Democratic leadership works well with competent and motivated employees.

The third leadership style is **laissez-faire leadership,** or permissive management. This style involves the least structure and control. The manager leaves the work group to set goals, make decisions, and take responsibility for their own management (Ellis & Hartley, 2000). Employees often function at high levels because of the independence. Decisions are not readily made because managers cannot or are unwilling to make them. Change is rare. This leadership works well with professional employees.

Each leadership style can be effective, depending on the particular situation. A good leader can determine which approach is best for a particular circumstance. Ellis and Hartley (2000) refer to this ability as **multicratic leadership,** which combines the best of all styles, mediated by the requirements of the situation at hand. The multicratic leader provides maximum structure when appropriate to the situation, asks for maximum group participation when needed, and gives support and encouragement to subordinates in all instances.

Stop, Think, and Respond ● BOX 65-1

A new LPN/LVN works on a long-term care unit where the nurse manager typically uses an autocratic style of leadership. What are the advantages and disadvantages of this style for the new LPN/LVN?

Power and Leadership

The leader/manager has the potential to provide guidance, direction, and support to coworkers, and also exerts a certain power. **Power** is the ability to control, influence, or hold authority over an individual or group. People in leadership/management positions are in a position to exert power in an organization. For leadership to be effective, a degree of power must support it.

Each type of power has a particular source or base. The first type is *reward power,* which a person attains through the ability to grant favors or rewards. For example, organizational leaders have the ability to grant financial rewards or special favors.

Coercive or *punishment power* is the ability to threaten or punish someone who fails to meet expectations. In using such power, a manager may threaten undesirable schedules, denial of vacation time, or layoff if an employee is not compliant.

A manager exercises *legitimate power* through a designated position, which also may be referred to as *authority*. A manager has legitimate power by virtue of the management position.

Expert power results from knowledge, expertise, or experience in a particular area. Managers typically possess expert power through education and work experience.

Referent power concerns the power a person has because of his or her association with others who are powerful. For example, society perceives that physicians are powerful. A new physician may use this referent power to his or her advantage. Referent power also may be called *charismatic* or *connection power*, referring to personal characteristics, such as charisma, the way a person talks or acts, the people he or she associates with, or the organizations to which he or she belongs.

Another type is *informational power*, which exists when a person has information that others need to accomplish certain goals. Examples may relate to budget preparation, planning for educational events, or making changes in an organization.

Leaders and managers may exercise power to accomplish assigned tasks. They also must have the authority or legitimate right to direct and guide work. A nurse in an authorized position (e.g., team leader, charge nurse) can exert power in a positive way.

THE LPN/LVN AS LEADER/MANAGER

Usually, managers are appointed to or hired for a specific management position. In healthcare, the term *manager* may be used more broadly, in that nurses manage care of clients. This role involves overseeing the care that a client receives. Other healthcare providers may actually care for the clients. In acute care settings, registered nurses (RNs) are assigned to a group of clients. An LPN/LVN and certified nurse's aide (CNA) may work with the RN and be responsible for certain aspects of client care. The RN, as manager of care, ensures that the LPN/LVN and CNA complete all assigned tasks, assess the clients, and evaluate the effects of all nursing interventions.

In other healthcare settings, the role of the LPN/LVN may be extended. For example, in long-term care settings LPN/LVNs may be team leaders and thus assigned to oversee the work of unlicensed assistive personnel (UAPs). In medical offices, an LPN/LVN may be the office manager, coordinating certain aspects of the office work, such as scheduling and coordinating work assignments. These roles require the LPN/LVN to delegate responsibility for certain tasks and then supervise the accomplishment of the work. The next sections delineate the terms *delegation, supervision, responsibility,* and *accountability.*

Delegation

The National Council of State Boards of Nursing (NCSBN) (1995) states that **delegation** is "transferring to a competent individual the authority to perform a selected nursing task in a selected situation. The nurse retains the accountability for the delegation" (p. 3). Delegation also is a means of accomplishing work through others (Marquis & Huston, 1998). The ability to guide, teach, and direct others is integral to the ability to delegate.

Nurses need to learn delegation skills. The NCSBN (1995) identified the Five Rights of Delegation: (1) right task, (2) right circumstances, (3) right person, (4) right direction/communication, and (5) right supervision/evaluation. Ellis and Hartley (2000) suggest that carrying out the five rights of delegation requires following certain steps similar to those of the nursing process:

- *Assess the situation*—know the client's needs, the skills of the UAPs, and the priorities. Match the UAPs' skills with the tasks to be completed.
- *Plan actions*—identify the UAPs who will best handle the delegated tasks.
- *Implement the plan*—communicate expectations clearly to UAPs, including what they need to do, what to watch for, and potential problems.
- *Evaluate the results*—ensure that tasks are completed according to standards.

Part of succeeding at delegating involves the process of supervision.

Supervision

Supervision is the process of guiding, directing, evaluating, and following-up on tasks delegated to others (NCSBN, 1995). Delegation and supervision are tightly connected, because once a nurse delegates a task, he or she is obligated to supervise the person to whom he or she assigns that task. In reviewing the steps of delegation, supervision begins when the LPN/LVN implements the plan. The implementation step includes giving instructions about what needs to be done, and when. The nurse must include any specific issues, such as telling the UAP that a client must complete morning care before going for physical therapy at 10:00 AM. In addition, the nurse needs to tell the UAP about any potential problems, such as a client who may experience dizziness when getting up secondary to antihypertensive medications.

Supervision also is necessary throughout the implementation step. The LPN/LVN must check with UAPs during the shift to assess if tasks are complete, the results, if something has changed that may interfere with the work, or if the UAP is having problems accomplishing the task safely.

The evaluation step of delegation also includes supervision of the UAP, in that the LPN/LVN ensures that the client received the appropriate care, all the client's needs were met, and that problems were addressed. Providing feedback to UAPs also is important, in terms of letting them know that they did a good job or asking questions about the client's response to the care provided.

Delegation and supervision imply that the people carrying out these functions assume responsibility and accountability for their actions as well as the actions of those to whom they delegate. The next section defines these concepts.

Responsibility and Accountability

Responsibility is a duty or assignment related to a specific job. It means being obligated to perform certain activities and duties. When a person is responsible for something, he or she is obligated to ensure that the task or job is completed (Ellis & Hartley, 2000).

Accountability means being answerable for the consequences of one's actions or inactions. The term *liability* is closely associated with accountability, because of the legal implications. "Although the tasks may be delegated, the nurse who delegates that task to others remains accountable—or legally liable—for the outcome" (Ellis & Hartley, 2000, p. 32).

An LPN/LVN who delegates to a UAP is responsible for ensuring that the task is appropriate for the UAP and that the UAP has the skills to complete the task. The LPN/LVN is accountable for determining if the task is accomplished, and if there are any issues associated with completing or not completing the task. In addition, the LPN/LVN also is accountable for evaluating results of the tasks. The UAP is responsible for performing the actual task. The following exercise clarifies these concepts.

Stop, Think, and Respond ● BOX 65-2

An LPN is the team leader for 20 clients on a long-term care unit. She delegates to a UAP the task of feeding supper to an older client. When the UAP feeds this client, the client begins to cough and choke, aspirating some food. The client eventually develops pneumonia and must be hospitalized for 1 week. Who is responsible for this incident?

Confronting Problems

LPN/LVNs may experience some problems with delegation and supervision of tasks. In part this is because LPN/LVNs may not be well prepared for the role of team leader. Schools of practical/vocational nursing traditionally have focused primarily on the direct caregiver role. In turn, employers may not plan for LPN/LVNs to be team leaders or other managers of care, but out of necessity place LPN/LVNs in these roles. Other factors that may interfere with effective delegation and supervision are:

- Reluctance to delegate from fear of overloading a coworker or desire to do everything
- Inability to move out of the role of direct caregiver: "It is easier to do it myself."
- Miscommunication regarding specific directions and desired outcomes
- Desire to be liked by coworkers, which interferes with ability to delegate, supervise, or both

In addition, LPN/LVNs are not strictly supervisors, in that they do not have authority to hire or fire. They may have responsibility for overseeing and directing the care that UAPs provide, but they do not have responsibility for disciplining them.

Solutions for improving one's ability to delegate and direct UAPs include obtaining education for this role. In addition, LPN/LVNs must focus on client care needs first, ensuring that the clients receive appropriate care and that tasks are carried out efficiently and in a caring manner. If an LPN/LVN remains responsible and accountable for his or her actions, it assists him or her to delegate and direct responsibly.

Other Functions

Although LPN/LVNs as team leaders have primary responsibility for delegating tasks to UAPs, other functions are important for the LPN/LVN leader/manager. These functions include collaboration, advocacy, resource management, and time management.

Collaboration

Collaboration involves a team effort to achieve client care outcomes. Although RNs often direct collaborative efforts, LPN/LVNs are responsible to direct the care of UAPs. As a team member and leader, LPN/LVNs maintain open and effective communication with all team members. They also assist in solving problems related to client care. LPN/LVNs may contribute to decisions about client care and unit activities by participating in client care conferences and unit meetings. Last, collaborative behavior for the LPN/LVN involves participating in the management of the unit by following the appropriate channels of communication and supporting the group in collaborative efforts.

Advocacy

Advocacy means promoting the cause of another person or organization. In healthcare, advocates support the needs of a client or organization. Nurses in general act on behalf of their clients. Ethically, nurses support a client's right to be autonomous and to make informed decisions

(American Nurses Association, 1998). LPN/LVNs function as client advocates by understanding the rights of all clients, remaining informed about diagnoses, treatments, prognoses, and choices; contributing to the provision of information and education; supporting the client's decisions; and communicating with other professionals (Ellis & Hartley, 2000).

Resource Management

Resource management, the responsibility of all who work in healthcare, means using resources, which include not only actual money but also supplies, equipment, buildings, and personnel, optimally. Nurses who provide direct care may not have a direct role in formulating budgets, but they are responsible for controlling the use of resources and recognizing when resources are inadequate. In addition, they must know the costs of resources and the importance of using cost-effective measures when caring for clients.

Many factors are related to the rising costs of healthcare. In general, new technologies increase costs, which leads to the need for better facilities and, it is hoped, better outcomes for client care. Related costs are salaries for healthcare personnel, newer and more expensive medications, and equipment. As a result of increased costs, healthcare providers are expected to be more cost-conscious. Cost-conscious measures, or resource management, include prudent use of expensive supplies, knowledgeable operation of medical equipment, careful monitoring of clients to reduce potential complications and lengths of stay, heightened awareness of practicing measures that reduce costs, essential knowledge of all costs of caring for clients, and deliberate reduction of waste of limited resources.

LPN/LVNs also may be involved in controlling costs by participation in a client acuity system. Acute care and long-term care facilities may use an acuity system to determine staffing needs. Acuity measures the degree of a client's illness and what care is required to meet the client's needs. Often systems use categories to designate the level of care needed. For example, one category may reflect the need for complex dressing changes, another the need for special monitoring, such as neurologic checks. Each category has assigned points—at the end, the points are totaled to ascertain the acuity level of the client. This information may then be used to determine what nursing staff is needed to provide adequately for the needs of the unit (Ellis & Hartley, 2000).

Time Management

Time is an essential resource, particularly in today's fast-paced healthcare environment. **Time management** involves organizing time, as well as delegating tasks to other personnel. There are three basic steps for managing time. In the first step the nurse makes time to plan and establish priorities. The second step involves completing the highest-priority task and moving from completing one task to beginning another. The final step requires that the nurse reassess and reprioritize tasks based on any changes.

The onset of managed care increased the focus on efficiency and productivity. Making the most of one's time is an important skill that takes effort to achieve. Although on chaotic days it may seem that nothing works, those most effective at managing time will have the most success in accomplishing the work that needs to be done. New nurses usually need to learn to organize their time. The following techniques are useful in learning to manage time:

- Assess expectations for the shift. Do so in a chart that identifies specific periods (e.g., 30-minute increments). This also can be done after a shift to determine how one spent time that particular day and how it might help to organize another shift.
- Use a worksheet to identify specific tasks and important assessments that need to be done for that particular shift. This works well with multiple client assignments. Organize the worksheet according to each client. Many nurses refer to this as a "to do" list or "brain sheet." They use the worksheet to identify tasks, but also to write quick notes to jog their memories for further tasks or assessments.
- Prioritize tasks that need to be accomplished (Box 65-1). Reprioritize as needed.

BOX 65-1 ● Criteria for Setting Priorities

1. Items critical to maintaining life: Think in terms of your cardiopulmonary resuscitation basics.
   - Essential assessment
   - Airway management
   - Breathing support
   - Circulation needs
   - Neurologic stability
2. Critical symptom management: What is important to the client?
   - Pain management
   - Relief of nausea
   - Relief of diarrhea
   - Relief of severe anxiety
3. Items needed to progress in health restoration: What orders has the physician written? What nursing plans have been developed?
   - Medication and intravenous fluid administration
   - Completing treatments
   - Preventing complications
   - Meeting nutritional needs
4. Items needed to move toward self-care
   - Teaching
   - Contacting referral needs
   - Meeting psychosocial needs
   - Creating comfort and feelings of well-being
   - Bathing
   - Changing linens

(Adapted from Ellis, J. R. & Hartley, C. L. [2000]. *Managing and coordinating nursing care* [3rd ed.]. Philadelphia: Lippincott Williams & Wilkins.)

- Write things down to remember later for charting and reporting. Many nurses use their worksheet as a report sheet for the oncoming shift.
- Develop efficiency and the ability to multitask, which means engaging in more than one task at a time. For example, if a client requests pain medication and you need to assess his roommate's vital signs, bring needed equipment as well as pain medication.
- Delegate appropriate tasks to appropriate personnel.

Most people readily admit that they do not always make good use of their time and then have to scramble to complete tasks. Reasons for this essentially include an inability to plan, procrastination, chatting, allowing low-priority tasks to take precedence, inability to delegate appropriately, and difficulty saying no. Assessing what wastes one's time is an important step in using time more effectively.

Critical Thinking Exercises

1. *An LPN is a team leader on a skilled care unit. When she returns from her dinner break, the UAP reports the following:*
   - *One client vomited after receiving her 6 PM medications.*
   - *A family member is upset that his mother pulled out her feeding tube and it is not replaced.*
   - *A client's catheter seems to be leaking.*
   - *A physician wants to order medications for the new client who had hip replacement surgery 2 weeks ago.*

Prioritize these tasks, and indicate what the LPN should attend to and what she can delegate.

2. *An LVN is planning to change jobs from acute care to long-term care. He is concerned about his role in the new job as a team leader. He knows that he will be working with UAPs. What should he know about his role in delegating tasks to UAPs if he takes this new job?*

• NCLEX-STYLE REVIEW QUESTIONS 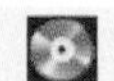

1. A nurse manager on a large medical unit is initiating a new staffing pattern. The manager sends a memo explaining the new pattern and produces the staff schedule, noting assignments. Which type of leadership is the nurse manager exhibiting?
   1. Autocratic
   2. Democratic
   3. Laissez-faire
   4. Multicratic
2. Before delegating activities to a member of the nursing team, the LPN is most correct to first:
   1. Give detailed instructions.
   2. Assess the situation.
   3. Plan the appropriate action.
   4. Inquire what others think.
3. An LPN at a nursing home delegates simple wound dressing care to the nurse's aide. If an attorney reviews the chart for upcoming legal action, who would be held accountable for the wound dressing care?
   1. The nurse's aide
   2. The LPN
   3. The physician
   4. The institution

connection

Visit the Connection site at **http://connection.lww.com/go/timbyEssentials** for links to chapter-related resources on the Internet.

References and Suggested Readings

A 10-step approach to better time management. (2003). *RN's TNT*, 35–38.

Ahmed, D. S. (2000). Practice errors: It's not my job. *American Journal of Nursing, 100*(6), 25.

American Nurses Association. (1998). *Standards of clinical nursing practice* (2nd ed.). Washington, DC: Author.

DeMarco, R. F., & Roberts, S. J. (2003). Negative behaviors in nursing. *American Journal of Nursing, 103*(3), 113–116.

Ellis, J. R., & Hartley, C. L. (2000). *Managing and coordinating nursing care* (3rd ed.). Philadelphia: Lippincott Williams & Wilkins.

Gardner, J. W. (1990). *On leadership.* New York: The Free Press.

Gokenbach, V. (January 2003). Infuse management with leadership. *Nursing Management*, 8–10.

Hamilton, J. (April 28, 2003). Managing conflict. *Advance for Nurses*, 20–23.

Harrington, N., & Terry, C. (2003). *LPN to RN transitions* (2nd ed.). Philadelphia: Lippincott Williams & Wilkins.

Keeling, B., Adair, J., Seider, D., & Kirksey, G. (2000). Appropriate delegation. *American Journal of Nursing, 100*(12), 24A–24D.

Lewin, K. (1951). *Field theory in social sciences.* New York: Harper & Row.

Malestic, S. (2003). A quick guide to verbal reports. *RN, 66*(2), 47–49.

Marquis, B. L., & Huston, C. J. (1998). *Management decision making for nurses* (3rd ed.). Philadelphia: Lippincott Williams & Wilkins.

Marquis, B. L., & Huston, C. J. (2002). *Leadership roles and management functions in nursing: Theory and application* (4th ed.). Philadelphia: Lippincott Williams & Wilkins.

Mooney, B. (May 27, 2002). Delegate with ease. *Advance for Nurses*, 28–30.

National Council of State Boards of Nursing. (1995). *Delegation: Concepts and decision making process.* Chicago: Author.

chapter 66

Career-Building Skills and Transition Issues

Words to Know 

burnout
competency
cover letter
long-term goals
reality shock
résumé
role transition
scope of practice
short-term goals

Learning Objectives

On completion of this chapter, the reader will:

- Summarize methods to become employed as a licensed practical/vocational nurse.
- Develop a list of personal short- and long-term goals.
- Examine issues related to role transition.
- Discuss workplace problems related to reality shock and burnout.
- Describe strategies to ease role transition.
- Define approaches for self-care.
- Explain the importance of maintaining competency.
- Review opportunities for future nursing education.

Finishing a practical/vocational nursing program represents the completion of an intense time of learning, studying, and practicing. It also marks the beginning of a new career transition. Many of the experiences of beginning and finishing school are similar to starting a career, but new licensed practical/vocational nurses (LPN/LVNs) face additional challenges and issues. This chapter presents an overview of methods for obtaining employment, issues that may potentially affect new LPN/LVNs, and strategies for self-care in the demanding workplace.

BEGINNING YOUR CAREER

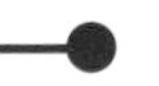

Employment Opportunities

A nursing shortage brought about economic and demographic changes in the 1990s. The push for cost containment led to restructurings of hospitals, downsizing of nursing staff, and shorter hospital stays. Clients in today's healthcare facilities are more acutely ill and older, with multiple health problems. In addition, the nursing workforce is aging; many nurses are expected to retire within the next 10 years. Demand for nurses will increase greatly in the next 2 decades, related to the same factors (Health Resources and Services Administration, 2002). Opportunities for LPN/LVNs are and will be available, particularly in long-term care facilities and ambulatory care settings. Jobs in acute care settings for LPN/LVNs are obtainable, but may be more competitive and require previous experience.

New Graduate Competencies

The National Council of State Boards of Nursing (NCSBN, 2001) identified particular competencies expected of new graduates from practical/vocational nursing programs. These competencies form the basis for the National Council Licensure Examination for Practical Nurses (NCLEX-PN). **Competency** refers to a person's ability to perform designated nursing skills effectively and safely (Ellis & Hartley, 2004). Employers' expectations, although different in various parts of the country and diverse work settings, center on passing the NCLEX-PN test and performing at an entry level that is safe. They also expect that new graduate LPN/LVNs will progress and function independently as permitted within the assigned **scope of practice**—activities that a person with a particular license can legally perform. Graduate LPN/LVNs need to demonstrate ability in communication, clinical, organizational, delegation, and priority-setting skills, and to practice according to standards set by the individual state boards of nursing, specific employers, and professional organizations.

Personal Career Goals

Setting personal goals is an important skill for career growth and mobility. Following the steps of the nursing process, the first step involves assessing your abilities and skills and comparing them to employment opportunities and expectations. It also involves looking at likes and dislikes, positive student clinical experiences, and particular needs, such as family, physical restrictions, and geographical considerations.

The next step is to determine **short-term goals**—those you anticipate accomplishing fairly quickly. An example is obtaining 2 years' experience on a skilled care unit.

Stop, Think, and Respond ● BOX 66-1

List short-term goals that you hope to accomplish in the first and second years following graduation.

After establishing short-term goals, develop a plan for meeting those goals. These goals help identify potential employers in the geographical area you would like to live. Many new graduates look at clinical sites where they had student experiences, where they have acquaintances with employees, or where they have worked in another capacity. New graduates also may be eager to find a place of employment that provides adequate orientation to the new position. Another source for seeking potential employment is through classified advertisements in local papers. The Internet has become an excellent place to look for job opportunities, both locally and in new locations. It is also important that you consider if a particular institution/job can help you meet your short-term goals.

The next step is to implement your plan. Several components are involved. The first involves sending a cover letter and résumé to potential employers. A well-written **cover letter** provides a positive overview of your attributes for a particular job (Fig. 66.1) and supplements the **résumé,** which summarizes your work and educational experiences, as well as specific skills and attributes you feel are important to highlight for employers (Fig. 66.2). Many resources are available for preparing a résumé—textbooks, the Internet, and career planning centers at schools and colleges.

Ellis and Hartley (2004, p. 422) suggest the following questions as you begin to prepare your résumé:

1. What educational institutions have you attended? Dates? Degrees or certificates?
2. What credentials do you have that may be useful in a nursing employment setting?
3. What jobs have you held that you want to highlight? Were any healthcare related?
4. What specific skills did you apply in your workplace that would be transferable to nursing?
5. To what skills, abilities, or personal characteristics do you want to draw the employer's attention?
6. Have you had volunteer or community experiences that demonstrate positive personal attributes?
7. Have you had any awards or recognition that identify your positive abilities or attributes?

Include references on a separate page and give them to the employer if requested. It is important to ask people to serve as references who can speak to your potential for employment in a healthcare facility in a positive way.

Another aspect of implementation includes preparing for the interview. Employers are concerned about if you have the appropriate skills and knowledge, if you have a positive work ethic, and if your personality and attitude are a good match for the institution. Appearance is very important, as first impressions are formed quickly. Make sure that you dress professionally and look neat and well groomed. Arrive on time, showing respect for the interviewer's schedule. If you are unavoidably delayed, call and reschedule the interview time.

Stop, Think, and Respond ● BOX 66-2

Select questions that an interviewer may ask. Practice interviewing with classmates (Box 66-1).

After an interview or a discussion with personnel in a human resources office, it is important to write a follow-up letter. This involves thanking the person for his or her time and again expressing your interest in the position or restating your understanding of any agreement reached. Figure 66.3 provides an example of a follow-up letter.

The last step of the process involves evaluating job choices and making decisions. The preceding steps hopefully provide the information needed to make a wise decision. It is important, as in any other major decision, to determine the pros and the cons and ascertain what characteristics of a job are the most important and the most compatible to what you are seeking. Box 66-2 provides a tool for making an employment decision.

Another important aspect of this step is the process of evaluating the job once you begin work. Hopefully, you will select a place that allows you to meet your short-term goals. **Long-term goals,** those that identify where you want to be or what you want to be doing in 5 to 10 years, become more significant as you gain work experience. It is important to review your goals at least annually, so that you can begin the assessment and planning process for your career again. If you decide to make a change, provide your employer with a letter of resignation within the appropriate amount of time—this is usually defined

Ellen Williams
248 Martin Street
Manchester, Massachusetts 02057
(508) 774-4821
e-mail: ewilli@aol.com

May 5, 2004

Janice M. Langton, MS, RN
Director of Nursing
Riverside Nursing Care Center
2 Antoine Avenue
Eddington, Massachusetts 02098

Dear Ms. Langton:

Enclosed please find a copy of my résumé, along with the application to Riverside Nursing Care Center. I will graduate from the practical nursing program at Welton Community College on June 10. I plan to take the NCLEX-PN exam in mid-July. I am particularly interested in a LPN position on the skilled care unit at your facility.

I feel that my past experiences will greatly contribute to your organization. I have six years of experience as a certified nurse's aide in long-term care. My most recent experience was on a skilled care unit at Dorrington Nursing and Rehabilitation Center in Centerville. I wish to continue working with the elderly and disabled population, particularly with clients requiring rehabilitation to improve their quality of life.

My student nurse experiences were in a variety of settings in the Welton area, including many adult health experiences in acute care and long-term care settings. My nursing instructors can attest to my strong interest in the elderly population. I believe my experiences contribute significantly to my knowledge of the care of the elderly and disabled population and my desire to maintain high standards.

I hope that you will agree to interview me for a position at your facility, and look forward to hearing from you. Please note my address, phone number, and email address at the top of the letter. If I do not hear from you within the next two weeks, I will contact the human resources office to determine the status of my application. Thank you for your consideration of my application.

Sincerely,

Ellen Williams

Ellen Williams

FIGURE 66.1 Example of a cover letter from a new PN graduate.

Ellen Williams
248 Martin Street
Manchester, Massachusetts 02057
(508) 774-4821

OBJECTIVE: A beginning LPN position on a skilled care unit that provides for opportunity to develop skills and advance in the nursing profession.

SKILLS:

- Work effectively with the elderly and disabled population
- Communicate well with co-workers, clients, and families
- Demonstrate strong work ethic
- Have experience working in a variety of assignments
- Participate well in client-care decisions
- Contribute to a positive work environment
- Provide safe and effective care to clients

EDUCATION:

Welton Community College
Diploma, Practical Nursing, June 2004

EXPERIENCE:

Dorrington Nursing and Rehabilitation Center, Centerville, MA
Certified Nursing Assistant: 2002-Present

- Provided direct care to elderly and disabled clients
- Developed effective relationships with clients, families, and co-workers
- Functioned as effective team member
- Oriented new certified nursing assistants

Townsend Nursing Home, Carlton, MA
Certified Nursing Assistant: 1998-2002

- Provided direct care to dependent elderly clients
- Adhered to standard procedures and protocols
- Functioned as integral team member

AWARDS:

- Welton Community College Scholastic Honor Award/Scholarship
- Townsend Nursing Home – Employee of the Month – April 2001

References available on request

FIGURE 66.2 Sample résumé for a new PN graduate.

within a contract and/or policy. The letter should be positive—if there are work-related problems, those should be addressed in a meeting with your supervisor. Negative approaches are not professional and may interfere with future references.

Stop, Think, and Respond ● BOX 66-3

Consider your long-term goals and write a list, prioritizing your goals.

BOX 66-1 ● Questions to Help You Prepare for a Job Interview

NURSING PHILOSOPHY AND BELIEFS

- What is your philosophy of nursing?
- Is there a nursing theorist that you use as a basis for your nursing practice?
- What do you believe is the most central concept to support excellence in nursing?

PERSONAL GOALS AND PLANNING

- Where do you see yourself in 1 year? 5 years? 10 years?
- Have you developed any professional goals? If so, would you share those with me?
- Why do you want to work here?
- What plans do you have for continuing education in nursing?
- What do you see as your weakest area in nursing?
- What do you see as your strengths in nursing?

YOUR EXPERIENCES

- What experience in your nursing education did you find the most rewarding? Why?
- What experience in your nursing education did you like the least? Why?
- In what kind of settings did you have an opportunity to work as a nursing student?
- What other job experiences have you had? What skills did you develop there that will be useful in nursing?

PROBLEM SOLVING

- Identify a problem in patient care that you encountered as a student and explain how you solved that problem.
- Describe a difficult patient with whom you worked. Include why you found that client difficult and how you managed the situation.
- Identify a situation in which you were involved in a conflict and describe how you handled that situation. If you had it to do over again, what would you do differently?
- Explain how you would use the nursing process in client care.
- A problem may be presented to you for your solution. Plan ahead to approach it in a systematic manner.

TECHNICAL SKILLS

- What technical nursing skills do you feel comfortable performing?
- What skills will you require assistance with?
- What do you do when you encounter a technical skill you have not performed before?

THE EMPLOYMENT SETTING

- In what type of unit do you wish to work?
- Why do you want to work here?
- Why do you think we should hire you for this position?

PROBLEMS NEW GRADUATES MAY EXPERIENCE IN THE WORKPLACE

Beginning a new job in a new role is both exciting and scary. New graduates experience many conflicting emotions, ranging from feelings of inadequacy to those of great accomplishment. The following sections review transition issues and strategies to assist with achieving success in the LPN/LVN role.

Role Transition

Moving from the role of student nurse to the role of LPN/LVN involves **role transition**—learning the functions and expectations for that role. You will build on the skills and behaviors that you learned in nursing school, expanding your knowledge and abilities, and gaining valuable experiential knowledge (Harrington & Terry, 2003). Role transition represents the process of change in the way one thinks and acts. It does not occur quickly, and is different for each person. During this transition you will experience anxiety and frustration. As a new LPN/LVN you want to be excellent at what you do, but it takes time to learn a new job, take on more responsibility and accountability, and continue to be safe in your practice.

Yoder-Wise (2003) uses the acronym "ROLES" to understand the process of role transition.

- **R**—represents *responsibility,* which entails the specific job description, including tasks that each person must carry out.
- **O**—stands for *opportunities,* which are the potential prospects of the job, such as professional development and committee work.
- **L**—denotes *lines* of communication that are important for each person within an organization; a new LPN/LVN needs to learn the appropriate channels for communicating information related to clients' care or employment issues.
- **E**—defines *expectations* for each role within the organization, and specifically for a person employed in a new role.
- **S**—depicts the *support* needed to meet expectations; a LPN/LVN needs the support of the RNs within the organization, and in particular the support of the unit supervisor.

Success for a new LPN/LVN is dependent on these elements.

Stop, Think, and Respond ● BOX 66-4

What concerns do you have as you prepare to begin your LPN/LVN career?

Reality Shock

New graduates often experience an overwhelming feeling that it is impossible to provide effective and safe care to clients in the manner in which they were taught. There also does not seem to be any way to change the system that prevents them from practicing as they had hoped to.

Ellen Williams
248 Martin Street
Manchester, Massachusetts 02057
(508) 774-4821
e-mail: ewilli@aol.com

May 22, 2004

Janice M. Langton, MS, RN
Director of Nursing
Riverside Nursing Care Center
2 Antoine Avenue
Eddington, Massachusetts 02098

Dear Ms. Langton:

Thank you for meeting with me today to discuss opportunities for LPNs at Riverside Nursing Care Center. I am particularly interested in the evening position on the skilled care unit, but I would consider another position.

My educational and clinical experiences appear to match your needs very well. I will be able to meet my desire to work with the elderly and disabled population at your facility.

Again, I hope that you will consider me for a position at Riverside Nursing Care Center. I am available to meet with the nurse manager of the skilled care unit, or with other nurse managers as needed. I understand that is the next step in the process. Please contact me at the phone number or email address listed above. I will check with you in a few weeks regarding the status of my application if I have not heard from you.

Thank you again for your time and consideration.

Sincerely,

Ellen Williams

Ellen Williams

FIGURE 66.3 Example of a follow-up letter.

This phenomenon, described by Marlene Kramer (1979), is known as **reality shock.** As a student nurse, you were taught not to give any medications until familiar with its actions and side effects. As a staff LPN/LVN, the priority is to give medications quickly, on time, and correctly. There is little or no time to look up all of the medications (Ellis & Hartley, 2004). Issues such as this one create anxiety and frustration for new graduates. Some nurses may become so discouraged and disillusioned that they do not want to remain in the profession. Others may change jobs frequently, trying to find the ideal job. And still others either become very critical of the system or passively accept the situation and make no attempt to remedy a poor situation.

Being aware that reality shock may occur assists new graduates to take steps to ease role transition issues and promote their success in the workplace. The following section provides possible strategies to alleviate reality shock.

Recognize Limitations

New graduates are not experts as they begin their work as new LPN/LVNs. Patricia Benner (1984) identified

BOX 66-2 ● Making a Decision About a Job

Use the following factors when making a decision about a future job:

- The facility adheres to standards of nursing practice.
- There is adequate staffing as evidenced by nurse–client ratios.
- There is adequate and organized orientation for new graduates/employees.
- The facility provides opportunities for professional development and job mobility.
- Salary and benefits are competitive.
- There is adequate nursing supervision at all times.

(Cherry, B., & Jacob, S. R. [2002]. *Contemporary nursing: Issues, trends, and management.* St. Louis, MO: Mosby, Inc.)

stages that new graduates experience when beginning their nursing careers. Although her work focused on registered nurses, the progressive stages are applicable to LPN/LVNs as well. There are five stages, including novice, advanced beginner, competent, proficient, and expert. The novice stage generally occurs when a person is in school, and the remaining stages take place when the student becomes a graduate. Each stage represents progressive acquisition and mastery of skills, socialization to the role of the LPN/LVN, and eventual ability to see the whole picture, anticipate problems, and demonstrate intuitive ability and knowledgeable competency. Although length of time for each stage is individual, it generally involves several years within the same setting.

Nurses experiencing these stages generally have stress. Charnley (1999) identified four categories that contribute to stress:

1. Reality of practice—new nurses think they should have all the answers, feel overwhelmed by the volume of work, and experience guilt because they are not practicing as they were taught.
2. Unfamiliarity with role and setting—new graduates lose time trying to find things and figure out roles in specific situations.
3. Lack of professional relationships and increased dependency on others.
4. Lack of clinical skills and judgment.

Recognizing that stress is typical leads to a reality of recognizing one's limitations. A new graduate cannot be an expert and needs time to learn, adapt, and develop self-confidence. Limitations can be turned into successes through asking questions, focusing on client needs, and accepting that learning requires time, practice, repetition, and patience (Vallano, 2002).

Celebrate Achievements

New graduates, in reference to Benner's (1984) work, need realistic expectations about their abilities in the work setting. Vallano (2002) suggests that new graduates celebrate their achievements, beginning with graduation, passing boards, and moving to successes at work. Self-congratulations are difficult but essential for survival. This process can actually assist in believing in oneself and developing self-confidence. Vallano (2002) asserts that affirmations do work. Instead of saying, "I'll never learn this" it is better to state, "Everyday, I am improving in my ability to _____" (p. 89). Using this process will assist new graduates to believe in themselves and accept their limitations, with a focus on small accomplishments.

Identify a Mentor

Finding a person who has more experience and knowledge is not difficult for a novice nurse. Identifying a person who can nurture a new graduate, however, may be more of a challenge. It is useful to seek advice and help from nurses who demonstrate a willingness to teach and support new graduates. Mentoring a new nurse requires sensitivity and patience, but can be very rewarding. The ideal mentor provides ongoing support and inspiration.

When looking for employment, it is important to ask about orientation, particularly to know if one or several people will be responsible for your orientation. It also will be important to know the length of the orientation and how soon the employer expects you to be able to work independently.

Mentors can be within the work setting, or may be other professionals from your school, former places of employment, or professional organizations or networks. Whatever the source, seek an experienced nurse you respect and who demonstrates respect for you. Mentors provide a perspective that assists new graduates to remain on track and to recognize that the new job is a learning process (Bensing, 2003). New nurses need to resist getting caught up in workplace politics and should be cautious in forming relationships with those who are quick to judge or complain. A positive mentor will help you adapt and grow in your role and, as you gain experience and expertise, nourish your ability to become a mentor to a future graduate.

Join or Form a Support Group

Some work settings organize a support group or network for new employees. In many instances, however, new graduates need to join a professional organization or form a group on their own. A nursing listserve through a professional organization is another way to get input from experienced nurses. Group networking provides a nonthreatening way to explore one's feelings and methods to cope in the workplace as a new LPN/LVN.

Stop, Think, and Respond ● BOX 66-5

Recall what strategies you used to cope with stress related to being a student nurse.

Burnout

Burnout occurs after a person has been working for awhile and is a type of chronic stress related to the job. A work environment with issues such as inadequate staff, high stress level related to client acuity, or poor staff relationships fosters feelings of being overwhelmed and disheartened. Symptoms of burnout include chronic physical ailments such as fatigue, headaches, and insomnia. Emotional responses involve anger, depression, and guilt. Causes of burnout are similar to reality shock in that there "is the conflict between ideals and reality" (Ellis & Hartley, 2004, p. 440). Nurses work harder and harder to achieve the ideal and increasingly are more critical of the work environment that prevents the ideal from being fulfilled. Poor staffing, high mortality rates, and highly critically ill clients contribute to nurses' inability to feel they are performing as well as they should.

Many strategies used to deal with reality shock are also effective in coping with or preventing burnout. Table 66.1 describes other strategies for managing chronic stress related to burnout. Often nurses may choose to change jobs or leave nursing without trying to deal with the issues related to burnout. Future success in nursing depends on self-care, reduction of stress, and meeting identified needs. When experiencing overwhelming feelings of failure or stress, having strategies to refocus priorities and ability to examine goals will decrease burnout.

MAINTAINING COMPETENCY

Licensure as an LPN/LVN signifies that a person demonstrates minimum competency requirements to practice in that role. Licensure is also a means of protecting the public. Some states have mandatory continuing education; others rely on employers to ensure that healthcare employees remain competent. Increased concern for client safety, advances in technology and medical practice, and an ever-increasing body of knowledge require that anyone caring for clients must maintain proficiency in skills and information needed for client care.

Methods to continue one's education include seminars, workshops, and conferences. Many employers provide short educational activities at work that focus on specific needs for a unit or facility. In addition, attending professional association meetings and regularly reading professional journals support a person's quest for continuing education.

"Each individual nurse must be committed to personal excellence and assume responsibility for maintaining competence" (Ellis & Hartley, 2004, p. 341). It is essential for each LPN/LVN to identify knowledge and practice deficits and then take steps to acquire needed information. Some facilities engage in self-evaluation for each employee, which provides time to determine goals for the coming year. Whether or not self-evaluation is required, return to the steps of the nursing process to make a determination of your learning needs and how you can best meet them. This process will enhance your ability to be a competent and safe LPN/LVN.

FUTURE NURSING EDUCATION

Education is a lifelong process and makes it possible for people to achieve career goals. Educational opportunities vary for graduates of practical nursing programs. Some states have excellent educational mobility paths, particularly if the practical nursing programs are connected with or located in community colleges. Table 66.2 summarizes educational programs in the United States. As LPN/LVNs consider continuing their formal education, it is important to thoroughly explore what options are available, what is needed prior to applying to a school for admission, and if a program fits with one's long-term goals.

TABLE 66.1 MANAGING STRESS RELATED TO BURNOUT

PHYSICAL	MENTAL	EMOTIONAL/SPIRITUAL
Accept physical limitations. Modify nutrition: high carbohydrate, low caffeine, low sugar. Exercise at least 30 minutes three times a week—select something that is enjoyable. Take breaks—do not skip meals. Arrange to get adequate sleep. Engage in relaxation through meditation, yoga, massage, or biofeedback.	Learn to say no! Use self-talk to rethink negative thoughts/feelings. Learn imagery techniques. Develop hobbies/activities outside of work. Plan and take vacations. Continue education. Learn skills to improve time management, communication, and conflict resolution.	Use meditation. Seek solace in prayer. Seek professional counseling. Participate in support groups and networking. Communicate feelings to appropriate people in an appropriate manner. Develop a relationship with a mentor. Ask for feedback and clarification.

(Adapted from Yoder-Wise, P. S. [2003]. *Leading and managing in nursing.* [3rd ed.]. St. Louis, MO: Mosby, Inc.)

TABLE 66.2 EDUCATIONAL OPPORTUNITIES FOR REGISTERED NURSING: A COMPARISON

	DIPLOMA	ASSOCIATE DEGREE	BACCALAUREATE
Location	Is usually conducted by and based in a hospital	Most often conducted in junior or community colleges, occasionally in senior colleges and universities	Located in senior colleges and universities
Length of study	Requires generally 24–30 months, but may require 3 academic years	Usually requires 2 academic or sometimes 2 calendar years	Requires 4 academic years
Requirements for admission	Requires graduation from high school or its equivalent, satisfactory general academic achievement, and successful completion of certain prerequisite courses	Requires that applicants meet entrance requirements of college as well as of program	Requires that applicants meet entrance requirements of the college or university as well as those of program
Program of learning	Includes courses in theory and practice of nursing and in biologic, physical, and behavioral sciences. May require that certain courses in the physical and social sciences be taken at a local college or university	Combines a balance of nursing courses and college courses in the basic natural and social sciences with courses in general education and the humanities	Frequently concentrates on courses in the theory and practice of nursing in the junior and senior years. Provides education in the theory and practice of nursing and courses in the liberal arts as well as the behavioral and physical sciences.
Clinical component	Provides early and substantial clinical learning experiences in the hospital and a variety of community agencies; these focus on an understanding of the hospital environment and the interrelationship of other health disciplines	Requires as a significant part of the program supervised clinical instruction in hospitals and other community health agencies	Provides clinical laboratory courses in a variety of settings where health and nursing care are given
Opportunity for educational advancement	Little or no transferability of courses unless affiliated with a community college or university	Is structured so that some credits may be applied to baccalaureate degree	Provides the basic academic preparation for advancement to higher positions in nursing and to master's degree
Competency on graduation	Graduate is prepared to plan for the care of clients with other members of the healthcare team, to develop and carry out plans for the care of individuals or groups of clients, and to direct selected members of the nursing team. Has an understanding of the hospital climate and the community health resources necessary for the extended care of clients.	Graduate is prepared to plan and give direct client care in hospitals, nursing homes, or similar healthcare agencies, and to participate with other members of the healthcare team, such as licensed practical nurses, nurses aides, physicians, and other registered nurses, in rendering care to clients.	Graduate is prepared to plan and give direct care to individuals and families, whether sick or well, to assume responsibility for directing other members of the healthcare team, and to take on beginning leadership positions. Practices in a variety of settings and emphasizes comprehensive healthcare, including preventive and rehabilitative services, health counseling and education, and care in acute and long-term illnesses. Has necessary education for graduate study toward a master's degree and may move rapidly to specialized leadership positions in nursing as teacher, administrator, clinical specialist, nurse practitioner, and nurse researcher.
Licensure	Must successfully complete state licensing examination	Must successfully complete state licensing examination	Must successfully complete state licensing examination

(Ellis, J. R., & Hartley, C. L. [2004]. *Nursing in today's world* [8th ed.]. Philadelphia: Lippincott Williams & Wilkins.)

LPN/LVNs with career goals and plans will find wonderful opportunities and challenges in nursing. There are few limits to what a person can achieve in a nursing career. Carefully planned job choices and education will ensure an exciting and rewarding nursing career.

Critical Thinking Exercises

1. *Should continuing education be mandatory for license renewal? Why? Why not?*
2. *Explore an associate degree nursing program in your area. What prerequisites are required before admission?*

● NCLEX-STYLE REVIEW QUESTIONS 

1. Which of the following statements from a seasoned nurse is most appropriate to give a new nurse?
   1. "New graduates need realistic expectations about their abilities in the work setting."
   2. "New graduates are up to date on the newest technologies with sharp clinical skills."
   3. "New graduates should trust their instincts and make decisions on their own."
   4. "New graduates need to rely on other nurses for the first year of practice."
2. Which statement by the nurse indicates burnout?
   1. "I have a lot of responsibility on the nursing unit."
   2. "I work hard during my shift to provide quality client care."
   3. "I am tired of being dumped on by the administration of this hospital."
   4. "I must prioritize my assignments to ensure the client is taken care of."

connection

Visit the Connection site at **http://connection.lww.com/go/timbyEssentials** for links to chapter-related resources on the Internet.

References and Suggested Readings

Bauzys, R. (April 28, 2003). Be prepared. *Advance for Nurses,* 42.

Benner, P. (1984). *From novice to expert.* Menlo Park, CA: Addison-Wesley.

Bensing, K. (May 12, 2003). Got mentors? *Advance for Nurses,* 33.

Charnley, E. (1999). Occupational stress in the newly qualified staff nurse. *Nursing Standard, 13*(29), 32–37.

Cherry, B., & Jacob, S. R. (2002). *Contemporary nursing: Issues, trends, and management.* St. Louis, MO: Mosby, Inc.

DeMarco, R. F., & Roberts, S. J. (2003). Negative behaviors in nursing. *American Journal of Nursing, 103*(3), 113–116.

Ellis, J. R., & Hartley, C. L. (2004). *Nursing in today's world* (8th ed.). Philadelphia: Lippincott Williams & Wilkins.

Fest, G. (Spring, 2003). Field of dreams. *Future Nurse,* 39–41.

Flynn, K. (May 26, 2003). Interview skills and tips. *Advance for Nurses,* 35.

Haffner, B. (2002). *Where do I go from here? Exploring your career alternatives within and beyond nursing.* Philadelphia: Lippincott Williams & Wilkins.

Harrington, N., & Terry, C. (2003). *LPN to RN transitions: Achieving success in your new role* (2nd ed.). Philadelphia: Lippincott Williams & Wilkins.

Haylock, P. J. (2003). Charting the course of your nursing career. *American Journal of Nursing Career Guide 2003,* 33–36.

Health Resources and Services Administration (2002). *Projected supply, demand, and shortages of registered nurses.* Author. [On-line]. Available: http://bhpr.hrsa.gov/healthworkforce/rnproject/report.htm.

Hugg, A. (Spring, 2003). Keys to the kingdom. *Future Nurse,* 56–60.

Into the fire. (Spring, 2003). *Future Nurse,* 46–47.

Kramer, M. (1979). *Reality shock.* St Louis, MO: CV Mosby.

LaDuke, S. (2003). Keeping up with standards: Your key to safe practice. *Nursing 2003, 33*(3), 45.

Malugani, M. (2003). Battling burnout: Health professionals are at high risk. Monster Healthcare. [On-line.] Available: http://healthcare.monster.com/articles/burnout.

McPeck, P. (Spring, 2003). Road map. *Future Nurse,* 84–85.

Miller, T. W. (2003). *Building and managing a career in nursing: Strategies for advancing your career.* Indianapolis, IN: Sigma Theta Tau International.

Monarch, K. (2003). Making informed employment decisions. *American Journal of Nursing Career Guide 2003,* 29–32.

Morgan, D. W. (2003). Going up the chain of command. *RN, 66*(6), 67–70.

National Council of State Boards of Nursing (2002). *Report of findings from the 2001 PN practice analysis update.* Chicago: NCSBN.

Sanford, K. (Spring, 2003). Getting to know you. *Future Nurse,* 13–15.

Tobin, S. (April 28, 2003). The burnout blues. *Advance for Nurses,* 25–26.

Vallano, A. T. (2002). *Your career in nursing.* New York: Kaplan Publishing.

Wray, R., & Williams, R. (2003). Negotiating a salary. *American Journal of Nursing, 102*(2), 71–73.

Yoder-Wise, P. S. (2003). *Leading and managing in nursing* (3rd ed.). St. Louis, MO: Mosby, Inc.

Index

Pages numbers followed by b indicate box; those followed by f indicate figure; those followed by t indicate table.

A

B

D

E

H

I

J

M

N

Q

R

S

V

W

X

Y

Z

NANDA-Approved Nursing Diagnoses

This list represents the NANDA-approved nursing diagnoses for clinical use and testing.

Activity Intolerance
Activity Intolerance, Risk for
Adjustment, Impaired
Airway Clearance, Ineffective
Allergy Response, Latex
Allergy Response, Risk for Latex
Anxiety
Anxiety, Death
Aspiration, Risk for
Attachment, Risk for Impaired Parent/Infant/Child
Autonomic Dysreflexia
Autonomic Dysreflexia, Risk for
Body Image, Disturbed
Body Temperature, Risk for Imbalanced
Bowel Incontinence
Breastfeeding, Effective
Breastfeeding, Ineffective
Breastfeeding, Interrupted
Breathing Pattern, Ineffective
Cardiac Output, Decreased
Caregiver Role Strain
Caregiver Role Strain, Risk for
Comfort, Impaired
Communication, Impaired Verbal
Conflict, Decisional
Conflict, Parental Role
Confusion, Acute
Confusion, Chronic
Constipation
Constipation, Perceived
Constipation, Risk for
Coping, Ineffective
Coping, Ineffective Community
Coping, Readiness for Enhanced Community
Coping, Defensive
Coping, Compromised Family
Coping, Disabled Family
Coping, Readiness for Enhanced Family
Denial, Ineffective
Dentition, Impaired
Development, Risk for Delayed
Diarrhea
Disuse Syndrome, Risk for
Diversional Activity, Deficient
Energy Field, Disturbed
Environmental Interpretation Syndrome, Impaired
Failure to Thrive, Adult
Falls, Risk for
Family Processes: Alcoholism, Dysfunctional
Family Processes: Interrupted
Fatigue
Fear
Fluid Volume, Deficient
Fluid Volume, Excess
Fluid Volume, Risk for Deficient
Fluid Volume, Risk for Imbalanced
Gas Exchange, Impaired
Grieving
Grieving, Anticipatory
Grieving, Dysfunctional
Growth and Development, Delayed
Growth, Risk for Disproportionate
Health Maintenance, Risk for Ineffective
Health-Seeking Behaviors
Home Maintenance, Impaired
Hopelessness
Hyperthermia
Hypothermia
Identity, Disturbed Personal
Incontinence, Functional Urinary
Incontinence, Reflex Urinary
Incontinence, Risk for Urge Urinary
Incontinence, Stress Urinary
Incontinence, Total Urinary
Incontinence, Urge Urinary
Infant Behavior, Disorganized
Infant Behavior, Readiness for Enhanced Organized
Infant Behavior, Risk for Disorganized
Infant Feeding Pattern, Ineffective
Infection, Risk for
Injury, Risk for
Injury, Risk for Perioperative-Positioning
Intracranial, Adaptive Capacity, Decreased
Knowledge, Deficient